brief contents

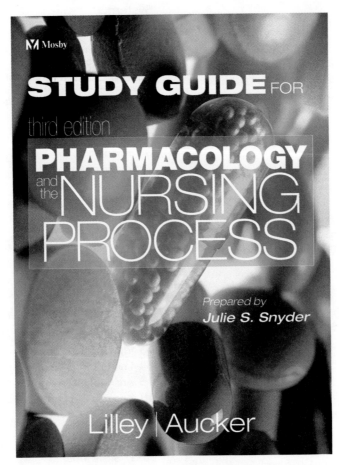

Attached is a
Pull-Out IV Incompatibility Chart

IV Compatibilities

The IV compatibility table provides data when two or more medications are given into a Y-site of administration. The data in this table largely represent physical incompatibilities (e.g., haze, precipitate, change in color). Therapeutic incompatibilities have not been included; therefore professional judgment should be exercised when using the table.

● = Physically compatible via Y-site administration;
✗ = physically incompatible.

From Hodgson BB, Kizior RJ: *Saunders nursing drug handbook 2002*, Philadelphia, 2002, WB Saunders

IV Incompatibility Chart — columns (left to right): heparin, gentamicin, furosemide, fluconazole, filgrastim, fentanyl, famotidine, esmolol, erythromycin, epinephrine, enalapril, droperidol, dopamine, dobutamine, diltiazem, digoxin, diazepam, dexamethasone, cyclophosphamide, cisplatin, ciprofloxacin, cimetidine, cefazolin, calcium gluconate, bumetanide, bretylium, aztreonam, ampicillin, amphotericin, amiodarone, aminophylline, amikacin, acyclovir.

Rows (top to bottom): acyclovir, amikacin, aminophylline, amiodarone, amphotericin, ampicillin, ampicillin/sulbactam, aztreonam, bretylium, bumetanide, calcium chloride, calcium gluconate, cefazolin, cefotaxime, ceftazidime, ceftizoxime, ceftriaxone, cefuroxime, chloramphenicol, cimetidine, ciprofloxacin, cisplatin, clindamycin, cyclophosphamide, dexamethasone, diazepam, digoxin, diltiazem, dobutamine, dopamine, doxycycline, droperidol, enalapril, epinephrine, erythromycin, esmolol, famotidine, fentanyl, filgrastim, fluconazole, furosemide, gentamicin, haloperidol, heparin, hetastarch, hydrocortisone, insulin, isoproterenol, labetalol, lidocaine, lorazepam, magnesium, mannitol, meperidine, methotrexate, methylprednisolone, metoclopramide, metronidazole, midazolam, milrinone, morphine, multivitamins, nalbuphine, nitroglycerin, nitroprusside, norepinephrine, ondansetron, oxytocin, penicillin G, phenylephrine, phenytoin, piperacillin, phosphate, potassium, procainamide, ranitidine, sodium bicarbonate, streptokinase, thiamine, ticarcillin, tobramycin, vancomycin, vasopressin, verapamil.

IV Compatibilities *(continued)*

The IV compatibility table provides data when two or more medications are given into a Y-site of administration. The data in this table largely represent physical incompatibilities (e.g., haze, precipitate, change in color). Therapeutic incompatibilities have not been included; therefore professional judgment should be exercised when using the table.

● = Physically compatible via Y-site administration;

X = physically incompatible.

From Hodgson BB, Kizior RJ: *Saunders nursing drug handbook 2002*, Philadelphia, 2002, WB Saunders

PHARMACOLOGY

and the

NURSING PROCESS

about the authors

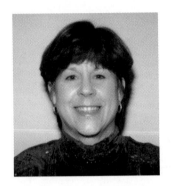

Linda Lane Lilley, RN, PhD

Linda Lilley received her diploma from Norfolk General School of Nursing, BSN from the University of Virginia, Master of Science (Nursing) from Old Dominion University, and PhD in Nursing from George Mason University. Her teaching experience spans over 22 years with the last 16 years at Old Dominion University School of Nursing. As an Associate Professor, Linda's areas of teaching expertise include pharmacology, adult nursing, physical assessment, fundamentals, oncology nursing, nursing theory, trends in health care and nursing, and role transition. Linda also has over 12 years of experience teaching RNs returning for their BSN via the "distance learning" mode. Her areas of research interests include retention of minority students in baccalaureate schools of nursing and human needs of patients with cervical or uterine cancer. She recently completed a 2-year term on the U.S. Pharmacopeia national advisory panel on medication errors. In August 1999, Linda received the University's most prestigious award of teaching excellence with the title of University Professor, an award for tenured faculty members. She has also been a two-time university nominee for the State Council of Higher Education in Virginia award for excellence in teaching, service, and scholarship.

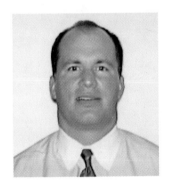

Robert S. Aucker, PharmD

Bob Aucker is currently a cardiovascular research specialist for a large pharmaceutical company. He has focused his career in the area of cardiology and critical care working in several large integrated health care systems over the past decade. He has had clinical, academic, and research responsibility in a variety of settings, including long-term care, general medicine clinics, operating rooms, and critical and intensive care. He has many years of experience teaching pharmacology as an adjunct professor at Mercer Southern School of Pharmacy and Kennesaw State College School of Nursing in Atlanta. He also speaks nationally on a variety of topics.

third edition

PHARMACOLOGY
and the
NURSING PROCESS

Linda Lane Lilley, RN, PhD

Associate Professor
School of Nursing
Old Dominion University
Norfolk, Virginia

Robert S. Aucker, PharmD

Regional Medical Research Specialist
Cardiovascular - Southeast Region
Pfizer Pharmaceuticals Group
New York, New York

With *Study Skills* content by:

Richard E. Lake, BS, MS, MLA

Director, Center for Student Success;
Professor, Reading Department
St. Louis Community College at Florissant Valley
St. Louis, Missouri

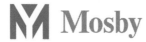

Mosby

An Affiliate of Elsevier Science

St. Louis   London   Philadelphia   Sydney   Toronto

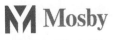

An Affiliate of Elsevier Science

Vice President, Publishing Director, Nursing: Sally Schrefer
Executive Editor: Robin Carter
Senior Developmental Editor: Kristin Geen
Project Manager: Catherine Jackson
Project Specialist: Jeff Patterson
Designer: Amy Buxton
For illustration credit information for the illustrations in Chapter 8,
please refer to the illustration credits at the end of the chapter.

NOTICE

Pharmacology is an ever-changing field. Standard safety precautions must be followed, but as new research and clinical experience broaden our knowledge, changes in treatment and drug therapy may become necessary or appropriate. Readers are advised to check the most current product information provided by the manufacturer of each drug to be administered to verify the recommended dose, the method and duration of administration, and contraindications. It is the responsibility of the licensed prescribers, relying on experience and knowledge of the patient, to determine dosages and the best treatment for each individual patient. Neither the Publisher nor the editor assumes any liability for any injury and/or damage to persons or property arising from this publication.

Mosby, Inc.
An Affiliate of Elsevier Science
11830 Westline Industrial Drive
St. Louis, Missouri 63146

Printed in the United States of America

ISBN   0-323-01267-1

02 03 04 05 GW/KPT 9 8 7 6 5 4 3

Valerie O'Toole Baker, RN, MSN, CS
Assistant Professor
Villa Maria School of Nursing
Gannon University
Erie, Pennsylvania

Nancy Henne Batchelor, MSN, RNC
Assistant Professor
Northern Kentucky University
Highland Heights, Kentucky

Linda P. Bolin, RN, MSN, ANP
Adult Nurse Practitioner, Student Health Service
Adjunct Faculty, School of Nursing
East Carolina University
Greenville, North Carolina

Bernadette M. Dragich, MSN, RN, CS, FNP
Associate Professor of Nursing
Bluefield State College
Bluefield, West Virginia

Sherry D. Ferki, RN, MSN
Instructor
Louise Obici School of Nursing
Suffolk, Virginia

Brian J. Gates, PharmD
Pharmacy Resident in Geriatrics and Clinical Instructor
Washington State University
Spokane, Washington

Roberta A. Goeckner, PharmD
Clinical Pharmacist
Managed Pharmacy Benefits
St. Louis, Missouri

Teresa D. Holimon, PharmD, BCPS
Assistant Professor and DUR Coordinator
University of Tennessee College of Pharmacy
Memphis, Tennessee

JaCinda L. Jones, PharmD
Manager, Pharmaceutical Care and Disease Management
Department of Professional Practice Initiatives
Medicine Shoppe International, Inc.
St. Louis, Missouri

Natasha Leskovsek, RN, MBA, JD
Nurse Attorney
Fox, Bennett, & Turner
Washington, D.C.

Patrick Leung, PharmD, BCPS
Assistant Professor of Pharmacy Practice,
College of Pharmacy
Washington State University
Pullman, Washington

Jane A. Madden, MSN, RN
Assistant Professor
Deaconness College of Nursing
St. Louis, Missouri

Dorothy M. Mathers, RN, MSN, ACLS
Associate Professor
Pennsylvania College of Technology
Williamsport, Pennsylvania

Lora McGuire, RN, MS
Professor of Nursing
Joliet Junior College
Joliet, Illinois

Lori Beth Mooberry, BSN, CMT
Faculty, Practical Nursing
Illinois Central College
Peoria, Illinois

Vicky K. Parker, RN, MSN, FNP
Assistant Professor
Ohio University, Chillicothe Campus
Chillicothe, Ohio

Robert G. Pendleton, PhD
Lecturer in Pharmacology
Thomas Jefferson University
Philadelphia, Pennsylvania

Elaine T. Princevalli, RN, BSN, MS
Instructor, Practical Nurse Education Program
Eli Whitney Regional Vocational-Technical School
Hamden, Connecticut

Willa Taite Sawyer, RN, BSN
Assistant Nurse Executive
Nursing/Infection Control, Employee Health
Memphis Mental Health Institute
Memphis, Tennessee

Stephen M. Setter, PharmD, DVM
Assistant Professor, Pharmacy Practice
College of Pharmacy, Washington State University
Spokane, Washington

Allen F. Shaughnessy, PharmD, BCPS, FCCP
Director of Research, Harrisburg Family Practice
Residency
Pinnacle Health System
Harrisburg, Pennsylvania

Linda R. Young, PharmD
Assistant Professor and Director, Pharmacy Practice and
Pharmacoeconomics
University of Tennessee at Memphis
Memphis, Tennessee

preface

INTRODUCTION

Pharmacology and the Nursing Process provides the most current and clinically relevant information in an appealing, understandable, and practical format. The accessible size, readable writing style, and full-color design are ideal for today's busy nursing student. This text takes a unique approach to the study of pharmacology by presenting study skills content that will help students understand and learn the particularly demanding subject of pharmacology. Each part begins with a Study Skills Tips section, which features a discussion of researched and proven study skills and applies the discussion to the content in that part. Students are therefore encouraged to use research-based study skills to enhance their study of pharmacology and nursing.

MARKET RESEARCH

This text incorporates many suggestions from focus group participants composed to nursing instructors from 2-, 3-, and 4-year degree programs in Chicago, Philadelphia, and Los Angeles. The focus groups assessed changes that have occurred in the teaching of pharmacology and determined what was needed to better teach pharmacology to nursing students. Based on faculty descriptions of their courses and students, these general recommendations were made:

- Accommodate the reading styles and abilities of the growing number of nontraditional nursing students.
- Increase the use of tables, boxes, illustrations, graphics, and other visually oriented approaches.
- Use color to increase interest and highlight important drug interactions and processes.

We have taken a truly collaborative approach with this text. The concerns raised by faculty members in market research have been addressed, as have additional improvements suggested by faculty members who served as reviewers or consultants, either formally or informally, throughout the manuscript's development and by the authors and editors of this text.

ORGANIZATION

This book includes 55 chapters presented in 10 parts organized by body system. The eight concepts chapters in

Part One lay a solid foundation for the subsequent drug units and address the following topics:

- Study skills applied to learning pharmacology
- The nursing process and drug therapy
- Pharmacologic principles
- Lifespan considerations related to pharmacology
- Legal, ethical, and cultural considerations
- Patient education and drug therapy
- Over-the-counter drugs and herbal remedies *(new to this edition!)*
- Substance abuse *(new to this edition!)*
- Photo atlas of medication administration techniques, including over 120 illustrations

Parts Two through Ten present pharmacology and nursing management in a traditional *body systems/drug function* framework. This accepted approach facilitates learning by grouping functionally related drugs and drug groups. It provides an effective means to integrate the content into medical-surgical or adult health nursing courses or for teaching pharmacology in a separate course.

The 47 drug chapters in these parts constitute the main portion of the book. Drugs are presented in a consistent format with an emphasis on drug groups and key similarities and differences among the drugs in each group. Each chapter is subdivided into two discussions, beginning with a complete, clear discussion of pharmacology, followed by a comprehensive yet succinct discussion of the nursing process. Pharmacology is presented for each drug group in a consistent format:

- Mechanism of Action
- Drug Effects
- Therapeutic Uses
- Side Effects and Adverse Effects
  - Toxicity and Management of Overdose
- Interactions
- Dosages

Drug group discussions are followed by **Drug Profiles,** or brief narrative capsules of individual drugs in the class or group, including **Pharmacokinetics** tables for each drug. **Key drugs,** or prototypical drugs within a class, are identified with the ⊶ symbol for easy identification. These individual drug profiles are followed by **Nursing**

Process discussions relating to the entire drug group. The nursing content is covered in a functional, six-step nursing process format of the following:
- Assessment
- Nursing Diagnoses
- Planning
  - Outcome Criteria
- Implementation
- Evaluation

At the end of each nursing process section is a **Patient Teaching Tips** box that summarizes key points to cover in educating the patient about the uses and effects of drugs within a given group. The role of the nurse as patient educator continues to grow in importance, so this text emphasizes this key content.

Each part begins with a **Study Skills Tips** section that presents a study skills topic and relates it to the unit being discussed. Topics include time management, note taking, studying, test taking, and others. This unique approach to teaching pharmacology is intended to aid those students who find pharmacology difficult and to provide a tool that may prove beneficial throughout their nursing school careers. Coverage of this study skills content is limited to the beginning of each part so that instructors who choose not to require their students to read this material can easily eliminate it. However, this arrangement of content may be very beneficial to those faculty members teaching pharmacology through an integrated approach because it helps the student identify key content and concepts. This arrangement also facilitates location of content for either required or optional reading.

FEATURES

This book includes various pedagogic features that prepare the student for important content covered in each chapter and encourage review and reinforcement of that content. Chapter opener pedagogy includes the following:
- **Learning Objectives**
- Box listing **Drug Profiles** in the chapter with page number references
- **Glossary** of key terms with pronunciations, definitions, and page number references. Glossary terms are bolded in the narrative to emphasize this essential terminology. Included at the end of the book is a list of glossary terms with page numbers for quick reference.

The following features appear at the end of each chapter:
- **Patient Teaching Tips** specific to the drug class or topic
- **Points to Remember** boxes summarizing key points and subdivided by key topic, drug group, or nursing management
- NCLEX-style multiple-choice **Review Questions** with answers provided on the MERLIN website
- **Critical Thinking Activities** with answers provided on the MERLIN website
- **Bibliography** listing references for more information

Special features that appear throughout the text include the following:
- **Cultural Implications** boxes
- **Home Health/Community Points** boxes
- **Herbal Interactions** boxes *(new to this edition!)*
- **Legal/Ethical Principles** boxes
- **Geriatric and Pediatric Considerations** boxes
- **Case Studies** with answers provided on the MERLIN website
- **Research** boxes
- Case-based **Nursing Care Plans** applying pharmacology to the nursing process
- Alphabetized **Dosages** tables listing drug generic and trade names, class, dosages, and purposes

Additional special features in the text include the following:
- **Online Worksheets** for each chapter, including answers, to provide additional review of challenging content and important concepts *(new to this edition!)*. This symbol appears in the text where there is a related question or activity in the Online Worksheet for that chapter.
- A tear-out **IV Incompatibility Chart** provides students with a portable reference on incompatible drugs administered intravenously *(new to this edition!)*.
- A separate **Disorders Index** is included that references disorders in the text. This unique feature aids in integrating the text with medical-surgical or adult health nursing course content.

COLOR

The first edition of this book was the first full-color pharmacology text for nursing students. Faculty members suggested that color be used in both a functionally and visually appealing manner to more fully engage students in this typically demanding yet important content. Full color is used throughout to do the following:
- Highlight important content
- Illustrate how drugs work in the body in numerous anatomic and drug process color figures
- Improve the visual appearance of the content to make it more engaging and appealing to today's more visually sophisticated reader

We believe that the use of color in these ways significantly improves students' involvement and understanding of pharmacology.

ANCILLARY PACKAGE

A carefully prepared ancillary package is available to students and instructors using *Pharmacology and the Nursing Process*. These materials, which have been thoroughly revised for this edition, can significantly assist teaching and learning of pharmacology. The ancillaries and their features include the following:

Study Guide

This popular student workbook includes the following:
- **Study Tips** guide that reinforces the study skills explained in the text and allows students to practice analyzing tests and applying test-taking strategies

- **Worksheets** for each chapter containing a variety of learning activities, including review and critical thinking questions, case studies, and crossword puzzles
- **Drug calculations overview,** including sample drug labels and practice problems *(new to this edition!)*
- **Answers** provided in the back to enable self-study

MERLIN Website

Located at www.harcourthealth.com/Merlin/Lilley/, the MERLIN website for this book includes the following:

- **Online Worksheets** for each chapter, including answers (to access this resource, use the passcode in the front of the textbook)
- A variety of **Online Resources,** including a list of Canadian trade names and generic equivalents, as well as helpful pharmacology abbreviations, weights and measures, and drug measurement conversion tables
- An updated library of pharmacology **WebLinks**
- **Frequently Asked Questions, Content Updates,** and **Case Studies** with answers
- **Teaching Tips** for instructors teaching pharmacology
- **Answers** to the Review Questions, Critical Thinking Activities, and Case Studies in the text

Mosby/Saunders ePharmacology Update

This e-mail publication is available free to students who purchase and instructors who adopt the third edition of this text. Delivered twice each semester, this newsletter helps students and instructors keep up-to-date on the latest new drugs, indications, warnings, and precautions. It also includes helpful questions and answers, information on common medication errors, and updates on herbal remedies.

Mosby's GenRx

This comprehensive online drug database is available free for 6 months to students who purchase and instructors who adopt the third edition of this text. To access this resource, use the passcode in the front of the textbook.

Instructor's Electronic Resource with Test Bank

This CD-ROM contains three components:

- **Instructor's Manual,** including Chapter Overviews, Key Terms, Chapter Outlines, Teaching Tips and Strategies (expanded and enhanced in this edition), references to related images on the Electronic Image Collection CD-ROM, and a guide on *How to Teach Pharmacology in an Integrated Curriculum.*
- **Test Bank** with over 350 multiple-choice NCLEX-format questions coded for cognitive level, nursing process, and client need categories *(new!).* Answers to test questions include rationales. The Test Bank is available in word processing files, enabling instructors to edit, add, and delete material.
- **Pharmacology Lecture Outlines in PowerPoint** developed by co-author Robert S. Aucker, PharmD, feature lecture outlines for various drug classes and body systems. These outlines can be used "as is" or customized by adding or deleting material.

Electronic Image Collection for Pharmacology on CD-ROM

This versatile CD-ROM contains 150 full-color images for use in lectures. Images can be printed or imported into PowerPoint.

acknowledgments

This book truly has been a collaborative effort. We wish to thank the instructors who provided input on an ongoing basis throughout the development of the first, second, and third editions. In addition, we would like to thank the following people: Chuck Dresner, Judith Myers, Julie Snyder, Ted Huff, Donald O'Connor, Linda Wendling, Ken Turnbough, Greg McVicar, Anthony Saranita, and Susan Orf. We thank Carolyn Duke and the Saint Louis University School of Nursing for their assistance and cooperation.

We thank our editors Robin Carter and Kristin Geen for their contributions and support throughout the third edition. We are grateful to Catherine Jackson and Jeff Patterson for very capably guiding the project through to publication and to Amy Buxton for her effective design. Richard Lake lent his study skills expertise and has created for us a unique and appropriate feature for students, and for his collaboration we are most grateful. Finally we thank Joe Albanese for his contributions to the first edition.

Linda would like to thank her husband Les and her daughter Karen for their constant support and encouragement. Family, friends, colleagues, and students have shown their support as well. Linda also wishes to acknowledge the students during all her years at Old Dominion University for their support and constructive feedback on the text with each edition. Linda is most gracious and thankful for a continued "sense" of humor and strong faith that she believes has really been at the backbone of all of her successes.

Bob would like to thank God, through whom all things are made possible. An endeavor of this magnitude requires divine intervention. The successful completion of this project required the support and guidance of many. To acknowledge the support of loved ones is not really adequately possible. They have had the patience and understanding of saints to put up with the demands placed on our personal lives by this project. Bob would also like to thank his wife Carol, whose love, support, and encouragement have no end.

Finally, to those who teach, although your work may seem to go unnoticed or unappreciated, your impact will always be remembered in the accomplishments of your students. Your inspiration and motivation shape the future.

We always welcome comments from instructors and students who use this book so that we may continue to make improvements and be responsive to your needs in future editions. Please send any comments you may have in care of the publisher.

Linda Lane Lilley, RN, PhD
Robert S. Aucker, PharmD

contents

Appendixes in Book

Appendixes on MERLIN website
(www.harcourthealth.com/MERLIN/Lilley/):

Part one
Pharmacology Basics: Study Skills Tips

- Introduction to Study Skills Concepts
- PURR
- Pharmacology Basics

INTRODUCTION TO STUDY SKILLS CONCEPTS

What to study? When to study? How much to study? How to study? In the best of worlds, every student would have all the skills necessary to be effective in all academic areas. Unfortunately, many students do not know how to study effectively or have developed techniques that work well in some circumstance but not in others. The purpose of this Study Skills Tips is to introduce you to the steps to follow in learning text and maintaining focus on the appropriate material. This section also offers some specific examples for selected chapters in Part One to help you apply the study techniques and strategies discussed here.

Extensive study skills covering time management, note taking, mastering of the text, preparation for and taking of examinations, and development of vocabulary are presented in the *Study Guide* that accompanies this text. These tools are important to any student, but in challenging technical areas such as nursing and pharmacology, they become even more valuable. The techniques described here and in the *Study Guide* will not necessarily make learning easy, but they will help you achieve your goals as a student.

PURR

PURR is a handy mnemonic device representing a four-step process that will lead to mastery of material. These steps are as follows:

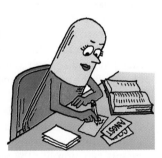

- *Prepare*
- *Understand*
- *Rehearse*
- *Review*

PURR has positive and negative aspects. The negative is that it requires that you go through every chapter four times. The good news is that you are not going to actually *read* the chapter four times. You are only going to *go through* it four times. Only one of those times is a slow, careful, intensive reading. The other trips through the chapter are much quicker. The first time you go through the chapter should only take 5 or 10 minutes. Each time you go through the chapter, you are processing the information in distinctly different ways. The PURR approach will enhance your learning, and if you use it from the first assignment on, you will find that it takes you less time than you were spending before you adopted the PURR approach to learn what you need.

Prepare

Reading the text, like any complex process, is not something to dive into without thought and planning. *Pharmacology and the Nursing Process* is organized to help you learn the material, but you have to take advantage of what the authors have done for you to facilitate this. Preparing to read means setting goals and objectives for your own learning, but the tools you need to help you do this are already in place. Look at the opening pages of any chapter in the text and you will see a standard structure.

Every chapter begins with a **title.** Learn to use the title as the first step in preparing to learn. Chapter 4 is entitled "Legal, Ethical, and Cultural Considerations." This instantly identifies what the chapter is about. Do not start reading immediately; instead think about the title for a few seconds. Are there any unfamiliar terms? If your answer is "no," great. If it is "yes," then you already have some focus for your reading because you know you will need to learn the unfamiliar terms and their meanings.

The next feature of every chapter is the **objectives.** You need objectives for learning, and the authors have anticipated this. Read the objectives actively. Do not just look at the words; think about the objectives. Ask yourself the following questions: What do I already know about this material? How do these objectives relate to earlier assignments? How do they relate to objectives the instructor has given? The chapter objectives identify things you should be able to do after you have read the material. Do not wait until you have read the chapter to start trying to respond. *Prepare* means getting the brain engaged from the beginning. Studying the chapter objectives establishes a direction and purpose for your reading. This will enable you to maintain concentration and focus while you read.

Another feature in the opening pages of each chapter is the **glossary.** This is one of the most valuable tools the authors have provided. They know that there are many terms to learn and are giving you a head start on learning them. Spend a few minutes with the glossary. Notice the terms that are also used in the chapter objectives. Go back and look at the objectives and think about what you have learned from the glossary. As you study the glossary, look for shared root words, prefixes, or suffixes. If words share such common word elements, these words also have a shared meaning. Learning the meaning of common word elements can simplify the whole process of learning vocabulary. Perhaps you remember in elementary school being told to "look for the little words in the big word." This is essentially the same technique—one that worked then and one that will work now.

Now make a quick pass through the chapter or the assigned pages from the chapter. Focus on the text conventions, which are described later in this chapter. Look for anything that stands out in the chapter, such as boldfaced text, boxed material, and tables. This provides a quick overview of the chapter, which will make the next steps in the PURR process much more effective and efficient.

The **chapter headings** show the major points to be covered. Study them and notice the major headings (topics) and the subordinate headings (subtopics). This is essentially a picture of the chapter, and using the picture is an essential step in preparing to read. As you read through the chapter headings, turn the topic and subtopics into a series of questions that you want to be able to answer when you finish reading. Think about the objectives and how these headings relate to them. Finally, in the headings devoted to specific classes of agents, notice there are elements that are common to every one. The last two headings are always "Implementation" and "Evaluation." This tells you that these are two common elements you will be expected to know at the end of every chapter. The minutes you spend *preparing* will pay off in a big way when you start to read.

Preparing makes the whole approach to learning an active one. It may not make the chapters the most exciting reading you will ever do, but it will help you accomplish your personal learning objectives as well as those set by the authors.

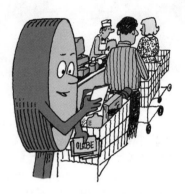

On-the-run Action. Preparing is great to do during "found" time. It should not take more than 5 or 10 minutes. Time between classes, time spent waiting for the coffee water to boil, or any other small block of time that usually just slips away can be used to accomplish this step.

Understand

The time has now come to read the assignment. Go to your desk, the library, or wherever you have chosen for serious study. Reading the assignment is where all your preparation pays off. If you did the *Prepare* step earlier in the day, it is not a bad idea to spend a minute or two going through the chapter features again to get your focus. As you read the assignment, remember the chapter objectives and notice the chapter headings in the body of the chapter. As you read, rephrase the chapter headings as questions to help keep you focused on the task at hand. Because this is the first time you are really focusing on the concepts and the details, this is not the time to do any text notations. Read and, as you read, think. Terms from the glossary are repeated, and their meanings are often expanded and clarified in the body of the text. Pay attention to these terms as you read. Think about what they mean and how you would define them to someone else. Read for meaning. Read to *understand*. Do not read just to get to the end of the assignment. That is a passive action. Ask yourself questions. Analyze, respond, and react as you read.

Often reading assignments are too long to be read with complete understanding in one session. If you find that your concentration is flagging or you do not remember anything you read on the previous page, it is time to take a break. All too often students have only one objective—to finish the assignment. You might be able to force yourself to continue reading, but you will not learn much. Mark your place and take a 5- or 10-minute break. Take a walk, read the daily comic strips, get a soda or a cup of coffee, and then go back to reading. When you come back to the assignment, spend the first 3 or 4 minutes reviewing. Look back at the previous chapter heading and think about what you were reading before the break. The chapter can be broken down into many small reading sessions, but it is critical that you do not lose sight of the chapter as a whole. Spending these minutes in review may seem like time that could be better spent continuing with the reading, but this quick review will save time in the long run.

There is no quick way to read a chapter. You will not find an "on-the-run action" for this step because it cannot be done in this way. However, if you do the *Prepare* step first, you will be surprised at how much more easily you get the reading done and how much more learning you have achieved in the process.

Rehearse

Rehearsing is the third step in the process. It starts the process of consolidating your learning and establishing a basis for long-term memory. Rehearsal accomplishes two things. First, it helps you find out what you understand from the reading. Knowing what you know is really important. Second, it identifies what you do not understand, and this may be an even more important benefit. Knowing what you do not know before it comes to light during an examination is critical.

How to Rehearse. Everything you do in the *Prepare* and *Understand* steps comes into play in the *Rehearse* step. Rehearsal should begin with the features at the beginning of the chapter. Open the text to the beginning of the chapter. Start with the chapter title and begin to quiz yourself on what you have read. Compose three or four questions pertaining to the chapter title, and then try to answer them to your satisfaction. The questions you ask yourself should be both literal (asking for specific information presented in the chapter) and interpretive (testing your comprehension of concepts and relationships). An example of a literal question using the Chapter 4 title might be, "What are the definitions of *legal, ethical,* and *cultural?*" This question would help you determine whether you can satisfactorily define these terms in your own words. Asking and answering such questions as this always serves to move learning from short-term to long-term memory. Literal questions are very important to help you grasp the factual information and terminology contained in the reading assignment. However, it is also necessary to ask questions that stimulate thought about the concepts and the relationships between the facts and concepts presented in the chapter. An example

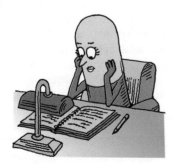

of an interpretive question regarding the Chapter 4 title might be: "What are the most important legal, ethical, and cultural concepts pertaining to the use of drugs?" Sometimes you will find that, even though the question is interpretive, the authors have anticipated the question and the text does contain the direct answer to your question. Other times you will need to formulate your own response by pulling together bits and pieces of information from the entire reading assignment.

Once you have exhausted the question potential for the chapter title, move on to the chapter objectives. Use the same process here. Rephrase the objectives as questions and try to answer them. Remember that the object of rehearsal is to reinforce what you have learned and to identify areas where you need to spend additional time (review).

Go to the glossary. Cover the definitions, and try to define each term in your own words. Another method is to cover the term, and on the basis of the definition, name the term. Do not just memorize the definition, because you may find the information presented differently on an examination, and you will then be unable to respond.

Now proceed to the chapter or assigned pages. The chapter headings are the main tools for rehearsal. Apply the same question-and-answer technique used for the title and objectives to test what you may already know about the chapter content. Turn the headings into questions and answer them. Look at the text for boldfaced and italicized items, lists, and other text conventions. These too can become the basis for questions. The tables and diagrams should also be used for this purpose. Keep in mind the importance of asking both literal and interpretive questions. Some of the questions you ask yourself should also tie different topic headings together. Ask yourself how topic A relates to topic B.

As you proceed through the chapter, do not worry if you cannot answer the questions you ask. As stated earlier, one of the goals of the rehearsal process is to identify what you need to spend more time on. If you can give no response to a particular question, put a mark in the margin of the pertinent place in the text to remind yourself to come back and spend more time on this material, but move on at this point. Rehearsal should be a relatively quick procedure. Once you become accustomed to the PURR

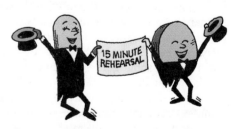

method, it should take no more than 15 or 20 minutes to rehearse 15 pages after doing the *Prepare* and *Understand* steps.

As you reach the end of the chapter, skim the *Implementation* and *Evaluation* sections. Make sure that the relationship between these sections and the information in the rest of the chapter is clear. If you have questions or concerns, note them in the margins and ask your instructor to clarify these points. Although the objective is to master the chapter content as an independent learner, sometimes it is essential to ask questions of the instructor to facilitate the process.

When to Rehearse. Ideally rehearsal should take place almost immediately after you finish reading the material. Take a 10- to 15-minute break, and then start the process. The longer the gap between reading and rehearsal, the more you will forget and the longer it will take to rehearse. If you are breaking a reading assignment down into smaller segments, do the rehearsal for each segment before you begin reading the new material. This helps maintain the sense of continuity in the chapter. This seems like a lot of work to do in a study session, but with practice it will go quickly and you will be pleasantly surprised at the quality and quantity of your learning.

Review

Review is the fourth and final step in the PURR process, and it is an essential step. No matter how well you have learned material in the preceding steps, forgetting will always occur. Reviewing is the only way to store what you have learned in long-term memory. The good news is that, using the PURR model, the review can be done for small segments of material and can be done relatively quickly.

How to Review. The basic review process is essentially the same as the rehearsal process, with some limited rereading as the only difference. When you cannot immediately answer a question, read the pertinent material again. *This does not mean you should read the entire chapter again.* Often the answer to the question will pop into your mind after you have read only a few lines. When this happens, stop reading and go back to responding to your question. The idea is to reread only as much material as is necessary to make the answer clear. One or two words or one or two sentences may trigger personal recall, but it may also take two or three paragraphs for this to happen.

Frequency of Review. How many times should you review material in this way? This actually depends on many factors, such as the difficulty of the material, the length of the assignment, and your personal background. Only you can determine how often you need to review, but there are some guidelines that will help you decide this for yourself.

First, consider the difficulty of the material. If it is very complex, contains many new terms and difficult concepts, and seems difficult to grasp, then you should review very frequently. On the other hand, if the material is straightforward and you are able to relate it well to what you have already learned, then less frequent reviews will serve to keep the material in your memory.

Second, consider how well the review went. If you had difficulty answering many questions to your satisfaction or had to do a lot of rereading, you should schedule another review soon (a day or two later at most).

The success of each review session should be used to help you determine when to schedule another session. The review step is a means of monitoring the success of the learning process. If reviews go well, limited rereading is necessary, and you are able to give clear answers to your questions, this tells you that you can wait several days (4 or 5) before reviewing this material again. A mediocre review, more extensive rereading, and poor answers indicate that you should only let 2 or 3 days go by before reviewing the material again. If the review goes very poorly, you should plan to review the material again the next day. It is up to you to judge the success of each review and to decide how often you need to review. The nice thing about PURR is that it enables you to monitor your success and to easily regulate the learning process.

Technique for Rehearsal and Review. Both rehearsal and review foster active learning, which helps you maintain interest in the material and strengthens your memory. For these benefits to occur, it is essential that the review and rehearsal processes be done orally. Simply talk aloud as you go through the material. Ask questions and give your answers out loud. This forces you to think about the material. It helps you organize it and translate it into your own words. The object is not to memorize everything you have read but to understand and be able to explain it. Eventually you will need to answer questions on an examination. Framing questions as a part of the learning process is a way to anticipate examination questions. The more questions you ask yourself during study time, the more likely some of the questions on the examination will be ones you have asked yourself. Further, by doing the rehearsal and review orally, you will find it easier to recall the answers during the examination, because this oral model requires more than just remembering seeing the material; you will actually be able to hear the rehearsed answers in your mind. Another advantage of doing the rehearsal and review processes orally is, as stated earlier, that it helps to identify what needs further study. When your oral answer is fragmentary, contains many "uhs," and is really disorganized, then you know that you need to devote more time to learning this term, fact, or concept.

The PURR system may seem like a lot of work at first. The idea of going through a chapter four times understandably seems daunting. Add to this the need for several review sessions, and the first reaction is likely to be: "This won't work," or "I don't have the time to do this." Don't take that attitude. This system does work. It cultivates interest, aids concentration, fosters mastery of the material, and ensures long-term memory of the material, which is important not just for doing well on examinations but also for doing well as a nurse with the safe care of patients at stake. The PURR system will work if you use it. It may take 3 or 4 weeks to get comfortable with the system, but if you keep at it, pretty soon it will become a good habit. After a while you will not be able to imagine studying in any other way.

Like all study systems, the PURR method is a model. As you use it, you may discover ways of changing it that work better for you. That is okay. Do not hesitate to make adjustments that better suit your learning style and strategies. Just remember as you start out that *Preparation, Understanding, Rehearsal,* and *Review* are solid learning principles and cannot be ignored.

Study skills tips are included on the two pages at the beginning of each part. These hints are directly applied to the content found within the chapters of the following unit. Detailed information on specialized study skills, such as time management, note taking, examination preparation, and vocabulary building, are present in the *Study Guide* that accompanies this text.

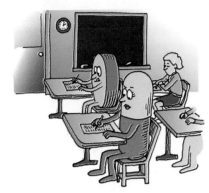

PHARMACOLOGY BASICS
Prepare

As you begin to work with individual chapters, consider how the first step in the PURR system can be used to help you set a purpose and become an active learner.

Chapter 1 Objectives

Consider Objective 1. *List the five phases of the nursing process.* Now turn the objective into a question. *What are the five phases of the nursing process?* Now move to Objective 2 and make it a question. *What are the functions and purposes of the nursing process as related to drug therapy?* Note that this question relates directly to Objective 1. By putting Objective 2 into a question format you will begin to expand and extend on the focus of the first objective, and you will begin to focus on active learning with a clear purpose.

When you begin to read Chapter 1 you will discover that the five phases of the nursing process are repeated as topic headings, and you have the Objective 2 question on which to focus your reading. Begin now to develop the habit of applying this strategy to the objectives in every chapter assigned before you begin to read. Remember to look at the chapter headings at this point as well. It is amazing how much can be learned by using the text structures provided.

Vocabulary Development

Turn to Chapter 2. Objective 1 makes an important point. "Define common terms used in pharmacology." Success depends heavily on knowledge of the "language." The objective makes it clear that this chapter contains a number of terms that the author views as important to be mastered. This is only Chapter 2, and now is the time to be-

gin to apply yourself to mastering the language of this content. Look at the glossary. There are six terms that share the common element *pharmaco.* Although each of these six words will have different meanings, they will have something in common. *Pharmaco* is an example of a group word. No matter what prefixes, group words, and/or suffixes are added to it, a part of the meaning of any word containing *pharmaco* will be "drug" or "medicine." Look up *pharmaco* in any dictionary and you will find "drug" or "medicine" to be the definition. Although you probably already knew that, it is always beneficial to start working on a new technique with something that is familiar. Look at four of the words that begin with *pharmaco,* and consider the rest of the word:

dynamics   genetics   gnosy   kinetics

What do each of these word parts mean? The meaning of *pharmacodynamics* is simply the combination of the meaning of *pharmaco* and *dynamics.* The definition, according to the glossary begins, "the study of the biochemical and physiologic interactions of drug action." You could simply memorize this definition, which would seem to accomplish Objective 1. However, memorization does not always equal understanding. Try another approach. What does *dynamics* mean. Think about the word, and relate it to your own experience and background. It appears to deal with movement or action. After looking it up in the dictionary, all the meanings given seem to relate in some fashion to the idea of motion and/or action. A simplistic definition of *pharmacodynamics* would be "drugs in action." Certainly this is not a technical or medical definition, but

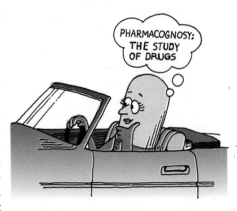

it contributes a great deal to an understanding of the definition provided in the glossary. This is the object of learning vocabulary. Do not memorize words without understanding. Apply a little thought, and relate the term and definition in a way that makes the meaning personal for you. When you do that, you will find that you understand the glossary definition better, and your ability to retain the meaning will be significantly improved. This means that the test item that asks you to select the definition for *pharmacodynamics* from a list of similar definitions will be much easier, because you will remember action and movement and look for the choice that best represents that concept.

Apply this same strategy to genetics. You already know what genetics means. Now you must determine how to connect that to the meaning in the text. After you have the

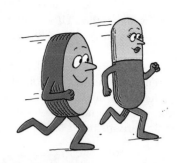

definitions of *gnosy* and *kinetics,* you can apply the same procedure. When you have done this with all four words, you will discover that you will not need to spend a great amount of time trying to memorize esoteric definitions. You will have personalized the meanings. Those meanings will stay with you much more readily than those learned by rote memorization. By the way, do you know what *biochemical* and *physiologic* mean? These terms are used in the glossary definition of *pharmacodynamics.* You need to know what they mean to fully understand pharmacodynamics.

The Nursing Process and Drug Therapy

www.harcourthealth.com/MERLIN/Lilley/

Look for this symbol for topics covered in the **Online Worksheet** Activity

When you reach the end of this chapter, you should be able to do the following:

1 List the five phases of the nursing process.

2 Discuss the function and purposes of the nursing process as related to drug therapy.

3 Describe how the nursing process would be specifically used in medication administration.

4 Identify the components of the assessment process for patients receiving medications, including collection of subjective and objective data.

5 Discuss the process of formulating nursing diagnoses for patients receiving medications.

6 Identify goals and outcome criteria for patients receiving medications and related nursing implementation.

7 Discuss the evaluation process as it relates to the administration of medications.

glossary

Goals Objective, measurable, and realistic changes of behavior in the patient, achieved through nursing care, with an established time period for achieving the outcome. (p. 7)

Nursing process An organizational framework for the practice of nursing. It encompasses all steps taken by the nurse in caring for a patient: assessment, nursing diagnosis, planning (with outcome criteria), implementation of the plan (with patient teaching), and evaluation. The rationale for each step is founded on nursing theory. (p. 7)

Outcome criteria Descriptions of patient goals that are succinct and well thought out. They include behavioral expectations to be met by specific deadlines and always bear in mind the ultimate goal of patient safety. (p. 7)

OVERVIEW

The **nursing process** is an orderly and systematic method of identifying the following components of patient care related to drug therapy:

- Specific health status
- Specific problems and alterations in human needs
- Plans to solve these problems through the establishment of **goals** and **outcome criteria**
- Implementation of the plans related to the above
- Evaluation of how effective, or ineffective, your plans were in promoting optimal wellness and health and in resolving the identified problems

The nursing process is central to all nursing care. It is flexible, adaptable, and adjustable to numerous situations, including the administration of medications. The nursing process has specific phases, including assessment, planning, implementation, and evaluation. Box 1-1 provides an example of the application of this nursing process to a particular patient care situation and its specific use in the administration of medications.

ASSESSMENT

During the assessment phase of the nursing process, subjective and objective data on the patient, drug, and environment are collected. The information on the patient and environment may be collected from the patient, family, or significant other. Data regarding the drug may be collected from authoritarian sources such as a reference textbook, drug manufacturer's insert, drug handbook, or a licensed pharmacist. All the information obtained will then be synthesized and analyzed by the nurse so appropriate nursing diagnoses and plan of care may be developed.

First, information regarding the patient and environment (both objective and subjective) can be collected through a drug history and nursing assessment. Often there are standardized forms for nurses to use with this process. A drug history may include information such as use of prescription and over-the-counter (OTC) medications, home remedies, or herbal or homeopathic treatments; intake of alcohol, tobacco, or caffeine; past and present health history; and family history. A nursing assessment should also include a head-to-toe assessment and a collection of information regarding the patient's

BOX 1-1 Nursing Process: Patient Care and Medication Administration

PATIENT CARE SITUATION AND THE NURSING PROCESS

Assessment

Objective data
43-year-old African-American male
Family history of DM
VS within normal limits (BP 130/70, R20, P84)
FBS 239
Diminished pedal pulses

Subjective data
c/o frequent urination, increase in thirst, weight loss, headache, lethargy, confusion.

Nursing diagnosis

Impaired urinary elimination, frequency, due to possible pathophysiologic changes from DM as evidenced by frequent trips to bathroom at night.

Planning/Outcome Criteria

Goal
Patient will regain normal urinary patterns.

Outcome Criteria
Patient will awaken to void no more than once per night and void per usual routine during the day.

Implementation

Monitor FBS as ordered.
Monitor fluid intake and output daily for excessive output or any other imbalance.
Assess skin turgor daily.
Assess pre-illness urinary elimination patterns.
Educate patient about the disease process and management of symptoms once therapy is initiated.

Evaluation

Sleeping most of the night; only gets up once during the night to void for the last few weeks since treatment.
Normal urinary patterns during the day.

MEDICATION ADMINISTRATION AND THE NURSING PROCESS

Assessment

Objective data
43-year-old male
Recent Dx of IDDM (Type 1 diabetes)
New insulin regimen of regular and NPH
No history of previous illnesses
No other health problems

Subjective data
States "uneasy with treatment plan"
States "knows very little about DM, its treatment and complications"
States "fearful of giving self injections"

Nursing diagnosis

Deficient knowledge related to newly diagnosed DM and new treatment regimen with insulin as evidenced by voicing fears and anxieties and asking many questions.

Planning/Outcome Criteria

Goal
Patient adheres to new insulin treatment regimen without complications.

Outcome Criteria
Patient will state reasons for taking insulin therapy to help regulate blood sugars.
Patient will state importance of daily glucometer testing to maintain consistent blood sugar levels.
Patient will state the S&S of hypoglycemia and means of treatment.
Patient understands importance of follow-up with physician for close monitoring.
Patient demonstrates safe "drawing-up" of insulin and injection technique with rotation of sites of injection.

Implementation

Educate patient and family about DM, its treatment with insulin, and side effects of therapy.
Use AV aids, films, pamphlets for education about insulin therapy, injection sites, etc.
Monitor FBS as ordered.
Assess patient's response to Dx of DM and to its treatment.
5 "Rs": right dose, right drug, right time, right patient, right route.

Evaluation

Has normal FBS and monitors blood sugar levels daily with glucometer.
Able to continue insulin therapy at home.
Has minimal to no complications related to insulin therapy.
Able to treat S&S of hypoglycemia, should they occur.

AV, Audiovisual; *c/o*, complains of; *DM*, diabetes mellitus; *Dx*, diagnosis; *FBS*, fasting blood sugar; *IDDM*, insulin-dependent diabetes mellitus; *NPH*, insulin; *S&S*, signs and symptoms; *VS*, vital signs.

religious preferences, health beliefs, sociocultural profile, lifestyle, stressors, storage capacities for medications (such as a refrigerator), socioeconomic status, educational level, motor skill abilities, and cognitive ability. Objective data may be obtained through physical assessment and include vital signs, weight, height, laboratory results, and results of diagnostic tests. A thorough medication history is important to ensure the safe use of medications in patients. The following information is just an exam-

ple of the type of information that would make up a complete medication history:
- OTC medications (aspirin, vitamins, acetaminophen products [Tylenol], laxatives, cold preparations, sinus medications, and antacids)
- Prescription medications (including birth control pills)
- Street drugs (marijuana, cocaine, angel dust, lysergic acid diethylamide [LSD])
- Herbals and homeopathic substances

- Problems with drug therapy in the past (allergies, adverse effects, side effects, diseases that may contraindicate or limit the use of some medications)
- Growth and development issues as related to the patient's age

Interviewing skills and establishment of a therapeutic relationship are important. Open-ended questions are preferred for collection of more thorough information about the patient. Direct questions that may be answered with a simple "yes" or "no" are not as helpful in collecting thorough responses to questions posed to the patient, family, or significant other. Some questions to ask the patient, significant other, caregiver, and yourself include the following:

- What is the patient's medical diagnosis?
- What are the laboratory and diagnostic test findings?
- What have been the patient's experiences with medicines and with hospital and health care facilities?
- What are the patient's vital signs?
- What are the medications ordered? What medications is the patient already taking? How is the patient taking the medications?
- What does the particular drug do? Is it really helping the patient?
- What are the drug's adverse effects, contraindications to its use, appropriate dosages, and routes of administration?
- What are the developmental concerns, issues, or implications related to the patient receiving the medication?
- What is the patient's cultural origin and its influence on drug therapy?

Information collection on the drug or medication must begin by obtaining a complete order from the physician or other licensed individual. The order has six elements:

- Patient's name
- Date order was written
- Name of medication
- Dosage (includes size, frequency, and number of doses)
- Route of delivery
- Signature of the prescriber

Once this information has been verified and transcribed appropriately, information about the medication should be researched. Use of a drug handbook, pharmacology textbook, *Mosby's GenRx*, or other authoritative sources are recommended for the review of drug information. Information to review includes classification, mechanism of action, dosage, routes, side effects, contraindications, drug incompatibilities, cautions, and nursing implications. If information is unavailable, you may contact a registered pharmacist for information about the medication. You should document the source of information, including the pharmacist's name. You should never give a medication with which you are unfamiliar unless you have researched it thoroughly.

It is also important during the assessment phase of the nursing process to consider the expanded and collaborative role of the nurse. Physicians and dentists are no longer the only health care prefessionals prescribing and writing medication orders. Nurse practitioners and physician assistants have also gained the professional privilege to legally prescribe medications. Nurses should always be aware of and obtain a copy of their state's nurse practice acts so they are informed of RN's limitations and any responsibilities and expanded roles of the nurse (i.e., nurse practitioner).

Analysis of Data

Once all the data regarding the patient, environment, and drug have been collected and reviewed, the nurse must make a critical evaluation of the information (analysis) and make decisions about its importance and implications to the patient. Effort should be made to ensure that all information is obtained and documented at this time.

NURSING DIAGNOSES

Once the assessment has been completed, the next step is to analyze the information before formulating the nursing diagnoses. A nursing diagnosis as it relates to drug therapy should be a judgment or conclusion about the risk for or actual need or problem of a particular patient. Remember, the two major tasks associated with the assessment phase are the collection of subjective and objective data and the formulation of nursing diagnoses. Nursing diagnoses related to drug therapy will most likely develop out of data such as knowledge deficit; risks for injury; noncompliance; and various deficits, excesses, or alterations, to name only a few.

The North American Nursing Diagnosis Association (NANDA) is the formal organization for the development of a classification system for nursing diagnoses and is recognized by the American Nurses Association. One recent change in the format of nursing diagnoses is the replacement of the phrase *potential for* with the phrase *risk for*. The phrase *risk for* represents the fact that a patient, family, or community may be more vulnerable to developing a particular problem than others in the same situation. Other terms in the NANDA Nursing Taxonomy II include impaired, deficient, ineffective, decreased, increased, imbalanced, etc. Altered and alteration are now outdated terms. In 2001, NANDA diagnoses were modified and updated by the organization.

Activity

PLANNING

After data are collected, the planning phase begins. Planning includes the identification of goals and outcome criteria.

The major aims of the planning phase are to prioritize all the nursing diagnoses and to specify the goals and outcome criteria with the time when these should be achieved. The planning phase provides time to get special equipment, review the possible procedures or techniques to be rendered, and gather information either for oneself or the patient. This step leads to the provision of safe care if professional judgment-making is combined with the acquisition of knowledge about the patient and the medication to be given.

Goals and Outcome Criteria

Goals are objective, measurable, and realistic, with an established time period for achievement of the outcome, which is more specifically stated in the outcome criteria. Patient goals are reflected in expected changes through nursing care. The outcome criteria, or description of goals, should be succinct, well thought out, and patient and nursing focused, and it should include behavioral expectations to be met by certain deadlines. The ultimate aim of these criteria is the safe and effective administration of medications. These criteria should relate to each nursing diagnosis and guide the implementation of the nursing care plan. The formulation of these criteria begins with the analysis of the judgments made about all the patient data and subsequent nursing diagnoses and ends with the development of a nursing care plan. Outcome criteria provide a standard of measure that can be used to move toward the goal. These criteria may address special storage and handling techniques, administration procedures, equipment needed, drug interactions, side effects, and contraindications. In this text, specific time frames are usually not included in the goals and outcome criteria because this process must be individualized for each patient situation and reflect such individual and specific planning and nursing judgment.

The patient-oriented outcome criteria must apply to any medications the patient will receive. For example, in the sample situation described in Box 1-1, the outcome criteria of the 43-year-old man with diabetes mellitus were focused on the administration and general aspects of insulin therapy. In this patient the nurse-oriented outcome criteria include specific patient education about insulin, its side effects, contraindications to its use, and injection techniques, as well as what you, as a nurse, should know about the medication before it is administered. If you have any questions about the order, its appropriateness, or safety in a given patient, you should get answers to these questions and then use professional judgment in the implementation of the order. During the planning phase, if the patient's condition is changing and could be worsened by the medication or the physician's order is

unclear or incorrect, the medication should be withheld, the physician should be contacted for clarification or further instructions, and the information should be documented. If the physician is unavailable, the nurse manager or nursing supervisor should be notified immediately about the problem. Nursing policy guidelines should also be checked to find out who else should be contacted.

Activity

IMPLEMENTATION

Implementation consists of initiation and completion of the nursing care plan as defined by the nursing diagnoses and outcome criteria. When it comes to medication administration, you need to know and understand all the information about your patient and each medication prescribed (see assessment questions on p. 9).

In addition, it is important to always go by the *five rights of medication administration:* right drug, right dose, right time, right route, and right patient.

Implementation is guided by the assessment and planning phases of the nursing process. It requires constant communication and collaboration with the patient and with members of the health care team who are involved in the patient's care. In addition to following the five rights of medication administration, you also need to be aware of the following:

- Constant system analysis (e.g., the system of the nursing unit or pharmacy department, patient education)
- Drug storage and documentation
- Preparation of the dosage of medication
- Use of all types of medication delivery systems
- Checking of transcription of orders
- Procedures and techniques of medication administration
- Routes of administration and specific implications
- Consideration of special situations (e.g., patient with difficulty swallowing, patient with a nasogastric tube, unconscious patient)
- Preventing and reporting of medication errors
- Patient teaching
- Monitoring of the patient for therapeutic effects, side effects, and toxic effects
- Documentation (format and forms vary; documentation may be in narrative form or SOAP [Subjective, Objective, Assessment, Planning] format). The nurse needs to document prns, stats, one-time orders, and responses, including adverse and therapeutic effects of medications.

The five rights of medication administration and system analysis should always be considered and integrated into drug therapy and the nursing process.

Right Drug

To ensure that the right drug is administered, attention must be paid to both the drug orders and the medication labels when preparing medications for administration. In addition, you should consider whether the drug is appropriate for the patient. To be sure that the right drug is being administered and is appropriate, you must obtain information about the patient, such as his or her past and present medical history and a thorough and updated medica-

---

legal & ethical principles

Five Rights of Medication Administration

We are legally responsible to administer the right drug, to the right patient, at the right time, right dose, and right route. In reflecting on this principle and standard-of-care issue, it is also important to know that dispensing the wrong drug is one of the most common medication errors that occurs. Some contributing factors are as follows:

- Labeling and packaging of products that look similar
- Products with similar names
- Storage of products in close proximity

One way to decrease the risk of these errors is to ensure that you read the label while double checking your orders and medications. Read and re-read all labels, name of the drug, and dosage, and obtain the medication immediately. Then re-check it with the order before administration. ∎

From Wiegman S, Cohem M: *ISMP Medication Safety Alert!* Warminster, Penn, 1997, Institute for Safe Medication Practices.

tion history, including OTC medications used. Information about the drug is also important. Sources of information include drug reference books, drug inserts (manufacturer's information), and a pharmacist. It is important to be familiar with the generic (nonproprietary) drug name and the trade name (proprietary name that belongs to a specific drug manufacturer). Be careful not to rely on information from your peers and co-workers because *you* are the one responsible for administering the right drug. Therefore always look to the appropriate authoritative sources.

Right Dose

Before administering any drug by any route, you must know the particulars about each drug given. No matter how busy you may be, you must check the order and the label on the medication and check for all the five rights at least *three* times before giving the medication to the patient. If you have any questions, contact the physician to clarify the order, and never assume anything when it comes to the dose of a drug. Always ask yourself if the dose is appropriate to the patient's age and size. Always recheck your mathematical calculations. Pay careful attention to decimal points because an error could cause massive overdosage. The patient's age may also require differences in dosages. Patient information to obtain before you administer a dose of a medication includes the patient's weight, height, vital signs, and age. Remember that neonates, pediatric patients, and elderly patients are more sensitive to medications as compared with other patient populations.

Right Time

When it comes to the right time of medication administration, often you will be confronted with a conflict between the pharmacokinetic and pharmacodynamic properties of the drugs prescribed and the patient's lifestyle and likelihood of compliance. For example, the right time for the administration of antihypertensive agents may be four times a day (qid), but for the active, working, 42-year-old newlywed man, taking a medication with side effects of impotency on time qid may lead to decreased compliance. This emphasis on and teaching about the right time for the administration of medications to your patients must be reflected in your own practice. No matter how busy you are with patients, you must concentrate on the patient and assess every patient individually to identify any special time considerations.

In addition, medications must be given either one-half hour before or after the actual time specified in the physician's orders (i.e., if a medication is ordered to be given at 9:00 every morning, you may give the drug any time between 8:30 and 9:30 AM), except for stat medications, which must be given within one-half hour of the order. Always check the hospital or facility policy and procedure for any other specific information concerning the "half hour before or after" rule.

If medications are ordered every day on a twice daily (bid), three times daily (tid), or even qid basis, the times may be changed if this is not harmful to the patient, if the medication and the patient's condition do not require adherence to an exact schedule, and with physician ap-

proval or notification. For example, an antacid is ordered to be given tid at 9:00 AM, 1:00 PM, and 5:00 PM, but the nurse has misread the order and gives it at 11:00 AM. Depending on the hospital or facility policy, the medication, and the patient's condition, this may not be considered an error. The dosing times can be changed to 11:00 AM, 3:00 PM, and 7:00 PM without harm to the patient and without incident to the nurse.

There are other factors to consider when it comes to the right time. These include multiple-drug therapy, drug-drug or drug-food compatibility, diagnostic studies, bioavailability of the drug (such as the need for consistent timing of doses around the clock to maintain blood levels), drug actions, and any biorhythm effects as occur with steroids.

Right Route

As previously stated, you must know the particulars about each medication before administering it to ensure that the right drug, dose, and routes are being used. Never assume the route for administration—always check with the physician if in doubt.

Right Patient

It is critical to the patient's safety that you check his or her identity each time before you give a medication. Ask for his or her name, and always check for an identification band or bracelet for clarification and confirmation of the patient's name, ID number, age, and allergies. Other areas to assess in reference to the right patient include assessment of the patient's cultural background, preexisting ideas and attitudes, and personal beliefs and religious affiliation. Although the standard five rights of medication administration hold true for safe nursing practice, they do not include *all* of the variables that affect medication administration. Therefore it is important to also consider a possible "sixth right"—the process of system analysis. System analysis looks at more than just the five rights. It also addresses the entire "system" of medication administration, including ordering, dispensing, preparing, administering, and documenting.

Medication Errors

While discussing the five rights of medication administration and system analysis, it is important to discuss medication errors. Medication errors are a major problem in all settings of health care today. The National Coordinating Council for Medication Error Reporting and Prevention (NCCMERP) defines *medication error* as "any preventable event that may cause or lead to inappropriate medication use or patient harm, while the medication is in the control of the health care professional, patient, or consumer. Such events may be related to professional practice, health care products, procedures, and systems including prescribing; order communication; product labeling, packaging, and nomenclature; compounding; dispensing; distribution; administration; education; monitoring; and use." This definition is important to understand and appreciate because it makes us look at not only the five rights of medication administration as contributors to a medication error but also at various systems involved in the medication administration process. The systems may involve any part of the process from where the order is received to where the medication is administered. It includes various health care professionals and ancillary personnel as well as unit stocking, transcription of orders, and how the medication order is verified and interpreted.

The goal of drug therapy is to achieve therapeutic outcomes without injury to the patient. Use of the five rights of medication administration and a system analysis perspective will help most units and facilities "catch" an error before it occurs if the proper safety checks are in place. Physicians, nurses, and pharmacists working collaboratively may help identify the prone "problem" errors and decrease the occurrence of medication errors.

Some medication errors that you should be aware of include the following:

- Similar product names (e.g., quinidine vs. quinine, cisplatin vs. carboplatin, Lanoxin vs. Levoxine, Lodine vs. codeine)
- Abbreviations (e.g., qid vs. qod because of poor handwriting, SC vs. SL)
- Labeling and packaging
- Medication orders not clearly written with nurses assuming what was intended
- Miscalculation and/or improper dosage
- Errors as a result of similar drug names and health care provider being rushed or tired
- Medication order written on the wrong patient's chart
- Wrong route, patient, or time
- Health care provider who administers the drug failing to document; another provider checks the chart, sees no documentation, and gives patient a second dose
- Poor use of assessment without attention to areas covered in a medication history, etc.
- Complications due to drug incompatibilities, etc.

Since we are aware that these are common medication errors, it is necessary that we are very cautious in all aspects of medication administration and these areas in particular.

A few suggestions for avoiding some of the common medication errors include the following:

- Repeat a verbal order, spell the drug name aloud, and speak slowly and clearly.
- Have computer entry of medication orders.
- Have the indication or purpose for use with each product.
- Avoid dosage abbreviations and product abbreviations since they can cause problems for those interpreting them.
- NEVER assume route of administration that a prescriber intends for a medication.
- ALWAYS read the label three times and check with the medication order before administering the medication.
- NEVER use trailing zeros with medication orders and transcription of orders (e.g., use 25 instead of 25.0).
- Carefully read all labels for the five rights of medication administration.
- When in doubt, always check an order with the prescriber, a pharmacist, or the literature.

- Do not assume anything.
- Do not try to decipher illegibly written orders.
- Always be alert; never be too busy to stop, learn, and inquire.
- Encourage the use of both brand name and generic name with orders for medications.
- Do not assume that the physician was correct if you question an order, dose, drug, or indication.
- Question the medication if the patient states, "That isn't what I usually take," "I already had that pill today," or "The doctor said he was changing my medication or dosage."

Reporting medication errors is also a professional responsibility. The steps to take with medication administration errors include the following:

- Check the patient by assessing all parameters (e.g., vital signs) and document accordingly.
- Assess for effects of the drug.
- Complete medication error forms after contacting the physician and nurse in charge.
- Monitor patient carefully.
- Think and act critically; modify nursing practice to prevent further errors.

There is a confidential and autonomous reporting system through the United States Pharmacopeia Medication Errors Reporting Program (USPMERP), which aids in the collection of a nationwide database about medication errors and their causes. It also looks at potential errors. Any health care professional can report a medication error by contacting the USPMERP at 1-800-23-ERROR. The data collected by this program have led to important changes in some serious areas leading to medication errors and will continue to do so if health care professionals report the errors.

EVALUATION

Evaluation occurs after the plan has been implemented but is actually an ongoing part of the nursing process and the drug therapy. Evaluation in the context of drug therapy is the monitoring of the patient's response to the drug—the expected and unexpected responses, therapeutic effects (produced intended effects), side effects, and toxic effects. An example of monitoring therapeutic effects and adverse effects is as follows: patient receives an antihypertensive agent to treat hypertension. The therapeutic effect is that blood pressure decreases to within normal limits (WNL). The adverse effect is that blood pressure is less than 100/60 mm Hg and/or the occurrence of postural hypotension.

Evaluation is also important in determining the status of educational goals and patient care goals regarding medication administration. Several standards are in place to help in evaluation of outcomes of care such as those standards established by nurse practice acts and the Joint Commission on Accreditation of Healthcare Organizations (JCAHO). Within the JACHO, guidelines are established for nursing services about policies and procedures. There are even specific standards regarding medication administration, which are established to protect both the patient and the nurse.

The nursing process is an ongoing and essentially circular process (see Box 1-1). The evaluation of the pa-

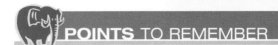

tient's response to previous therapy and other components of his or her medical or surgical regimen is an important facet of the safe and effective delivery of drug therapy. The documentation of any findings and cautions regarding medication use and the continuous assessment of patients are critical aspects of safe and effective nursing care. The nursing process as it relates to drug therapy is the way you organize and provide drug therapy in the context of prudent nursing care. Astute assessments, the establishment of outcome criteria, a correct administration technique and procedure related to the drug, and continual evaluation will become easier and more comprehensible with additional experience and knowledge.

POINTS TO REMEMBER

Nursing Considerations

- Nurses are entrusted with confidential information and with the lives of their patients during all facets of patient care, including drug therapy.
- Safe, therapeutic, and effective medication administration is a major responsibility of professional nurses.
- Nurses are responsible for safe and prudent decision making in the nursing care of their patients, including the provision of drug therapy.

REVIEW QUESTIONS

1. Your 86-year-old patient is being discharged to home on digitalis and has very little information on the medication. Which of the following statements best reflects a realistic goal or outcome of patient teaching activities?
   a. Include significant others in the teaching of the medication.
   b. Provide client with only written instructions about the medication.
   c. Provide client with instruction about monitoring at home with an electrocardiogram at least once monthly.
   d. Client will immediately identify three parameters to use in assessing whether they need to adjust their dosage.
2. Many medications commonly lead to clinically significant drug-drug interactions. Of the following, which one would be less likely to result in such a drug-drug interaction?
   a. Vitamins
   b. Antidepressants
   c. Antihypertensives
   d. Coumadin preparations
3. The nurse would opt for a different site for subcutaneous injections if the skin were:
   a. Pale.
   b. Hairy.
   c. Shiny.
   d. Bruised.
4. Which of the following statements would be more effective in compiling a drug history from a patient?
   a. "Do you frequently take analgesics?"
   b. "Do you experience diarrhea when taking antibiotics?"
   c. "Have you ever had an allergic or anaphylactic reaction?"
   d. "Do you always have your prescriptions filled at the same pharmacy?"
5. Mr. H is a 77-year-old male with newly diagnosed hypertension. His medical history includes a 2-year history of cerebrovascular accident and use of Coumadin. He smokes two packs of cigarettes a day and has for 15 years. He states to you that he is "allergic" to penicillin because he has "vomiting and diarrhea." Your best response to him would be:
   a. "All gastrointestinal reactions to medications are of an allergic nature."
   b. "These are very common allergic reactions, so don't be so concerned."
   c. "Nausea and vomiting are not symptoms of allergic reactions but are common side effects of this drug."
   d. "These symptoms are characteristic of a systemic anaphylactic reaction, and you must seek immediate treatment."

For Answers see www.harcourthealth.com/MERLIN/Lilley/.

CRITICAL THINKING Activities

1. Because of the changes in the ordering, distribution, and administration of drugs; the advances in technology; and the increased potency of medications, what is the *crucial* responsibility of the nurse when implementing drug therapy?
2. When administering medications during the night shift, a patient refused to take his 2 AM dose of an antibiotic, claiming that he had just taken it. What actions by the nurse would ensure sound decision making and maintain patient safety?
3. What are the implications of biotransformation on drug therapy?

For Answers see www.harcourthealth.com/MERLIN/Lilley/.

bibliography

Dirksen SR, Lewis SM, Heitkemper MM: *Clinical companion to medical-surgical nursing,* ed 2, St Louis, 2000, Mosby.

Katz J: Back to basics: providing effecting patient teaching, *Am J Nurs* 5:33, 1997.

Kowalski K, Horner M: A legal nightmare: Denver nurses indicted, *MCN Am J Matern Child Nurse* 23(3):125, 1998.

Lilley LL, Guanci R: Med errors: the new antihistamines, *Am J Nurs* 95(5):14, 1995.

Skidmore-Roth L: *Mosby's 2001 nursing drug reference,* St Louis, 2001, Mosby.

United States Pharmacopeial Convention: *USP DI drug information for the health care professional,* vol 1, ed 20, Englewood, Colo, 2000, Micromedex.

Wilkinson A: Nursing malpractice, *Nursing 98* 6:34, 1998.

Activity

Remember to check the **Online Worksheet** for additional learning opportunities: **www.harcourthealth.com/MERLIN/Lilley/**

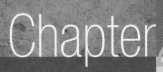

Chapter 2

Pharmacologic Principles

www.harcourthealth.com/MERLIN/Lilley/

Look for this symbol for
topics covered in the
Online Worksheet
Activity

When you reach the end of this chapter, you should be able to do the following:

1 Define common terms used in pharmacology.

2 Understand the role of pharmacokinetics and pharmacodynamics in medication administration.

3 Discuss the application of the four principles of pharmacotherapeutics to everyday nursing practice as related to drug therapy.

4 Discuss the use of natural drug sources in the development of new drugs.

glossary

Additive effect Result of a drug interaction that occurs when two drugs with similar actions are given together. (p. 27)

Adverse drug events (ADEs) Preventable medication errors resulting in harm to patient. (p. 28)

Adverse drug reaction (ADR) An inherent, nonpreventable event that results in hospital admission, prolongation of hospital stay, change in drug therapy, initiation of supportive treatment, and complication of diagnosed disease state. (p. 28)

Antagonistic effect Drug interaction that results in combined drug effects that are lesser than those that could have been achieved if either drug was given alone. (p. 27)

Bioavailability A term used to quantify the extent of drug absorption. (p. 18)

Chemical name The name that describes a drug's chemical composition and molecular structure. (p. 16)

Dissolution The process of how solid forms of drugs disintegrate, become soluble, and get absorbed into circulation. (p. 17)

Drug Any chemical that affects the physiologic processes of a living organism. (p. 16)

Drug-induced teratogenesis (ter ə to jen′ ə sis) The study of drug-induced congenital anomalies. It deals with the toxic effects that drugs can have on the developing fetus. (p. 29)

Drug interaction The alteration of one drug by another drug. (p. 27)

Generic name The name given to a drug by the United States Adopted Names (USAN) council. Also called the *nonproprietary name*. The generic name is much shorter and simpler than the chemical name and is not protected by a trademark. (p. 16)

Iatrogenic responses (i a trə jen′ ik) Unintentional adverse effects that are physician or health-care-professional induced or treatment induced. (p. 29)

Incompatibility Reaction that occurs when two parenteral drugs or solutions are mixed together, resulting in chemical deterioration of the drug. (p. 27)

Medication errors Errors that occur during the administration, dispensing, monitoring, or prescribing of a medication (p. 28)

Medication misadventures The adverse reactions to drugs as a result of medication errors, drug interactions, drug allergies, and unknown causes. (p. 28)

Medication use process The administration, dispensing, monitoring, and prescribing of medications (p. 28)

Pharmaceutics The science of pharmaceutical systems (i.e., preparations, dosage forms, etc.). (p. 16)

Pharmacodynamics (fahr mə ko di na′ miks) The study of the biochemical and physiologic interactions of drugs. It examines the physicochemical properties of drugs and their pharmacologic interactions with suitable body receptors. (p. 16)

Pharmacogenetics (fahr mə kō ge ne′ tiks) The study of genetic factors and their influence on drug response. It investigates the nature of genetic aberrations that result in the absence, overabundance, or insufficiency of drug metabolizing enzymes. (p. 28)

Pharmacognosy (fahr mə kog′ nə sē) The study of drugs that are obtained from natural plant and animal sources. This science was formerly called *materia medica* (materials of medicines) and is concerned with the botanical or zoological origin, biochemical composition, and therapeutic effects of natural drugs, their derivatives, and constituents. (p. 17)

Pharmacokinetics (fahr mə kō ki ne′ tiks) The study of drug distribution rates between various body compartments. It deals with the absorption, distribution, metabolism, and excretion of drugs. (p. 16)

Pharmacology The study or science of drugs. (p. 16)

Pharmacotherapeutics (fahr mə kō ther ə pu′ tiks) The treatment of pathologic conditions through the use of drugs. There are two forms of therapeutics: empirical and rational. In empirical therapeutics there is no suitable explanation for effectiveness of the drugs involved. In rational therapeutics the drugs have known mechanisms of action. Pharmacotherapeutics has also been called *therapeutics*. (p. 16)

Side effects Expected, well-known reactions that result in little or no change in patient management. Intensity and occurrence of side effects are related to the size of the dose. These are unwanted or undesirable effects and may be harmful. (p. 26)

Steady state The physiologic state in which the amount of drug removed via elimination is equal to the amount of drug absorbed with each dose. (p. 24)

Synergistic effect (sin er jis' tik) Drug interaction that results in combined drug effects that are greater than those that could have been achieved if either drug was given alone. (p. 27)

Therapeutic effect The desired effect or intended effect of a particular medication. (p. 24)

Therapeutic index The difference between the minimum therapeutic and minimum toxic concentrations of a drug. If the index is narrow, the range between the therapeutic and toxic drug concentrations is small. (p. 26)

Toxic The state of being poisonous (i.e., injurious to health or dangerous to life). (p. 16)

Toxicology (tok si kol' ə jē) The study of poisons. It deals with the effects of drugs and chemicals in living systems, their detection, and the treatment to counteract their poisonous effects. (p. 16)

Trade name The final name given to a drug; also called the *proprietary name.* Indicates that a drug is registered and that its use is restricted to the owner of that drug. (p. 16)

OVERVIEW

Any chemical that affects the processes of a living organism can broadly be defined as a **drug.** The study or science of drugs is known as **pharmacology.** This study of drugs may incorporate knowledge from a variety of areas. There are many areas of focus in the field of pharmacology:

- Drug history
- Drug origin
- Physical and chemical properties
- Biochemical effects
- Physical effects
- Mechanisms of action
- Absorption
- Distribution
- Biotransformation
- Excretion
- Therapeutic (beneficial) effects
- **Toxic** (harmful) effects

Study in any one of these areas can be defined as pharmacology. Knowledge of these various aspects of pharmacology will enable you to better understand how drugs affect human beings. Without a sound understanding of basic pharmacologic principles, you cannot appreciate the therapeutic benefits and potential toxicity of drugs. Pharmacology is an extensive science that incorporates five interrelated sciences: pharmacokinetics, pharmacodynamics, pharmacotherapeutics, toxicology, and pharmacognosy. The various pharmacologic agents discussed within each chapter are described from the standpoint of these five interrelated sciences. Other commonly used terms such as *therapeutic index, tolerance, dependence,* and *dose-response curves* are also discussed within this chapter.

Throughout the process of drug development, a drug will acquire at least three different names. The **chemical name** describes the drug's chemical composition and molecular structure. The **generic name,** or nonproprietary name, is given to the drug by the United States Adopted Name (USAN) council. It is often much shorter and simpler than the chemical name. The generic name is used in most official drug compendiums to list drugs. The **trade name,** or proprietary name, indicates that the drug has a registered trademark and that its use is restricted to the owner of the drug. The owner is usually the manufacturer of the drug (Fig. 2-1).

Three basic areas of pharmacology describe the relationship between the dose of a drug given to a patient and the effectiveness of that drug in treating the patient's disease: pharmaceutics, pharmacokinetics, and pharmacodynamics. **Pharmaceutics** is the study of how various dosage forms influence various pharmacokinetic and pharmacodynamic properties. **Pharmacokinetics** is the study of what the body does to the drug. **Pharmacodynamics** is the study of what the drug does to the body. Fig. 2-2 illustrates the various phases that affect drug activity, starting with the pharmaceutical phase, proceeding to the pharmacokinetic phase, and finishing with the pharmacodynamic phase.

Pharmacokinetics examines four characteristics of drugs in the body: drug absorption, distribution, metabolism, and excretion. These four characteristics and their relationship to drug and drug metabolite concentrations are then determined for various body sites over specified periods. The onset of action, the peak effect of a drug, and the duration of a drug's effect are also properties studied by pharmacokinetics. Pharmacodynamics investigates the biochemical and physical effects of drugs in the body. More specifically, it determines a drug's mechanism of action. The use of drugs and the clinical indications for drugs to prevent and treat diseases constitute the focus of **pharmacotherapeutics.** Pharmacotherapeutics incorporates the principles of drug actions. An understanding of pharmacotherapeutics is essential for nurses in implementing drug therapy. The study of the adverse effects of drugs on living systems is **toxicology.** Such toxicologic effects are often an extension of a drug's therapeutic action. Therefore toxicology often involves overlapping principles of both pharmacotherapy and toxicology. Plants are the source for

Chemical name	
(+/−)-2-(p-isobutylphenyl) propionic acid	
Generic name	
ibuprofen	
Trade name	
Motrin	

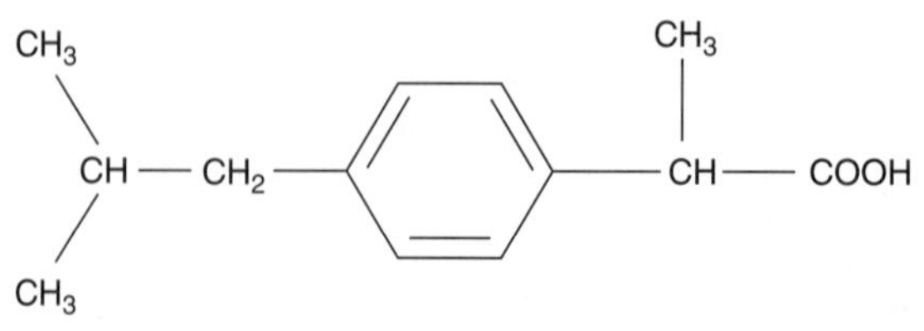

Fig. 2-1 The chemical, generic, and trade names for the common analgesic ibuprofen are listed next to the chemical structure of the drug.

many drugs, and the study of these natural drug sources (plants, animals) is called **pharmacognosy.**

Pharmacology is very dynamic, incorporating several different disciplines. Traditionally, chemistry is seen as the primary basis of pharmacology, but pharmacology also relies heavily on the physical, biologic, and social sciences.

PHARMACEUTICS

Drug preparations are considered pharmaceutical-related properties. Drug preparations can determine the rate at which **dissolution** and thus absorption occurs. Multiple pharmaceutical-related changes in a dosage formulation can affect drug dissolution. When a drug is ingested orally it may come in either a solid form (tablet, capsule, or powder) or liquid form (solution or suspension). The process of dissolution describes how solid forms of drugs disintegrate, become soluble, and get absorbed into the blood stream. Table 2-1 shows various drug preparations and the rate at which they are absorbed. Oral drugs that are liquids, elixirs, or syrups are already dissolved and therefore quickly get absorbed. Enteric-coated tablets, on the other hand, have a coating that prevents them from being broken down and therefore absorbed until they reach the lower pH of the intestines. This pharamceutical property results in slower dissolution and therefore slower absorption. Sometimes the size of the particles

within a capsule can make different capsules containing the same drug dissolve at different rates, get absorbed at different rates, and thus have different onsets of action. A prime example of this is the difference between micronized (Glynase) and nonmicronized (DiaBeta and Micronase) forms of glyburide. The micronized formulation of glyburide reaches a maximum concentration peak more quickly than the nonmicronized formulation.

A variety of dosage forms exists to provide both accurate and convenient drug delivery systems (Table 2-2). These delivery systems are designed to achieve a desired therapeutic response with minimal side effects. Many dosage forms have been developed with patient compliance in mind. Convenience of administration tends to correlate with medication compliance. Many of the extended-release oral dosage forms were designed with this in mind.

The specific characteristics of various dosage forms have a large impact on how and to what extent the drug is absorbed. If a drug is to work at a specific site in the body, it must either be applied directly at that site in an active from or it must have a way of getting to that site. A drug's dosage form influences this placement. Oral dosage forms rely on the stomach's enzymes or pH to break them down into particles that are small enough to be absorbed into the circulation. Once dissolved through

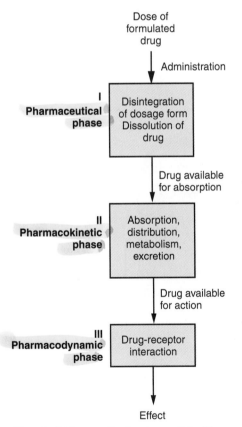

Fig. 2-2 Phases affecting drug activity. (From McKenry LM, Salerno E: *Mosby's pharmacology in nursing*, ed 21, St Louis, 2001, Mosby.)

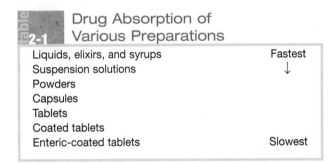

Table 2-1 Drug Absorption of Various Preparations

Liquids, elixirs, and syrups	Fastest
Suspension solutions	↓
Powders	
Capsules	
Tablets	
Coated tablets	
Enteric-coated tablets	Slowest

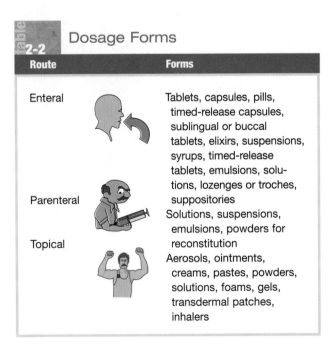

Table 2-2 Dosage Forms

Route	Forms
Enteral	Tablets, capsules, pills, timed-release capsules, sublingual or buccal tablets, elixirs, suspensions, syrups, timed-release tablets, emulsions, solutions, lozenges or troches, suppositories
Parenteral	Solutions, suspensions, emulsions, powders for reconstitution
Topical	Aerosols, ointments, creams, pastes, powders, solutions, foams, gels, transdermal patches, inhalers

the mucosa of the stomach, the drug is then transported to the site of action by blood or lymph.

Many topically applied dosage forms work directly on the surface of the skin. Therefore when the drug is applied, it is already in a dosage form that allows it to work immediately. To other topical dosage forms the skin acts as a barrier through which the drug must pass to get to the circulation, which then carries the drug to the site of action.

Dosage forms that are administered via injection are called *parenteral dosage forms.* They must have certain characteristics to be safe and effective. The arteries and veins that carry drugs throughout the body can easily be damaged if certain drug characteristics are not appropriate. The solutions used in these dosage forms must be very similar to the blood to be safely administered. Unlike oral and topical dosage forms, parenteral dosage forms do not have to be dissolved and absorbed before they can be carried to the site of action.

PHARMACOKINETICS

A particular drug's onset of action, time to peak effect, and duration of action are all characteristics defined by pharmacokinetics. Pharmacokinetics is the study of what actually happens to a drug from the time it is put into the body until the time all of it and its metabolites have left the body. Therefore drug absorption into, distribution to, metabolism within, and excretion from a living organism represent the combined focus of pharmacokinetics.

Absorption
Process
Absorption describes the rate at which a drug leaves its site of administration and the extent to which it occurs. A term used to quantify the extent of drug absorption is **bioavailability.** For example, drug that is absorbed from the intestine must first pass through the liver before it reaches the systemic circulation. If the drug is metabolized in the liver or excreted in the bile, some of the active drug will be inactivated or diverted before it can reach the general circulation and its sites of action. This makes its bioavailablity less than 100%. Many drugs administered by mouth have bioavailabilities less than 100%, whereas drugs administered by the intravenous

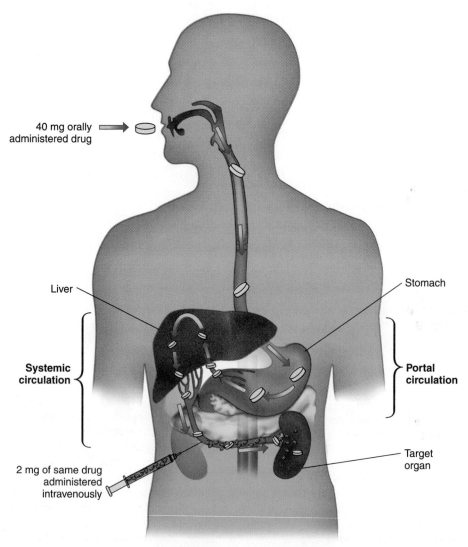

40 mg orally administered drug

Liver

Stomach

Systemic circulation

Portal circulation

2 mg of same drug administered intravenously

Target organ

Fig. 2-3 First-pass effect is the metabolism of a drug by the liver before its systemic availability.

(IV) route are 100% bioavailable. If two medications have the same bioavailability, they are said to be bioequivalent.

There are various factors affecting the rate of drug absorption. These include the administration route of the drug; food, or fluids administered with the drug; dosage formulation; status of the absorptive surface; rate of blood flow to the small intestine; acidity of the stomach; and status of gastrointestinal motility.

Route

How a drug is administered, or its route of administration, affects the rate and extent of absorption of that drug. Although there are several dosage formulations available for delivering medications to the body, they can all be broken down into three basic categories, or routes of administration: enteral (oral), parenteral, and topical. Absorption characteristics vary depending on the dosage form and category.

Enteral. In enteral drug administration the drug is absorbed into the systemic circulation through the oral or gastric mucosa, small intestine, or rectum. The rate of absorption of these drugs can be altered by many factors. When drugs are taken orally, they are absorbed from the gastrointestinal tract into the portal circulation (liver). Depending on the particular drug, it may be extensively metabolized in the liver before it reaches the systemic circulation. Normally, orally administered drugs are absorbed from the intestinal lumen into the mesenteric blood system and conveyed by the portal vein to the liver. Once the drug is in the liver, the enzyme system metabolizes it and it is passed into the general circulation. The initial metabolism of a drug and its passage from the liver into the circulation is called the *first-pass effect* (Fig. 2-3).

If a large percentage of a drug is metabolized into inactive metabolites in the liver, less active drug will make it into circulation. The drug would have a high first-pass effect (e.g., oral nitrates).

When drugs with a high first-pass effect are administered orally, a large amount of drug may be metabolized before it reaches the systemic circulation. The same drug given intravenously will bypass the liver. This prevents the first-pass effect from taking place, and therefore more drug reaches the circulation. Parenteral doses of drugs with a high first-pass effect are much smaller than enterally administered oral doses, yet they produce the same pharmacologic response.

Oral. There are many factors that can alter the absorption of orally (enterally) administered drugs. Acid changes within the stomach, absorption changes in the intestines, and the presence or absence of food and fluid can alter the rate and extent of absorption of drugs administered enterally. Various factors that affect the acidity of the stomach are the time of day, the age of the patient, the presence of food, and the type of food. If there is food in the stomach during the dissolution of an orally administered medication, this may interfere with its dissolution and absorption and delay its transit from the stomach to the small intestine, where most drugs are absorbed. On the other hand, food may enhance the absorption of some fat-soluble drugs or drugs that are easily broken down in an acidic environment.

Before orally administered drugs are passed into the portal circulation of the liver, they are absorbed in the small intestine, which has an enormous surface area. Drug absorption may be altered in patients who have had portions of their small intestine removed because of disease. Anticholinergic drugs may slow down the gastrointestinal transit time, or the time it takes substances in the stomach to be dissolved and passed into the intestines. This may allow more time for an acid-susceptible drug to be in contact with the acid in the stomach and subsequently broken down.

The stomach and small intestine are highly vascularized. When blood flow to that area is decreased, absorption may also be decreased. Sepsis and exercise are examples of conditions in which blood flow is decreased. In both cases, blood is shunted away from the gastrointestinal tract to other areas.

Sublingual. Drugs administered by the sublingual route are absorbed into the highly vascularized tissue under the tongue—the oral mucosa. Sublingual nitroglycerin is an example. These drugs are absorbed rapidly because this area has a large blood supply, and such drugs bypass the liver. Drugs administered by the buccal, sublingual, vaginal, and IV routes bypass the liver. By doing so, drugs like sublingual nitroglycerin are absorbed rapidly into the bloodstream and delivered to their site of action, in this case coronary arteries. These same characteristics are true for rectally administered medications. Most enemas and suppositories (rectal and

---

home health/community points

Drugs to Be Taken on an Empty Stomach and with Food

Numerous medications are generally taken on an empty stomach with at least 6 ounces of water. The nurse must educate patients about taking the following drugs on an empty stomach, mainly because these agents are used so commonly: acetaminophen (analgesic); cephalosporins (all generations); sulfonamides, tetracyclines, penicillins, and erythromycins (antibiotics); isoniazid and rifampin (antituberculin agents); and quinidine (antidysrhythmic).

Medications that are generally taken with food include carbamazepine (anticonvulsant), cimetidine (H₂ receptor antagonist), hydralazine (antihypertensive), lithium (antimanic), propanolol (beta-blocker), spironolactone (potassium-sparing diuretic), NSAIDs (antiinflammatory agents) to decrease GI irritation; and theophylline (xanthine bronchodilator).

Erythromycins, tetracyclines, and theophylline are often taken with food (even though it is indicated to take with a full glass of water and on an empty stomach) to minimize the GI irritation associated with these agents. If in doubt, consult your licensed pharmacist or an authoritative resource. An Internet source to use is www.usp.org.

vaginal) are absorbed directly into the bloodstream, thus bypassing the liver and the first-pass effect. The various drug routes according to whether they are affected by first-pass effects in the liver is given in Box 2-1.

Parenteral. With most medications, the parenteral route is the fastest route by which a drug can be absorbed, followed by the enteral and the topical routes. Intravenous (IV) injections deliver the drug directly into the circulation, where it is distributed with the blood throughout the body. An IV drug formulation is absorbed the fastest. At the other end of the spectrum are transdermal patches, intramuscular (IM) injections, and subcutaneous (SC) injections. These drug formulations may take several hours to days before they are totally absorbed by the body.

Parenterally administered drugs can be given intradermally, subcutaneously, intramuscularly, intrathecally, intraarticularly, and intravenously. The medications that are commonly given by the parenteral route offer the advantage of bypassing the first-pass effect and are in general quickly absorbed. The parenteral route of administration offers an alternative route of delivery for those medications that cannot be given orally. The problems posed by acid changes within the stomach, absorption changes in the intestines, and the presence or absence of food and fluid are not then a concern. There are fewer obstacles to absorption in parenteral administration than in enteral administration of drugs. However, drugs that are administered by the parenteral route must still be absorbed into cells and tissues before they can exert their pharmacologic effect.

Subcutaneous and Intramuscular. Parenteral injections under the skin are referred to as SC injections, and parenteral injections into the muscle are called IM injections. Muscles have a greater blood supply than the skin does, therefore drugs injected intramuscularly are typically absorbed faster than ones injected subcutaneously. Absorption from either of these sites may be increased by applying heat to the injection site or by massaging the site. This increases the blood flow to the area and therefore enhances absorption.

Absorption can be decreased by administering cold packs to the site of injection. This is typically done to localize an injection. This would be done, for example, if an intravenously administered vasopressor, like epinephrine, has extravasated or leaked out of the vein and into the surrounding tissue and has begun to cause ischemia and tissue damage. Cool compresses produce vasoconstriction, which reduces cellular activity and in turn may limit tissue injury. Sometimes injections may be given with a vasoconstrictor such as epinephrine to confine an injected drug to the site of injection, thereby limiting its pharmacologic action to that area.

Some intramuscularly and subcutaneously administered drugs are suspensions and are poorly absorbed. This is by design. The slow absorption of the IM suspension allows for delivery over a longer time. Such injections are commonly called *depot injections.*

Topical. Topical routes of drug administration involve the application of medications to body surfaces. Several different drug delivery systems exist for doing this. Topically administered drugs can be applied to the skin, eyes, ears, nose, and lungs, to name just a few. As with the other routes (enteral and parenteral), there are both benefits and drawbacks to using the topical route of administration. Topically applied drugs deliver a constant amount of drug over long periods, but the drug's effects are usually very slow in their onset and very prolonged in their offset. This can be a problem if the patient begins to experience side effects from the drug and there is already a considerable amount of drug in the subcutaneous tissues. Exceptions are some inhaled drugs such as aerolized albuterol for acute treatment of an asthma attack.

Topical ointments, gels, and creams are examples of topically administered drugs. They are commonly used for their local effects, and they include sunscreens, antibiotics, and nitroglycerin paste and ointment. The drawback to their use is that their systemic absorption is very unreliable. Therefore topically applied ointments, gels, and creams are seldom used for the treatment of any systemic illnesses.

Topically applied drugs can also be utilized in the treatment of various illnesses of the eye, ear, and sinuses. In such conditions, most frequently the required drug is delivered topically to the actual site of illness and bypasses the first-pass effect in the liver.

Transdermal. Transdermal drug delivery is a topical route of drug administration that has been used commonly. Some examples of drugs administered by this route are fentanyl, nitroglycerin, nicotine, estrogen, and clonidine. This method of drug delivery offers the advantage of bypassing the liver and its first-pass effects. It is suitable for patients who cannot tolerate orally administered medications or when it is a practical or convenient method for drug delivery. The various drug delivery systems of specific transdermal patches determine their length of effect.

BOX 2-1 Drug Routes and First-Pass Effects

FIRST-PASS ROUTES
Oral
*Rectal
Hepatic artery
Portal vein

NON-FIRST-PASS ROUTES

Intravenous	Intraocular
Subcutaneous	Transdermal
Inhalation	Intramuscular
Intranasal	Buccal
Intraarterial	Intravaginal
Sublingual	Otic

*Undergoes both first- and non-first-pass effects.

Inhalation. Inhaled drugs are delivered to the lungs as micron-size drug particles. This small drug size is necessary to get the drug to the small airways within the lungs (alveoli). Once the small particle of drug is in the alveolus, drug absorption is fairly easy. At this site the thin-walled pulmonary alveolus is in contact with the capillaries, where the drug can be absorbed quickly. Many pulmonary-related diseases can be treated with such topically applied (inhaled) drugs. Examples of inhaled drugs include pentamidine, which is used to treat *Pneumocystis carinii* infections in the lung; albuterol, which is used for the treatment of bronchial constriction in asthmatics; and vasopressin, which is used to treat diabetes insipidus.

Distribution

The transport of a drug in the body by the bloodstream to its site of action is referred to as *distribution* (Fig. 2-4). Once a drug enters the bloodstream (circulation), it is distributed throughout the body. At this point it is also beginning to be eliminated by the organs that metabolize and excrete drugs—the liver and the kidney. A drug can be freely distributed to extravascular tissue only if it is not bound to protein. If a drug is bound to protein, it is generally too large to pass through blood vessels into tissues. There are three primary proteins that bind to and carry drugs throughout the body. They are albumin, alpha-1-acid glycoprotein, and corticosteroid-binding globulin. By far the most important of these is albumin.

When a patient has a low albumin level, for instance when he or she is malnourished or burned, there is more free, unbound drug as a result.

When an individual is taking two medications that are highly protein bound, the medications compete for binding to these proteins. This competition results in either less of both or less of one of the drugs binding to the proteins. Consequently, this leaves more free, unbound drug. This process can lead to an unexpected drug response called *drug-drug interaction.* A drug-drug interaction occurs when a drug decreases or increases the response of another concomitantly administered drug.

The areas where the drug is distributed first are those that are most extensively supplied with blood. Areas of rapid distribution are the heart, liver, kidneys, and brain. Areas of slow distribution are muscle, skin, and fat.

A theoretical volume, called the *volume of distribution,* is sometimes used to describe the various areas where drugs may be distributed. These areas, or compartments, can be the blood, total body water, or fat. Typically a drug that is highly water soluble will have a small volume of distribution and high blood concentrations. The opposite is true for drugs that are highly fat soluble. Fat-soluble drugs have a large volume of distribution and low blood concentrations. Drugs that are water soluble and highly protein bound are more strongly bound to proteins in the blood and less likely to be absorbed into tissues. Because of this, their distribution and onset of action can be slow.

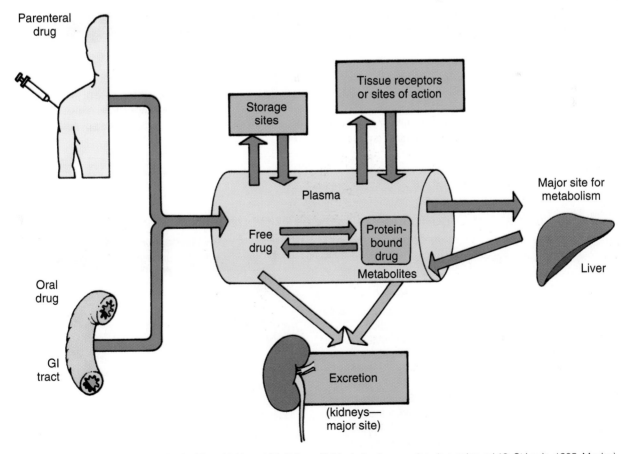

Fig. 2-4 Drug transport in the body. (From McKenry LM, Salerno E: *Mosby's pharmacology in nursing,* ed 19, St Louis, 1995, Mosby.)

Drugs that are highly lipid soluble and poorly bound to protein are easily taken up into tissues and distributed throughout the body. They may even be resorbed back into the circulation from fatty tissue.

There are some sites in the body where it may be very difficult to distribute a drug. These sites typically either have a poor blood supply (e.g., bone) or have barriers that make it difficult for drugs to pass through (e.g., the blood-brain barrier).

Metabolism

Metabolism is also referred to as *biotransformation* because it involves the biologic transformation of a drug into an inactive metabolite, a more soluble compound, or a more potent metabolite. Biotransformation is the next step after absorption and distribution. The organ most responsible for the biotransformation or metabolism of drugs is the liver. Other tissues and organs that aid in the metabolism of drugs are the kidneys, lungs, plasma, and intestinal mucosa.

Hepatic biotransformation involves the use of an enormous variety of microsomal enzymes that control a variety of chemical reactions and aid in transforming medications. These microsomal enzymes are targeted against lipid-soluble, nonpolar (no charge) drugs, which are typi-

cally very difficult to eliminate. Some of the ways in which the liver can metabolize drugs are listed in Table 2-3.

The biotransformation capabilities of the liver can vary considerably from patient to patient. Various factors, diseases, conditions, and medications that can alter biotransformation are listed in Table 2-4.

Delayed drug metabolism results in the accumulation of drugs and a prolonged action of the effects or responses to drugs. Stimulating drug metabolism can thus cause diminishing pharmacologic effects. This is often the case with the repeated administration of some drugs that may stimulate the formation of new microsomal enzymes.

Excretion

The elimination of drugs from the body is referred to as *excretion.* Whether they are active, metabolized, or changed, all drugs must eventually be removed from the body. The primary organ responsible for this is the kidney. Two other organs that also play an important role in the excretion of drugs are the liver and bowel. Most drugs are metabolized or biotransformed in the liver by various glucuronidases and by hydroxylation and acetylation. Therefore, by the time most drugs reach the kidneys, they have been extensively metabolized and only a small fraction of the original drug is excreted as the original com-

Table 2-3 Mechanisms of Biotransformation

Type of Biotransformation	Mechanism	Result
Oxidation Reduction Hydrolysis	Chemical reactions	Increase polarity of chemical, making it more water soluble and more easily excretable. Often this results in a loss of pharmacologic activity.
Conjugation	Combination with another substance (e.g., glucuronide, glycine, methyl, or alkyl groups)	

Table 2-4 Conditions and Drug-Induced Changes in Biotransformation

Condition or Drug-Induced	Actual Disease or Drug	Biotransformation Increased	Biotransformation Decreased
Diseases	Cardiovascular dysfunction		X
	Renal insufficiency		X
Condition	Starvation		X
	Obstructive jaundice		X
	Genetics		X
	Fast acetylator	X	
	Slow acetylator		X
Drugs	Barbiturates	X	
	rifampin	X	
	erythromycin		X
	ketoconazole		X

pound. Other drugs may circumvent metabolism and reach the kidneys in their original form. Drugs that have been metabolized by the liver become very polar and water soluble. This makes elimination by the kidney much easier. The kidney itself is capable of forming glucuronides and sulfates from various drugs and their metabolites.

The actual act of excretion is accomplished through glomerular filtration, reabsorption, and tubular secretion. Free, unbound, water-soluble drugs and metabolites go through passive glomerular filtration, which takes place between the blood vessels of the afferent arterioles and the glomeruli. Many substances present in the nephrons go through active tubular reabsorption. Reabsorption occurs at the level of the tubules, where substances are taken back up into the circulation and transported away from the kidney. This is an attempt by the body to retain needed substances. These substances are actively resorbed back into the systemic circulation. Some sub-

stances may also be secreted into the nephron from the vasculature surrounding it. The processes of filtration, reabsorption, and secretion are shown in Fig. 2-5.

The excretion of drugs by the intestines is another common route of elimination. This is also referred to as *biliary excretion.* Drugs that are eliminated by this route are taken up by the liver, released into the bile, and eliminated in the feces. Once certain drugs, like fat-soluble drugs, are in the bile, they may be resorbed into the bloodstream, returned to the liver, and again secreted into the bile. This process is called *enterohepatic circulation.* Enterohepatic-recycled drugs persist in the body for much longer periods.

Less common routes of elimination are the lungs and the sweat, salivary, and mammary glands. Depending on the drug, these organs can be highly effective eliminators.

Half-life

Another pharmacokinetic variable is the half-life of the drug. It is the time it takes for one half of the original

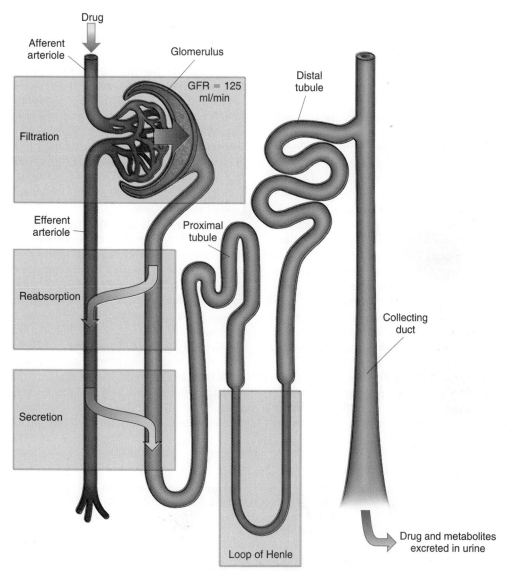

Fig. 2-5 Renal drug excretion. The primary processes involved in drug excretion and the approximate location that these processes take place in the kidney are illustrated.

amount of a drug in the body to be removed and is a measure of the rate at which drugs are removed from the body. For instance, if the maximum level that a particular dosage could achieve in the body is 100 mg/L, and in 8 hours the measured drug level is 50 mg/L, the estimated half-life for that drug is 8 hours. The concept of drug half-life from several perspectives is illustrated in Table 2-5.

After about five half-lives, most drugs are considered removed from the body. At that time approximately 97% of the drug has been removed, and what little is remaining is too small to have any beneficial or toxic effects.

The concept of half-life is clinically useful in determining when a patient taking a particular drug will be at **steady state.** Steady state blood levels of a drug refer to a physiologic state in which the amount of drug removed via elimination (i.e., clearance) is equal to the amount of drug absorbed with each dose. The physiologic phenomenon typically occurs after four half-lives of a drug. Therefore if a drug has an extremely long half-life, it will take much longer for the drug to reach steady-state blood levels. Once an individual has reached steady-state blood levels, there are consistent levels of drug in the body that correspond to maximum therapeutic benefits.

Onset, Peak, and Duration

The pharmacokinetic terms *absorption, distribution, metabolism,* and *excretion* are all used to describe the movement of drugs through the body. Drug actions are the cellular processes involved in the drug and cell interaction (e.g., a drug's action on a receptor). This is in contrast to a *drug effect,* which is the physiologic reaction of the body to the drug. It is similar to a drug's therapeutic effect in that it constitutes how the function of the body is affected as a whole by the drug. The terms *onset, peak,* and *duration* are used to describe drug effects.

A drug's onset of action is the time it takes for the drug to elicit a therapeutic response. The time it takes for a drug to reach its maximum therapeutic response is its peak effect. Physiologically, this corresponds to increasing drug concentrations at the site of action. The duration of action of a drug is the time that drug concentration is sufficient to elicit a therapeutic response.

As with aminoglycoside antibiotics, onset, peak, and duration often play an important part in determining peak (highest blood level) and trough (lowest blood level). If the peak blood level is too high, then toxicity may occur. If the trough blood level is too low, then the drug may not be at therapeutic levels. Therefore peak and trough levels are important monitoring parameters for some medications. The processes of drug absorption, distribution, and elimination directly determine the duration of action of a drug.

PHARMACODYNAMICS

The study of the mechanism of drug actions in living tissues is called *pharmacodynamics.* Anatomy and physiology study body structure and why the body functions the way it does. Drug-induced alterations in these normal physiologic functions are explained by the concept of pharmacodynamics. A positive change in a faulty physiologic system is called the **therapeutic effect** of a drug, and this is the goal of drug therapy. Understanding the pharmacodynamic characteristics of a drug can aid in assessing a drug's therapeutic effect.

Mechanism of Action

There are several ways by which drugs can produce therapeutic effects called *mechanisms of action.* The effects that a particular drug has depend on the cells or tissue targeted by the drug. Once the drug is at the site of action, it can modify the rate (increase or decrease) at which that cell or tissue functions, or it can modify the function of that cell or tissue. A drug cannot, however, make a cell or tissue perform a function that it was not designed to perform.

There are three basic ways by which drugs can exert their mechanism of action: receptor, enzyme, and nonspecific interactions.

Receptor Interaction

If a drug's mechanism of action is the result of a receptor interaction, then the drug's structure is essential. This drug-receptor interaction involves the selective joining of the drug molecule with a reactive site on the surface of a cell or tissue. This in turn elicits a biologic effect. Therefore a receptor is a reactive site on the surface of a cell or tissue. Once a substance (drug or chemical) binds to and interacts with the receptor, a pharmacologic response is produced (Fig. 2-6). The degree to which a drug attacks and binds with a receptor is called its *affinity.* The drug with the best "fit" and strongest affinity for the receptor will elicit the greatest response from the cell or tissue. A drug becomes bound to the receptor through the formation of chemical bonds between receptors on the cell and

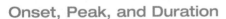

Table 2-5 The Concept of Drug Half-Life

Different Perspectives	Changing Values					
Drug concentration (mg/L)	100	50	25	12.5	6.25	3.125
Hours after peak concentration	0	8	16	24	32	40
Number of half-lives	0	1	2	3	4	5
Percentage of drug removed	0	50	75	88	94	97

the active site of the drug. Drugs that bind to receptors interact with receptors in different ways to either elicit or block a physiologic response. Table 2-6 lists the different types of drug-receptor interactions and their definitions. Drugs that are most effective at eliciting a response from a receptor are those drugs that most closely resemble the body's endogenous substances, which normally bind to that receptor.

Enzyme Interaction

Enzymes are substances that catalyze nearly every biochemical reaction in a cell. The second way drugs can produce effects is by interacting with these enzyme systems. For a drug to alter a physiologic response this way, it must inhibit the action of a specific enzyme. To do this, the drug "fools" the enzyme into binding to it instead of its normal target cell. This protects these target cells from the actions of the enzymes. For example, angiotensin-converting enzyme (ACE) causes an enzymatic reaction that results in the production of a substance called *angiotensin II*, which is a potent vasoconstrictor and mediator of several other processes. The group of drugs called *ACE inhibitors* fools the ACE into binding to it rather than the angiotensin I and thereby prevents the formation of angiotensin II. This in turn causes vasodilation and helps reduce blood pressure.

Nonspecific Interactions

Nonspecific mechanisms of drug action do *not* involve a receptor or an enzyme in the alteration of a physiologic or biologic function of the body. Instead, cell membranes and various cellular processes such as metabolic processes are their main sites of action. Such drugs can either physically interfere with or chemically alter these cellular processes. Some cancer drugs and antibiotics have this mechanism of action. By incorporating themselves into the normal metabolic process, they alter the final product, causing the formation of a defective final product. This final product could be a cell wall that, if not properly formed, results in cell death caused by cell lysis, or it could be the lack of a needed energy substrate that leads to cell starvation and death.

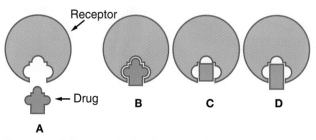

Fig. 2-6 A, Drugs act by forming a chemical bond with specific receptor sites, similar to a key and lock. **B,** The better the "fit," the better the response. Those with complete attachment and response are called *agonists*. **C,** Drugs that attach but do not elicit a response are called *antagonists*. **D,** Drugs that attach, elicit a small response, and also block other responses are called *partial agonists*. (From Clayton BD, Stock YN: *Basic pharmacology for nurses,* ed 12, St Louis, 2001, Mosby.)

PHARMACOTHERAPEUTICS

Before the initiation of a drug therapy, an endpoint or expected outcome of therapy should be established. This desired therapeutic outcome should be patient specific and should be established in collaboration with the patient and, if appropriate, with other members of the health care team. Outcomes must be clearly defined and either measurable or observable by the patient or caregiver. There should also be a specified time line for these outcomes. The progress being made toward the targeted objective should also be monitored. These outcomes should be realistic and should be prioritized so they begin with interventions that are essential to the patient's acute well-being or those that the patient perceives to be important. Examples of such outomes are cure of a disease, elimination or reduction of a preexisting symptom, arresting or slowing of a disease process, preventing a disease or other unwanted condition, or improving the quality of life.

Assessment

Patient therapy assessment is the process whereby a practitioner integrates his or her knowledge of medical and drug-related facts with information about a specific patient's medical and social history. Items that should be considered in the assessment are current medications (prescription, over-the-counter [OTC], and illicit), pregnancy and breast-feeding status, and concurrent illnesses that could contradict beginning a medication. This process ensures an optimal therapeutic plan for the patient.

Implementation

The implementation of a treatment plan can involve several types and combinations of therapies. Therapy can be acute, maintenance, supplemental (or replacement), palliative, supportive, or prophylactic.

Table 2-6 Drug-Receptor Interactions: Definitions

Interaction Term	Definition
Agonist	Drug binds to receptor, and there is a response.
Partial agonist	Drug binds to receptor, and there is a diminished response compared with that elicited by the agonist.
Antagonist	Drug binds to receptor, but there is no response. Drug prevents binding of agonists.
Competitive antagonist	Drug competes with the agonist for binding to receptor. If it binds, there is no response.
Noncompetitive antagonist	Drug combines with different parts of receptor and inactivates it, so agonist has no effect.

Acute Therapy

Acute therapy involves intensive drug therapy and is typically implemented in the critically ill patient. It is generally needed to sustain life. Examples are the administration of vasopressors to maintain blood pressure and cardiac output after open heart surgery, use of volume expanders in a patient who is in shock or even antibiotics in high-risk trauma patients.

Maintenance Therapy

Maintenance therapy typically does not eradicate the problems the patient may have but does prevent progression of the disease. It is used for the treatment of chronic illnesses such as hypertension. The drug therapy maintains the patient's blood pressure within certain limits, which prevents certain end-organ damage. Another example includes use of oral contraception for birth control.

Supplemental Therapy

Supplemental or replacement therapy supplies the body with a substance needed to maintain normal function. This substance may be needed either because it cannot be made or because it is deficient in quantity. Examples are the administration of insulin to diabetic patients or iron to patients with iron-deficiency anemia.

Palliative Therapy

The goal of palliative therapy is to make the patient as comfortable as possible. It is typically used in the end stages of an illness when all possible therapy has failed. The use of high-dose opioid analgesics to relieve pain in the final stages of cancer is an example. The use of oxygen in end-stage pulmonary disease is another.

Supportive Therapy

Supportive therapy maintains the integrity of body functions while the patient is recovering. Providing fluids and electrolytes to prevent dehydration in a patient with influenza who is vomiting and has diarrhea is an example. Giving fluids, volume expanders, or blood products to a patient who has lost blood during surgery is another.

Prophylactic Therapy

Prophylactic therapy is drug therapy provided on the basis of practical experience. It is based on scientific knowledge often acquired during years of observation of a disease and its causes. For example, based on practical experience a surgeon knows that when he or she makes an incision through the skin there is the possibility that skin bacteria are present that can later infect that incision.

Prophylactic therapy is also used with dental procedures for women with mitral valve prolapse or for a patient with prosthetic valves or joints or teflon grafts. IV antibiotic therapy may also be used to prevent infections in a high-risk surgery and is considered prophylactic.

Based on this knowledge, the surgeon administers an antibiotic before making the incision. The antibiotic is also chosen on the basis of experience. Empiric therapy, on the other hand, is not founded on a scientific or rational basis. It is the administration of a drug when a certain pathologic process is suspected on the basis of the patient's symptoms. For example, acetaminophen is given to a patient who has a fever. The cause of the fever may not be known, but empirically the patient is given acetaminophen because it is believed to lower the temperature.

Monitoring

Once the appropriate therapy has been implemented, the effectiveness of that therapy must be evaluated. This constitutes the clinical response of the patient to the therapy. Evaluating this clinical response requires that the evaluator be familiar with both the drug's intended therapeutic action (beneficial effects) and its unintended but potential **side effects** (predictable, adverse drug reactions).

All drugs are potentially toxic and can have cumulative effects. Recognizing them and knowing their effect on the patient are integral components of this monitoring process. *A drug accumulates when it is being absorbed more quickly than it can be eliminated, or when it is administered before the previous dose has been metabolized or cleared from the body.* Knowledge of the function of the organs responsible for metabolizing and eliminating a drug combined with knowledge of how a particular drug is metabolized and excreted will enable the nurse to anticipate problems or treat them appropriately if they occur.

Therapeutic Index

The ratio between a drug's therapeutic benefits and its toxic effects is referred to as its **therapeutic index.** The safety of a particular drug therapy is determined by this index. If a drug has a low therapeutic index, there is a narrow range between a therapeutically active dose of the drug and a toxic dose. Such a drug has a greater likelihood of causing an adverse reaction and therefore requires closer monitoring. Some examples of drugs with narrow therapeutic indexes are warfarin and digoxin.

Drug Concentration

Drug concentrations in patients can also be an important tool for evaluating the clinical response to drug therapy. Certain drug levels correspond to therapeutic responses, whereas others correspond to toxic effects. Toxic drug levels are typically seen when the body's normal mechanisms for metabolizing and excreting drugs are impaired. This commonly occurs when liver and kidney functions are impaired or in persons such as neonates who have an immature liver or kidneys. Dosage adjustments should be made in these patients to appropriately accommodate their impaired metabolism and excretion.

Patient's Condition

Another patient-specific factor to be considered when monitoring drug therapy is a patient's concurrent diseases or other medical conditions. A patient's response to a drug may vary greatly depending on his or her physiologic and psychologic demands. Disease, infection, cardiovascular function, and gastrointestinal function are just a few such physiologic factors. Stress, depression, and anxiety are some psychologic factors that can alter a patient's therapeutic response.

Tolerance and Dependence

The monitoring of drug therapy requires a knowledge of tolerance and dependence and an understanding of the difference. *Tolerance* is a decreasing response to repetitive drug doses, whereas *dependence* is a physiologic or psychologic need for a drug. *Physical dependence* is the physiologic need for a drug (e.g., an opioid in a patient with cancer-related pain). *Psychologic dependence* is the desire for the euphoric effects of drugs and typically involves the recreational use of various drugs such as benzodiazepines, narcotics, and amphetamines.

Interactions

Drugs may interact with other drugs, foods, or agents administered as part of laboratory tests. Knowledge of drug interactions is vital to the appropriate monitoring of drug therapy. The more drugs a patient receives, the more likely a drug interaction will occur. This is especially true in the elderly, who typically have an increased sensitivity to drug effects and are receiving several medications. The patient's use of OTC medications and herbal therapies also carries significant interactions with other medications.

The alteration of the action of one drug by another is referred to as **drug interaction.** A drug interaction can either increase or decrease the actions of another drug and can be either beneficial or harmful. Drug interactions increase in frequency with the number of concomitant drugs taken by a patient. Careful patient care and knowledge of all drugs being administered can decrease the likelihood of a harmful drug interaction.

Understanding the mechanism by which drug interactions occur can help prevent them. There are four methods by which concomitantly administered drugs may interact with each other and alter the pharmacokinetics of one another (absorption, distribution, metabolism, and excretion). Table 2-7 provides examples of these mechanisms for drug interactions. It also illustrates how many drug interactions can be beneficial.

Many terms are used to describe these drug interactions. When two drugs with similar actions are given together, the result is an **additive effect.** Examples of this are the many combinations of analgesic products, such as aspirin and opioid combinations (aspirin and codeine) or acetaminophen and opioid combinations (acetaminophen and oxycodone). Drugs used together for their additive effects are often done so that smaller doses of each drug can be given. This avoids toxic effects while maintaining adequate drug action.

Synergistic effects differ from additive effects in that synergism describes a drug interaction that results in combined drug effects that are greater than those that could have been achieved if either drug was given alone. The combination of hydrochlorothiazide with enalapril (Vaseretic) for the treatment of hypertension is an example.

The term used to describe the drug effect that is close to the opposite of the synergistic effect is **antagonistic effect.** Antagonist effects result when the combination of two drugs results in drug effects that are less than if the drugs were given separately. Antagonistic effects are experienced when antacids are given with tetracycline resulting in decreased absorption of tetracycline.

Incompatibility is a term that most commonly involves parenteral drugs. An incompatibility occurs when two parenteral drugs or solutions are mixed together resulting in chemical deterioration of the drug. The combination of these two drugs usually produces a precipitate, haziness, or a change in color in the solution. The combination of parenteral furosemide (Lasix) and heparin will result in an incompatibility.

Drug Misadventures

Adverse patient outcomes associated with medication use vary from mild discomfort to death. The most serious outcomes are death, permanent disability, and life-threatening complications. These outcomes are caused

Examples of Drug Interactions and Their Effects on Pharmacokinetics

Table 2-7

Pharmacokinetic Factor	Drug	Mechanism	Result
Absorption	Antacids with ketoconazole	Increases gastric pH, preventing the breakdown of ketoconazole	Decreased effectiveness of ketoconazole, resulting from decreased blood levels (harmful)
Distribution	warfarin with amiodarone	Both drugs compete for protein-binding sites	Higher free-unbound warfarin and amiodarone, increasing actions of both drugs (harmful)
Metabolism	erythromycin with cimetidine	Both drugs compete for the same hepatic enzymes	Decreased metabolism of astemizole, resulting in toxic levels of astemizole (harmful)
Excretion	amoxicillin with probenecid	Inhibits the secretion of amoxicillin into the kidneys	Elevates and prolongs the plasma levels of amoxicillin

by adverse reactions to drugs. Adverse reactions to drugs as a result of medication errors, drug interactions, drug allergies, and unknown causes can broadly be termed **medication misadventures.** The two broad categories of drug or medication misadventures are adverse drug events (ADEs) and adverse drug reactions (ADRs). The main difference between an ADE and an ADR is that ADEs are preventable and ADRs are not. The main reason for an expansion in terminology is the growing realization that harmful consequences associated with medication use and misuse extend beyond ADRs and may include therapeutic appropriateness (or misuse), medication errors, patient compliance, and other problems that result in suboptimal outcomes.

Adverse drug events (ADEs) are medication errors that result in patient harm. All ADEs are preventable. **Medication errors** occur during the administration, dispensing, monitoring, or prescribing of a medication, which is known as the **medication use process.** Other terms used for ADEs are *therapeutic misadventures* and *medication-related problems.* ADEs are noxious and unintended. They occur at doses used for prophylaxis, diagnosis, therapy, or modification of physiologic function. ADEs are also defined as an injury resulting from medical intervention related to a drug.

Two other more specific ADE subcategories are *potential adverse drug events (PADEs)* and *adverse drug withdrawal events (ADWEs).* A PADE is an elevated laboratory value of a narrow therapeutic index drug known to predispose a patient to increased risk of death or injury but not resulting in an adverse event. A common example of a PADE is an elevated bleeding time (INR) in a patient on warfarin (Coumadin) that has not yet resulted in any adverse outcome. An ADWE is associated with discontinuation of therapy that results in an adverse outcome. An example of an ADWE is hypertension after abrupt discontinuation of clonidine therapy.

As mentioned previously, ADRs are not preventable. An **adverse drug reaction (ADR)** is an inherent, nonpreventable event occurring in the normal therapeutic use of a drug. An ADR is any reaction to a drug that is unexpected, is undesirable, and occurs at doses normally used for prophylaxis, diagnosis, or therapy and may result in hospital admission, prolongation of hospital stay, change in drug therapy, initiation of supportive treatment, and complication of diagnosed disease state. Some ADRs can be classified as side effects. *Side effects* are defined as expected, well-known reactions that result in little or no change in patient management. It is an expected, well-known reaction resulting in little or no change in patient management, an effect with a predictable frequency, and an effect whose intensity and occurrence are related to the size of the dose. Side effects are dose-related and predictable events. ADRs can lead to serious adverse events. *Serious adverse events* are defined as serious events that are fatal, life-threatening, or permanently or significantly disabling; require or prolong hospitalization; cause congenital anomalies; or require intervention to prevent permanent impairment or damage.

Adverse Drug Events. Knowledge of adverse drug reactions is an essential component of pharmacotherapy. An adverse drug reaction is an undesirable response to drug therapy. The study of poisons and unwanted responses to therapeutic agents is commonly referred to as *toxicology.* An adverse drug reaction can be either a side effect or a harmful effect. Many are extensions of the drug's normal pharmacologic actions. Adverse drug reactions can be broken down into four basic categories: pharmacologic, idiosyncratic, and hypersensitivity reactions and drug interaction.

Pharmacologic adverse drug reactions are extensions of the drug's effects in the body. For example, a drug that is used to lower blood pressure in a patient with hypertension causes a pharmacologic adverse drug reaction when it lowers the blood pressure to the point where the patient becomes unconscious.

Idiosyncratic reactions are not the result of a known pharmacologic property of a drug or patient allergy but are peculiar to that patient. Such a reaction is a genetically determined abnormal response to ordinary doses of a drug. Genetically inherited traits that result in the abnormal metabolism of drugs are universally distributed throughout the population. The study of such traits that are solely revealed by drug administration is called **pharmacogenetics.** Idiosyncratic drug reactions are usually caused by abnormal levels of drug-metabolizing enzymes (a complete absence, a deficiency, or an overabundance of the enzyme).

There are many pharmacogenetic disorders. A common one is glucose-6-phosphate dehydrogenase (G6PD) deficiency. This pharmacogenetic disease is transmitted as a sex-linked trait and affects approximately 100 million people. People who lack proper levels of G6PD have idiosyncratic reactions to a wide range of drugs. There are more than 80 variations of the disease, and all produce varying degrees of drug-induced hemolysis. Drugs capable of inducing hemolysis in such patients are listed in Box 2-2.

Hypersensitivity reactions involve the patient's immune system. The patient's immune system recognizes

---

BOX 2-2

Drugs to Avoid in Patients with Glucose-6-Phosphate Dehydrogenase Deficiency

- para-aminosalicylic acid
- furazolidone
- Sulfonamides
- Antimalarials
- nitrofurantoin
- Sulfones
- aspirin
- phenacetin
- All oxidants
- chloramphenicol
- probenecid

the drug, a drug metabolite, or an ingredient in a drug formulation as a dangerous foreign substance. This foreign substance is then attacked, neutralized, or destroyed by the immune system, causing a hypersensitivity reaction.

The final type of adverse drug reaction is a *drug interaction* and results when two drugs interact and produce an unwanted effect. This unwanted effect can be the result of one drug either making the other more potent and accentuating its effects or diminishing the effectiveness of another. As previously mentioned, in some instances drug interactions are intentional and beneficial.

Iatrogenic Responses. Unintentional adverse effects that are physician- or health care professional-induced or treatment-induced are referred to as **iatrogenic responses.** There are a variety of iatrogenic responses that may occur to therapy:

- Treatment-induced dermatologic (e.g., rash, hives, acne, psoriasis, and erythema)
- Renal damage (e.g., aminoglycoside antibiotics, nonsteroidal antiinflammatory drugs [NSAIDs], and contrast agents)
- Blood dyscrasias (e.g., a total destruction of all cells produced by the bone marrow or just a particular cell line, such as platelets); most common after therapy with antineoplastic agents
- Hepatic toxicity (although not as common, the hepatic response will take the form of elevated hepatic enzymes, presenting as a hepatitislike syndrome)

Other Drug Effects

Other drug-related effects that need to be monitored during therapy are teratogenic, mutagenic, and carcinogenic effects. These can result in devastating patient outcomes and can be prevented in many instances by appropriate monitoring.

Teratogenic. The teratogenic effects of drugs result in structural defects in the unborn fetus. Such agents are called *teratogens.* There are three major categories of exogenous human teratogens: viral diseases, radiation, and drugs or chemicals. Fetal development involves a delicate programmed sequence of interrelated embryologic events. Any significant disruption in embryogenesis can result in a teratogenic effect. Drugs that are capable of crossing the placenta can act as teratogens and cause **drug-induced teratogenesis.** Drugs administered during pregnancy can produce different types of congenital anomalies. The period when the fetus is most vulnerable to teratogenic effects begins with the third week of fetal development and usually ends after the third month.

Mutagenic. Mutagenic effects are changes in the genetic composition of living organisms (permanent changes) and consist of alterations in the chromosome structure, the number of chromosomes, and the genetic code of the deoxyribonucleic acid (DNA) molecule. Agents capable of inducing mutations are called mutagens. Radiation, chemicals, and drugs can act as mutagenic agents in human beings. The largest genetic unit that can be involved in a mutation is a chromosome. The smallest is a base pair in a DNA molecule. Agents that affect genetic processes are active only during cell reproduction.

Carcinogenic. The carcinogenic effects of drugs cause cancer, and such chemicals and drugs are called *carcinogens.* There are several exogenous factors that contribute to the development of cancer besides drugs, and the list grows daily. Some of the more notable ones are listed in Box 2-3.

Chemically induced carcinogenesis usually requires lengthy exposure to carcinogens. Even brief exposures to potent carcinogens will involve a long latent period before cancer develops.

Reassessment

The data collected during assessment, implementation, and evaluation should be reassessed regularly. In this reassessment the nurse should appraise a patient's clinical symptoms in the context of the efficacy of drug therapy. This should be done regularly throughout the course of therapy. It is also a dynamic process that should change to reflect the changes in a patient's status. As the patient's condition improves or worsens, the treatment plan (pharmacotherapy) should be changed to accommodate the

---

cultural implications

Glucose-6-Phosphate Dehydrogenase Deficiency

Glucose-6-phosphate dehydrogenase (G6PD) is an enzyme found in abundant amounts in tissues in most individuals. It reduces the risk of hemolysis of red blood cells (RBCs) when they are exposed to oxidizing agents such as aspirin. Approximately 13% of African-American men and 20% of African-American women may carry the gene that results in G6PD deficiency. Approximately 14% of Sardinians and more than 50% of the Kurdish Jewish populations also show G6PD deficiencies. When exposed to agents such as sulfonamides, antimalarials, and aspirin, patients with this deficiency may suffer life-threatening hemolysis of the RBCs, whereas individuals with the enzyme have no problems taking these drugs.

BOX 2-3 ## Exogenous Carcinogens

- Dietary customs
- Environmental pollution
- Food-production procedures
- Oncogenic viruses
- Food-processing procedures
- Smoking
- Drug abuse

new therapeutic needs of the patient. Neglecting the re-assessment component of pharmacotherapy heightens the risk of inappropriate and ineffective therapy being rendered.

PHARMACOGNOSY

The source of all early drugs was nature, and the study of these natural drug sources (plants and animals) is called *pharmacognosy*. Although many current drugs are synthetically derived, most were first isolated in nature. By studying the composition of the natural substance and its physiologic effects in living systems, researchers can identify the exact chemical features of a substance that produce the desired response. Armed with this knowledge, they can then go to the laboratory and produce that exact substance, but it is devoid of the unwanted effects that many naturally occurring substances may have. Although most new drug products are synthetic, the underlying principle of pharmacognosy is that an understanding of the actions and effects of natural drug sources is essential to new drug development. The principles of pharmacognosy have enabled isolation of the naturally occurring hormone insulin, determination of its exact genetic sequence, and synthesization of that exact sequence over and over again. This has enabled the production of human insulin synthetically.

The four main sources for drugs are plants, animals, minerals, and laboratory synthesis. An example of a plant from which a drug is derived is foxglove. It is the source of cardiac glycosides and has yielded the present-day drug digoxin. The plant family also provides alkaloids, which are very useful and potent drugs. Examples include atropine (belladonna), caffeine (coffee), and nicotine (tobacco). Animals are the source of many hormone therapies. Premarin (conjugated estrogen) is derived from the urine of pregnant female horses (*pregnant mares*). Insulin comes from three sources: beef (cow), pork (pig), and human. Human insulin is either semisynthetic (converting pork to human insulin by changing one amino acid) or is made by recombinant DNA techniques. Heparin is another commonly used drug that is derived from cows and pigs (bovine and porcine heparin). Some common mineral sources of currently used drugs are salicylic acid, aluminum hydroxide, and sodium chloride. Recombinant DNA techniques provide many laboratory-derived drug products, such as erythropoietin (Epogen and Procrit), granulocyte-macrophage-colony stimulating factor (Sargramostim), granulocyte-colony stimulating factor (Filgrastim), and human insulin (Humulin and Novolin).

The interrelated pharmacologic principles of pharmacokinetics, pharmacodynamics, pharmacotherapeutics, toxicology, and pharmacognosy are essential to a sound understanding of pharmacology and the nursing practice. Medications are very powerful and effective. Without a thorough knowledge and appreciation of these principles, a potentially very useful treatment modality could become a very harmful and dangerous one in your hands. Therefore an understanding of pharmacologic principles ensures the provision of safe and effective drug therapy.

POINTS TO REMEMBER

Pharmacology
- Study of all interactions between drugs and living things.
- Drug origin, nature, chemistry, effects, and uses.
- Essential to understanding medicines and how they work.

Pharmacokinetics
- Involves drug absorption, distribution, metabolism, and excretion.
- Used to explain a drug's actions in the body, such as its onset, peak, and duration.

Pharmacodynamics
- Effects of drugs in the body (biochemical and physical).
- Example: receptor stimulation by a drug and the resulting biologic response.
- The way the drug works (mechanism of action).

Pharmacotherapy
- Use of a drug to treat a disease.
- Includes assessment, implementation, monitoring, and reassessment.

Prophylactic Therapy
- Starting drug therapy based on prior knowledge and experience.
- Based on scientific knowledge and years of observation.

Drug Actions
- Its pharmaceutical, pharmacokinetic, and pharmacodynamic properties—each having a specific effect on the overall way a drug works within a patient.

Adverse Reactions
- Predictable and unpredictable.
- Iatrogenic, carcinogenic, and teratogenic.

Nurse's Role
- More than just the memorization of the names of pharmacologic agents, their use, and associated interventions is required in drug therapy because it requires a sound comprehension and application of drug knowledge to a variety of clinical situations.

REVIEW QUESTIONS

1. Pharmacologic principles of drug therapy important for the nurse to understand include which of the following about drugs?
   a. Drugs often need receptors with which to interact.
   b. Drugs produce only agonistic reactions in the body.
   c. Drugs result in unwanted effects that are not desirable.
   d. Drugs create all new responses in target organ or body systems.
2. Patients with liver failure who have problems with drug metabolism would also have abnormalities with which of the following laboratory values?
   a. CPK and LDH
   b. BUN and RBC
   c. Creatine clearance
   d. Complete blood counts
3. Patients with disorders of the peripheral circulation would have problems in which phase of pharmacokinetics?
   a. Excretion
   b. Absorption
   c. Distribution
   d. Metabolism
4. A patient in shock would most likely not respond to intramuscular injections of medications because of:
   a. Altered biliary functioning.
   b. Altered glomerular filtration.
   c. Diminished liver metabolism.
   d. Diminished peripheral circulation.
5. Your patient just received a prescription for an enteric-coated stool softener. Instructions to the patient should include which of the following statements?
   a. Take the tablet with 2 to 3 ounces of orange juice.
   b. Avoid taking all other medications with any enteric-coated tablet.
   c. Crush the tablet before swallowing if you have problems with swallowing.
   d. To achieve maximal absorption, take the enteric-coated tablet with a minimum of 6 to 8 ounces of fluid.

For Answers see www.harcourthealth.com/MERLIN/Lilley/.

CRITICAL THINKING Activities

1. Your patient is inquiring about the benefits that transdermal medication offer over the administration of some oral medications. In relation to the pharmacologic principle of absorption, what is one major benefit of transdermal patches vs. oral medication administration?
2. Your patient relates to you during the nursing assessment that he experiences some "strange" problem with drug metabolism that he was born with, so he is not to take certain medications. What type of disorder do you think this patient is referring to, and what are the problems it can cause in the patient when taking specific medications?
3. Mr. LL is admitted to the burn trauma unit with multisystem injury from an auto accident. He presents with multiple abnormal findings including shock, decreased cardiac output, and less than 30 ml-hr urinary output. Which route of administration would be indicated for any medications in this patient? Explain your rationale.
4. Explain the difference between a medication's action and its effect.
5. Explain the importance of each phase of pharmacokinetics.

For Answers see www.harcourthealth.com/MERLIN/Lilley/.

bibliography

American Hospital Formulary Service: *AHFS drug information*, Bethesda, Md, 2000, American Society of Health-System Pharmacists.

Anderson PO, Knoben JE, Troutman WG: *Handbook of critical drug data 1999-2000*, ed 9, New York, 1999, McGraw-Hill.

DiPiro JT et al: *Pharmacotherapy: a pathophysiologic approach*, ed 4, New York, 1999, Elsevier Science.

Edwards J: Guarding against adverse drug events, *Am J Nurs* 97(5):26, 1999.

Johns Hopkins Hospital, Department of Pediatrics et al: *The Harriet Lane handbook*, ed 15, St Louis, 2000, Mosby.

Keen JH: *Critical care and emergency drug reference*, ed 3, St Louis, 1996, Mosby.

McKenry LM, Salerno E: *Mosby's pharmacology in nursing*, ed 21, St Louis, 2001, Mosby.

Mosby's GenRx: a comprehensive reference for generic and brand drugs, ed 10, St Louis, 2000, Mosby.

Ross TW: Adverse drug reactions and events: what, why, and how? Inet-CE article #146-000-98-004-H04. Available at www.inetce.org/articles/146-000-98-004-H04.html.

Skidmore-Roth L: *Mosby's 2001 nursing drug reference*, St Louis, 2001, Mosby.

United States Pharmacopeial Convention: *USP DI: drug information for the healthcare professional*, vol 1, ed 20, Englewood, Colo, 2000, Micromedex.

Remember to check the **Online Worksheet** for additional learning opportunities: **www.harcourthealth.com/MERLIN/Lilley/**

Activity

Chapter 3

Lifespan Considerations

www.harcourthealth.com/MERLIN/Lilley/

objectives

When you reach the end of this chapter, you should be able to do the following:

1 Discuss the influence of age on the effects of medications in a patient, including both the pediatric or geriatric patient.

2 Identify medication-related concerns during pregnancy.

3 Identify age-related considerations specific to drug administration.

4 Discuss the process of pharmacokinetics in relation to lifespan considerations and other physiologic concerns.

5 Calculate a drug dosage for a pediatric patient.

6 Identify the importance of a body surface area (BSA) nomogram in pediatric patients.

7 Develop a nursing care plan for the administration of medications to the pediatric or geriatric patient.

Look for this symbol for topics covered in the **Online Worksheet**

glossary

Geriatric (jer ē a' trik) Pertaining to a person who is 65 years of age or older. (p. 35)

Pediatric (pē dē a' trik) Pertaining to a person who is 12 years of age or younger. (p. 34)

Polypharmacy (pol ē fahr' mə sē) The use of many different drugs in treating a patient who may have one or several health problems. (p. 35)

Most of our experience with drugs and pharmacology has been gained from the adult population, and by far the greater majority of drug studies and articles on drugs have focused on the population between 13 and 65 years of age. To further compound the problem, it has been estimated that 75% of our currently approved drugs lack Food and Drug Administration (FDA) approval for pediatric use and therefore lack specific dosage guidelines for use in neonates and children. Drug usage, however, extends far beyond patients between 13 and 65 years of age. Most drugs are also effective in younger and older patients, but drugs often behave very differently in these patients at the opposite ends of the age spectrum. It is therefore vitally important from the standpoint of the safe and effective administration of drugs to understand what these differences are and how to adjust for them.

During the time from the beginning to the end of life, our bodies change in many ways. These changes have a dramatic effect on the four pharmacokinetic factors of drugs: absorption, distribution, metabolism, and excretion. Newborn, pediatric, and geriatric patients each have special needs, which are discussed in this chapter. Drug therapy at the two ends of the spectrum of life is more likely to result in adverse effects and toxicity. This is especially true if certain basic principles are not understood and followed. However, an individual's response to drug therapy changes in a reasonably predictable manner in younger and older patients. Knowing the effect that age has on the pharmacokinetic factors of drugs helps predict these changes.

DRUG THERAPY DURING PREGNANCY

Exposure to drugs occurs across the entire life span. The life span begins before birth. A fetus is exposed to many of the same substances as the mother, including drugs. Therefore it is important to know and understand drug effects during gestational life. The first trimester of pregnancy is the period of greatest danger for drug-induced developmental defects. Also of importance is the fact that an average of four or more drugs is taken by the child-bearing patient during pregnancy.

Transfer of drugs and nutrients to the fetus occurs primarily by diffusion across the placenta. Active transport plays a lesser role. The factors that contribute to the safety or potential harm of drug therapy during pregnancy can be broadly broken down into three areas: drug properties, fetal gestational age, and maternal factors.

Drug properties that impact drug transfer to the fetus are a drug's chemical properties and dosage. The important chemical properties are molecular weight, protein binding, lipid solubility, and chemical structure. Important drug dosage variables are dose, duration of therapy, and concomitantly administered drugs.

Fetal gestational age is an important factor in determining the potential for harmful drug effects to the fetus. During the first trimester of pregnancy the fetus is at the greatest risk for drug-induced developmental defects. During this period the fetus undergoes rapid cell proliferation, and the skeleton, muscles, limbs, and organs are developing at their most rapid rate. Self-treatment of any minor illness should be strongly discouraged, especially during the first trimester. Gestational age is also important in determining when a drug can most easily cross the placenta to the fetus. During the last trimester the greatest percentage of maternally absorbed drug will get to the fetus.

Maternal factors can also play a role in determining drug effects to the fetus. Any change in the mother's physiology that could impact the pharmacokinetic factors of drugs (absorption, distribution, metabolism, excretion) can impact the amount of drug to which the fetus may be exposed. Maternal kidney and liver function play a major role in drug metabolism and excretion. Impairment in either kidney or liver function may result in higher drug levels than normal and/or prolonged drug exposure. Maternal genotype may also affect how and to what extent certain drugs are metabolized, which in turn affects drug exposure to the fetus. The lack of certain enzyme systems, as seen in the pharmacogenetic disease glucose-6-phosphate dehydrogenase (G6PD) deficiency, may result in adverse drug effects to the fetus when the mother is exposed to a susceptible drug.

Although drug exposure to the fetus is most detrimental during the first trimester, drug transfer to the fetus is more likely during the last trimester. This is the result of enhanced blood flow, increased surface area, thinner membranes separating maternal blood and the fetus, and an increased amount of free drug in the mother's circulation.

As important as it is to judiciously use drugs during pregnancy, there are certain situations that require their use. Without drugs, such maternal conditions as hypertension, epilepsy, diabetes, and infection could seriously endanger both the mother and the fetus.

The FDA classifies drugs according to their safety for use during pregnancy. The basis for this system of drug classification is rooted primarily in animal studies and limited human studies. This is due in part to ethical dilemmas surrounding the study of potential adverse effects in fetuses. We have also learned from some unfortunate mistakes, such as thalidomide-induced birth defects and maternal use of diethylstilbestrol (DES) causing a high occurrence of gynecologic malignancy in female offspring. Currently the best method for determining potential fetal risk is by using the FDA's pregnancy safety categories listed in Table 3-1.

Table 3-1   Pregnancy Safety Categories

Category	Description
Category A	Studies indicate no risk to the fetus.
Category B	Studies indicate no risk to animal fetus; information in humans is not available.
Category C	Adverse effects reported in animal fetus; information in humans is not available.
Category D	Possible fetal risk in humans reported; however, considering potential benefit versus risk may, in selected cases, warrant the use of these drugs in pregnant women.
Category X	Fetal abnormalities reported and positive evidence of fetal risk in humans is available from animal and/or human studies. These drugs should not be used in pregnant women.

DRUG THERAPY DURING BREAST FEEDING

Breast-fed infants are also at risk for exposure to drugs consumed by the mother. A wide variety of drugs easily cross from the mother's circulation to the breast milk and subsequently to the breast-feeding infant. Drug characteristics similar to those discussed in the section on drug therapy during pregnancy apply to drugs that are taken by the mother who breast feeds. The primary drug characteristics that increase the likelihood that a drug given to a breast-feeding mother will end up in her breast milk are fat solubility, low molecular weight, nonionized drugs, and drugs present in high concentrations.

In general, breast milk is not the primary route for maternal drug excretion. Drug levels in breast milk are usually lower than those in the maternal circulation. The actual amount of drug that a breast-feeding infant is exposed to depends largely on the volume of milk consumed. The ultimate decision as to whether a breast-feeding mother should take a particular drug depends upon the risk-to-benefit ratio. The risks of transfer of maternal medication to the infant versus the benefits of continuing breast feeding and the therapeutic benefits to the mother must be considered on a case-by-case basis.

NEONATAL AND PEDIATRIC CONSIDERATIONS

The definition of a *child* in terms of age is vastly different from that of a neonate or infant. Therefore *child* (i.e., the age ranges) should not be mistakenly used to refer to a patient younger than 2 years of age. Definitions of the terms used to refer to the patient are given in Table 3-2. This is the classification that applies throughout this chapter.

Physiology and Pharmacokinetics

The physiology unique to neonates accounts for most of the differences in the pharmacokinetic and pharmacodynamic

Table 3-2 Classification of Young Patients

Age Range	Classification
<38 wk gestation	Premature or preterm infant
<1 mo	Neonate or newborn infant
1 mo to <1 yr	Infant
1 to <12 yr	Child

pediatric considerations

Pharmacokinetic Changes in the Neonate and Pediatric Patient

ABSORPTION
- Gastric pH is less acidic because acid-producing cells in the stomach are immature until approximately 3 years of age.
- Gastric emptying is slowed because of slow or irregular peristalsis.
- First-pass elimination by liver is reduced because of immaturity of liver and reduced levels of microsomal enzymes.
- Topical absorption is faster because of a proportionally greater body surface area and thin skin.
- Intramuscular absorption is faster and irregular.

DISTRIBUTION
- In infants, total body water (TBW) is 70% to 80% in full-term infants, 85% in premature newborns, and 64% in children 1 to 12 years of age.
- Fat content is less in young patients because of the greater TBW content.
- Protein binding is decreased because of decreased production of protein by immature liver.
- More drugs enter the brain because of an immature blood-brain barrier.

METABOLISM
- The levels of microsomal enzymes are decreased because the immature liver has not yet started producing enough.
- Older children may have increased metabolism and require higher doses once hepatic enzymes are produced.
- There are many variables that affect metabolism in premature infants, infants, and children, including the status of liver enzyme production, genetic differences, and what the mother has been exposed to during pregnancy.

EXCRETION
- Glomerular filtration rate as well as tubular secretion and resorption are all decreased in young patients because of the immaturity of the kidney.
- Perfusion to the kidneys is often low, resulting in immature glomeruli and renal tubules and a shorter loop of Henle. This causes reduced renal function and concentrating ability.

behavior of drugs between neonates and adults. The immaturity of organs is the physiologic factor most responsible for these differences. The various physiologic characteristics of the neonatal population also apply to the total **pediatric** population but to a lesser extent. In both groups, anatomic structures and physiologic systems and functions are still in the process of developing. The Pediatric Considerations box lists those physiologic factors responsible for altering the pharmacokinetic properties of drugs.

Pharmacodynamics

As previously mentioned, drug actions (or pharmacodynamics) are altered in young patients, and the maturity of various organs plays a role in how drugs act in the body. Certain drugs may be more toxic, whereas others may be less toxic in young patients. Drugs that are more toxic in children are phenobarbital, morphine, and aspirin. Drugs that children tolerate the same as or better than adults are atropine, codeine, digoxin, and phenylephrine. The sensitivity of receptor sites may also vary with age, thus higher or lower doses are required depending on the drug. In addition, rapidly developing tissues may be more sensitive to certain drugs, and therefore smaller doses are required. Drugs may also be contraindicated during the growth years. For instance, tetracycline may discolor teeth, corticosteroids may suppress growth, and fluoroquinolone antibiotics may damage cartilage, leading to deformities in gait.

Dose Calculations

Many drugs commonly used in adults have not been sufficiently investigated to ensure their safety and effectiveness in children. Most drugs administered in children are given on an empirical basis with little in the way of formal studies supporting their use. Because newborns are small and immature in many respects, this makes them very susceptible to many insults. They lack many of the protective mechanisms that allow adults to resist these same stressors in the environment.
- Skin is thin and permeable
- Stomach lacks acid to kill bacteria and other invaders
- Lungs lack mucous barriers
- Body temperatures are poorly regulated and they can easily become dehydrated
- Liver and kidneys are immature and cannot manage foreign substances as well as in older patients

Because of such factors, the doses used in young patients must differ from those used in adults. The most common method for calculating doses for pediatric patients is weight-based (i.e., mg/kg). However, several formulas for calculating drug doses in young patients have been devised, as noted in the following:
- Height and weight (based on BSA*—for any child)

$$\text{BSA (m}^2) / 1.73 \text{ (m}^2) \times \text{Adult dose} = \text{Child's dose}$$

*BSA is considered more accurate than age or weight as a basis for calculating a child's dose.

- Clark's rule (based on weight—for children >2 years old)

    Weight (lb) \ 150 × Adult dose = Child's dose

- Young's rule (based on age*—for children >2 years old)

    Age (yr)/Age (yr) + 12 × Adult dose = Child's dose

- Fried's rule (based on age—for children <1 year old)

    Age (mo)/150 × Adult dose = Child's dose

These four methods are used to calculate a starting dose from which to work. Dose calculations based on the BSA are the most accurate because this method takes into consideration the relationship between the child's height and weight and more precisely gauges the maturity of a child's organs and metabolic rate. Dose calculations based on weight alone make the assumption that a child is a miniature adult, which is incorrect. Some medications have precalculated dosage recommendations.

BSA is used for chemotherapeutic regimens, and mg/kg is used for most other pediatric medications.

The surface area nomogram in Fig. 3-1 is an example of how to determine BSA. The nomogram represents the relationship between height, weight, and BSA in adults and children. To use the nomogram, a ruler is aligned with the appropriate height for the child (left column) and the appropriate weight (right column). The point where the ruler crosses the BSA column corresponds to the value for surface area. For example, using Fig. 3-1, a child with a height of 25 inches weighing 25 pounds has a BSA of 0.45 m². If the child falls within normal standards for height and weight, the green bar labeled *For children of normal height for weight* can be used. Next, to determine the actual dose that should be given, take the calculated BSA (0.45 m²) and insert it into the height and weight equation. Also insert the adult dose (e.g., for codeine an adult dose is 15 to 30 mg every 4 to 6 hours):

$$BSA \ (m^2) \ / \ 1.73 \ m^2 \times Adult \ dose = Child's \ dose$$

0.45 m² / 1.73 m² × 15-30 mg every 4-6 hr =
3.9-7.8 mg every 4-6 hours

The child's response to the dose calculated is ultimately the most important dosing tool, and titrating to the desired response should be the goal. The potential problems in younger patients are many, so dose calculations and the drug preparation should always be double-checked. Small mistakes can translate into far greater consequences in these fragile human systems.

To accurately administer medications to pediatric patients, the weight, height, age, maturity of organs (kidney and liver), and their response to the medication must all be taken into account. If this is done, safe and effective administration of medications is enhanced. De-

velopmental considerations must also be part of the decision-making process in drug administration to pediatric patients (Box 3-1).

GERIATRIC CONSIDERATIONS

Between the beginning and end of life, our bodies change in many ways. These changes have a dramatic effect on the pharmacokinetics of drugs. The geriatric patient has special needs, and drug therapy at this end of the spectrum of life is much more likely to result in adverse effects and toxicity. This is especially true if certain basic principles are not understood and followed.

For the sake of this discussion, a **geriatric** patient is defined as a person who is 65 years of age or older. This segment of the population is growing at a dramatic pace (see Geriatric Considerations box). At the beginning of the twentieth century, geriatric persons constituted a mere 4% of the total population. At that time more people died of infections than of degenerative, chronic illnesses such as heart disease, cancer, and diabetes. As medical technology has advanced, so has our ability to prolong life, oftentimes by treating and curing illnesses that at one time people commonly died of. This has resulted in a growing population of older adults. Today patients over the age of 65 constitute 12% of the population. Life expectancy is approximately 74.9 years, and it is estimated that by the year 2020, 20% of the population will reach 65 years of age. The elderly represent the fastest growing segment of the population, increasing by about 2% a year. This is only expected to continue as new disease prevention and treatment methods are developed.

Polypharmacy and Drug Use

The growing geriatric population also consumes a larger proportion of all medications. The geriatric patient population consumes approximately 35% of all prescription drugs and over 40% of over-the-counter (OTC) drugs. Drugs commonly prescribed include antihypertensives, beta-blockers, digitalis, diuretics, insulin, and potassium supplements. The most commonly used OTC drugs include analgesics, laxatives, and nonsteroidal antiinflammatory drugs (NSAIDs). For this and many physiologic reasons, the elderly are at a greater risk (three to seven times greater) for suffering adverse drug reactions and drug interactions.

Not only does the geriatric population consume a greater proportion of prescription and OTC medications, they frequently take multiple medications on a daily basis. One third of all people in the geriatric age group take more than 8 different drugs a day, and some take as many as 15. More than 80% of these patients have one or more chronic illnesses. In this age of medical specialization, patients may see several physicians for their many illnesses. These specialists may all prescribe medications for the illness they are treating, which often explains why a patient is taking 8 to 15 medications plus OTC drugs. This practice is called **polypharmacy**. The risk of drug interactions, adverse reactions, and potentially a hospitalization or prolonged hospitalization is far greater in this setting. As the number of medications a person takes increases, so

*Age is considered less desirable than weight or BSA as a basis for calculating a child's dose.

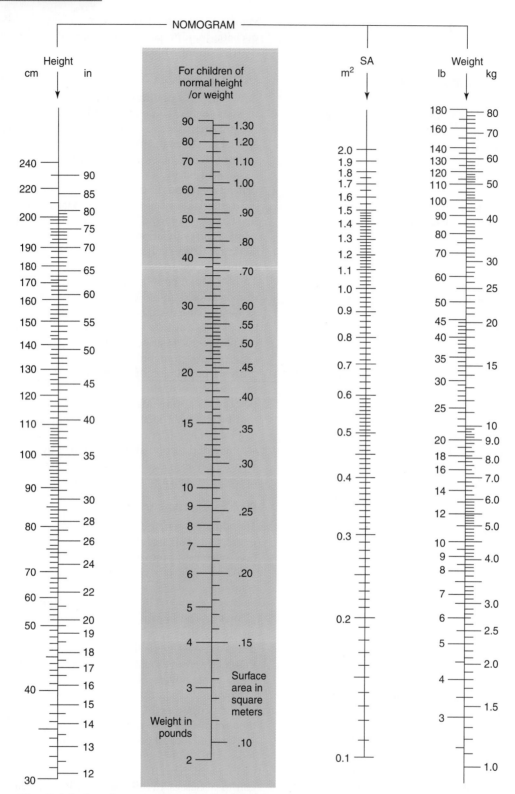

NOMOGRAM

Fig. 3-1 Body surface area nomogram. (Modified from Behrman RE, Kliegman RM, Jenson HB: *Nelson textbook of pediatrics*, ed 16, Philadelphia, 2001, W.B. Saunders.)

does the risk of a drug interaction (Box 3-2). For example, a patient receiving two medications has approximately a 6% chance of suffering a drug interaction. This risk drastically increases as the number of drugs the patient is taking increases. A patient taking five medications has a

50% chance of a drug interaction. This chance rises to 100% if he or she is taking eight medications.

Along with the risk of drug interactions come other risks. More hospitalizations for the treatment of adverse drug effects, greater likelihood of drug-induced falls that

BOX 3-1   Nursing Process: Patient Care and Medication Administration

GENERAL INTERVENTIONS

Always come prepared for procedure with all equipment and assistance necessary.

Ask the parent and/or child if parent should or should not remain for procedure (for in-hospital administration).

Assess comfort methods appropriate before and after administration.

INFANTS

Perform procedure swiftly, then offer comfort measures (e.g., parent holding, rocking, cuddling, soothing).

Allow self-comforting measures (e.g., use of pacifier, fingers in mouth, self-movement).

TODDLERS

Offer brief, concrete explanation of procedure, then perform it.

Accept aggressive behavior, within reasonable limits, as a healthy response.

Provide comfort measures immediately after procedure (e.g., touch, holding).

Help the child understand the treatment and his feelings through puppet play, stuffed animals, or play with hospital equipment such as needleless syringes and water.

Provide for ways to release aggression with such play as hammering or water play.

PRESCHOOLERS

Offer brief, concrete explanation.

Provide comfort measures after procedure (e.g., touch, holding).

Accept aggressive responses and provide outlets for them.

Make use of magical thinking—use "ointments" or "special medicines" to make discomfort go away.

Role of parent is very important for comfort and understanding.

SCHOOL-AGE CHILDREN

Explain procedure, allowing for some control over body and situation.

Provide comfort measures.

Explore feelings and concepts by therapeutic play, drawings of own body and self in hospital; use books and realistic hospital equipment.

Set appropriate behavior limits (e.g., okay to cry or scream, but not bite).

Provide activities for releasing aggression and anger.

Use opportunity to teach about relation of getting medication to body function and structure (e.g., what a seizure is and how medication helps prevents the seizure).

Offer the complete picture (e.g., need to take medication, relax with deep breaths, medication will help prevent pain).

ADOLESCENTS

Prepare in advance for procedure.

Allow for expression in a way that does not cause "losing face," such as giving the adolescent time alone after the procedure (once the seizure is controlled) and giving him time to discuss his discomfort if he wants to verbalize his feelings.

Explore current concepts of self, hospitalization, and illness, and correct any misconceptions.

Encourage self-expression, individuality, and self-care.

Encourage participation in procedure to a preagreed-upon extent. Increased participation should be discussed after procedure.

Modified from Blaber M: Related to nursing intervention in pain, *Newington Children's Hospital Manual for Global Pediatric Nursing Assessment* (unpublished), 1990, pp. 52-53. In McKenry LM, Salerno E: *Mosby's pharmacology in nursing,* ed 21, St Louis, 2001, Mosby.

geriatric considerations

Percentage of Population Over 65 Years of Age

Year	Percentage >65 Years
1900	4%
1990	12%
2000	20%

BOX 3-2   Risk of Polypharmacy-Induced Drug Interactions

Number of Drugs	Risk
2	6%
5	50%
8	100%

lead to hip fractures, and heightened risk of addiction are just a few. All of these are preventable. Recognizing polypharmacy in a patient and taking steps to reduce it by seeing to it that drugs are eliminated or changed or the dosages altered can dramatically lower the incidence of these undesirable drug effects.

Physiologic Changes

The physiologic changes that geriatric people undergo also affect how many drugs act. An understanding of these physiologic changes and how they affect pharmacokinetics and pharmacodynamics (drug action) will help ensure the provision of safe and effective drug therapy.

The body ages and the function of several organ systems slowly deteriorates after many years of wear and tear. The collective physiologic changes associated with the aging process have a major effect on the disposition of drugs. Table 3-3 lists four of the most important body systems affected by the aging process.

geriatric considerations

Alzheimer's Disease

Alzheimer's disease afflicts approximately 4 million Americans, and this figure might reach 14 million by the middle of the twenty-first century. It is presently the fourth leading cause of death in adults preceded by heart disease, cancer, and cerebrovascular accidents, or strokes. Unfortunately, approximately 1 in 10 families in the United States has a loved one with Alzheimer's disease.

■

Physiologic Changes in the Geriatric Patient

Table 3-3

System	Physiologic Change
Cardiovascular	↓ Cardiac output = ↓ absorption and distribution
	↓ Blood flow = ↓ absorption and distribution
Gastrointestinal	↑ pH (alkaline gastric secretions)
	↓ Peristalsis = delayed gastric emptying
Hepatic	↓ Enzyme production = ↓ metabolism
	↓ Blood flow = ↓ metabolism
Renal	↓ Blood flow = ↓ excretion
	↓ Function = ↓ excretion
	↓ Glomerular filtration rate = ↓ excretion

These and other physiologic changes that take place in the elderly directly affect drug action. The sensitivity of the elderly patient to many drugs is altered as a result of these physiologic changes, and therefore drug usage should be adjusted to accommodate these changes. For instance, there is a general decrease in body weight. However, the drug doses administered in the elderly are often the same as those administered to healthy adults. The criteria for drug doses in the elderly should therefore be based more on weight and less on age (i.e., adult versus pediatric doses).

Laboratory values are important to monitor in the elderly. They can serve as a gauge of organ function. The two most important organs from the standpoint of how drugs are broken down and eliminated are the liver and the kidneys. Assessment of kidney function is done by testing urine for levels of blood urea nitrogen (BUN) and serum creatinine. Assessment of liver function is done testing liver enzymes for levels of aspartate aminotransferase (SGOT) and alanine aminotransferase (SGPT). These laboratory values can help in the assessment of an elderly patient's ability to metabolize and eliminate medications.

Pharmacokinetics

The pharmacokinetic properties of absorption, distribution, metabolism, and excretion may be different in the elderly than in the younger adult. An awareness of these helps in the appropriate administration of drugs and monitoring of the geriatric patient taking medications. The Geriatric Considerations box lists the four pharmacokinetic phases and summarizes how they are altered by the aging process.

Absorption

Absorption in the elderly can be altered by many mechanisms. Advancing age not only results in a reduction in the absorption of nutrients from the elderly patient's diet but also in the absorption of drugs. There are several physiologic changes that account for this. There is a gradual reduction in the stomach's ability to produce hydrochloric acid, which results in a decrease in gastric acidity. This may alter the absorption of weakly acidic drugs like barbiturates and aspirin. The combination of decreased cardiac output and advancing atherosclerosis results in a general reduction in the flow of blood to major organs such as the stomach. By 65 years of age there is

an approximate 50% reduction in blood flow to the gastrointestinal (GI) tract. Absorption, whether nutrient or drug, is dependent on good blood supply to the stomach and intestine. Once the drug is absorbed it must be carried by the bloodstream to its eventual site of action.

GI motility is important not only for moving substances out of the stomach but also for moving them throughout the GI tract. Muscle tone and motor activity in the GI tract are reduced, and this often results in constipation in geriatric patients, for which they frequently take laxatives. This use of laxatives may accelerate GI motility and reduce the absorption of drugs. One particular category of laxatives, bulk-forming laxatives, has been shown to reduce the absorption of certain medications such as cardiac glycosides (digoxin). Bran and high-fiber foods may have the same effect. Another consequence of aging is an overall reduction in the absorptive surface area of the GI tract. The aging process also causes the villi to become flattened and blunted, reducing their overall absorptive capabilities.

Distribution

The distribution of medications throughout the body is vastly different in the elderly than it is in younger adults. There seems to be a gradual reduction in the total body water content with aging. Therefore the concentrations of highly water-soluble drugs may be higher in geriatric patients because they have less water in which the drugs can be diluted. The composition of the body also changes with aging. The lean muscle mass decreases, resulting in increased body fat. In both men and women there is an approximate 20% reduction in muscle mass between 25 and 65 years of age and a corresponding 20% increase in the fat content. Drugs such as hypnotics and sedatives that are primarily distributed to the fat will therefore have a prolonged effect.

Many drugs distributed by means of the blood are carried by proteins. By far the most important of these is al-

geriatric considerations

Pharmacokinetic Changes in the Geriatric Patient

ABSORPTION
- Gastric pH is less acidic because of a gradual reduction in the production of hydrochloric acid in the stomach.
- Gastric emptying is slowed because of a decline in muscle tone and motor activity.
- Movement throughout the gastrointestinal (GI) tract is slower because of decreased smooth muscle tone and motor activity.
- Blood flow to GI tract is reduced by 40% to 50% because of decreased cardiac output and decreased blood flow.
- The absorptive surface area is decreased because the aging process blunts and flattens villi.

DISTRIBUTION
- TBW in adults from 40 to 60 years of age is 55% (male) and 47% (female); for those over 60 years of age, 52% (male) and 46% (female).
- Fat content is increased because of decreased lean body mass.
- Protein (albumin) binding sites are reduced because of decreased production of proteins by aging liver and reduced intake.

METABOLISM
- The levels of microsomal enzymes are decreased because the capacity of the aging liver to produce them is reduced.
- Liver blood flow is reduced by approximately 1.5% per year after age of 25, decreasing hepatic metabolism.

EXCRETION
- Glomerular filtration rate is decreased by 40% to 50% primarily because of decreased blood flow.
- Number of intact nephrons is decreased.

bumin. Reduced protein concentrations, including that of albumin, result from aging. This may be due in part to reduced liver function (which produces many of these proteins), to decreased intake or poor absorption despite adequate intake, or to a combination of these factors. Whatever the cause, a reduced number of protein-binding sites for highly protein-bound drugs results in higher levels of unbound drug. Drugs that are not bound to proteins are active. Therefore the effects of highly protein-bound drugs may be enhanced if their doses are not adjusted in keeping with the albumin concentrations.

Metabolism

Metabolism declines with advancing age. The transformation of active drugs into inactive metabolites is primarily performed by the liver, but the liver slowly loses its ability to metabolize drugs effectively because the production of microsomal enzymes is reduced. There is also a reduction in blood flow to the liver because of reduced cardiac output and atherosclerosis. A reduction in the he-

patic blood flow of approximately 1.5% per year occurs after the age of 25. All these factors contribute to prolonging the half-life of many drugs, which can potentially result in drug accumulation if drug intervals are not adjusted accordingly.

Excretion

The excretion of drugs is reduced in the geriatric population. A reduction in the glomerular filtration of 40% to 50% in the elderly combined with a reduction in blood flow (for the same reasons that apply to the liver) can result in extremely delayed drug excretion and hence drug accumulation. Renal function should be monitored frequently in the elderly to prevent drug accumulation. Appropriate dose and interval adjustments can be made easily based on a patient's renal function, and the potentially dangerous complications that can result from inappropriate dosing can thereby be prevented.

Problematic Geriatric Medications

Drugs in certain classes are more likely to cause problems in the elderly because of many of the physiologic alterations and pharmacokinetic changes already discussed. Table 3-4 lists the most common problematic geriatric medications.

Knowledge of the physiologic changes in the elderly combined with an understanding of the various pharmacokinetic changes that occur is extremely useful in the management of the geriatric patient. It can lead to improvements in drug therapy and thereby the prevention of unwanted consequences of inappropriate dosing.

nursing process

● Assessment

Before administering any medication to a pediatric patient, a thorough health and medication history must be obtained (often from parents or caregivers) that includes the following:
- Age
- Allergies to drugs and food
- Medical and medication history (including adverse drug reactions)
- Head-to-toe assessment findings
- Baseline vital signs
- Weight (important because many doses are calculated per kilogram of body weight)
- Height
- Usual response to medications
- Use of prescription and OTC medications
- State of anxiety
- Fears
- Age-related concerns
- Level of growth and development

The prescriber's orders should be triple-checked because there is no room for error when working with pediatric patients. The medication dosage should be calculated and re-checked for safety purposes.

General assessment data to be gathered in the elderly patient include the following:

- Age
- Allergies to drugs and food
- Present and past medical and medication history (especially prescription and OTC medications being taken)
- Use of polypharmacy
- Use of home remedies
- Dietary habits
- List of all physicians
- Self-medication practices
- Limitations (sensory, visual, hearing, cognitive/motor skills, financial status)
- Results of renal and liver function studies

Just because patients appear to be alert does not mean they understand what you are saying or can self-administer medications without difficulty or without causing themselves harm. It is important to realize that while most geriatric patients are able to provide their own information, some geriatric patients might be confused or poorly informed about their medications. In this case, it is recommended that you seek additional information or confirm information with significant others, family, or friends.

With both age groups, you should assess the family support systems and the patient's ability to take medications safely. Whenever possible, always opt, unless ordered otherwise, to use a nonpharmacologic approach to treatment in pediatric or geriatric patients. The patient's financial status is also important to assess because this may affect compliance.

Other general questions that should be posed to both the pediatric patient (most likely to their caregiver or parent) and the geriatric patient include: Are there any chronic illnesses, nutritional problems, or GI tract disorders? Are there certain attitudes toward medical treatment? What is ability of the patient or family to understand information about the medication, instructions concerning its use, and the importance of medication compliance?

● Nursing Diagnoses

Nursing diagnoses related to the administration of medications to pediatric and geriatric patients include the following:

- Risk for injury related to side effects of medications
- Risk for imbalanced nutrition, less than body requirements, related to age or medication therapy
- Risk for injury related to idiosyncratic reactions because of age
- Deficient knowledge related to information about medications and their side effects or about when to contact the physician

● Planning

Goals related to the pediatric or geriatric patient (or parent/legal guardian/caregiver) include the following:

- Patient is free of complications associated with the adverse effects of medications.
- Patient remains compliant (or takes medication as prescribed with assistance) until medication is discontinued by physician.
- Patient contacts physician when appropriate as related to medication therapy.

Outcome Criteria

Outcome criteria related to the administration of medications to the pediatric or geriatric patient (or parent/legal guardian/caregiver) include the following:

- Patient will state the importance of taking medication as prescribed (e.g., improved condition, decreased symptoms).
- Patient will follow instructions specific to the administration of the medication ordered (e.g., the special application of an ointment, taking of liquid, dosaging).
- Patient will state therapeutic and side effects of specific medication therapy.
- Patient will show improvement in condition related to compliance and successful medication therapy.
- Patient will take or receive medications safely and without injury.

Table 3-4 Problematic Geriatric Medications

Medication	Common Geriatric Complications
Analgesics	
Opioids	Confusion, constipation, urinary retention, nausea, vomiting, and respiratory depression
NSAIDs	Edema, nausea, abdominal distress, gastric ulceration, and bleeding
Anticoagulants (heparin and warfarin)	Major and minor bleeding episodes, many drug interactions, and dietary interactions
Anticholinergics	Blurred vision, dry mouth, constipation, confusion, urinary retention, and tachycardia
Antihypertensives	Nausea, hypotension, diarrhea, bradycardia, and heart failure
Cardiac glycosides (digoxin)	Visual disorders, nausea, diarrhea, dysrhythmias, hallucinations, decreased appetite, and weight loss
Sedatives and hypnotics	Confusion, daytime sedation, ataxia, lethargy, forgetfulness, and increased risk of falls
Thiazide diuretics	Electrolyte imbalance, rashes, fatigue, leg cramps, and dehydration

NSAIDs, Nonsteroidal antiinflammatory drugs.

- Patient will state specific situations when the physician must be contacted (e.g., occurrence of fever, pain, vomiting, rash or diarrhea, worsening of condition, bronchospasms, dyspnea).

Implementation

In general, it is always important to emphasize and practice the five rights concerning the administration of medications and follow the label and medication instructions. Patients should be encouraged to take medications as directed and not to discontinue them, "double-up" on doses, or take any OTC medications unless they clear this with the prescriber *first*. In general, when it comes to pediatric or geriatric patients, be sure the patient, parents, or caregiver understands instructions specific to the medication and understands that all medications should be kept out of the reach of small children. Provide written and oral instructions concerning the drug name, action, purpose, dose, time of administration, route, side effects, safety of administration, storage, interactions, and any cautions about or contraindications to its use. Specific guidelines for administration are given in Chapter 8 and are discussed throughout the book where appropriate. The Home Health/Community Points box lists some home health points for the pediatric patient.

Evaluation

In general, when dealing with pediatric or geriatric patients, the nurse should be constantly observing for the expected and therapeutic effects of the medication. Side effects should also be watched for, and the nurse should know when the effects represent toxicity or overdosage and inform the prescriber immediately. The patient, parent, legal guardian, or caregiver should also be aware of these points of monitoring.

home health/community points

Pediatric Patient

- Avoid disguising medications in essential foods such as milk, orange juice, or cereal, because the child may develop a dislike for the food in the future.
- Always document what was successful so that the method may be communicated to others (e.g., a frozen popsickle before administration of an unpleasant tasting pill or liquid).
- Unless contraindicated, adding small amounts of water to elixirs may help in the child's tolerance of the medication.
- Avoid using the word "candy" in place of "medications." Medications should be called medicines and their dangers made known to children.
- Keep all medications out of the reach of children of all ages. Secure medications at all times to prevent accidental poisoning.
- Request child-resistant medication containers when children are in the home.
- Most medications are better tolerated with 6 to 8 ounces of fluids such as juices, water, or milk.

POINTS TO REMEMBER

Age-Related Pharmacokinetic Effect
- Dramatic differences in drug absorption, distribution, metabolism, and excretion at the beginning and end of life.
- At one end neonates and pediatrics; at the other end geriatric patients.

Preterm, Newborn, Infant, and Child
- Preterm = <38 weeks.
- Newborn = <1 month.
- Infant = 1 month to <1 year.
- Child = 1 to <12 years.

Dose Calculations in Children
- Most commonly calculated by mg/kg formula, but body surface area (BSA) is also still used for drug calculations.

Geriatric Patients
- >65 years of age.
- In 1990, 12% of total population; in 2000, 20% of total population.

- Fastest-growing segment of the population.
- Consume >25% of all medications and >70% of OTC medications.

Polypharmacy
- One patient may have several illnesses and be taking many drugs.
- Drastically increases the risk of drug interactions, adverse reactions, and hospitalization.
- One patient on five medications has 50% chance of a drug interaction, a 100% chance if on eight.

Nurse's Role
- Nurse must be well informed and knowledgeable about growth and development principles and the effects of various agents during each life phase and in various phases of illness.
- Always follow the five "rights" of medication administration to prevent drug errors and harm to patients of all ages.
- Thorough patient education for all involved in the patient's care should include written and oral instructions.

REVIEW QUESTIONS

1. Which of the following factors place the neonate at risk as related to pharmacokinetics and drug therapy?
   a. Immature renal system
   b. Hyperperistalsis in the GI tract
   c. Functional temperature regulation
   d. Dysfunctional musculoskeletal movement

2. The physiologic differences in the infant as compared with the adult patient affect the amount of drug needed to produce a therapeutic effect. One of the main differences is that infants have:
   a. A lesser water composition.
   b. Fat composition less than 0.001%.
   c. Greater body muscular composition.
   d. Water composition of approximately 75%.

3. You must encourage Mr. Y, a 76-year-old patient, to keep a journal of side effects experienced from his medications. This intervention may be critical to the elderly patient because of alterations in pharmacokinetics, such as:
   a. Increased renal excretion of protein-bound drugs.
   b. More alkaline gastric pH, resulting in more side effects.
   c. Decreased liver blood perfusion with altered metabolism.
   d. Less adipose tissue and therefore more distribution of fat-soluble drugs.

4. Of the following medications that this same 76-year-old patient is taking, which may result in hypotension, postural orthostatic blood pressures, and possible syncope?
   a. NSAIDs
   b. Adrenaline
   c. Epinephrine
   d. Antihypertensives

5. One of the most important phases of the nursing process for the elderly patient is the nurse's ability to:
   a. Communicate with patience, empathy, dignity, and understanding.
   b. Suggest to the family that the patient needs to be institutionalized.
   c. Refer the patient to several health care providers for a multiprovider plan.
   d. Develop a detailed instruction and plan for self-medication administration.

For Answers see www.harcourthealth.com/MERLIN/Lilley/.

CRITICAL THINKING Activities

1. Select either phenytoin or tetracycline, and discuss its potential risks to the fetus or breast-feeding newborn in relation to the needed benefits to the mother.

2. A 73-year-old nursing home resident is experiencing problems that you think are indicative of some absorption problems when taking his oral medications. In particular, you notice that he is experiencing unusual bleeding tendencies since taking warfarin; however, he tolerated the medication very well over the last 3 years. Which of the following physiological changes is probably the basis of his untoward reaction to the warfarin:
   a. Increased cardiac output and cardiac volume
   b. Increased glomerular filtration and renin excretion
   c. Decreased GI pH with increased peristalsis
   d. Decreased hepatic enzyme production and altered liver perfusion

3. List medications that are particularly problematic for the geriatric patient. Discuss the problem or complication associated with these drugs or drug classifications.

For Answers see www.harcourthealth.com/MERLIN/Lilley/.

bibliography

American Hospital Formulary Service: *AHFS drug information,* Bethesda, Md, 2000, American Society of Health-System Pharmacists.

Anderson PO, Knoben JE, Troutman WG: *Handbook of clinical drug data 1999-2000,* ed 9, New York, 1999, McGraw-Hill.

Broussard MC, Pitre S: Medication problems in the elderly: a home healthcare nurse's perspective, *Home Healthcare Nurse* 14(6):44, 1996.

DiPiro JT et al: *Pharmacotherapy: a pathophysiologic approach,* ed 4, New York, 1999, Elsevier Science.

Johns Hopkins Hospital, Department of Pediatrics et al: *The Harriet Lane handbook,* ed 15, St Louis, 2000, Mosby.

Keen JH: *Critical care and emergency drug reference,* ed 3, St Louis, 1996, Mosby.

Lee M: Drugs and the elderly: do you know the risks? *AJN* 96(7):25, 1996.

McKenry LM, Salerno E: *Mosby's pharmacology in nursing,* ed 21, St Louis, 2001, Mosby.

Mosby's GenRx: a comprehensive reference for generic and brand drugs, ed 10, St Louis, 2000, Mosby.

Nadler-Moodie M, Wilson MF: Best approaches in Alzheimer's care, *RN,* July 1998.

Skidmore-Roth L: *Mosby's 2001 nursing drug reference,* St Louis, 2001, Mosby.

Activity

Remember to check the **Online Worksheet** for additional learning opportunities: **www.harcourthealth.com/MERLIN/Lilley/**

Chapter 4

Legal, Ethical, and Cultural Considerations

objectives

www.harcourthealth.com/MERLIN/Lilley/

Look for this symbol for
topics covered in the
Online Worksheet
Activity

When you reach the end of this chapter, you should be able to do the following:

1 Identify important drug legislation passed at the state and federal levels.

2 Discuss the impact of drug legislation on drug therapy and nursing.

3 Provide examples of the scheduled categories for controlled substances.

4 Identify the process involved in the development of new drugs, including investigational new drug application, phases of investigational drug studies, and informed consent.

5 Discuss the nurse's role in the development of new and investigational drugs.

6 Discuss the ethical aspects of drug administration and the nurse's role.

7 Explain the effect of culture on a patient's response to and compliance with drug therapy.

glossary

Blinded investigational drug study A research method in which the subject taking the drug under study is purposely unaware of a key element or elements in the study (e.g., which administered substance is the drug under study versus a placebo). This method eliminates bias on the part of the subject. (p. 46)

Canadian Food and Drugs Act Amended many times since its inception in 1953, this act is the main piece of drug legislation in Canada. It protects consumers from contaminated, adulterated, or unsafe drugs and unsafe labeling practices; and addresses appropriate advertising and selling of drugs, food, cosmetics, or devices. (p. 47)

Canadian Narcotic Control Act Addresses the possession, sale, manufacture, production, and distribution of narcotics. It was enacted in response to increasing misuse and abuse of drugs in the mid to late 1960s. (p. 47)

Controlled Substance Act of 1970 Also known as the Comprehensive Drug Abuse Prevention and Control Act, it promotes research on drug abuse; the prevention of drug abuse through education, treatment, and rehabilitation for drug-addicted persons; and enhancement of law enforcement. It also created the classification system for controlled substances that is used to regulate the manufacture, distribution, and dispensing of drugs. (p. 45)

Double-blind, placebo-controlled study A research method in which both the investigator and subject are purposely unaware of key elements in the study (e.g., which administered substance is the drug under study versus a placebo). This method eliminates bias on the part of both the investigator and the subject. (p. 46)

Drug polymorphism (pol ē mor′ fizm) Variation in response to a drug because of a patient's age, gender, size, and body composition. (p. 49)

Durham-Humphrey Amendment A modification of the Food, Drug, and Cosmetic Act of 1938 that differentiated between prescription (i.e., legend) drugs and over-the-counter medications. Also identified were medications that could and could not be refilled without another prescription and which original prescriptions and refills could be authorized over the telephone. (p. 44)

Expedited drug approval A hastening of the usual investigational new drug approval process by the Food and Drug Administration and pharmaceutical companies in response to a public health threat (e.g., AIDS). Drugs showing promise in phase I and II clinical trials are given to qualified patients, and the drug approval process is shortened if the drug continues to show promise. (p. 46)

Food, Drug, and Cosmetic Act of 1938 This act required drug manufacturers to apply for an investigational new drug exemption for a safety review before marketing new drugs. (p. 44)

Informed consent Permission obtained from a patient consenting to the performance of a specific test or procedure. Informed consent is required before most invasive procedures can be performed and before a patient can be admitted into a research study. The document must be written in a language understood by the patient and be dated and signed by the patient and at least one witness. Included in the document are clear, rational descriptions of the procedure or test. Also required is a statement that care will not be withheld if the patient does not consent to this; informed consent is voluntary. By law, informed consent must be obtained more than a given number of days or hours before certain procedures are performed and must always be obtained when the patient is fully mentally competent. (p. 46)

Investigational new drug A drug not approved for marketing by the Food and Drug Administration but available for use in experiments to determine its safety and efficacy. (p. 46)

Kefauver-Harris Amendment of 1962 This act required drugs to be proved both safe and effective before being granted an approved status. Because of this act many drugs found to be ineffective have been removed from the market. (p. 44)

Legend drugs Another name for prescription drugs. The Durham-Humphrey Amendment required that prescription drug labels include the legend stating, "Caution—Federal law prohibits dispensing without prescription." (p. 44)

New drug application Once a drug successfully completes the first three phases of an investigational new drug study, the drug manufacturer may submit a new drug application to the Food and Drug Administration. If this application is approved, the company may sell the drug exclusively. (p. 46)

Over-the-counter (OTC) drugs Drugs that are available to consumers without a prescription. Also called *nonprescription drugs.* (p. 44)

Placebo (pla sē' bo) An inactive substance (e.g., saline, distilled water, starch, or sugar) or a less-than-effective dose of a harmless substance (e.g., a water-soluble vitamin). Placebos are used in experimental drug studies to compare the "effects" of the inactive substance with the bona fide effects of the experimental drug. They are also prescribed to satisfy the requests of patients who cannot be given the medication they request or who, in the judgment of the health care provider, do not need this medication. (p. 46)

Pure Food and Drug Act of 1906 The first federal law that attempted to protect the public from dangerous, adulterated, and mislabeled products. It established the *United States Pharmacopeia* and the *National Formulary* and gave the federal government authority to enforce the standards these contained. The act applied only to drugs sold in interstate commerce. (p. 44)

U.S. DRUG LEGISLATION

Until the beginning of the 20th century there were no federal rules and regulations in the United States to protect consumers from the dangers of medications. Not until numerous devastating, drug-induced catastrophes occurred did the government intervene. The first act passed by the federal government in response to these catastrophes was the **Pure Food and Drug Act of 1906.** Since 1906, several acts have been passed to further ensure the safe and effective use of drugs. This federal legislation protects the public from drugs that are impure, toxic, or ineffective, or that have not been tested before public sale. The primary purpose of this federal legislation is to ensure safety. A brief understanding of the most important acts provides both an overview of the past and a view into the possible future of drug development and usage.

Pure Food and Drug Act of 1906

In 1906 the federal government passed the Pure Food and Drug Act to protect the public from adulterated or mislabeled drugs. It required drug companies to declare on the package label the presence of identified dangerous and possibly addicting drugs. This act designated *The United States Pharmacopeia* and *The National Formulary* as official standards for therapeutic use, patient safety, quality, purity, strength, packaging safety, and dosage form. "USP" can be placed after the names of drugs that meet these

standards. This act also empowered the federal government to enforce these standards and to take legal action against those companies that do not comply with the provisions of the act.

Food, Drug, and Cosmetic Act of 1938

There were several shortcomings to the 1906 act that resulted in new legislation. The Food and Drug Act only specified that drug labeling not contain false or misleading claims about the therapeutic benefits of a particular drug. It did not address the issue of proper testing for safety before a drug could be marketed. In 1937 more than 100 deaths occurred as a result of the ingestion of a diethyleneglycol solution of sulfanilamide. This product had been marketed as an "elixir of sulfanilamide" without its toxicity being investigated. This stimulated the government to enact the **Food, Drug, and Cosmetic Act of 1938,** which prohibited the marketing of new drugs before proper testing of their safety had been done. Pharmaceutical companies now had to submit an investigational new drug exemption to the government for review of a drug's safety before they could sell the product.

1952: Durham-Humphrey Amendment of the 1938 Act

To provide further safety to the consumers of drugs, the **Durham-Humphrey Amendment** was passed. This amendment distinguished between drugs that could be sold with or without a prescription and identified those that should not be refilled without a new prescription. Drugs for which a prescription is needed before they can be sold are called **legend drugs** because the labels have to carry the legend: "Caution—Federal law prohibits dispensing without a prescription." These drugs are also called *prescription drugs.* Drugs for which a prescription is not needed are referred to as *nonprescription,* or **over-the-counter (OTC) drugs.** This act also specified that certain drugs such as opioids, hypnotics, and tranquilizers could not be refilled without a new prescription from a physician.

1962: Kefauver-Harris Amendment of the 1938 Act

The **Kefauver-Harris Amendment of 1962** was initiated partly because of concern on the part of a senator from Tennessee and also in response to the thalidomide tragedy. In 1958 Senator Estes Kefauver began a Senate investigation into the drug industry. Drug companies were making huge profits through the use of false or misleading promotions. Not much attention was paid to Senator Kefauver's concerns until the thalidomide tragedy occurred in Europe. Thalidomide was a widely used sedative-hypnotic marketed in Europe at this time that was found to cause severe deformities in the babies of mothers who took the drug during pregnancy. The European thalidomide experience prompted the United States to enact the Kefauver-Harris Amendment of 1962. Before 1962 the safety but not the efficacy of a new drug had be

Table 4-1   Controlled Substances: Schedule Categories

Schedule	Abuse Potential	Medical Use	Dependency
C-I	High	None	Severe
C-II	High	Accepted	Severe physical and/or psychologic
C-III	<C-II	Accepted	Moderate/low physical or high psychologic
C-IV	<C-III	Accepted	Limited physical or psychologic
C-V	<C-IV	Accepted	Limited physical or psychologic

Table 4-2   Controlled Substances: Categories, Dispensing Restrictions, and Examples

Schedule	Dispensing Restrictions	Examples
C-I	• Only with approved protocol	Heroin, LSD, marijuana, mescaline, peyote, psilocybin, and methaqualone
C-II	• Written prescription only (if telephoned in, need written prescription within 24 hours) • No prescription refills • Container must have warning label	Codeine, cocaine, hydromorphone, meperidine, morphine, methadone, secobarbital, pentobarbital, amphetamine, methylphenidate, and others
C-III	• Written or oral prescription that expires in 6 months • No more than five refills in 6-month period • Container must have warning label	Codeine, hydrocodone, oxycodone, morphine, and dihydrocodeine combination products; paregoric and nonopioid preparations of pentazocine and propoxyphene
C-IV	• Written or oral prescription that expires in 6 months • No more than five refills in 6-month period • Container must have warning label	Barbital, phenobarbital, chloral hydrate, meprobamate, the benzodiazepines (e.g., diazepam, temazepam, lorazepam), dextropropoxyphene, pentazocine, and others
C-V	• Written prescription or over-the-counter varies with each state law	Medications generally for relief of coughs or diarrhea containing limited quantities of certain opioid-controlled substances

proved before its approval and marketing. After this amendment was passed, both safety and efficacy had to be proved before a new drug could be approved for use.

1970: Comprehensive Drug Abuse Prevention and Control Act

Much like the previous acts, the Comprehensive Drug Abuse Prevention and Control Act was enacted by Congress in response to the growing misuse and abuse of drugs in the middle and late 1960s. This act is also known as the **Controlled Substance Act of 1970** and was designed to address the problem of drug abuse at that time. It promoted drug education and research into the prevention and treatment of drug dependence, strengthened enforcement authority, established treatment and rehabilitation facilities, and designed schedules or categories for controlled substances. These categories of drugs were defined according to their abuse potential and are listed in Table 4-1. Each controlled substance category has specific dispensing restrictions, which are listed in Table 4-2. Examples of drugs that fall into the various controlled substance categories are also given in Table 4-2.

Activity

NEW DRUG DEVELOPMENT

The research into and development of new drugs is an ongoing process. The pharmaceutical industry is a multibillion-dollar industry that must continuously develop new and better drugs to maintain a competitive edge. The research required for the development of new and better drugs may take several years. Hundreds of substances are isolated that never make it to market. Once a potentially beneficial drug has been isolated, there is a very regulated, systematic process that the pharmaceutical company must go through before the drug can be used in the open market. This highly sophisticated, systematic process is regulated and carefully monitored by the United States Food and Drug Administration (FDA). The primary purpose of the FDA is to ensure patient safety and drug efficacy.

This system of drug research and development is one of the most stringent in the world. There are many benefits and drawbacks to it. It was developed out of concern for patient safety and drug efficacy. To ensure that these two very important objectives are met with some degree of certainty requires much time and paperwork. This is the downside to the system. Many drugs are marketed and used in foreign countries long before they get approval for use in the United States. However, many drug-related tragedies are averted by this strict system. The thalidomide tragedy, which occurred in Europe but not in the United States, proves this. There must be a balance between making new lifesaving therapies available and protecting consumers from potential drug-induced adverse effects.

Investigational New Drug Application

A pharmaceutical company must prove both the safety and efficacy of a newly isolated drug before it can be used in the general population. Testing begins in animal models. The new medication must be tested for its pharmacologic use, dosage ranges, and possible toxic effects. After extensive animal testing that proves the safety and efficacy of the new drug, the pharmaceutical company can then submit an application for an **investigational new drug** (IND). Only after the FDA reviews and approves this application can the pharmaceutical company proceed with investigational studies of the IND in human subjects. There are four phases to this clinical evaluation process in human subjects. The collective goal of these phases is to provide information on the safety, toxicity, efficacy, potency, bioavailability, and purity of the IND. Informed consent must be obtained of all patients before they can be enrolled in an IND study.

Informed Consent

Informed consent involves the careful explanation of the purpose of the study, procedures to be used, and risks involved. Participants in experimental drug studies should be informed volunteers and not uninformed, coerced subjects. Some patients may have unrealistic expectations of the IND's usefulness. Often they have the misconception that because an investigational drug is "new," it must automatically be better than existing forms of therapy. To prevent any bias introduced by such thinking, many studies are designed to incorporate a **placebo.** A placebo is an inert substance that is not a drug (e.g., normal saline). A study incorporating a placebo is called a *placebo-controlled study.* It attempts to eliminate any bias that an IND study volunteer may have toward the new drug. Other volunteers may be reluctant to enter the study because they think they will be treated like "guinea pigs." Whatever the circumstances of the study, the study volunteers must be informed of all the potential hazards as well as the possible benefits of the new therapy. It should be stressed to the study volunteer that involvement in IND studies is truly voluntary and that the subject can quit the study at any time.

Four Phases of Investigational Drug Studies

Phase I

Phase I studies involve small numbers of healthy volunteers as opposed to volunteers afflicted with the disease or ailment that the new drug is meant to treat. The purpose of these studies is to determine the optimal

dosage range and the pharmacokinetics of the drug (absorption, distribution, metabolism, and excretion). Also performed are blood tests, urinalyses, assessments of vital signs, and specific monitoring tests.

Phase II

Phase II studies involve small numbers of volunteers that have the disease or ailment that the drug is designed to diagnose or treat. Study participants are closely monitored for the drug's effectiveness and any side effects. If no serious side effects occur, the study can progress to phase III.

Phase III

Phase III studies involve large numbers of patients at medical research centers. The purpose of this larger sample size is to provide information about infrequent or rare adverse effects that may have been selected out in the studies consisting of small numbers of patients. Information obtained during this clinical phase helps identify any risks associated with the new drug. Placebo-controlled studies are employed during this phase to eliminate any patient bias. Since the study subject does not know whether the drug being administered is a placebo or the IND, this is referred to as a **blinded investigational drug study.** To eliminate any bias on the part of the investigator, he or she is also blinded to the identity of the investigational substance. This type of study is called a **double-blind, placebo-controlled study.** The three objectives of this phase are to establish the drug's clinical effectiveness, safety, and dosage range.

Phase IV

Phase IV studies are postmarketing studies voluntarily conducted by pharmaceutical companies to obtain further proof of the therapeutic effects of the new drug. Often these studies compare the safety and efficacy of the new drug with that of another drug in the same therapeutic category. An example would be a comparison of a new nonsteroidal antiinflammatory drug (NSAID) with ibuprofen in the treatment of osteoarthritis. Some medications make it through all phases of clinical trials without any problems. However, when they are used in the general population, sometimes severe adverse effects show up.

New Drug Application

After the first three phases are completed, the FDA reviews all the results. If these are favorable, the pharmaceutical company may submit a **new drug application** (NDA). Once the FDA has reviewed and approved the NDA, the pharmaceutical company is free to market the new drug exclusively.

Expedited Drug Approval

The FDA has attempted to make lifesaving, investigational drug therapies available to the population sooner by offering an **expedited drug approval** process. The public health threat posed by the acquired immunodeficiency syndrome (AIDS) has motivated the FDA and pharmaceutical companies to shorten the IND approval process, allowing physicians to give qualified AIDS patients medications that have shown promise during early phase I and II clinical trials. If the drug then continues to show favorable results, the overall process of drug approval is hastened as much as possible.

Activity

CANADIAN LEGISLATION

In Canada, concerns over the sale and use of foods, drugs, cosmetics, and medical devices began long before these concerns arose in the United States. Canadian drug legislation began in 1875 when the Parliament of Canada passed an act to prevent the sale of adulterated food, drink, and drugs. Since that time foods and drugs have been controlled on a national basis.

Canadian Food and Drugs Act

The **Canadian Food and Drugs Act** is the primary piece of legislation concerning drugs in Canada. The act has been amended several times since its beginning in 1953 and has two main purposes.

1. To protect the consumer from drugs that are contaminated, adulterated, or unsafe for use
2. To address drugs that are labeled falsely, may be misleading, or are deceptive

To determine if drugs comply with this act, one of six recognized pharmacopeias and formularies can be used as a reference. These are listed in one of the many "schedules" contained in this act, Schedule B. The references contained in Schedule B are listed below:

- Pharmacopoeia Internationalis
- The United States Pharmacopeia/National Formulary
- British Pharmaceutical Codex
- The British Pharmacopoeia
- Pharmacopee Francaise
- The Canadian Formulary

The second purpose of the Canadian Food and Drugs Act is to address appropriate advertising and selling of drugs, food, cosmetics, and devices. The Act stipulates that no food, drug, cosmetic, or device is to be advertised or sold to the general public as a treatment, preventive, or cure for certain diseases listed in Schedule A of the Act. Some examples of these diseases are alcoholism, arteriosclerosis, and cancer. When a drug meets these standards it is labeled with the legend *Canadian Standard Drug,* or CSD, on its inner and outer labels.

This particular Act has many more amendments or schedules that have been added over the years. Some of the more important ones are listed in Table 4-3.

Canadian Narcotic Control Act

The regulations that address the possession, sale, manufacture, production, and distribution of opioids are covered in the **Canadian Narcotic Control Act.** This act was passed in 1961 and replaced the previous act, the Canadian Opium and Narcotic Act of 1952. The Canadian Narcotic Control Act is similar in its purpose to the Comprehensive Drug Abuse Prevention and Control Act of 1970

in the United States, which was enacted in response to the growing misuse and abuse of drugs in the middle and late 1960s.

The administrative responsibility for this Act belongs to the Department of National Health and Welfare. The enforcement of this Act belongs to the members of the Royal Canadian Mounted Police.

NURSING IMPLICATIONS
Legal Issues

It is within the framework of the standards of nursing care and nurse practice acts that the nurse's role and responsibility are defined. Besides these standards, there are specific institutional policies and procedures with which nurses must be familiar to fulfill their legal obligation and responsibility to their patients. Some of the legal issues and concepts are listed and defined in the box on p. 48. The five "rights" of medication and the law provide necessary standards for safe patient care and should never be ignored. The law should be viewed as helpful and as a framework for practice, not as an impediment to care.

Ethical Practice

Ethical nursing practice is based on the basic ethical principles of beneficence, nonmalfeasance, autonomy, justice, veracity, and confidentiality. The American Nurses Association Code of Ethics and Canadian Nurses Association Code of Ethics (Boxes 4-1 and 4-2) should be a familiar

Table 4-3 Additional Schedules to the Canadian Food and Drug Act

Schedule	Description
Schedules C and D	Drugs in these schedules must list where the drug was manufactured and the process and conditions of manufacturing.
Schedule F	List of drugs that can be sold and refilled only on prescription; refills cannot exceed 6 mo; labels on these drugs are marked *Pr,* or prescription required. *Examples:* Antibiotics, hormones, and tranquilizers.
Schedule G	These drugs, also known as controlled drugs, affect the CNS; identified by *C* on the label. *Examples:* Amphetamines, barbiturates, and phenmetrazine.
Schedule H	These are restricted drugs; only available to institutions for research; have dangerous physiologic and psychologic side effects; have no recognized medical use.

legal & ethical principles

Ethical Principles and Nursing Implications

- *Beneficence:* The doing or active promotion of good; implications include "how the patient is best served."
- *Nonmaleficence:* The duty to do no harm to a client; implications include avoiding doing any deliberate harm while rendering nursing care.
- *Autonomy:* Self-determination and ability to act on one's own; implications include promoting a patient's decision-making process, supporting informed consent, and assisting in decisions or making a decision when a patient is posing harm to himself or herself.
- *Justice:* Being fair or equal in one's actions; implications include the fair distribution of resources for the care of the patient and determination of when to treat.
- *Veracity:* Duty to tell the truth; implications include telling the truth with regard to investigational new drugs and informed consent.
- *Confidentiality:* The duty to respect privileged information about a patient; implications include not talking about a patient in public or outside the context of the health care setting.

Activity

box 4-1 American Nurses Association Code of Ethics

- The nurse provides services with respect for human dignity and the uniqueness of the patient unrestricted by considerations of social or economic status, personal attributes, or the nature of health problems.
- The nurse safeguards the patient's right to privacy by judiciously protecting information of a confidential nature.
- The nurse acts to safeguard the patient and the public when health care and safety are affected by the incompetent, unethical, or illegal practice of any person.
- The nurse assumes responsibility and accountability for individual nursing judgments and actions.
- The nurse maintains competence in nursing.
- The nurse exercises informed judgment and uses individual competence and qualifications as criteria in seeking consultation, accepting responsibilities, and delegating nursing activities to others.
- The nurse participates in activities that contribute to the ongoing development of the profession's body of knowledge.
- The nurse participates in the profession's efforts to implement and improve standards of nursing.
- The nurse participates in the profession's efforts to establish and maintain conditions of employment conducive to high-quality nursing care.
- The nurse participates in the profession's effort to protect the public from misinformation and misrepresentation and to maintain the integrity of nursing.
- The nurse collaborates with members of the health professions and other citizens in promoting community and national efforts to meet the health needs of the public.

Reprinted with permission from *Code for Nurses with Interpretive Statements,* © 1985, American Nurses Publishing, American Nurses Foundation/American Nurses Association, Washington, DC.

framework of practice to all nurses and serve as an ethical guideline for nursing care. These ethical principles and code of ethics ensure that the nurse is acting on behalf of the patient and with his or her best interests at heart.

As a professional, the nurse has the responsibility to provide safe nursing care to patients regardless of the setting, person, group, community, or family involved. Although it is not within the nurse's realm of ethical and professional responsibility to impose his or her own values or standards on the patient, it is within his or her realm to provide information and assist the patient in facing decisions regarding health care.

The nurse also has the right to refuse to participate in any treatment or aspect of a patient's care that violates personal ethical principles. However, this should be done without deserting the patient. Should this situation arise, it is the nurse's responsibility to inform the appropriate persons about the conflict and to transfer the patient to the safe care of another professional nurse before the start of treatment.

It is a nurse's responsibility to always provide the highest-quality nursing care and practice within the standards of care. The American Nurses Association Code of Ethics, Canadian Nurses Association Code of Ethics, and the previously mentioned ethical principles should constitute the framework for the professional practice of nursing.

CULTURAL CONSIDERATIONS

The United States is a tremendously culturally diverse nation. With a health care system emphasizing cure, pre-

scribed drugs are often a major part of a patient's therapeutic regimen with an emphasis on high medication doses unless adverse effects occur. The U.S. health care system also advocates a "one size fits all" type of treatment; there needs to be more consideration of all the variances within the diverse population in the United States. In addition, the demographics in the United States continue to change. In 1997, the Statistical Abstracts of the United States estimated that, between the years 2000 and 2010, the number of Hispanics will increase by 31.2%, African-Americans by 11.6%, Native Americans by 12.9%, Asian-Americans and Pacific Islanders by 36.1%, and Caucasians by 2.7%. These changes in the nation's demographics will demand that the approach to health care—including prescribing of medications—will need to be individualized to the patient with specific attention to cultural background. Nurses need to then continue to be familiar with medications and how culture influences

Canadian Nurses Association Code of Ethics

BOX 4-2

The Canadian Nurses Association Code of Ethics contains four divisions, including *patients, health team, social context of nursing,* and *responsibilities of the profession.* In this code, the nurse views the *patient* as someone deserving of respect and who has individual needs and values. The patient is also to have his or her control respected at all times; confidentiality of *all* information about the patient is demanded. The patient's dignity is of utmost importance in nursing care, as is the role of the nurse as an advocate. Regarding the *health team,* all patients should be treated in a comprehensive and individualized approach. Patients are treated with the assistance of experts around the nurse, who should acknowledge his or her own limitations when appropriate. The *social context of nursing* aspect specifies that nurses should work in a setting that contributes to patient care and to their own professional satisfaction. *Responsibilities of the profession* holds that nurses are to always sustain ethical conduct and remain true to the patient and his or her rights, needs, and interests.

Data from the Canadian Nurses Association: *Code of ethics for registered nurses,* Ottawa, 1997, The Association.

cultural implications

Cultural Practices

Culture	Practice
African	People of African ancestry in the West Indies, Haiti, Jamaica, and Dominican Republic as well as natives of the continent of Africa practice folk medicine and employ "root workers" as healers.
Asian	Believe in traditional medicine and use physicians and herbalists in their health care.
European	Traditional health beliefs are held, and there are some people who still practice folk medicine.
Western	Increased participation in health care; demand more explanation about diseases and treatment, as well as the prevention of diseases.

a particular drug response or the way a specific patient uses or responds to a medication.

Cultural factors are important to holistic nursing care because they affect the patient's health, health beliefs, and health care practices, including drug therapy. The nurse needs to acknowledge and accept the influences of a patient's cultural beliefs, values, and customs to prevent a conflict from arising between the goals of nursing and health care and the dictates of a patient's cultural background. Some examples of cultural influences are presented in the Cultural Implications box.

In reference to specific drug therapy and a patient's response, the concept of polymorphism is critical to further understanding how the same drug can result in a different response. For example, why does a Chinese patient require lower doses of an antianxiety drug than a Caucasian individual? Why does an African-American respond differently to antihypertensives than a Caucasian? **Drug polymorphism** refers to the effect of a patient's age, gender, size, body composition, and other variables such as ethnicity with associated changes in how an individual absorbs or metabolizes specific drugs. Factors contributing to drug polymorphism may be loosely categorized into environmental (such as diet and nutritional status as the body's environment), cultural (values and beliefs), and genetics (inherited factors).

Specifically in reference to cultural influences and drug therapy, medication response depends greatly upon one's compliance level with the therapy. Compliance may vary depending on a patient's cultural beliefs, experiences with medications, expectations, family expectations, family influence, and level of education. However, compliance is not the only factor influencing the cultural influence on drug therapy. Health care providers need to also be aware that some patients subscribe to other therapies, such as herbal and homeopathic remedies, that can inhibit or accelerate drug metabolism and therefore alter a drug response.

Environmental considerations that play an important part in drug responses and their variance depending on culture include factors such as diet. For example, a diet high in fat has been documented to increase the absorption of the agent griseofulvin (an antifungal agent). Malnutrition with deficiencies in protein, vitamins, and minerals may alter the functioning of metabolic enzymes that may alter the body's ability to absorb or eliminate a medication.

Genetic factors also influence how different cultures respond to drugs. Some patients of European and African descent are slow acetylators, which causes elevated drug concentrations because of changes in metabolism. Some patients of Japanese and Inuit descent are more rapid acetylators and metabolize drugs more aggressively, resulting in decreased drug concentrations. Chinese, Japanese, Malaysians, and Thais are poor metabolizers of debrisoquine; therefore agents such as codeine are likely to be more effective in Chinese, Japanese, Malaysian, and Thai patients than in those of European descent. Several major drug classifications are relatively well researched with regard to responses in different cultures; these are outlined in Table 4-4.

Individuals throughout the world share common views and beliefs regarding health practices and taking of medications. However, some specific cultural influences, beliefs, and practices related to medication administration affect different individuals. These cultural differences are even more critical in the care of patients

Table 4-4   Examples of Varying Responses of Drug Classifications on Cultural Groups

Racial or Ethnic Group	Drug Classification	Response
African-American	Antihypertensive agents	• African-Americans respond better to diuretics than to beta-blockers and ACE inhibitors. • African-Americans respond less effectively to beta-blockers than Caucasians. • African-Americans respond best to calcium channel blockers, especially diltiazem. • African-Americans respond less effectively to single drug therapy.
Asian and Hispanic	Antipsychotic and antianxiety agents	• Asians need lower doses of certain drugs such as haloperidol. • Japanese and Chinese are more prone to rapid build-up of mephenytoin and so are at risk for sedation and over-dosage. • Asians and Hispanics respond better to lower doses of antidepressants than Caucasians. • Chinese require lower doses of antipsychotics. • Japanese require lower doses of antimanic agents than Caucasians.

today as the demographics of the United States are constantly changing. As previously mentioned, the minority composition of the United States will continue to change drastically between the years 2000 and 2010. In addition, the Caucasian majority is not only shrinking but also aging, whereas the Asian, Native American, and Hispanic populations are growing and young. With these cultural differences compounded with rapidly changing demographics, nurses need to be astute to and concerned with each patient's cultural background to ensure safe and quality nursing care, including medication administration.

Specifically, some African-Americans have a variety of health belief practices such as proper diet and rest; the use of herbal teas, laxatives, and protective bracelets; and the use of folk medicine, prayer, and the "laying on of hands." Home remedies are also an important component of their health practices.

Some Asian Americans, especially the Chinese, believe in the yin and yang, which are opposing forces leading to illness or health, depending on which force is in balance. The yin represents the female and represents negative energies of darkness and cold, and the yang represents the male and positive energies of light and warmth. The yin and yang beliefs must be respected by all who participate in the care of the Chinese. Other health practices for Asian Americans include the beliefs in acupuncture, herbal remedies, and the use of heat. All of these beliefs need to be strongly considered—especially when there are strong beliefs toward their use versus use of medications.

Some Native Americans have always held the belief of harmony with nature or keeping a balance between the body, mind, and the environment to maintain

health. Ill spirits are seen as the causation of disease. The traditional healer for this culture is the medicine man, and treatments vary from massage and heat to acts of purification.

Some Hispanic individuals view health as good luck and living right versus illness as bad luck or the result of a bad deed. To restore health, these individuals seek out a balance between the body and mind through use of cold remedies or foods for "hot" illness (of blood or yellow bile) or hot remedies for "cold" illnesses (phlegm or black bile). It is important to remember, though, that these beliefs still vary from patient to patient, so always consult with the patient first! Hispanics also use a variety of religious rituals for healing (e.g., lighting of candles).

Barriers to adequate health care for our culturally diverse patient population include language, poverty, access, pride, and beliefs regarding medical practices. Medications may represent different meanings to different cultures as would any aspect of medical treatment. Therefore, before any medication administration, a thorough cultural assessment should be completed, including questions regarding the following:
• Health beliefs and practices
• Past uses of medicine
• Folk remedies
• Home remedies
• Use of nonprescription drugs and herbal remedies
• OTC treatments
• Usual responses to illness
• Responsiveness to medical treatment
• Religious practices and beliefs (for example, Christian Scientists believe in taking no medications at all)
• Dietary habits

POINTS TO REMEMBER

Food and Drug Act of 1906

- Enacted to protect public from adulterated or mislabeled drugs.
- Designated the *United States Pharmacopeia* and the *National Formulary* as official standards for therapeutic use, patient safety, quality, purity, strength, packaging safety, and dosage form.

Durham-Humphrey Amendment

- Specified which drugs need a prescription to be sold and which do not.
- Do need a prescription: legend drugs; do not need a prescription: over-the-counter drugs.

Controlled Substance Act

- Passed in 1971 in response to growing misuse and abuse of drugs in the middle and late 1960s.
- Provides for increased research into, and prevention of, drug abuse and "drug dependence."
- Provides for treatment and rehabilitation of drug abusers and drug-dependent persons.
- Strengthens law enforcement authority.
- Controlled substances schedule (C-I through C-V).
- C-I: high abuse potential and no medical use.
- C-V: low abuse potential and accepted medical use.

Informed Consent

- Careful explanation of the purpose of a study.
- Describes procedures used and risk involved.

- Informed volunteers are not uninformed, coerced subjects.

FDA Drug Approval Process

- IND: investigation new drug; NDA: new drug application.
- Clinical phases I, II, and III (to determine safety, dose, and efficacy).
- Experimental phases: IND phases I, II, and III; put on market if NDA approved by FDA.
- Takes several years.

Canadian Food and Drugs Act

- Main piece of drug legislation in Canada.
- Enacted to protect consumer from adulterated or mislabeled drugs.
- Regulates advertising and selling of drugs, food, cosmetics, or devices.

Nurse's Role

- The five "rights" of medication administration include the right drug, patient, route, time, and dose.
- Nurses involved in drug research need to be knowledgeable about the research process, patient's rights, and informed consent.
- Legal guidelines, ethical principles, and the ANA Code of Ethics ensure that the nurse is acting on sound foundations of nursing care.

REVIEW QUESTIONS

1. Your patient states that she has been taking six or more aspirin per day for her "bad bones." You inform her that one of the most serious problems associated with the use of aspirin is:
   a. Cystitis.
   b. Polyuria.
   c. Bleeding.
   d. Dependency.
2. Barriers to health care for your 59-year-old Chinese patient would most likely include which of the following?
   a. X-rays are seen as a break in the soul's integrity.
   b. Hospital diets are interpreted as being healing and healthful.
   c. Being hospitalized is a source of peace and socialization for this culture.
   d. Intrusive procedures are seen as contrary to holding the body in high regard and respect.
3. A 39-year-old female Muslim was just admitted to the labor and delivery unit for preterm labor. Perceived barriers to health care for this patient about "self-care" include which of the following? Individuals of Muslim faith:
   a. Cannot consume pork.
   b. Do not believe in self-help.

   c. Do not believe in self-discipline.
   d. Cannot value good health because of beliefs.
4. This same 39-year-old female Muslim is diagnosed as having type 1 (insulin-dependent) diabetes mellitus. Which of her beliefs may pose a problem for her because of beef allergy?
   a. The beef allergy is not problematic because insulins are only available in pork origin.
   b. She cannot consume pork, so she cannot take two different forms of insulin, which she needs.
   c. Her belief of not helping herself because it may be perceived as weakness will not allow her to take insulin.
   d. She does not believe in self-help, so she will not inquire about other options available to her for treatment.
5. What symbolic meaning do drugs have for some patients?
   a. Help
   b. Addiction
   c. Dependence
   d. Purity of the soul

CRITICAL THINKING Activities

1. Discuss the impact of cultural practices as they relate to safe and effective drug therapy.
2. Medication errors have been occurring with increasing frequency in the unit where you are employed. A committee has been appointed to look at why the medication errors occur and how to resolve the problems. In consideration of this and of the drug administration process, is it always safe to only go by the guidelines of using the five rights of drug administration? Why or why not and explain your answer.
3. One of your psychiatric patients is an Alaskan Native youth with a problem of alcohol abuse. He is 17 years of age and has a history of repeated problems with being drunk, coming to school with alcohol detected on his breath, and acting as if under the influence. What is of particular concern for this patient and why?

For Answers see www.harcourthealth.com/MERLIN/Lilley/.

bibliography

American Hospital Formulary Service: *AHFS drug information,* Bethesda, Md, 2000, American Society of Health-System Pharmacists.

American Nurses Association: *Code for nurses with interpretive statements,* Kansas City, Mo, 1985, The Association.

Canadian Nurses Association: *Code of ethics for nursing,* Ottawa, 1995, The Association.

Eskreis TR: Seven common legal pitfalls in nursing, *Am J Nurs* 98(4):34, 1998.

Kudzma EC: Culturally competent, *Am J Nurs* 99(8):46, 1999.

Lilley LL et al: Getting back to basics—"5 rights" of medication administration, *Am J Nurs* 94(9):15, 1994.

McKenry LM, Salerno E: *Mosby's pharmacology in nursing,* ed 21, St Louis, 2001, Mosby.

Pharmaceutical Research Manufacturers Association, annual report, 1998.

Skidmore-Roth L: *Mosby's 2001 nursing drug reference,* St Louis, 2001, Mosby.

Remember to check the **Online Worksheet** for additional learning opportunities: **www.harcourthealth.com/MERLIN/Lilley/**

Chapter 5

Patient Education and Drug Therapy

objectives

www.harcourthealth.com/MERLIN/Lilley/

Look for this symbol for
topics covered in the
Online Worksheet
Activity

When you reach the end of this chapter, you should be able to do the following:

1 Discuss the importance of patient education in the administration of medications.

2 Discuss patient education as related to drug therapy and the nursing process.

3 Identify the impact of the various developmental phases (as per Erikson) on patient education and drug therapy.

With the everchanging arena of health care today and the increasing emphasis on consumer awareness, the role of nurses as educators is expanding and increasing. Because of the changes in health care and patients being managed more frequently in the home setting, education is an essential component of the health care system and in providing quality patient care. In addition, patient education is crucial for patients to adapt to illness, prevent illness, maintain wellness, and care for self. Patient education is identified as a process, similar to the nursing process, whereby the patient is assisted to learn and assimilate healthy behaviors into their lifestyle. Learning is then defined as a change in behavior, and teaching is the sharing of knowledge. Although nurses can never be certain that patients will take medications as prescribed, they can be sure to carefully assess, plan, implement, and evaluate the teaching provided to patients about their medications.

ASSESSMENT OF LEARNING NEEDS RELATED TO DRUG THERAPY

Similar to the nursing process, in the patient education process, a thorough assessment of learning needs must be completed before educating the patient about their medications. A thorough assessment would include the gathering of subjective and objective data about the following:
- Level of education
- Cognitive abilities
- Nutritional status
- Self-care ability
- Mobility
- Social support
- Financial status
- Sensory status
- Past health behaviors
- Health beliefs
- Emotional status
- Adaptation to any illnesses
- Growth and development level as per Erikson's stages of development (Box 5-1)
- Coping mechanisms
- Language(s) spoken
- Limitations (physical, psychologic, cognitive, motor)
- Environments at home and work
- Family relationships
- Cultural background
- Medications currently being taken (over-the-counter [OTC] and prescription)
- Information the patient understands about past and present medical condition, medical therapy, and medications.

The nurse needs to also inquire about any drug misinformation and use of folk medicine, home remedies, or herbal treatments. Other questions may need to focus on the patient's beliefs about their illness, its treatment, past experiences with health care regimens, compliance history, and barriers to learning (language, finances, cultural beliefs, previous negative or limited experiences with the health care system/team, denial of illness or need for health care intervention). During the assessment of learning needs, the nurse needs to be astutely aware of verbal and nonverbal communications. Often a patient's feelings are much different than the spoken word. This may be a clue to the nurse that the patient's emotional state may need to be further assessed in relation to the patient's readiness for learning. With assessment of patients, use of open-ended questions is recommended, because these questions will encourage more clarification and discussion from the patient. The use of closed-ended questions that require only a "yes" or "no" answer provide limited information and insight about the patient.

BOX 5-1

Erickson's Stages of Development

Infant (birth to 1 year of age): Trust vs mistrust. Infant learns to trust himself, others, and the environment; learns to love and be loved.

Toddler (1 to 3 years of age): Autonomy vs shame and doubt. Toddler learns independence; learns to master the physical environment and maintain self-esteem.

Preschooler (3 to 6 years of age): Initiative vs guilt. Preschooler learns basic problem-solving; develops conscience and sexual identity; initiates activities as well as imitates.

School-age child (6 to 12 years of age): Industry vs inferiority. School-age child learns to do things well; develops a sense of self-worth.

Adolescent (12 to 18 years of age): Identity vs role confusion. Adolescent integrates many roles into self-identity through role models and peer pressure.

Young adult (18 to 45 years of age): Intimacy vs isolation. Young adult establishes deep and lasting relationships; learns to make commitment as spouse, parent, partner.

Middle-age adult (45 to 65 years of age): Generativity vs stagnation. Adult learns commitment to community and world; is productive in career, family, civic interests.

Older adult (over 65 years of age): Integrity vs despair. Older adult appreciates life role and status; deals with loss and prepares for death.

From McKenry LM, Salerno E: *Mosby's pharmacology in nursing*, ed 21, St Louis, 2001, Mosby.

NURSING DIAGNOSES APPROPRIATE TO DRUG THERAPY

Some of the most commonly used nursing diagnoses related to patient education and drug therapy include deficient knowledge, risk for injury, altered health, noncompliance, and maintenance, to name only a few. Deficient knowledge essentially refers to the state in which the patient (caregiver, significant other) has limited cognitive knowledge base or skills related to or about the medication. A nursing diagnosis of deficient knowledge evolves from data collected that proves that the patient has a lack of or limited understanding regarding the medication, its action, side effects, or cautions and related administration techniques. Deficient knowledge may also pertain to the lack of motor skills needed to self-administer the medication safely. Deficient knowledge differs from noncompliance in that the latter occurs when the patient does not take the medication as prescribed or at all—in other words, the patient does not adhere to the instructions given about the medication. A nursing diagnosis of noncompliance evolves from data collected from the patient that shows that a condition or symptoms of "reason for taking the medication" has re-occurred or was never resolved because of the patient not taking the medication per physician's orders or not taking the medication at all.

Patient Education

You must research various cultures to enhance your individualized approach to nursing care. For example, the Mexican-American patient and all other aspects of nursing care need to be approached during drug administration in a sensitive manner with strong consideration to the family, communication needs, and religion. Some 90% of native Mexicans are Roman Catholic. Therefore to help meet their needs more effectively, you must speak with them about having visits from the clergy, if they so desire while in the hospital. Family members are generally involved and they have large extended families, so you should take time to include them in the patient's care, discharge instructions, and medication instructions.

Other nursing diagnoses as listed by the North American Nursing Diagnosis Association (NANDA) (see Chapter 1) may also be used, when applicable, with patients as related to medication administration.

PLANNING RELATED TO LEARNING NEEDS AND DRUG THERAPY

The planning phase of the teaching/learning process occurs as soon as a learning need has been identified in a patient or caregiver. With mutual understanding, the nurse and patient identify goals and outcome criteria related to the specific medication the patient is taking as associated with the identified nursing diagnosis. An example of a measurable goal with outcome criteria related to a nursing diagnosis of knowledge deficit is as follows:

A patient who is undergoing self-administration of an oral antidiabetic agent has many questions about the medication.

- *Goal:* The patient safely self-administers the prescribed oral antidiabetic agent.
- *Outcome criteria:* The patient remains without signs and symptoms of over-medication with oral antidiabetic agents, such as hypoglycemia with tachycardia, palpitations, diaphoresis, hunger, and fatigue.

When writing and developing goals and outcome criteria related to drug therapy, appropriate time frames for outcome criteria should be identified (see Chapter 1 for more information on the nursing process and related phases). Measurable verbs should also be used and some examples of words that reflect measurable terms include *list, identify, demonstrate, self-administer, state, describe,* and *discuss.* Goals and outcome criteria should also be realistic and in patient terms as related to drug therapy and with time frames.

IMPLEMENTATION RELATED TO DRUG THERAPY

After the assessment phase has been thoroughly completed with identification of nursing diagnoses and a plan of care identified, the implementation phase of the

BOX 5-2 Selected Aging Changes and Educational Strategies Appropriate to Pharmacology Content

CHANGES ASSOCIATED WITH AGING THAT MAY INFLUENCE LEARNING

Altered thought processes
Slowed cognitive function
Decreased short-term memory
Decreased ability to think abstractly
Decreased ability to concentrate
Increased reaction time (slower to respond)

Altered sensory-perceptual status
Hearing
  Decreased ability to distinguish sounds (i.e., words beginning with S, Z, T, D, F, and G)
  Decreased conduction of sound
  Loss of ability to hear high frequency sounds
Vision
  Decreased visual acuity
  Decreased ability to read fine detail
  Decreased ability to discriminate between blue, violet, and green; all colors tend to fade, with red fading the least
  Lens become thicker and yellower with decreased accommodation
  Pupil smaller; decreased amount of light reaching retina
  Decreased depth perception
  Peripheral vision decreased
Touch and vibration
  Sense of touch decreased
  Decreased sense of vibration

NURSING INTERVENTIONS

Slow pace of presentation.
Provide smaller amounts of information at one time.
Repeat information frequently.
Use examples to illustrate information.
Decrease external stimuli as much as possible.
Allow more time for feedback from elderly learners.
Use a variety of methods—audiovisuals and practice sessions.
Provide written instructions for home use.
Speak distinctly.
Sit on side of learner's "best" ear.
Do not shout; speak in a normal voice, but lower its pitch.
Face the client so that lip reading is possible.
Use visual aids to reinforce verbal instruction.
Reinforce teaching with easy-to-read materials.
Decrease extraneous noise.
Ensure glasses are clean and in place.
Use printed material with large print.
Use high-contrast materials (i.e., black on white).
Avoid use of blue, violet, and green in type or graphics; use red instead.
Use nonglare lighting and avoid contrasts of light (i.e., darkened room with single light).
Adjust teaching to allow for the use of touch to gauge depth.
Increase time for the teaching of psychomotor skills, repetitions, and return demonstration.
Teach to palpate more prominent pulse sites (i.e., carotid and radial).

Adapted from Weinrich SP et al: Continuing education: adapting strategies to teach the elderly, *J Gerontol Nurs* 15(11):17, 1989; From McKenry LM, Salerno E: *Mosby's pharmacology in nursing*, ed 21, St Louis, 2001, Mosby.

teaching/learning process occurs and includes the specific information to be conveyed to the patient by the nurse about the medication. Teaching-learning sessions should be conducted with the sharing of information enhanced with any learning aids such as films, written instructions, oral instructions, pamphlets, or any other strategy that will help in the acquisition of learning per the patient's specific learning needs. It may be necessary to conduct several short learning sessions, but each patient should be approached individually with consideration of all factors as related to learning (Box 5-2). It may also be necessary for the nurse to identify aids to help in the safe administration of medications at home, such as the use of medication day and time calendars, pill reminder stickers, daily medication containers with alarms, and a method of documenting doses taken to avoid overdosage or omitting of doses.

Teaching of manual skills for specific medication administration is also part of the teaching/learning session. Sufficient time (each patient has different needs) should be allowed for the patient to become familiar with any equipment and also for several return demonstrations to the nurse. Any family members, significant others, or caregivers should also be included in teaching sessions

for reinforcement purposes. Audio-visual aids may also be used in the teaching of manual skills.

Resources for information about medications may also be shared with the patient, such as the *USP DI: Advice for the Patient* volume. This type of resource may be helpful to the patient when inquiring about a medication, its purpose, side effects, and method of administration.

The following are some definite pointers to help ensure the effectiveness of the teaching/learning session:
• Individualizing the teaching session
• Using positive rewards or reinforcement for accurate administration or compliance
• Completing a medication calendar with times of the day and medications to take
• Using audio-visual aids
• Involving family members or significant others
• Keeping learning on a level that is most meaningful to that patient.

Box 5-3 lists some general teaching and learning principles to remember.

Documentation of learning with specific information about what was taught (content), strategies used, patient's response, and evaluation of learning should occur after the teaching/learning process has been completed.

Throughout this textbook, Patient Teaching Tips boxes are specific to a particular class of medications or for a specific drug.

EVALUATION RELATED TO DRUG THERAPY

Evaluation of learning is crucial to safe patient drug administration. Nurses should always validate whether learning has occurred by asking questions related to the teaching session as well as requesting the patient to provide a return demonstration of skills. Most importantly, the patient's behavior is the key to whether learning has occurred and teaching is successful, such as compliance and adherence to a schedule for medication adminis-

tration with few or no complications of therapy. If a patient's behavior is evidence of noncompliance or decreased learning, a new plan of teaching should be developed and implemented.

In summary, patient education is a critical part of patient care, and medication administration is no exception. From the time of initial contact with the patient throughout the time the nurse works with the patient, the patient is entitled to all information about the medication as well as all aspects of their patient care. Evaluation of learning and compliance to the medication regimen should be a continual process, and the nurse should always be willing to listen to the patient about any aspects of their drug therapy.

BOX 5-3   **General Teaching and Learning Principles**

- Make learning patient-centered and individualized to each patient's needs, including his or her learning needs. This includes assessment of cultural beliefs, educational level, previous experience with medications, level of growth and development (to best match a teaching learning strategy), age, gender, family support systems, resources, ability to learn and how he or she learns best, and level of sophistication in regard to health care and the patient's own health care treatment.
- Assess the patient's ability to use and interpret label information on medication containers.
- Remember that a patient's ability to interpret drug instructions is more culturally based and somewhat consistent regardless of age, gender, or educational background.
- Some studies have shown that up to 20% of the population is functionally illiterate, and so the nurse should ensure that those educational strategies and materials are at a level that the patient is able to

understand and that this consideration is done subtly so as to not lead to embarrassment on the patient's behalf.
- If a patient is illiterate, he or she still needs to be instructed on safe medication administration. Pictures may be used to re-emphasize instructions.
- Language and ethnicity should be considered, assessed, and appreciated during education about medications.
- Assessment of the family support system is important for adequate patient teaching. Family living arrangements, financial status, resources, communication patterns, the roles of family members, and the power and authority of different family members should always be considered.
- Learning should be simple, easy, fun, thorough without being monotonous, applicable to daily life, and done at a time when the patient is "ready" to learn.
- Learning occurs better with repetition and often with periods of demonstration and use of audiovisuals and other educational aids.

---

patient teaching tips

Teaching and Learning as Related to Drug Therapy

➤ Teaching may need to focus on either the cognitive, affective, or psychomotor domain or a combination of all three.
➤ The cognitive domain refers to behaviors such as thought processes and problem-solving abilities and may involve recall to synthesis of facts.
➤ The affective domain refers to values and beliefs and may involve behaviors such as responding, valuing, and organizing.
➤ The psychomotor domain refers to gross motor movements, speech, and nonverbal communication

and may involve behaviors such as learning how to perform a procedure.
➤ A thorough assessment of the patient (and/or significant other(s), family, spouse, etc.) and their readiness to learn is crucial to effective patient education.
➤ Establish realistic patient teaching goals and involve the patient in these goals.
➤ Emphasize to patients the importance of knowing about their medications in preventing errors and in maximizing therapeutic benefits.

POINTS TO REMEMBER

- Patient teaching is a very important nursing function during the implementation phase of the nursing process.
- Patient teaching should occur after a thorough patient assessment of their readiness to learn and should include all aspects of the patient or a holistic approach.

- Patients need to receive information through as many senses as possible, such as verbally, visually (as with pamphlets, videos, diagrams) to maximize their learning.
- Always involve the patient and any significant others in the teaching process.

REVIEW QUESTIONS

1. Mr. SL is a 47-year-old diabetic being discharged on insulin injections bid. Which of the following statements is most accurate regarding proper storage and handling of insulin?
   a. "Make sure when you travel to have enough insulin with you to allow for any extended stays."
   b. "Make sure you put the medication vial on the kitchen counter at all times to remind you to take it."
   c. "You can store the insulin in a dark, warm closet or drawer and throw away the vial with each dosing."
   d. "You should keep the insulin vial in your medicine cabinet in the bathroom because it needs moisture and heat."

2. Other discharge instructions for this diabetic patient about expired insulin dates include which of the following?
   a. Always add 3 months to the expired date for safety reasons.
   b. Replace the vial in the refrigerator to prolong its effectiveness.
   c. Mix the insulin with dextrose to increase its absorbency and duration of action.
   d. Make arrangements to contact your health care provider for a new order of insulin if no extra vials are on hand.

3. You are responsible for the preoperative teaching for one of your patients who is mildly anxious about receiving narcotics postoperatively. As a nurse, you acknowledge that this patient's level of anxiety may:
   a. Impede learning because no anxiety is helpful.
   b. Lead to major unsteadiness of emotional status.
   c. Result in learning by increasing one's willingness to learn.
   d. Reorganize one's thoughts with inadequate potential for learning.

4. How do you as a professional nurse assess the patient's learning needs?
   a. Quiz the patient daily on all medications.
   b. Validate the patient's present level of knowledge.
   c. Assess the family's knowledge of the medication.
   d. Question other caregivers about their experience with drugs.

5. Which of the following techniques would be most appropriate for teaching patients who have a language barrier?
   a. Speak slowly.
   b. Use detailed and lengthy explanations.
   c. Always assume that if no questions are asked the patient understands.
   d. Use any type of jargon to help explain the specific type of medication regimen.

For Answers see www.harcourthealth.com/MERLIN/Lilley/.

CRITICAL THINKING Activities

1. Develop a teaching plan for the patient who is 65 years old and is to begin treatment for her diabetes mellitus with insulin injections. Your task is to develop a 10-minute teaching plan on the basics of self-administration of subcutaneous insulin.

2. Develop a teaching plan for a 69-year-old male patient who has experienced a left sided stroke (brain attack or cerebrovascular accident [CVA]), is aphasic, and is paralyzed on the right side. He is going to be returning home to have his wife care for him. Your discharge teaching will occur with him and his wife, and you are to teach them about safety measures for a patient with slight difficulty in swallowing who is going to be sent home on oral medications. He tolerates liquids and soft foods fairly well.

3. Your patient does not speak English or understand any of your communication techniques thus far. Develop a plan of care that addresses the patient's need for medication information on digitalis drugs, specifically their potential for toxicity.

For Answers see www.harcourthealth.com/MERLIN/Lilley/.

bibliography

Craven RF, Hirnle CJ: *Fundamentals of nursing: human health and functioning*, ed 3, Philadelphia, 2000, Lippincott.

Facts and comparisons, St Louis, September, 17, 1999.

Hansen M, Fisher JC: Patient-centered teaching from theory to practice, *AJN* 98(1):56, 1998.

Katz J: Back to basics: providing effective patient teaching, *AJN* 97(5):33, 1997.

Keegan L: Alternative and complementary therapies, *Nursing 98* 28(4):50, 1998.

Kelley M: Medications and the visually impaired elderly, *Geriatric Nursing* 17(2):60, 1996.

McKenry LM, Salerno E: *Mosby's pharmacology in nursing*, ed 21, St Louis, 2001, Mosby.

United States Pharmacopeia: *USP DI: advice for your patient*, Rockville, Md, 2001, The Author.

Remember to check the **Online Worksheet** for additional learning opportunities: **www.harcourthealth.com/MERLIN/Lilley/**

Chapter 6

Over-the-Counter Drugs and Herbal Remedies

objectives

www.harcourthealth.com/MERLIN/Lilley/

Look for this symbol for
topics covered in the
Online Worksheet
Activity

When you reach the end of this chapter, you should be able to do the following:

1 Discuss the differences between prescription, over-the-counter (OTC), and herbal medications.

2 Explain the differences in federal legislation that govern the promotion and sale of prescription versus OTC and herbal medications.

3 Describe the advantages and disadvantages of OTC and herbal medications.

4 Explain the proper use of OTC and herbal medications.

5 Discuss the potential dangers associated with OTC and herbal medications.

6 Develop a nursing care plan for the patient who is self-administering OTC or herbal medications.

herbal remedy profiles*

Aloe, p. 68	**Ginseng,** p. 69
Echinacea, p. 68	**Kava,** p. 70
Ephedra, p. 69	**St. John's Wort,** p. 70
Garlic, p. 69	**Saw Palmetto,** p. 70
Ginko, p. 69	**Valerian,** p. 70

*Over-the-counter (OTC) drugs are profiled in later chapters organized by drug category.

glossary

Alternative medicine Refers to herbal medicine, chiropractics, acupuncture, reflexology, or any other therapies not taught in a medical school but used for health care. (p. 66)

Commission E Monographs Comprehensive published herbal recommendations from the German equivalent of the Food and Drug Administration (FDA). (p. 66)

Conventional medicine The practice of medicine as taught in a western medical school. (p. 66)

Herbs Refers not only to herbaceous plants but also to bark; roots; leaves; seeds; flowers and fruit of trees, shrubs, and woody vines; and extracts of the same that are valued for their savory, aromatic, or medicinal qualities. (p. 66)

Herbal medicine The practice of using herbs to heal. (p. 66)

Iatrogenic effects Unintentional adverse effects that are physician- or health-care professional–induced or treatment-induced. (p. 66)

Legend drugs Drugs that require a prescription to purchase. (p. 66)

Phytochemicals The pharmacologically active ingredients in an herbal remedy. (p. 67)

OVER-THE-COUNTER REMEDIES

Health care consumers are becoming increasingly involved in the diagnosis and treatment of common ailments. This has led to a great increase in the use of nonprescription, or over-the-counter (OTC), drug products. OTC medications now account for about 60% of all medications used in the United States. Health care consumers use OTCs to treat or cure more than 400 different ailments. About 30% of new OTCs marketed between 1975 and 1994 were products that had been changed from prescription to OTC status.

Some history on the Food and Drug Administration (FDA) approval process is helpful in understanding current OTC classification. Table 6-1 lists the major events in the drug approval process. The purpose of the 1972 OTC Drug Review was to ensure appropriate safety, effectiveness, and labeling standards for the OTC products at that time. As a result of this review, approximately one third of the over 500 OTC products available at that time were determined to be safe and effective for their intended uses and one third were found to be ineffective. A small number were considered to be unsafe, and the remainder-required submission of additional data before safety and effectiveness could be established.

Another result of the OTC Drug Review was the reclassification from prescription to OTC status of more than 40 primary product ingredients. The FDA's Nonprescription Drugs Advisory Committee is responsible for reclassification of prescription drug products to OTC status. A drug must meet the three criteria listed in Table 6-2 to be considered for reclassification. This information is obtained from clinical trial results and postmarketing safety

Events in the FDA Approval Process

6-1

Food, Drug, and Cosmetic Act (1938)	Durham-Humphrey Amendments (1951)	Kefauver-Harris Amendments (1962)	OTC Drug Review (1972)
Required that drugs be cleared by the U.S. FDA before being marketed for human use	Established the distinction between prescription and OTC drugs	Established that drugs must not only prove safety but also effectiveness for their intended uses	FDA-initiated scientific review of OTC product ingredients in use at that time (>500)

Criteria for OTC Status

6-2

Indication for Use	Safety Profile	Practical for OTC Use
Consumer must be able to easily: • Diagnose condition • Monitor effectiveness	Drug should have: • Favorable adverse-event profile • Limited drug-interaction profile • Low potential for abuse	Drug should be: • Easy to use • Easy to monitor

Reclassified OTC Products

6-1

ANALGESICS
ibuprofen
ketoprofen
naproxen sodium

ANTIFUNGAL MEDICATIONS
butoconazole
clotrimazole
miconazole

HISTAMINE-BLOCKERS
cimetidine
clemastine fumarate
famotidine
nizatidine
ranitidine

MAST CELL STABILIZERS
cromolyn sodium

SMOKING DETERRENTS
nicotine polacrilex gum
nicotine transdermal systems

TOPICAL MEDICATIONS
minoxidil solution and hydrocortisone acetate 1% cream

Some professionals argue that allowing patients to self-treat minor illnesses enables physicians to spend more time caring for patients with more serious health problems. Others argue that it delays patients from seeking medical care until they are really sick. The financial influence of this status change is enormous; by the year 2010, OTC sales will reach an estimated $22 billion. Manufacturers often benefit as well by prolonging market exclusivity without generic competition.

Reclassification of a prescription drug to an OTC drug may increase out-of-pocket costs for many patients. This is due to refusal of third-party health insurance payers to pay for OTC products. However, overall health care costs tend to decrease when reclassification occurs due to a direct reduction in drug costs, elimination of physician office visits, and elimination of pharmacy dispensing fees. A case in point is the reclassification of cough and cold products to OTC status. This reclassification resulted in annual consumer health care savings of approximately $1 billion. Some recent examples of drugs that have been reclassified as OTC products are listed in Box 6-1.

The importance of patient counseling cannot be overstated. Many patients are inexperienced in the interpretation of medication labels, resulting in misuse of the product (Fig. 6-1). This often leads to adverse events or drug interactions with prescription medications or other OTC medications. Another common complaint of reclassification of prescription products to OTC is that their use may delay effective treatment of more serious medical disorders. This is because symptoms of a disorder are relieved by the OTC medication but the cause of the disorder has not been addressed.

Health care professionals have an excellent opportunity to prevent common problems associated with the use of reclassified drugs. Up to 60% of patients consult a health care professional when selecting an OTC product. Pa-

surveillance data, which is submitted to the FDA by the manufacturer of the product. Although this procedure has been criticized as overly time consuming, it is structured to ensure that products reclassified to OTC status are safe and effective when used by the average consumer.

Changing drugs from prescription to OTC status has many favorable advantages. Patients are allowed to conveniently and effectively self-treat many minor ailments.

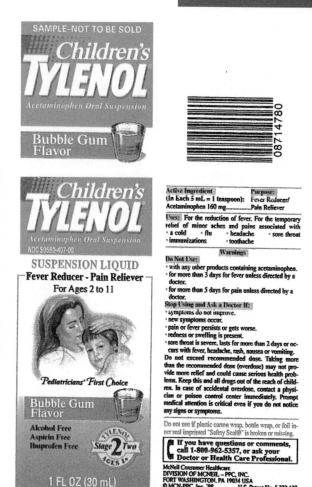

Fig. 6-1 Example of an OTC drug label.

tients should be provided with verbal information about choosing an appropriate product, correct dosing, common side effects, and drug interactions with other medications.

nursing process

● Assessment

Assessment criteria for patients taking OTC *nonsteroidal antiinflammatory drugs* (NSAIDs) should be screened carefully and warned about cautions and contraindications for use of these agents (and all other OTC agents). (For further discussion of NSAIDs, see Chapter 42). Cautious use is recommended in individuals who are elderly, pregnant, or lactating. Cautious use is also necessary with patients who have bleeding, gastrointestinal (GI), or cardiac disorders and with children. OTC NSAIDs are also contraindicated in individuals who are allergic to NSAIDs or aspirin, have asthma, or have severe renal or liver disease. Drug interactions with these agents include alcohol, aspirin and aspirin-containing products, acetaminophen, and other OTC medications unless the patient consults with a health care professional.

Other important assessment areas are a patient's knowledge about the medication, frequency of use, and whether NSAIDs are going to be used on a long-term basis because many patients have the misconception that OTC medication cannot be harmful, which is not true. Assessment of a patient's level of knowledge and circumstances of self-medication with NSAID use is therefore crucial to his or her safety and safe use of these agents because overdosage and overuse can lead to serious complications such as GI bleeding, bleeding disorders, hepatotoxicity, and nephrotoxicity. If patients are going to be taking NSAIDs for long periods of time or are categorized in any of the cautious situations mentioned previously, the health care provider should encourage them to seek the advice of a health care professional and have the following laboratory studies performed before initiation of therapy: blood urea nitrogen (BUN), creatinine, aspartate aminotransferase (AST, or serum glutamic-oxaloacetic transaminase [SGOT]), alanine transaminase (ALT, or serum glutamate pyruvate transaminase [SGPT]), and hemoglobin (Hgb).

Before the use of *histamine-blocking agents* for a variety of GI complaints (hyperacidity, indigestion, heartburn, gastroesophageal disease [GERD], ulcer disease), the health care provider should assess the patient for his or her level of knowledge about the specific agent and the patient should be aware of cautions and contraindications to their use. Drug interactions vary according to the specific agent but include agents such as theophylline, warfarin, sulfonylureas, anticholinergics, diazepam, metoclopramides, lidocaine, phenytoin, and ketoconazole. The histamine-blocking agents should be taken 1 hour before antacids. Cautions include patients who are confused, elderly, or disoriented. Histamine-blocking agents or H_2 receptor antagonists are contraindicated in patients with known hypersensitivity and in patients with impaired renal or hepatic function.

Antifungals are like many other OTC agents; they can be used safely, but complications may occur if they are overused or if directions are not followed. To try to prevent problems or complications, the patient should be aware of conditions, specific situations, and diseases that should be assessed for before taking the antifungal agent. Cautions to their use include renal or hepatic diseases, pregnancy, and hypersensitivity to penicillin. Antifungals are contraindicated in patients with severe bone marrow suppression or allergic reactions to antifungals. Many drug interactions occur, so the patient should be aware of them to prevent adverse reactions. Because miconazole interacts with alcohol, antacids, cyclosporine, anticholinergics, H_2 blockers, and antitubercular agents, a potential exists for many complications. Butoconazole, clotrimazole, and miconazole are indicated for vaginal fungal infections and should not be used by patients who are experiencing severe burning and severe discharge and pain of the vagina because they should seek medical help.

Before a patient begins a *nicotine smoking deterrent* system, he or she should be aware of cautions, contraindications, and drug interactions. Cautions include angina, cardiac disease, myocardial infarction (MI), renal or liver insufficiency, peptic ulcer disease, hypertension, cardiac dysrhythmias, diabetes, and advanced age. Nicotine smoking deterrents are contraindicated in patients who have an allergy to the product, are pregnant, are nonsmokers, have had life-threatening cardiac dysrhythmias, have had severe angina, and have had a recent MI. These nicotinic systems are also contraindicated in children. Some drug interactions include caffeine, theophylline, insulin, and adrenergic agonists; however, patients should always check the packaging label for other drug interactions.

Patients self-administering the topical dosage form of minoxidil should be aware of contraindications. Minoxidil is contraindicated in patients who have dermatologic inflammation or open sores, rash, irritated areas of the scalp, or an allergy to the product.

Cautious use of *topical steroid OTC* products is recommended with pregnant or lactating women because these groups have not been studied. These products are contraindicated in patients with herpetic lesions of the skin or varicella or with hypersensitivity to these products. The health care provider must assess reactions to any topical agent (OTC or prescribed) because patients may be allergic to certain preservatives found in the product. Infants should not be treated with these agents unless prescribed by their health care provider.

Cromolyn is contraindicated in individuals who are hypersensitive to the cromolyn or lactose or who suffer from status asthmaticus. Cautious use is recommended in patients who are pregnant, have renal or liver disease, and are age 5 years of age. Patients using OTC cromolyn should self-assess their respiratory status and keep a journal of the incidence and severity of their asthmatic attacks, respiratory rate, cough, wheezing, and shortness of breath. If the patient is not used to performing peak flows, then the health care provider should give instructions because monitoring of peak flow changes and implementation of other treatments may be beneficial to the patient's overall treatment. The health care provider should also assess the patient's understanding of the delayed onset of the true therapeutic effects (possibly 4 weeks) and its preventive nature. The health care provider should also assess the patient's level of education, knowledge base, and learning needs so that he or she can individualize teaching.

• Nursing Diagnoses

Nursing diagnoses relevant to the use of OTC drugs include the following:

NSAIDs:
- Chronic pain related to various disease processes or injury.
- Impaired physical mobility related to disease processes or injury.
- Deficient knowledge related to first-time drug therapy with OTC NSAIDs.

H_2 histamine-blocking agents:
- Acute pain related to GI hyperacidity and other GI complaints.
- Constipation or diarrhea related to side effects of the H_2 blockers.
- Risk for injury related to CNS side effects such as confusion and dizziness.
- Deficient knowledge related to lack of information about use of H_2-blocking agents and their potential side effects.

Antifungal medications:
- Acute pain related to symptoms of a fungal infection.
- Deficient knowledge related to the lack of information about the agents and their use.
- Risk for injury related to potential adverse effects of the antifungals.

Nicotine smoking deterrent medications:
- Risk for injury related to withdrawal effects from quitting smoking.
- Constipation and/or diarrhea related to the side effects of nicotine systems.
- Deficient knowledge related to lack of experience and information about the smoking deterrent systems.

Use of topical minoxidil for baldness:
- Disturbed body image related to perceived poor image from baldness.
- Deficient knowledge related to limited use with medication regimen of long-term nature.

Topical forms of hydrocortisone acetate:
- Deficient knowledge related to lack of information about the use, adverse effects, and cautions and contraindications of topical antiinflammatory agents.
  For cromolyn:
- Deficient knowledge related to lack of experience with preventive management of asthma and lack of information on proper inhalation technique.
- Risk of injury related to adverse reactions to the medication.

● Planning

Goals pertinent to patients taking OTC NSAIDs include the following:
- Patient is able to describe the use of the NSAID as related to the relief of pain or inflammation.
- Patient experiences pain relief or relief of the symptoms of the disease process or injury within the expected period of time.
- Patient uses nonpharmacologic measures to enhance the effect of OTC NSAIDs.
- Patient reports adverse effects to the appropriate health care professional.
- Patient safely self-administers the NSAID.

Topical steroid antiinflammatory agents such as hydrocortisone acetate:
- Patient states the rationale and adverse effects associated with hydrocortisone acetate.

H_2 histamine-blocking agents include the following:
- Patient's complaints of GI symptoms decrease while on H_2 blockers.
- Patient experiences minimal GI complaints, such as constipation or diarrhea, with self-administration of the H_2 blockers.
- Patient remains free from injury as related to the improper use of H_2 blockers and/or the experience of their side effects.
- Patient states the rationale for use, dosing, cautions, drug interactions, and side effects of H_2 blockers.

Antifungal medications:
- Patient experiences improvement of fungal infection because of proper medication dosing and use.
- Patient states action, use, side effects, drug interactions, and cautions related to the use of antifungal agents.
- Patient remains injury free while self-administering antifungals.

Nicotine smoking deterrent medications:
- Patient remains without withdrawal symptoms or experiences minimal withdrawal related to discontinuation of smoking.
- Patient experiences minimal side effects of the smoking deterrent system.
- Patient shares information about the use, proper dosing, side effects, symptoms, and other relevant information related to the smoking deterrent symptoms.

Use of topical minoxidil for baldness:
- Patient expresses improved body image.
- Patient discusses the need for long-term use of minoxidil for baldness.

Topical forms of hydrocortisone acetate:
- Patient discusses the proper use of, adverse effects of, and cautions and contraindications related to topical antiinflammatory agents.
- Patient states the purpose of the need for long-term treatment.

Cromolyn:
- Patient states the importance of using medication on a long-term basis.
- Patient understands the process of self-administration and the proper dosing and frequency of medication.

Outcome Criteria

Outcome criteria for patients taking OTC drugs include the following:

NSAIDs
- Patient will state the actions of NSAIDs that make it appropriate for use with pain and inflammatory disease processes and the decrease of pain and/or inflammation related to the therapy.
- Patient will identify factors that aggravate or alleviate the pain and/or inflammation and evidence of relief of the pain and/or inflammation such as decreased complaints of pain, increased mobility, sense of well-being, and ability to carry out activities of daily living (ADLs).
- Patient will describe the nonpharmacologic measures such as hot or cold packs, physical therapy, massage, relaxation therapy, biofeedback, imagery, and hypnosis that are appropriate for the pain and/or inflammation.
- Patient will state the importance of immediately reporting GI upset, epigastric pain, heartburn, nausea, vomiting, bleeding tendencies, or GI bleeding to a health care provider.
- Patient will state the importance of proper self-administration of NSAIDs, such as taking with meals, taking only the recommended dose, and adhering to frequency of dosing.
- Patient will experience relief in pain (GI pain such as heartburn, epigastric pain, burning pain, abdominal discomfort, and nausea) within the appropriate time frame (related to onset, peak, and duration of the specific agent) and that continued use over a period of time may be needed for maximal therapeutic effects.
- Patient experiences minimal side effects such as diarrhea, constipation, nausea, vomiting, abdominal pain, confusion, insomnia, and palpitations but will report severe forms of these side effects to his or her health care provider.

H_2 histamine-blocking agents:
- Patient reports to the health care provider adverse effects such as confusion, hallucinations, and dizziness that may indicate complications related to the histamine-blocking agent.
- Patient states the proper dosing regimen, such as bid dosing or other specifically recommended dosages/dosing on the packaging label as well as taking the medication for recommended length of time and in divided doses.

- Patient avoids driving and other hazardous activities until drowsiness or dizziness related to most of these agents has been stabilized to avoid injury.
- Patient avoids OTC preparations such as aspirin, NSAIDs, cough and cold preparations, and others listed on the label while taking OTC H$_2$ blockers.

For antifungal medications:

- Patient experiences a decrease in vaginal (or topical if fungal infections of the skin) discomfort, itching, discharge and swelling.
- Patient uses vaginal antifungal agent for 1, 3, or 7 days as per manufacturer guidelines, adheres to dosing/dosage, and inserts one full applicator or vaginal suppository high into vagina as noted.
- Patient adheres to instructions, washes hands before and after use, washes reusable applicators with warm soapy water, and abstains from sexual intercourse until no further symptoms of infections.
- Patient applies topical antifungal to affected area, covering all lesions while using gloved hands to prevent further spread of dermal infection as recommended by instructions.
- Patient reports to health care provider any symptoms that persist such as the following: continued itching, swelling, discharge, and discomfort (for vaginal infections) and burning, itching, blistering, swelling, and oozing at the site (for skin infections).

Nicotine smoking deterrent medications:

- Patient reports increased toleration to discontinuation of smoking with minimal withdrawal symptoms, such as headache, tremors, shakiness, irritability, nausea, tachycardia, insomnia, hypertension, and anxiety.
- Patient doses medication as instructed and chews gum (if route used) slowly for 30 minutes to enhance buccal absorption or applies to nonhairy, clean, dry area of upper outer arm with rotation of sites daily as indicated in dosage directions with use of appropriate dosage and frequency.
- Patient reports severe headache, abdominal pain, vomiting, erythema and burning at patch site, or severe diarrhea or constipation to health care provider.
- Patient acknowledges that the patch is as toxic as cigarettes and should only be used to deter smoking and stop smoking immediately after treatment has begun with the patch or other deterrent system dosing form.

Topical minoxidil:

- Patient experiences increased socialization, self-worth, and body image with minimal feelings of self-consciousness.
- Patient prepares for long-term treatment with minoxidil because hair loss will occur once topical drug is discontinued.

Topical forms of hydrocortisone acetate:

- Patient states how to apply medication only to affected areas, leave site uncovered, and wash hands before and after application.
- Patient continues treatment with topical agent even up to a few days after area has cleared and is careful not to use medication on any open, weeping, or infected skin lesions.

- Patient states that treatment is for up to 14 days and uses only as directed on packaging label to prevent adverse effects of atrophy or epidermal thinning.

Cromolyn:

- Patient explains the importance of daily use (or as indicated by health care provider) for long-term therapy to prevent asthmatic attacks.
- Patient demonstrates proper use of inhalation technique by using inhaler—exhales and then inhales deeply using the inhaler with head tipped back, holds breath as long as possible, and then exhales and repeats as instructed with mouth care (rising with mouthwash) after each treatment.
- Patient reports severe headache, dizziness, syncope, neuritis, severe throat irritation, wheezing, cough, and burning eyes to health care provider and withholds next dose until further instructions from health care provider.

Implementation

Most important in the safe self-administration of any OTC product is thorough and individualized patient education. For NSAIDs, it is important to inform the patient to take NSAIDs with food to decrease the incidence and occurrence of GI symptoms and to report blurred vision and tinnitus (ringing in the ears), which may indicate toxicity. (For further discussion of NSAIDs, see Chapter 42). Patients taking NSAIDs should also be instructed to report any change in urinary patterns and the occurrence of edema or blood in the urine, which indicates renal toxicity.

Another important emphasis in teaching is that antiinflammatory effects may take up to one month of drug administration versus the onset of action for just the analgesic effects (peak effects of about 2 hours with most of these agents). Patients should also be told not to crush, chew, or break apart caplets or capsules. Patients need to receive as much information as possible about OTC NSAIDs and their safe use, and they should understand that just because they are OTC does *not* automatically mean that they are completely safe and without toxicity. NSAIDs may be very toxic to many organs and, if taken improperly, may result in damage to the liver and kidneys or precipitate GI bleeding. However, instructions about their safe use, frequency of dosing and dosage, specifics about how to take the medication (e.g., with food), cautions, contraindications, side effects to report to a health care provider, and interactions with other OTC and prescription medications may help prevent complications and toxic effects.

With so many H$_2$ antagonist agents available OTC, it its critical to patient safety that patients receive adequate instructions about the use of the medication. For example, cimetidine and ranitidine should be given with meals, and if given with antacids the antacids should be given 1 hour before or after the drugs. Also, the patient should be cautioned about possible drug interactions such as with oral anticoagulants. Any OTC H$_2$-blocking agent should be taken cautiously with other OTC products with careful attention to the instructions and interactions on the label.

Antifungal vaginal agents should be administered as outlined on the label of the medication. Generally one full applicator is recommended every night high into the vagina for 3 to 7 days depending on the product. The medication should be kept at room temperature. Patients should follow instructions for insertion, including directions to wash hands before and after each application, apply medication with applicator only, and wash the applicator thoroughly with warm soap and water after insertion. The patient may also want to wear sanitary napkins to prevent soiling of undergarments. Sexual intercourse should be avoided until the medication treatment is completed because reinfection and further irritation may occur. If symptoms persist after treatment, the health care provider should be contacted.

Patients using the transdermal nicotine smoking deterrent system should be informed that they are to apply the patch to a nonhairy site on the upper part of the body or upper outer arm daily as instructed and to rotate sites to prevent skin irritation. Once the protective covering over the patch is removed, the patient needs to apply the patch immediately to prevent a decrease in the strength of the patch. All patches and gum should be kept out of the reach of children and pets. Patients must be aware that these systems (patches or gums) are just as toxic as cigarettes and should be used *only* to deter smoking. Patients should be encouraged to always check for potential drug interactions if taking any other OTC or prescribed medication.

Dosages for the transdermal systems range from 7 mg/day to 21 mg/day, other patches vary between 5 mg/day and 15 mg/day, and some are available in 11 mg/day to 22 mg/day dosages. The Nicoderm system recommends that if a patient weighs less than 100 pounds or smokes less than 10 cigarettes a day, he or she should begin with the 14 mg/day patches. Dosages and recommendations vary depending on the specific system used. The nicotine gum is 2 or 4 mg (1 piece of gum) as needed, and generally the initial requirement is 20 mg/day of the 2 mg strength or 80 mg/day of the 4 mg strength. The amount of gum that is needed is individually based and on a fixed schedule of every 1 to 2 hours. The gum should be chewed slowly until a tingling sensation is felt, and then the gum is placed between the gums or cheek without chewing until the tingling sensation disappears, which is usually about 1 minute. Regardless of the system used (patch or gum), patients should avoid overuse of the product and follow the instructions closely.

With minoxidil, as with any medication, patient education is critical to its safe and effective use, whether OTC or prescribed. However, the patient should follow specific instructions listed on the label. He or she should be aware that the minoxidil topical solution is only to be used on the scalp area and must be continued over a long-term time period because new hair growth will be lost. The action of enhancing hair growth will be reversed once the drug is discontinued. Topical dosing is generally 1 ml regardless of the degree of balding, and it is important to inform the patient that hair growth does not increase if he or she increases the dose more than what is recommended. The patient should also report itching,

rash, or abnormal skin reactions to his or her health care provider and not continue with further dosing if the irritation or inflammation continues.

With hydrocortisone acetate, the patient must use the medication exactly as instructed on the label. Most common adverse effects of steroid-type antiinflammatory medications used topically include overgrowth of organisms, delayed healing, and contact dermatitis. Often instructions on these OTC products suggest limiting the drug's use to 4 days to help prevent these problems. In addition, if strong antiinflammatory topical agents are being used, a rebound in the skin disorder is possible. Although this may occur more commonly with more potent prescription agents, the less potent OTC steroid topicals may be used as the patient is being weaned from the stronger to the weaker product (OTC most likely) to no steroid topical at all. Education for patients using these products should emphasize following instructions, avoiding overuse, and reporting unusual reactions, allergic reactions, or lack of resolution of the disorder to their health care provider immediately.

Patients taking cromolyn should be educated about how it is used as a preventive agent only and that it takes up to 4 weeks for the therapeutic effect. This drug is not for acute attacks and must be taken daily according to packaging directions and year round for it to be effective in preventing asthma. Patients should also be informed about the possibility of adverse reactions, such as burning eyes, irritated or sore throat, wheezing, nausea, vomiting, nasal congestion, and changes in taste, and they should report them to the health care provider. After each dose of the cromolyn nebulizer or inhaler, patients must perform oral hygiene. Patient education should also emphasize the need to take this medication exactly as ordered and year round to prevent asthma attacks.

Patient teaching tips for OTC drugs and herbal remedies are presented on p. 72.

● Evaluation

Patients taking OTC medications should carefully monitor themselves for unusual or adverse reactions and therapeutic responses to the medication to prevent overuse. With NSAIDs, patients should be informed about the therapeutic responses for which to monitor, including decreased pain, decreased stiffness and swelling in joints, increased ability to carry out ADLs, and ability to move around with more ease. Patients should be educated about effects that warrant discontinuation of the drug, including nephrotoxicity (dysuria, hematuria, oliguria), blood disorders, and liver dysfunction, including cholestatic hepatitis. Patients should be aware of the therapeutic responses to the H_2 antagonists, which include a decrease in GI symptoms related to either ulcer disease, hyperacidity, gastroesophageal reflux disease (GERD), epigastric pain, and abdominal pain. Side effects for which to monitor include nausea, abdominal pain, constipation, diarrhea, headache, confusion, palpitations, impotence, gynecomastia, and hepatotoxicity.

Therapeutic responses to the antifungal medication include a decrease in vaginal itching, discharge, swelling, and discomfort. Adverse reactions for which to monitor include vaginal itching and burning and abdominal or pelvic cramps. Therapeutic responses to nicotine smoking deterrents include a decrease in the urge to smoke and absence of nicotine withdrawal symptoms. Adverse effects include headache, nausea, vomiting, tachycardia, palpitations, and irritability. Therapeutic responses to cromolyn include a decrease in asthmatic symptoms, such as improved lung sounds and less wheezing. The health care provider must monitor for adverse effects during therapy, including bronchospasms, irritated throat, cough, nasal congestion, and burning of the eyes.

HERBAL REMEDIES

History

Herbs have been an integral part of society since the beginning of human civilization. Use of plants for healing purposes dates back to the Neanderthal period. Herbs are valued for their culinary and medicinal properties. **Herbal medicine** has made many contributions to commercial drug preparations that are currently manufactured (Box 6-2). About 30% of all modern drugs are derived from plants. In the early nineteenth century, scientific methods became more advanced and preferred and the practice of botanical healing was dismissed as quackery. Herbal medicine lost ground to new synthetic medicines as the development of patent medicines took off in the early part of the twentieth century. These new synthetically derived medicines were touted by scientists and physicians to be more effective and reliable.

In the 1960s, concerns were expressed over the **iatrogenic effects** of **conventional medicine**. Along with a desire for more self-reliance, this lead to a renewed interest in "natural health" and the use of herbal products increased. In 1974 the World Health Organization (WHO) encouraged developing countries to use traditional plant medicine to "fulfill a need unmet by modern systems." In 1978 the German equivalent of the FDA published a series of herb recommendations known as the **Commission E Monographs**. These monographs focus on herbs, which are supported by literature to be effective for specific indications. Worldwide herbal use again became popular. Recognition of the rising use of herbal medicines and other nontraditional remedies, called **alternative medicine**, led to the establishment of the Office of Alternative Medicine by the National Institutes of Health in 1992. This office would later come to be called The National Center for Complementary and Alternative Medicine (NCCAM). NCCAM is classified into seven categories:

1. Alternative systems of medical practice (e.g., traditional Chinese medicine)
2. Bioelectromagnetic applications
3. Diet, nutrition, and lifestyle changes
4. Herbal medicine
5. Manual healing
6. Mind-body control
7. Pharmacologic and biologic treatments

BOX 6-2 Conventional Medicines Derived From Plants

Medicine	Plant
atropine	*Atropa belladonna*
capsaicin	*Capsicum frutescens*
cocaine	*Erythroxyion coca*
codeine	*Papaver somniferum*
ephedrine	*Ephedra sinica*
ipecac	*Cephaelis ipecacuanha*
quinine	*Cinchona officinalis*
reserpine	*Rauvolfia serpentina*
scopolamine	*Datura fastuosa*
senna	*Cassia acutifolia*
taxol	*Taxus brevifolia*
vincristine	*Catharanthus roseus*

In 1993 the FDA Commissioner David Kessler threatened to remove herbal products from the market. The American public responded with a massive effort, writing more letters to Congress than during the entire war in Vietnam. In October 1994 the 103rd Congress passed the Dietary Supplement and Health Education Act (DSHEA). One of the responsibilities of DSHEA is to define dietary supplements and provide the regulatory framework for their sale. A major difference between **legend drugs** and herbal medicines is that DSHEA requires no proof of efficacy or safety and sets no standards for quality control for products labeled as supplements. The FDA has specific and stringent requirements for manufacturers of legend drugs. Manufacturers of supplements must claim effect but do not have to promise a specific cure on the label. The burden lies with the FDA to prove a product unsafe rather than a company proving that its product is safe. The FDA posts recent warnings on herbal products on their Internet page (www.fda.gov). In contrast, regulating agencies in Germany, France, the United Kingdom, and Canada enforce standards of herb quality and safety assessment on manufacturers.

Consumer Use of Herbs

In general, consumers use herbal products as therapeutic agents for treatment and cure of diseases and pathologic conditions, as prophylactic agents for long-term prevention of disease, and as proactive agents to maintain health and wellness. Additionally, herbs and *phytomedicinals* can be used as adjunct therapy to support conventional pharmaceutical therapies. This last use is usually found in societies in which *phytotherapy*, the use of herbal medicines in clinical practice, is considerably more integrated with conventional medicine, as in Germany. Box 6-3 lists helpful Internet sites that provide information on herbal remedies.

Many herbal products are used to treat minor conditions and illnesses (coughs, colds, stomach upset) in much the same manner as conventional FDA-approved OTC nonprescription drugs are used. In addition a growing number of health consumers use herbs and other di-

Resources for Information on Herbal Remedies

box 6-3

ALTERNATIVE MEDICINE FOUNDATION

www.amfoundation.org
5411 W. Cedar Lane, Suite 205-A
Bethesda, MD 20814
Tel: 301-581-0116 or 888-258-4420
Fax: 301-581-0119
E-mail: amfi@amfoundation.org

AMERICAN BOTANICAL COUNCIL/DIRECTORY

www.herbalgram.org
P.O. Box 1443454
Austin, TX 78714-4345
Tel: 512-926-4900
Fax: 512-926-2344

AMERICAN HERBAL PHARMACOPOEIA

www.herbal-ahp.org
Box 5159
Santa Cruz, CA 95063
Tel: 831-461-6317
Fax: 831-475-6219
E-mail: herbal@got.net

HERBMED

www.amfoundation.org/herbmed.htm
A database listing evidence-based information on the scientific data underlying the use of herbs for health. Each herb monograph includes information on evidence for activity, warnings, preparations, mixtures, and mechanisms of action.

NATIONAL CENTER FOR COMPLEMENTARY AND ALTERNATIVE MEDICINE (NCCAM)

nccam.nih.gov
NCCAM Clearinghouse
P.O. Box 8218
Silver Spring, MD 20907-8218
Tel: 888-644-6226
Fax: 301-495-4957

cultural implications

Drug Responses and Cultural Factors

Drug responses may be affected by beliefs, values, and genetic factors associated with specific cultures. An example of cultural beliefs affecting drug response or administration is that in Japan, nausea, vomiting, and bowel changes as side effects to medications often go unreported. Because this culture finds it unacceptable to complain about GI-related symptoms, adverse reactions or toxicity may go unreported.

Use of herbal and homeopathic drugs may also be widely used in some cultures. A problem with this type of an approach to health care is that many herbals may interact significantly with prescribed medications. For example, the Chinese herb ginseng may inhibit or even accelerate the metabolism of a specific medication and significantly affect the drug's absorption or elimination.

Genetic factors associated with specific cultures that have an influence on drug response include concepts such as *acetylation polymorphism,* which means that drug metabolism is genetically determined or race may also affect drug metabolism. For example, patients of European or African descent have been shown to have equal ratios of rapid or slow acetylators (affecting drug metabolism), and those of Japanese or Inuit populations may have more rapid acetylators.

Another cultural variation with metabolism and subsequent drug response is found in how specific cultures respond to different drug classes. For example, patients of Chinese or Japanese descent are more likely to respond to codeine more favorably than those of European descent.

From Kudzma EC: Culturally competent drug administration, *AJN* 99(8):47, 1999.

herbal remedies compared with synthetic drug treatments. For some herbal remedies the risk may be less than that for conventional drugs. The discriminate and proper use of some herbal products is safe and may provide some therapeutic benefits, but the indiscriminate or excessive use of herbs can be unsafe and even dangerous. The FDA has implemented MEDWATCH, a toll-free number to which adverse effects of herbs can be reported (800-332-1088).

Epidemiology

Over 20,000 herbal remedies are currently used in the United States. These many different herbs have a wide variety of active **phytochemicals**. Some of the more common are listed in Box 6-4. A great deal of public interest exists in the use of herbal remedies. Estimates of the prevalence of herbal medicine use differ, with studies concluding that between 3% and 93% of the U.S. population uses herbs. The variability of these estimates is due to discrepant definitions of herbs and different inclusion of the length of use (i.e., ever vs. in the last 12 months). Internationally, the use of botanical medicines is generally

etary supplements as preventive measures to increase the body's general wellness and strengthen the immune system (e.g., reduction of cardiovascular risk factors, increase in liver and immune system functions, increase in feelings of wellness).

Safety

Herbal medicines are often perceived as being natural and therefore harmless; however, this is not the case. Many examples exist of allergic reactions, toxic reactions, and adverse effects related to herbs. Herbs have been shown to have possible mutagenic effects, drug interactions, and drug contamination. Cases also exist in which whole plants or parts of plants have not been identified properly and thus mislabeled. Because of underreporting, our present knowledge may well be just the "tip of the iceberg." Little is known about the relative safety of

BOX 6-4 — Common Phytochemicals in Herbal Remedies

Cartenoids
Coumarins
Curcumins
Flavonoids
Lignans
Phthalides
Plant sterols
Polyphenolics
Saponins
Sulfides
Terpenoids

BOX 6-5 — Common Ailments Treated with Herbal Remedies

Anxiety
Arthritis
Colds
Constipation
Coughs
Fever
Headache
Infection
Insomnia
Intestinal disorders
Premenstrual syndrome (PMS)
Stress
Ulcers
Weakness

higher than in the United States. According to one study performed in 1997, 60 million Americans stated that they had used herbs in the previous year. This use accounted for $3.24 billion in sales.

Herbal medicine is based on the premise that plants contain natural substances that can promote health and alleviate illness. Some of the more common ailments and conditions treated with herbs are listed in Box 6-5.

Herbal products constitute the largest growth area in retail pharmacy. They are growing at a rate of 20% to 25% a year, far exceeding growth in the conventional drug category. Insurance plans and managed care orga-nization (MCOs) are beginning to offer reimbursement for alternative treatments. One MCO made the decision to cover herbal remedies based on a survey that showed that 33% of its 1.5 million members had sought alterna-tive treatment in the previous 2 years. Ten of the more commonly used herbal remedies are aloe, Echinacea, ephedra, garlic, ginko, ginseng, kava, St. John's Wort, Saw Palmetto, and valerian. These agents are covered in detail in the following tables.

Common Name: Aloe	Scientific Name: Aloe vera L.

Overview: The dried leaves of the aloe plant contain anthranoids, which give aloe a laxative effect when taken orally. The topical application of the plant has been known for years to help aid in wound healing.

Therapeutic Use(s)	Dosage	Adverse Effects
Wound healing, constipation	20-30 mg hydroxyanthracene derivatives/day, calculated as anhydrous aloin	Diarrhea, nephritis, abdominal pain, dermatitis when used topically

Drug Interactions: Digoxin, antidysrhythmics, diuretics, steroids

Common Name: Echinacea	Scientific Name: Echinacea

Overview: The three kinds of Echinacea are *E. angustifolia*, *E. pallida*, and *E. purpurea*. They are most commonly used to treat colds and chronic infections of the respiratory and lower urinary tract.

Therapeutic Use(s)	Dosage	Adverse Effects
Antiseptic, antiviral, influenza-like infections, poorly healing wounds and chronic ulcerations	900 mg/day	Dermatitis, hepatotoxicity

Drug Interactions: Anabolic steroids, amiodarone, methotrexate, ketoconazole; tachyphylaxis likely to develop if used for more than 8 weeks

Common Name: Ephedra

Scientific Name: Ephedra vulgaris

Overview: Ephedra, ephedrae herba, and ma huang contain alkaloids such as ephedrine and pseudoephedrine. Ephedra (ma huang) is commonly found in herbal weight-loss products referred to as "herbal fen-fen." Promoted as an alternative to the use of fenfluramine (Pondimin) and dexfenfluramine (Redux), the prescription anorexiants that were recently removed from the U.S. market.

Therapeutic Use(s)	Dosage	Adverse Effects
Weight loss, decongestant, bronchodilator, stimulant	300 mg/day	Hypertension, insomnia, dysrhythmia, nervousness, nausea, vomiting, tremor, headache, seizure, cerebrovascular events, myocardial infarction, kidney stones

Drug Interactions: Digoxin, monoamine oxidase inhibitors (MAOIs), caffeine, decongestants, stimulants

Common Name: Garlic

Scientific Name: Allium sativum

Overview: Garlic obtains its pharmacologic effects from the active ingredient allinin.

Therapeutic Use(s)	Dosage	Adverse Effects
Antispasmodic, antiseptic, antibacterial and antiviral, antihypertensive, antiplatelet, lipid-lowering activity	4 g/day	Dermatitis, vomiting, diarrhea, anorexia, flatulence, antiplatelet activity

Drug Interactions: May inhibit iodine uptake, warfarin

Common Name: Ginko

Scientific Name: Ginkgo biloba

Overview: The dried leaf of the plant contains flavonoids, terpenoids, and organic acids, which help Ginko preparations exert their positive effects as an antioxidant and inhibitor of platelet aggregation.

Therapeutic Use(s)	Dosage	Adverse Effects
• Organic brain syndrome • Peripheral arterial occlusive disease • Vertigo and tinnitus	• 120-240 mg in 2 or 3 doses • 120-160 mg in 2 or 3 doses • 120-160 mg in 2 or 3 doses	Stomach or intestinal upset, headache, bleeding, allergic skin reaction

Drug Interactions: Aspirin, NSAIDs, warfarin, heparin, anticonvulsants, ticlopidine, clopidegrel, dipyridamole, tricyclic antidepressants

Common Name: Ginseng

Scientific Name: Panax ginseng

Overview: Ginsenosides are the active component in *Panax ginseng*. The roots of this plant are used as a tonic for invigoration, fortification, and concentration. It is believed to inhibit platelet aggregation by potently inhibiting thromboxane A_2 production.

Therapeutic Use(s)	Dosage	Adverse Effects
Stimulant, analgesic, hemostasis, angina, coronary artery disease	1-2 g/day	Hypertension, diarrhea, nervousness, depression, headache, amenorrhea, insomnia, skin rashes

Drug Interactions: Warfarin, heparin, aspirin, NSAIDs

Activity

Common Name: Kava	Scientific Name: *Piper methysticum Forst.f*

Overview: Kava kava rhizome consists of the dried rhizomes of *Piper methysticum G*. The drug contains kava-pyrones (kawain). Extended continuous intake can cause a temporary yellow discoloration of skin, hair, and nails.

Therapeutic Use(s)	Dosage	Adverse Effects
Anxiety, stress, restlessness	60-120 mg/day	Skin discoloration, possible accommodative disturbances such as enlargement of the pupils

Drug Interactions: Alcohol, barbiturates, psychoactive agents

Common Name: St. John's Wort	Scientific Name: *Hypericum perforatum L.*

Overview: St. John's Wort consists of the dried, above-ground parts of *Hypericum perforatum L.* gathered during flowering season, as well as their preparations in effective dosage. St. John's Wort is sometimes referred to as the "herbal Prozac."

Therapeutic Use(s)	Dosage	Adverse Effects
Depression, anxiety, sleep disorders, nervousness	2-4 g/day	GI upset, allergic reactions, fatigue, dizziness, confusion, dry mouth, possible photosensitization (especially in fair-skinned individuals)

Drug Interactions: MAOIs, selective serotonin reuptake inhibitors (SSRIs), sympathomimetic amines, piroxicam, tetracycline, tyramine-containing foods

Activity

Common Name: Saw Palmetto	Scientific Name: *Serenoa serrulata and repens*

Overview: Saw Palmetto is used as a diuretic, as a urinary antiseptic, and for its anabolic properties. The most common use for Saw Palmetto is for benign prostatic hypertrophy. It is believed to inhibit dihydrotestosterone and 5-alpha-reductase.

Therapeutic Use(s)	Dosage	Adverse Effects
Diuretic, urinary antiseptic, benign prostatic hypertrophy	1-2 g/day	GI upset

Drug Interactions: Estrogen replacement therapy, oral contraceptives

Activity

Common Name: Valerian	Scientific Name: *Valeriana officinalis*

Overview: Valerian root, consisting of fresh underground plant parts, contains essential oil with monoterpenes and sesquiterpenes (valerenic acids). This preparation is used to treat restlessness and sleeping disorders.

Therapeutic Use(s)	Dosage	Adverse Effects
Restlessness, sleeping disorders	2-3 g/day	CNS depression

Drug Interactions: Barbiturates

nursing process

● Assessment

Aloe may precipitate a dermatitis when used topically, and nephritis has been reported with its systemic use. Therefore patients with kidney dysfunction should be careful with this agent and seek medical advice before using it. Aloe also has many drug interactions, including digoxin, antidysrhythmics, diuretics, and steroids; therefore the patient should not take aloe if he or she is on any of these medications.

Echinacea may result in liver toxicity and should be used cautiously or not at all in patients with liver dysfunction. Drug interactions include anabolic steroids, and tachyphylaxis may develop in patients who use Echinacea for more than 8 weeks.

Many areas of concern exist in assessing patients who are taking Ephedra. Some adverse effects, such as cardiac stimulation and CNS stimulation, pose a caution to its use for patients with seizure disorders, myocardial infarction, hypertension, dysrhythmias, history of cerebrovascular accident (CVA), and any other type of cardiovascular disease. Patients with a history of any of these types of health problems should be cautious and even possibly not take Ephedra because of potential complications. Drug interactions for which to assess in patients taking Ephedra include digoxin, MAO inhibitors, OTC and prescriptive cold and cough preparations (decongestants), caffeine, and any other CNS or cardiac stimulant.

Garlic use is associated with antiplatelet activity, so it should be used cautiously in patients with bleeding disorders or platelet dysfunction. Garlic also interacts with warfarin.

Before using Ginko, the patient should be assessed for any GI disorders and bleeding tendencies because these are adverse effects of the drug and may worsen these conditions. Drugs that interact with Ginko include aspirin, NSAIDs, anticoagulants, anticonvulsants, and tricyclic antidepressants, so these should not be taken with Ginko.

Ginseng is not without cautions and drug interactions. Because this herbal product can cause hypertension, it is not recommended for patients with cardiovascular diseases and hypertension. Drug interactions with ginseng include anticoagulants, aspirin, and NSAIDs.

Patients taking Kava should be assessed for possible drug interactions such as alcohol, barbiturates, and psychoactive drugs.

St. John's Wort is often used for depression and for patients who desire effects similar to those of fluoxetine (Prozac); however, it may result in allergic reactions and even seizures have been reported. Patients with any type of allergic response to the drug should not take the drug again, and those with a history of convulsive disorders should not take it either. Many drug interactions exist that patients should be aware of, including MAO inhibitors, SSRIs, sympathomimetics, tetracyclines, and tyramine-containing foods such as beer, nuts, avocados, cheeses, and wines.

Saw Palmetto carries drug interactions with estrogen hormonal replacements and oral contraceptives.

Valerian may lead to CNS depression; therefore it should not be taken with other agents that are CNS depressing, such as narcotics, antidepressants, and sedative hypnotics. The major drug interaction is with barbiturates.

● Nursing Diagnoses

Nursing diagnoses pertinent to patients who self-administer herbal products are as follows:
- Deficient knowledge related to lack of information about self-medication
- Risk for injury related to potential drug interactions and adverse reactions of herbal products

● Planning

Goals related to the use of herbal products include the following:
- Patient states rationale for uses and potential problems related to the various herbal agents.
- Patient remains free of injury related to occurrence of adverse effects.

Outcome Criteria

Outcome criteria related to the use of herbal products include the following:
- Patient will experience relief of symptoms (indication for use of herbal product) without the various side effects and complications.
- Patient will take herbal products as indicated, and no more than what is directed, stops medication once adverse or untoward effects occur, and contacts a health care provider if any unusual reactions or side effects occur.

● Implementation

For herbal products, as with other OTC medications, patient education is of utmost importance for safe and effective use. The health care provider must inform the patient that the Dietary Supplement Health and Education Act of 1994 does not require the manufacturers of herbal remedies to provide evidence of safety and effectiveness. Unfortunately, many patients believe that no risks exist if a medication is herbal and "natural." As health care providers, we need to ensure that patients realize that even if it is a "natural" product, herbal products still need to be taken as cautiously as any other medication. The health care provider must also emphasize that herbals are not FDA-approved drugs, so even their labeling cannot be relied upon to provide adequate instructions for use or even information about warnings. Just because an agent is an herbal or a "dietary supplement" does not mean it can be safely administered to children, infants, pregnant or lactating women, or patients with other conditions that may result in harm.

Patient teaching tips for OTC drugs and herbal remedies are presented on p. 72.

● Evaluation

Patients taking herbal products should monitor themselves for improvement in symptoms for which they first initiated treatment with an herbal product and for presence of adverse reactions or side effects.

patient teaching tips

Over-the-Counter Drugs and Herbal Remedies

➤ Patients should be provided with verbal and written information about choosing an appropriate OTC and herbal product, correct dosing, common side effects, and drug interactions with other medications.

➤ The health care provider must inform the patient that the Dietary Supplement Health and Education Act of 1994 does not require the manufacturers of herbal remedies to provide evidence of safety and effectiveness.

➤ Many patients believe that no risks exist if a medication is herbal and "natural" or if it is sold OTC. Therefore education about the pros and cons of these agents is crucial to patient safety.

➤ Patients should be instructed on how to read the OTC and herbal labels. They should ask questions of their pharmacist or health care provider about the specific agents that they are beginning to take.

➤ Patients should take all herbal and OTC medications with caution and contact their health care provider if adverse effects occur.

➤ Patients taking herbal or OTC products should monitor themselves for improvement in symptoms or adverse effects for which they first initiated treatment.

➤ Elderly patients and children should be cautious taking OTC NSAIDs because of the risk of toxicity and adverse reactions in these age groups.

➤ Directions on all OTC products should be read carefully with particular attention to drug interactions, cautions and contraindications, and specific instructions for self-administration.

➤ H_2-blocking agents have many drug interactions that should be emphasized with patients, including theopylline, warfarin, sulfonylureas, anticholinergics, diazepam, metoclopramide, lidocaine, phenytoin, and ketoconazole.

➤ If the patient is also taking antacids, histamine-blocking agents should be taken 1 hour before antacids are taken.

➤ The transdermal nicotine smoking deterrent system may be applied to any nonhairy site on the upper part of the body or upper outer arm daily. Rotation of sites is encouraged to prevent skin irritation.

➤ All OTC products should be kept out of the reach of children and pets.

POINTS TO REMEMBER

• In general, consumers use herbal products as therapeutic agents for treatment and cure of diseases and pathologic conditions, as prophylactic agents for long-term prevention of disease, and as proactive agents to maintain health and wellness.

• About 30% of new OTCs marketed between 1975 and 1994 were products that had been changed from prescription to OTC status.

• The FDA has implemented MEDWATCH, a toll-free number to which adverse effects of herbs can be reported (800-332-1088).

• The term *phytotherapy* refers to the use of herbal medicines in clinical practice.

• Ten of the more commonly used herbal remedies are aloe, Echinacea, ephedra, garlic, ginko, ginseng, kava, St. John's Wort, Saw Palmetto, and valerian.

• Herbal products are not FDA-approved drugs, so the labeling cannot be relied upon to provide adequate instructions for use or even information about warnings.

• Just because an agent is an herbal product, "dietary supplement," or OTC medication does not mean that it can be safely administered to children, infants, pregnant or lactating women, or patients with other conditions that may result in harm.

REVIEW QUESTIONS

1. The most commonly used OTC products currently available include which of the following drugs?
   a. Mild antihypertensives
   b. Topical antiinfective agents
   c. Acetaminophen (Tylenol) with codeine
   d. Ibuprofen (Advil) mixed with low doses of codeine

2. For the safe use of herbal products, it is important to educate your patient that:

   a. Herbal and OTC products are both approved by the FDA.
   b. These products are safely scrutinized and tested repeatedly by the FDA.
   c. No side effects are associated with these agents because they are natural.
   d. Labeling is not reliable for the provision of proper instructions or any warnings.

3. OTC antifungals are used for which of the following?
   a. Anemia
   b. Hypertension
   c. Hypokalemia
   d. Vaginal fungal infection
4. Contraindications associated with the various OTC histamine-blocking agents include which of the following?
   a. GERD
   b. GI upset
   c. Heartburn
   d. Impaired renal failure

5. Which of the following characteristics is associated with current legislation about herbal products?
   a. Herbals were regulated in the early 1900s in reference to their efficacy and toxicity.
   b. The Dietary Supplement Health and Education Act permits the sale of herbal remedies as dietary supplements.
   c. The Kefauver-Harris Amendment was passed to help with prevention of carcinogenic effects related to herbal products.
   d. The Durham-Humphrey Amendment was specifically designed to control the safety and efficacy of OTC and herbal agents.

For Answers see www.harcourthealth.com/MERLIN/Lilley/.

CRITICAL THINKING Activities

1. Indicate whether this statement is true or false, and explain your answer: OTC agents and herbal products may be safely taken in the recommended amounts without concern of adverse effects.

2. From which law have current laws regulating OTC medications evolved?
3. Discuss some important points to include when teaching patients about analgesia and pain control for "at-home" management with OTC products.

For Answers see www.harcourthealth.com/MERLIN/Lilley/.

bibliography

Borins MB: The dangers of using herbs: what your patients need to know, *Postgrad Med* 104(1):91, 1998.

Craig WJ: Health-promoting properties of common herbs, *Am J Clin Nutr* 70(3 suppl):491S, 1999.

Cupp MJ: Herbal remedies: adverse effects and drug interactions, *Am Fam Physician* 59:1239, 1999.

Ernst E: Harmless herbs? A review of the recent literature, *Am J Med* 104:170, 1998.

Jacobs LR: Prescription to over-the-counter drug reclassification, *Am Fam Physician* 57(9):2209, 1998.

Johnson JE: Insomnia, alcohol, and over-the-counter drug use in old-old urban women, *J Community Health Nurs* 14(3):181, 1997.

Kurtzweil PA: FDA guide to dietary supplements. *FDA Consumer* Sept-Oct:1, 1998. Available at www.fda/gov/fdac/features/1998/598_guid/html.

Mashour NH, Lin GI, Frishman WH: Herbal medicine for the treatment of cardiovascular disease, *Arch Intern Med* 158:2225, 1998.

Miller LG: Herbal medicinals: selected clinical considerations focusing on known or potential drug-herb interaction, *Arch Intern Med* 158:2200, 1998.

Mosby GenRx: A comprehensive reference for generic and brand drugs, ed 10, St Louis, 2000, Mosby.

Skidmore-Roth L: *Mosby's 2001 nursing drug reference*, St Louis, 2001, Mosby.

United States Pharmacopeia: Available at www.usp.org.

Winslow LC, Kroll DJ: Herbs as medicines, *Arch Intern Med* 158:2192, 1998.

Activity

Remember to check the **Online Worksheet** for additional learning opportunities: **www.harcourthealth.com/MERLIN/Lilley/**

Chapter 7

Substance Abuse

objectives

When you reach the end of this chapter, you should be able to do the following:

www.harcourthealth.com/MERLIN/Lilley/

Look for this symbol for topics covered in the **Online Worksheet**

1 Define *substance abuse.*

2 Discuss the significance of the substance abuse problem in health care.

3 Identify the major drug categories for substance abuse and the major individual agents in each category.

4 Identify the signs and symptoms of opiate withdrawal and drugs used for opiod withdrawal.

5 Identify the commonly abused stimulants and treatment of their abusive syndromes.

6 Describe the signs and symptoms of depressant abuse and the treatment process for benzodiazepine and barbiturate withdrawal.

7 Describe the alcohol abuse syndrome and its treatment.

8 Identify the signs and symptoms of ethanol withdrawal, ranging from mild to severe withdrawal, and medications used to treat the various stages of withdrawal.

9 Develop a nursing care plan including all phases of the nursing process for the patient who is suffering from abusive disorders.

10 Identify the various resources, including websites, for substance abuse information.

glossary

Amphetamines Drugs that stimulate the CNS. (p. 76)

Enuresis Urinary incontinence. (p. 77)

Illicit drug use The use of a drug or substance that is not intended to be used in the manner in which it is being used or the use of a drug that is not legally approved for human consumption. (p. 76)

Micturition Urination, the desire to urinate, or the frequency of urination. (p. 77)

Narcolepsy A sleep disorder characterized by sleeping during the day, disrupted nighttime sleep, cataplexy, sleep paralysis, and hypnagogic hallucinations. (p. 77)

Opioid analgesics Pain-relieving substances that originated from the opium plant. (p. 75)

Physical dependence A condition characterized by physiologic reliance upon a substance; usually indicated by tolerance to the effects of the substance and withdrawal symptoms that develop when use of the substance is terminated. (p. 74)

Psychoactive properties Mood, anxiety, behavior, cognitive processes, and mental tension. (p. 76)

Psychologic dependence A condition characterized by behaviors related to obtaining and using a substance. (p. 74)

Raves Increasingly popular all-night parties that typically involve dancing, drinking, and the use of various illicit drugs. (p. 76)

Roofies Pills that are classified as benzodiazepines. They have recently gained popularity as a recreational drug; chemically known as flunitrazepam (Rohypnol). (p. 78)

Substance abuse affects people of all ages, sexes, and ethnic and socioeconomic groups. **Physical dependence** and **psychologic dependence** upon a substance are chronic disorders with remissions and relapses like any other chronic disease. Exacerbations should not be seen as failures but as times to intensify treatment. Recognition of physical or psychologic dependence, guidelines for treatment, and withdrawal of various drugs of abuse are important skills for the individual caring for these patients.

Nearly 50% of the patients who visit a family practice have an alcohol or drug disorder. Approximately 25% to 40% of hospital admissions are related to substance abuse and its sequelae. Of outpatients seen in a general medicine practice, 10% to 16% are suffering from problems related to substance abuse. Assessment, intervention, prescription of medications, participation in specific addiction treatment strategies, and monitoring of recovery are essential to the care of this patient population.

This chapter focuses on three major classes of commonly abused substances and two commonly abused individual agents. A description of the category or the individual agent, possible effects, signs and symptoms of intoxication and withdrawal, peak period and duration of withdrawal symptoms, and agents used to treat withdrawal are discussed. Box 7-1 is not an all-inclusive list of substances that are abused, but it lists some of the most commonly abused substances at this time.

The specific agents used to treat withdrawal are discussed with the major category or individual agent for which it is used to treat. Pharmacologic therapies are indicated for use in patients with addictive disorders to prevent life-threatening withdrawal complications, such as seizures and delirium tremens, and to increase compliance with psychosocial forms of addiction treatment.

OPIOIDS

Opioid analgesics are pain-relieving substances that originated from the opium plant. More than 20 different alkaloids are obtained from the unripe seed of the opium poppy plant, only a few of which are clinically useful. Morphine and codeine are the only two that are useful as analgesics. The multitude of other opioid analgesics that are currently used in medical practice are synthetic or semisynthetic derivatives of these two agents.

Diacetylmorphine, better known as *heroin*, and *opium* are also opioids. Heroin and opium are considered Schedule I agents and are not available in the United States for therapeutic use. Heroin was banned in 1924 because of its high potential for abuse and an increasing number of heroin addicts. Currently it is still one of the top 10 drugs abused in the United States and often is used in combination with cocaine. Heroin is one of the most commonly abused opioids. When heroin is injected (mainlining or skin-popping), sniffed (snorted), or smoked, it binds with opiate receptors found in many regions of the brain. The result is intense euphoria, often referred to as a "rush." The rush lasts only briefly and is followed by a couple of hours of a relaxed, contented state. In large doses, heroin can reduce or eliminate respiration. Some classify cocaine as a narcotic and therefore include it when talking about opioids. It is discussed with "stimulants" in this chapter. Some of the more commonly abused substances within this category are listed in Box 7-2.

Mechanism of Action

Opioids work by blocking receptors in the central nervous system (CNS). By blocking these receptors, the perception of pain is blocked. There are three main receptor types to which they bind. These various receptors and their physiologic effects when stimulated are discussed in Chapter 9. The unique mixture of receptor affinities that

a specific opioid possesses determines therapeutic and toxic effects. One of the reasons that the opioids are abused is their ability to produce euphoria that is a mu-receptor response to stimulation by an opioid.

Drug Effects

The drug effects of opioids are primarily centered on the CNS. However, they also act outside the CNS and many of their unwanted effects stem from these actions. Opioids produce analgesia, drowsiness, euphoria, tranquility, and other alterations of mood. The mechanism by which opioids produce their effects is also not entirely clear. Areas outside the CNS that are affected by opioids are the skin, gastrointestinal (GI) tract, and genitourinary (GU) tract.

Therapeutic Uses

The intended drug effects of opioids are to relieve pain, reduce cough, relieve diarrhea, and induce anesthesia. Many have a high potential for abuse and are therefore classified as Schedule II controlled substances. The drug effects of relaxation and euphoria are the most common drug effects that lead to abuse and psychologic dependence.

Side Effects and Adverse Effects

The side effects and adverse effects of opioids can be broken down into two areas—CNS and all other. The primary side effects and adverse effects of opioids are related to their actions in the CNS. The primary CNS-related side effects and adverse effects are diuresis, miosis, convulsions, nausea, vomiting, and respiratory depression. Many of the side effects and adverse effects that occur outside the CNS are secondary to the release of histamine caused by opioids. This histamine release can cause vasodilation leading to hypotension; spasms of the colon leading to constipation; increased contractions of the ureter resulting in decreased urine flow; and dilation of cutaneous blood vessels leading to skin of the face, neck, and upper thorax becoming flushed. This release of histamine is also thought to cause sweating, urticaria, and pruritus.

Toxicity and Management of Overdose

Box 7-3 lists the signs and symptoms of substance abuse and withdrawal from opioids. The box also lists the time when these symptoms are most likely to occur and their duration. Management of acute intoxication and discussion

---

box 7-1	Drug Categories for Substance Abuse

MAJOR CATEGORIES
Opioids
Stimulants
Depressants
INDIVIDUAL AGENTS
Alcohol
Nicotine

---

box 7-2	Commonly Abused Opioids

codeine
heroin
hydromorphone
meperidine
morphine
opium
oxycodone
propoxyphene

BOX 7-3 Signs and Symptoms of Opiate Withdrawal

PEAK PERIOD
1 to 3 days

DURATION
5 to 7 days

SIGNS
Drug seeking, mydriasis, piloerection, diaphoresis, rhinorrhea, lacrimation, diarrhea, insomnia, elevated blood pressure and pulse

SYMPTOMS
Intense desire for drugs, muscle cramps, arthralgia, anxiety, nausea, vomiting, malaise

---

BOX 7-4 Medications for Opioid Withdrawal

CLONIDINE (CATAPRES) SUBSTITUTION
Clonidine, 0.1 or 0.2 mg orally, is given every 4 to 6 hours as needed for signs and symptoms of withdrawal for 5 to 7 days. Days 2 through 4 are typically the toughest days in detoxification. Check blood pressure before each dose, and do not give medication if patient is hypotensive.

METHADONE SUBSTITUTION
Methadone test dose of 10 mg is given orally in liquid or crushed tablet. Additional 10 to 20 mg doses are given for signs and symptoms of withdrawal every 4 to 6 hours for 24 hours after initial dose. Range for daily dose is 15 to 30 mg. Repeat total first day dose in two divided doses (stabilization dose) for 2 to 3 days, then reduce dosage by 5 to 10 mg per day until medication is completely withdrawn.

BOX 7-5 Commonly Abused Stimulants

amphetamine
benzedrine
benzphetamine
butyl nitrite
cocaine
dextroamphetamine
methamphetamine
methylphenidate
phenmetrazine

---

on physical dependence are discussed in detail in Chapter 9. Withdrawal symptoms include nausea, dysphoria, muscle aches, lacrimation or rhinorrhea, pupillary dilation, piloerection or sweating, diarrhea, yawning, fever, and insomnia. The medications listed in Box 7-4 are intended to help reduce the desire for the abused opioid and the severity of these withdrawal symptoms.

Medications are sometimes used to prevent relapse to drug use once an initial remission is secured. These medications are only useful when used with concurrent counseling and provide an additional insurance against return to **illicit drug use**. For opioid abuse or dependence, naltrexone (ReVia), an opioid antagonist, is used (50 mg/day). Naltrexone works by blocking the opioid receptors so that use of opioid drugs does not produce euphoria. When euphoria is eliminated, the reinforcing effect of the drug is lost. The patient should be free from opioids for at least 1 week before beginning this medication because naltrexone can produce withdrawal symptoms if given too soon. Naltrexone is also approved for alcohol-dependent patients. The same dose of naltrexone as used with opioid-dependent patients, 50 mg/day, decreases craving for alcohol and reduces the likelihood of a full relapse if a slip occurs.

STIMULANTS

Amphetamines are examples of commonly abused stimulants. Chemically, three types of amphetamines exist: salts of racemic amphetamine, dextroamphetamine, and methamphetamine. All three classes vary with respect to their potency and peripheral effects. Some of the properties of the stimulants that have led to their abuse are elevation in mode, reduction of fatigue, a sense of increased alertness, and "invigorating aggressiveness." Another social recreational drug of abuse is cocaine. It also produces strong CNS stimulation. Box 7-5 lists some of the more commonly abused substances within this category.

One of the most commonly abused classes of amphetamines is methamphetamine. Multiple slight chemical derivations of methamphetamines exist. Table 7-1 lists commonly abused forms of amphetamines and their street names. These "designer drugs" have **psychoactive properties** along with their stimulant properties, further enhancing their abuse potential. Along with cocaine, they are two of the most commonly abused stimulants. Although these agents have many therapeutic benefits, they are often abused and can lead to physical and psychologic dependence. Methamphetamine is a stimulant drug chemically related to amphetamine, but it has much stronger effects on the CNS.

Methamphetamine is used in pill form or in powdered form by snorting or injecting. Crystallized methamphetamine, known as "ice," "crystal," or "glass," is a smokable and more powerful form of the drug. Methamphetamine users who inject the drug and share needles are at risk for acquiring human immunodeficiency virus (HIV) and acquired immunodeficiency syndrome (AIDS). Methamphetamine is an increasingly popular drug at **raves** (all-night dancing parties) and as part of several drugs used by college-age students. Marijuana and alcohol are commonly listed as additional drugs of abuse among methamphetamine treatment admissions. Most of the methamphetamine-related deaths (92%) reported in 1994 involved methamphetamine in combination with at least one other drug, most often alcohol (30%), heroin (23%), or cocaine (21%).

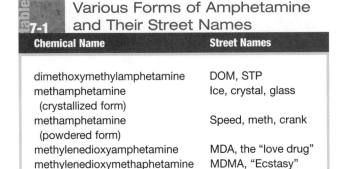

Table 7-1 Various Forms of Amphetamine and Their Street Names

Chemical Name	Street Names
dimethoxymethylamphetamine	DOM, STP
methamphetamine (crystallized form)	Ice, crystal, glass
methamphetamine (powdered form)	Speed, meth, crank
methylenedioxyamphetamine	MDA, the "love drug"
methylenedioxymethaphetamine	MDMA, "Ecstasy"

Table 7-2 Various Forms of Cocaine and Their Street Names

Chemical Name	Street Names
cocaine (powdered form)	coke, dust, snow, flake, blow, girl
cocaine (crystallized form)	crack, crack cocaine, freebase rocks, rock

Cocaine is a white powder that comes from the leaves of the South American coca plant. Cocaine is either "snorted" through the nasal passages or injected intravenously. Cocaine tends to give a temporary illusion of limitless power and energy that leave the user feeling depressed, edgy, and craving more. Crack is a smokable form of cocaine that has been chemically altered. Cocaine and crack are highly addictive. This psychologic and physical dependence can erode physical and mental health and can become so strong that these drugs dominate all aspects of an addict's life. Table 7-2 lists commonly abused forms of cocaine and their street names.

Mechanism of Action

Stimulants work by releasing biogenic amines from their storage sites in the nerve terminals. The primary biogenic amine released is norepinephrine. This release results in stimulation of the CNS.

Drug Effects

The drug effects of stimulants are typically cardiovascular stimulation resulting in increased blood pressure and slowed heart rate, possibly leading to cardiac dysrhythmias. The effect on smooth muscle is primarily seen in the urinary bladder, resulting in contraction of the sphincter. This is helpful in treating **enuresis** and incontinence but results in pain and difficulty in **micturition** otherwise. Stimulants, particularly amphetamines, are very potent CNS stimulants. This CNS stimulation frequently results in wakefulness, alertness, and a decreased sense of fatigue; elevation of mood, with increased initiative, self-confidence, and ability to concentrate; often elation and euphoria; and an increase in motor and speech activity. Physical performance in athletes is improved, leading to abuse.

Therapeutic Uses

Many therapeutic uses of stimulants exist. Stimulants may be used to prevent or reverse fatigue and sleep as when they are used for **narcolepsy**. They also have a slight analgesic effect and may be used to enhance the analgesic effects of other more potent analgesics and limit the CNS-depressant effects of stronger analgesics, such as opioids. Another therapeutic effect of amphetamines is their ability to stimulate the respiratory center. Occasionally they

Box 7-6 Signs and Symptoms of Stimulant Withdrawal

PEAK PERIOD
1 to 3 days
DURATION
5 to 7 days
SIGNS
Social withdrawal, psychomotor retardation, hypersomnia, hyperphagia
SYMPTOMS
Depression, anhedonia, suicidal thoughts and behavior, paranoid delusions

are used after anesthesia to stimulate the respiratory center in individuals whose respirations are slowed. Stimulants are also used to reduce food intake and treat obesity. This therapeutic effect is limited because of rapid development of tolerance. Stimulants have also shown benefits in the treatment of attention deficit disorders.

Side Effects and Adverse Effects

The side effects and adverse effects of stimulants are commonly an extension of their therapeutic effects. The CNS-related side effects are restlessness, dizziness, tremor, hyperactive reflexes, talkativeness, tenseness, irritability, weakness, insomnia, fever, and sometimes euphoria. Confusion, aggression, increased libido, anxiety, delirium, paranoid hallucinations, panic states, and suicidal or homicidal tendencies occur, especially in mentally ill patients. Fatigue and depression usually follow the CNS stimulation. Cardiovascular effects are common and include headache, chilliness, pallor or flushing, palpitations, cardiac dysrhythmias, anginal pain, hypertension or hypotension, and circulatory collapse. Excessive sweating can also occur. GI effects include dry mouth, metallic taste, anorexia, nausea, vomiting, diarrhea, and abdominal cramps.

Toxicity and Management of Overdose

Box 7-6 lists the signs and symptoms of substance abuse and withdrawal from stimulants. The box also lists the time when these symptoms are most likely to occur and their duration. Fatal poisoning is usually due to convulsions, coma, or cerebral hemorrhages.

DEPRESSANTS

Depressants are drugs that relieve anxiety, irritability, and tension when used as they are intended. They are also used to treat seizure disorders and induce anesthesia. The two main pharmacologic classes are benzodiazepines and barbiturates. Benzodiazepines are relatively safe. They offer many advantages over older agents that used to be used to relieve anxiety and insomnia. However, they are often intentionally and unintentionally misused. When they are co-ingested with alcohol, they can become a fatal combination. A benzodiazepine that has recently gained popularity as a recreational drug is flunitrazepam (Rohypnol). Flunitrazepam is not legally available for prescription in the United States, but is legal in over 60 countries worldwide for treatment of insomnia.

Flunitrazepam has gained popularity in the last few years as a recreational drug called "**roofies**" among young people. The drug creates a sleepy, relaxed, and drunk feeling that lasts 2 to 8 hours, and a single dose costs from $1.50 to $5.00. "Roofies" are frequently used in combination with alcohol and other drugs. They are sometimes taken to enhance a heroin high or to mellow or ease the experience of coming down from a cocaine or crack high. Used with alcohol, "roofies" produce disinhibition and amnesia.

"Roofies" have recently gained a reputation as the "date rape" drug. Girls and women around the country have reported being raped after being involuntarily sedated with "roofies," which were often slipped into their drink by an attacker. The drug has no taste or odor, so the victims do not realize what is happening. About 10 minutes after ingesting the drug, the woman may feel dizzy and disoriented, simultaneously too hot and too cold, and nauseated. She may experience difficulty speaking and moving and then pass out. Such a victim will have no memories of what happened while under the drug's influence.

Flunitrazepam is sold under the trade name Rohypnol, from which the street name "Rophy" is derived. In South Florida, street names include "circles," "Mexican valium," "rib," "roach-2," "roofies," "roopies," "rope," "ropies," and "ruffies." Being under the influence of the drug is referred to as being "roached out." In Texas, flunitrazepam is called "R-2" or "roaches."

Mechanism of Action

Benzodiazepines and barbiturates work by increasing the action of gamma-aminobutyric acid (GABA). GABA is an inhibitory amino acid in the brain that functions to inhibit nerve transmission in the CNS. The alteration of GABA in the CNS results in relieved anxiety, sedation, and muscle relaxation.

Drug Effects

The drug effects of depressants are primarily limited to the CNS. Their CNS drug effects include sedation, amnesia, muscle relaxation, unconsciousness, and reduced anxiety. They have moderate drug effects outside of the CNS, only causing slight blood pressure decreases.

BOX 7-7 Signs, Symptoms, and Treatment of Depressant Withdrawal

PEAK PERIOD
2 to 4 days for short-acting agents
4 to 7 days for long-acting agents

DURATION
4 to 7 days for short-acting agents
7 to 12 days for long-acting agents

SIGNS
Increased psychomotor activity; agitation; muscular weakness; hyperpyrexia; diaphoresis; delirium; convulsions; elevated blood pressure, pulse, and temperature; tremors of eyelids, tongue, and hands

SYMPTOMS
Anxiety, depression, euphoria, incoherent thoughts, hostility, grandiosity, disorientation, tactile, auditory and visual hallucinations, suicidal thoughts

TREATMENT

Benzodiazepine Withdrawal
7- to 10-day taper (10- to 14-day taper with long-acting benzodiazepines). Treat with diazepam (Valium) 10 to 20 mg four times daily on day 1, then taper until the dosage is 5 to 10 mg orally on last day. Avoid giving the drug "as needed." Adjustments in dosage according to the patient's clinical state may be indicated.

Barbiturate Withdrawal
7- to 10-day taper or 10- to 14-day taper. Calculate barbiturate equivalence and give 50% of the original dosage; taper (if actual dosage is known before detoxification). Avoid giving the drug "as needed."

Therapeutic Uses

Many therapeutic uses of the depressants exist. Benzodiazepines are more widely used and abused than barbiturates. Benzodiazepines are more commonly prescribed because they are felt by many to be safer than barbiturates. Benzodiazepines are used primarily to relieve anxiety, to induce sleep, to sedate, and as anticonvulsants. Barbiturates are used as hypnotics, as sedatives, as anticonvulsants, and to induce anesthesia.

Side Effects and Adverse Effects

The most common undesirable effect of benzodiazepines and barbiturates is an overexpression of their therapeutic effects. The CNS is the primary area of the body adversely affected by them. Drowsiness, sedation, loss of coordination, dizziness, blurred vision, headaches, and paradoxical reactions (insomnia, increases excitability, and hallucinations) are the primary CNS side effects. Occasional GI effects include nausea, vomiting, constipation, dry mouth, and abdominal cramping. Other possible side effects include pruritus and skin rash.

Table 7-3 Barbiturate Equivalencies

Drug	Dose (mg)	Phenobarbital Dose (mg)	Conversion Factor
BARBITURATES			
butabarbital (Butisol)	600	180	0.3
pentobarbital (Nembutal)	600	180	0.3
phenobarbital	180	180	1
secobarbital (Seconal)	600	180	0.3
OTHERS			
glutethimide (Doriden)	1500	180	0.12
meprobamate (Equanil)	2400	180	0.075
methaqualone	1800	180	0.1

Toxicity and Management of Overdose

Box 7-7 lists the signs and symptoms of substance abuse and withdrawal from depressants. The box also lists the time when these symptoms are most likely to occur and their duration. Fatal poisoning is unusual with benzodiazepines when they are ingested alone. However, when benzodiazepines are ingested with ethanol or barbiturates the combination can be lethal. Death is typically due to respiratory arrest. Abrupt withdrawal of benzodiazepines that have been taken for several months to years has resulted in autonomic withdrawal symptoms, seizures, delirium, rebound anxiety, myoclonus, myalgia, and sleep disturbances.

Table 7-3 should be used for conversion from various barbiturates to phenobarbital, which is less addicting and easier to withdrawal from. To use this table, determine the total dose of the barbiturate that the patient is dependent upon. Take this dose and multiply it times the conversion factor to get the equivalent dose of phenobarbital. Then taper from there as described in Box 7-7.

Flumazenil (Romazicon) can be used to acutely reverse the sedative effects of benzodiazepines. Flumazenil antagonizes the action of benzodiazepines on the CNS by directly competing with benzodiazepines for binding at the benzodiazepine receptor in the CNS. However, it has a stronger affinity for the receptor and knocks the benzodiazepine off from the receptor, reversing the sedative action of the benzodiazepine. The dosage regimen to be followed for the reversal of conscious sedation or general anesthesia induced by benzodiazepines and the management of suspected benzodiazepine overdoses are summarized in Table 9-7 on page 126.

Limiting depressant abuse is important. Barbiturates and benzodiazepines are frequently implicated in suicides, especially when combined with alcohol. None of the depressants should be regularly prescribed over a long period of time. Relatively safe hypnotic agents such as benzodiazepines should be preferentially used whenever possible, especially in emotionally disturbed patients. Combinations of sedative-hypnotic compounds and the single use of these drugs with alcohol should be avoided. Chronic hypnotic drug use leads to ineffective control of insomnia, decreased rapid eye movement (REM) sleep, dependence, and drug withdrawal symptomatology.

ALCOHOL

Alcoholic beverages have been used since the beginning of time. The Arabs introduced the technique of distilling to Europe in the Middle Ages. Alcohol has been termed the *elixir of life* and has been a remedy for practically all diseases, which leads to the term *whisky*, which is Gaelic for 'water of life.' It has been determined that the therapeutic value of ethanol is extremely limited, and chronic ingestion of excessive amounts is a major social and medical problem.

Mechanism of Action

Alcohol, more accurately known as *ethanol*, causes CNS depression by dissolving in lipid membranes in the CNS. The latest hypothesis is that ethanol causes a local disordering in the lipid matrix of the brain. This has been termed *membrane fluidization*. Some also believe that ethanol may augment GABA-mediated synaptic inhibition and fluxes of chloride. By enhancing GABA, an inhibitory neurotransmitter in the brain, CNS depression occurs.

Drug Effects

Many drug effects of ethanol exist. The CNS is continuously depressed in the presence of ethanol. Moderate amounts of ethanol may stimulate or depress respirations. Effects of ethanol on the circulation are relatively minor. In moderate doses, ethanol causes vasodilatation, especially of the cutaneous vessels, and produces warm, flushed skin. Ingestion of ethanol causes a feeling of warmth because alcohol enhances cutaneous and gastric blood flow. Increased sweating may also occur. Heat is therefore lost more rapidly, and the internal temperature consequently falls. The acute ingestion of ethanol even in intoxicating doses probably produces little lasting change in hepatic function. Ethanol exerts a diuretic effect by virtue of inhibition of antidiuretic hormone (ADH) secretion and a resultant decrease in renal tubular reabsorption of water.

Therapeutic Uses

Few legitimate uses of ethanol and alcoholic beverages exist. Ethanol is an excellent solvent for many drugs and is frequently employed as a vehicle for medicinal mixtures. When applied topically to the skin, ethanol acts as a coolant. Ethanol sponges are therefore used to treat fever. Ethanol may also be used in liniments. High concentrations (50% to 70%) may be used as a rubbing agent on the skin of bedridden patients to prevent decubitus ulcers. Applied topically, ethanol is still the most popular skin disinfectant.

Ethanol is still widely employed for its hypnotic and antipyretic effects in various cold and cough products. Dehydrated alcohol is injected in the close proximity of nerves or sympathetic ganglia for the relief of the long-lasting pain that occurs in trigeminal neuralgia, inoperable carcinoma, and other conditions. Systemic uses of ethanol are primarily limited to the treatment of methyl alcohol and ethylene glycol intoxication.

Side Effects and Adverse Effects

Chronic excessive ingestion of ethanol is directly associated with serious neurologic and mental disorders. These neurologic disorders can result in seizures. Nutritional and vitamin deficiencies can occur, resulting in Wernicke's encephalopathy, Korsakoff's psychosis, polyneuritis, and nicotinic acid deficiency encephalopathy.

Moderate amounts of ethanol may stimulate or depress respirations. Large amounts produce dangerous or lethal depression of respiration. Although circulatory effects of ethanol are relatively minor, acute severe alcoholic intoxication may cause cardiovascular depression. Long-term excessive use of ethanol has largely irreversible effects on the heart, such as cardiomyopathy.

When consumed on a regular basis in large quantities, ethanol produces a constellation of dose-related deleterious effects, such as alcoholic hepatitis or its progression to cirrhosis. Teratogenic effects can be devastating and are due to a direct action of ethanol inhibiting embryonic cellular proliferation early in gestation.

Toxicity and Management of Overdose

Box 7-8 lists the common signs and symptoms of ethanol withdrawal. Signs and symptoms may vary depending on the individual's usage pattern, his or her preferred type of ethanol, and the existence of other comorbidities.

One pharmacologic option for the treatment of alcoholism is disulfiram (Antabuse). Disulfiram is not a cure for alcoholism; it helps a patient who has a sincere desire to stop drinking. The rationale for its use is that patients know if they are to avoid the devastating experience of the acetaldehyde syndrome, they cannot drink for at least 3 or 4 days after taking disulfiram. Table 7-4 outlines the acetaldehyde syndrome.

BOX 7-8 Treatment of Ethanol Withdrawal

MILD WITHDRAWAL
Systolic blood pressure >150 mm Hg, diastolic blood pressure >90 mm Hg, pulse >110 beats/min, temperature >37.7° C (100° F), tremors, insomnia, and agitation
Treat with the following:
diazepam (Valium), 5-10 mg orally as needed
lorazepam (Ativan), 1-2 mg orally every 4-6 hours as needed for 1-3 days

MODERATE WITHDRAWAL
Systolic blood pressure 150 to 200 mm Hg, diastolic blood pressure 100 to 140 mm Hg, pulse 110 to 140 beats/min, temperature 37.7° to 38.3° C (100° to 101° F), tremors, insomnia, and agitation
Treat with the following:
diazepam (Valium)
day 1: 15-20 mg orally four times daily
day 2: 10-20 mg orally four times daily
day 3: 5-15 mg orally four times daily
day 4: 10 mg orally four times daily
day 5: 5 mg orally four times daily
lorazepam (Ativan)
days 1 and 2: 2-4 mg orally four times daily
day 3 and 4: 1-2 mg orally four times daily
day 5: 1 mg twice daily

SEVERE WITHDRAWAL (DELIRIUM TREMENS)*
Systolic blood pressure >200 mm Hg, diastolic blood pressure >140 mm Hg, pulse >140 beats/min, temperature >38.3° C (101° F), tremors, insomnia, and agitation
Treat with the following:
diazepam (Valium), 10-25 mg orally as needed every hour while awake until sedation occurs
lorazepam (Ativan), 1-2 mg IV as needed every hour while awake for 3 to 5 days

---

*Monitoring in an intensive care unit is recommended for cardiac and respiratory function, fluid and nutrition replacement, vital signs, and mental status. Restraints are indicated in patients who are confused or agitated to protect the patient from self and others (delirium tremens can be a terrifying and life-threatening state). Thiamine (100 mg IM or orally every day for 3 to 7 days), hydration, and magnesium replacement may be indicated according to the severity of the withdrawal state.

Disulfiram works by altering the metabolism of alcohol. When ethanol is given to an individual previously treated with disulfiram, the blood acetaldehyde concentrations rises 5 to 10 times higher than in an untreated individual. Within about 5 to 10 minutes of ingesting alcohol, the face feels hot, and soon afterward it is flushed and scarlet in appearance. After this, throbbing in the head and neck, nausea, copious vomiting, diaphoresis, dyspnea, hyperventilation, vertigo, blurred vision, and confusion appear. As little as 7 ml of alcohol will cause mild symptoms in a sensitive person. The effects last between 30 minutes and several hours. After the symptoms wear off, the patient is exhausted and may sleep for several hours. Most of the

Table 7-4	Acetaldehyde Syndrome	
Body System Affected	**Result**
Cardiovascular	Vasodilation over the entire body, hypotension, orthostatic syncope, chest pain
Central nervous system	Intense throbbing of the head and neck leading to a pulsating headache, sweating, marked uneasiness, weakness, vertigo, blurred vision, and confusion
Gastrointestinal	Nausea, copious vomiting, thirst
Respiratory	Difficulty breathing

signs and symptoms observed after the ingestion of disulfiram plus alcohol are attributable to the resulting increase in the concentration of acetaldehyde in the body. The usual dosage of disulfiram is 250 mg per day, or 125 mg per day in patients who experience side effects such as sedation, sexual dysfunction, and elevated liver enzymes.

NICOTINE

Nicotine was first isolated from leaves of tobacco by Posselt and Reiman in 1828. The medical significance of nicotine can be attributed to its toxicity, presence in tobacco, and propensity for conferring a dependence on its users. The chronic effects of nicotine and the untoward effects of the chronic use of tobacco are considerable. Although many people smoke because they believe cigarettes calm their nerves, smoking releases epinephrine, a hormone which creates physiologic stress in the smoker rather than relaxation. The use of tobacco is addictive. Most users develop tolerance for nicotine and need greater amounts to produce a desired effect. Smokers become physically and psychologically dependent and will suffer withdrawal symptoms. Smoking is particularly dangerous in adolescents because their bodies are still developing and changing. The 4000 chemicals, including 200 known poisons, in cigarette smoke can adversely affect this process. Cigarettes are highly addictive. One-third of young people who are just "experimenting" end up being addicted by the time they are 20 years of age.

Mechanism of Action

Nicotine works by directly stimulating the autonomic ganglia. Its site of action is the ganglion itself rather than the preganglionic or postganglionic nerve fiber. The organs throughout the body that are innervated with nerves that are stimulated by nicotine actually have on them "nicotinic receptors." These receptors are named such because they were originally tested with nicotine to measure their response. Nicotine can have multiple, unpredictable, and dramatic affects on the body.

Drug Effects

The major action of nicotine is initially transient stimulation followed by more persistent depression of all autonomic ganglia. Small doses of nicotine stimulate the ganglion cells directly and facilitate the transmission of impulses. When larger doses of the drug are applied, the initial stimulation is followed quickly by a blockade of transmission.

Nicotine markedly stimulates the CNS. Respiratory stimulation is also common. This stimulation of the CNS is followed by depression. Nicotine can have dramatic effects on the cardiovascular system as well, resulting in increases in heart rate and blood pressure. The GI system is generally stimulated by nicotine, resulting in increased tone and activity in the bowel. This often leads to nausea and vomiting and occassionally diarrhea.

Therapeutic Uses

Nicotine has no therapeutic uses. It has significance primarily because of its medical significance secondary to its toxicity.

Side Effects and Adverse Effects

Nicotine primarily affects the CNS. Large doses can produce tremors and even convulsions. Respiratory stimulation is also common. The initial stimulation of the CNS induced by nicotine is quickly followed by depression. Death can even result from respiratory failure, which is thought to be due to both central paralysis and peripheral blockade of respiratory muscles.

Cardiovascular effects of nicotine are an increase in heart rate and blood pressure. Nicotine stimulates sympathetic ganglia with the discharge of catecholamines from the sympathetic nerve endings.

The effects of nicotine on the GI system are largely due to parasympathetic stimulation, which results in increased tone and motor activity of the bowel. Nicotine induces vomiting by both central and peripheral actions. Centrally, nicotine's emetic effects are due to stimulation of the chemoreceptor trigger zone (CTZ).

Toxicity and Management of Overdose

Smoking cessation is the primary cause for nicotine withdrawal, although discontinuation of any tobacco product can lead to this syndrome. An important and often overlooked problem in hospitalized patients is nicotine withdrawal. Nicotine withdrawal manifests largely as cigarette craving. Irritability, restlessness, and a decrease in heart rate and blood pressure occur. Cardiac symptoms resolve over 3 to 4 weeks, but cigarette craving may persist for months to years.

The nicotine transdermal system (patch) and nicotine polacrilex (gum) can be used to provide nicotine without the carcinogens in tobacco and are now available over-the-counter (OTC). The patches use a stepwise reduction in subcutaneous delivery to gradually decrease the nicotine dose and appear to have greater compliance than the gum. Acute relief from withdrawal symptoms

Table 7-5 Nicotine Withdrawal Therapies

Drug	Dosage Per Patch	Recommended Duration of Use
TRANSDERMAL NICOTINE SYSTEMS		
Habitrol	7 mg/24 hr, 14 mg/24 hr, 21 mg/24 hr	2-4 wk, 2-4 wk, 4-8 wk
Nicoderm	7 mg/24 hr, 14 mg/24 hr, 21 mg/24 hr	2-4 wk, 2-4 wk, 4-8 wk
Nicotrol	5 mg/16 hr, 10 mg/16 hr, 15 mg/16 hr	2-4 wk, 2-4 wk, 4-12 wk
Prostep	11 mg/24 hr, 22 mg/24 hr	2-4 wk, 4-8 wk
NICOTINE GUM (RESIN)		
	When the client has a strong urge to smoke, a stick of gum is chewed; gradually reducing over a 2- to 3-month period.	
ANTIDEPRESSANT		
bupropion (Zyban)	150 mg sustained release tablets	150 mg on days 1-3, then 150 mg twice a day for 7-12 weeks

is most easily achieved with use of the gum because rapid chewing releases an immediate dose of nicotine. However, the dose is approximately half of that which the average smoker receives in one cigarette, and the onset of action is 30 minutes instead of 10 minutes or less with smoking. These pharmacologic changes in delivery minimize the reinforcement and self-reward effects that are prominent with the rapid nicotine delivery of cigarette smoking.

A sustained-release form of bupropion called Zyban has been approved as first-line therapy to aid in smoking cessation treatment. Zyban is an innovative treatment because it is the first nicotine-free prescription medicine to treat nicotine dependence. Table 7-5 lists the currently available agents for nicotine withdrawal.

Box 7-9 lists helpful resources containing information on substance abuse.

Activity

nursing process

• Assessment

The nurse must include questions about substance abuse in any medication history or assessment process to identify problems or the potential for withdrawal. In patients who are suspected of or diagnosed with substance abuse, the nurse must assess them thoroughly and be astute to every detail so as to avoid withdrawal symptoms, assist with appropriate medications as ordered, and determine and develop an appropriate plan of care. In patients with possible substance abuse, honesty may be problematic when it comes to answering questions about their drug use, so use open-ended questions and maintain a nonjudgmental approach. List all current medications on the medication history (OTC, prescription, illegal, etc.) and include their names, dosages, and frequency and duration of dosing. Remember that when a patient states that he or she has multiple prescribed drugs or multiple prescribers, this may be an "alert" to the fact of drug abuse. Always be alert to the patient's behavior and mental status for "cues."

The most dangerous substances to be aware of for withdrawal are CNS depressants, which include alcohol, barbiturates, and benzodiazepines. Delerium tremens (DTs) may begin with tremors and agitation and may progress to hallucinations and sometimes death. Careful assessment of vital signs and mental status is once again critical to the safe care of these patients because early withdrawal symptoms may be reflected by an increase in blood pressure and pulse with an alteration in mental status.

• Nursing Diagnoses

Nursing diagnoses related to the individual with substance abuse are as follows:

- Risk for injury and falls related to substance abuse and abrupt withdrawal.
- Situational low self-esteem related to the influence of substance abuse on the person and his or her life.
- Disturbed thought process related to impaired mental status as a result of the abuse and its treatment.
- Deficient knowledge related to lack of information about the process of abuse and its long-term management.

• Planning

Goals related to management of the patient with substance abuse include the following:

- Patient will remain without injury during treatment for substance abuse.
- Patient will regain an improved self-esteem during treatment.
- Patient will discuss drug abuse problem and its management openly with the health care team.

Outcome Criteria

Outcome criteria related to substance abuse are as follows:

- Patient will be safely withdrawn from drugs with stabilization of physical state that was aggravated by the substance abuse (see the specific drug and related signs and symptoms).
- Patient will have appropriate referrals and humane treatment for the substance abuse problem in a safe, nonthreatening, and healthy environment.

BOX 7-9 Resources for information on Substance Abuse

Addiction Research Foundation (ARF)
www.arf.org
Library, Addiction Research Foundation
33 Russell Street
Toronto, Ontario M5S 2S1
Tel: 416-595-6144
Fax: 416-595-6601
E-mail: isd@arf.org

American Psychiatric Association: APA Online
www.psych.org/main.html
1400 K Street, NW
Washington, DC 20005
Tel: 202-682-6000
Fax: 202-682-6850
E-mail: apa@psych.org

American Society of Addiction Medicine (ASAM)
www.asam.org/asam50.htm
4601 North Park Ave, Arcade Suite 101
Chevy Chase, MD 20815
Tel: 301-656-3920
Fax: 301-656-3815

National Association of Alcoholism and Drug Abuse
Counselors (NAADAC)
www.naadac.org
1911 N Fort Myer Drive, Suite 900
Arlington, VA 22209
Tel: 703-741-7686 or 800-548-0497
Fax: 703-741-7698 or 800-377-1136

National Council on Alcoholism and Drug Dependence
(NCADD)
www.ncadd.org
12 West 21 Street
New York, NY 10010
Tel: 212-206-6770
Fax: 212-645-1690
Hope Line: 800-NCA-CALL

National Institute on Drug Abuse
www.nida.nih.gov
    Contains summary information on commonly abused
drugs, including links to research reports and updates and
related publications

National Nurses Society on Addictions (NNSA)
www.nnsa.org
4101 Lake Boone Trail, Suite 201
Raleigh, NC 27607
Tel: 919-783-5871
Fax: 919-787-4916

PREVLINE Prevention Online
www.health.org
    A resource for research in the field of substance abuse
prevention, including research briefs, information on
workplace issues, online forums, and facts about drugs
and alcohol

Substance Abuse & Mental Health Services Administration
(SAMHSA)
www.samhsa.gov
Room 12-105 Parklawn Building
5600 Fishers Lane
Rockville, MD 20857
Tel: 301-443-4795
Fax: 301-443-0284

Implementation

Nurses working with substance abuse patients need a special understanding and empathy, beginning with the nurse's knowledge about the substance abuse process and understanding of the patient's lifestyle. Once a therapeutic rapport has been established, the patient may then need to have information about the drug being abused, its characteristics, and problems associated with the use of the drug and its withdrawal. The withdrawal process also needs to be discussed with the patient if appropriate, and then the nurse closely monitors the patient through the parameters of vital signs and mental status. Family members and significant others should be encouraged to lend their support and assistance during treatment. Life-long treatment is often indicated, and support for the long-term process of recovery should be emphasized and recommended. Education about the particular recovery process and medication regimen for promoting abstinence (if recommended) should be thorough and reinforced to the patient and family members or significant others.

Patient teaching tips for drug abuse are presented on p. 84.

Evaluation

The patient should realize a feeling of safety and security during treatment and should understand the symptoms that he or she may experience during withdrawal of the drug and associated substance abuse treatment. Any change in mental status or in any parameter (vital sign) should be reported to the physician or health care provider immediately.

patient teaching tips

Substance Abuse

➤ The patient and family members or significant others must receive current and accurate information about their treatment regimen to make a more informed and individualized decision about their treatment plan.

➤ Education of family members or significant others about support groups and community resources is important for success during and after a treatment program.

➤ The health care provider should include information about any medication the patient may be receiving with an emphasis on timing of doses, consequences of missed doses, and side effects.

➤ The health care provider should emphasize the danger of multiple drug use and the combination of drugs with alcohol.

POINTS TO REMEMBER

Overview Of Substance Abuse

• Nurses and all other health care providers continually encounter a variety of substance abuse problems and may play a significant part in the patient's recovery.

• Thorough assessment of a patient's past and present medical history with a medication history is also crucial to the successful treatment of patients with substance abuse problems.

• Withdrawal symptoms are characteristic of the drug class and may even be opposite of the drug's action, such as with alcohol (a CNS depressant), which produces withdrawal symptoms that are typically characterized by hyperactivity.

Nursing Considerations

• Nurses and their response to a patient with substance abuse must include an understanding of the pathology of the disease of abuse and how the drug has become a lifestyle for the particular patient.

• Family members or support systems should be included in any treatment regimen for a more successful treatment.

REVIEW QUESTIONS

1. Your patient in the emergency room has been diagnosed with an overdosage of opiates. Which of the following is most commonly associated with "acute" opiate overdosage?
   a. Polyuria
   b. Psychosis
   c. Bradypnea
   d. Dysphagia

2. Any patient who drinks alcohol while taking disulfiram (Antabuse) is most likely to suffer from which of the following?
   a. Euphoria
   b. Hypotension
   c. Severe vomiting
   d. Urinary frequency

3. One of your patients in the emergency room is a 16-year-old female being admitted to the intensive care unit after a suicide attempt. Your initial assessment shows the following: blood pressure 88/44 mm Hg, pulse 110 beats/min, and respiratory rate

8 breaths/min. Her thought processes are also altered. Which of the following agents is most likely the "culprit" of the overdosage?
   a. Alcohol
   b. Adrenaline
   c. Barbiturates
   d. Amphetamines

4. Which of the following symptoms would make you suspicious of a young lady for abusing inhalants?
   a. Dysphagia
   b. Tachycardia
   c. Mental acuity
   d. Tubular necrosis

5. Which of the following would you look for while assessing an individual for use of amphetamines?
   a. Lethargy
   b. Vomiting
   c. Nephrotoxicity
   d. Aggressiveness

CRITICAL THINKING Activities

1. Your patient has been admittted to labor and delivery, has a history of heavy use of alcohol, and appears to be intoxicated. What are the potential complications of alcohol on a fetus, and what would be some concerns during the first few months of the newborn's life?

2. Explain how any substance that may be ingested or abused by the pregnant female can have effects on the fetus.

3. Your patient presents to the emergency room with symptoms of weakness, tremulousness, restlessness, anxiety, insomnia, orthostatic hypotension, and a variety of GI complaints. From these symptoms, what do you think is occurring with the patient?

For Answers see www.harcourthealth.com/MERLIN/Lilley/.

bibliography

Kinney J: *Clinical manual of substance abuse*, ed 2, St Louis, 1996, Mosby.

Kowalski SD: Self-esteem and self-efficacy as predictors of success in smoking cessation, *J Holistic Nurs* 15(2):128, 1997.

Johnson JE: Insomnia, alcohol, and over-the-counter drug use in old-old urban women, *J Community Health Nurs* 14(3):181, 1997.

McKenry LM, Salerno E: *Mosby's pharmacology in nursing*, ed 21, St Louis, 2001, Mosby.

Miller NS, Gold MS: Management of withdrawal syndromes and relapse prevention in drug and alcohol dependence, *Am Fam Physician* 58(1):139, 1998.

Mosby's GenRx: a comprehensive reference for generic and brand drugs, ed 10, St Louis, 2000, Mosby.

Skidmore-Roth L: *Mosby's 2001 nursing drug reference*, St Louis, 2001, Mosby.

Smith DE, Seymour RB: Cannabis and cannabis withdrawal, *J Substance Misuse Nurse Health Society Care* 2(1):49, 1997.

Weaver MF, Jarvis MA, Schnoll SH: Role of the primary care physician in problems of substance abuse, *Arch Intern Med* 159:913, 1999.

Remember to check the **Online Worksheet** for additional learning opportunities: **www.harcourthealth.com/MERLIN/Lilley/**

Chapter 8

Photo Atlas of Drug Administration

www.harcourthealth.com/MERLIN/Lilley/

MEDICATION ORDERS AND DOCUMENTATION

- Computer-controlled dispensing system **(1)**.
- Unit dose cabinet **(2)**.
- Example of a medication administration record **(3)**.
- The nurse is responsible for checking the label of the medication with the transcribed medication order **(4)**.
- Before administering any medication, the nurse should check the patient's identification and allergy bracelet **(5)**.

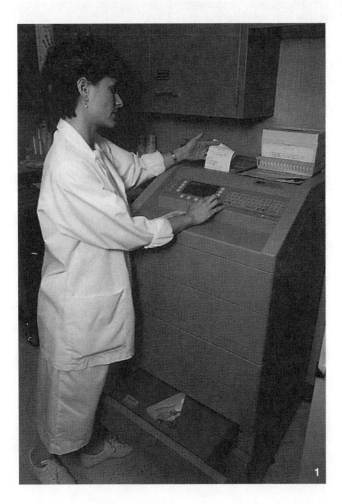

PARENTERAL ADMINISTRATION

PREPARING PARENTERAL MEDICATIONS

Syringes

- Parts of a syringe and hypodermic needle **(6)**.
- Close-up view of the bevel of a needle **(7)**.
- Types of syringes **(8)**. *Top to bottom:* disposable 3-ml hypodermic syringe (intramuscular), 3-ml hypodermic syringe (subcutaneous), tuberculin syringe, and insulin syringe.
- Hypodermic needles arranged in order of gauge **(9)**. *Top to bottom:* 19-, 20-, 21-, 23-, and 25-gauge.
- A prefilled sterile cartridge with needle may be used. The Carpuject prefilled syringe **(10)** is one example of a prefilled syringe.
- Assembling the Carpuject **(11)**.
- The cartridge slides into the syringe barrel, turns, and locks at the needle end. The plunger then screws into the cartridge end **(12)**.

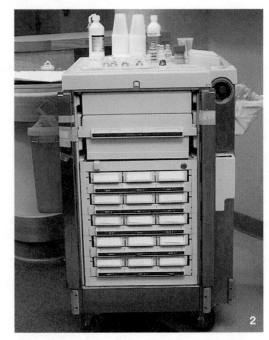

SMITHVILLE HOMETOWN HOSPITAL
MEDICATION ADMINISTRATION RECORD

NAME:	Julie Byrne		RM-BD:	520-1
ID NO.	454-98-7800		AGE:	49
DIAGNOSIS:	Myocardial infarction		SEX:	F
PHYSICIAN:	L. Sparring, M.D.		HT:	5'4" Wt: 136 lb

DATE	INIT	MEDICATION (STRENGTH, FORM)	RTE	SCHEDULE	SHIFT	TIME	TIME	TIME
10/5	JJJ	Fiorinal # 3	oral	every 6 hr prn	~~NIGHT~~ (DAY) EVENING	1100		
10/5	JJJ	Acyclovir ointment +- 5%	topical	apply every 6 hr 6x/day for 7 days	~~NIGHT~~ (DAY) (EVENING)	1000, 1500 1800		
10/6	JJJ	Claritin 10 mg	oral	½ tab every 12 hr	~~NIGHT~~ (DAY) (EVENING)			09 21
					NIGHT DAY EVENING			
					NIGHT DAY EVENING			

AGE/SEX	HT	WT	DATE	ALLERGIES:
49/F	5'4"	136 lb	10/5	NKDA

NAME	ROOM/BED
Julie Byrne	520-1

3

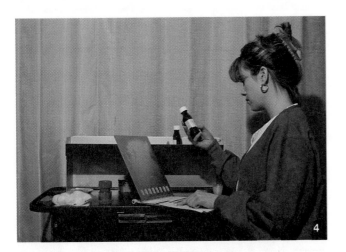

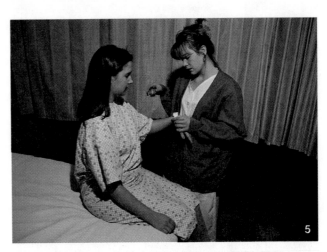

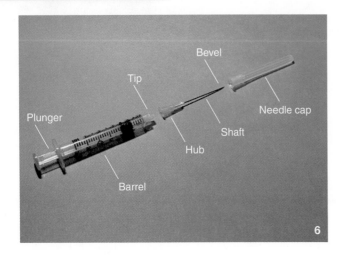

Bevel
Tip
Plunger
Needle cap
Shaft
Hub
Barrel

6

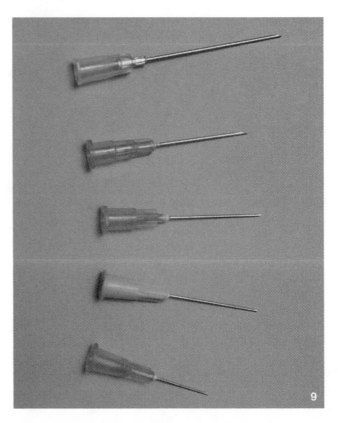

9

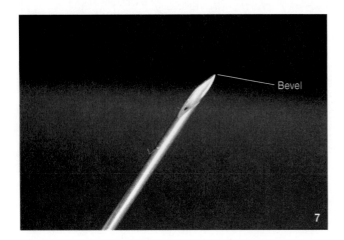

Bevel

7

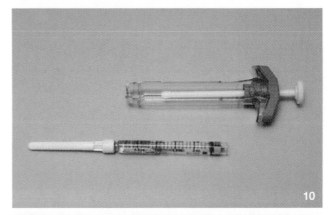

10

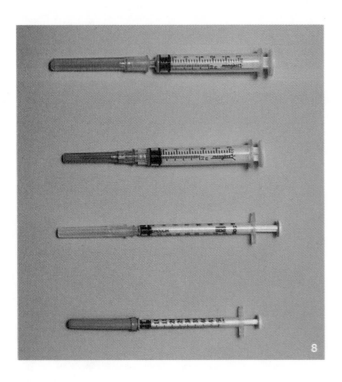

8

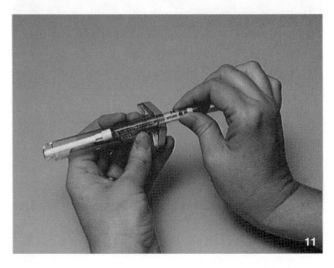

11

- Needle with plastic guard to prevent needle sticks **(13).** Position of guard before injection.
- After injection, the guard locks in place and covers the needle **(14).**
- Special container for the disposal of contaminated syringes **(15).**
- Example of a needleless syringe system used in some institutions to reduce needle-stick injuries **(16).**

Catheters

The following are examples of types of central venous catheters.
- Hickman catheter **(17).**
- Broviac catheter **(18).**
- Groshong catheter **(19).**
- Implantable infusion ports with catheters **(20).**

Preparing Injections from Ampules and Vials

- Prepare needed equipment and supplies.
  1. Ampules **(21)**
     a. Ampule containing medication
     b. Syringe and needle
     c. Small gauze pad or alcohol swab
     d. Container for disposing of glass
     e. Filter for glass particles
  2. Vials **(22)**
     a. Vial with medication
     b. Syringe and needle
     c. Alcohol swab
     d. Solvent (e.g., normal saline or sterile water)

3. Medication cards, forms, or computer printouts
- Assemble supplies at work area in medicine room.
- Check each medication card, form, or printout against label on each ampule or vial.

Prepare Injections from Ampule

- Tap top of ampule lightly and quickly with finger until fluid leaves neck **(23).**
- Place small gauze pad or dry alcohol swab around neck of ampule.
- Snap neck quickly and firmly away from hands **(24).**
- Draw up medication quickly. Hold ampule upside down or set it on flat surface. Insert syringe needle into center of ampule opening **(25).** Do not allow needle tip or shaft to touch rim of ampule.
- Aspirate medication into syringe by gently pulling back on plunger **(26).**
- Keep needle tip below surface of liquid. Tip ampule to bring all fluid within reach of needle.
- If air bubbles are aspirated, do not expel air into ampule.
- To expel excess air bubbles, remove needle. Hold syringe with needle pointing up. Tap side of syringe to cause bubbles to rise toward needle **(27).** Draw back slightly on plunger, and push plunger upward to eject air. *Do not eject fluid.*
- If syringe contains excess fluid, use sink for disposal. Hold syringe vertically with needle tip up and slanted slightly toward sink. Slowly eject excess fluid into sink. Recheck fluid level in syringe by holding it vertically.

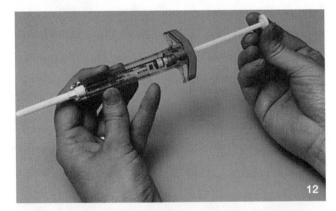

12

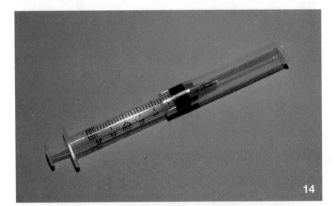

14

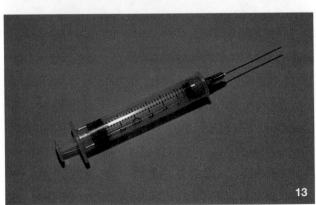

13

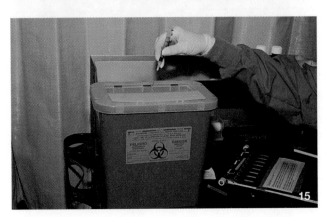

15

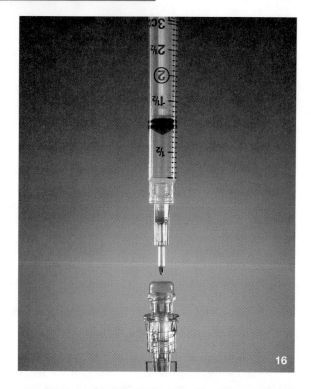

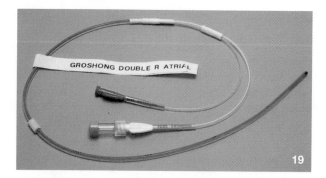

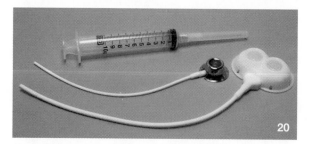

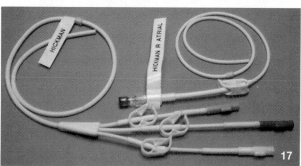

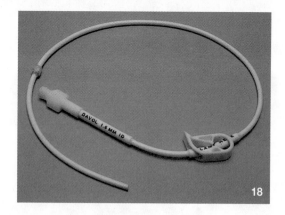

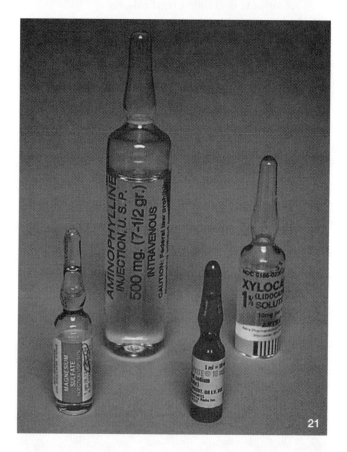

- Cover needle with sheath or cap. Change needle on syringe.
- Dispose of soiled supplies. Place broken ampule in special container for glass.

Prepare Injections from Vial
- Remove metal cap covering top of unused vial. Expose rubber seal.

- Wipe off surface of rubber seal with alcohol swab if vial had been previously opened.
- Take syringe and remove needle cap. Pull back on plunger to draw amount of air into syringe equivalent to volume of medication to be aspirated from vial (28).
- Insert tip of needle, with bevel pointing up, through center of rubber seal.
- Apply pressure to tip of needle during insertion.

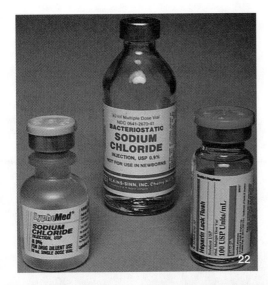

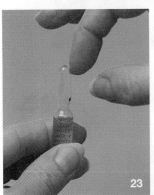
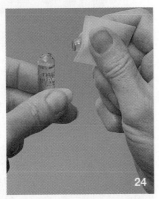

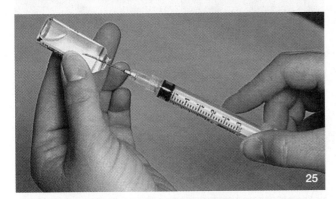

- Inject air into vial, holding onto plunger.
- Invert vial while keeping firm hold on syringe and plunger **(29)**. Hold vial between thumb and middle fingers of nondominant hand. Grasp end of syringe barrel and plunger with thumb and forefinger of dominant hand.
- Clean work area. Wash hands.
- Once again, check fluid level in syringe and compare with desired dose.

Prepare Injections in one Syringe by Mixing Two Vials

- Do not contaminate one medication with another.
- Ensure that the final dosage is accurate.

- Maintain aseptic technique.
- Take a syringe **(30)** and aspirate the volume of air equivalent to the first drug's dosage (vial A).
- Inject air into vial A, making sure that the needle does not touch the solution **(31)**.
- Withdraw the needle, aspirate air equivalent to the second drug's dose (vial B) **(32)**, then inject the volume of air into vial B.
- Immediately withdraw the required medication from vial B into the syringe **(33)**. At this point the drug from vial A has not contaminated vial B. When preparing insulin injections, always withdraw the unmodified (Regular) insulin first.
- Apply a new, sterile needle to the syringe and insert it into vial A, being careful not to push the plunger and expel the drug within the syringe into the vial.
- Withdraw the desired amount of drug from vial A into the syringe **(34)**. (*Note:* If a vial has excess positive pressure, the plunger may begin to move, causing an accidental withdrawal of too much of the drug.)
- Withdraw the needle, apply a new needle, and sheath the syringe.

Injection Sites

- Common sites for SC injections **(35)**. Note how sites might be rotated.
- A comparison of the angles of insertion for IM (90 degrees), SC (90 or 45 degrees), and ID (15 degrees) injections **(36)**. NOTE: SC injections are usually inserted at a 90-degree angle using a 25- to 29-gauge needle that has a length of ⅜, ½, or ⅝ inch. However, institutions may vary on angle (45 or 90 degrees), so always consult the institution's policy. A 45-degree angle is often used in thin or emaciated patients.
- Injection site into the vastus lateralis muscle **(37)**.
- Anatomic view of the site for IM injection into the vastus lateralis muscle **(38)**.
- The vastus lateralis muscle is the site of choice for IM injections for children under 3 years of age. This site is found on the anterior outer aspect in the center third of the thigh **(39)**.
- Injection site into ventrogluteal muscle avoids major nerves and blood vessels **(40)**.
- Anatomic view of ventrogluteal muscle injection site **(41)**.
- Site of injection into the left dorsogluteal muscle **(42)**.
- Imaginary diagonal line extending from the posterior superior iliac spine to the greater trochanter is the landmark for selecting the dorsogluteal injection site **(43)**.
- Site of IM injection into the deltoid muscle **(44)**.
- Site of deltoid muscle injection below acromion process **(45)**.
- The Z-track method of injection prevents the deposit of medication through sensitive tissues **(46)**.
- Administering IM injection by the air-lock technique prevents tracking of medication through SC tissues **(47)**.

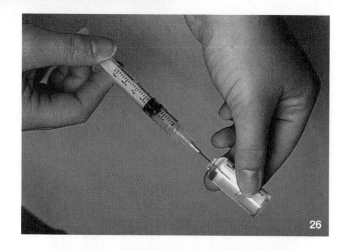

26

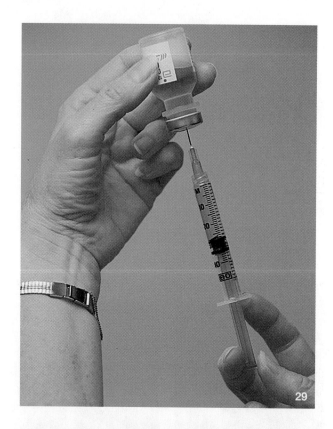

29

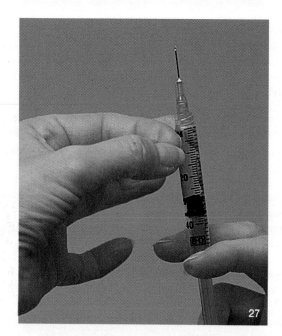

27

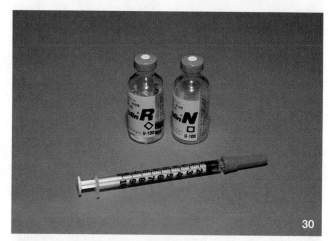

30

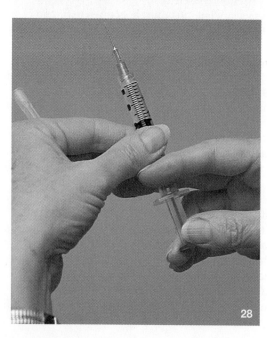

28

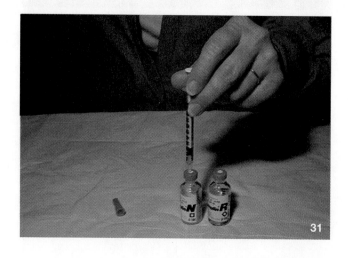

31

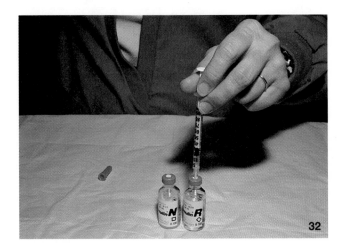

32

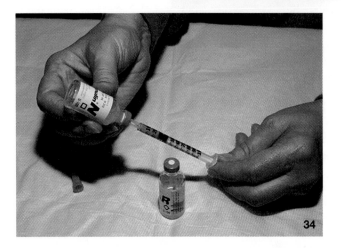

34

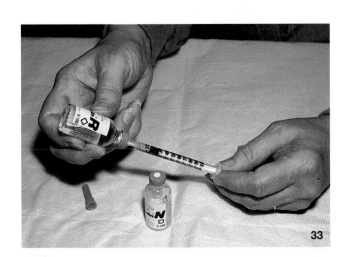

33

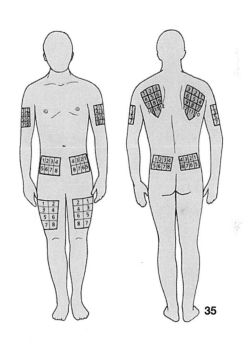

35

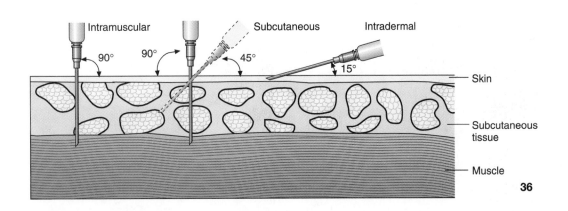

36

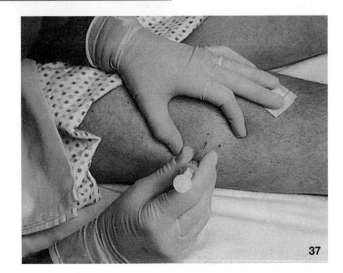

37

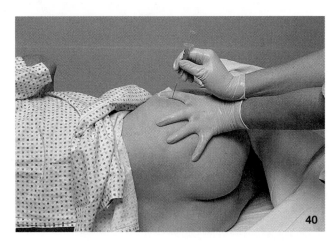

40

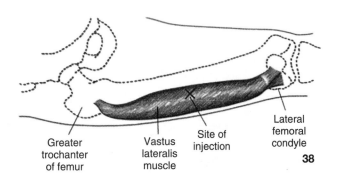

Greater
trochanter
of femur

Vastus
lateralis
muscle

Site of
injection

Lateral
femoral
condyle

38

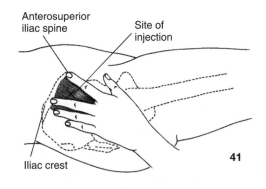

Anterosuperior
iliac spine

Site of
injection

Iliac crest

41

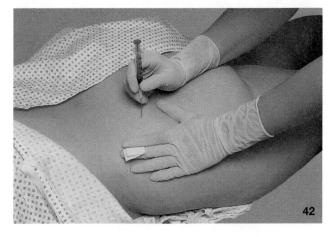

42

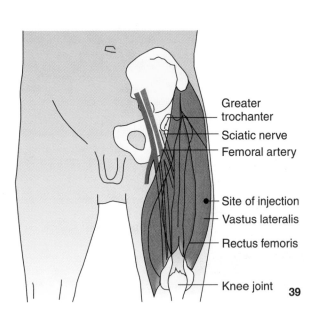

Greater
trochanter

Sciatic nerve

Femoral artery

Site of injection

Vastus lateralis

Rectus femoris

Knee joint **39**

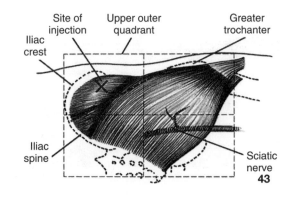

Site of
injection

Upper outer
quadrant

Greater
trochanter

Iliac
crest

Iliac
spine

Sciatic
nerve

43

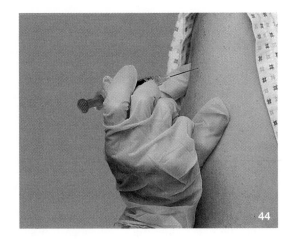

44

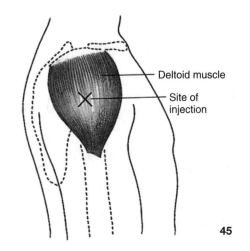

Deltoid muscle

Site of injection

45

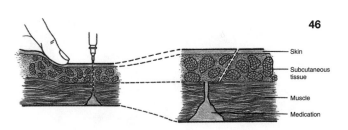

46

Skin

Subcutaneous tissue

Muscle

Medication

47

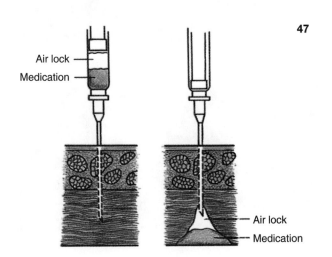

Air lock

Medication

Air lock

Medication

ADMINISTERING PARENTERAL MEDICATIONS

Administering Injections

Always adhere to Standard Precautions, including the following:

- *Wear clean gloves when exposed or when there is potential exposure to blood, body fluids, secretions, excretions, and any items that may contain these substances. Always wash hands immediately when there is direct contact with these substances or any item contaminated with blood, body fluids, secretions, and excretions.*
- *Wash hands after removing gloves and between patient contacts.*
- *Wear masks, eye protective gear, and face shields during any procedure or patient care situation with the potential for splashes or spraying of blood, body fluids, secretions, and excretions. A gown may also be indicated for these situations.*
- *While administering medications (not only parenterally but with all routes) once the exposure or procedure is completed and exposure risk is eliminated or no longer a danger, remove soiled protective garments or gear.*
- *Never remove, recap, cap, bend, or break any used needle or needle system. Make sure to discard any disposable syringes and needles in the appropriate puncture-resistant containers.*
- *If during drug administration you are handling or transporting soiled and contaminated items from the patient, dispose of them in the appropriately labeled containers for contaminated wastes.*

Administering Subcutaneous (SC) and Intramuscular (IM) Injections

- Prepare needed equipment and supplies **(48).**
  1. Proper size syringe
     a. SC: 1 to 2 ml
     b. IM: 2 to 3 ml for adult; 1 to 2 ml for children
  2. Proper size needle:
     a. SC: 25- to 27-gauge and ⅜ to ⅝ inches in length
     b. IM: 18- to 23-gauge and 1 to 1 ½ inches in length for adults; 25- to 27-gauge and ½ to 1 inch in length for children and ⅝ for newborn
  3. Antiseptic swab (Betadine or alcohol)
  4. Disposable gloves
  5. Medication ampule or vial
  6. Medication card, forms, or printouts
- Check medication order again. (Three checks promotes safety!)
- Prepare correct medication dose from ampule or vial **(49).** Check carefully. Be sure all air is expelled. (For IM medications that are particularly irritating to tissues, draw 0.2 cc of air into syringe, being careful not to expel drug dose.)
- For IM injection, change needle if medication is irritating to SC tissue.
- Apply disposable gloves. *Always adhere to Standard Precautions with patient contact.*
- Identify patient by checking identification armband and asking name.

- Explain procedure to patient and proceed in a calm, confident manner.
- Close room curtains or door.
- Keep sheet or gown draped over body parts not requiring exposure.
- Select appropriate injection site. Inspect skin surfaces over sites for bruises, inflammation, or edema.
  1. SC: Palpate sites for masses of tenderness.
  2. IM: Note integrity and size of muscle and palpate for tenderness.
- If injections are given frequently, rotate sites.
- Assist the patient to a comfortable position.
  1. SC: Have patient relax arm, leg, or abdomen, depending on the site chosen.
  2. IM: Have patient lie flat, on side, or prone, or have client sit, depending on site chosen.
- Relocate site using anatomical landmarks.
- Remove antiseptic swab from package **(50)** and cleanse site with swab **(51)**. Apply swab at center of site and rotate outward in circular direction for about 5 cm (2 inches).
- Hold swab between third and fourth fingers of nondominant hand.
- Remove cap from needle by pulling it straight off.
- Hold syringe correctly between thumb and forefinger of dominant hand.
  1. SC: Hold as dart **(52)** at 90-degree angle. (Inject needle at 45-degree angle only if patient is emaciated.)
  2. IM: Hold as dart.
- Administer injection.

1. SC
   a. For average-size patient, spread skin tightly across injection site or pinch skin with nondominant hand.
   b. Inject needle quickly and firmly at 90-degree angle **(53)**. Then release skin if pinched.
   c. For obese patient, pinch skin at site and inject needle below tissue fold.
2. IM
   a. Position nondominant hand at proper anatomic landmarks and spread skin tightly **(54)**. Inject needle quickly at 90-degree angle into muscle.
   b. If client's muscle mass is small, grasp body of muscle between thumb and other fingers.
   c. If medication is irritating, use Z-track method.
- After needle enters site, grasp lower end of syringe barrel with nondominant hand. Move dominant hand to end of plunger. Avoid moving syringe while slowly pulling back on plunger to aspirate drug. If blood appears in syringe, remove needle, discard medication and syringe, and repeat procedure.
- Inject medication slowly.
- Withdraw needle while applying alcohol swab gently above or over injection site.
- Massage skin lightly. (Do not massage with subcu heparin!)
- Assist patient to comfortable position.
- Discard unsheathed needle and attached syringe into appropriately labeled receptacles.
- Remove disposable gloves. Wash hands.
- Chart medication dose, route, site and time, and date given in medication record. Correctly sign according to institutional policy.

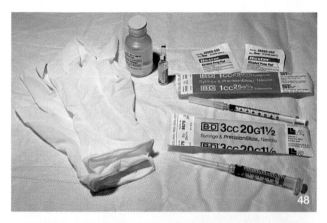

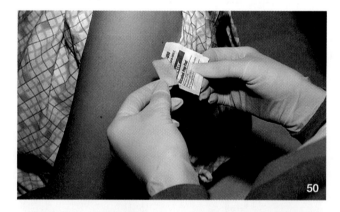

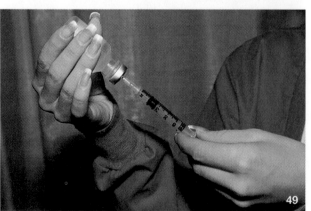

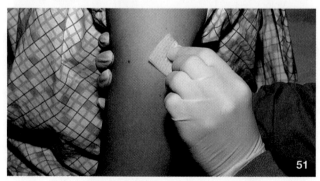

Administering Intradermal (ID) Injections

- Prepare needed equipment and supplies.
  1. Proper size syringe: 1 ml tuberculin
  2. Proper size needle: preattached 26- to 27-gauge
  3. Antiseptic swab (Betadine or alcohol)
  4. Disposable gloves
  5. Medication ampule or vial
  6. Medication card, forms, or printouts
- Check medication order again. (Three checks promotes safety!)
- Prepare correct medication dose from ampule or vial. Check carefully. Be sure all air is expelled.
- Apply disposable gloves. (*Note: always adhere to Standard Precautions with patient contact. See discussion on p. 95*)
- Identify patient by checking identification armband and asking name.
- Explain procedure to patient and proceed in a calm, confident manner.
- Close room curtains or door.
- Keep sheet or gown draped over body parts not requiring exposure.
- Select appropriate injection site. Inspect skin surfaces over sites for bruises, inflammation, or edema. Note lesions or discoloration of forearm.
- If injections are given frequently, rotate sites.
- Assist patient to comfortable position. Have patient extend elbow and support it and forearm on flat surface.
- Relocate site using anatomic landmarks.
- Cleanse site with antiseptic swab. Apply swab at center of site and rotate outward in circular direction for about 5 cm (2 inches).
- Hold swab between third and fourth fingers of nondominant hand.
- Remove cap from needle by pulling it straight off.
- Hold syringe correctly between thumb and forefinger of dominant hand **(55)**. Hold bevel of needle pointing up.
- Administer injection.
  1. With nondominant hand, stretch skin over site with forefinger or thumb.
  2. With needle almost against client's skin, insert it slowly at 5- to 15-degree angle until resistance is felt. Then advance needle through epidermis to approximately 3 mm (⅛ inch) below surface. Needle tip can be seen through skin.
- Inject medication slowly. It is normal to feel resistance; if not, needle is too deep.
- Note formation of a small bleb on skin's surface **(56).**

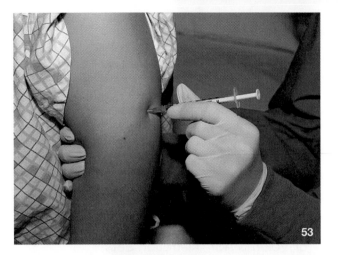

53

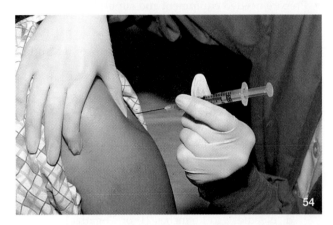

54

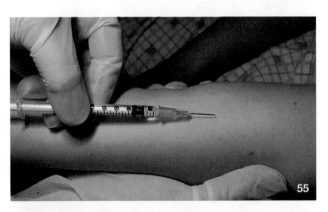

55

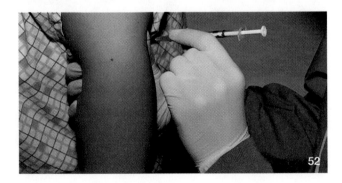

52

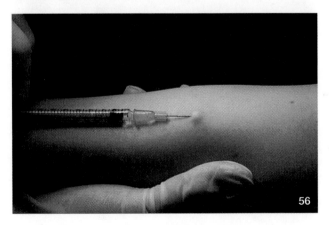

56

- Withdraw needle while applying alcohol swab gently above or over injection site.
- OPTIONAL: Apply bandage. *Do not massage site.*
- Assist patient to comfortable position.
- Discard unsheathed needle and attached syringe into appropriately labeled receptacles.
- Remove disposable gloves. Wash hands.
- Draw circle around perimeter of injection site with skin pencil.
- Record areas of injection, amount and type of testing substance, and date and time on medication record **(57)**.

Administering Intravenous (IV) Medications

Administering IV Medications by Piggyback or Volume Administration Sets

- Prepare needed equipment and supplies:
  1. Piggyback set
     a. Medication prepared in a 50 to 100 ml labeled infusion bag with IV line, microdrip, or macrodrip infusion tubing set
     b. Needle (21- or 23-gauge)
     c. Adhesive tape (optional)
     d. Antiseptic swab
     e. Metal hook (optional)
     f. Disposable gloves
  2. Volume-control administration set
     a. Volutrol, Pediatrol, or Burette
     b. Infusion tubing
     c. Syringe (5 to 20 ml)
     d. Needle (1 to 1.5 inches 21- or 23-gauge)
     e. Vial or ampule of ordered medication
     f. Medication label

- Wash hands and apply gloves.
- Administer medications by piggyback set.
  1. Assemble supplies at bedside.
  2. Connect infusion tubing to medication bag. Allow solution to fill tubing by opening regulator flow clamp.
  3. Hang medication bag at or above level of main fluid bag. Hook may be used to lower main bag **(58)**.
  4. Connect covered sterile needle to end of infusion tubing.
  5. Check patient's identification by looking at armband and asking name.
  6. Clean injection Y-port of main line with antiseptic swab.
  7. Remove cover and insert needle of secondary piggyback line through injection port of main line. Secure with strip of adhesive tape if necessary. If available, use needle-lock devices to secure needle of secondary piggyback line through injection port of main line **(59, 60, 61)**.
- Administer medication by volume-control administration set (e.g., Volutrol).
  1. Assemble supplies in medication room.
  2. Prepare medication from vial or ampule.
  3. Check patient's identification by looking at armband and asking name.
  4. Fill Volutrol with desired amount of fluid (50 to 100 ml) by opening, clamp between Volutrol and main IV bag **(62)**.
  5. Close clamp and check to be sure clamp in air vent of Volutrol chamber is open.
  6. Clean injection port on top of Volutrol with antiseptic swab.

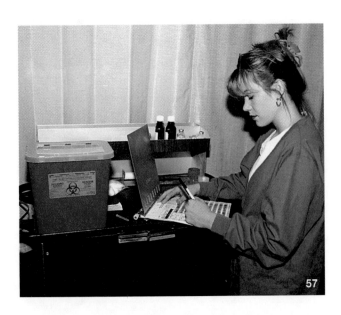

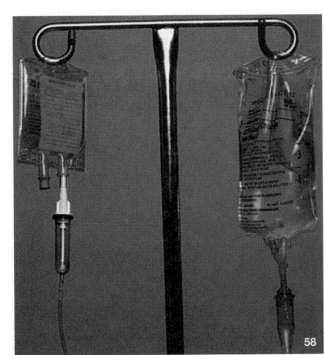

7. Remove needle cap and insert syringe needle through port and then inject medication **(63).** Gently rotate Volutrol between hands.

8. Regulate IV infusion rate appropriate for medication. Follow physician, pharmacist, or manufacturer recommendations for infusion rates. Label Volutrol with name of drug, dose, total volume including diluent, and time of administration.

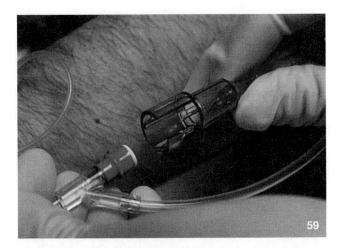

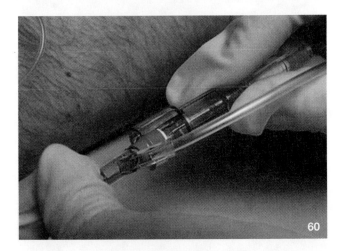

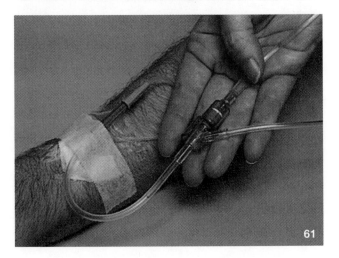

9. Dispose of uncapped needle and syringe in proper container.

- Remove and dispose of gloves. Wash hands. Document.
- Record drug, dose, route, and time administered on medication form. Record volume of fluid in medication bag or Volutrol on intake and output form.

Administering Medications by IV Bolus (Push)

- Prepare needed equipment and supplies.
  1. IV push (existing line)
     a. Medication in vial or ampule
     b. Syringe (3 to 5 ml)
     c. Sterile needles (21- and 25-gauge)
     d. Antiseptic swab
     e. Watch with second hand or digital readout
  2. IV push (IV lock)
     a. Medication in vial or ampule
     b. Syringe (3 to 5 ml)
     c. Syringe (3 ml)
     d. Vial of heparin flush solution (1 ml = 100 units or 1 ml = 10 units) or vial of normal saline (depending on agency policy)
     e. Sterile needles (21- and 25-gauge)
     f. Antiseptic swab
     g. Watch with second hand or digital readout
     h. Disposable gloves
- Wash hands. Apply gloves.
- After preparing medication, apply small-gauge needle to syringe.

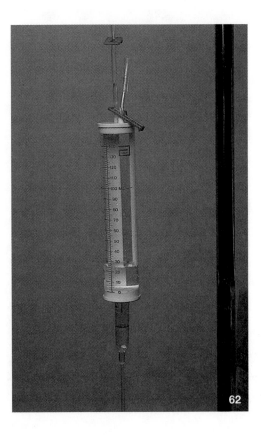

- Administer medication by IV push (existing line).
  1. Check patient's identification by looking at armband and asking name.
  2. Select injection port of IV tubing closest to patient (64). (Circle on port may indicate site for needle insertion.)
  3. Clean off injection port with antiseptic swab (65).
  4. Insert small-gauge needle of syringe containing prepared drug through center of port (66).
  5. Occlude IV line by pinching tubing just above injection port (67). Pull back gently on syringe's plunger to aspirate for blood return.
  6. After noting blood return, inject medication slowly over several minutes or as indicated. The IV tubing above the injection site is clamped off. (Read directions on drug package). Use watch to time administration.
  7. After injecting medication, release tubing, withdraw syringe, and recheck fluid infusion rate.
- Administer medications by IV push (IV lock).
  1. Check patient's identification by looking at armband and asking full name.
  2. Heparin flush:
     a. Prepare syringe with 1 ml of heparin flush solution.
     b. Prepare syringe with 3 ml of normal saline. Attach 25-gauge needle to syringe.
  3. Saline only:
     Prepare 2 syringes with 2 ml of normal saline each. Attach 25-gauge needle to each syringe.
  4. Heparin and saline:
     a. Clean lock's rubber diaphragm with antiseptic swab.

  b. Insert needle of syringe containing normal saline through center of diaphragm. Pull back gently on syringe plunger and look for blood return.
  c. Flush reservoir with 1 ml saline by pushing slowly on plunger.
  d. Remove needle and saline-filled syringe.
  e. Clean lock's diaphragm with antiseptic swab.
  f. Insert needle of syringe containing prepared drug through center of diaphragm (68).
  g. Inject medication bolus slowly over several minutes. (Each medication has recommended rate

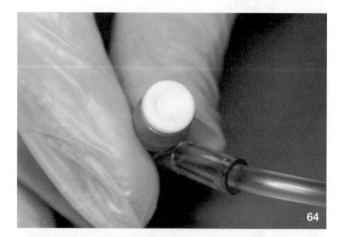

64

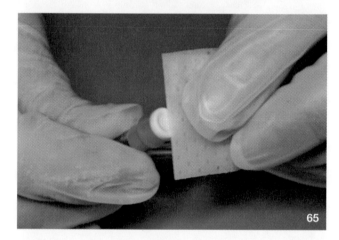

65

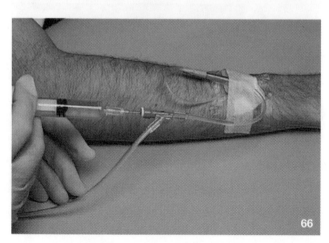

66

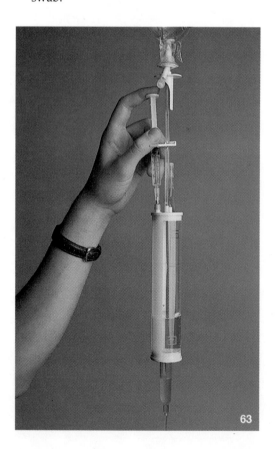

63

for bolus administration. Check package directions.) Use watch to time administration.

  h. After administering bolus, withdraw syringe.

  i. Clean lock's diaphragm with antiseptic swab.

  j. Repeat injection of 1 ml of normal saline.

  k. *Heparin flush:* Insert needle of syringe containing heparin through diaphragm. Inject heparin slowly, and remove syringe.

  l. *Saline flush:* If using only saline to flush reservoir, use 2 ml of saline before and after each use of IV lock.

- Dispose of uncapped needles and syringes in proper receptacle.
- Remove and dispose of gloves and sharps. Wash hands. Document.
- Record drug, dose, route, and time administered on medication form. Also note adverse reactions. (NOTE: Institutions may use needle-less systems; consult manufacturer's guidelines and instructions.)

Adding Medications to IV Fluid Containers

- Prepare needle equipment and supplies.
  1. Vial or ampule of prescribed medication
  2. Syringe of appropriate size (5 to 20 ml)
  3. Sterile needle (1 to 1½ in, 19- to 21-gauge) with special filters (optional)
  4. Correct solvent (e.g., sterile water or normal saline)

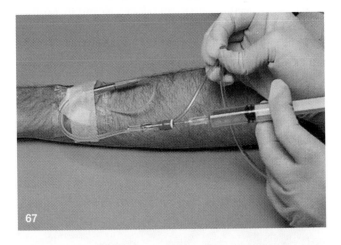

67

  5. Sterile IV fluid container (bag or bottle, 500 to 1000 ml in volume)
  6. Alcohol or antiseptic swab
  7. Label to attach to IV bag or bottle
- Wash hands thoroughly.
- Assemble supplies in medication room.
- Prepare prescribed medication from vial or ampule. With an ampule, use a filter needle. Replace it with regular needle before injecting medication into IV fluid container.
- Identify patient by reading identification band and asking name.
- Prepare patient by explaining that medication is to be given through existing IV line or one to be started. Explain that no discomfort should be felt during infusion. Encourage patient to report symptoms of discomfort.
- Add medication to new container.
  1. Locate medication injection port on IV solution bag. Remove plastic cover over port. Port has small rubber stopper at end. Do not select port for IV tubing insertion or air vent.
  2. Locate injection site on IV solution bottle.
     a. Remove metal or plastic cap and rubber disk. Place cap upside down on counter top.
     b. Locate medication injection site on bottle's rubber stopper. Site is usually marked by X, circle, or triangle.
  3. Wipe off port or injection site with alcohol or antiseptic swab **(69)**.
  4. Remove needle cap from syringe and insert needle of syringe through center of injection port or site and inject medication **(70)**.
  5. Withdraw syringe from bag or bottle **(71)**. Cover glass bottle top with antiseptic swab and sterile bottle cap.
  6. Mix medication and IV solution by holding bag or bottle and turning it gently end to end **(72)**.
  7. Complete medication label with name and dose of medication, date, time, and your initials. Stick it upside down on bottle or bag.
  8. Spike bag or bottle with IV tubing **(73)** and hang. Regulate infusion at ordered rate.
- Add medication to existing container.
  1. Prepare vented IV bottle or plastic bag.
     a. Check volume of solution remaining in bottle.

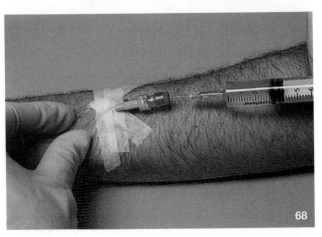

68

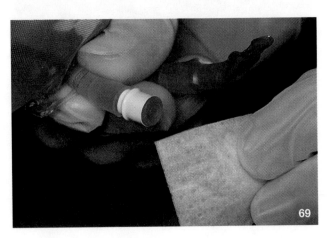

69

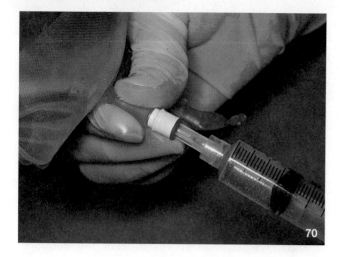

70

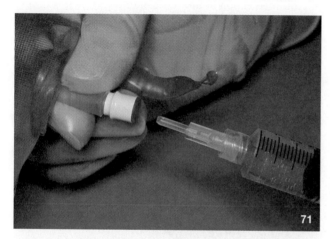

71

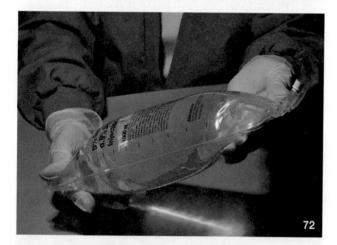

72

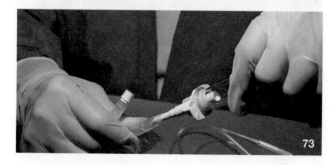

73

b. Verify dilution of medication desired (amount of medication per milliliter).

c. Close off IV infusion clamp.

d. Wipe medication port with alcohol or antiseptic swab.

e. Lower bag or bottle from IV pole. Insert syringe needle through injection port and inject medication.

f. Gently mix bottle or bag.

g. Rehang bag and regulate infusion to desired rate.

2. Complete medication label and stick it to bag or bottle.

• Properly dispose of equipment and supplies and chart appropriate places in patient's chart.

• Record solution and medication added to parenteral fluid on appropriate form.

Initiation of Patient-Controlled Analgesia (PCA)

• Once you have verified the physician's order, check to see what is available on the unit and be sure to have all tubing, medication needed (checking calculations), filters, syringes, patent IV, and pump (with appropriate and functioning parts and equipment) at the bedside **(74).** Note that there are various models used for PCA; shown here is one example.

• Always identify the patient before administering any medication or procedure, and recheck for the 5 "Rs" of medication administration. In addition, explain to the patient everything that will take place and its purpose and how this will help in the management of pain.

• Make sure you snap off the caps of the plunger or the injector piece and the prefilled vial. Connect the injector to the prefilled vial. This can be done with most pumps by screwing them together **(75).**

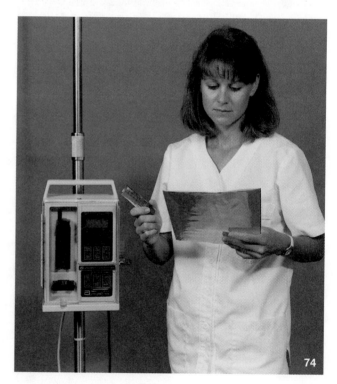

74

- You must prime and remove all air from the pump and all of the corresponding equipment by pushing down on the injector **(76).**
- Attach the female connector found on the long end of the PCA tubing to the male end of the injector located in the vial **(77).**
- It is then recommended to flush the tubing up to the Y-branch or Y-injection site at the backcheck valve port. It is important to remember that flushing ALL the tubing would cause an excess dose of IV narcotic to be administered when first attached to the patient. Once this is completed, close off the slide clamp located on the PCA tubing **(78).**
- You may now activate the drive release mechanism of the machine after you have opened the machine door and pinched the spring-loading device **(79).**
- Now load the vial of medication into the space provided. Be sure to clamp it securely into place and then pinch the drive release mechanism AGAIN by pinching the spring-loaded level and slide it down until it locks into place. It is important to remember that you may hear a "CLICK" once the flange of the injector or syringe locks **(80, 81).** Close the door to the pump and plug it into a safe outlet in the patient's room, unless battery-driven operation is needed.
- Once you are in the patient's room, remove the protective cap from the Y-site of the PCA tubing and connect it (keeping ends sterile) to the distal end of the patient's IV (maintenance fluids for patient) fluid tubing **(82).**
- You must now prime (clear the tubing of all air) the remainder of the PCA tubing using the roller clamp on the maintenance tubing infusion to control and regulate flow **(83).**
- You are now ready to attach the male end of the PCA tubing to the female end of the patient's connector tubing and open all slide clamps on the main IV infusion tubing, PCA tubing, and the patient's connector tubing. In some cases the PCA tubing may fit directly into the patient's angiocath hub site. If you have any questions, consult a procedure manual or contact the IV team for assistance.
- At this time you may want to press the ON/OFF button on the IV pump. Several messages will appear **(84, 85)** such as DOOR OPEN, VOLUME DELIVERED, CHECK SYRINGE, ALARM (especially if the injector is not positioned or secured properly.) FOUR-HOUR DOSE LIMIT will appear once the machine is turned on. Set the

FOUR-HOUR DOSE LIMIT as prescribed by the patient's physician. This represents the maximum amount of medication the patient can receive in a 4-hour period and as prescribed in the designated INCREMENTS of 50 cc (such as 1 cc every 10 minutes or 20 cc limit within 4 hours). If a loading dose has been prescribed by the physician, use the LOCKOUT LIMIT setting and place at 00 minutes. Then, using the DOSE VOLUME setting, dial in the prescribed volume to be delivered and press LOADING DOSE. The volume will appear on the pump's screen. If there is no loading dose ordered, use the setting DOSE VOLUME and put in the prescribed amount in tenths of a cc and use the LOCKOUT INTERVAL for the interval between doses given in minutes. Remember that 9 minutes will be designated as 09 and 15 minutes as 15.

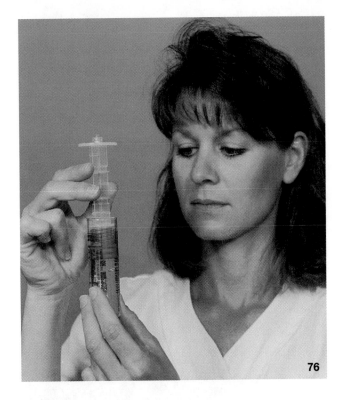

76

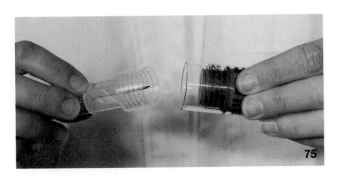

75

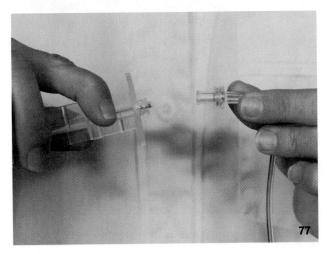

77

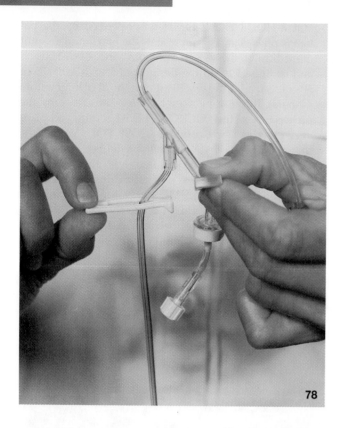

78

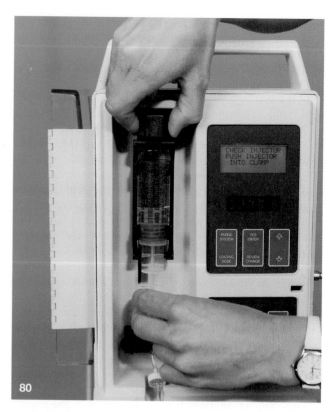

80

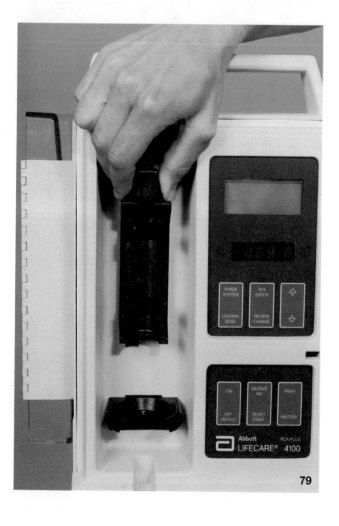

79

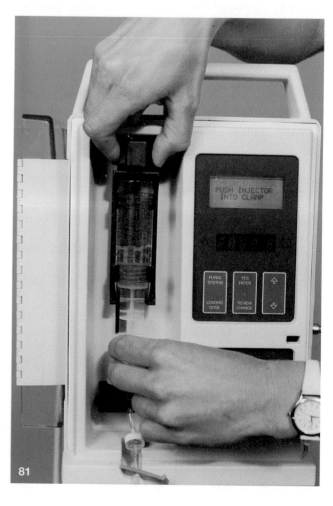

81

- Once these steps have been implemented, the pump's door is closed and locked securely and agency protocol regarding use of this equipment, documentation, and use of narcotics has been followed, write the time and date when the medication vial was inserted on a piece of tape or provided tag, and place in a visible area of the pump for the benefit of co-workers and for patient safety (document appropriate notes in the chart and medication administration record [MAR] as well).
- Provide instructions to the patient and attach the hand-held control button to the siderail or area of convenient access to the patient. Have the patient do a mock demonstration for you **(86)**. A READY message on the pump signals that it is in the patient mode and the first dose is available. Once the patient presses the button, a beep is heard acknowledging request and READY will disappear once the dose is delivered. Reemphasize these points to the patient.

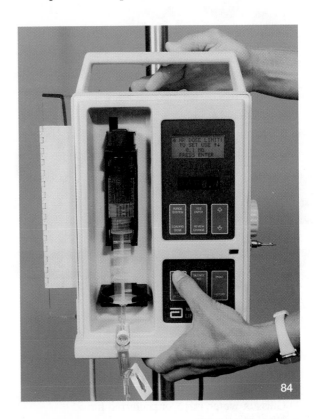

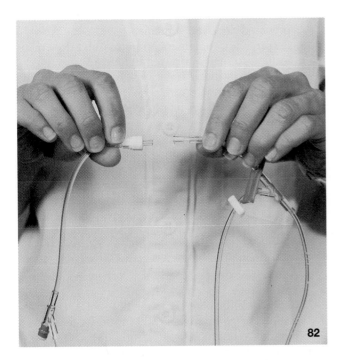

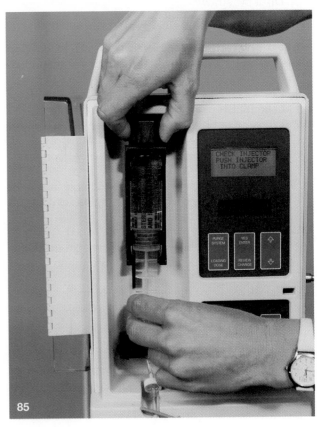

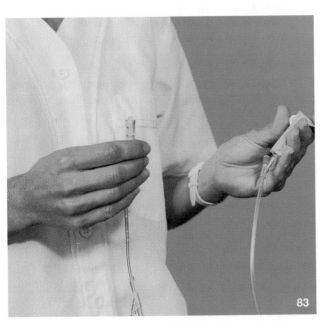

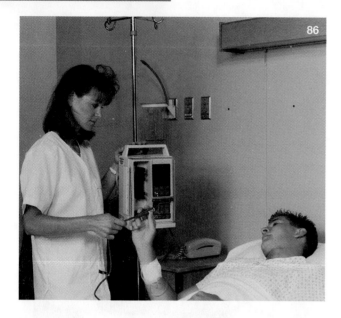

ENTERAL ADMINISTRATION

ADMINISTERING ORAL MEDICATIONS: LIQUIDS
Adult or Child

- Prepare needed equipment and supplies.
  1. Medication cards, record forms, or printout
  2. Medication cart or tray
  3. Disposable medication cups
  4. Glass of water, juice, or preferred liquid
  5. Drinking straw
  6. Syringe without needle
  7. Paper towels
- Check accuracy and completeness of each medication card, form, or printout with physician's written medication order.
  1. Check patient's name and drug name, dosage, route of administration, and time for administration.
  2. When preparing narcotic, check narcotic record for previous drug count, compare with supply available, remove drug, complete necessary information on narcotic form, and sign.
  3. Report discrepancy in order to charge nurse or physician. (Three checks to five "rights" of drug administration enhance safety.)
- Wash hands and prepare drug.
  1. Arrange medication tray and cups in medicine room or move medication cart to position outside patient's room.
  2. Unlock medicine drawer or cart. (Narcotics are generally stored in double-locked box separate from medicine drawers or carts.)
  3. Prepare medications for one patient at a time. Keep medication tickets or forms for each patient together.
  4. Select correct drug from stock supply or unit-dose drawer Compare label of medication with medication form, card, or printout.
  5. Calculate correct drug dose. Take time. Double check calculation.

- Prepare liquids (87).
  1. Remove bottle cap from container and place cap upside down.
  2. Hold bottle with label against palm of hand while pouring.
  3. Hold medication cup at eye level and fill to desired level on scale (88). (Scale should be even with fluid level at its surface or base of meniscus, not edges.)
  4. Discard excess liquid in cup into sink. Wipe lip of bottle with paper towel.
  5. Draw volumes of less than 10 ml in syringe (without needle). To prevent accidental ingestion during administration, never use needle to draw up oral medication.
  6. Dilute medication as recommended by manufacturer.
  7. Compare medication form, card, or printout with prepared drug and container.
  8. Return stock containers or unused unit-dose medications to shelf or drawer and reread label.
  9. Place medications and cards, forms, or printouts together on tray or cart.
  10. Do not leave drugs unattended.
- Administer medications.
  1. Take medications to patient at correct time (89).
  2. Identify patient by comparing name on card, form, or printout with name on patient's identification bracelet. Ask client to state full name.
  3. Perform necessary preadmistration assessment for specific medications (e.g., blood pressure or pulse).
  4. Explain purpose of each medication and its action to patient. Allow patient to ask questions about drugs.
  5. Assist patient to sitting or side-lying position.
  6. Administer drug properly and adhere to Standard Precautions.
  7. If patient is unable to hold medications, place medication cup to lips and gently introduce liquid into mouth. Do not rush.
  8. Stay with patient until medication has been swallowed. If uncertain whether medication has been swallowed, ask patient to open mouth.
  9. Assist the patient in returning to a comfortable position.
- Dispose of soiled supplies and wash hands.
- Return medication cards, forms, or printouts to appropriate file for next administration time.
- Replenish stock such as cups and straws, return cart to medicine room, and clean work area.

Infant

- Since infants cannot take oral pills or capsules, liquids are usually ordered. For administration of liquids to infants, note the following considerations:
  1. A plastic disposable syringe is recommended for measuring small amounts of medications.
  2. Position infant so that the head is at least slightly elevated (90) to prevent aspiration. Not all infants will be cooperative, and many may need safe securing.
  3. Place plastic dropper or syringe inside infant's mouth next to the tongue and administer in small amounts while allowing the infant to swallow as needed. (*Note:*

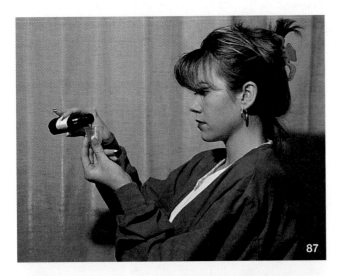

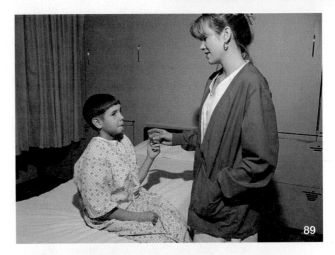

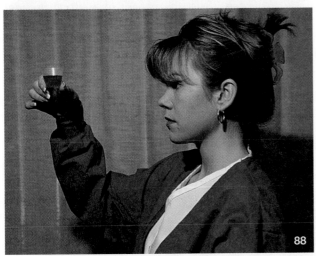

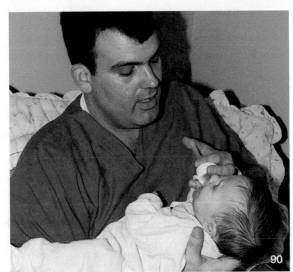

If desired, allow infant to suck medication placed inside an empty nipple from a bottle or insert syringe or dropper parallel to nipple to elicit sucking response.) Rinse with only a few milliliters of water unless contraindicated. Be sure all the medication is used.
4. Adhere to Standard Precautions (see discussion on p. 95).
5. After making sure all oral medicine has been taken, return infant to a safe, comfortable position. Complete documentation as necessary.

ADMINISTERING ORAL MEDICATIONS: CAPSULES AND TABLETS

- Prepare needed equipment and supplies **(91).**
  1. Medication forms, record forms, or printout
  2. Medication cart or tray
  3. Disposable medication cups
  4. Glass of water, juice, or preferred liquid
  5. Drinking straw
  6. Pill crusher or mortar and pestle
  7. Paper towels
- Assess the patient's medication profile, and compare it with the physician's order and patient's identification band. Assess for accuracy and completeness of the order.

1. When preparing a narcotic, always check narcotic record and documentation for previous drug counts. Be sure to compare the supply available with what should be available based on the latest count. Complete the necessary information on the narcotic documentation sheet, and regardless of institution, always follow the specific guidelines for administration of narcotics and narcotic sign outs. If an automated system is used, follow institutional policy for dispensing narcotics.
2. Once the count is confirmed to be accurate (always count with another nurse), check patient's name, drug name, dosage, route of administration, and time for administration against the order. Report any discrepancy in the order to the nurse in charge, a registered nurse, or a nurse supervisor.
- Wash your hands, maintain Standard Precautions (see p. 95), and prepare the drug.
  1. Only prepare one medication at a time for one patient, not multiple patients. Avoid using a tray of medications for multiple patients; this will help prevent medication errors.
  2. For an automated system, unlock or access the patient's medication drawer. After obtaining the right drug, check the drug, use the five rights of drug administration, and check three times against the

medication order. Check the label of the medication and the medication profile against the order. If mathematic calculations are necessary, be careful in the process and always double-check your calculations.

3. Look up information on the medication if you are the least bit unfamiliar with the drug.

- Administer medication.

1. Place required number of capsules or tablets into a medication cup, being careful not to touch the medication with your hands **(92).** Leaving them in their packaging until you get into the patient's room is often recommended to avoid contamination and wasting of medication should the patient refuse the medication.

2. Ensure that medications that require special nursing assessments, such as digitalis medications (need to take apical pulse for 1 full minute and document pulse rate), are placed in a separate medication cup to remind you of special assessment. This also applies to situations where blood pressure measurement is needed.

3. If the patient is experiencing difficulty swallowing (dysphagia), crush and grind tablets with a mortar and pestle and make sure that they are completely crushed into very minute fragments. If a mortar and pestle are not available, you may use a medication crusher, which is available at most outpatient pharmacies **(93-95),** or you may use two medication cups and crush the medication between the cups. Mix the crushed medication in a small amount of food, such as applesauce, pudding, or ice cream. Wash out the

container after use. CAUTION: Do not crush enteric-coated or sustained- or long-release tablets or capsules (these medications often have the abbreviations EC, LA, SA, SR).

4. While preparing a narcotic, check count as mentioned above.

5. Once the medications are ready to administer, place all stock containers or unused unit-dose medications to the shelf or patient's medication drawer. Re-read and check the order against the label when placing medications back into the patient's drawer. Never leave medications unattended.

6. Take medications to the patient's room, and explain the purpose of each medication, its action, possible side effects, and any other pertinent information, such as drug-drug or drug-food interactions. This is particularly important for oral medications.

7. If needed, assist the patient to a sitting or side-lying position. This is the most cautious and safe positioning for patients taking oral substances.

8. Administer medications safely, and always adhere to Standard Precautions, regardless of route (see p. 95).

   a. Ask the patient if he or she wishes to self-administer solid or liquid medications. If the patient requests, you may place the solid medication in his or her mouth using gloves. If you are placing the oral solid medication on the patient's tongue or to the buccal area, be sure to always take your time and not rush the patient.

   b. Offer the patient a full glass of water or other fluids (check interactions with juices for specific

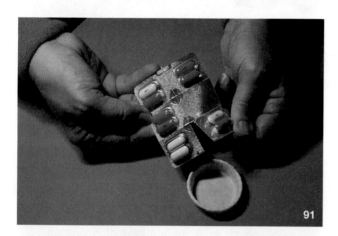

91

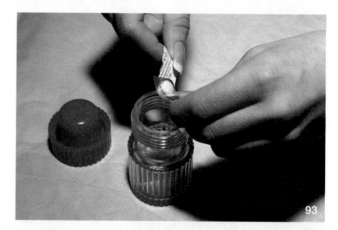

93

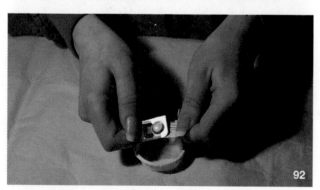

92

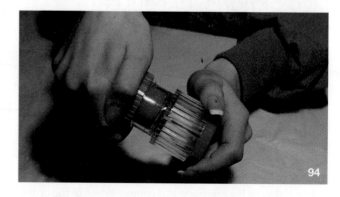

94

oral medications). Four to six ounces of water or fluid is recommended for the best dissolution and absorption.

c. Sublingual medications should be placed under the tongue **(96).** In most cases (e.g., nitroglycerine) the drug should be allowed to completely dissolve before swallowing. This should be explained to the patient. This route of medication administration should not include taking fluids with the medication.

d. For buccal medications, the medication should be placed between the upper molar teeth and cheek area, and the patient is often instructed, depending on the medication, not to swallow until the medication is completely dissolved. Do not use with fluids.

e. Powdered medications should be given with liquids and followed with liquids to ensure that the medication has been completely swallowed.

f. Lozenges should not be chewed unless specifically instructed.

g. Effervescent powders and tablets are mixed with water or fluids and should be given immediately after they are dissolved.

9. Discard any medications that should fall to the floor or become contaminated by other means.

10. Remain with the patient until all medication has been swallowed. Ask the patient to open his or her mouth so you can inspect to see that all medication is gone.

11. Once the medication has been taken, return the patient to a comfortable position with the call light or bell at bedside and the side rails up.

- Dispose of all contaminated or soiled items and supplies, and be sure to wash your hands. Return the medication profile to the medication cart or automated dispensing system. Always consider your colleagues by leaving the medication drawer or cabinet stocked appropriately. Document as needed in the nurse's notes, and be sure to sign off that you gave the dose of medication on the medication profile. Document therapeutic responses, adverse effects, and any other problems.

ADMINISTERING MEDICATIONS VIA A NASOGASTRIC (NG) TUBE

- Gather all equipment needed for the procedure such as a large bulb or piston syringe, an emesis basin, protective blue pad, towels, 30 to 60 cc tap water, and disposable gloves. Adhere to Standard Precautions (see p. 95).

1. Identify your patient and position with head of the bed elevated. Place protective pad under patient's head and on the chest area.

2. FOR SMALL-BORE TUBES, after obtaining and setting-up a piston syringe of at least 10 to 20 cc in volume (to minimize pressure and damage to the tube) **(97),** confirm placement of tube (confirmed for the first time by radiology). (*Note:* After the position of the

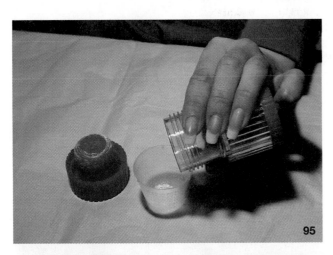

95

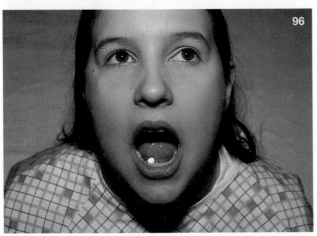

96

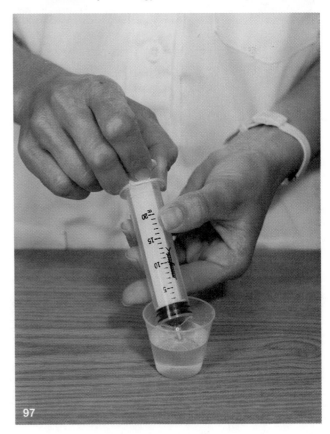

97

NG tube has been confirmed [98], a three-way stop-cock may be used to help control flow of solution.)

- Attach the small medication syringe to the tube after it has been uncapped and infuse the medication while applying gentle pressure on the syringe's piston (99). Once medication is instilled, flush with approximately 10 cc tap water. Cap the tube with the plug and position patient in a high-Fowler's position or a slightly elevated right side-lying position.

- With large-bore NG tubes, leave medication in the medication cup and confirm placement of the tube. With the piston removed from the syringe, uncap the NG tube, pour in 30 cc of water to clear tubing, and pour the medication from the dosage cup into the barrel of the syringe, followed by 30 cc of tap water to ensure that the medication is cleared from the tube. ALWAYS allow any fluid to flow via gravity in the NG tubes—NEVER force any fluid into the tube (100).

- Once completed, close the tube with the cap and position patient in high-Fowler's position or slightly elevated right side-lying position (101).

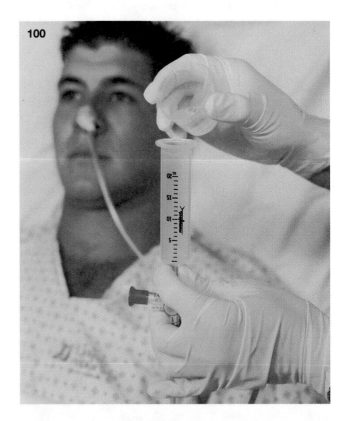

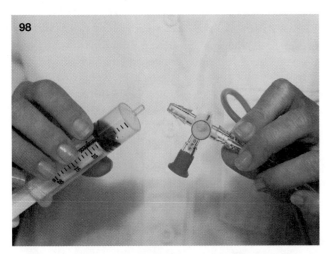

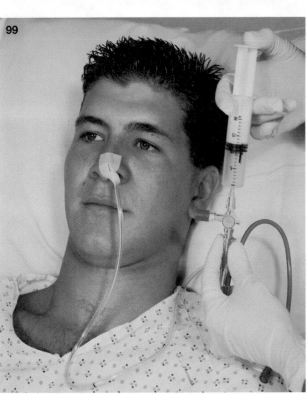

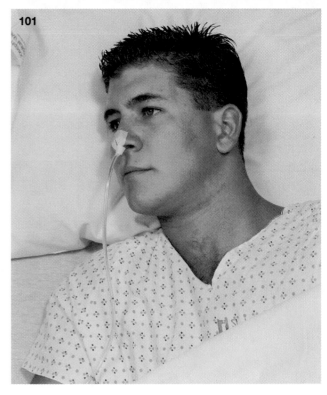

ADMINISTERING RECTAL SUPPOSITORIES

- Prepare needed equipment and supplies.
  1. Rectal suppository (102)
  2. Water-soluble lubricant
  3. Finger cot or gloves
  4. Patient drape
  5. Medication card, forms, or printout
  6. Medication cart
  7. Disposable gloves
- Check accuracy and completeness of each medication card with physician's order. Check patient's name, drug name, route, dose, and time.
- Wash hands and prepare drug. Arrange medication and prepare medication for one patient at a time.
- Administer medication.
  1. Explain procedure to patient.
  2. Provide privacy and drape.
  3. Have patient defecate, if possible.
  4. Position patient on left side unless contraindicated (103).
  5. Use finger cot or gloves (index finger for adult or fourth finger for infants).

6. Patient should bend the uppermost leg toward the waist.
7. Apply a small amount of water-soluble lubricant to an unwrapped suppository (104).
8. Insert tip of the suppository into the rectum while having the patient take a deep breath and exhale through the mouth.
9. Gently insert suppository about 1 inch past the internal sphincter (beyond orifice) (105).
10. Have the patient remain lying on left side for 15 to 20 minutes to allow absorption of the medication.
11. With children, it may be necessary to gently but firmly hold the buttocks in place for 15 to 20 minutes to prevent expulsion.

- Remove disposable gloves and wash hands thoroughly.
- Chart medication dose, route, site and time, and date in medication record. Correctly sign according to institutional policy.

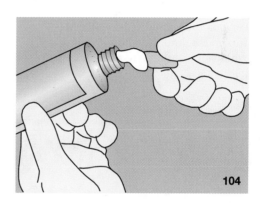

104

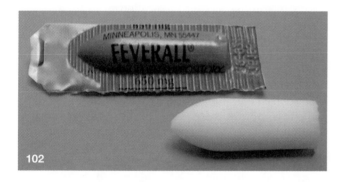

102

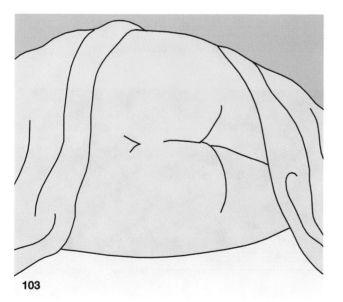

103

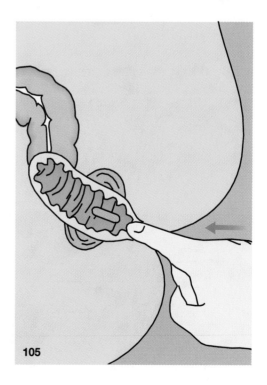

105

ADMINISTERING DISPOSABLE ENEMAS

- Prepare needed equipment and supplies.
  1. Water-soluble lubricant
  2. Wash cloth and towel
  3. Chux or underpad
  4. Patient drape
  5. Enema kit or package
  6. Bedpan or access to bathroom
  7. Medication card, forms, or printout
  8. Medication cart
  9. Disposable gloves
- Check accuracy and completeness of each medication card with physician's order. Check patient's name, drug name, route, dose, and time.
- Wash hands and prepare drug.
- Administer medication.
  1. Explain procedure to patient
  2. Provide privacy and drape
  3. Position patient on left side (106).
  4. Put on gloves, remove protective covering from rectal enema tube, and lubricate (107).
  5. Insert enema into the rectum.
  6. Administer solution by compressing plastic container (108).

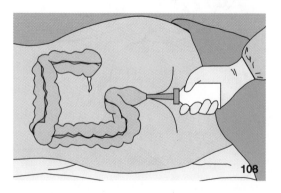

106

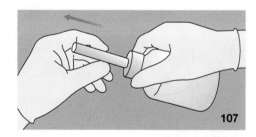

107

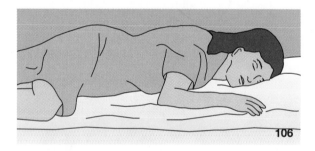

108

  7. Encourage patient to hold solution for at least 30 minutes before defecating.
  8. Assist patient with a bedpan or to the bathroom.
  9. Tell patient not to flush the toilet until results are checked by the nurse.
- Remove disposable gloves and wash hands thoroughly.
- Chart medication dose, route, site and time, and date in medication record. Correctly sign according to institutional policy.

PERCUTANEOUS ADMINISTRATION

INSTILLING OPHTHALMIC MEDICATIONS

Administering Ointment

- Gather medication (109) and all necessary equipment such as sterile 2 × 2 gauze. Gather gloves.
- Put on gloves and adhere to Standard Precautions (see p. 95). Position patient in either a sitting or supine position and place the head so that it is slightly tilted back. Remove any secretions from the eye by wiping the area with a sterile 2 × 2 gauze from inner to outer canthus. Have the patient look upward, and instill the medication into the conjunctival sac by exerting only gentle traction to keep the conjunctival sac open. Gently squeeze the tube of medication to instill an even strip (about 1 to 2 cm) of medication along the border of the conjunctival sac starting at the inner canthus and working toward the outer canthus. Be careful not to touch the tip of the medication container to the eye to help minimize irritation and possible infection.
- Once the medication is instilled, release the lower lid of the eye and ask the patient to close eye and move it around to help distribute the medication. Remove any excess medication with a sterile 2 × 2 gauze, wiping from inner to outer canthus. Document on appropriate parts of the chart and medication record.

Instilling Eyedrops

- With dominant hand resting on patient's forehead, hold filled medication eye dropper approximately 1 to 2 cm (½ to ¾ inch) above conjunctival sac.

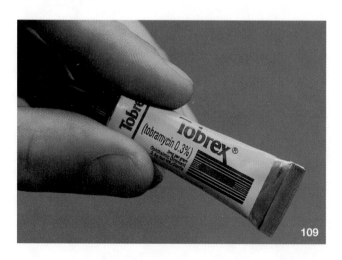

109

- Drop prescribed number of drops into conjunctival sac **(110)**.
- If patient blinks or closes eye or if drops land on outer lid margin, repeat procedure.
- When administering drugs that cause systemic effects, protect your finger with clean tissue and apply gentle pressure to patient's nasolacrimal duct for 30 to 60 seconds **(111)**.
- After instilling drops, ask patient to close eye gently.

ADMINISTERING EARDROPS

- Prepare needed equipment and supplies.
  1. Medication bottle and dropper
  2. Medication card, form, or printout
  3. Cotton-tipped applicator
  4. Tissue
  5. Cotton ball (optional)
  6. Disposable gloves (adhere to Standard Precautions; see p. 95).
- Apply gloves.
- Assess the patient's external ear structures and ear canal.
- Explain the procedure to the patient, and place him or her in a side-lying position with the affected ear facing up. If cerumen (ear wax) or drainage is seen in the outermost part of the ear canal, carefully remove without

pushing the substance back into the ear if unable to easily remove it. Contact the physician and document.
- If you are administering the ear drops to a child under 3 years of age, the child must be in a side-lying or sitting position with the auricle of the ear pulled down and back **(112)**. If the patient is an adult or a child over 3 years of age, the auricle should be pulled up and outward **(113)**.
- Administer the number of prescribed drops and let the patient remain in the side-lying position for 2 to 3 minutes. Gentle massage or pressure to the tragus of the ear after administration may be helpful.
- If cotton is ordered to be placed into the ear canal, be sure to place it into the outermost part of the canal and never press or push it into the innermost part of the canal.
- After about 15 minutes, the cotton (if ordered) should be removed and discarded.
- Dispose of all soiled or contaminated supplies, wash hands, and record.
- Ensure that the patient is positioned comfortably after drop administration.

ADMINISTERING NASAL DROPS AND SPRAY

- Wash hands and adhere to Standard Precautions, (see p. 95).
- Prepare needed equipment and supplies.
  1. Prepared medication with clean dropper or spray
  2. Medication card, form, or printout
  3. Facial tissue

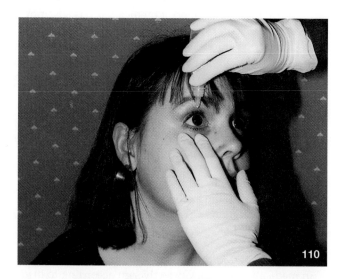

110

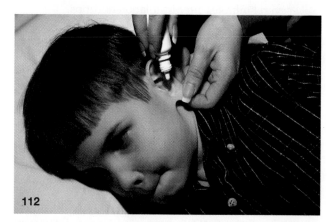

112

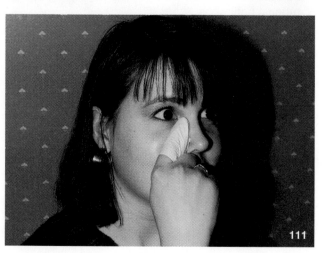

111

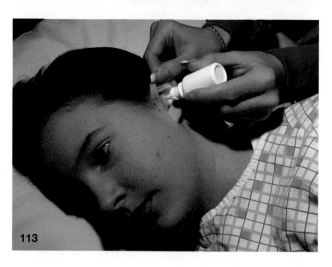

113

4. Small pillow (optional)
5. Washcloth (optional)
6. Disposable gloves
- Check the patient's identification by comparing the medication card with his or her identification band.
- Explain the procedure to the patient, and let him or her know that burning or stinging may occur.
- Educate the patient that is it important to clear the nasal passages by blowing his or her nose, unless contraindicated (patients with increased ICP), before administering the medication.
- Administer nasal drops.
  1. Place or assist patient to a supine position.
  2. Position head backward for posterior pharynx. For the ethmoid or sphenoid sinus areas, place head gently over the top edge of the bed or with a pillow under the shoulders and tilt head back. For frontal or maxillary sinus areas, place the head back and turned toward the side receiving the treatment.
  3. Support the patient's head as needed.
  4. Have the patient breathe through his or her mouth during instillation.
  5. Hold the nose dropper approximately ½ inch above the nasal passages. Administer the proper number of drops toward the midline of the ethmoid bone.
  6. Keep the patient in a supine position for approximately 5 minutes.
  7. Have tissues available to offer the patient to blot his or her nose, but have the patient avoid blowing for several minutes after instillation of drops.
- Administer nasal spray.
  1. Patient should be placed in the upright sitting position with one nostril occluded. After shaking the nasal spray container, insert the tip into the nostril. As the patient inhales through the open nostril **(114),** the spray should be squeezed into the affected nostril at the same time.
  2. Repeat the administration if and as ordered.
- After the medication has been absorbed, assist the patient to a comfortable position.
- Discard all soiled and contaminated items, and wash your hands.
- Record the medication administration, and document any significant findings, such as drainage. Document the therapeutic response if it occurs.

ADMINISTERING VAGINAL MEDICATIONS

- Prepare needed equipment and supplies.
  1. Vaginal applicator
  2. Patient drape
  3. Disposable gloves
  4. Paper towels
  5. Water-soluble lubricant (for suppository)
  6. Perineal pads (for suppository)
  7. Medication card, forms, or printout
- Check accuracy and completeness of order. Check patient's name, drug, route, dose, and time.
- Wash hands and prepare medication.

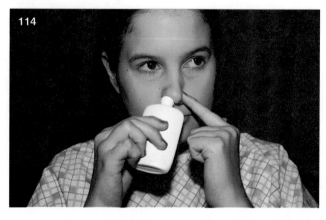

114

- Administer medication.
  1. Provide privacy.
  2. Explain the procedure to the patient.
  3. Have the patient void to empty the bladder.
  4. Put on gloves and fill applicator with prescribed tablet, jelly, cream, or foam.
  5. Place patient in the lithotomy position and elevate the hips with a pillow. Drape patient.
  6. For creams, foams, and jellies, use the gloved, nondominant hand to spread the labia and expose the vagina. Gently insert the applicator as far as possible into the vagina.
  7. Push plunger to deposit medication **(115).** Remove applicator and wrap in paper towel for cleaning.
  8. For suppositories, unwrap vaginal suppository that has warmed to room temperature.
  9. Lubricate with water-soluble lubricant. Insert the suppository (rounded end first) as far into the vagina as possible with the dominant index finger.
  10. Remove glove by turning inside out; place on paper towel for disposal.
  11. Apply a perineal pad.
  12. Have patient remain in supine position with hips elevated for 5 to 10 minutes to allow melting and spreading of the medication. Try to administer vaginal medications at bedtime to allow the solution to remain in place as much as possible, if ordered.
- Dispose of all waste and wash hands thoroughly.
- Chart medication dose, route, site and time, and date in medication record. Correctly sign according to institutional policy.

ADMINISTERING MEDICATIONS VIA METERED-DOSE INHALERS (MDIs)

- Prepare needed equipment and supplies and have patient demonstrate the same.
  1. MDI with medication canister
  2. Facial tissues
  3. Paper towels
  4. Wash basin or sink with warm water
  5. Medication card, forms, or printout
- Check accuracy and completeness of order. Check patient's name, drug, route, dose, and time.
- Wash hands and have patient wash hands and prepare medication.

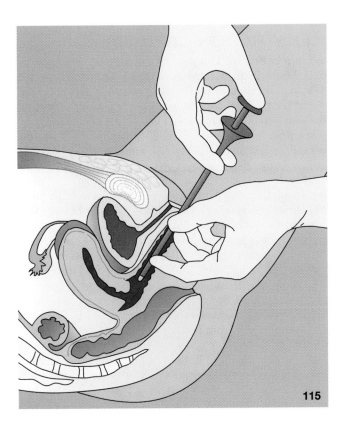

115

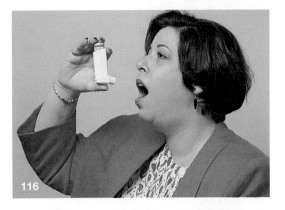

116

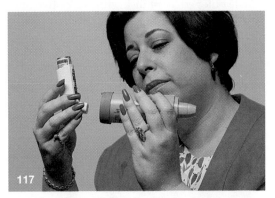

117

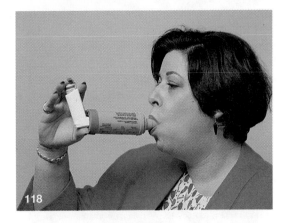

118

- Administer medication and have patient demonstrate.
  1. Remove cap, hold inhaler upright, and grasp with thumb and first two fingers.
  2. Shake inhaler.
  3. Tilt head back slightly. Breathe out.
  4. Position inhaler in one of the following ways:
     a. Open mouth with inhaler 1 to 2 inches away from mouth **(116).**
     b. Attach spacer to mouthpiece of inhaler **(117).**
     c. Place mouthpiece in mouth **(118).**
  5. Press down on inhaler to release medication (one puff) while inhaling slowly **(119).**
  6. Continue to breathe in slowly for 2 to 3 seconds.
  7. Hold breath for approximately 10 seconds.
  8. If repeat puffs are ordered, wait 1 minute between puffs.
- Chart medication dose, route, site and time, and date in medication record. Correctly sign according to institutional policy. Note that spacers are not always ordered.

ADMINISTERING MEDICATIONS VIA TRANSDERMAL DRUG DELIVERY SYSTEM

- Prepare needed equipment and supplies.
  1. Wash cloth
  2. Medication card, forms, or printout
  3. Medication cart
  4. Disposable gloves
- Check accuracy and completeness of order. Check patient's name, drug, route, dose, and time.
- Wash hands and prepare medication.
- Administer medication.

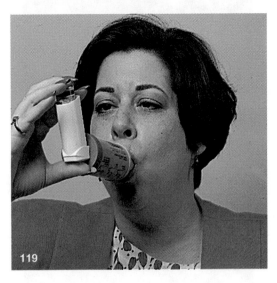

119

1. Provide privacy.
2. Place patient in a position so that the surface on which the topical materials are to be applied is exposed and that ensures patient comfort.
3. If reapplying a transdermal disk, remove the old disk and cleanse thoroughly.
4. Select a new site for application.
5. Once located, the old disk can be encased in the glove as the nurse removes it and should be disposed of in a receptacle on the medication cart.
6. Remove backing from new disk **(120)**.
7. Place adhesive of disk on skin site and press firmly **(121)**.
8. Circle outer edges of disk with one or two fingers to ensure adequate disk contact with skin **(122)**.

- Remove disposable gloves and wash hands thoroughly.
- Chart medication dose, route, site and time, and date in the medication record. Correctly sign according to institutional policy.

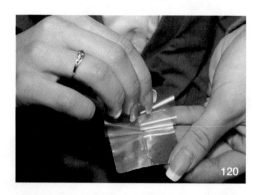

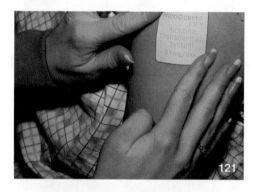

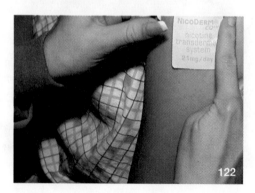

ILLUSTRATION CREDITS

1, From Potter PA, Perry AG: *Fundamentals of nursing,* ed 5, St Louis, 2001, Mosby; **2,** Courtesy Chuck Dresner. In Clayton BD, Stock YN: *Basic pharmacology for nurses,* ed 12, St Louis, 2001, Mosby; **4-7,** Courtesy Chuck Dresner; **8,** From Potter PA, Perry AG: *Fundamentals of nursing: concepts, process, and practice,* ed 3, St Louis, 1993, Mosby; **9-12,** From Potter PA, Perry AG: *Fundamentals of nursing,* ed 5, St Louis, 2001, Mosby; **13-15,** Courtesy Chuck Dresner; **16,** Courtesy Becton Dickinson and Co, Franklin Lakes, NJ; **17-19,** Courtesy Chuck Dresner. In Clayton BD, Stock YN: *Basic pharmacology for nurses,* ed 12, St Louis, 2001, Mosby; **20,** From Potter PA, Perry AG: *Fundamentals of nursing: concepts, process, and practice,* ed 3, St Louis, 1993, Mosby; **21-24,** From Potter PA, Perry AG: *Fundamentals of nursing,* ed 5, St Louis, 2001, Mosby; **25-26,** From Potter PA, Perry AG: *Fundamentals of nursing: concepts, process, and practice,* ed 3, St Louis, 1993, Mosby; **27,** From Potter PA, Perry AG: *Fundamentals of nursing,* ed 5, St Louis, 2001, Mosby; **28,** From Potter PA, Perry AG: *Fundamentals of nursing: concepts, process, and practice,* ed 4, St Louis, 1997, Mosby; **29,** From Potter PA, Perry AG: *Fundamentals of nursing,* ed 5, St Louis, 2001, Mosby; **30-34,** Courtesy Chuck Dresner; **35,** From Potter PA, Perry AG: *Fundamentals of nursing: concepts, process, and practice,* ed 4, St Louis, 1997, Mosby; **36,** Courtesy Nadine Sokol; **37,** From Potter PA, Perry AG: *Basic nursing: a critical thinking approach,* ed 4, St Louis, 1999, Mosby; **38,** From Potter PA, Perry AG: *Fundamentals of nursing: concepts, process, and practice,* ed 3, St Louis, 1993, Mosby; **39,** Courtesy Nadine Sokol; **40,** From Potter PA, Perry AG: *Basic nursing: a critical thinking approach,* ed 4, St Louis, 1999, Mosby; **41,** From Potter PA, Perry AG: *Fundamentals of nursing: concepts, process, and practice,* ed 3, St Louis, 1993, Mosby; **42-43,** From Potter PA, Perry AG: *Fundamentals of nursing: concepts, process, and practice,* ed 4, St Louis, 1997, Mosby; **44,** From Potter PA, Perry AG: *Basic nursing: a critical thinking approach,* ed 4, St Louis, 1999, Mosby; **45-46,** From Potter PA, Perry AG: *Fundamentals of nursing: concepts, process, and practice,* ed 3, St Louis, 1993, Mosby; **47,** From Potter PA, Perry AG: *Fundamentals of nursing: concepts, process, and practice,* ed 4, St Louis, 1997, Mosby; **48-57,** Courtesy Chuck Dresner; **58-60,** From Potter PA, Perry AG: *Fundamentals of nursing,* ed 5, St Louis, 2001, Mosby; **61,** From Potter PA, Perry AG: *Fundamentals of nursing: concepts, process, and practice,* ed 3, St Louis, 1993, Mosby; **62-63,** From Potter PA, Perry AG: *Fundamentals of nursing,* ed 5, St Louis, 2001, Mosby; **64-65,** Courtesy Chuck Dresner; **66-68,** From Potter PA, Perry AG: *Fundamentals of nursing: concepts, process, and practice,* ed 3, St Louis, 1993, Mosby; **69-89,** Courtesy Chuck Dresner; **90,** Courtesy Oscar H. Allison, Jr. In Clayton BD, Stock YN: *Basic pharmacology for nurses,* ed 12, St Louis, 2001, Mosby; **91-96,** Courtesy Chuck Dresner; **102,** Courtesy Chuck Dresner. In Clayton BD, Stock YN: *Basic pharmacology for nurses,* ed 12, St Louis, 2001, Mosby; **103-108,** Courtesy Nadine Sokol; **110-111,** Courtesy Oscar H. Allison, Jr. In Clayton BD, Stock YN: *Basic pharmacology for nurses,* ed 12, St Louis, 2000, Mosby; **112-114,** Courtesy Chuck Dresner; **115,** Courtesy Nadine Sokol; **116-119,** From Potter PA, Perry AG: *Basic nursing: theory and practice,* ed 3, St Louis, 1995, Mosby; **120-122,** Courtesy Chuck Dresner.

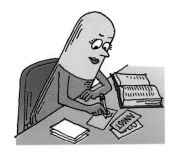

Part two

Drugs Affecting the Central Nervous System: Study Skills Tips

- Vocabulary
- Text Notation
- Language Conventions

VOCABULARY

In any subject matter, mastering the vocabulary is essential to mastering the content. But in a complex, technical subject such as nursing pharmacology, if the vocabulary is not mastered, understanding the content will be almost impossible. Each chapter in this text contains a glossary of unfamiliar terms at the beginning and, as an independent learner, you should spend some time and energy on the vocabulary contained in the glossary. Do not expect to completely understand and master the terms from the glossary alone. The terms are further defined and explained in the body of the chapter, and it is when you read the chapter that you should expect to fully master the vocabulary. However, the time you spend working on the glossary will pay off when you read the chapter.

Consider the terms *agonist* and *antagonist* in the Chapter 9 glossary. These terms share a common word part, which means the words are related in meaning. This is an important first step in mastering them. What does *agonist* mean? What is the similarity between *agonist* and *antagonist*? What is the essential difference between the two? Asking these questions as you start to work on Chapter 9 is a valuable technique for beginning to master the language of the content. Do not simply memorize the terms. Learn what they mean, and link relationships between words with common elements. As you practice this technique it will become easier to retain the meaning.

The Chapter 9 glossary has another group of words that should be viewed as a group that shares an important relationship. The first of these words is *pain*. The definition provided is clear and relatively easy to understand, but your focus should be not just on that single word because there are 12 other words that relate to pain: *acute, cancer, central, chronic, neuropathic, phantom, psychogenic, referred, somatic, superficial, vascular,* and *visceral.* Each of these words defines and categorizes pain in very specific ways. As you go about setting up vocabulary cards, look at the opening pages in this chapter. You will find considerable discussion of these terms, which is useful in helping you obtain the fullest understanding of these terms. Do not simply focus on a meaning of each term, but also ask what the similarities and/or differences are and how these words relate to one another.

TEXT NOTATION

The Study Skills Tips for Part One discussed a method for text underlining. If it is done carefully, this strategy is particularly useful for later review of text material.

The object of text underlining is to pick out important terms, ideas, and key information so you can come back to it later for quick review. The three key elements in successful text notation are as follows: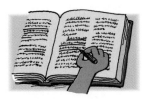

1. You must read the material once before attempting any underlining.
2. You must be acutely aware of the author's language.

3. You must be highly selective in underlining. The most common fault in underlining is to mark too much material.

The following are two paragraphs from Chapter 9 that have been underlined. The underlining should be viewed as an example of what can be done. Each reader will mark the text somewhat differently based on his or her background and experience. As you study this example, think not only about what has been underlined but also about *why* that material was chosen.

To fully understand how analgesics work, it is necessary to know what pain is and what its characteristics are. **Pain** is most commonly defined as an unpleasant sensory and emotional experience associated with either actual or potential tissue damage. It is a very personal and individual experience. Pain can be defined as whatever a patient says it is, and it exists whenever he or she says it does. Although the mechanisms of pain and the nature of pain pathways are becoming better understood, an individual patient's perception of pain and appreciation of its meaning are complex processes. Pain involves psychologic and emotional processes. Because pain is a very individual experience and cannot be quantified, for a caregiver to effectively manage a patient suffering from pain, he or she must cultivate a relationship with the patient that is built on trust and faith. There is no single approach to effective pain management. Instead pain management has to be individualized and must take into account the cause of the pain, if known; the existence of concurrent medical conditions; the characteristics of the pain; and the psychologic and cultural characteristics of the patient. It also requires ongoing reassessment of the pain and the effectiveness of treatment. Therefore pain is often described as having two elements—a physical element and a psychologic element.

The physical element of pain involves the patient's actual sensation of pain. This involves various nerve pathways and the brain and is often referred to as the **pain threshold,** or the level of stimulus needed to produce the perception of pain. This is a measure of the physiologic response of the nervous system and is therefore similar for most persons. The psychologic element represents the patient's emotional response to the pain. These responses are greatly molded by the patient's age, sex, culture, previous pain experience, and anxiety level. This psychologic element of pain is also called **pain tolerance,** or the amount of pain a patient can endure without its interfering with normal function. Pain tolerance can vary from patient to patient because it is a subjective response to pain, not a physiologic function. As a result, the patient's personality, environment, culture, or ethnic background can separately or collectively alter this response. Relatively speaking, a constant pain threshold exists in all people under normal circumstances. However, pain tolerance, or the point beyond which pain becomes unbearable, varies widely. It can even vary within the patient depending on the circumstance involved. Table 9-1 lists the various conditions that can cause a person's pain threshold to be altered.

LANGUAGE CONVENTIONS

Certain words and phrases are like signal lights at an intersection. They serve to tell the reader that something special, important, or noteworthy is happening. To the attentive, active reader these conventions contribute significantly to understanding what the author is trying to convey. Whether you are highlighting, underlining, writing margin notes, or studying the material using the PURR model, it is important that you become sensitive to these conventions.

The text following the topic heading *Opioid Analgesics: Chemical Structure* contains several examples. The second sentence contains the phrase *classified by.* Whenever an author says that something is being classified it means there are at least two (and perhaps several more) elements of the term or idea that are being classified. This means that you should immediately ask a question about the reading, "What is being classified? How many classifications are there for this?" These questions will help you focus on what to learn and keep your attention firmly fixed on the process of learning.

As you read this chapter, or any other chapter, try to become aware of words and phrases like these that are intended to draw your attention to something the author especially wanted to emphasize. The more aware of language conventions you become, the easier it will be to become a selective reader. Selective readers do not try to remember everything they read but are able to select from the mass of information those concepts and/or terms that the writers tried to stress.

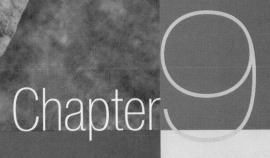
Analgesic Agents

objectives

www.harcourthealth.com/MERLIN/Lilley/

Look for this symbol for
topics covered in the
Online Worksheet

When you reach the end of this chapter, you should be able to do the following:

1 Define *analgesia*.

2 Discuss the use of opioids in pain management.

3 Discuss the difference between an opioid agonist, agonist-antagonist, and antagonist.

4 List the different drugs in the groupings of opioid analgesics.

5 Compare the mechanisms of action, drug effects, therapeutic uses, side effects, adverse effects, and interactions of the opioid agonists and agonist-antagonists.

6 Discuss the different "special" pain situations such as cancer pain and its management.

7 Develop a nursing care plan that includes all phases of the nursing process related to the administration of opioids to the patient experiencing pain.

drug profiles

acetaminophen, p. 132
codeine sulfate, p. 128
fentanyl, p. 128
meperidine
 hydrochloride, p. 129
methadone
 hydrochloride, p. 129
morphine sulfate, p. 128

naloxone hydrochloride,
 p. 130
naltrexone
 hydrochloride, p. 130
propoxyphene
 hydrochloride/
 napsylate, p. 129
tramadol hydrochloride,
 p. 130

Key drug

glossary

Acute pain Pain that is sudden in onset and usually subsides when treated. (p. 121)

Adjuvant agent A drug that is not a primary analgesic but has been shown to have independent or additive analgesic properties. (p. 124)

Agonist A substance that binds to a receptor and causes a response. (p. 124)

Agonist-antagonist A substance that binds to a receptor and causes the receptor to be stimulated and a response to occur while simultaneously binding to another receptor, occupying it but not stimulating it. (p. 126)

Analgesics Medications that relieve pain without causing loss of consciousness (sometimes referred to as *painkillers*). (p. 120)

Antagonist An agent that binds to a receptor and prevents a response. (p. 124)

Cancer pain Pain related to a variety of causes as a result of cancer and/or the metastasis of cancer. (p. 121)

Central pain Pain resulting from any disorder that causes CNS damage. (p. 121)

Chronic pain Persistent or recurring pain that is often difficult to treat. Typically it is pain that lasts longer than 3 months. (p. 121)

Gate theory The most common and well-described theory of pain transmission and pain relief. It uses a gate model to explain how impulses from damaged tissues are sensed in the brain. (p. 121)

Neuropathic pain Pain that results from a disturbance of function or pathologic change in a nerve. (p. 121)

Opioid analgesics Narcotic agents that bind to the mu, kappa, and delta receptors to relieve pain. (p. 123)

Opioid tolerance A physiologic result of long-term opioid use in which larger doses of opioids are required to maintain the same level of analgesia. (p. 126)

Opioid withdrawal (opioid abstinence syndrome) The signs and symptoms associated with the abstinence from or withdrawal of opioid analgesics when the body has become physically dependent on the substance. (p. 126)

Pain An unpleasant sensory and emotional experience associated with actual or potential tissue damage. Pain is a subjective and individual experience; it can be defined as whatever the experiencing person says it is and it exists whenever he or she says it does. (p. 120)

Pain threshold The level of stimulus that results in the perception of pain. (p. 120)

Pain tolerance The amount of pain a patient can endure without it interfering with normal function. (p. 120)

Partial agonist A substance that binds to a receptor and causes effects similar to but less pronounced than those of a pure agonist. (p. 124)

Phantom pain Pain experience in a body part that has been surgically or traumatically removed. (p. 121)

Physical dependence The physical adaptation of the body to the presence of an opioid or other substance. (p. 126)

Psychogenic pain Pain that is psychologic in nature but is truly real pain. (p. 121)

Psychologic dependence (addiction) A pattern of compulsive opioid use characterized by a continuous craving for the substance and the need to use it for effects other than pain relief. (p. 125)

Referred pain Pain occurring in an area away from the organ of origin. (p. 121)

Somatic pain Pain that originates from skeletal muscles, ligaments, or joints. (p. 121)

Superficial pain Pain that originates from the skin or mucous membranes. (p. 121)

Vascular pain Pain that results from a pathology of the vascular or perivascular tissues. (p. 121)

Visceral pain Pain that originates from organs or smooth muscles. (p. 121)

Medications that relieve pain without causing loss of consciousness are referred to as **analgesics** but are also often called *painkillers.* There are various classes of analgesics. These classes are determined by the chemical structures and mechanisms of action of the agents. This chapter focuses on those agents commonly used to relieve moderate to severe pain. These agents are called *opioid analgesics.* The next most common analgesic class consists of nonsteroidal antiinflammatory drugs (NSAIDs), which are discussed in Chapter 42.

PHYSIOLOGY AND PSYCHOLOGY OF PAIN

To fully understand how analgesics work, it is necessary to know what pain is and what its characteristics are. **Pain** is most commonly defined as an unpleasant sensory and emotional experience associated with either actual or potential tissue damage. It is a very personal and individual experience. Pain can be defined as whatever the patient says it is, and it exists whenever he or she says it does. Although the mechanisms of pain and the nature of pain pathways are becoming better understood, an individual patient's perception of pain and appreciation of its meaning are complex processes. Pain involves psychologic and emotional processes. Because pain is a very individual experience and cannot be quantified, for a caregiver to effectively manage a patient suffering from pain, he or she must cultivate a relationship with the patient that is built on trust and faith. There is no single approach to effective pain management. Instead pain management has to be individualized and must take into account the cause of the pain, if known; the existence of concurrent medical conditions; the characteristics of the pain; and the psychologic and cultural characteristics of the patient (see the Cultural Implications box). It also requires ongoing reassessment of the pain and the effectiveness of treatment. Therefore pain is often described as having two elements—a physical element and a psychologic element.

The physical element of pain involves the patient's actual sensation of pain. This involves various nerve pathways and the brain and is often referred to as the **pain threshold,** or the level of stimulus needed to produce the perception of pain. This is a measure of the physiologic response of the nervous system and is therefore similar for most persons. The psychologic element represents the patient's emotional response to the pain. These responses are greatly molded by the patient's age, sex, culture, previous pain experience, and anxiety level. This psychologic element of pain is also called **pain tolerance,** or the amount of pain a patient can endure without it interfering with normal function. Pain tolerance can vary from patient to patient because it is a subjective response to pain, not a physiologic function. As a result, the patient's personality, environment, culture, or ethnic background can separately or collectively alter this response. Relatively speaking, a constant pain threshold exists in all people under normal circumstances. However, pain tolerance, or the point beyond which pain becomes unbearable, varies widely. It can even vary within the patient depending on the circumstance involved. Table 9-1 lists the various conditions that can cause a person's pain threshold to be altered.

cultural implications

Pain and Pain Management

- Each culture has its own beliefs, thoughts, and ways of approaching, defining, and managing pain.
- Attitudes, meanings, and perceptions of pain vary with each culture.
- Many African-Americans believe in the power of healers who rely strongly on the religious faith of the people and often use prayer and the laying on of hands.
- Hispanic-Americans believe in prayer, the wearing of amulets, and the use of herbs and spices in maintaining health and states of wellness. Specific herbs are used in teas, and therapies often include religious practices, massage, and "cleansings" such as the passing of herbs over the body.
- The traditional methods of healing for the Chinese include acupuncture, herbal remedies, yin and yang, and cold treatment. Moxibustion is another form of healing and involves placing pulverized wormwood on the skin over specific meridian points.
- For Native Americans, treatments include massage, the application of heat, sweatbaths, herbal remedies, and being in harmony with nature.
- Nurses should be aware of all the cultural influences on health-related behaviors, on patients' attitudes toward medication therapy, and ultimately on its effectiveness. A thorough assessment with questions about the patient's cultural background and practices is important to the effective and individualized delivery of nursing care.

Pain can also be further classified in terms of its onset and duration as either acute or chronic. Acute and chronic pain differ not only in their onset and duration but also in how they are treated. They are also associated with various diseases or conditions. **Acute pain** is sudden in onset and usually subsides when treated. **Chronic pain** is persistent or recurring and is often very difficult to treat. Table 9-2 gives the different characteristics of acute and chronic pain and lists various diseases and conditions associated with each.

Pain can be further classified according to its source. The two most commonly mentioned sources of pain are somatic and visceral pain. **Somatic pain** originates from skeletal muscles, ligaments, or joints. **Visceral pain** originates from organs or smooth muscles. Sometimes pain is described as superficial. This type of pain originates from the skin or mucous membranes and is called **superficial pain.** Pain treatment can be more appropriately selected when the source of the pain is known. Visceral and superficial pain usually require opioids for relief, whereas somatic pain usually responds better to nonopioid analgesics like NSAIDs.

Another type of pain is **vascular pain,** which possibly originates from some pathology of the vascular or perivascular tissues and is thought to account for a large percentage of migraine headaches. **Referred pain** happens as a result of visceral nerve fibers synapsing at a level in the spinal cord close to fibers that supply specific subcutaneous tissues in the body. An example of referred pain

is with cholecystitis, which is often referred to the back and scapula areas. **Neuropathic pain** results from injury or damage to peripheral nerve fibers or damage to the CNS and is often present in the absence of disease or pathologic processes that generally result in pain. **Phantom pain** occurs in a body part that has been removed—surgically or traumatically—and is characterized as burning, itching, tingling, or stabbing. **Cancer pain** is to be taken seriously, as with all types of pain, and has many causes such as pressure on nerves, organs, or tissues. Other causes include hypoxia, blockage to an organ, metastasis, pathologic fractures, muscle spasms, and side effects of radiation, surgery or chemotherapy. **Psychogenic pain** is a very real pain to a patient and is due to psychologic factors, not physical conditions or disorders. **Central pain** occurs with tumors, trauma, or inflammation of the brain and may occur with any condition that yields CNS damage, such as with cancer, diabetes, cerebrovascular accident, and multiple sclerosis.

Several theories explain pain transmission and pain relief. The most common and well described is the **gate theory.** This theory, proposed by Melzack and Wall in 1965, uses the analogy of a gate to describe how impulses from damaged tissues are sensed in the brain. First, the tissue injury causes the release of several substances such as bradykinin, histamine, potassium, prostaglandins, and serotonin. Many of our current pain management strategies are aimed at altering the actions and levels of these substances. Once these substances are released by the damaged tissue, an action potential is initiated. This action potential travels along a sensory nerve fiber and activates a pain receptor. There are two basic types of these nerve fibers—A and C. Table 9-3 summarizes the differences in the size and function in these two types of nerve fibers. The different types of pain experienced are believed to be related to the relative proportions of A and C fibers in a particular area of the body.

These pain fibers, along with other sensory nerve fibers, enter the spinal cord and travel up to the brain. The site where these fibers enter the spinal cord is referred to as the *dorsal (posterior) horn of the spinal cord.* It is here that the so-called gates are located. These gates regulate the flow

Table 9-1 Conditions That Alter Pain Threshold

Pain Threshold	Conditions
Lowered	Anger, anxiety, depression, discomfort, fear, isolation, chronic pain, sleeplessness, and tiredness
Raised	Diversion, empathy, rest, sympathy, and medications (analgesics, anti-anxiety agents, and antidepressants)

Table 9-2 Acute versus Chronic Pain

Type of Pain	Onset	Duration	Examples
Acute	Sudden (minutes to hours) Usually sharp, localized Physiologic response (SNS: tachycardia, sweating, pallor, increased blood pressure)	Limited (has an end)	Myocardial infarction Appendicitis Dental procedures Kidney stones Surgical procedures
Chronic	Slow (days to months) Long duration Dull, persistent aching	Persistent or recurring (endless)	Arthritis Cancer Lower back pain Peripheral neuropathy

SNS, Sympathetic nervous system.

Table 9-3   A and C Nerve Fibers

Type of Fiber	Myelin Sheath	Fiber Size	Conduction Speed	Type of Pain
A	Yes	Large	Fast	Sharp and well localized
C	No	Small	Slow	Dull and nonlocalized

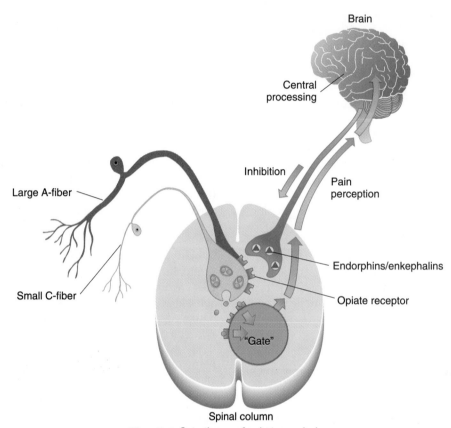

Fig. 9-1 Gate theory of pain transmission.

of sensory impulses. If impulses are stopped by the gate at this junction, no impulses are transmitted to the higher centers of the brain. Because it is at these higher centers where impulses are consciously perceived by the patient, in this instance there would be no perception of pain. Figure 9-1 depicts the gate theory of pain transmission.

The opening and closing of this gate are influenced by the relative activation of the large-diameter A-fibers and the small-diameter C-fibers. The closing of the gate seems to be effected by the activation of A-fibers. This causes the inhibition of impulse transmission to the brain and thus no perception of pain. Opening of the gate is effected by stimulation of the C-fibers. This allows impulses to be transmitted to the brain and pain to be perceived. This gate is also connected to (innervated) nerve fibers that originate in the brain as opposed to fibers that originate from the gate and go to the brain. The nerve fibers that go from the brain to the gate allow the brain to have some control over this gate. They enable the brain to evaluate, identify, and localize the pain. Thus the brain can control the gate, either keeping the gate closed or allowing it to

open so that the brain is stimulated and pain is perceived. The cells that control the gate have a threshold. Impulses that reach these cells must overcome this threshold before an impulse is permitted to travel up to the brain.

The body is equipped with certain endogenous neurotransmitters known as *enkephalins* and *endorphins*. These substances are produced within the body to fight pain and are considered the body's painkillers. They are capable of binding with opioid receptors and inhibiting the transmission of pain impulses by closing the gate. These endogenous analgesic substances are released whenever the body experiences pain. They are responsible for the phenomenon of a runner's high. Figure 9-1 depicts this entire process.

Another phenomenon of pain relief that can be explained by the gate theory is that of massaging or of applying liniment to a painful area. Typically this reduces pain. When rubbing or applying liniment to an area, large sensory fibers from peripheral receptors carry impulses to the spinal cord. This causes impulse transmission to be inhibited and the gate to be closed. This in turn reduces the recognition of the pain impulses arriv-

pediatric considerations

Opioid Administration and Implications

- Assessment of the pediatric patient is challenging, and all types of behavior that may indicate pain, such as muscular rigidity, restlessness, screaming, fear of moving, and withdrawn behavior, have to be carefully considered.
- Assessment of pain is very important in pediatric patients because they are often undermedicated. Always thoroughly assess the pediatric patient and do not underestimate the child's complaints.
- When the pediatric patient is to receive opioids, the nurse should be very careful to recheck dosages against the physician's order and pharmacy references and to double-check the fractions and decimals to minimize and prevent errors.
- If suppositories are used, be careful to administer the exact dose and do not split, halve, or divide the adult dose into a child's dose, because this may result in the administration of an unknown dose.
- Always monitor pediatric patients very closely for any unusual behavior or signs and symptoms while they are receiving opioids.
- Central nervous system changes such as dizziness, light-headedness, drowsiness, hallucinations, changes in the level of consciousness, and a sluggish pupil reaction should be reported immediately to the physician and no further medication given until further orders are received from the physician.
- Always monitor and document vital signs before, during, and after the administration of opioid analgesics. Withhold the medication if respirations are <12 breaths/min or if there are any changes in the level of consciousness.
- Respiratory status—respiratory rate, rhythm, character, rate, and difficulty—should be carefully assessed in pediatric patients.
- Generally speaking, smaller doses of opioids are indicated for the pediatric patient.
- Keep bed or crib side rails up and the bed in a low position at all times!
- Meperidine should be used cautiously in patients younger than 18 years of age.
- Oral opium derivatives should be given with meals or milk to decrease gastrointestinal tract distress.
- With opiates, the therapeutic response is a decrease in pain.
- Allergic reactions may include a rash or urticaria.
- Withdrawal symptoms include nausea, vomiting, cramps, faintness, fever, and anorexia.

geriatric considerations

Opioid Administration and Implications

- Assess patient carefully before administration of opioids because a dose and interval adjustment may be necessary, depending on the development of undesirable adverse reactions such as confusion, decreased respirations, and excessive central nervous system depression.
- Height and weight should be recorded and noted before the start of opioid treatment.
- Carefully monitor elderly patients who are receiving opioids because they are generally more sensitive to these agents. This includes frequent monitoring of vital signs, respiratory function, and central nervous system status. Document any changes.
- Smaller doses of opioids are generally indicated for the aged patient, and idiosyncratic or unexpected reactions may occur in patients of this age group.
- Polypharmacy is often a problem in the elderly, so it is important to have a complete list of all medications the patient is currently taking.
- Keep side rails up and bed in low position with call bell/light at bedside.
- With possible decreased circulation, the absorption of IM or IV dosage forms will vary, and often result in a slower absorption of parenteral forms of opioids.
- Encourage elderly patients to ask for medications because they often hesitate to ask for pain medication because they do not want to "bother" the nurse or give in to pain.
- Note, report, and document any unusual reactions to the opioid agents.

ing by means of the small fibers. This is the same pathway that the opioid analgesics use to alleviate pain.

Treatment of Pain in Special Situations

In situations such as pain associated with malignancies, the main consideration in pain management is for patient comfort and not prevention of drug addiction. Often this means aggressive treatment with large doses of fre-

quently administered narcotic analgesics to relieve the pain and prevent it from recurring. As the disease progresses, the patient may develop tolerance and then require larger doses and more frequent medication administration using oral, rectal, and transdermal routes. These routes are preferred over long-term use of injections. Also, if patients are taking long-acting narcotic analgesics, "breakthrough" pain may be problematic and need to be resolved with shorter-acting or fast-acting forms on a regular schedule. In this case, if a patient is requiring larger doses for "breakthrough" pain, the baseline dose of the narcotic may need to be titrated upward, or increased in increments. Other medications, such as antidepressants, antiemetics, and laxatives, may be used in special situations such as cancer pain and severe chronic pain to prevent or relieve associated constipation.

OPIOID ANALGESICS

The analgesics currently known as **opioid analgesics** originated from the opium plant. The word *opium* is a Greek word that means "juice." More than 20 different alkaloids are obtained from the unripe seed of the opium poppy plant. The properties of opium and its many alkaloids have been known for centuries. As early as the third century BC, reference to poppy juice is found in the writings of Theophrastus. Arabian physicians were well versed in the uses of opium as well. It was Arabian traders who introduced the drug to East Asia. Opium-smoking immigrants brought opium to the United States where unrestricted availablility of opium prevailed until the early twentieth century.

Chemical Structure

Opioid analgesics are very strong pain relievers. They can be classified according to their chemical structure or by their action at specific receptors (see Mechanism of Action). Of the 20 different alkaloids available from the opium poppy plant, only a few are clinically useful—morphine, codeine, and papaverine. Of these three only morphine and codeine are considered pain relievers, whereas papaverine is a smooth muscle relaxant. Relatively simple chemical modifications of these opium alkaloids have produced the three different chemical classes of opioids:

- Morphine-like drugs
- Meperidine-like drugs
- Methadone-like drugs

Table 9-4 lists the various opioid analgesics and their respective chemical categories.

Mechanism of Action

Opioid analgesics can also be characterized according to their mechanism of action. They can be agonists, partial agonists, or antagonists. An **agonist** binds to a receptor and causes a response. A **partial agonist** binds to a receptor and causes only limited actions. The physiologic response produced by the binding of a partial agonist is not as pronounced as that produced by an agonist. **Antagonists** are substances that reverse the effects of these agents on pain receptors. Antagonists bind to a receptor and exert no response. They may also be referred to as *competitive antagonists* because they compete with the substance that normally binds to that receptor.

The actual receptors to which opioids bind to relieve pain are listed and their characteristics are summarized in Table 9-5. Five types of opioid receptors have been identified to date: mu, kappa, sigma, delta, and epsilon. Mu, kappa, and delta, are the primary receptors. Many of the characteristics of a particular opioid, such as its abil-

ity to sedate, its potency, or its ability to cause hallucinations, can be attributed to the particular opioid's affinity for these various receptors.

Drug Effects

Opioid analgesics achieve their beneficial effects by their actions in the central nervous system (CNS). However, they also act outside the CNS, and many of their unwanted effects stem from these actions.

Therapeutic Uses

The main effect of opioids is to alleviate moderate to severe pain. The degree to which pain is relieved or unwanted side effects occur depends on the specific agent, the receptors to which it binds, and its chemical structure. Often drugs from other chemical categories are added to the opioid regimen as **adjuvant agents.** These assist the primary agents in relieving pain. NSAIDs are commonly used in this capacity. This allows the use of smaller doses of opioids, which accomplishes two important functions. First, it diminishes some of the side effects that are seen with higher doses of opioids, such as respiratory depression, constipation, and urinary retention. Second, it approaches the pain stimulus from another mechanism and has a resulting synergistic beneficial effect in reducing the pain.

Many opioids have an affinity for the CNS. Once there, they suppress the medullary cough center, which results in cough suppression. The most commonly used opioid for this is codeine. Hydrocodone has also been used in many cough suppressants either alone or in combination with other agents. Sometimes the opioid-related cough suppressants have a depressant effect on the CNS and cause sedation. To avoid this problem, dextromethorphan, a nonopioid cough suppressant, is often given instead.

Decreased gastrointestinal motility (constipation) is an unwanted side effect of opioids that is sometimes used therapeutically to treat diarrhea. Some of the most common opioid-containing antidiarrhea preparations are camphorated opium tincture (paregoric) and diphenoxylate (Lomotil).

Strong opioid analgesics like fentanyl, sufentanil, and alfentanil are commonly used in combination with anesthetics during surgery. These agents are used not only to

Table 9-4	Chemical Classification of Opioids	
Chemical Category	**Opioid Agents**	
meperidine-like agents	meperidine, fentanyl, remifentanil, sufentanil, alfentanil	
methadone-like agents	methadone, propoxyphene	
morphine-like agents	morphine, heroin, hydromorphone, oxymorphone, levorphanol, codeine, hydrocodone, oxycodone	
Other	tramadol	

Table 9-5	Opioid Receptors and Their Characteristics	
Receptor Type	**Prototypical Agonist**	**Effects**
Mu	morphine	Supraspinal analgesia Respiratory depression Euphoria ++Sedation
Kappa	ketocyclazocine	Spinal analgesia ++++Sedation Miosis
Delta	enkephalins	Analgesia

relieve pain but to also maintain a balanced state of anesthesia. This practice of using combinations of drugs rather than a single agent to produce anesthesia is referred to as *balanced anesthesia*.

Side Effects and Adverse Effects

As previously mentioned, many of the unwanted effects of opioid analgesics are related to their effects on parts of the body other than the CNS. Some of these unwanted effects can be explained by the respective agent's selectivity for the receptors listed in Table 9-5. The various body systems that the opioids affect and their side effects and adverse effects are summarized in Table 9-6.

Opioids that have an affinity for mu receptors and have rapid onset of action produce marked euphoria. These are the opioids that are most likely to be abused and used for recreational use. The person taking them to alter his or her mental status will soon become psychologically dependent on them. **Psychologic dependence (addiction)** is a pattern of compulsive drug use characterized by a continuous craving for an opioid and the need to use it for effects other than pain relief.

All opioids cause some histamine release. It is thought that this histamine release is responsible for many of the unwanted side effects, such as itching or pruritus, rash, and hemodynamic changes. The histamine release causes peripheral arteries and veins to dilate, which leads to flushing and orthostatic hypotension. The amount of histamine release that an opioid analgesic causes is related to its chemical class. The naturally occurring opiates elicit the most histamine release; the synthetic opioids elicit the least histamine release. (See Table 9-4 for the various opioids and their respective chemical classes.)

The most serious side effect of opioids is CNS depression, which may lead to respiratory depression. When opioids are given, care should be taken to titrate the dose so that the patient's pain is controlled without respiratory function being affected. Individual responses to opioids vary, and patients may occasionally suffer respiratory compromise or the loss of airway reflexes despite careful dose titration. Respiratory depression can be prevented in part by using agents with very short durations of action and no active metabolites. It seems to be more common in patients with a preexisting condition causing respiratory compromise such as asthma or chronic obstructive pulmonary disease (COPD). Respiratory depression is strongly related to the degree of sedation. Stimulation of the patient may be adequate to reverse mild hypoventilation. If this is unsuccessful, assisted ventilation by bag and mask or, if needed, by endotracheal intubation may be needed to support respiration. It may also be necessary to administer naloxone, an opioid reversal agent, to reverse severe respiratory depression. However, keep in mind that naloxone will not only reverse the patient's respiratory depression but will also reverse the pain control. Careful, slow titration of naloxone will prevent over-reversal of the opioid-induced respiratory depression and pain relief. The effects of naloxone are short-lived, usually lasting about 1 hour. With long-acting opioids the respiratory depressant effects can reappear after the naloxone has worn off, and redosing may be needed.

Gastrointestinal tract side effects are common in patients receiving opioids. Nausea, vomiting, and constipation are the most common side effects associated with opioid analgesics. Opioids irritate the gastrointestinal tract, stimulating the chemoreceptor trigger zone in the CNS, which in turn causes nausea and vomiting. Opioids slow peristalsis and increase water absorption from intestinal contents. These two actions combine to produce

---

legal & ethical principles

Falls, Restraints, and Medication Use

Many medications have adverse effects that put the patient at risk for falls and possible injury, including dizziness, hypotension, postural hypotension, sedation, altered sensorium, and level of consciousness. Patient falls and resultant injuries are the most common cause of litigation against nurses. Numerous lawsuits have consistently shown the importance of assessing patients for the potential for falls or who is at risk for falls. Make sure that you are cautious and prudent in preventing falls whether it is as simple as leaving the side rails of the bed up, leaving the call light at the bedside, placing a patient on a frequent "watch" program, or attaining an order for restraints. As the professional nurse, if you assess and make the decision to restrain a patient to prevent falls, remember that you must follow the facility's policy and procedure regarding orders for and application of restraints and subsequent nursing care. Restraints themselves can cause many adverse injuries, so be sure to follow procedure. Assess, monitor, evaluate, and document the reason for the restraint. Document the patient's behavior, type of restraint, and the assessment of the patient after placement of restraints. Provide fluids and toileting care as needed, and *always* document your nursing interventions. ■

Table 9-6 Opioid-Induced Side Effects and Adverse Effects by Body System

Body System	Side Effect or Adverse Effect
Cardiovascular system	Hypotension, palpitations, and flushing
Central nervous system	Sedation, disorientation, euphoria, light-headedness, dysphoria, lowered seizure threshold, and tremors
Gastrointestinal tract	Nausea, vomiting, constipation, and biliary tract spasm
Genitourinary tract	Urinary retention
Respiratory tract	Respiratory depression and aggravation of asthma
Other	Itching, rash, and wheal formation

constipation. This is more pronounced in a hospitalized patient who is nonambulatory, because lack of daily activity also causes constipation.

Urinary retention, or the inability to void, is another unwanted side effect of opioid analgesics. They cause this by increasing bladder tone. This is sometimes treated with low doses of an opioid **agonist-antagonist** like nalbuphine or with an opioid antagonist like naloxone.

Severe hypersensitivity or anaphylaxis to opioid analgesics is rare. Most patients will experience gastrointestinal tract or histamine-mediated reactions to opioids and call these "allergic reactions." True anaphylaxis is rare, even with intravenously administered opioids. Some patients may complain of flushing, itching, or wheal formation at the injection site, but this is usually local and histamine mediated.

Toxicity and Management of Overdose. Opioid analgesics produce both beneficial effects and toxic or unwanted effects by means of receptors. These receptors and the positive and negative effects they bring about are listed in Table 9-5. The opioid antagonists naloxone and naltrexone bind to and occupy all these receptor sites (mu, kappa, and sigma). They are competitive antagonists with a strong affinity for these binding sites. In doing so they can reverse the adverse effects induced by the opioid such as respiratory depression. These agents are used in the management of both opioid overdose and opioid addiction. The commonly used opioid antagonists (reversal agents) are listed in Table 9-7.

In the management of opioid overdose or toxicity, it is important to recognize the signs and symptoms of withdrawal. **Opioid tolerance** may be a physiologic result of long-term opioid use; patients with opioid tolerance require larger doses of the opioid agent to maintain the same level of analgesia. The physiologic adaptation of the body to the effects of an opioid is referred to as **physical dependence.** Opioid tolerance and physical dependence are expected in patients undergoing long-term opioid treatment and should not be confused with psychologic dependence (addiction), manifested by drug abuse behavior. Confusing these terms in relation to opioid therapy leads to ineffective pain management and contributes to the problem of undertreatment. Physical dependence on opioids is seen when an agent is discontinued abruptly or when an opioid antagonist is administered. This physiologic response is referred to as **opioid withdrawal,** or **opioid abstinence syndrome.** It is manifested by anxiety, irritability, chills and hot flashes, joint pain, lacrimation, rhinorrhea, diaphoresis, nausea, vomiting, and abdominal cramps and diarrhea.

The timing of the onset of withdrawal symptoms is directly related to the half-life of the opioid analgesic being used. The withdrawal symptoms resulting from the discontinuance or reversal of short-acting opioid therapy (codeine, hydrocodone, morphine, and hydromorphone) will arise within 6 to 12 hours and peak at 24 to 72 hours. The withdrawal symptoms associated with the long half-life agents (methadone, levorphanol, and transdermal fentanyl) may not appear for 24 hours or more after drug discontinuation and may be milder. The appearance of abstinence syndrome indicates physical dependence on the opioids, which may occur after just 2 weeks of therapy. It does not, however, imply the existence of psychologic dependence or addiction. Most patients with cancer take opioid analgesics for more than 2 weeks, and only very rarely do they exhibit the drug abuse behavior and psychologic dependence that characterize addiction.

Interactions

Potential drug interactions with opioids are significant. Coadministration of opioids with alcohol, antihistamines, barbiturates, benzodiazepines, phenothiazine, and other CNS depressants can result in additive respiratory depressant effects. The combined use of monoamine oxidase inhibitors (MAOIs) with opioids can result in respiratory depression and hypotension. This is especially true with meperidine and MAOIs.

Dosages

For the recommended dosages of selected analgesic agents, see the dosages table on p. 127.

Table 9-7 Opioid Antagonists (Reversal Agents)

Generic Name	Trade Name	Dosage	Cautions
nalmefene	Revex	0.5 mg/70 kg; if needed a second dose of 1.0 mg/70 kg 2-5 minutes later (for nonopioid dependent patients)	
naloxone (IV)	Narcan	0.4-2 mg q2-3/min (<10 mg) IV infusion: 2 mg in 500 ml (titrate to response)	Raised or lowered blood pressure Dysrhythmias Pulmonary edema Withdrawal
naltrexone (PO)	ReVia	25-50 mg qd	Nervousness Headache Nausea/vomiting Pulmonary edema Withdrawal

DOSAGES Selected Analgesic Agents

agent	pharmacologic class	dosage range		purpose
Opioid				
codeine sulfate	Opioid Opiate Opium alkaloid	*Pediatric* PO/SC/IM: 2.5 y/o, 2.5-5 mg q4-6h—do not exceed 30 mg/day *Adult/Children >12 y/o* 10-20 mg q4-6h—do not exceed 120 mg/day *Pediatric* 6-11 y/o, 5-10 mg q4-6h *Adult* 15-60 mg 3-4 times/day		Antitussive Antitussive Antitussive Opioid analgesic

meperidine HCl
(Demerol, Pethidine)
	Opioid
	Synthetic opioid
		Pediatric
		PO/IM/SC: 1-1.5 mg/kg q2-3h prn (max 100 mg/dose)
		IM/SC: 0.5-1 mg/kg 30-90 min before anesthesia
		  (max 100 mg/day)
		Adult
		PO/IM/SC: 50-150 mg q2-3 prn
		IM/SC: 50-100 mg
		IM/SC: 50-100 mg 30-90 min before anesthesia
				Opioid analgesic
				Preop sedation
				
				Obstetric analgesia,
				  preop sedation

methadone HCl
(Dolophine)
	Opioid
	Synthetic opioid
		Adult
		PO/IM/SC: 2.5-10 mg q3-4h; ≥40 mg once/day, reduced
		  doses every few days; ≥40-120 mg once/day
				Opioid analgesic,
				  opioid detoxification,
				  opioid addiction
				  maintenance

morphine sulfate (Astramorph, Duramorph, Infumorph, MS Contin, MSIR, Oramorph, Roxanol, and others)	Opioid Opiate Opium alkaloid	*Pediatric* SC: 0.1-0.2 mg/kg dose—do not exceed a 15-mg single dose *Adult* PO/IM/SC: 5-30 mg q4h; rectal: 10-20 mg q4h; IV: 2.5-15 mg.		Opioid analgesic Opioid analgesic

naloxone HCl
(Narcan)
	Opioid antagonist	*Pediatric*
		IM/IV/SC: 0.01 mg/kg IV followed by 0.1 mg/kg if needed;
		  0.0005-0.01 mg/kg IV—repeat in 2-3 min intervals
		Adult
		IM/IV/SC: 0.4-2 mg IV—repeat in 2-8 min if needed;
		  0.1-0.2 mg IV—repeat in 2-3 min intervals.
				Opioid overdose,
				  postop reversal
				
				Opioid overdose,
				  postop reversal

naltrexone HCl (Trexan)	Opioid antagonist	*Adult* PO: 50 mg q24h or 100 mg qod		Maintenance of opioid-free state
propoxyphene HCl/napsylate (Darvon, Pulvules, Dolene)	Analgesic	*Adult* PO: 65 mg q4h prn—do not exceed 340 mg/day; 100 mg q4h prn—do not exceed 600 mg/day		Analgesic
Nonopioid				
acetaminophen (Tylenol and many others)	Nonopioid	*Pediatric* PO/PR for:		Mild to moderate pain relief
		0-3 mo	40 mg q4-6 hr	
		4-11 mo	80 mg q4-6 hr	
		1-2 yr	120 mg q4-6 hr	
		2-3 yr	160 mg q4-6 hr	
		4-5 yr	245 mg q4-6 hr	
		6-8 yr	320 mg q4-6 hr	
		9-10 yr	400 mg q4-6 hr	
		11-12 yr	480 mg q4-6 hr	
		Adult PO/PR	325- 650 mg q4-6 hr; do not exceed 4 g/day. In alcoholics, do not exceed 2 g.	

case study Opioid Administration

Ms. MB is 67 years of age and has recently undergone surgery, chemotherapy, and irradiation for breast cancer. She has been in pain after her therapy, for which she has been taking oxycodone and acetaminophen (Percocet), two tablets PO q3h prn, and extended-release morphine (MS Contin), 30 mg q12h.

She has been taking the Percocet every 3 hours and the MS Contin continuously every 12 hours but is still in pain. Oral thrush has also developed as a result of her chemotherapy, and she can no longer tolerate swallowing. It is decided that her oral medications should be changed. The physician wants to know her total daily dose of opioids so that this can be converted to the equivalent dose of transdermal fentanyl and to supplement with prn morphine injections.

- *What is her total daily dose of oxycodone and morphine?*
- *What dose of morphine is equivalent to her total daily dose of combined oxycodone and morphine?*
- *What dose of transdermal fentanyl should this patient receive?*

For Answers see www.harcourthealth.com/MERLIN/Lilley/.

Laboratory Results. Opioids can cause an abnormal increase in the serum levels of amylase, alanine aminotransferase, alkaline phosphatase, bilirubin, lipase, creatinine kinase, and lactic acid dehydrogenase. Other abnormal results include a decrease in urinary 17-ketosteroid level and an increase in the urinary alkaloid and glucose concentrations.

drug profiles

morphine sulfate

Morphine is an alkaloid obtained from opium and is the prototype opioid drug. Opium is the dried juice of the poppy plant *Papaver somniferum* and is a mixture of opioid and nonopioid alkaloids. A potential for morphine misuse exists, as with other narcotics. However, fear of opioids that cause addiction should not result in the patient not having adequate pain relief. Gradual withdrawal with chronic use may minimize the development of withdrawal symptoms after long-term use. It is considered a C-II scheduled substance. It is also highly constipating.

The drug is contraindicated in patients showing hypersensitivity to it, and extreme caution is required when administering it to patients with head injuries. It is indicated for treatment of severe pain and may be administered by a variety of routes (oral, IM, sustained release tabs, IV, SC, rectal, epidural, and intrathecal) depending on the patient's condition. Continuous infusions of morphine may also be initiated through a patient-controlled analgesia (PCA) pump.

PHARMACOKINETICS

HALF-LIFE	ONSET	PEAK	DURATION
1.7-4.5 hr	Rapid	IM: 30-60 min	IM: 6-7 hr

codeine sulfate

Codeine sulfate methylmorphine is the second opioid alkaloid obtained from opium. However, the yield is low, and the high medical consumption of codeine necessitates its synthesis by methylating morphine. Codeine is similar to morphine in terms of its pharmacokinetic and pharmacodynamic properties. However, codeine is less effective as an analgesic and is widely used as an antitussive agent in an array of cough preparations. It is currently listed on schedule C-II of controlled substances, which would imply a high physical and psychologic dependence. Fixed-combinations using codeine are classified as schedule C-III controlled substances. Codeine is combined with many other drugs. These combination codeine products have differing controlled substance schedules.

PHARMACOKINETICS

HALF-LIFE	ONSET	PEAK	DURATION
2.5-4 hr	15-30 min	35-45 min	4-6 hr

fentanyl

Fentanyl (Duragesic, Fentanyl Oralet, Sublimaze) is a synthetic opioid used to treat moderate to severe pain. It is also used as an adjunct to general anesthetics. It is available in several dosage forms: transdermal patches (Duragesic), buccal lozenges (Fentanyl Oralet), and parenteral injections (Sublimaze). It is also available as a combination product called Innovar, in which it is combined with droperidol. Fentanyl is a very potent analgesic. The potencies of some of the more common opioids as compared with 10 mg of both IM and oral forms of morphine are listed in Table 9-8. Fentanyl at a dose of 100 μg (0.10 mg) given intravenously is equivalent to 10 mg of morphine given intramuscularly.

One of the new ways of administering fentanyl is the transdermal delivery system, or the Duragesic patch. It has been shown to be highly effective in the treatment of various chronic types of pain syndromes such as cancer-induced pain. It is recommended that patients never before exposed to opioids be started on the lowest-strength patch of 25 μg/hr (2.5 mg/10 cm^2). However, prior exposure to opioids is common in many patients. In these patients it is necessary to know the appropriate dose (the equipment dose) of transdermal fentanyl to which to convert the patient. Table 9-9 is provided to aid in this conversion.

The analgesic potency of 10 mg of IM morphine relative to that of 100 μg of IV fentanyl was used by the manufacturer to derive the equivalent potency dose of transdermal fentanyl. Thus, a 10-mg IM or 60-mg oral dose of morphine given every 4 hours for 24 hours (60 mg daily intramuscularly or 360 mg daily orally) was considered by the manufacturer to be approximately equivalent to a transdermal fentanyl system that delivered 100 μg/hr. The transdermal fentanyl doses that should be used and the estimated daily equivalent doses of morphine are given in Table 9-9. (The table was arranged in this manner to avoid the need to prepare a table for every dosage range.) To perform the conversion shown in this table, first you should determine the daily (24-hour) opioid requirement of your patient. Second, if the opioid is not morphine, you should convert its dose to the equianalgesic dose of morphine using Table 9-8. Finally, the equipotent transdermal fentanyl dose can be calculated using Table 9-9.

Most patients will experience adequate pain control for 72 hours with this method of fentanyl delivery. A new patch should be applied every 72 hours.

Fentanyl is classified as a pregnancy category C agent and is contraindicated in patients who have shown a hypersensitivity reaction to opioid analgesics and in those with myasthenia gravis. It is available in transdermal doses of 25 μg/hr (2.5 mg/ 10 cm^2), 50 μg/hr (5 mg/20 cm^2), 75 μg/hr (7.5 mg/ 30 cm^2), and 100 μg/hr (10 mg/40 cm^2); as a buccal lozenge in doses of 200, 300, and 400 μg; as a 50-μg/ml parenteral injection; and as a combination product (Innovar) consisting of 50 μg/ml of fentanyl and 2.5 mg/ml of droperidol. The commonly recommended transdermal dosages are determined on the basis of a patient's prior opioid use. If a patient has no such history, then a 25 μg patch should be used. If he or she has been treated with other opioids, then Table 9-9 should be used to determine the equivalent transdermal fentanyl dose. This table is conservative in its doses for achieving pain relief, and often supplemental, short-acting opioid analgesics should be added as needed. Dosage titration in patients with fentanyl patches should be done as needed every 72 hours.

PHARMACOKINETICS

HALF-LIFE	ONSET	PEAK	DURATION
IV: 1.5-6 hr	Rapid	Minutes	30-60 min
IM: 1.5-6 hr	7-15 min	20-30 min	1-2 hr
Transdermal: 13-40 hr	Delayed	12-24 hr	48-72 hr

meperidine hydrochloride

Meperidine hydrochloride (Demerol, Pethidine) is a widely used synthetic opioid analgesic. The misuse potential and addiction liability associated with its use are both high. Meperidine should be used with caution, if at all, in the elderly and in patients who require chronic analgesia with meperidine or who have kidney dysfunction. A metabolite, normeperidine, can accumulate and lead to seizures. After 48 hours, meperidine accumulates in the body and is toxic. The drug is contraindicated in patients showing a hypersensitivity to it and in patients currently or recently treated with MAOIs. The concurrent use of MAOIs and meperidine can lead to deep coma and death.

PHARMACOKINETICS

HALF-LIFE	ONSET	PEAK	DURATION
3-5 hr	Rapid	30-60 min	2-4 hr

methadone hydrochloride

Methadone hydrochloride (Dolophine) is a synthetic opioid analgesic. The potential for misuse and the addiction liability are both high for this agent. It is the opioid of choice for the detoxification treatment of opioid addicts. The drug has seen widespread use in the methadone maintenance program. The usual dose for methadone maintenance ranges from 40 to 120 mg or higher, given once daily. Concurrent use of agonist-antagonist opioids (pentazocine and the like) in heroin-addicted or methadone-maintenance patients can induce significant withdrawal symptoms.

PHARMACOKINETICS

HALF-LIFE	ONSET	PEAK	DURATION
25 hr	30-60 min	1.5-2 hr	22-48 hr

propoxyphene hydrochloride/napsylate

Propoxyphene hydrochloride (Darvon, Pulvules, Dolene) is an analgesic agent that is structurally related to methadone. Although it is not as potent as methadone, its misuse potential and addiction liability must be considered. It is used for the relief of mild to moderate pain.

Propoxyphene napsylate is more insoluble than propoxyphene hydrochloride, and this makes for more stable liquid and solid (tablets and the like) dosage formulations.

PHARMACOKINETICS

HALF-LIFE	ONSET	PEAK	DURATION
6-12 hr	.25-1 hr	2-2.5 hr	4-6 hr

OPIOIDS WITH MIXED ACTIONS

Drugs discussed in this section bind to the mu receptor and can therefore compete with other substances for these sites. However, they either exert no actions (i.e., they are competitive antagonists) or only limited actions (i.e., they are partial agonists). Buprenorphine is a partial agonist. Butophanol, dezocine, nalbuphine, and pentazocine (Talwin) are agonist-antagonists.

PARTIAL AGONIST OPIOID ANALGESICS

The partial agonist opioid analgesics include buprenorphine, butophanol, dezocine, nalbuphine, and pentazocine. They are also known as the agonist-antagonist opioids. These agents are very similar to the agonist opioid agents from the standpoint of their therapeutic indications. They are potent synthetic analgesics, but their misuse potential and addiction liability are both low.

The antagonistic activity of this group can produce withdrawal symptoms in opioid-dependent patients. They are also contraindicated in patients who have shown hypersensitivity reactions to the drugs.

OPIOID ANTAGONISTS

Opioid antagonists are synthetic derivatives of oxymorphone, a potent semisynthetic opioid. They produce their opioid antagonistic activity by competing with opioids for CNS receptor sites.

naloxone hydrochloride

Naloxone hydrochloride (Narcan) is a pure opioid antagonist because it possesses no agonist morphine-like properties. Accordingly, the drug does not produce analgesia or respiratory depression. Naloxone is the drug of choice for the complete or partial reversal of opioid-induced respiratory depression. It is also indicated in the diagnosis of suspected acute opioid overdose. If its administration does not significantly reverse the opioid overdose, this indicates the condition may be due to an overdose of non-opioid drugs or a dosing process.

The drug is contraindicated in patients with a history of hypersensitivity to it.

PHARMACOKINETICS

HALF-LIFE	ONSET	PEAK	DURATION
64 min	<2 min	Rapid	Variable with dose and route

naltrexone hydrochloride

Naltrexone hydrochloride (Revia, Trexan) is an opioid antagonist used as an adjunct for the maintenance of an opioid-free state in former opioid addicts. It recently received approval from the FDA as a safe and effective adjunct to psychosocial treatments for alcoholism.

The drug is contraindicated in patients with acute hepatitis or liver failure, a demonstrated hypersensitivity to the drug, or opioid dependency in patients currently receiving opioids; and in patients suffering from acute opioid withdrawal.

PHARMACOKINETICS

HALF-LIFE	ONSET	PEAK	DURATION
3.9-12.9 hr	Rapid	1 hr	24-72 hr

The most serious adverse effect is dose-related hepatocellular toxicity. Other adverse effects include nasal congestion, nosebleeds, phlebitis, depression, nightmares, and photophobia.

Nalmefene (Revex) is an IV opioid antagonist indicated for treatment of opioid overdose and the management of postoperative respiratory depression. Its longer duration of action offers an advantage over naloxone. It is recommended for reversal of postoperative opioid depression. Nausea and tachycardia are the most common adverse effects, and they occur at an incidence similar to naloxone.

OTHER OPIOIDS

tramadol hydrochloride

Tramadol hydrochloride (Ultram) is a centrally acting analgesic with a dual mechanism of action. It creates a weak bond to opioid receptors and inhibits the reuptake of both norepinephrine and serotonin. Tramadol is indicated for the treatment of moderate to moderately-severe pain. The usual dose is 50 to 100 mg every 4 to 6 hours, up to a maximum of 400 mg daily. Tramadol is available as 50 mg tablets. It is rapidly absorbed, with peak serum levels occurring within 2 hours. Tramadol absorption is unaffected by food. It is metabolized in the liver to an active metabolite (O-dimethyl tramadol) and eliminated via renal excretion. The half-life of tramadol and its active metabolite is 5 to 8 hours. Adverse effects include drowsiness, dizziness, headache, nausea, and constipation. Tramadol is contraindicated in patients who have previously demonstrated hypersensitivity to tramadol, another component of this product, or opioids. It is also contraindicated in cases of acute intoxication with alcohol, hypnotics, centrally acting analgesics, opioids, or psychotropic drugs.

Seizures have been reported in patients taking Ultram. These seizures have occurred in patients taking normal doses and doses exceeding normal recommended dosages. Patients who may be at risk are those patients taking tricyclic antidepressants, selective-serotonin reuptake inhibitors, MAOIs, neuroleptics, or other drugs that reduce the seizure threshold.

Equianalgesic Opioid Potency

Table 9-8

Opioid Analgesic	Equianalgesic Dose (MG)	
	Intramuscular	Oral
codeine	130	200
hydromorphone	1.5	7.5
meperidine	75	300
methadone	10	20
morphine	10	30
oxycodone	15	30
oxymorphone	1	10 (rectal)

Transdermal Fentanyl Dose

Table 9-9

Oral 24-Hour Morphine (IN mg/day)	Intramuscular 24-Hour Morphine (IN mg/day)	Transdermal Fentanyl (IN μg/h)
45-134	8-22	25
135-224	23-37	50
225-314	38-52	75
315-404	53-67	100
405-494	68-82	125
495-584	83-97	150
585-674	98-112	175
675-764	113-127	200
765-854	128-142	225
855-944	143-157	250

NONOPIOID ANALGESICS

The primary compound considered a nonopioid analgesic is acetaminophen. The entire class of NSAIDs are also analgesics that are not opioids; these agents are discussed in greater depth in Chapter 42. Acetaminophen is a nonopioid drug that has both analgesic as well as antipyretic effects. It is available in a variety of dosage formulations, and is available both over-the-counter (OTC) and by prescription. It is also a component of many combination products with opioids. Tramadol (Ultram) and nabumetone are both marketed as nonopioid pain relievers, also known as nonopioid analgesics. However, a closer look at the chemical structure of these agents reveals that they belong to existing drug categories. Tramadol is structurally very similar to codeine. It may have some pain relieving properties that are different from those of the opioids. Nabumetone is an NSAID. This section will focus primarily on the nonopioid analgesic acetaminophen.

Mechanism of Action

The mechanism of action of acetaminophen is similar to that of the salicylates. It is believed to cause pain impulses to be blocked peripherally. This is in response to

case study Pain Management for Terminal Illness

You are assigned to a patient who is in the terminal phases of breast cancer. As a home health care nurse, you have many responsibilities; however, you have not cared for many patients who are in the terminal phases of their illness. In fact, most of your patients are post-operative and have only required assessments, dressing changes, and wound care.

Ms. OD is 56 years of age and underwent bilateral mastectomy 4 years ago. She had lymph node involvement at the time of surgery, and recently metastasis to the bone has been diagnosed. She has been taking oxycodone (one 5-mg tablet every 6 hours) at home but is not sleeping through the night and is now complaining of increasing pain to the point that her quality of life has decreased significantly. She wants to stay at home during the terminal phases of her illness but needs to have adequate and safe pain control. Her husband of 28 years is very supportive, and they have no children. They are both college graduates and have medical insurance.

(Provide references from within this chapter for the selection of the specific opioid agent.)

- *Ms. OD's recent increase in pain has been attributed to bone metastasis in the area of the lumbar spine. At this time the oxyodone is not beneficial, and you as the home health care nurse need to recommend another pain medication to the physician. What medication would you recommend to relieve the bone pain, and what is your rationale for this recommendation?*
- *Identify the patient education guidelines for the specific medication you recommended to the physician.*
- *Outline a comprehensive nursing care plan appropriate to the specific agent used or recommended.*

For Answers see www.harcourthealth.com/MERLIN/Lilley/.

the inhibition of prostaglandin synthesis that is produced by acetaminophen. Acetaminophen is believed to lower the body temperature in patients with fever, but it rarely does so in patients with normal body temperatures. Acetaminophen accomplishes this by acting on the hypothalamus, the structure in the brain that regulates body temperature. Heat is dissipated as the result of the vasodilation and increased peripheral blood flow that occur.

Drug Effects

The drug effects of acetaminophen are limited primarily to its ability to alter the perception of pain and to lower temperature. It has only weak antiinflammatory effects. Although acetaminophen shares some of the same effects as the salicylates, it does not have many of the unwanted effects. Acetaminophen has no drug effects on the cardiovascular or respiratory systems. It does not cause acid-base changes, gastric irritation, erosion, or bleeding. It does not adversely effect platelets, prolong bleeding time, or increase the excretion of uric acid.

Therapeutic Uses

Acetaminophen is indicated for the treatment of mild to moderate pain and fever. It is an appropriate substitute for aspirin because of its analgesic and antipyretic uses. Acetaminophen is a valuable alternative for those patients who cannot tolerate aspirin or in whom aspirin may be contraindicated.

Side Effects and Adverse Effects

Acetaminophen is an effective and relatively safe agent. It is therefore available OTC and in many combination prescription drugs. The ingestion of large amounts, as in an acute overdose, can cause hepatic necrosis. This is the most serious acute toxic effect. Acute ingestion of acetaminophen doses of 150 mg/kg or more may result in hepatic toxicity. The long-term ingestion of large doses is more likely to result in nephropathy. Because the reported or estimated quantity of drug ingested is often inaccurate and not a reliable guide to the therapeutic management of the overdose, a serum acetaminophen concentration should be determined for this purpose no sooner than 4 hours after the ingestion. If a serum acetaminophen level cannot be determined, it should be assumed that the overdose is potentially toxic, and treatment with acetylcysteine (the recommended antidote for acetaminophen toxicity) should be started. Acetylcysteine works by preventing the hepatotoxic metabolites of acetaminophen from forming. The treatment regimen consists of an initial loading dose of 140 mg/kg orally, followed by 70 mg/kg every 4 hours for 17 additional doses. If the patient vomits within 1 hour of receiving a dose of acetylcysteine, then that dose should be given again immediately. All 17 doses must be given to prevent hepatotoxicity, regardless of what the subsequent acetaminophen serum levels are.

Interactions

There is a variety of substances that may interact with acetaminophen. Alcohol is potentially the most dangerous. Other drugs only mildly affect acetaminophen's action. Chronic, heavy alcohol abusers may be at increased risk of liver toxicity from excessive acetaminophen use. The majority of reports involve cases of severe chronic alcoholics taking large dosages of acetaminophen. Most often these dosages of acetaminophen exceed recommended doses and often involve substantial overdose. Professionals should alert their patients who regularly consume large amounts of alcohol to not exceed recommended doses of acetaminophen.

Dosages

For dosage information on acetaminophen, see the dosages table on p. 127.

drug profiles

There is a variety of drugs that could be classified as nonopioid analgesics. Acetaminophen, tramadol, nabumetone, and ketorolac are just a few of the more commonly used nonopioid analgesics. Nabumetone and ketorolac are both NSAIDs (discussed in Chapter 42), whereas tramadol is structurally very similar to codeine. Acetaminophen is one of the most widely used nonopioid analgesics, available both OTC and prescription.

⊸acetaminophen

Acetaminophen (Tylenol and others) is an effective and relatively safe nonopioid analgesic used for mild to moderate pain relief. It is classified as a pregnancy category B agent and is contraindicated in patients with a hypersensitivity to it or an intolerance to tartrazine (yellow dye no. 5), alcohol, sugar, or saccharin. Its use should be avoided in patients who are anemic or who have renal or hepatic disease.

Acetaminophen is available in many oral and rectal dosage formulations. It is available in the form of capsules, solution, granules, suspension, tablets, chewable tablets, film-coated tablets, tablets for solution, and rectal suppositories. It is available in numerous strengths, depending on whether it is intended for use in children or adults.

PHARMACOKINETICS*

HALF-LIFE	ONSET	PEAK	DURATION
1-4 hr	10-30 min	0.5-2 hr	3-4 hr

*For orally administered acetaminophen.

nursing process

Patients experiencing pain pose many challenges to the nurse and other health care providers who are involved in their health care. Adequate analgesia, pain relief without complications, and patient teaching are all goals of the health care overseen by the nurse in this context. Nurses need to adequately and accurately assess the nature of the patient's pain (Box 9-1). Assessment of pain is now being considered as a fifth vital sign (BP, P, T, R, and pain assessment) so that pain management is adequate and effective. They should also evaluate and monitor the patient's response to the analgesic (regardless of whether opioid or nonopioid analgesics are used) to provide safe and effective nursing care.

● Assessment

Before you administer an opioid agonist or agonist-antagonist, you must obtain an accurate and thorough medication history. This ensures the safe use of these medications, meaning analgesic treatment that is free of complications or injury to the patient. The nurse should ask about and document information regarding the following:
• Allergies
• Use of other opiates (the use of other opioids with agonists can lead to toxicity and overdosage; their use

BOX 9-1
Assessment of Pain

- Assess factors influencing pain, such as individual reaction, pain tolerance, underlying cause of pain, pain quality, pain intensity, pain duration, type of pain, pain experience, pain threshold, age, physical influences such as sleep and stress, and psychologic influences (family roles, spiritual system, meaning of pain, cultural influences, stereotypes, level and stage of growth and development, motivations, personality, fatigue, stress, anxiety, and fear). This approach to assessing pain embraces the *gate theory* of pain because it addresses the emotional and psychologic components of pain and how they are intertwined with the physiologic, perceptual, and reflexive pain components.
- Use a variety of scales to assess pain, such as numeric rating scales (0 = no pain, 10 = worst possible pain), visual analog scales, and adjective rating scales (e.g., no pain, little pain, large pain, etc.).
- In children under 5 years of age, consider level and stage of growth and development; pain often characterized by anger, hostility, and aggressiveness; use of pictures with happy (no pain with a scale of "0") and sad faces (pain is "bad" with scale of "5"); and tools that the pediatric patient can relate to, such as 6-inch ruler, to show level of pain.
- In your assessment of the geriatric patient, never assume that elderly patients do not feel pain as they did when they were younger because even though there may be barriers to pain (dementia, cognitive impairment), the older individual still experiences pain.
- Chronic pain assessment should consider that pain can occur with or without evident tissue damage and serves

no useful purpose. It is a complex and multifactoral problem that requires consideration of the holistic approach to patient care with consideration of not just physical factors but also psychologic factors (insomnia, depression, withdrawal, anxiety, personality changes, and changes in lifestyle) because chronic pain is generally characterized not by physical changes but by psychologic and functional ability changes.
- Assessment of chronic pain is challenging, but health care providers must go the "extra mile" to assess and then act. Remember that chronic pain is difficult to describe and manage and often not responsive to conventional measures.
- Cancer pain should be managed as individually as all other aspects of patient care with full belief in the patient's pain and suffering. Treatment may include narcotics and possibly high doses; however, addiction should not be the concern in this situation but rather *quality of life* for the patient. Remember this with your assessment.
- Ask for the patient with acute or chronic pain (or any type of pain) to keep a daily journal of his or her pain experience inclusive of precipitating and aggravating factors; measures that alleviate or help the pain; duration of pain and degree of intensity; referred pain, character, onset, and pattern; an assessment of his or her meaning of pain; and psychologic factors.
- Chronic and cancer pain may be perceived as an actual or potential loss to a patient, including a loss of control.

---

with agonist-antagonists can lead to an effect antagonistic to the analgesic)
- Alcohol use
- Nature of the pain including its severity (perhaps graded on a scale of 1 to 10, with 10 being the worst)
- Type of pain (stabbing, throbbing, dull ache, sharp, diffuse, localized, referred, or knifelike)
- Precipitating and relieving factors
- Home or herbal remedies used and the response to them
- Other pain treatments (pharmacologic and nonpharmacologic).

Vital signs (blood pressure, pulse, and respirations) should also be noted, determined, and documented. Do not forget that during the acute pain response, the stimulation to the sympathetic nervous system (SNS) may result in elevated vital sign values (blood pressure, >120/80 mm Hg, pulse >100 beats/min, respiration >20 breaths/min), and opioids will depress vital signs. Always document baseline intake and output measurements and continue to monitor and document these throughout the opioid treatment because of the associated urinary retention.

Before administering an opioid (pure or partial) agent, it is also essential to check the route and time of the previous analgesic administration and the patient's response. Always check the patient's chart, physician's order,

nurses' notes, and medication administration record before administering any additional doses of an analgesic.

With regard to the administration of the synthetic agonist-antagonist drugs, it is important to determine whether the patient is in an addictive state, because the administration of an adjunctive opioid may well precipitate withdrawal in such patients. Opioid antagonists such as naloxone hydrochloride and naltrexone have an

herbal interactions

Feverfew

BENEFIT OF HERB
Relieves headache, migraine; can be used to treat fever and menstrual irregularities

POTENTIAL INTERACTIONS
Can increase bleeding with use of aspirin, dipyridamole, and warfarin

CAUTIONS AND NOTES
Contraindicated in pregnant patients (may stimulate menstruation), breastfeeding patients, or patients 2 years of age or younger

antagonistic effect on opioid agonists and are used to reverse their effects in the event of toxicity or overdosage.

Drug interactions (increased effects) with opioid agonists and agonist-antagonists occur with the following agents: alcohol, other CNS depressants, sedative-hypnotics, muscle relaxants, major tranquilizers, and antipsychotic agents. Opioids are contraindicated in patients with allergies to them, bronchial asthma, opioid addiction, head injuries, and increased intracranial pressure. Cautious use, meaning close monitoring of the patient's response, reaction, and vital signs during opioid treatment, is called for in patients with any disease or altered state of the liver or kidneys. Refer to each opioid agonist agent for specific contraindications and cautions.

Contraindications to the use of acetaminophen include intolerance to yellow dye no. 5 (tartrazine), alcohol, table sugar, and saccharin. Cautious use is recommended in patients who have anemia, hepatic disease, and chronic alcoholism. You should also include a monitor of liver function studies if long-term therapy is indicated and assess for chronic poisoning such as rapid, weak pulse; dyspnea; or cold, clammy extremities. Drug interactions include alcohol, caffeine, colestipol, and cholestyramine.

● Nursing Diagnoses

Nursing diagnoses appropriate for the patient who is taking analgesics include the following:
- Acute or chronic pain related to etiology and need for analgesia.
- Acute or chronic pain related to nausea, vomiting, and constipation from side effects of opioids and other analgesics.
- Risk for injury and falls related to decreased sensorium from opioid agents.
- Risk for injury related to possible overdosage and adverse reactions to drug interactions associated with opioids.
- Risk for injury related to physical or psychological dependency of opioids.
- Impaired gas exchange related to possible respiratory depression from opioids.
- Constipation related to side effects of opioid analgesics.
- Risk for infection related to bladder retention and opioids on the CNS.

- Deficient knowledge related to unfamiliarity of opioids, their use, and side effects.

● Planning

Goals appropriate to the use of analgesics include the following:
- Patient identifies the rationale and therapeutic and side effects associated with the use of analgesics.
- Patient states measures that will enhance the effectiveness of the analgesic.
- Patient states measures that will decrease the occurrence of commonly associated side effects.

Outcome Criteria

Outcome criteria related to the use of analgesics are as follows:
- Patient will experience minimal side effects and complications associated with the use of analgesics such as nausea, vomiting, or constipation.
- Patient will demonstrate increased comfort levels as seen by decreased use of analgesics, increased activity, decreased complaints of pain, and decreased rating of pain.
- Patient will use nonpharmacologic measures to enhance comfort such as relaxation therapy, distraction, and music therapy.
- Patient manage side effects associated wth analgesics through fluid intake and possible antiemetic therapy.

● Implementation

Once the cause of pain has been diagnosed, pain management should begin immediately and aggressively. Pain management is varied, multifaceted, and inclusive of not only pharmacologic but also nonpharmacologic and alternative approaches to pain relief (Box 9-2). If it is time for the patient to receive another dose of a opioid medication, then you should administer the opioid, record it in the nurses' notes and medication record, and sign with a full signature. The medication, amount, site, and response should all be documented (see Chapter 8). When using opioids, both pure and mixed agents, you must always be sure to medicate patients before the pain becomes severe or when the pain is beginning to return so as to provide adequate analgesia and pain control. It is often recommended that the oral

---

Box 9-2 Treatment Options for Pain

Acupressure	Hot or cold packs	Reduction of fear
Acupuncture	Hypnosis	Relaxation
Art therapy	Imagery	Surgery
Behavioral therapy	Massage	Therapeutic baths
Comfort measures	Meditation	Therapeutic communication
Counseling	Music therapy	Therapeutic touch
Cutaneous stimulation	Over-the-counter drugs	Transcutaneous electric nerve
Distraction	Pet therapy	stimulation (TENS)
Herbals	Prescription drugs	Yoga

forms of opioids be taken with food to minimize gastrointestinal tract upset, specifically nausea. Antiemetic therapy may be needed should such nausea and vomiting prove uncontrollable. Safety measures, such as keeping the side rails up and having the call bell within the patient's reach, are crucial in preventing falls stemming from possible confusion, hypotension, and decreased sensorium, especially in the elderly patient. When administering morphine, meperidine, and similiar drugs, you should withhold the dose and contact the physician if there is any decline in the patient's condition or if the vital signs are abnormal (see normal values given earlier), especially a respiratory rate of less than 12 breaths/min. When administering IM injections of analgesics, sites should be adequately and accurately oriented and cleansed with an antiseptic, a needle in the proper size and gauge used (see Chapter 8), the injectant aspirated before injection, and the site and other information documented as with any prn medication.

With the IV administration of analgesics, always follow the insert instructions regarding the diluent and time over which the amount ordered should be delivered. When patient-controlled analgesia is being used, the amounts and times of dosing should be noted in the appropriate records. When an opioid is used, *always* check and recheck the opioid count and immediately report any errors in counting to the charge nurse, nurse manager, or supervisor. Never assume that someone else will report

or detect the error. Another point to remember when administering analgesics is that each medication has a different onset of action, peak, and duration of action, and these differences apply to the route of administration as well. In addition, each patient responds differently. See Box 9-3 for opioid administration guidelines.

home health/community points

Analgesics

- With most opioids, the patient's mental and physical abilities may be impaired, so every effort should be made to instruct the patient, family members, and caregivers about the need for safety measures such as not allowing the patient to engage in activities requiring mental alertness (e.g., driving a car or operating any type of machinery).
- Remind patients that different opioids should not be mixed in any form or manner.
- Instruct persons caring for the patient and the patient proper about careful and accurate pain assessment and the need to keep a journal containing information about the patient's pain, precipitating factors, alleviating factors, and the response to pain medication and nonpharmacologic measures.

BOX 9-3   Opioid Administration Guidelines

Narcotic	Nursing Administration
buprenorphine and butorphanol	When giving IV, infuse over 3 to 5 minutes; always assess respirations. Give IM butorphanol in deep gluteal muscle mass.
codeine	Give PO doses with food to minimize gastrointestinal tract upset; ceiling effects with oral codeine.
dezocine	Mixed agonist-antagonist; short duration of action; IM: deep gluteal muscle mass.
fentanyl	IM and IV dosages to be administered slowly and per package insert instructions to prevent muscular rigidity and cardiac arrest; when administered IV or epidurally, should have resuscitative equipment nearby and naloxone at the bedside; patches come in various strengths, so watch dosing versus order very carefully to prevent overdosage; fentanyl will also soon be available in lozenge form for anesthetic premedication in children and adults.
hydromorphone	May be given SC, rectally, IV, PO, or IM.
levorphanol	May be given PO, SC, or IV; IV forms to be given over 5 minutes or adhere to manufacturer guidelines; longer acting (6-8 hours).
meperidine methadone	Given by a variety of routes; IV, IM, or PO; highly protein bound, so watch for interactions and toxicity with PO, or IM forms.
morphine	In a variety of forms: SC, IM, IV, extended and immediate release, and morphine sulfate (Duramorph) for epidural infusion; morphine sulfate (MS Contin) now available in a 200-mg, sustained-release tablet.
nalbuphine	IV dosages of 10 mg undiluted over 5 minutes.
naloxone	Antagonist given for opioid overdose; 0.4 mg usually given IV over 15 seconds or less.
propoxyphene	Oral dosing only; high abuse potential.
oxycodone	Often mixed with acetaminophen or aspirin; oral and suppository dosage forms.
oxymorphone	Oral, IM, IV, SC, and rectal suppository dosage forms.
pentazocine	SC, IV, and IM forms; mixed agent; 5 mg IV to be given over 1 minute.
sufentanil	Used as adjunct to anesthesia and so given with oxygen.

To reverse an opioid overdose or opioid-induced respiratory depression, an opioid antagonist such as naloxone must be administered. If naloxone is the antagonist used in your unit, 0.4 to 2 mg should be given either intravenously in its undiluted form and administered over 15 seconds (or as ordered), or the dose should be given as an injection diluted in water, 5% dextrose in water, or normal saline solution (see Table 9-7). The guidelines in the package insert should also be followed. Emergency resuscitative equipment should be nearby in the event of respiratory or cardiac arrest.

When administering opioid agonist-antagonist agents such as buprenorphine and nalbuphine, remember that they are very similar to the pure opioids when given by themselves, so the same nursing interventions apply. Be careful to always check the dosages and routes. Their misuse potential and addiction, however, are lower than with pure opioids. Also remember the possibility of withdrawal symptoms in individuals who are opioid dependent.

Acetaminophen should be taken as prescribed by all patients, especially pediatric and elderly patients. This medication may be given with meals if gastrointestinal upset is problematic. Patient teaching should focus on the emphasis of taking the medication as indicated to avoid liver damage and acute toxicity. If taking other OTC medications, patients should read the labels very carefully for any other interactions. Teaching signs of overdose is also important and includes bleeding, malaise, fever, sore throat and easy bruising. It is also important to inform the patient to report a fever or pain lasting longer than 3 days since this individual should be re-evaluated. Many community resources are often available within one's community or at least at a nearby health care facility. Phone calls may be placed to area hospitals in reference to availability of a pain clinic. Internet sites that may be helpful to patients include www.unitedpainclinic.com, www.pain.com, and www.mayohealth.org. Many other pain sites are available on the Internet using the keyword "pain" or "pain clinic."

Patient teaching tips for analgesic agents are presented below.

Activity

● Evaluation

After and during the administration of opioid or nonopioid analgesics, it is important to monitor the patient for both therapeutic and side effects. Therapeutic effects include decreased complaints of pain and increased periods of comfort, with improved activities of daily living, appetite, and sense of well-being. Side effects vary with each drug (see earlier discussion in this chapter) but often consist of nausea, vomiting, constipation, dizziness, headache, blurred vision, decreased urinary output, drowsiness, lethargy, sedation, palpitations, bradycardia, bradypnea, dyspnea, and hypotension. Should vital signs change, the patient's condition decline, or pain continue, the nurse should contact the physician immediately. Respiratory depression may be manifested by a rate of less than 12 breaths/min, dyspnea, diminished breath sounds, or shallow breathing.

A positive therapeutic outcome to acetaminophen includes a decrease in the symptomatology, decreased fever or decreased pain. Adverse reactions for which to monitor include the previously mentioned liver problems with hepatotoxicity, anemias. In addition, abdominal pain and vomiting should be reported to the physician.

⬧ patient teaching tips

Analgesic Agents

➤ Encourage patients to keep a record or journal of their pain experience and all methods of treatment, both pharmacologic and nonpharmacologic.

➤ Patients should follow instructions on the medication vial or bottle regarding the dose, route, and frequency of the medication. Following instructions closely is essential to preventing toxicity or overdose that may result in cardiac or respiratory arrest.

➤ The physician or health care provider should be contacted if emesis occurs while the patient is taking the opioid, because nausea and vomiting are common side effects; often medication is needed to alleviate the nausea.

➤ Constipation is a common side effect of opioid use and may be prevented with forced fluids (unless contraindicated) and a high-fiber diet.

➤ The physician should be contacted should the patient show symptoms of allergic reaction such as wheezing, difficulty breathing, itching, hives, or central nervous system changes such as weakness, dizziness, or fainting.

➤ Withdrawal symptoms associated with opioids include nausea, vomiting, cramps, fainting spells, and fever.

➤ Patients should be instructed to carefully read the directions on the opioids prescription container as well as on any over-the-counter medications so that they are alerted to possible contraindications or drug interactions.

➤ Side effects patients should be alerted to include gastrointestinal tract upset, constipation, drowsiness, dizziness, headache, sleepiness, tinnitus (ringing of the ears), blurred vision, palpitations, bradycardia, and hypotension.

➤ Patients should be encouraged to change positions slowly to prevent possible orthostatic hypotension.

POINTS TO REMEMBER

Pain

- Involves senses and emotions that are unpleasant.
- Is associated with actual or potential tissue damage.
- Is a personal and individual experience.
- Can be made worse or better by many conditions.

Analgesic

- Relieves pain without causing loss of consciousness.
- Includes painkillers.

Types of Pain

- Acute (sudden in onset and severe) versus chronic (persistent or recurring pain lasting more than 6 months).
- Somatic (skeletal muscles, ligaments, or joints) versus visceral (organs or smooth muscle).
- Superficial (skin or mucous membranes).

Gate Theory

- Gate in dorsal horn of spinal column allows pain sensation from damaged tissues to travel to brain.
- If sensation gets to brain, we feel pain. If not, we do not feel pain.
- Brain can, in return, send inhibitory signals to gate to turn it down or close it.

Physical versus Psychologic Dependence

- Physical: adaptation of body to opioid analgesic (expected).
- Psychologic: compulsive drug use with intent to alter mental status (unexpected).

Types of Analgesics

- NSAIDS: nonopioid, nonsteroidal analgesics used for acute and chronic pain.
- Opioids are natural or synthetic agents that either contain or are derived from morphine (opiates) or have opiate-like effects or activities (opioids).

Mechanism of Action

- Agonist: binds to receptor and causes response.
- Agonist-antagonist: acts as an agonist at one type of receptor and as an antagonist at another type of receptor.
- Antagonist: binds to receptor and prevents response.

Nursing Considerations

- Pain must be managed before it gets uncontrollable.
- A nonopioid agent is used first in most situations depending on the pain rating.
- Stronger analgesics are used as the next step to pain control.

REVIEW QUESTIONS

1. A nonsteroidal antiinflammatory agent is often added to narcotic pain regimens for treatment of bone cancer pain. Which of the following actions is the reason for its use as an adjunct in this type of pain?
   a. Antiseptic
   b. Antipyretic
   c. Anticoagulant
   d. Antiinflammatory

2. Which of the following drugs has a known interaction with NSAIDs?
   a. Aspirin
   b. Acetaminophen
   c. Antihypertensives
   d. Oral hypoglycemics

3. Which of the following is a benefit of using the narcotic agonist-antagonist agents to treat pain?
   a. More analgesia
   b. Less constipation
   c. Greater CNS stimulation
   d. Lower dependency potential

4. You suspect that your patient is toxic to the narcotic being administered and is showing signs of respiratory depression. Which of the following drugs is used for narcotic overdosage?
   a. Naloxone (Narcan)
   b. Meperidine (Demerol)
   c. Methadone (Dolophine)
   d. Levorphanol (Levo-Dromoran)

5. Meperidine (Demerol) would generally not be recommended for use in a patient suffering from moderate to severe pain related to ovarian cancer. Which of the following statements best describes the rationale for not using Demerol in cancer patients?
   a. Mood alterations and euphoria are minimal.
   b. It is longer acting on the gamma, kappa, and mu receptors.
   c. It is similar to ultra–long-acting barbiturates and, as such, works well for these patients.
   d. It has a duration of action that is shorter than that of other desirable agents, such as morphine.

For Answers see www.harcourthealth.com/MERLIN/Lilley/.

CRITICAL THINKING Activities

1. What is the purpose of a "drug holiday" with patients who are taking narcotics on a long-term basis?
2. Indicate whether this statement is true or false, and explain your answer: Cancer patients should never receive strong narcotics at the beginning of any pain experience because of the fear of addiction.
3. You administer 100 mg meperidine (Demerol) IM to a patient in severe postoperative pain, as ordered. What assessment data should be gathered before and after administering this drug? Explain your answer.
4. Your patient complains that the drugs he is receiving for severe pain are really not helping. What would be the most appropriate response to this patient?
5. Compare and contrast the effectiveness of the following routes for narcotic administration, including their ease of self-preparation and administration, onset of therapeutic serum concentrations, degree of sedation, side effects, and ease of management in the home setting: oral, intramuscular, transdermal.

For Answers see www.harcourthealth.com/MERLIN/Lilley/.

bibliography

Albanese J, Nutz P: *Mosby's 2001 nursing drug reference and review cards,* St Louis, 2001, Mosby.

American Hospital Formulary Service: *AHFS drug information,* Bethesda, Md, 2000, American Society of Health-System Pharmacists.

American Society of Pain Management Nursing (ASPMN), ASPMN @aol.com.

Anderson PO, Knoben JE, Troutman WG: *Handbook of clinical drug data 1999-2000,* ed 9, New York, 1999, McGraw-Hill.

Bral EE: Caring for adults with chronic cancer pain, *AJN* 98(4):26, 1998.

Johns Hopkins Hospital, Department of Pediatrics et al: *The Harriet Lane handbook,* ed 15, St Louis, 2000, Mosby.

Keen JH: *Critical care and emergency drug reference,* ed 3, St Louis, 1996, Mosby.

McCaffery M, Pasero C: *Pain: clinical manual,* ed 2, St Louis, 1999, Mosby.

McCaffery M: Pain management handbook, *Nursing 97* 27(4);42, 1997.

Mosby's GenRx: A comprehensive reference for generic and brand drugs, ed 10, St Louis, 2000, Mosby.

Pasero C: Transdermal fentanyl for chronic pain, *AJN* 97(11):17, 1997.

Purdue Pharma LP: *Symposium spotlight,* Stamford, Conn, 2000, One Stamford Forum.

Skidmore-Roth L: *Mosby's 2001 nursing drug reference,* St Louis, 2001, Mosby.

Remember to check the **Online Worksheet** for additional learning opportunities: **www.harcourthealth.com/MERLIN/Lilley/**

Activity

General and Local Anesthetics

objectives

When you reach the end of this chapter, you should be able to do the following:

Look for this symbol for topics covered in the **Online Worksheet**

1 Define *anesthesia.*

2 Discuss the differences between and indications of general and local anesthetics.

3 List the most commonly used general and local anesthetics with their associated risk factors.

4 Discuss what occurs in anesthesia, including the stages of anesthesia.

5 Discuss the differences between depolarizing neuromuscular blocking agents (NMBAs) and nondepolarizing NMBAs.

6 Compare the mechanism of action, side effects, cautions, contraindications, nursing implementations, and indications for general anesthesia (including depolarizing NMBAs and nonpolarizing NMBAs) and local anesthesia.

7 Develop a nursing care plan that includes preanesthesia and postanesthesia care for patients receiving either general or local anesthesia.

drug profiles

enflurane, p. 143
halothane, p. 143
o━ isoflurane, p. 144
o━ lidocaine, p. 147
methoxyflurane, p. 144
nitrous oxide, p. 144

pancuronium, p. 150
propofol, p. 144
rapacuronium, p. 150
succinylcholine, p. 150
vecuronium, p. 150

o━ Key drug.

glossary

Adjunctive agents (ad junk′ tiv) Agents used in combination with anesthetic agents to control the side effects of anesthetics or to help maintain the anesthetic state in the patient. (p. 141)

Anesthesia (an′ es the zhə) A drug-induced state in which the CNS is altered to produce varying degrees of pain relief, depression of consciousness, skeletal muscle relaxation, and diminished or absent reflexes. (p. 139)

Anesthetics (an′ əs the′ tiks) Agents that depress the CNS to produce depression of consciousness, loss of responsiveness to sensory stimulation, or muscle relaxation. (p. 139)

Balanced anesthesia The practice of using combinations of drugs to produce anesthesia rather than using a single agent. Common combinations include a sedative-hypnotic, an antianxiety agent, an analgesic, an antiemetic, and an anticholinergic. (p. 141)

General anesthetics Agents that induce the state of anesthesia. Their effects are global in that they affect the whole body, with loss of consciousness being one of those effects. (p. 140)

Local anesthetics Agents that render a specific portion of the body insensitive to pain without affecting consciousness. Also called *regional anesthetics.* (p. 144)

Overton-Meyer theory A theory that describes the relationship between the lipid solubility of anesthetic agents and their potency. It is often used to explain how anesthetic agents are believed to work. (p. 141)

Parenteral anesthetics (pə ren′ tər əl) Agents that can be administered directly into the CNS by various spinal injection techniques. In addition, they can be injected adjacent to main nerves to accomplish anesthesia of the peripheral nervous system. (p. 144)

Topical anesthetics A class of local anesthetics that are applied directly to the skin and mucous membranes. They consist of solutions, ointments, gels, creams, powders, ophthalmic drops, and suppositories. (p. 144)

Anesthetics are agents that depress the central nervous system (CNS), which in turn produces depression of consciousness, loss of responsiveness to sensory stimulation (including pain), or muscle relaxation. This state of depressed CNS activity is called **anesthesia.** There are many mechanisms by which anesthetics accomplish these responses, but in general they all do so by interfering with nerve conduction. Anesthetics can produce one or all of the actions just mentioned, depending on the agent. Anesthetics are most commonly classified as either general anesthetics or local anesthetics, depending on where in the CNS the particular anesthetic agent works.

GENERAL ANESTHETICS

A **general anesthetic** is an agent that induces a state in which the CNS is altered so that varying degrees of pain relief, depression of consciousness, skeletal muscle relaxation, and reflex reduction are produced. General anesthesia can be achieved by the use of one drug or a combination of drugs. Often a combination of drugs is used to accomplish general anesthesia, allowing less of each of the agents to be used and a more balanced, controlled state of anesthesia to be achieved. General anesthetic agents are used most commonly to produce deep muscle relaxation and loss of consciousness during surgical procedures.

There are two main categories of general anesthetics that are determined by their respective routes of administration. The first group, inhaled anesthetics, are volatile

Table 10-1 Inhaled General Anesthetics

Agents	
Generic Name	**Trade Name**
INHALED GAS	
cyclopropane	(many)
nitrous oxide	("laughing gas")
INHALED VOLATILE LIQUID	
desflurane	Suprane
enflurane	Ethrane
halothane	Fluothane, Somnothane*
isoflurane	Forane
methoxyflurane	Penthrane
sevoflurane	Ultane

*Canadian trade name.

Table 10-2 Intravenous Anesthetic Agents

Agents		
Generic Name	**Trade Name**	**Dosage**
etomidate	Amidate	0.2-0.6 mg/kg IV
ketamine	Ketalar	1-4.5 mg/kg IV; 6.5-13 mg/kg IM
methohexital	Brevital, Brietal*	50-120 mg IV (induction); 20-40 mg IV (maintenance)
propofol†	Diprivan	1-2.5 mg/kg IV (induction); 50-200 μg/kg/min IV (maintenance)
thiamylal	Surital	Titrate to response IV
thiopental	Pentothal	25-75 mg IV as needed

*Canadian trade name.
†Dosages for propofol are typically 5 to 50 mg/kg/min for initiation and maintenance of ICU sedation.

Table 10-3 Adjunctive Anesthetic Agents

Agent	Pharmacologic Class	Dosage Range	Purpose
alfentanil (Alfenta) fentanyl (Sublimaze) sufentanil (Sufenta)	Opioid analgesic	130-245 μg/kg IV 50-100 μg/kg IV 8-30 μg/kg IV	Anesthesia induction
diazepam (Valium, Meval*) midazolam (Versed)	Benzodiazepine	2-20 mg PO/IV/IM 0.05-0.35 mg/kg IV	Amnesia and anxiety
atropine glycopyrrolate (Robinul) scopolamine	Anticholinergic	0.1-0.6 mg IM/IV/SC 0.0044 mg/kg IM 0.3-0.6 mg SC/IM	To dry up excessive secretions
meperidine (Demerol) morphine	Opioid analgesic	50-100 mg IM/SC 5-20 mg IM/SC	Pain prevention and pain relief
hydroxyzine (Atarax, Vistaril, Multipax*) pentobarbital (Nembutal) promethazine (Phenergan, Histanil*) secobarbital (Seconal)	Sedative-hypnotic	25-100 mg IM 150-200 mg IM 25-50 mg IM 100-250 mg IV	Amnesia and sedation

*Canadian trade name.

liquids or gases that are vaporized in oxygen and inhaled to induce anesthesia. The second group, injectable anesthetics, are administered intravenously. The different inhaled gases and volatile liquids used as general anesthetics are listed in Table 10-1.

Intravenously administered anesthetic agents are used to induce or maintain general anesthesia, to induce amnesia, and as an adjunct to inhalation-type anesthetics. These agents are commonly used in combination with **adjunctive agents,** which are sedative-hypnotics, antianxiety agents, opioid and nonopioid analgesics, antiemetics, and anticholinergics that can minimize some of the undesirable after-effects of excessive doses of the inhaled anesthetics. This practice is called **balanced anesthesia.** Some of the after-effects are excessive salivation, bradycardia, and vomiting. This combining of several different agents makes it possible for general anesthesia to be accomplished with smaller amounts of anesthetic gases, thereby lessening the side effects. The IV anesthetics, their dosage forms, and the usual doses are given in Table 10-2. A brief list of the adjunctive agents is given in Table 10-3. These agents are discussed in greater detail in chapters devoted to discussion of the respective classes of agents.

Mechanism of Action

Many theories have been proposed to explain the actual mechanism of action of general anesthetics. However, the agents vary widely in their chemical structure, and therefore their mechanism of action is not easily explained by a structure—receptor relationship. The concentrations required for different anesthetics to produce a given state of anesthesia also differ greatly. The **Overton-Meyer theory** explains some of the properties of anesthetic agents that may make the mechanism of action of these agents easier to understand. This theory states that there is a relationship between the lipid solubility of an anesthetic agent and its potency: the greater the solubility of the agent in fat, the greater the effect. Nerve cell membranes have a high lipid content, as does the blood-brain barrier. Anesthetic agents can therefore easily cross this blood-brain barrier and concentrate in nerve cell membranes. Initially this produces a loss of the senses of sight, touch, taste, smell, awareness, and hearing, and usually the patient becomes unconscious. Even though the heart and lungs (the vital centers responsible for blood pressure and breathing) are controlled by the medulla, they usually can be spared because the medullary center is depressed last.

Drug Effects

The main effect of general anesthetics is an orderly and systematic paralysis of the CNS. They produce a progressive depression of cerebral and spinal cord functions. Therapeutic (anesthetic) doses cause minimal depression of the medullary centers that govern vital functions. However, an anesthetic overdose paralyzes the medullary centers. This can lead to death stemming from circulatory and respiratory failure.

The progressive paralysis of nervous system functions produced by general anesthetics can be categorized into four distinct stages (Table 10-4). These stages vary greatly depending on the anesthetics used.

Therapeutic Uses

General anesthetics are used to produce unconsciousness, skeletal muscular relaxation, and visceral smooth muscle relaxation for surgical procedures.

Side Effects and Adverse Effects

The adverse effects of general anesthetics are dose dependent and vary with the individual agents. The heart, peripheral circulation, liver, kidneys, and respiratory tract

pediatric considerations

Anesthesia

- The premature infant, neonate, or pediatric patient is more affected by anesthesia than the young or middle-age adult patient. All of their body systems are very sensitive to the effects of anesthesia, so the nurse must take all precautions to protect the patient and ensure his or her safety during all phases of surgery and all phases of anesthesia, whether general or regional.
- The pediatric patient's hepatic, cardiac, respiratory, and renal systems are either not fully developed or they are not yet fully functional, which makes these patients more susceptible to problems such as CNS depression, toxicity, atelectasis, pneumonia, and cardiac abnormalities.
- It is important to assess for the presence of any disease of the cardiac, renal, hepatic, or respiratory systems and to document any pertinent findings because of the attendant increased risk of complications during anesthesia in such settings. Add to this the risk associated with a very young age or with being a newborn or preemie, and the possible complications of surgery and adverse effects of anesthesia become even more problematic and more likely to occur.
- The neonate is at a higher risk of upper airway obstruction of laryngospasms during general anesthesia because of the airway physical characteristics in this age group.
- A more rapid metabolic rate and small airway diameter also put the neonate at greater risk of suffering complications during general anesthesia.
- Carefully calculated doses must consider the neonate's weight and/or body surface area.
- Nitrous oxide is commonly used in pediatric patients because of the decreased risk of hepatitis associated with this agent.
- Resuscitative equipment should be nearby in any neonatal or pediatric unit.
- Any change in the level of consciousness should be assessed, noted, documented, and reported immediately to a physician, even if it occurs during the postoperative period.

Table 10-4 Stages of Anesthesia

CNS Effects	Stage 1	Stage 2	Stage 3 Plane 1	Stage 3 Plane 2	Stage 3 Plane 3	Stage 3 Plane 4	Stage 4
Consciousness	Maintained / Analgesia / Euphoria / Some distortion of perceptions / Variable amnesia	Lost	Absent	Absent	Absent	Absent	Absent
Respiration	No alteration, or increased rate with some irregularity	Rapid, irregular	Regular	Regular, but expirations longer than inspirations	Diaphragmatic	Thoracic ceased / Diaphragmatic depressed	No respiratory movement / Respiratory paralysis / Diaphragm paralyzed
Skeletal muscles	Normal tone	Tone increased	Small muscles relaxed	Large muscles relaxed	Complete relaxation	Complete relaxation	
Eyes							
Pupils	Reaction to light	Dilated	Constricted	Mid-dilation	Increasing dilatation	Dilated	Dilated
Movements	Unchanged	Increased	Increased	None	None	None	None
Tear secretion				Decreased	Decreased	Absent	Absent
Reflexes							
Lid	Present	Present	Absent	Absent	Absent	Absent	Absent
Corneal	Present	Present	Present	Absent	Absent	Absent	Absent
Pharyngeal or "gag"	Absent		Absent				
Laryngeal				Absent			
Cough					Absent in large bronchi	Absent in small bronchi	
Heart rate		Increased	Decreased	Normal	Decreased	Decreased	
Blood pressure	Unchanged	Increased	Normal				Decreased
Venous pressure	Unchanged	Increased	Unchanged				Increased

From McKenry LM, Salerno E: *Mosby's pharmacology in nursing*, ed 19, St Louis, 1995, Mosby.

DOSAGES Selected General Anesthetic Agents

agent	pharmacologic class	dosage range	purpose
enflurane (Ethrane)	Inhalation general anesthetic (halogenated ether)	0.5%-3% concentration	General anesthesia
halothane (Fluothane)	Halogenated inhalation general anesthetic	0.5%-1.5% concentration	General anesthesia
isoflurane (Forane)	Inhalation general anesthetic (enflurane isomer)	1.5%-3% concentration	General anesthesia
methoxyflurane (Penthrane)	Inhalation general anesthetic (halogenated ether)	0.1%-2% concentration with appropriate drugs	General anesthesia
nitrous oxide ("laughing gas")	Inorganic inhalation general anesthetic	20%-40% with oxygen 70% with 30% oxygen	Analgesia Anesthesia

are the sites primarily affected. Myocardial depression is a common side effect. All of the halogenated anesthetics are capable of causing hepatotoxicity, and methoxyflurane can cause significant respiratory depression.

With the development and use of newer agents, many of the unwanted side effects of the older agents (such as hepatotoxicity and myocardial depression) are now a thing of the past. In addition, many of the bothersome side effects such as nausea, vomiting, and confusion have become less common as balanced anesthesia has been more widely used. This practice prevents many of the unwanted, dose-dependent side effects and toxicity associated with the anesthetic agents while simultaneously achieving a more balanced general anesthesia.

Toxicity and Management of Overdose

In large doses all anesthetics are potentially life-threatening, with cardiac and respiratory arrest the ultimate causes of death. However, these agents are almost exclusively administered in a very controlled environment by personnel trained in advanced cardiac life support. These agents are also very quickly metabolized. In addition, the medullary center, which governs the vital centers, is the last area of the brain to be affected by the anesthetics and the first to regain function if it is lost. These factors combined make an anesthetic overdose rare and easily reversible.

Symptomatic and supportive therapy is usually all that is needed in the event of an anesthetic overdose.

Interactions

Because general anesthetics produce both desired and adverse effects on so many body systems, they are associated with a wide array of drug interactions that also vary widely in severity. Some of the more common drug-drug interactions are antihypertensives, beta-blockers, and tetracycline. These agents will have additive effects when given with general anesthetics. When given with antihypertensives, general anesthetics may result in increased hypotensive effects; with beta-blockers increased myocardial depression; and with tetracycline increased renal

toxicity. No significant laboratory test interactions have been reported.

Dosages

For the recommended dosages of selected general anesthetic agents, see the dosages table above.

drug profiles

All of the agents used for general anesthesia are, of course, prescription-only drugs. Desflurane, enflurane, sevoflurane, halothane, isoflurane, and methoxyflurane are all volatile liquids; nitrous oxide is a gas. The dose of each agent depends on the surgical procedure to be performed and the physical characteristics of the patient. All of the general anesthetics have a rapid onset of activity that is maintained for the duration of the surgical procedure by continuous administration of the agent. Propofol is chemically unrelated to the other intravenous anesthetic agents. Its favorable pharmacokinetics, quick onset of anesthesia, and quick offset have made it a widely used and attractive agent.

enflurane

Enflurane (Ethrane) is a fluorinated ether that produces good muscular relaxation and minimal cardiac sensitivity to catecholamines. The drug can produce seizures in the setting of low carbon dioxide blood levels and should not be used in patients with convulsive disorders. The dosage information is given in the table above.

Activity

halothane

Halothane (Fluothane) is a halogenated hydrocarbon (containing three molecules of fluoride and one each of chlorine and bromine) that is frequently used with nitrous oxide. It causes considerable cardiac sensitivity to catecholamines, it produces poor muscular relaxation when used alone, and its high halogen content can result in significant liver toxicity. The dosage information is given in the table on p. 143.

isoflurane

Isoflurane (Forane) is very similar to enflurane in its chemical structure. However, the differences in its chemical structure give it some favorable characteristics that distinguish it from its chemical relative. Isoflurane has a more rapid onset of action, causes less cardiovascular depression, and overall has been associated with little or no toxicity. The dosage information is given in the table on p. 143.

methoxyflurane

Methoxyflurane (Penthrane) is a fluorinated and chlorinated ether that produces excellent muscular relaxation without causing any significant cardiac sensitivity to catecholamines. However, the biotransformation of this agent produces free halogen ions that can cause significant liver toxicity, and its use is therefore contraindicated in patients with liver disease. In addition, methoxyflurane produces respiratory depression, which limits its use to patients undergoing short operations. The dosage information is given in the table on p. 143.

nitrous oxide

Nitrous oxide, also known as *laughing gas,* is the only inhaled gas currently used as a general anesthetic. It is the weakest of the general anesthetic agents and is primarily used for dental procedures or as a useful supplement to other more potent anesthetics. The dosage information is given in the table on p. 143.

propofol

Propofol (Diprivan) is an intravenous sedative-hypnotic agent for use in the induction and maintenance of anesthesia or sedation. Propofol has many favorable characteristics that have lead to its widespread use. It produces its effects very rapidly, and when it is turned off its effects subside very quickly. Propofol also is typically well-tolerated, producing few undesirable effects. Propofol can be used to initiate and maintain monitored anesthesia care (MAC) sedation during diagnostic procedures in adults. It is also used in intubated, mechanically ventilated adult patients in the intensive care unit (ICU) to provide continuous sedation and control of stress responses. When used in the ICU, typical dosages are 5 to 50 $\mu g/kg/min$. At higher doses it can be used for induction and maintenance of general anesthesia. Dosage information is provided in Table 10-2 on p. 140.

LOCAL ANESTHETICS

Local anesthetics are the second class of anesthetics. They are also called *regional anesthetics* because they render a specific portion of the body insensitive to pain. They do this by interfering with nerve transmission in specific areas of the body, blocking nerve conduction only in the area where they are applied without causing loss of consciousness. They are most commonly used in those clinical settings in which loss of consciousness, whole body muscle relaxation, and loss of responsiveness are either undesirable or unnecessary (e.g., during childbirth). Other uses for local anesthetics include dental procedures, the suturing of skin lacerations, spinal anesthesia, and diagnostic procedures such as lumbar puncture or thoracentesis.

Local anesthetics belong to several different groups of organic compounds and are classified as either topical or parenteral anesthetics. **Topical anesthetics** are applied directly to the skin and mucous membranes. They are available in the form of solutions, ointments, gels, creams, powders, ophthalmic drops, lozenges, and suppositories. These agents, the route of administration, and the dosages are listed in Table 10-5. **Parenteral anesthetics** can be administered directly into the CNS by various spinal injection techniques. Anesthesia of specific areas of the peripheral nervous system is accomplished either by injecting the agents adjacent to main nerves (to produce a large body area of anesthesia) or by infiltrating it (for a more limited area of anesthesia). Some of the common types of local anesthesia are described in Box 10-1. The parenteral anesthetic agents and the pharmacokinetics are summarized in Table 10-6.

Mechanism of Action

Local anesthetics work by rendering a specific portion of the body insensitive to pain by interfering with nerve transmission in specific areas of the body. Nerve conduction is blocked only in the area where they are applied without loss of consciousness.

Local anesthetics block both the generation and conduction of impulses through all nerve fibers (sensory, motor, and autonomic) by blocking the movement of certain ions (sodium, potassium, and calcium) important to this process. They do this by making it more difficult for these ions to move in and out of the nerve fiber. For this reason, some of these agents are also described as *membrane stabilizing* because they stabilize the nerve fiber cell membrane so that it is less permeable to the free movement of ions.

Drug Effects

As stated previously, local anesthetics have effects on all nerve fibers (sensory, motor, and autonomic). The membrane-stabilizing effects occur first in the small fibers, then in the large fibers. In terms of paralysis, usually autonomic activity is affected first, then pain and other sensory functions are lost. Motor activity is the last to be lost. When the effects of the local anesthetics wear off, they do so in reverse order, as function returns to motor activity, then sensory functions, and last autonomic activity.

Topical Anesthetics

table 10-5

Agent	Route	Dosage Strength
benzocaine (Dermoplast, Lanacaine, Solarcaine)	Topical Aerosol and spray	0.5%-20% ointment or cream
butamben (Butesin)	Topical	1% ointment
cocaine	Topical	1%-10% solution, jelly
dibrecaine (Nupecainal)	Injection and topical	0.5%-1% solution, ointment, or cream
dibucaine	Topical	1% ointment
dyclonine (Dyclone, Sucrets)	Topical	0.5%-1% solution, 0.1% spray, 1, 2 and 3 mg oral lozenges
ethyl chloride (Chlorethane)	Topical	Spray
lidocaine	Topical	5% patch
proparacaine (Alcaine, Ophthetic)	Ophthalmic	0.5% solution
pramoxine (Tronolane)	Topical	1% jelly, cream, or lotion
prilocaine (Emla)	Topical	2.5% prilocaine and 2.5% lidocaine cream
tetracaine (Pontocaine)	Injection, topical, and ophthalmic	0.5%-2% solution, ointment, or cream

Types of Local Anesthesia

box 10-1

EPIDURAL
The anesthetic agent is injected via a small catheter into the epidural space, which is just outside of the dura mata of the spinal column. This route is becoming more popular for the administration of opioids for pain management.

INFILTRATION
Small amounts of anesthetic solution are injected into the tissue that surrounds the operative site. This approach to anesthesia is commonly used for such procedures as suturing wounds or dental surgery. Often agents that cause constriction of local blood vessels are also administered to limit the site of action locally.

NERVE BLOCK
Anesthetic solution is injected at the site where a nerve innervates a specific area such as a tissue. This allows large amounts of anesthetic agent to be delivered to a very specific area without affecting the whole body. It is often reserved for more difficult to treat pain syndromes such as those seen with various cancers.

SPINAL
Anesthetic solution is injected into the epidural space or the subarachnoid space that surrounds the spinal cord. Different nerves can be anesthetized depending on the location of the injection. This type of local anesthesia is frequently used for obstetric procedures.

TOPICAL
The anesthetic agent is applied directly onto the surface of the skin, eye, or any other mucous membrane to relieve pain or prevent it from being sensed. It is frequently used for diagnostic eye examinations and suturing of skin.

Parenteral Anesthetic Agents*

table 10-6

Properties	Lidocaine	Mepivacaine	Procaine	Tetracaine
Trade name	Xylocaine	Carbocaine	Novocain	Pontocaine
Potency†	2nd	2nd	3rd	1st
Onset	Immediate	<5 min	2-5 min	5-10 min
Duration	60-90 min	120-150 min	30-60 min	90-120 min
Dose	0.5%-4% injection	1%, 1½%, 2%, 3% injection	1%, 2%, 10% injection	0.2%, 0.3%, 1% injection

*Other common parenteral anesthetic agents include bupivacaine (Marcaine, Sensoricaine), chloroprocaine (Nesacaine), etodocaine (Duranest), propoxycaine (Ravocaine), and ropi-vacaine (Nacropin).
†Denotes order of potency from the most (1st) to the least (5th) potent.

Other prominent effects of local anesthetics are their circulatory and respiratory effects. Local anesthetics produce sympathetic blockade, which means that the two neurotransmitters of the sympathetic nervous system (SNS), norepinephrine and epinephrine, are blocked. The cardiac drug effects of this sympathetic blockade result in decreased stroke volume, cardiac output, and peripheral resistance. The respiratory drug effects cause normal respiratory function to be interfered with. Tachyphylaxis, the rapid appearance of a progressive decrease in response to a pharmacologically or physiologically active substance after its repetitive administration, is another bothersome drug effect.

Therapeutic Uses

Local anesthetics are used for surgical, dental, or diagnostic procedures as well as for the treatment of certain types of pain. They are administered by two techniques: infiltration anesthesia and nerve block anesthesia. Infiltration anesthesia is commonly used for minor surgical and dental procedures. It involves injecting the local anesthetic solution intradermally, subcutaneously, or submucosally across the path of nerves supplying the area to be anesthetized. The local anesthetic may be administered in a circular pattern around the operative field. Nerve block anesthesia is used for surgical, dental, and diagnostic procedures and in the therapeutic management of pain. It involves injecting the local anesthetic directly into or around the nerve trunks or nerve ganglia that supply the area to be numbed.

Some local anesthetics, for either infiltration or nerve block anesthesia, are combined with vasoconstrictors such as epinephrine, phenylephrine, and norepinephrine to help confine the local anesthetic to the injected area and prevent systemic absorption.

Side Effects and Adverse Effects

The side effects and adverse effects of the local anesthetics are, under most circumstances, limited and of little clinical importance. The undesirable effects usually result from high plasma concentrations of the drug, which results from inadvertent intravascular injection, an excessive dose or rate of injection, slow metabolic breakdown, or injection into a highly vascular tissue. In addition, when a local anesthetic gets absorbed into the circulation, it can result in adverse reactions similar to those produced by general anesthetics.

True allergic reactions to local anesthetics are rare. However, allergic reactions can occur. They may appear as skin lesions, urticaria, or edema, or they may be acutely anaphylactic. These rare allergic reactions are generally limited to a particular chemical class of anesthetics called the *ester type*. Table 10-7 separates the local anesthetic agents into their two chemical families of local anesthetics. These two groups have different enzymes that are responsible for their breakdown in the body. Anesthetics belonging to the ester family are metabolized by cholinesterases in the plasma and liver. They are metabolized to a para-aminobenzoic acid (PABA) compound. This compound is mainly responsible for allergic reactions. The *amide type* of anesthetics are metabolized in the liver by other enzymes to active and inactive metabolites. Often, when an individual has an undesirable experience after the administration of one of the local anesthetics, changing from one chemical class to another can prevent these experiences.

Toxicity and Management of Overdose

Local anesthetics have little opportunity to cause toxicity under most circumstances. However, as just mentioned, they can become just as toxic as the general anesthetics if they become systemically absorbed. To prevent this from occurring, vasoconstrictors such as epinephrine are coadministered with local anesthetics to keep the anesthetic at its local site of action. Another reason for the lower incidence of toxic effects with local anesthetics is that the doses of local anesthetics are on average much smaller than those of the general anesthetics. If for some reason significant amounts of the locally administered anesthetic get absorbed systemically, cardiovascular and respiratory func-

---

geriatric considerations

Anesthesia

- The elderly patient is more affected by anesthesia than the young or middle-age adult patient. Body systems are very sensitive to the effects of anesthesia, so the nurse must take all precautions to protect the patient and ensure his or her safety during all phases of surgery and all phases of anesthesia, whether general, regional, or local.
- The elderly patient's hepatic, cardiac, respiratory, and renal systems are all affected by aging, and these age-related changes make the patients more susceptible to problems such as CNS depression, toxicity, atelectasis, pneumonia, and cardiac abnormalities.
- It is important to assess for the presence of any disease of the cardiac, renal, hepatic, or respiratory systems and to document any pertinent findings because of the increased risk of complications during anesthesia in such settings. Add to this the risk associated with advanced age, and the possible complications of surgery and adverse effects of anesthesia become even more problematic and more likely to occur. ∎

Table 10-7 Local Anesthetic Chemical Groups

Ester Type	Amide Type
benzocaine	bupivacaine
chloroprocaine	etidocaine
cocaine	dibucaine
procaine	lidocaine
proparacaine	mepivacaine
propoxycaine	prilocaine
tetracaine	

tion may be compromised. Symptomatic and supportive therapy is usually all that is needed to reverse the toxic effects stemming from systemic absorption of the agent.

Interactions

Few clinically significant drug interactions occur with the local anesthetics. Some of the more important drug-drug interactions are bupivacaine, chloroprocaine, and etidocaine. When given with enflurane, halothane, or epinephrine, they can lead to dysrhythmias.

drug profiles

Besides lidocaine (described in detail here) other local anesthetics include bupivacaine, chloroprocaine, etidocaine, mepivacaine, prilocaine, procaine, propoxycaine, and tetracaine. There are two types of local anesthetics, as determined by their chemical structure: amide and ester. This refers to the type of linkage between the aromatic ring and the amino group of the agent, two of the structural components that make an anesthetic an anesthetic. Lidocaine belongs to the amide type of local anesthetics. Some patients may report that they have allergic or anaphylactic types of reactions to "caines," as they may refer to lidocaine and the other amide agents. In these situations it may be wise to try a local anesthetic of the ester type.

lidocaine

Lidocaine (Xylocaine) is one of the most commonly used local anesthetics. It is available in several strengths and in many combinations with epinephrine and is used for both infiltration and nerve block anesthesia. It is available as a 0.5%, 1%, 1.5%, 2%, and 4% parenteral injection as well as in a 0.5% 1%, 1.5%, and 2% concentration in combination with epinephrine in a parenteral injection. Lidocaine is now available as a 5% patch for relief from the pain of postherapeutic neuralgia. Lidocaine is classified as a pregnancy category B agent and is contraindicated in those who have a hypersensitivity to it. Commonly recommended dosages are listed in the table below.

NEUROMUSCULAR BLOCKING AGENTS

Neuromuscular blocking agents (NMBAs) prevent nerve transmission in certain muscles, leading to paralysis of the muscle. They are often used with anesthetics to perform surgery. Use of NMBAs requires artificial mechanical ventilation because these drugs paralyze respiratory and skeletal muscles. The patient is left unable to breathe on his or her own. The drugs do not cause sedation or relieve pain; therefore the health care provider should assume that the paralyzed patient is in pain and anxious and should take steps to relieve this with analgesics and anxiolytics.

Snakes and plants played a large role in the discovery of the receptor and the chemical structure of a substance that would cause paralysis. The beginning steps involved in the identification of the receptor involved study of the seemingly irreversible antagonism of neuromuscular transmission by toxins from krait venoms (*Bungarus multicinctus*) and the venoms of certain varieties of the cobra (*Naja naja*). Once the receptor at which these venoms work was identified, pharmacologic agents that would mimic the venoms and produce paralysis were studied.

Curare, a nondepolarizing NMBA, has a long and romantic history. It has been used for centuries by natives of South America along the Amazon and Orinoco rivers and in other parts of that continent for killing wild animals used for food. Animals shot with arrows soaked in this plant substance would die from paralysis of skeletal muscles. Curare is actually a generic term for various South American arrow poisons. The most potent of all curare alkaloids are the toxiferines, obtained from *Strychnos toxifera*. The seeds of the trees and shrubs of the genus *Erythrina*, widely distributed in tropical and subtropical areas, contain substances with curare-like activity.

NMBAs are traditionally classified as depolarizing or nondepolarizing agents. Succinylcholine is the only commonly used depolarizing drug. Nondepolarizing NMBAs prevent acetylcholine (ACh) from acting at neuromuscular junctions. Consequently, the nerve cell membrane is not depolarized, the muscle fibers are not stimulated, and skeletal muscle contraction does not occur. Nondepolarizing NMBAs are typically broken

DOSAGES Selected Local Anesthetic Agent

agent	pharmacologic class	dosage range	purpose
lidocaine (Xylocaine)	Amide local anesthetic	0.5%, 1% solution: 5-300 mg	Percutaneous infiltration
		1% solution: 200-300 mg	Caudal obstetric analgesia, thoracic nerve block
		1% solution: 100 mg/each side	Paracervical obstetric analgesia
		1% solution: 50-100 mg	Sympathetic lumbar nerve block
		1% solution: 30-50 mg	Paravertebral nerve block
		1% solution: 30 mg	Intercostal nerve block
		1% solution: 50 mg	Sympathetic cervical nerve block
		1.5% solution: 225-300 mg	Brachial nerve block, caudal surgical anesthesia
		2% solution: 20-100 mg	Dental procedures
		2% solution: 200-300 mg	Lumbar anesthesia

down into three groups based on their duration of action—short-, intermediate-, and long-acting agents.

Mechanism of Action

Succinylcholine works similar to the neurotransmitter ACh. Initially succinylcholine combines with cholinergic receptors at the motor endplate to produce depolarization and muscle contraction. Repolarization and further muscle contraction are then inhibited as long as an adequate concentration of drug remains at the receptor site. Unlike ACh, succinylcholine is metabolized much more slowly. Because of this slower metabolism, succinylcholine persistently subjects the motor end plate to ongoing depolarizing stimulation and repolarization cannot occur. As long as sufficient succinylcholine concentrations are present, the muscle loses its ability to contract and a flaccid muscle paralysis results. This muscle paralysis is preceded by muscle spasms, which may damage muscles. These muscle spasms are termed *muscle fasciculations* and are most pronounced in the muscle groups of the hands, feet, and face. Injury to muscle cells may cause postoperative muscle pain and release potassium into the circulation. If hyperkalemia develops, it is usually mild and insignificant. Rarely cardiac dysrhythmias or even cardiac arrest have occurred. Succinylcholine is normally deactivated by plasma pseudocholinesterase. This enzyme breaks down succinylcholine, freeing up the receptor site and allowing repolarization of the motor end plate. Succinylcholine's duration of action after a single intubating dose is about 5 to 9 minutes as a result of the rapid breakdown of the drug by this enzyme.

Nondepolarizing NMBAs prevent ACh from acting at neuromuscular junctions. They act as antagonists blocking ACh from binding to the postsynaptic receptors. Conse-

quently, the nerve cell membrane is not depolarized, the muscle fibers are not stimulated, and skeletal muscle contraction does not occur. The prototype drug d-Tubocurarine (dTC), the active ingredient of curare, is a naturally occurring plant alkaloid that causes skeletal muscle relaxation or paralysis. Most of the newer drugs are synthetic preparations. Anticholinesterase drugs, such as neostigmine, pyridostigmine, and edrophonium, are antidotes and are used to reverse muscle paralysis. They work by preventing the enzyme cholinesterase from breaking down ACh. This causes ACh to build up at the muscle endplate and eventually knocks off the nondepolarizing NMBA, returning the nerve to its original state.

Drug Effects

Skeletal muscle effects of depolarizing and nondepolarizing NMBAs are described in the mechanism of action section. The first sensation that is typically felt is muscle weakness. This is usually followed by a total flaccid paralysis. Small rapidly moving muscles such as those of the fingers and eyes are typically the first to be paralyzed. The next muscles to be paralyzed are those of the limbs, neck, and trunk. Finally the intercostal muscles and the diaphragm are paralyzed. Respirations stop as a result; the patient can no longer breathe on his or her own. Recovery of muscles usually occurs in the reverse order to that of their paralysis, and thus the diaphragm is ordinarily the first to regain function. Before causing paralysis, depolarizing agents such as succinylcholine evoke transient muscular fasciculations. Muscle soreness may follow the administration of succinylcholine. Small doses of nondepolarizing NMBAs have been used to minimize these muscle fasciculations. This reduces the muscle pain caused by depolarizing agents like succinylcholine.

Table 10-8 Effects of Ganglionic Blockade by Neuromuscular Blocking Agents

Site	Nervous System Stimulated by Ganglionic Blockade	Physiologic Effect of Ganglionic Blockade
Arterioles	Sympathetic	Vasodilation and hypotension
Veins	Sympathetic	Dilation
Heart	Parasympathetic	Tachycardia
Gastrointestinal tract	Parasympathetic	Reduced tone and motility; constipation
Urinary bladder	Parasympathetic	Urinary retention
Salivary glands	Parasympathetic	Dry mouth

Box 10-2 Conditions that Predispose Patients to Toxic Effects from Neuromuscular Blocking Agents

Acidosis	Myasthenia gravis
Amyotrophic lateral sclerosis	Myasthenic syndrome
Hypermagnesemia	Neonates
Hypocalcemia	Neurofibromatosis
Hypokalemia	Paraplegia
Hypothermia	Poliomyelitis

Central nervous system effects are usually minimal because of the chemical structure of most of the nondepolarizing agents. They are quaternary ammonium compounds and are not able to penetrate the bloodbrain barrier. The effects on the cardiovascular system vary depending on the NMBA used and the individual patient. Increases and decreases in blood pressure and heart rate have been seen. Some NMBAs cause a release of histamine, which can result in bronchospasm, hypotension, and excessive bronchial and salivary secretion. The gastrointestinal tract is seldom affected by NMBAs. When it is affected, decreased tone and motility typically result, which can lead to constipation or even ileus.

Therapeutic Uses

The main therapeutic use of NMBAs is in maintaining controlled ventilation during surgical procedures. When respiratory muscles are paralyzed by NMBAs, mechanical ventilation is easier because the body's desire to control respirations is eliminated by the NMBAs ability to allow the ventilator to have total control of the respirations.

NMBAs may also be used for endotracheal intubation and to reduce muscle contraction in an area that needs surgery. Short-acting NMBAs are often used to facilitate intubation with an endotracheal tube. This is commonly done to facilitate a variety of diagnostic procedures such as laryngoscopy, bronchoscopy, and esophagoscopy. When used for this purpose NMBAs are often combined with anxiolytics or anesthetics. Additional nonsurgical applications include reduction of laryngeal or general muscle spasms, reduction of spasticity from tetanus in neurological diseases and multiple sclerosis, and prevention of bone fractures during electroconvulsive therapy. These drugs are also used as diagnostic agents for myasthenia gravis.

Side Effects and Adverse Effects

The key to limiting side effects and adverse effects with most NMBAs is to use enough of the agent to block the neuromuscular receptors. If too much is used, the risk is increased that other ganglionic receptors will be affected. Blockade of these other ganglionic receptors leads to most of the undesirable effects of NMBAs.

The effects of ganglionic blockade in various areas of the body are listed in Table 10-8.

Nondepolarizing NMBAs have relatively few side effects when used appropriately. Their cardiovascular effects include blockade of autonomic ganglia resulting in hypotension, blockade of muscarinic receptors resulting in tachycardia, and release of histamine resulting in hypotension. The depolarizing agent succinylcholine has been associated with hypokalemia, dysrhythmias, fasciulations, muscle pain, myoglobinuria, and increased intraocular, intragastric, and intracranial pressure.

Toxicity and Management of Overdose

The primary concern when NMBAs are overdosed is prolonged paralysis requiring prolonged mechanical ventilation. Cardiovascular collapse can also be seen and is thought to be the result of histamine release. Multiple medical conditions can predispose an individual to toxicity. These conditions increase the sensitivity of an individual to NMBAs and prolong their effects. The conditions are listed in Box 10-2.

Some conditions make it more difficult for NMBAs to work and therefore require higher doses of NMBAs. Although these conditions do not result in toxicity or overdose they are worthy of mentioning and are listed in Box 10-3.

Interactions

Many drugs can interact with NMBAs, resulting in either synergistic or opposing effects. Some of the antibiotics when given concomitantly with an NMBA can result in additive effects. The aminoglycoside antibiotics are a common example. They produce neuromuscular blockade by inhibiting ACh release from the preganglionic terminal. The tetracycline antibiotics can also produce neuromuscular blockade, possibly by chelation of calcium. Calcium channel blockers have also been shown to enhance neuromuscular blockade. Some of the more notable drugs that interact with NMBAs are listed in Table 10-9.

BOX 10-3 Conditions that Oppose Effects of Neuromuscular Blocking Agents

Cirrhosis with ascites
Clostridial infections
Hemiplegia
Hypercalcemia
Hyperkalemia
Peripheral nerve transection
Peripheral neuropathies
Thermal burns

Table 10-9 Drugs that Interact with Neuromuscular Blocking Agents

Additive Effects	Opposing Effects
Aminoglycosides	carbamazepine
Calcium channel blockers	Corticosteroids
clindamycin	phenytoin
cyclophosphamide	
cyclosporine	
dantrolene	
furosemide	
Inhalation anesthetics	
Local anesthetics	
magnesium	
polymyxin	
procainamide	
quinidine	
trimethaphan	

drug profiles

NMBAs are one of the most frequently used classes of drugs in the operating room. They are used primarily with general anesthetics to facilitate endotracheal intubation and to relax skeletal muscles during surgery. In addition to their use in the operating room, NMBAs frequently are used in the ICU to paralyze mechanically ventilated patients. The two basic types of NMBAs are depolarizing and nondepolarizing agents. The only depolarizing agent is succinylcholine. Nondepolarizing agents can be classified in a variety of ways but are typically classified by their chemical structure or their duration of action. Table 10-10 lists some nondepolarizing agents currently in use.

DEPOLARIZING NEUROMUSCULAR BLOCKING AGENTS

As mentioned previously, succinylcholine is the only agent in this subclass of NMBAs. Succinylcholine has a structure similar to the parasympathetic neurotransmitter ACh. It stimulates the same neurons as ACh and produces the same physiologic responses initially. Unlike ACh, succinylcholine is metabolized much more slowly. Because of this slower metabolism, succinylcholine persistently subjects the motor end plate to ongoing depolarizing stimulation. Repolarization cannot occur. As long as sufficient succinylcholine concentrations are present the muscle loses its ability to contract and flaccid muscle paralysis results. Because of succinylcholine's quick onset it is most commonly used to facilitate endotracheal intubation. It is seldom used over long periods of time because of the unwanted effects that develop with continuous infusions.

succinylcholine

Succinylcholine (Anectine) is the only currently available depolarizing NMBA. It is an ultra–short-acting, depolarizing-type, skeletal muscle relaxant for intravenous administration. Succinylcholine is indicated as an adjunct to general anesthesia, to facilitate tracheal intubation, and to provide skeletal muscle relaxation during surgery or mechanical ventilation. It is contraindicated in patients with personal or familial history of malignant hyperthermia, skeletal muscle myopathies, and known hypersensitivity to the drug. The FDA rates succinylcholine as a pregnancy category C agent. It is available as a 20-mg/ml 20-ml solution, a 500-mg sterile powder, and a 1000-mg sterile powder. The recommended dosage is given in the table on p. 151.

PHARMACOKINETICS

HALF-LIFE	ONSET	PEAK	DURATION
Seconds	Rapid ≈ 1 min	Rapid	4-6 min

NONDEPOLARIZING NEUROMUSCULAR BLOCKING AGENTS

Nondepolarizing NMBAs are commonly used to facilitate endotracheal intubation, reduce muscle contraction in an area that needs surgery, and facilitate a variety of diagnostic procedures. They are often combined with anxiolytics or anesthetics. They may also be used to induce respiratory arrest in patients on mechanical ventilation. Nondepolarizing NMBAs can be classified in a variety of ways but are typically classified by their chemical structure or their duration of action.

pancuronium

Pancuronium (Pavulon) is a long-acting nondepolarizing NMBA. It is indicated as an adjunct to general anesthesia to facilitate tracheal intubation and to provide skeletal muscle relaxation during surgery or mechanical ventilation. It is most commonly used for long surgical procedures that require prolonged muscle paralysis. Pancuronium is contraindicated in patients with known hypersensitivity to pancuronium. The FDA rates pancuronium as a pregnancy category C agent. It is available as 1 mg/ml 10-ml vials and 2 mg/ml 2- and 5-ml ampules. The recommended dosage is given in the table on p. 151.

PHARMACOKINETICS

HALF-LIFE	ONSET	PEAK	DURATION
80-120 min	3-5 min	Rapid	60-100 min

rapacuronium

Rapacuronium (Raplon) is a short-acting nondepolarizing NMBA. It is indicated as an adjunct to general anesthesia to facilitate tracheal intubation and to provide skeletal muscle relaxation during surgical procedures. Its main advantages are its rapid onset and short duration. The most common side effects are hypotension (5.2%), tachycardia (3.2%), and bronchospasm (3.2%). Rapacuronium is contraindicated in patients with known hypersensitivity to rapacuronium. The FDA rates rapacuronium as a pregnancy category C agent. It is available as a 100- and 200-mg sterile powder. The recommended dosage is given in the table on p. 151.

PHARMACOKINETICS

HALF-LIFE	ONSET	PEAK	DURATION
Unknown	60 sec	90 sec	15-18 min

vecuronium

Vecuronium (Norcuron) is an intermediate-acting nondepolarizing NMBA. It is indicated as an adjunct to general anesthesia to facilitate tracheal intubation and to provide skeletal muscle relaxation during surgery or mechanical ventilation. It is one of the most commonly used NMBAs. Long-term use in the ICU setting has resulted in prolonged paralysis and consequently difficulty weaning from mechanical ventilation. This is believed to be due to an active metabolite, 3-desacetyl vecuronium, which tends to accumulate with prolonged use. Vecuronium is contraindicated in patients with known hypersensitivity to vecuronium. The FDA rates vecuronium as a pregnancy category C agent. It is available as 1 mg/ml 10- and 20-ml vials and 1 mg/ml 10-ml syringes. The recommended dosage is given in the table below.

PHARMACOKINETICS

HALF-LIFE	ONSET	PEAK	DURATION
65-75 min	2.5-3 min	3-5 min	25-40 min

nursing process

● Assessment

Assessment of patients about to undergo general anesthesia with NMBAs should indicate a head-to-toe assessment and a medical and medication history. Cautious use is necessary when patients have disorders such as hypothermia, hypokalemia, and hypocalcemia. Conditions that may require higher doses of NMBAs include burns, hyperkalemia, hypercalcemia and cirrhosis. Drug interactions are common with NMBAs and include corticosteroids, carbamazepine, phenytoin, quinidine, magnesium, tri-

methaphan, cyclophosphamide, cyclosporine, furosemide, dantrolene, inhalation anesthetics, local anesthetics, aminoglycosides, clindamycin, polymyxin, calcium channel blockers, and procainamide. Some agents, such as succinylcholine, may also cause an increase in intraocular and intracranial pressure and should be used cautiously, if at all, in patients with glaucoma or head injuries.

Succinylcholine, a depolarizing NMBA, is contraindicated in patients with personal or familial history of malignant hyperthermia, skeletal muscle myopathies, and known hypersensitivity to the drug. Rapacuronium, a short-acting nondepolarizing NMBA, carries the same contraindications and should be used cautiously in patients with hypotension and history of bronchospasms. Vecuronium is an intermediate-acting nondepolarizing NMBA and is the most commonly used agent for surgery

Table 10-10 Classification of Neuromuscular Blocking Agents

Agent	Structure
SHORT-ACTING AGENTS	
mivacurium (Mivacron)	Benzylisoquinolinium
rapacuronium (Raplon)	Steroidal
INTERMEDIATE-ACTING AGENTS	
atracurium (Tracrium)	Benzylisoquinolinium
rocuronium (Zemuron)	Steroidal
vecuronium (Norcuron)	Steroidal
LONG-ACTING AGENTS	
doxacurium (Nuromax)	Benzylisoquinolinium
pancuronium (Pavulon)	Steroidal
tubocurarine (dTC)	Benzylisoquinolinium

DOSAGES Selected Neuromuscular Blocking Agents

agent	pharmacologic class	dosage range	purpose
pancuronium (Pavulon)	Nondepolarizing NMBA (long-acting)	*Pediatric* IV: 0.02 mg/kg *Adult* IV: 0.04-0.1 mg/kg Continuous infusion: 0.1 mg/kg/hr	Intubation Mechanical ventilation
rapacuronium (Raplon)	Nondepolarizing NMBA (short-acting)	*Pediatric* IV: 2-3 mg/kg *Adult* IV: 1.5 mg/kg	Intubation Mechanical ventilation
succinylcholine (Anectine, Quelicin, and others)	Depolarizing NMBA (short-acting)	*Pediatric* IV: 1-2 mg/kg IM: 3-4 mg/kg *Adult* IV: 0.3-1.1 mg/kg IM: 3-4 mg/kg	Intubation Mechanical ventilation
vecuronium (Norcuron)	Nondepolarizing NMBA (intermediate-acting)	*Pediatric* IV: 0.08-0.1 mg/kg *Adult* IV: 0.08-0.1 mg/kg Continuous infusion: 0.1 mg/kg/hr	Intubation Mechanical ventilation

and for mechanical ventilation. However, long-term use may create difficulty with prolonged paralysis and problems weaning off the mechanical ventilator; therefore it should be used cautiously in these situations. Vecuronium is contraindicated in patients allergic to these types of medications. Pancuronium is a long-acting nondepolarizing NMBA and is most commonly used for long surgical procedures or mechanical ventilation and is contraindicated in patients with allergy to the drug and during pregnancy.

With the use of neuromuscular blocking agents, the medication vials should never be on hand on a nursing unit so as to avoid errors and possible death. Since they produce apnea, it is important to have the mechanical ventilation and resuscitation equipment in the patient's room. These agents cause paralysis, not anesthesia, so if the patient is receiving this agent for paralysis induction for mechanical ventilation, he or she can still hear and feel your touch. Remain professional at all times, and take time to orient the patient to his or her surroundings, the noises, and what you are going to be doing to them. A reversing agent or antidote should always be on hand. Peripheral nerve stimulators are often used to monitor drug effectiveness with some of the NMBAs and may help avoid overdosage. Depolarizing NMBAs, such as succinylcholine chloride, must be administered carefully by highly qualified individuals, such as a nurse anesthetist, because administration that is too rapid may result in bradycardia and cardiac arrest (rare). The antidote is atropine and neostigmine.

One of the most important responsibilities of the nurse involving a patient receiving general anesthesia is to assess the patient's status during the four stages of anesthesia. These responsibilities are summarized in Table 10-11.

After the conclusion of the procedure and the termination of general anesthesia, the nurse's next main concern is summarized by the general rule of ABCs (airway, breathing, and circulation). Once the patient is quickly assessed from head to toe and all vital signs are checked, the nurse needs to collect data about the specific anesthetic used, the procedure done, the allergies the patient may have, the patient's medical history, and any complications that may have occurred during anesthesia. In addition, the nurse must review current laboratory results and assess the status of any tubes, dressings, IV catheters, and equipment. All body systems, including the integumentary system, need to be assessed frequently and thoroughly and the findings documented. The intake and output amounts, wound drainage amounts, secretion amounts, and the patient's pain level and level of consciousness are also important data to note. Allergic reactions and either CNS stimulation or depression may occur if access of the agent to the circulation has occurred. Frequent assessments will help detect any changes in the patient, no matter how small.

In assessing patients receiving NMBAs, the nurse must be aware of the influence of these agents on the respiratory system. Patients receiving NMBAs (often used to induce respiratory arrest in patients requiring mechanical ventilation) will require artificial mechanical ventilation because of the resultant paralysis on the respiratory muscles. In addition, the patient needs to be assessed for electrolyte imbalances, especially with potassium and magnesium, because these may lead to increased action of the NMBA. Allergic reactions to NMBAs are characterized by rash, fever, respiratory distress, and pruritus. Drug interactions include aminoglycosides, clindamycin, linocomycin, quinidine, polymyxin antibiotics, lithium, narcotics, thiazide diuretics, enflurane, isoflurane, magnesium salts, and oxytocin. These drugs will result in increased neuromuscular blockade, and the physician and/or anesthesiologist should be contacted and informed about the interaction.

Local anesthesia still carries with it some potential for causing complications, such as diminished sensation and motor responses and postural hypotension. However, unlike general anesthesia, the nurse may be the one responsible for administering a topical local anesthetic. In this event, the nurse should be sure to assess whether the patient has any preexisting illnesses and allergies; whether the patient uses OTC medications, alcohol, or any prescriptive medications; and whether the patient is or has been a smoker.

Table 10-11 Stages of General Anesthesia: Nursing Responsibilities

Stages of Anesthesia	Assessment	Responsibilities
Stage 1: analgesia	Patient unconscious; HR> and BP> to normal; R> to normal	Assess vital signs; keep environment quiet; safety measures
Stage 2: excitement	Loss of consciousness occurs; VS are increased	Monitor VS; protect patient from injury; quiet to ease induction process
Stage 3: surgical	Patient unconscious	Assess VS; assess environment and patient's safety; reflexes absent; prevent injury
Stage 4: medullary	Do not want patients in this state; this is a toxic and dangerous phase	Have resuscitative equipment nearby; have emergency drugs nearby for treating respiratory or cardiac arrest

BP, Blood pressure; *HR,* heart rate; *R,* respiration; *VS,* vital signs.

Nursing Diagnoses

Nursing diagnoses appropriate to the patient receiving either general or local anesthesia are as follows:

- Risk for injury related to decreased sensorium resulting from general anesthesia or related to decreased sensation resulting from local anesthesia.
- Decreased cardiac output related to systemic effects of general anesthesia.
- Impaired gas exchange related to CNS depression produced by general anesthesia.
- Anxiety related to the use of an anesthetic and the prospect of surgery.
- Deficient knowledge related to lack of information regarding and experience with anesthesia and surgery.

Planning

Goals related to the care of the patient receiving general or local anesthesia are as follows:

- Patient will state the side effects of general or local anesthesia (depending on situation).
- Patient will state potential complications of both general and local anesthesia.
- Patient will experience minimal to no injury related to anesthesia.
- Patient will describe what to expect during the recovery period of anesthesia.
- Patient will comply with care to decrease the chances of complications after anesthesia.
- Patient will follow preoperative instructions regarding his or her care during the postoperative period (see Home Health/Community Points box).
- Patient will verbalize anxiety prn regarding surgery and anesthesia.

Outcome Criteria

Outcome criteria related to the use of general or local anesthesia are as follows:

- Patient will experience minimal to no side effects of general or local anesthesia such as myocardial depression during operative period.
- Patient will remain free of complications such as injury, falls, and hepatotoxicity during the perioperative period (preoperative, intraoperative, and postoperative).
- Patient will be free of or experience minimal anxiety as evidenced by fewer complaints, better relaxation ability, and decreased postoperative pain.
- Patient will be compliant with all measures and treatments such as turning, coughing, and deep breathing during the perioperative period.

Implementation

Regardless of the type of anesthesia a patient is receiving, one of the most important points the nurse must consider during this time is close and frequent observation of the patient and all body systems with specific attention to the ABCs of nursing care and vital signs. This should be done as frequently as necessary or in conformance with the protocol. If any sudden elevation in body temperature occurs while a patient is receiving general anesthesia, this

should be reported to the anesthesiologist immediately because it may indicate the occurrence of malignant hyperthermia. Malignant hyperthermia is a life-threatening emergency and requires prompt medical attention. Other nursing actions to be carried out after a patient has received general anesthesia include monitoring all aspects of body functions, instituting safety measures, and implementing the physician's orders.

Oxygen is generally administered after a patient has received general anesthesia to compensate for the respiratory depression that occurred during surgery. In addition, hypotension and orthostatic hypotension are a problem after anesthesia because of the vasodilation it produces. In addition, when administering pain medication postoperatively, it is important to remember that the dose of any sedative or analgesic administered after surgery when the patient returns to the room or is in the recovery room is often decreased by one-half to one-fourth so that CNS depression does not occur. For IV anesthesia, all resuscitative equipment should be kept nearby.

In general, any sudden elevation in body temperature immediately postoperatively should be reported to the physician immediately because of the continued risk of malignant hyperthermia associated with general anesthesia that includes succinylcholine. Additional nursing observations during and after general (as well as local and spinal) anesthesia include the status of breath sounds assessed by auscultation (hypoventilation may be a complication of general anesthesia); any changes in neurologic status (no matter how minute); and any changes in sensation in body parts distal to the site of local anesthesia or distal to where the safety restraints were placed during the surgery. Improper positioning during surgery may lead to the damage of arteries and nerves. When caring for a client who has received either general or local anesthesia, all body functions should be monitored and safety

---

home health/community points

Anesthesia

- Home health care plays an important role in the recovery of any patient being discharged from the hospital to home. Home health care is a resource for all phases of the rehabilitation and recovery process in any aged patient.
- Community resources are available for the use of all aged patients during their recovery and rehabilitation at home after surgery. Contacting a home health care agency and city-sponsored social service agencies is a starting point to the receipt of these services.
- Meals on Wheels are often available for the elderly patient, and senior citizen resources and agencies are available through most city governments. Elderly patients are also encouraged to contact city-sponsored or church-related transportation services to meet their transportation needs.

measures implemented. Reorientation of the patient to his or her surroundings and implementation of the physician's orders should also be part of the patient's care during the postoperative phase. See Table 10-11 for more information regarding nursing interventions during the stages of anesthesia.

Patients receiving NMBAs should be monitored closely during and after the anesthesia or induction to mechanical ventilation. Vital signs are constantly monitored during and after the recovery from the administration of either of these agents with frequent measurement of blood pressure, pulse, respirations (rate, depth, pattern, quality), and hand grasp strength. Intake and output are also monitored every hour. Recovery from the NMBA is manifested by a decrease in paralysis of the face, diaphragm, leg, arm, and rest of the body. The health care provider must reassure the patient of his or her condition as he or she begins to recover because the patient may become frightened if communication is difficult during the recovery process or during intubation.

A local anesthetic solution that is cloudy or discolored or that contains any sort of crystalloids should not be used. Some anesthesiologists mix the solution with sodium bicarbonate to minimize the local pain during infiltration, but this also causes a more rapid onset of action and a longer duration of sensory analgesia. Resuscitative equipment should be kept close by. If an anesthetic ointment or cream is used, thoroughly cleanse the area to be anesthetized and dry it before application. If a suppository is being used, refrigerate it before use, remove the wrapper, moisten the suppository with water or water-soluble lubricant, and then insert it.

If a local anesthetic is being used in the nose or throat, it is important to remember that it may lead to paralysis of the structures of the upper respiratory tract, leading to possible aspiration. Exact amounts of the agent should be used and administered only at the prescribed times. Local anesthetics are not to be swallowed unless the physician has instructed this. If this is to be done, the nurse should then constantly observe the patient and check his or her gag reflex after administration of the agent, withholding food or drink until the gag reflex has returned.

Local anesthesia produces paralysis of certain areas, such as the area below the waist, so it is important to protect the patient from injury resulting from this loss of sensation. Bed side rails should be kept up, and there should be no untoward pressure on the affected skin area because the body's normal sensation and protective mechanisms have been diminished. After a spinal anesthetic, patients must remain flat in bed for up to 12 hours to prevent a spinal headache. They should also be well hydrated during this period.

Teaching tips important for patients receiving either local or general anesthesia are given in the box below.

● Evaluation

The therapeutic effects of any general or local anesthetic include loss of sensation during the procedure (such as loss of sensation in the eye for corneal surgery) or loss of consciousness and other reflexes (such as pain for abdominal or other major procedures). The patient who has received general anesthesia should be constantly monitored for the occurrence of adverse effects of the anesthesia. These effects include myocardial depression, convulsions, respiratory depression, allergic rhinitis, and decreased renal or liver function. Patients who have received a local anesthetic also need to be constantly monitored for the occurrence of adverse effects of the anesthesia (mostly stemming from the systemic absorption of the specific agent). These effects include bradycardia, myocardial depression, hypotension, and dysrhythmias. As mentioned earlier in this chapter, significant overdoses of local agents or direct injection into a blood vessel may result in cardiovascular collapse or cardiac or respiratory depression.

---

patient teaching tips

General and Local Anesthetics

General Anesthesia

➤ Obtain a listing of all prescription and OTC medications the patient may be taking so that any possible drug interactions can be averted by discontinuance of the medication before surgery. Encourage patient to have a list of all medications currently taken—on person—at all times.

➤ Obesity, smoking, and cardiac or respiratory disease are all factors that heighten the risks associated with anesthesia and should be identified preoperatively so that proper preparations can be made.

➤ Patient teaching about the procedure and the care before, during, and after surgery help to alleviate anxiety and promote recovery.

➤ Explain the rationale for the use of preoperative medications as well as the need to be NPO (to prevent aspiration).

➤ Patient teaching on turning, coughing, and deep breathing is also important for the promotion of healing and recovery.

➤ Patient teaching about postoperative pain control methods is also important to alleviating anxiety and promoting healing.

➤ Explain the rationale for any other treatments, such as the use of drainage tubes, catheters, intravenous lines, and so on.

➤ The importance of frequent vital sign monitoring should be discussed with the patient to minimize anxiety and fear postoperatively.

➤ Always ask patients whether they have any allergies to medications or foods.

➤ Instruct patients about the importance of safety features such as keeping side rails up and using the call light during the postoperative phase.

➤ Always tell patients about how some of these agents may make them feel. For example, with NMBAs the patient may be paralyzed but can also hear and feel because he or she is not anesthetized unless an anesthetic is also used.

Local Anesthesia

➤ Always perform a thorough patient assessment, including questions about allergies, prescribed and OTC medications, and any medical problems.

➤ Make sure patients understand how local anesthetics work, their side effects, and why the specific local agent was selected.

➤ For those patients receiving epidural or spinal anesthesia, vital sign and systems assessments should be done frequently during and after the procedure so as to monitor for and assess any complications. Inform patient of this to help decrease anxiety.

➤ Remind patients about decreased motor and sensory status so they know what to expect.

POINTS TO REMEMBER

Anesthesia

- CNS altered so that pain perception and consciousness are lost; also includes skeletal muscle relaxation and loss of reflexes.
- Drug-induced state of altered nerve conduction.
- Can be either general or local.
- Allows exposure to the surgical area so the surgeon can carry out specific and often very sophisticated procedures.

General Anesthetics

- Agents that induce a state of anesthesia.
- Global—affect the whole body.
- NMBAs, if given in high doses, may block neuromuscular receptors and other ganglionic receptors, leading to hypotension, tachycardia, decreased GI and GU tone, and dry mouth.

Balanced Anesthesia

- Combinations of drugs to produce anesthesia.
- Sedative-hypnotic, anxiolytic, analgesic, antiemetic, anticholinergic, and a neuromuscular blocking agent.

Local Anesthetics

- Also called *regional anesthetics*.
- Render specific portion of body insensitive to pain without affecting consciousness.
- Include spinal and epidural anesthesia.

Topical Anesthetics

- Applied to skin and mucous membranes.
- Solutions, ointments, gels, creams, powders, ophthalmic drops, and suppositories.

Nursing Considerations

- The perioperative phase includes the preoperative, intraoperative, and postoperative stages.
- Each stage calls for a complex and specific plan of care.
- NMBAs have many cautions and contraindications and should be used only if mechanical ventilation is being used or is on hand.
- NMBAs should not be kept on hand on any nursing unit because of careless use and possible induction of apnea.

REVIEW QUESTIONS

1. Your patient is in for a lymph node removal from his arm under local anesthesia. The physician has requested "lidocaine WITH epinephrine." Which of the following provides the most accurate rationale for adding epinephrine?
   a. Helps calm the patient before the procedure
   b. Helps minimize the risk of an allergic reaction
   c. Enhances the effect of the local lidocaine
   d. Causes vasoconstriction and keeps the anesthetic local

2. During your patient's surgery he experiences a sudden elevation in body temperature to about 105° F. What is mostly likely occurring with this patient?
   a. Malignant hyperthermia
   b. Spontaneous pneumothorax

   c. Severe intraoperative infection
   d. Malignant hypermetabolic syndrome

3. Of the following patients, which one is more prone to complications to general anesthesia?
   a. 79-year-old female about to have her gallbladder removed
   b. 49-year-old male athlete who quit heavy smoking 12 years ago
   c. 30-year-old female, in perfect health, but has never had anesthesia
   d. 50-year-old female scheduled for outpatient laser surgery for vision correction

4. Which of the following nursing diagnoses is most appropriate for a patient who is under general anesthesia for 3 to 4 hours for abdominal-thoracic surgery?
   a. Decreased urine output from use of vasopressants as anesthetics
   b. Increased cardiac output related to the effects of general anesthesia
   c. Risk for injury (fall) related to decreased sensorium 2 to 4 days postoperative

   d. Decreased gaseous exchange from the CNS depression of general anesthesia

5. What should be the nurse's main concern for the patient, during the immediate postoperative period, recovering from general anesthesia?
   a. Airway
   b. Pupilary reflexes
   c. Return of sensations
   d. Level of consciousness

For Answers see www.harcourthealth.com/MERLIN/Lilley/.

CRITICAL THINKING Activities

1. When would spinal anesthesia be the method of choice?
2. What is the purpose of adding epinephrine to the local anesthetic epinephrine?

3. What are potential complications of local anesthetics used in dental offices, such as xylocaine with epinephrine, in a patient with a variety of cardiac or vessel diseases?

For Answers see www.harcourthealth.com/MERLIN/Lilley/.

bibliography

Albanese J, Nutz P: *Mosby's 2001 nursing drug reference and review cards,* St Louis, 2001, Mosby.

American Hospital Formulary Service: *AHFS drug information,* Bethesda, Md, 2000, American Society for Health-System Pharmacists.

Anderson PO: Knoben JE, Troutman WG: *Handbook of clinical drug data 1999-2000,* ed 9, New York, 1999, McGraw-Hill.

Johns Hopkins Hospital, Department of Pediatrics: *The Harriet Lane handbook et al,* ed 15, St Louis, 2000, Mosby.

Keen JH: *Critical care and emergency drug reference,* ed 3, St Louis, 1996, Mosby.

McKenry L, Salerno E: *Mosby's pharmacology in nursing,* ed 21, St Louis, 2001, Mosby.

Mosby's GenRx: a comprehensive reference for generic and brand drugs, ed 10, St Louis, 2000, Mosby.

Skidmore-Roth L: *Mosby's 2001 nursing drug reference,* St Louis, 2001, Mosby.

Vermette E: Malignant hyperthermia, *AJN* 98(4):45, 1998.

Walker JR: What is new with inhaled anesthetics, Part 1, *J Perianesth Nurs* 11(5):330, 1996.

Remember to check the **Online Worksheet** for additional learning opportunities: **www.harcourthealth.com/MERLIN/Lilley/**

Activity

Chapter 11

Central Nervous System Depressants and Muscle Relaxants

www.harcourthealth.com/MERLIN/Lilley/

Look for this symbol for topics covered in the **Online Worksheet**

objectives

When you reach the end of this chapter, you should be able to do the following:

1 Differentiate between a sedative and a hypnotic agent.

2 Describe the differences between benzodiazepines and barbiturates as sedative-hypnotic agents.

3 Identify specific benzodiazepine and barbiturate agents.

4 Discuss the nursing process as it relates to the nursing care of patients receiving sedative-hypnotic agents.

5 Understand the importance of using nonpharmacologic approaches to treat sleep disturbances.

6 Develop patient education guidelines for patients receiving sedative-hypnotic agents.

7 Identify mechanisms of action, drug effects, therapeutic uses, interactions, and side and toxic effects of skeletal muscle relaxants.

8 Discuss the nursing process, including patient education, for skeletal muscle relaxants.

---

drug profiles

aprobarbital, p. 162	**pentobarbital**, p. 162
baclofen, p. 167	**phenobarbital**, p. 162
butabarbital, p. 162	**quazepam**, p. 165
cyclobenzaprine, p. 168	**secobarbital**, p. 162
dantrolene, p. 168	**temazepam**, p. 165
estazolam, p. 165	**triazolam**, p. 166
flurazepam, p. 165	**zolpidem**, p. 166

---

glossary

Anxiolytic (ang zi o lit′ ik) A medication that relieves anxiety. (p. 162)

Barbiturates (bahr bich′ ər əts) A class of drugs that are chemical derivatives of barbituric acid. They can induce sedation and sleep. (p. 158)

Benzodiazepines (ben zo di az ə penz) A chemical category of drugs most frequently prescribed as sedative-hypnotic and anxiolytic agents. (p. 162)

Gamma-aminobutyric acid (GABA) (ə me no bu ter′ ik) An inhibitory neurotransmitter found in the brain. (p. 159)

Hypnotics Drugs that, when given at low doses, calm or soothe the CNS without inducing sleep but when given at high doses may cause sleep. (p. 158)

Non–rapid eye movement (non–REM) One of the stages of the sleep cycle. It characteristically has four stages and pre-

cedes rapid eye movement sleep. Most of a normal sleep cycle consists of non–rapid eye movement sleep. (p. 158)

Rapid eye movement (REM) One of the stages of the sleep cycle. One of the characteristics of rapid eye movement sleep is the rapid movement of the eyes, vivid dreams, and irregular breathing. (p. 158)

Sedatives Drugs that have an inhibitory effect on the CNS to the degree that they reduce nervousness, excitability, or irritability without causing sleep. (p. 157)

Sedative-hypnotics Drugs that can act in the body either as a sedative or hypnotic. (p. 158)

Sleep A transient, reversible, and periodic state of rest in which there is a decrease in physical activity and consciousness. (p. 158)

Sleep architecture The various steps involved in the sleep cycle, including normal and abnormal patterns of sleep. (p. 158)

Tachyphylaxis (tak e fe lak sis) The rapid appearance of a progressive decrease in response to a drug after repetitive administration of the drug. (p. 168)

Therapeutic index The level of drug in the blood that provides a therapeutic effect without causing toxicity. (p. 158)

Drugs that have a calming effect or that depress the central nervous system (CNS) are referred to as *sedatives* and *hypnotics*. A drug is classified as either a sedative or a hypnotic agent depending on the degree to which it inhibits the transmission of nerve impulses to the CNS. **Sedatives** reduce nervousness, excitability, and irritability without causing sleep, but a sedative can become a hypnotic if it is given in large enough doses. **Hypnotics** cause sleep. They have a much more potent effect on the CNS than sedatives do. Many drugs can act in the body as either a sedative or a hypnotic, and for this reason are called **sedative-hypnotics.** Listed in Box 11-1 are some points of interest relating to sedative-hypnotics.

Sedative-hypnotics can be classified chemically into three main groups: barbiturates, benzodiazepines, and nonbarbiturates or miscellaneous agents. Before discussing the sedative-hypnotics in depth, it is important that the physiology of normal sleep is understood because of the significant effects these agents can have on normal sleep patterns.

SLEEP

Sleep is defined as a transient, reversible, and periodic state of rest in which there is a decrease in physical activity and consciousness. Normal sleep is cyclic and repetitive, and a person's responses to stimuli are markedly reduced during sleep. During waking hours the body is bombarded with stimuli that provoke the senses of sight, hearing, touch, smell, and taste. These stimuli elicit voluntary and involuntary movements or functions. During sleep a person is no longer aware of the sensory stimuli within his or her immediate environment.

Sleep research involves studying the patterns of sleep, or what is sometimes referred to as **sleep architecture.** The architecture of sleep consists of two basic stages that occur cyclically: **rapid eye movement (REM)** sleep and **non–rapid eye movement (non–REM)** sleep. The normal cyclic progression of the stages of sleep is summarized in Table 11-1. Various sedative-hypnotics affect different stages of the normal sleep pattern. If usage is prolonged, emotional and psychologic changes can occur. An appreciation of this will help prevent the inappropriate use of long-term sleeping agents.

BARBITURATES

Barbiturates were first introduced into clinical use in 1903 and were the standard agents for treating insomnia and producing sedation. Chemically they are derivatives of barbituric acid. Although there are close to 50 different barbiturates approved for clinical use in the United States, only a handful are in common clinical use today. This is in part due to the favorable safety profile and proven efficacy of the class of drugs commonly referred to as *benzodiazepines.* Barbiturates can produce many unwanted side effects. They are habit-forming and have a narrow **therapeutic index** (the dosage range within which the drug is effective but above which it is rapidly toxic). Barbiturates can be classified into four groups based on their onset and duration of action. Table 11-2 lists the agents within each category and summarizes their pharmacokinetic characteristics.

---

research

Sedative Hypnotics

An article by Tabloski, Cooke, and Thoman presents significant information about the use of sedative-hypnotics in elderly women who have been on sleep medication for prolonged periods of time. The authors explain the physiology of the elderly person that exacerbates difficulty with sleep. These changes include difficulty falling asleep, problems staying asleep, more awakenings, decreased amount of nocturnal sleep, and more daytime napping. ■

Box 11-1 Sedative-Hypnotic Agents: Points of Interest

Agent	Point
aprobarbital	Intermediate acting; onset in about 20 minutes; with oral dosing give with meals to decrease nausea and vomiting.
butabarbital	Effects last about 6-8 hours; cautious use in the elderly; keep tablets in an airtight container.
estazolam	Take with food to minimize gastrointestinal upset; *always* make sure patients have swallowed medication.
flurazepam	Causes less REM rebound versus that caused by the other benzodiazepines; cautious use in the elderly patient; give 15-30 minutes before bedtime.
pentobarbital	Short acting; can be given PO, by rectal suppository, or IM; IM injection given deep in large muscle mass; as with any of these agents, patients should avoid caffeine intake 4 hours around the time of dosing because of the decreased effectiveness that results.
phenobarbital	Long acting (up to 16 hours' duration); in the body longer and thus can react with other medications such as alcohol and other CNS depressants; because of long duration, use cautiously in the elderly patient who has decreased liver and renal function.
quazepam	Give 15 to 30 minutes before bedtime; hangover common in elderly patients.
secobarbital	Same as for pentobarbital; also given IM, PO, and as suppository; as with any sedative-hypnotic agent, do not mix with alcohol.
temazepam	Induces sleep within 20-40 minutes; give 20-30 minutes before bedtime.
triazolam	Short-term use only; try other medications in this category, as ordered by a physician; cautious use with elderly and causes confusion, so protect from injury.

Mechanism of Action

Barbiturates are CNS depressants that act primarily on the brainstem in an area called the *reticular formation.* Their sedative and hypnotic effects are dose related, and they act by reducing the nerve impulses traveling to the area in the brain called the *cerebral cortex.* Their ability to inhibit nerve impulse transmission is in part due to their ability to potentiate an inhibitory amino acid known as **gamma-aminobutyric acid (GABA),** which is found in high concentrations in the CNS. Barbiturates are capable of raising the convulsive or seizure threshold and are therefore also effective in treating status epilepticus and tetanus- or drug-induced convulsions. In addition, selected barbiturates are used as prophylaxis for epileptic seizures.

Drug Effects

In low doses, barbiturates act as sedatives. Increasing the dose produces a hypnotic effect, but this also decreases the respiratory rate. In normal doses they have little effect on the circulation. Barbiturates as a class are notorious enzyme inducers. They stimulate the enzymes in the liver that are responsible for the metabolism or breakdown of drugs. By stimulating these enzymes they cause drugs to be converted more quickly into active substances so they have a faster onset of action. However, the drugs are also broken down more quickly to inactive substances, therefore shortening their duration of effect. Warfarin, theophylline, and phenytoin are three such drugs. They are very commonly prescribed and potentially very dangerous drugs.

Therapeutic Uses

All barbiturates have the same sedative-hypnotic efficacy but differ in their potency, onset, and duration of action. They are used as hypnotics, sedatives, and anticonvulsants and also for anesthesia during surgical procedures. They are used for the following therapeutic reasons:

- *Ultrashort:* Anesthetic for short surgical procedures, anesthesia induction, control of convulsions, narcoanalysis, and reduction in intracranial pressure in neurosurgical patients.
- *Short:* Sedative-hypnotic and control of convulsive conditions.

Table 11-1 Stages of Sleep

Stage	Characteristics	Average Time in Each Stage (For Young Adult)
NON-REM SLEEP		
1	Dozing or feelings of drifting off to sleep. Persons can be easily awakened. Insomniacs have longer stage 1 periods than normal.	2%-5%
2	Person is relaxed but can be easily awakened. Has occasional REMs and also slight eye movements.	50%
3	Deep sleep; difficult to wake person up. Respiratory rates, pulse, and blood pressure may decrease.	5%
4	Sleepwalking or bedwetting may occur. Very difficult to wake person up; may be very groggy if done. Dreaming, especially about daily events.	15%
REM SLEEP	REMs occur. Vivid dreams occur. Breathing may be irregular.	25%-35%

Modified from McKenry LM, Salerno E: *Mosby's pharmacology in nursing,* ed 21, St Louis, 2001, Mosby.
REM, Rapid eye movement.

Table 11-2 Barbiturates: Onset and Duration

Category	Pharmacokinetics		Barbiturates
	Onset	Duration	
Ultrashort	IV: <15 min	IV: <2 hr	mephobexital, thiamylal, thiopental
Short	PO: 15-20 min	PO: 2-4 hr	pentobarbital, secobarbital
Intermediate	PO: 20-30 min	PO: 2-4 hr	aprobarbital, butabarbital
Long	PO: 30-60 min	PO: 6-8 hr	phenobarbital

- *Intermediate:* Sedative-hypnotic and control of convulsive conditions.
- *Long:* Sedative-hypnotic, epileptic seizure prophylaxis, and treatment of neonatal hyperbilirubinemia.

Side Effects and Adverse Effects

The main side effects of barbiturates affect the CNS and include drowsiness, lethargy, dizziness, hangover, and paradoxical restlessness or excitement. Their chronic effects on normal sleep architecture can be detrimental. Sleep research has shown that adequate rest from the sleep process is obtained only when there are proper amounts of REM sleep, which is sometimes referred to as *dreaming sleep.* Barbiturates deprive people of REM sleep, which can result in agitation and an inability to deal with normal stress. When the barbiturate is stopped and REM sleep once again occurs, a rebound phenomenon can occur. During this rebound the proportion of REM sleep is increased, the patient's dream time constitutes a larger percentage of the total sleep pattern, and the dreams are often nightmares. The adverse effects of barbiturates relative to the body systems affected are listed in Table 11-3.

Toxicity and Management of Overdose

Overdose frequently results in respiratory depression, leading to respiratory arrest. Often this is done therapeutically to induce anesthesia. In this situation, however, the patient is ventilated mechanically and respiration is controlled or assisted mechanically. Another situation in which intentional overdoses are given for therapeutic reasons is in the management of uncontrollable seizures. Such patients are sometimes put into what is called a *phenobarbital coma.* Because of the inhibitory effects of barbiturates on nerve transmission in the brain (possibly GABA mediated), the uncontrollable seizures can be stopped until appropriate drug levels of anticonvulsant drugs are achieved.

An overdose of barbiturates produces CNS depression ranging from sleep to profound coma and death. Respiratory depression progresses to Cheyne-Stokes respiration, hypoventilation, and cyanosis. Affected patients often have cold, clammy skin or are hypothermic; or later they can exhibit fever, areflexia, tachycardia, and hypotension. Pupils are usually slightly constricted but may be dilated in the event of severe poisoning.

Treatment of an overdose is mainly symptomatic and supportive. The mainstays of therapy should consist of maintenance of an adequate airway, assisted respiration, and oxygen administration if needed, along with fluid and pressor support as indicated. The multiple-dose (every 4 hours) nasogastric administration of activated charcoal is highly effective in removing barbiturates from the stomach as well as the circulation. Barbiturates are highly metabolized by the liver, and they increase enzyme activity there. In an overdose, however, the amount of barbiturate may overwhelm the liver's ability to metabolize it. This is where activated charcoal may be helpful. Activated charcoal helps pull the drug from the circulation and eliminate it by means of the gastrointestinal system. Some of the barbiturates (phenobarbital, aprobarbital, and mephobarbital) can be eliminated more quickly by the kidneys when the urine is alkalized. This keeps the drug in the urine and prevents it from being resorbed back into the circulation. Alkalization, along with forced diuresis, can hasten elimination of the barbiturate.

Interactions

The potential drug interactions with barbiturates are considerable in their intensity and often dramatic. The risk encountered in the coadministration of barbiturates with alcohol, antihistamines, benzodiazepines, opioids, and tranquilizers is additive CNS depression. Most of the drug-drug interactions involving barbiturates are secondary to their effects on the hepatic enzyme system. As mentioned previously, the barbiturates increase the activity of hepatic microsomal enzymes. This is called *enzyme induction.* Induction of this enzyme system results in increased drug metabolism and breakdown. However, if the two drugs are competing for the same enzyme system for metabolism, this can lead to inhibited drug metabolism or breakdown. Two examples are coadministration of monoamine oxidase inhibitors (MAOIs) or anticoagulants with barbiturates. Coadministration of MAOIs with barbiturates can result in prolonged barbiturate effects. Coadministration of anticoagulants with barbiturates can result in decreased anticoagulation response and possible clot formation.

Laboratory Test Interactions

Barbiturates can also interact with body substances and affect the results of various laboratory tests. Barbitu-

Table 11-3	Barbiturates: Adverse Effects
Body System	**Side/Adverse Effects**
Blood	Agranulocytosis, thrombocytopenia, and megaloblastic anemia
Cardiovascular	Vasodilation and hypotension, especially if given too rapidly
Gastrointestinal	Nausea, vomiting, diarrhea, and constipation
Nervous system	Drowsiness, lethargy, vertigo, headache, mental depression, and myalgic, neuralgic, or arthralgic pain
Respiratory	Respiratory depression, apnea, laryngospasm, bronchospasm, and coughing
Other	Hypersensitivity reactions: urticaria, angioedema, rash, fever, serum sickness, or Stevens-Johnson syndrome

rates can cause an increase in the serum levels of bilirubin, serum glutamate pyruvate transaminase (SGPT), serum glutamic-oxaloacetic transaminase (SGOT), and alkaline phosphatase.

Dosages

As previously mentioned, barbiturates can act as either sedatives or hypnotics depending on their dosage. The various barbiturates and their recommended sedative and hypnotic dosages are listed in the dosages table below.

drug profiles

Barbiturates are available in a variety of dosage forms, including tablets, capsules, elixirs, injections, and suppositories. They are all rated as pregnancy category D drugs by the Food and Drug Administration (FDA). (The inside back cover lists a description of what each pregnancy category means.) All barbiturates are considered prescription-only drugs because of the potential for misuse and the severe effects that result if they are not used appropriately. From a legal standpoint they are con-

DOSAGES Selected Barbiturates

agent	onset and duration	dosage range	purpose
aprobarbital (Alurate)	Intermediate acting	*Adult* PO: 40 mg tid 40-100 mg HS	Sedative Hypnotic
butabarbital (Buticaps, Butisol, Butalan)	Intermediate acting	*Pediatric* PO: 2-6 mg/kg before surgery *Adult* PO: 15-30 mg 3-4 times/day 50-100 mg before surgery 50-100 mg HS	Preop sedative Sedative Preop sedative Hypnotic
pentobarbital (Nembutal)	Short acting	*Pediatric* IM/IV/PO: 2-6 mg/kg Rectal: 2 mo-1 y/o, 30 mg; 1-4 y/o, 30-60 mg; 5-12 y/o, 60 mg; 12-14 y/o, 60-120 mg HS *Adult* PO/rectal: 100-200 mg HS IM: 150-200 mg IV: 100 mg	Anticonvulsant, preop sedative, sedative Hypnotic Anticonvulsant, preop sedative, hypnotic Anticonvulsant, preop sedative, hypnotic
phenobarbital (Solfoton)	Long acting	*Neonatal* PO: 5-10 mg/kg/day *Pediatric* PO: 6 mg/kg in 3 equally divided doses IM/IV: 1-3 mg/kg *Adult* PO: 30-120 mg/day divided 100-320 mg HS *Adult* IM/IV: 100-200 mg 60-90 min before surgery	Hyperbilirubinemia Sedative Preop sedative Sedative Hypnotic Preop sedative
secobarbital (Seconal)	Short acting	*Pediatric* PO: 2-6 mg/kg IM: 4-5 mg/kg 2 mg/kg several times/day PR: 3-5 mg/kg *Adult* PO: 100 mg HS 200-300 mg 1-2 hr before surgery IM: 100-200 mg HS 1 mg/kg 10-15 min before surgery IV: 50-250 mg 100-150 mg PR: 5.5 mg/kg	Preop sedative Preop sedative Sedative Anticonvulsant Hypnotic Preop sedative Hypnotic Preop sedative Hypnotic Dental sedative before nerve block Anticonvulsant

sidered controlled substances. As discussed in Chapter 4, controlled substances are medications that the U.S. Drug Enforcement Administration has identified as drugs that have a high abuse potential. State laws are often more stringent than federal laws in terms of the way in which these drugs are dispensed, so health care providers must be careful to comply with both federal and state laws. A detailed description of controlled substance schedules I through V can be found on the inside back cover. The various barbiturates are listed in Table 11-4 according to the controlled substance schedule.

Barbiturates are contraindicated in patients with known hypersensitivity reactions to them, latent porphyria, significant liver dysfunction, and known previous addiction.

aprobarbital

Aprobarbital is used for routine sedation and as a hypnotic in the short-term treatment of insomnia for periods of up to 2 weeks. The common dosages for achieving the sedative and hypnotic effects of aprobarbital are given in the dosages table on p. 161. Pregnancy category D.

PHARMACOKINETICS

HALF-LIFE	ONSET	PEAK	DURATION
14-34 hr	30-45 min	3 hr	8-12 hr

butabarbital

Butabarbital as a single agent is used for routine sedation and as a hypnotic in the short-term management of insomnia. It is also combined with aspirin, acetaminophen, and caffeine in various formulations used to treat migraine headaches. The common dosages of butabarbital that apply when it is administered as a single agent are given in the dosages table on p. 161. Pregnancy category D.

PHARMACOKINETICS

HALF-LIFE	ONSET	PEAK	DURATION
100 hr	30-45 min	3-4 hr	6-8 hr

pentobarbital

Pentobarbital is principally used as a hypnotic agent for the short-term management of insomnia. It is also used preoperatively to relieve anxiety and provide sedation. In addition, it is used for sedation and occasionally to control status epilepticus or acute seizure episodes resulting from meningitis, poisons, eclampsia, alcohol withdrawal, tetanus, or chorea. Pentobarbital may also be used to treat withdrawal symptoms in patients who are physically dependent on barbiturates or nonbarbiturate hypnotics. The sedative and hypnotic dosages are given in the dosages table on p. 161. Pregnancy category D.

Activity

PHARMACOKINETICS

HALF-LIFE	ONSET	PEAK	DURATION
PO/IV: 35-50 hr	PO: 15-60 min	PO: 30-60 min	PO: 1-4 hr
	IV: <1 min	IV: <30 min	IV: 15 min

phenobarbital

Phenobarbital is the most frequently prescribed barbiturate, either alone or in combination with other drugs. It is considered the *prototypical* barbiturate and is classified as a long-acting agent. Phenobarbital is used for the prevention of grand mal seizures and fever-induced convulsions. In addition, it has been useful in the treatment of hyperbilirubinemia in neonates. It has also been used for the treatment of Gilbert's syndrome. It is most commonly used, however, as a sedative-hypnotic agent. See the dosages table on p. 161 for dosages. Pregnancy category D.

PHARMACOKINETICS

HALF-LIFE	ONSET	PEAK	DURATION
PO/IV: 53-118 hr	PO: 30 min	PO: 8-12 hr	PO: 10-12 hr
	IV: 5 min	IV: 30 min	IV: 4-10 hr

secobarbital

Secobarbital is used primarily as a hypnotic agent to induce sleep. It may be administered intravenously to control status epilepticus or acute seizures, similar to the way in which pentobarbital is used. It may also be used to maintain a steady state of unconsciousness during general, spinal, or regional anesthesia or to facilitate intubation procedures. The common sedative and hypnotic dosages are given in the dosages table on p. 161. Pregnancy category D.

PHARMACOKINETICS

HALF-LIFE	ONSET	PEAK	DURATION
PO/IV: 30 hr	PO: 15 min	PO: 2-4 hr	PO: 1-4 hr
	IV: 1-3 min	IV: <30 min	IV: 15 min

BENZODIAZEPINES

Benzodiazepines are the most frequently prescribed sedative-hypnotic agents and one of the most commonly prescribed classes of drugs. This is directly attributed to their favorable side effect profiles, efficacy, and safety. Even when a drug in this class is taken as the sole agent in an overdose (i.e., not with alcohol), it is relatively benign, resulting in little more than sedation. Benzodiazepines are classified as either anxiolytics or sedative-hypnotics depending on their primary usage. An **anxiolytic** relieves anxiety, and the benzodiazepine anxiolytics are discussed in Chapter 14. Benzodiazepines discussed in this chapter, however, are the ones that work primarily to produce sedation or sleep. There are five such agents commonly used

TABLE 11-4 Barbiturates: Controlled Substance Schedule

Schedule	Barbiturates
C-II	pentobarbital, secobarbital
C-III	aprobarbital, butabarbital
C-IV	phenobarbital

TABLE 11-5 Sedative-Hypnotic Benzodiazepines

Generic Name	Trade Name
LONG ACTING	
flurazepam	Dalmane
quazepam	Doral
SHORT ACTING	
estazolam	Prosom
temazepam	Restoril
triazolam	Halcion
zaleplon*	Sonata
zolpidem*	Ambien

*Zolpidem and zalephon share many characteristics with the benzodiazepines but are classified as nonbenzodiazepine hypnotic agents.

The benzodiazepines discussed in Chapter 14 and those discussed here all have similar pharmacologic properties. They all act as anxiolytics and sedative-hypnotics. Different benzodiazepines are just more effective at one or the other pharmacologic effect.

as sedative-hypnotics. They are listed in Table 11-5 and can be further classified on the basis of their duration of action as either long acting or short acting.

Mechanism of Action

As mentioned previously, the sedative and hypnotic action of benzodiazepines is related to their ability to depress activity in the CNS. The specific areas they affect in the CNS appear to be the hypothalamic, thalamic, and limbic systems of the brain. Recent research has indicated that there are specific receptors in the brain for benzodiazepines. These receptors are thought to be the same as those of the CNS inhibitory transmitter GABA. If they are not the same, then they are adjacent to the GABA receptors. Their depressant action on the CNS appears to be related to their ability to inhibit stimulation of the brain. They have many favorable effects compared with the barbiturates. They do not suppress REM sleep to the same extent as barbiturates. They also do not induce hepatic microsomal enzyme activity and are therefore safe to administer to patients who are taking medications that are metabolized by this enzyme system.

Drug Effects

Benzodiazepines have a calming effect on the CNS. This causes the inhibition of hyperexcitable nerves in the CNS that might be responsible for causing seizure activity. Similarly, this calming effect on the CNS makes benzodiazepines useful in controlling agitation and anxiety. It also reduces excessive sensory stimulation and induces sleep. Benzodiazepines have also been shown to induce skeletal muscle relaxation. Their receptors in the CNS are in the same area as those that play a role in alcohol addiction. Therefore they are used in the treatment and prevention of the symptoms of alcohol withdrawal (see Chapter 14).

Therapeutic Uses

Benzodiazepines have a variety of therapeutic applications. They are most frequently used for sedation, sleep induction, skeletal muscle relaxation, and anxiety relief. They have also been used in the treatment of alcohol withdrawal, agitation, depression, and epilepsy. They are often combined with anesthetics, analgesics, and neuromuscular-blocking agents in what is called *balanced anesthesia*. Their use in this setting is mostly for their amnesiac properties, because most persons undergoing surgery would rather not remember the events of their procedure.

Side Effects and Adverse Effects

As a class, benzodiazepines have a relatively safe side effect profile. The side effects and adverse effects associated with their use are mild and infrequently reported, and they primarily involve the CNS. The more commonly reported undesirable effects are headache, drowsiness, paradoxical excitement or nervousness, dizziness or vertigo, and lethargy. Because of the benzodiazepines' effect on the normal sleep cycle, a hangover effect is sometimes reported. Other less common side effects and adverse effects are palpitations, dry mouth, nausea, vomiting, hypokinesia, and occasional nightmares.

Toxicity and Management of Overdose

An overdose of benzodiazepines may result in one or all of the following symptoms: somnolence, confusion, coma, and diminished reflexes. An overdose of just benzodiazepines rarely results in hypotension and respiratory depression. These are more commonly seen when benzodiazepines are coingested with other CNS depressants such as alcohol or barbiturates. The same holds true for their lethal effects. In the absence of the concurrent ingestion of alcohol or other CNS depressants, benzodiazepine overdoses rarely result in death.

The treatment of benzodiazepine intoxication is generally symptomatic and supportive. If ingestion is recent, decontamination of the gastrointestinal system is indicated. As a rule of thumb, the administration of syrup of ipecac (an emetic agent used to induce vomiting in overdoses) to produce gastric decontamination is contraindicated in patients who have ingested medications that cause sedation. The concern is that an unconscious patient induced to vomit could easily aspirate stomach contents. Therefore gastric lavage is generally the best and most effective means of gastric decontamination. Activated charcoal and a saline cathartic may be administered after gastric lavage to remove any remaining drug. Hemodialysis is not useful in the treatment of benzodiazepine overdose.

Flumazenil Treatment Regimen

11-6

Indication	Recommended Regimen	Duration
Reversal of conscious sedation or general anesthesia	0.2 mg (2 ml) given IV over 15 sec, wait 45 sec, then give 0.2 mg if consciousness does not occur; may be repeated at 60-sec intervals as needed up to four additional times (maximum total dose, 1 mg)	1-4 hr
Management of suspected benzodiazepine overdose	0.2 mg (2 ml) given IV over 30 sec; wait 30 sec; then give 0.3 mg (3 ml) over 30 sec if consciousness does not occur; further doses of 0.5 mg (5 ml) can be given over 30 sec at intervals of 1 min up to a cumulative dose of 3 mg.	1-4 hr

Important note: Flumazenil has a relatively short half-life and duration of effect of 1 to 4 hours; therefore if using flumazenil to reverse the effects of a long-acting benzodiazepine, the dose of the reversal agent may wear off and the patient may become sedated again, requiring more flumazenil.

Benzodiazepines: Drug Interactions

11-7

Drug	Mechanism	Result
cimetidine	Decreased benzodiazepine metabolism	Prolonged benzodiazepine action
CNS depressants	Additive effects	Increased CNS depression
Monoamine oxidase inhibitors	Decreased metabolism	Increased benzodiazepine effects
Protease inhibitors	Decreased metabolism	Increased benzodiazepine effects

Flumazenil can be used to acutely reverse the sedative effects of benzodiazepines. It formerly went by the product name Mazicon but was renamed and is now called Romazicon. This was done to prevent its confusion with Mevacron, which is a nondepolarizing neuromuscular-blocking agent used to paralyze patients. Flumazenil antagonizes the action of benzodiazepines on the CNS by directly competing with benzodiazepines for binding at the benzodiazepine receptor in the CNS. However, it has a stronger affinity for the receptor and knocks the benzodiazepine off from the receptor, reversing the sedative action of the benzodiazepine. The dosage regimen to be followed for the reversal of conscious sedation or general anesthesia induced by benzodiazepines and the management of suspected benzodiazepine overdose are summarized in Table 11-6.

Interactions

The potential drug interactions with the benzodiazepines are significant in their intensity, particularly when they are taken in combination with other CNS depressants and MAOIs. The risks associated with the coadministration of other agents are listed and described in Table 11-7.

Laboratory Test Interactions

There are no laboratory test interactions that occur with the five benzodiazepines that are typically used as either sedatives or hypnotics.

Dosages

The benzodiazepines discussed in this chapter are those that are commonly used to treat insomnia. Therefore the dosage recommendations given in the dosages table on p. 165 are those for achieving hypnotic effects. All agents used for the treatment of insomnia should be limited to a short-term usage of less than 2 to 4 weeks. With long-term usage, rebound insomnia and severe withdrawal can develop. Geriatric patients should also be started on lower doses because they generally experience a more pronounced effect from benzodiazepines.

Activity

drug profiles

Benzodiazepines are all prescription-only drugs, and they are designated as C-IV controlled substances. All five benzodiazepines discussed here have active metabolites, which can accumulate during long-term use, especially in patients who have altered metabolic function (hepatic dysfunction) or altered excretion capabilities (renal dysfunction). There are several other benzodiazepines, but they are more commonly used to treat anxiety or agitation, to produce amnesia, and to relax skeletal muscles. These other benzodiazepines are discussed in detail in the appropriate chapters. All benzodiazepines are rated pregnancy category X agents. They are all also contraindicated in patients who have shown a hypersensitivity reaction to them and in pregnant women.

Zolpidem (Ambien) and zaleplon (Sonata) share many characteristics with the benzodiazepines but are classified as nonbenzodiazepine hypnotic agents. Zolpidem is a nonbenzodiazepine hypnotic of the imidazopyridine class, and zaleplon is a nonbenzodiazepine hypnotic of the pyrazolopyrimidine class. Their pharmacologic properties are similar to the

DOSAGES Benzodiazepines: Selected Hypnotic Agents

agent	onset and duration	dosage range	purpose
estazolam (Prosom)	Short acting	*Adult* PO: 1-2 mg HS *Geriatric* PO: 0.5 mg HS	
flurazepam (Dalmane)	Long acting	*Adult* PO: 15-30 mg HS	
quazepam (Doral)	Long acting	*Adult* PO: 7.5 or 15 mg HS	
temazepam (Restoril)	Short acting	*Adult* PO: 15-30 mg HS *Geriatric* PO: 7.5 mg HS	Hypnotic
triazolam (Halcion)	Short acting	*Adult* PO: 0.25-0.5 mg HS *Geriatric* PO: 0.125-0.25 mg HS	
zolpidem* (Ambien)	Short acting	*Adult* PO: 10 mg HS *Geriatric* PO: 5 mg HS	

*Zolpidem is classified as a nonbenzodiazepine hypnotic agent.
HS, At bed time.

benzodiazepines in that they both have sedative, anxiolytic, muscle relaxant, and anticonvulsive effects. They are both indicated for the short-term (7 to 10 day) treatment of insomnia, only available orally, and designated as C-IV controlled substances. Zolpidem is classified as a pregnancy category B agent, zaleplon is a category C agent.

estazolam

Estazolam (Prosom) is available in 1- and 2-mg tablets. The usual adult dosage is 1 to 2 mg at bedtime; the geriatric dosage is usually 0.5 mg at bedtime (see dosage table above). Pregnancy category X.

PHARMACOKINETICS			
HALF-LIFE	ONSET	PEAK	DURATION
10-24 hr	20 min	2 hr	24 hr

flurazepam

Flurazepam (Dalmane) is available in 15- and 30-mg capsules. It is considered a long-acting hypnotic agent and is indicated for the short-term treatment of insomnia for periods of up to 4 weeks. Flurazepam has two active metabolites that account for its hypnotic effects. These active metabolites have also been shown to be responsible for inducing a "hangover" effect, causing lethargy or grogginess the morning after the medication has been taken. The recommended dosages for adult and geriatric patients are given in the dosages table above. Pregnancy category X.

Activity

PHARMACOKINETICS			
HALF-LIFE	ONSET	PEAK	DURATION
50-100 hr	15-45 min	30-60 min	7-8 hr

quazepam

Quazepam (Doral) is available in 7.5- and 15-mg tablets. Quazepam is considered a long-acting hypnotic agent and is indicated for the short-term treatment of insomnia for periods of up to 4 weeks. The recommended dosages for adult and geriatric patients are given in the dosages table above. Pregnancy category X.

PHARMACOKINETICS			
HALF-LIFE	ONSET	PEAK	DURATION
25-41 hr	30 min	2 hr	20 hr

temazepam

Temazepam (Restoril) is available in 7.5-, 15- and 30-mg tablets. It is contraindicated in patients who have narrow-angle glaucoma because it can exacerbate the glaucoma. It is indicated for the short-term treatment of insomnia. The common dosages are given in the dosages table above. Pregnancy category X.

PHARMACOKINETICS			
HALF-LIFE	ONSET	PEAK	DURATION
9.5-12.4 hr	30-60 min	2-3 hr	7-8 hr

triazolam

Triazolam (Halcion) is available in 0.125- and 0.25-mg tablets, and it is indicated for the short-term treatment of insomnia. The smallest effective dose given for the shortest time needed is generally the best approach to take. The common dosages for adult and geriatric patients are given in the dosages table on p. 165. Pregnancy category X.

PHARMACOKINETICS

HALF-LIFE	ONSET	PEAK	DURATION
2-5 hr	15-30 min	0.5-1.5 hr	6-7 hr

zolpidem

Zolpidem (Ambien) is a short-acting nonbenzodiazepine hypnotic agent. It is indicated for the short-term treatment of insomnia and, as with all benzodiazepines, should be limited to 7 to 10 days of treatment. Zolpidem has no contraindications. Zolpidem has a relatively short half-life compared with other benzodiazepines and no active metabolites. These two characteristics may account for less lethargy or grogginess the morning after the medication has been taken compared with other hypnotic benzodiazepines. The FDA rates zolpidem as a pregnancy category B agent. It is available in 5- and 10-mg tablets. The recommended dosage is given in the table on p. 165.

PHARMACOKINETICS

HALF-LIFE	ONSET	PEAK	DURATION
1.4-4.5 hr	Unknown	1.6 hr	Unknown

MUSCULOSKELETAL RELAXANTS

A variety of conditions such as trauma, inflammation, anxiety, and pain can be associated with acute muscle spasms. Although there is no completely satisfactory form of therapy available for relief of skeletal muscle spasticity, musculoskeletal relaxants are capable of providing some relief. The musculoskeletal relaxants are a group of compounds that act predominantly within the CNS to relieve pain associated with skeletal muscle spasms. The majority of musculoskeletal relaxants are called central-acting skeletal muscle relaxants because they have as their site of action the CNS. Central-acting skeletal muscle relaxants are similar in structure and action to other CNS depressants such as diazepam and therefore act within the CNS. It is believed the musculoskeletal relaxant effects of these agents are related to this CNS depressant activity. Only one of these compounds, dantrolene, acts directly on skeletal muscle. It belongs to a group of relaxants known as direct-acting skeletal muscle relaxants. It closely resembles GABA.

When these agents are used in conjunction with rest and physical therapy they are most effective. When mus-

culoskeletal agents are taken with alcohol, other CNS depressants, or opioid analgesics, enhanced CNS depressant effects are seen. Close monitoring and dosage reduction of one or both drugs should be considered.

Mechanism of Action

The majority of the musculoskeletal relaxants work within the CNS. Their beneficial effects are believed to come from their sedative effects rather than from direct muscle relaxation. Dantrolene has direct effects on skeletal muscle. All others have no direct effects on muscles, nerve conduction, or muscle-nerve junctions. One of the more effective agents in this class of drugs, baclofen, is a derivative of GABA. It is believed to work by depressing nerve transmission in the spinal cord. The other agents in this class of drugs are not derivatives of GABA but act by enhancing GABA's central inhibitory effects at the level of the spinal cord. These agents are generally less effective than baclofen. The only agent in the class to act directly on skeletal muscle in dantrolene. Dantrolene acts directly on the excitation-contraction coupling of muscle fibers and not at the level of the CNS. It appears to do this by decreasing the amount of calcium released from their storage sites in the sarcoplasmic reticulum.

Drug Effects

Musculoskeletal relaxants have a depressant effect on the CNS. Their effects are the result of CNS depression in the brain primarily at the level of the brainstem, thalamus, and basal ganglia but also at the spinal cord. Dantrolene has the additive effect of directly effecting skeletal muscles by decreasing the response of the muscle to stimuli. The effects of musculoskeletal relaxants are relaxation of striated muscles, mild weakness of skeletal muscles, decreased force of muscle contraction, and muscle stiffness. Other drug effects that may be experienced are generalized CNS depression seen as sedation, somnolence, ataxia, respiratory, and cardiovascular depression.

Therapeutic Uses

Musculoskeletal relaxants are primarily used for the relief of painful musculoskeletal conditions such as muscle spasms. They are most effective when used in conjunction with physical therapy. They may also be used in the management of spasticity associated with severe chronic disorders such as multiple sclerosis and other types of cerebral lesions, cerebral palsy, or rheumatic disorders. Some relaxants are used to reduce choreiform movement in patients with Huntington's chorea, to reduce rigidity in patients with parkinsonian syndrome, or in the relief of pain associated with trigeminal neuralgia. Intravenous dantrolene is used for the management of full blown hypermetabolism of skeletal muscle that is characteristic of a malignant hyperthermia crisis. Another muscle relaxant, baclofen, has been shown to be effective in relieving hiccups.

Side Effects and Adverse Effects

The primary side effects of musculoskeletal relaxants are an extension of their effects on the CNS and skeletal mus-

DOSAGES Selected Musculoskeletal Relaxants

agent	pharmacologic class	dosage range	purpose
baclofen (Lioresal)	Central acting	*Adult* PO: 5 mg tid × 3 days, then 10 mg tid × 3 days, then 15 mg tid, then titrated to response. Intrathecal: 12-1500 μg/day	Spasticity
cyclobenzaprine (Flexeril)	Central acting	*Adult* PO: 10 mg tid	Spasticity
dantrolene (Dantrium)	Direct acting	*Pediatric* PO: 1 mg/kg/day given in divided doses bid-qid *Adult* PO: 25 mg/day; may increase by 25-100 mg bid-qid *Pediatric and Adult* IV: 1 mg/kg, may repeat to total dose of 10 mg/kg	Spasticity and malignant hyperthermia

cles. Euphoria, lightheadedness, dizziness, drowsiness, fatigue, and muscle weakness are often experienced early in treatment. These side effects are generally short-lived with patients growing tolerant to them over time. Some less common side effects seen with the musculoskeletal relaxants are diarrhea, gastrointestinal upset, headache, slurred speech, muscle stiffness, constipation, sexual difficulties in males, hypotension, tachycardia, and weight gain. Dantrolene has a serious potential to cause hepatoxicity. This is however rare, occurring in 0.1% to 0.2% of patients treated with the drug for more than 60 days.

Toxicity and Management of Overdose

The toxicities and consequences of an overdose of musculoskeletal relaxants primarily involve the CNS. There is no specific antidote or reversal agent for musculoskeletal relaxant overdoses. They are best treated with conservative supportive measures. More aggressive therapies are generally needed when muscle relaxants are taken along with other CNS depressant drugs as an overdose. Gastric lavage and close observation of the patient are recommended. An adequate airway should be maintained and artificial respiration should be readily available. ECG monitoring and large quantities of IV fluids to avoid crystalluria should be instituted.

Interactions

When musculoskeletal relaxants are administered concomitantly with other depressant drugs such as alcohol and benzodiazepines, caution should be used to avoid overdosage. The combination of propoxyphene and orphenadrine has resulted in additive CNS effects. Mental confusion, anxiety, tremors, and additive hypoglycemic activity have been reported as well with this combination. A dosage reduction and/or discontinuance of one or both drugs is recommended.

Laboratory Test Interactions

A reducing substance in the urine of patients receiving metaxalone may produce false-positive results for glucose determination utilizing cupric sulfate (Benedict's solution, Clinitest, Fehling's solution) but does not interfere with glucose tests using glucose oxidase (Clinistix, Diastix, TesTape).

Dosages

For an overview of dosages for the more commonly used musculoskeletal relaxants see the dosages table above.

drug profiles

Musculoskeletal relaxants are all prescription-only drugs. There are over ten different musculoskeletal relaxants available. All but one of these agents are central-acting relaxants because of their site of action in the CNS. They are baclofen (Lioresal), carisoprodol (Rela, Soma), chlorphenesin (Maolate), chlorzoxazone (Paraflex), cyclobenzaprine (Flexeril), metaxalone (Skelaxin), methocarbamol (Robaxin, Marbaxin), and orphenadrine (Disipal, Norflex). Only dantrolene (Dantrium) works directly on skeletal muscle and is referred to as a direct-acting relaxant. All musculoskeletal relaxants are unclassified by the FDA as to their pregnancy category. The exception is cyclobenzaprine which is rated as a pregnancy category B agent. They are all contraindicated in patients who have shown a hypersensitivity reaction to them or have compromised pulmonary function, active hepatic disease, or impaired myocardial function.

baclofen

Baclofen (Lioresal, Atrofen) is available in 10-and 20-mg tablets as well as a 0.5-and a 2-mg/ml concentration for injection. The usual oral dosage is 5 mg three times a day for three days. It is then recommended to increase the dose by 5 mg every three days until a maximum of 20 mg three times a day is reached titrating to desired response. When given via intrathecal route a compatible pump must be implanted. With this administration route a test dose should be administered initially to test for a positive response. For patients who experience a positive response, continual dosing of 12-1500 μg/day is indicated. Pregnancy category C.

PHARMACOKINETICS

HALF-LIFE	ONSET	PEAK	DURATION
2.5-4 hr	0.5-1 hr	2-3 hr	>8 hr

cyclobenzaprine

Cyclobenzaprine (Flexeril) is available in a 10-mg dose. Cyclobenzaprine is a central-acting musculoskeletal relaxant that is structurally and pharmacologically related to the tricyclic antidepressants. The usual oral dosage is 10 mg three times a day for 1 week. It can be increased to a maximum of 60 mg daily. Pregnancy category B.

PHARMACOKINETICS

HALF-LIFE	ONSET	PEAK	DURATION
1-3 days	1 hr	3-8 hr	12-24 hr

dantrolene

Dantrolene (Dantrium) is available in 25-, 50-, and 100-mg capsules as well as a 20 mg parenteral injection. Dantrolene is a direct-acting musculoskeletal relaxant that is pharmacologically different than the central-acting relaxants in that it can work directly on the skeletal muscles. It can be administered orally to children at a dosage of 1 mg/kg/day in two to three divided doses or to an adult at a dosage of 25 mg/day. In adults dantrolene can be increased to 25-100 mg twice to four times a day when given orally. Dantrolene is also indicated for the acute management of malignant hyperthermia. When dantrolene is given for malignant hyperthermia it is administered intravenously at a dosage of 1 mg/kg and may be repeated until a total dose of 10 mg/kg has been given. Pregnancy category C.

PHARMACOKINETICS

HALF-LIFE	ONSET	PEAK	DURATION
PO: 8 hr	0.5-1 hr	5 hr	12-24 hr

MISCELLANEOUS AGENTS

There are several other miscellaneous medications that do not fall into the barbiturate or benzodiazepine drug class. These agents include chloral hydrate, glutethimide, methyprylon, ethchlorvynol, tizanidine, and paraldehyde. These are all prescription-only drugs. Of these six sedative-hypnotic agents, chloral hydrate and tizanidine are the ones most commonly prescribed because the other four are associated with severe side effects and are extremely toxic if taken inappropriately or in an overdose.

Chloral hydrate (Noctec) is one of the oldest nonbarbiturate sedative-hypnotic agents. It has the favorable

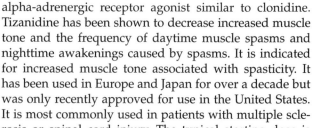

characteristic of not suppressing REM sleep at the usual therapeutic doses, and the incidence of hangover effects associated with its use is low because of its relatively short duration of action. One potential disadvantage to its use is that tachyphylaxis can develop rather quickly. **Tachyphylaxis** is the rapid appearance of a progressive decrease in response to a pharmacologically or physiologically active substance after its repetitive administration. This makes chloral hydrate only useful for short-term therapy. High doses lead to dependence and cause gastrointestinal tract irritation. The combination of alcohol and chloral hydrate leads to rapid loss of consciousness. This combination is commonly referred to as a Mickey Finn.

Tizanidine (Zanaflex) is a short-acting, centrally active alpha-adrenergic receptor agonist similar to clonidine. Tizanidine has been shown to decrease increased muscle tone and the frequency of daytime muscle spasms and nighttime awakenings caused by spasms. It is indicated for increased muscle tone associated with spasticity. It has been used in Europe and Japan for over a decade but was only recently approved for use in the United States. It is most commonly used in patients with multiple sclerosis or spinal cord injury. The typical starting dose is 4 mg at bedtime. It is then slowly titrated to a maintenance dose of 18 mg three times a day. Patients are less likely to suffer from hypotension and bradycardia when it is slowly titrated.

Nonprescription sleeping aids often contain antihistamines, and some may also contain analgesics such as aspirin or acetaminophen. The most common antihistamines contained in over-the-counter (OTC) sleeping aids are doxylamine, diphenhydramine, and pyrilamine. Besides having antihistaminic effects, these agents are heavily sedating. They have a depressant effect on the CNS. The analgesics are sometimes added to offer some pain relief if that is a component of the sleep disturbance or insomnia. As with other CNS depressants such as barbiturates and benzodiazepines, patients should avoid the consumption of alcohol when taking them. The combination can result in respiratory depression and death.

nursing process

● Assessment

Before administering any hypnotic or sedative agent, be it a barbiturate, benzodiazepine, or musculoskeletal relaxant, you need to determine whether the patient has or has had any of the following conditions or disorders:
- Allergies
- CNS disorders
- Sleep disorders (and the previous treatments for these)
- Diabetes
- Addictive disorders
- Personality disorders
- Thyroid conditions
- Depression
- Anxiety
- Suicidal thoughts or tendencies
- Mental disorders
  You also need to find out the following:
- Whether the patient consumes alcohol
- Whether the patient takes any other CNS depressants or other OTC medications
- Patient's renal and liver function status
- Patient's age (because of the increased effects of these agents in elderly persons and young children)
- Nature of the patient's sleep patterns
- Patient's stress level
- Patient's respiratory and cardiac status.

Interactions with musculoskeletal relaxants include other CNS depressing agents. It is a known fact that sedative-hypnotic agents, when combined with other drugs affecting the CNS, such as anticonvulsants, neuroleptics, and analgesics, have a 90% chance of causing adverse drug reactions.

Zolpidem is a newer agent in the nonbenzodiazepine sedative hypnotic category. Patients receiving this medication should be assessed for allergic reactions to benzodiazepines because this would be a contraindication. Cautious use is indicated in patients who are anemic, are suicidal, have a history of substance abuse, are elderly, are under the age of 18, have seizure disorders, are pregnant, are lactating, and have liver or renal disease. Before initiating therapy with zolpidem, the physician may order blood studies (Hct, Hgb, RBC) or renal or liver function studies to rule out any problems that might be exacerbated by the drug. The patient's mental status (mood, affect, level of consciousness, memory) should be assessed and documented, and a journal of the patient's type of sleep problems should be kept.

In addition, it is important to assess the patient's vital signs, including supine and erect blood pressures, especially if the intravenous use of any of these agents is planned. For instance, if diazepam is to be administered, hold the drug if the systolic blood pressure drops 20 mm Hg or more or if the pulse or respiratory rate declines. Also survey the laboratory data, such as the complete blood count and the results of hepatic studies (lactate dehydrogenase, creatine kinase, and bilirubin) and renal studies (blood urea nitrogen and creatinine). Patients receiving metaxalone may have false-positive results for glucose tests using Clinitest or Benedict's solution but not with tests using glucose oxidase.

● Nursing Diagnoses

Nursing diagnoses appropriate to the patient taking sedative-hypnotic agents include the following:
- Risk for injury or falls related to decreased sensorium.
- Sleep deprivation related to the drug's interference with REM sleep.
- Risk for injury, drug overdose, or adverse reactions related to the combined use of the agent with alcohol or other medications such as tranquilizers and analgesics.
- Risk for injury or addiction related to physical or psychologic dependency.
- Impaired gas exchange related to possible respiratory depression.
- Deficient knowledge related to inadequate information about CNS depressants.

● Planning

Goals related to the administration of sedative-hypnotic agents are as follows:
- Patient remains free of self-injury and falls related to decreased sensorium.
- Patient remains free of further sleep deprivation.
- Patient experiences little or no rebound insomnia.
- Patient remains free of or experiences minimal side effects and toxic effects from sedative-hypnotic agents or musculoskeletal relaxants.
- Patient remains free of drug interaction effects.
- Patient experiences no problems with addiction.
- Patient remains free of respiratory depression.
- Patient complies with drug therapy as ordered.
- Patient keeps follow-up visits as ordered by the physician.

Outcome Criteria

Outcome criteria related to the administration of sedative-hypnotic agents are as follows:
- Patient will state ways to minimize self-injury and falls related to decreased sensorium such as changing positions slowly.
- Patient will state pharmacologic and nonpharmacologic (relaxation therapy, massage) measures to enhance sleep patterns or enhance relaxation.
- Patient will state risk for REM interference from sedative-hypnotic agents with associated sleep hangovers and use nonpharmacologic measures as appropriate.

- Patient will state the common side effects, toxic effects, and the symptoms to be reported to the physician related to sedative-hypnotic agents such as drowsiness, confusion, and respiratory depression.
- Patient will state common side effects related to musculoskeletal relaxants such as euphoria, dizziness, drowsiness, and fatigue.
- Patient will minimize side effects and toxic effects by taking medications as prescribed.
- Patient will state the common drug interactions with alcohol and other medications, such as tranquilizers and analgesics, that may be life-threatening.
- Patient will state importance of measures to minimize problems with addiction such as taking medication only as needed.
- Patient, family, or significant other will state need to contact physician about possible complications, such as respiratory depression.
- Patient will demonstrate increased knowledge related to inadequate information about treatment, drug and nondrug, and regimen for sleeping disturbance.

● Implementation

Benzodiazepines generally have an onset of action of about 30 to 60 minutes (see the pharmacokinetics tables for respective agents) and must therefore be given 15 to 30 minutes before bedtime to maximize their effectiveness in inducing sleep. Most benzodiazepines, with the exception of flurazepam, interfere with REM sleep and produce REM rebound, and all of these agents should be given cautiously in elderly patients. Zolpidem should only be used after conservative and nondrug therapies for sleep. It should be taken on an empty stomach for a faster onset, but patients often take it with food to decrease GI upset. Patients may become sedated and sleepy and should be safely monitored with side rails up and assistance with ambulation. Patient education should include that dependence is possible with long-term use and that he or she should avoid driving or other activities that require mental alertness until drug levels are stable. Patients should also be instructed to avoid alcohol and any

other type of sedative hypnotic. It may take up to 2 nights before the full benefits of zolpidem are noticed, and the patient should also try other nondrug measures to help induce sleep. Hangover effects are less common than with barbiturates, but they may occur, especially in the elderly. Patients should also be informed that rebound insomnia may occur for a few nights after zolpidem has been discontinued. Nondrug therapy such as relaxation, music, and back massage should be encouraged when possible. See the herbal interactions boxes for kava kava and valerian, herbal agents used to promote sleep and relaxation.

Barbiturates differ in their onset of action, duration, and potency. Short-acting barbiturates (secobarbital) should be given 15 to 30 minutes before bedtime, as should some of the intermediate-acting agents (butabarbital). The longer-acting agents such as phenobarbital have an onset of action of 60 minutes. When administering any of these agents by intramuscular injection, the injection should be given deep into a large muscle mass to prevent tissue sloughing.

Toxicities associated with musculoskeletal relaxants are usually treated with supportive measures; therefore early identification of toxicity is critical to prompt treatment and to prevent respiratory depression and related CNS depression. Most of the agents previously discussed are given orally for spasticity with Dantrolene indicated intravenously (1 mg/kg; may repeat to total dose of 10 mg/kg) for malignant hyperthermia. Close monitoring of all vital parameters and level of consciousness is needed with all the CNS depressants.

Regardless of the agent given, for the safety of the patient and the prevention of injury stemming from decreased sensorium, it is crucial to keep the side rails of the bed up, to not allow smoking, to assist the patient with ambulation (especially the elderly), and to have the call light at the patient's bedside. Documentation of the dose, route, and time of administration along with the safety measures taken is also important. Patient teaching tips for benzodiazepines and barbiturates and listed on p. 171.

● Evaluation

Some of the criteria by which to determine a patient's therapeutic response to a sedative-hypnotic agent are an

---

herbal interactions

Kava Kava

BENEFIT OF HERB
Relieves anxiety, reduces stress, promotes sleep

POTENTIAL INTERACTIONS
Can increase central nervous system depression when taken with alcohol or sedatives

CAUTIONS AND NOTES
Contraindicated in pregnant or breastfeeding patients; can cause stomach disturbances, pupil dilation (affecting vision), or hair, skin, or nail discoloration; long-term use can cause scaly skin

---

herbal interactions

Valerian

BENEFIT OF HERB
Promotes sleep and relaxation

POTENTIAL INTERACTIONS
None known

CAUTIONS AND NOTES
Can cause heart palpitations, headaches, nervousness, stomach disturbances

increased ability to sleep at night, fewer awakenings, shorter sleep induction time, few side effects such as hangover effects, and an improved sense of well-being because of improved sleep. Therapeutic effects related to musculoskeletal relaxants include decreased spasticity, reduction of choreiform movements in patients with Huntington's chorea, decreased rigidity of parkinsonian syndrome, and relief of pain from trigeminal neuralgia. You must constantly watch for and document the occurrence of any of the side effects of benzodiazepines or barbiturates. The side effects of benzodiazepines include lethargy, confusion, drowsiness, dizziness, lightheaded-

ness, headache, a hangover effect, sedation during the day, nausea, and vomiting. The side effects of barbiturates include paradoxical excitement in children and the elderly, lethargy, confusion, headache, drowsiness, a hangover effect, rash, nausea, vomiting, Stevens-Johnson syndrome (with agents like phenobarbital), and respiratory depression. Side effects related to musculoskeletal relaxants range from short-term euphoria, dizziness, and drowsiness to less common side effects including slurred speech, gastroinstestinal upset, hypotension, and tachycardia.

---

patient teaching tips

Benzodiazepines and Barbiturates

➤ Take medication only as prescribed. If one dose does not work, you should *not* take a double dose. Follow the physician's orders in regard to the dosing of the medication. Overdosage, with muscle relaxants in particular, is usually treated by supportive measures.

➤ Keep a journal of your sleep habits and response to both drug and nondrug therapy.

➤ Avoid driving or operating heavy machinery or equipment, and avoid activities requiring mental alertness while on this medication.

➤ Avoid any other type of CNS-altering medications, especially CNS depressants such as tranquilizers, opioids, and alcohol.

➤ Always try measures other than medications to help you sleep because the REM rebound they cause, which results in your feeling more tired and not rested or in "hangover" effects the morning after. This hangover effect is more common in elderly patients and is less common with barbiturates.

➤ Keep all medications away from children.

➤ Because of the different characteristics of the benzodiazepines, such as flurazepam, it may take a night or two before you notice an improvement in your sleep patterns.

➤ Always check with your physician first or with the pharmacist before taking any over-the-counter medications because of the many drug interactions associated with sedative-hypnotic agents.

➤ It often takes 2 to 3 weeks for the therapeutic effects (improved sleep) of the oral forms of barbiturates to occur.

➤ Never stop taking these medications abruptly, especially the barbiturates, because of their highly addicting potential and because of the rebound insomnia you may experience.

➤ These agents should not be used every night or for more than a few days at a time (if possible) because of their potential to cause side effects, their interference with REM sleep, and their addicting properties.

 POINTS TO REMEMBER

Sedatives

• Reduce nervousness, excitability, or irritability by producing a calming effect without causing sleep.
• Can become hypnotic if given in large enough doses—major difference between sedatives and hypnotics.
• Inhibit transmission of nerve impulses to the CNS.

Hypnotics

• Calm or soothe the CNS to the point of sleep.
• More potent effect on inhibition of the CNS than sedatives have.
• Induce sleep.

Benzodiazepines

• Family of drugs that reduce nervousness, excitability, or irritability of CNS.
• Commonly prescribed as sedative-hypnotics and anxiolytics.

Muscle Relaxants

• Used for treatment of muscle spasms, spasticity and rigidity.
• Dantrolene is used to manage the occurrence of malignant hyperthermia.

Anxiolytics

- Drugs that relieve anxiety (increased nerve stimulation to the brain).
- Calm the CNS.

Sleep Architecture

- Stages in sleep cycle.
- Composed of non–REM and REM sleep.

- Non–REM: 4 stages; REM: vivid dreams occur here.
- The phases of sleep are affected by sedative-hypnotic agents.

Nonpharmacologic Approaches to Inducing Sleep

- Establish set sleep patterns.
- Avoid exercise before bedtime.
- Avoid heavy meals late in the evening.
- Drink warm decaffeinated drinks such as warm milk before bedtime.

REVIEW QUESTIONS

1. Which of the following is an important nursing action for the administration of a benzodiazepine as a sedative-hypnotic agent?
   a. Use IM dosage forms for longer duration.
   b. Administer safely with other CNS depressants for insomnia.
   c. Monitor elderly clients for the common occurrence of paradoxical reactions.
   d. Evaluate for physical dependence that occurs within 48 hours of beginning the drug.

2. Children and the elderly often react with more sensitivity to the drug group of CNS depressants. Therefore this type of sensitivity manifests itself in the development of which type of reaction?
   a. Idiopathic
   b. Teratogenic
   c. Paradoxical
   d. Psychomimenogenic

3. Your patient has a history of epilepsy and has been taking barbiturates for a few weeks because of difficulty sleeping. Your main concern for the patient who has then stopped taking the barbiturate would be the occurrence of:
   a. Seizures.
   b. Euphoria.
   c. Delirium tremors.
   d. Excessive sedation.

4. The most common adverse effect related to the use of barbiturates for sleep is:
   a. Tachycardia.
   b. Hypertension.
   c. Polyuria with a protein diuresis.
   d. Altered REM sleep with "hangover" effect.

5. Which of the following is an appropriate nursing diagnosis for patients taking muscle relaxants?
   a. Risk of injury related to ataxia
   b. Risk of injury related to tachypnea
   c. Altered thought processes related to CNS stimulation
   d. Altered thought processes related to cardiovascular degeneration

For Answers see www.harcourthealth.com/MERLIN/Lilley/.

CRITICAL THINKING Activities

1. Mrs. S.L. is a 65-year-old woman who underwent total hip replacement 6 days earlier. She is suffering from a lack of sleep and has tried all the nondrug therapy techniques. The physician has now ordered chloral hydrate, 250 mg at bedtime prn, for sleep.
   a. What are some of the home health care tips pertinent to the administration of sedative-hypnotic agents in an aged patient?
   b. Why would chloral hydrate be preferred in this patient over the other classes of sedative-hypnotic agents?

2. What instructions should be given to a 31-year-old registered nurse who was found unresponsive after drinking beer all day at a rock concert and who has a 6-year history of grand mal seizures, but these have been adequately controlled with phenytoin and diazepam?

3. Explain the need for monitoring AST (SGOT), ALT (SGPT), bilirubin, LDH, CBC, HCT, HGB, platelet studies, BUN, and creatine when patients are taking long-term barbiturates.

4. One of your patients has been told to discontinue her flurazepam (Dalmane) that she has been taking for about 1 year. The health care provider gave no other instructions. As her home health nurse, does this cause you concern? Why or why not?

5. True or false: IV diazepam may be used without any concern. If this is a false statement, explain your answer and discuss supportive nursing actions. If true, explain.

For Answers see www.harcourthealth.com/MERLIN/Lilley/.

bibliography

Albanese J, Nutz P: *Mosby's 2001 nursing drug reference and review cards,* St Louis, 2001, Mosby.

American Hospital Formulary Service: *AHFS drug information,* Bethesday, Md, 2000, American Society of Health-System Pharmacists.

Anderson PO, Knoben JE, Troutman WG: *Handbook of critical drug data 1999-2000,* ed 9, New York, 1999, McGraw-Hill.

Drug Facts and Comparisons 2000, St Louis, 2000, Facts and Comparisons.

Glod CA: Xanax: pros and cons, *J Psychosoc Nurs Ment Health Serv* 30(6):36, 1992.

Johns Hopkins Hospital, Department of Pediatrics et al: *The Harriet Lane handbook,* ed 15, St Louis, 2000, Mosby.

Keen JH: *Critical care and emergency drug reference,* ed 3, St Louis, 1996, Mosby.

Lammon CA, Adams AH: Recognizing benzodiazepine overdose, *Nursing* 23(1):33, 1993.

Mosby's GenRx: a comprehensive reference for generic and brand drugs, ed 10, St Louis, 2000, Mosby.

Sherman D: Evaluation and treatment of sleep disorders, *Contemp Longterm Care* 14:70, 1991.

Skidmore-Roth L: *Mosby's 2001 nursing drug reference,* St Louis, 2001, Mosby.

Sweetwyne K: Neonatal sedation and analgesia, *Neonat Pharmacol Q* 2:5, 1993.

Tabloski P, Cooke K, Thoman E: A procedure for withdrawal of sleep medication in elderly women who have been long-term users, *J Gerontol Nurs* 24(9):20, 1998.

Tizanidine for spasticity: *The Medical Letter* 39:1004, 1997.

Remember to check the **Online Worksheet** for additional learning opportunities: **www.harcourthealth.com/MERLIN/Lilley/**

Activity

Chapter 12

Antiepileptic Agents

objectives

www.harcourthealth.com/MERLIN/Lilley/

When you reach the end of this chapter, you should be able to do the following:

Look for this symbol for topics covered in the **Online Worksheet**

1 Discuss the rationale for the use of the various agents in the treatment of the various forms of epilepsy.

2 List the anticonvulsant agents according to their classification and the drug of choice.

3 Identify the mechanisms of action, contraindications, dosages, routes of administration, side effects, and toxic effects associated with the various anticonvulsants.

4 Discuss the importance of patient education and compliance in the control of seizure activity.

5 Develop a nursing care plan that includes all phases of the nursing process for patients receiving anticonvulsants.

drug profiles

carbamazepine, p. 183
clonazepam, p. 181
clorazepate dipotassium, p. 181
○━ **ethosuximide,** p. 182

gabapentin, p. 183
phenobarbital, p. 182
○━ **phenytoin,** p. 182
valproic acid, p. 183

○━ Key drug.

glossary

Anticonvulsant (an ti kən vul′ sənt) A substance or procedure that prevents or reduces the severity of epileptic or other convulsive seizures. (p. 175)

Autoinduction (aw to in dək′ shən) A metabolic process that occurs when a drug increases its own metabolism over time, leading to lower-than-expected drug concentrations. (p. 183)

Convulsion (kən vul′ sh ən) A type of seizure involving excessive stimulation of neurons in the brain and characterized by the spasmodic contraction of voluntary muscles. See also *seizure.* (p. 174)

Epilepsy (ep i lep′ se) A group of neurologic disorders characterized by recurrent episodes of convulsive seizures, sensory disturbances, abnormal behavior, loss of consciousness, or any combination of these. (p. 174)

International Classification of Seizures The most extensively used system of classifying seizures. Both the symptoms and characteristics of the various types of seizures are described. (p. 175)

Narrow therapeutic index (NTI) drugs Drugs that are characterized by a narrow difference between their therapeutic and toxic doses. (p. 179)

Primary or idiopathic epilepsy (id e o path′ ik) Epilepsy that develops without an apparent cause. More than 50% of cases of epilepsy are of unknown origin. (p. 175)

Secondary epilepsy Epilepsy that has a distinct cause (e.g., trauma). (p. 175)

Seizure (se′ zhər) Excessive stimulation of neurons in the brain leading to a sudden burst of abnormal neuron activity that results in temporary changes in brain function. (p. 174)

Status epilepticus (sta′ təs ep i lep′ ti kəs) A common seizure disorder characterized by generalized tonic-clonic convulsions that occur in succession. (p. 175)

Tonic-clonic seizure (tan′ ik klan′ ik) Formerly called grand mal seizure, this type of epilepsy is characterized by a series of generalized movements of tonic (stiffening) and clonic (rapid, synchronized jerking) muscular contraction. (p. 175)

Unclassified seizures Seizures that are not described by any of the seizure classifications. (p. 175)

EPILEPSY

A seizure disorder, or what is more commonly referred to as **epilepsy,** is not a specific disease like cancer or diabetes. It is a disorder of the brain that is a symptom of a disease. Most likely it involves the generation of excessive electrical discharges from nerves located in the area of the brain known as the *cerebral cortex.*

The terms *convulsion, seizure,* and *epilepsy* are often used interchangeably, but they do not have the same meaning. A **seizure** is a brief episode of abnormal electrical activity in the nerve cells of the brain. A **convulsion** is characterized by spasmodic contractions of voluntary muscles. Epilepsy is a chronic, recurrent pattern of seizures. These excessive electrical discharges can often be detected by an electroencephalogram (EEG), which is frequently obtained to help diagnose epilepsy. Other diagnostic aids that are helpful in the diagnosis of epilepsy are computerized tomography (CT) and magnetic resonance imaging (MRI). The information yielded by these diagnostic aids in conjunction with the common symptoms of the particular seizure disorder help establish the diagnosis. Commonly reported symptoms are abnormal motor function, loss of consciousness, altered sensory awareness, and psychic changes.

The cause of most cases of epilepsy is unknown, and this is true for more than 50% of the cases of epilepsy. That type of epilepsy for which a cause cannot be identified is called **primary** or **idiopathic epilepsy.** Other types of epilepsy have a distinct cause such as trauma, infection, a cerebrovascular disorder, or other illnesses. These types of epilepsy are termed **secondary epilepsy.** The chief causes of secondary epilepsy in children and infants are developmental defects, metabolic disease, or injury at birth. Acquired brain disorders account for the major causes of secondary epilepsy in adults. Some examples are head injury, disease or infection of the brain and spinal cord, a cerebrovascular accident (or stroke), a metabolic disorder, a primary or metastatic brain tumor, or some other recognizable neurologic disease.

The accurate diagnosis of a seizure disorder requires careful patient observation, a reliable patient history, and an EEG. Other diagnostic tests that are often used in revealing structural lesions of the central nervous system (CNS) as the cause of the seizure disorder are CT and MRI (which are superior to the clinical examination), EEG, and routine skull radiographs. Of MRI and CT, MRI is more sensitive and is now preferred in the evaluation of a patient with seizures.

Seizures can be classified into distinct categories based on their characteristics. In traditional classifications, seizures were categorized as grand mal seizures **(tonic-clonic seizures),** petit mal seizures, jacksonian epilepsy, and psychomotor attacks. In a newer classification system a more systematic approach is used, which breaks down seizures into two main types: partial seizures and generalized seizures. This system of classification is called the **International Classification of Seizures.** It is more extensively used because it more adequately describes the symptoms and characteristics of the various types of seizures. The various types of partial and generalized seizures are listed in Box 12-1. Under this new nomenclature, two other classifications of seizures exist—**unclassified seizures** and **status epilepticus.** Status epilepticus seizures start out as either partial or generalized seizures and become status epilepticus when there is no recovery between attacks.

ANTICONVULSANTS

Anticonvulsants are medications that are used to prevent the seizures typically associated with epilepsy. Anticonvulsant drugs are very commonly referred to as *antiepileptic drugs* (AEDs). This is probably a more appropriate term because many of these medications are indicated for the management of all types of epilepsy, not just convulsions.

The combined goal of AED therapy is to control or prevent seizures while maintaining a reasonable quality of life. Many AEDs have side effects, and balancing seizure control with side effects is often a difficult task. In most cases the therapeutic goal is not to eliminate seizure activity but rather to maximally reduce the incidence of seizures while minimizing drug-induced toxicity. Many patients must take AEDs for their entire life. Treatment may eventually be stopped in some, but others will suffer repeated seizures if constant levels of AEDs are not maintained in their blood. In both children and adults there is only a 40% chance of recurrence after the first partial or generalized seizure; therefore many physicians choose not to initiate treatment after the first seizure. However, it is the consensus that AED therapy should be implemented in patients who have had two or more seizures.

There are several AEDs available. Sometimes a combination of agents must be used to control the disorder. However, most seizure disorders can be controlled. Generally, single-drug therapy must fail before two-drug and

---

BOX 12-1   International Classification of Seizures

PARTIAL SEIZURES

Description

Short alterations in consciousness, repetitive unusual movements (chewing or swallowing movements), psychologic changes, and confusion.

Simple seizures
- No impaired consciousness
- Motor symptoms (most commonly face, arm, or leg)
- Hallucinations of sight, hearing, or taste along with somatosensory changes (tingling)
- Autonomic nervous system responses
- Personality changes

Complex seizures
- Impaired consciousness
- Memory impairment
- Behavioral effects
- Purposeless behaviors
- Aura, chewing and swallowing movements, unreal feelings, bizarre behavior
- Tonic, clonic, or tonic-clonic seizures

GENERALIZED SEIZURES

Description

Most often seen in children and commonly characterized by temporary lapses in consciousness lasting a few seconds. Staring off into space, daydreaming, and inattentive look are common symptoms. Patients may exhibit rhythmic movements of their eyes, head, or hands but do not convulse. May have several attacks per day.

- Both cerebral hemispheres involved
- Tonic, clonic, myoclonic, atonic or tonic-clonic seizures and infantile spasms possible
- Brief loss of consciousness for a few seconds with no confusion
- Head drop or falling-down symptoms

then multiple-drug therapy are implemented. A patient should always be started on a single AED and the dosage slowly increased until the seizures are controlled or until clinical toxicity occurs. If the first AED does not work, the drug should be tapered slowly while a second AED is introduced. AEDs should never be stopped abruptly unless a severe adverse effect occurs. It is sometimes difficult to control a patient's seizures using a single AED, but monotherapy is likely to result in higher serum drug concentrations, fewer adverse effects, and better control.

Serum drug concentrations are useful guides in assessing the effectiveness of therapy. They should, however, be only guidelines. The goal should be to slowly titrate to the lowest effective serum drug level that controls the seizure disorder. This decreases the risk of medication-induced adverse effects and interactions. The serum concentrations of phenytoin, phenobarbital, carbamazepine, and primidone correlate better with seizure control and toxicity than do those of valproic acid, ethosuximide, and clonazepam. Emphasis should be placed primarily on the clinical symptoms and patient's history rather than on strict adherence to established drug concentration ranges.

There are six traditional classes of AEDs, and many new agents have been marketed recently. These newer agents were developed with the goal of eliminating many of the drug interactions and side effects associated with the older agents. Successful control of a seizure disorder hinges on selecting the appropriate drug class and drug dosage, the patient complying with the treatment regimen, and limiting toxicity. Maintaining serum drug levels within therapeutic ranges helps not only to control seizures but also to reduce side effects. There are established normal therapeutic ranges for many AEDs, but these are useful only as guidelines. Each patient should be monitored individually and the dosages adjusted based on the individual case. Many patients are maintained successfully below or above the usual therapeutic range.

The underlying cause of most cases of epilepsy is an excessive electrical discharge from nerves within the CNS. The object of AED therapy is to prevent the generation and spread of these excessive discharges while simultaneously protecting surrounding normal cells.

Mechanism of Action

Like many classes of drugs, the exact mechanism of action of the AEDs is not known. The AEDs may act in a couple of ways to control epilepsy. Some researchers believe they act directly on abnormal neurons, decreasing their excitability and responsiveness to abnormal stimuli. Seizure activity may also be reduced by raising the seizure threshold, which is the amount of stimulation needed to stimulate a nerve and cause a response. Others believe that AEDs prevent the spread of abnormal impulses to normal neurons near the area of damaged or abnormal nerves. This may help limit the seizure activity to a small portion of the brain by confining excessive electrical activity. There is strong evidence, however, showing that they alter the movement of sodium, potassium, calcium, and magnesium ions. The normal conduction of

nerve impulses relies heavily on the movement of ions like sodium, potassium, calcium, and magnesium. The changes in the movement of these ions induced by AEDs result in stabilized and less responsive cell membranes. This ion theory may explain how AEDs decrease excitability and responsiveness.

Drug Effects

AEDs stabilize nerve cells and keep them from becoming hyperexcited. AEDs prevent hyperactive neuron discharges from being generated in areas of the brain that are dysfunctional. They also prevent the spread of these abnormal impulses to neurons located near the abnormal neurons. The primary pharmacologic effects of AEDs are threefold. First, they increase the threshold of activity in the area of the brain called the *motor cortex.* In other words, they make it more difficult for a nerve to be excited or they reduce the nerve's response to incoming electrical or chemical stimulation. Second, they act to depress or limit the spread of a seizure discharge from its origin. They do this by suppressing the transmission of impulses from one nerve to the next. Third, they can decrease nerve conduction. AEDs may also have effects outside the neuron, indirectly affecting the

---

pediatric considerations

Anticonvulsant Therapy

- When a skin rash develops in a child or infant taking phenytoin, the drug should be discontinued immediately and the physician notified.
- Chewable dosage forms should **not** be used for once-a-day administration, and IM injections of phenytoin should be avoided.
- Family members, parents, significant others, or caregivers should be encouraged to keep a record of the signs and symptoms, response to therapy, and any adverse reactions.
- Wearing of a MedicAlert bracelet or necklace should be encouraged and information on this given.
- Suspension forms should always be shaken thoroughly before use and an exact graduated device or oral syringe used for more accurate dosing.
- Pediatric patients are much more sensitive to barbiturates and may respond to lower-than-expected doses, show more profound CNS depressive effects, or exhibit depression, confusion, or excitement (paradoxical reactions).
- Safe response of neonates to benzodiazepines has not been established. Prolonged CNS depression has been associated with use of these agents in pediatric patients.
- Oral forms of valproic acid should not be given with milk because this may cause them to dissolve early and irritate local mucosa.
- Report excessive sedation, confusion, lethargy, or decreased movement in pediatric patients taking any AED.

area in the brain responsible for the problem by altering, for instance, the blood supply to that area.

Therapeutic Uses

The major therapeutic indication for AEDs is the prevention or control of seizure activity. They are especially useful for maintenance therapy in patients with the chronic recurring type of seizures that are commonly associated with epilepsy. As evidenced by the wide range of seizure disorders listed in Box 12-1, epilepsy is a very diverse disorder. As a result, no one drug can control all types of epilepsy. Although our understanding of epilepsy is still growing, we have a good idea of the primary causes of many of the various seizure disorders. Each involves a distinct area of dysfunction and has certain characteristics that make certain drugs more effective than others in treating it. Therefore particular drugs are indicated for the control of specific seizures. Some of the AEDs and the seizure disorders they are used to treat are listed in Table 12-1.

AEDs are chiefly used for the long-term maintenance treatment of epilepsy. However, AEDs are also useful for the acute treatment of convulsions and status epilepticus. Status epilepticus is a common seizure disorder that is a life-threatening emergency; it is characterized by generalized tonic-clonic convulsions that occur in succession. Affected patients typically do not regain consciousness between the many convulsions. Hypotension, hypoxia, and cardiac dysrhythmias complicate the disorder, and brain damage and death quickly ensue if prompt, appropriate therapy is not started. This typically is done with diazepam (Valium), which is considered by many to be the drug of choice. There are, however, other agents that are also useful for the treatment of status epilepticus. The agents most commonly used are listed in Table 12-2.

Once status epilepticus is controlled, long-term drug therapy is begun with other agents for prevention. Patients who undergo brain surgery or who have suffered severe head injuries may receive prophylactic AED therapy. These patients are at high risk for acquiring a seizure disorder, and frequently severe complications will arise if seizures are not controlled.

Side Effects and Adverse Effects

AEDs are plagued by many side effects, which often limit their usefulness. Agents must be withdrawn from many patients because of some of these effects. Each AED is associated with its own diverse set of side effects, which makes it difficult to categorize all the classes of AEDs according to their common side effects. The various AEDs and their most common side effects are listed in Table 12-3.

Table 12-1 Antiepileptic Drugs of Choice

Partial Seizures		Generalized Seizures						
Simple	Complex	GTC	Absence	Myoclonic	Clonic	Tonic	Atonic
FIRST CHOICE							
CBZ	CBZ	CBZ	ESX	VPA	VPA	VPA	VPA
PHB	PHB	PHB	PHB				
PHT	PHT	PHT	VPA				
PMD	PMD	PMD					
VPA	VPA	VPA					
SECOND CHOICE							
CNZ	CNZ	CNZ	AZM	CNZ	CNZ	CBZ	CNZ
CRZ	CRZ	CZP	CNZ			CNZ	
						PHT	

AZM, Acetazolamide; *CBZ*, carbamazepine; *CNZ*, clonazepam; *CRZ*, clorazepate; *ESX*, ethosuximide; *GTC*, generalized tonic-clonic; *PHB*, phenobarbital; *PHT*, phenytoin; *PMD*, primidone; *VPA*, valproic acid.

Table 12-2 Antiepileptic Drugs Used for Treatment of Status Epilepticus

Property	Diazepam	Lorazepam*	Phenytoin	Phenobarbital
Dose (mg/kg)	0.3-0.5 (<20 mg)	0.05-0.1	15-20	15-20
Onset (min)	3-10	1-20	5-30	10-30
Duration	Minutes	Hours	12-24 hr	Days
Half-life (hr)	35	15	10-60	96
Adverse effects	Hypotension, apnea, somnolence	Hypotension, apnea, somnolence	Cardiac dysrhythmias, hypotension	Hypotension, apnea, somnolence

*Nonlabeled use.

Antiepileptic Drug Side Effects

12-3

Drug or Drug Class		Side Effects
Barbiturates	CNS:	Drowsiness, dizziness, lethargy, paradoxical restlessness, excitement
	GI:	Nausea, vomiting
	Other:	Rash, Stevens-Johnson syndrome, urticaria
carbamazepine	Blood:	Bone marrow suppression (aplastic anemia, agranulocytosis, thrombocytopenia)
	Skin:	Exfoliative dermatitis, erythema multiforme, Stevens-Johnson syndrome
	Heart:	Dysrhythmias, congestive heart failure
	Other:	Thrombophelebitis, vision and hearing disturbances, acute urinary retention, dyspnea, pneumonitis, pneumonia
divalproex (valproic acid)	Other:	Pancreatitis, irregular menses, secondary amenorrhea, galactorrhea, rare breast enlargement, weight gain
	Blood:	Thrombocytopenia
felbamate	GI:	Anorexia, nausea, vomiting
	Other:	Headache, intramenstrual bleeding, respiratory and urinary tract infections
	Pediatric:	Fever, purpura, nervousness, somnolence
Hydantoins	Heart:	Dysrhythmias
	Skin:	Exfoliative dermatitis, lupus erythematosus, Stevens-Johnson syndrome
	Blood:	Bone marrow suppression (agranulocytosis, thrombocytopenia, megaloblastic anemia)
	Other:	Neuropathies, gingival hyperplasia
Oxazolidinediones	Blood:	Bone marrow suppression (thrombocytopenia, agranulocytosis, aplastic anemia)
	CNS:	Vsual disturbances, drowsiness
	Skin:	Lupus erythematosus, malignant lymphoma syndrome
	Other:	Myasthenia gravis, nephrosis, gingival and vaginal bleeding
Succinimides	Blood:	Agranulocytosis, aplastic anemia, leukopenia, vaginal bleeding
	Skin:	Stevens-Johnson syndrome, lupus erythematosus
	Other:	Drowsiness, headache, swollen tongue, gingival hyperplasia

CNS, Central nervous system; *GI,* gastrointestinal.

Antiepileptic Agents: Drug Interactions

12-4

Drug or Drug Class	Mechanism	Results
CARBAMAZEPINE		
Bone marrow depressants	Additive effect	Increased bone marrow toxicity
doxycycline, phenytoin, theophylline, warfarin	Alters metabolism	Significant decrease in their half-lives
DIVALPROEX (VALPROIC ACID)		
Barbiturates	Additive effect	Increased CNS depression
clonazepam	Not determined	May produce absence status
phenytoin	Not determined	May produce breakthrough seizures
FELBATOL		
carbamazepine	Alters clearance	Decreased Felbatol levels
phenytoin	Inhibits hepatic enzymes	Increased phenytoin levels
HYDANTOINS		
disulfiram, isoniazid, valproic acid	Inhibits hepatic enzymes	Increased hydantoin levels
Tricyclic antidepressants	Not determined	Possible seizures
OXAZOLIDINEDIONES		
Bone marrow depressants	Additive effect	Increased bone marrow toxicity
PHENACEMIDE		
ethotoin	Not determined	Paranoid symptoms
SUCCINIMIDES		
Bone marrow depressants	Additive effects	Increased bone marrow toxicity

Table 12-5 Therapeutic Plasma Levels of NTI Antiepileptic Drugs

AED	Therapeutic Plasma Level (μg/ml)
carbamazepine	5-12
clonazepam	0.02-0.07
divalproex	50-100
ethosuximide	40-100
phenobarbital	10-40
phenytoin	5-20
primidone	5-12
valproic acid	50-100

Table 12-6 Anticonvulsants: FDA Pregnancy Risk Classification

Pregnancy Class	Anticonvulsant
C	acetazolamide, carbamazepine, clonazepam, ethosuximide, gabapentin
D	Barbiturates, clorazepate, diazepam, divalproex, hydantoin, paramethadione, phenytoin, primidone, valproic acid
Unclassified	Succinimides, tiagabine, topiramate, trimethadione

Interactions

The drug interactions that can occur with the AEDs are many and varied, and these are summarized in Table 12-4. Significant drug interactions for selected agents are also listed in Table 12-4.

Dosages

With certain AEDs, the safe levels and toxic levels are very close. Drugs that have a narrow difference between safe and toxic levels are called **narrow therapeutic index (NTI) drugs.** Table 12-5 lists the various AEDs that require monitoring of therapeutic plasma levels and their corresponding therapeutic levels. For an overview of dosages, see the dosages table on p. 180.

drug profiles

AEDs are prescription-only drugs. These drugs are associated with many characteristics that make it undesirable for patients to be taking them without the supervision of a qualified medical specialist. They are available in many oral, injectable, and rectal formulations. The FDA's pregnancy risk classification of the AEDs is summarized in Table 12-6.

In most children and adults, epilepsy can be controlled with a first-line AED such as carbamazepine, ethosuximide, phenobarbital, primidone, phenytoin, or valproic acid. For patients who do not respond to the first-line AEDs, there are a number of second-line AEDs that are used occasionally, such as clonazepam, clorazepate, methsuximide, and acetazolamide. These are considered second-line agents because their efficacy or adverse effect profiles are not as favorable as those of the first-line agents.

Until the 1990s no major new drugs for the treatment of epilepsy had been introduced in the United States since 1978, when valproic acid was introduced. In recent years, at least 22 investigational AEDs have undergone clinical testing. A few of these have already been recommended for approval by an FDA advisory subcommittee, and others have

recently been approved and are being marketed. These new drugs show promise, offering possibly better efficacy and toxicity profiles than the older agents. Of these newer agents, four have shown great promise: felbamate, gabapentin, lamotrigine, and vigabatrin.

All four of these have received FDA approval. Gabapentin has been available in the United States since 1994. Gabapentin and lamotrigine are primarily used as add-on drugs in adults who have partial seizures alone or with secondary generalized seizures. Both drugs will probably see use in children. The FDA currently recommends that felbamate be given only to patients who have seizures that are refractory to treatment with all other medications and in whom risk-benefit considerations warrant its use. Reports of aplastic anemia and acute liver failure necessitate that weekly or biweekly complete blood counts and liver-function tests be performed.

AEDs that have most recently been approved are levetiracetam (Keppra), topiramate (Topamax), zonisamide (Zonegran), and tiagabine (Gabitril). These agents fall under the miscellaneous category of AEDs and have greatly expanded the options currently available to patients with seizure disorders. Topiramate is a structurally unique agent chemically related to fructose. It is presently approved as an add-on AED for partial seizures. Topiramate has teratogenic effects in animals and should be avoided during pregnancy if possible. It offers another add-on option for the large number of patients with partial seizures not controlled on first-line AEDs, but cognitive impairment may be troublesome. It has been shown to cause mental slowing (difficulty in word finding, impaired concentration) and fatigue or somnolence.

Another AED that falls under the miscellaneous class of AEDs is tiagabine. It has similar indications and side effects as topiramate. It is used as an adjunct to other drugs for treatment of partial seizures in

DOSAGES Selected Anticonvulsant Agents

agent	pharmacologic class	dosage range	purpose
carbamazepine (Tegretol, Tegretol XR)	Miscellaneous	*Pediatric* PO: <6 y/o, 10-35 mgkg/day PO: 6-12 y/o, 200-1000 mg/day PO: >12 y/o, 400-1600 mg/day	Partial seizures with complex symptoms; tonic-clonic, mixed seizures; trigeminal-glossopharyngeal neuralgia
clonazepam (Klonopin)	Benzodiazepine	*Pediatric* PO: ≤10 y/o or 30 kg, 0.1-0.2 mg/kg/day divided 3 times/day *Adult* PO: 4-20 mg/day	Lennox-Gastaut; absence, akinetic, and myoclonic seizures
clorazepate dipotassium (Gen-Xene, Tranxene)	Benzodiazepine	*Pediatric* PO: 9-12 y/o, 15-60 mg/day *Adult/children* PO: >12 y/o, 22-90 mg/day	Partial seizures
ethosuximide (Zarontin)	Succinimide	*Pediatric* PO: 3-6 y/o, 250 mg/day then adjust; >6 y/o, 500 mg/day then adjust *Adult* PO: 500 mg/day then adjust	Absence seizures
gabapentin (Neurontin)	Miscellaneous	*Adult* PO: >18 y/o, 900-1800 mg/day	Add-on therapy for partial seizures and neuropathic pain
phenobarbital (Solfoton)	Barbiturate	*Pediatric* PO: 3-5 mg/kg/day IM/IV: 10-20 mg/kg load, may repeat 5 mg/kg; max 40 mg/kg *Adult* PO: 100-300 mg/day IM/IV: 200-600 mg *Adult/Pediatric* PO: 3-4 mg/kg/day	Partial, tonic-clonic seizures Convulsions Partial, tone-clonic seizures Convulsions Prophylaxis for febrile convulsions
phenytoin (Dilantin)	Hydantoin	*Pediatric* PO: 4-8 mg/kg/day IV: 15-20 mg/kg *Adult:* PO: 300-600 mg/day IV: 15-20 mg/kg	Tonic-clonic, psychomotor seizures Convulsions Tonic-clonic, psychomotor seizures Convulsions
primidone (Mysoline)	Barbiturate	*Pediatric* PO: <8 y/o, 125-250 mg/tid *Adult/Pediatric* PO: >8 y/o, 250 mg 4-6 times/day; max 2 g/day	Partial seizures Tonic-clonic seizures
valproic acid (Depakene, Depakote)	Miscellaneous	*Adult/Pediatric* PO: 15-60 mg/kg/day divided 2-3 doses/day	Multiple seizures

patients over 12 years of age. Carbamazepine, phenytoin, and valproate remain the first-line drugs for treatment of partial seizures. Tiagabine exerts its beneficial effects by prolonging the action of gamma-aminobutyric acid (GABA). The uptake of this major inhibitory neurotransmitter is inhibited by tiagabine. Tiagabine has also been shown to cause cognitive problems such as confusion, abnormal thinking,

and difficulty in concentrating. Withdrawal seizures have been reported with sudden discontinuation of tiagabine. Withdrawal should be gradual and accompanied by substitution of another anticonvulsant. Tiagabine appears to be effective as an add-on AED in patients with refractory complex partial seizures.

Dilantin (USP) is a ready-mixed solution of phenytoin sodium in a vehicle containing 40% propylene glycol and 10% alcohol in water for injection, adjusted to pH 12 with sodium hydroxide. It is very irritating to veins when injected. Parenteral Dilantin should be injected slowly (not exceeding 50 mg per minute in adults), directly into a large vein through a large-gauge needle (preferably >20-gauge) or IV catheter. Each injection of IV Dilantin should be followed by an injection of sterile saline through the same needle or IV catheter to avoid local venous irritation caused by the alkalinity of the solution. Continuous infusion should be avoided.

Soft tissue irritation and inflammation has occurred at the site of injection with and without extravasation of IV phenytoin. Soft tissue irritation may vary from slight tenderness to extensive necrosis, sloughing, and in rare instances amputation. Improper administration including SC or perivascular injection should be avoided to help prevent the possibility of the above. Local irritation, inflammation, tenderness, necrosis, and sloughing have been reported with or without extravasation of IV phenytoin.

Fosphenytoin (Cerebyx) was developed in an attempt to overcome some of the physical shortcomings of phenytoin sodium. The physical characteristics of phenytoin sodium were changed to help reduce the tissue irritation and inflammation commonly associated with its IV administration (Table 12-7).

New formulations of already available AEDs have also been marketed. Fosphenytoin is a water-soluble, phosphorylated phenytoin derivative that can be given intramuscularly or intravenously without causing the pain associated with the present product. An intravenous formulation of valproate has also been released. A new controlled-release system, called the *osmotically released oral system* (OROS), is now available for another effective first-line AED carbamazepine. This system offers the combined advantage of providing long-duration, steady carbamazepine serum levels and ensuring increased patient compliance.

Activity

BENZODIAZEPINES

Benzodiazepines are used as first-line agents in the treatment of status epilepticus and generally as second-line agents for the treatment of epilepsy. The prototypical benzodiazepine for the treatment of status epilepticus is diazepam (Valium), although lorazepam (Ativan) has also been used for this purpose. (See Table 11-2 for a list of all the agents that are commonly used in the treatment of status epilepticus and their important pharmacodynamic and pharmacokinetic properties.) Diazepam remains the drug of choice for the treatment of status epilepticus because of its quick onset. Diazepam can be administered via a variety of routes—IM, IV, and a new rectal gel. The IV and rectal gel provide

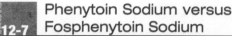

	Phenytoin Sodium (Dilantin IV)	Fosphenytoin Sodium (Cerebyx IM/IV)
pH	12	8.6-9
Maximum infusion rate	50 mg/min	150 mg PE*/min
Admixtures	None	0.9% saline or 5% dextrose

PE, Phenytoin sodium equivalents.

Activity

for quick onset of action. Oral tablets and solutions are available as well. Diazepam has a longer biologic half-life, approximately 20 to 80 hours, and therefore has a longer duration of action. It is more lipophilic and stays in the CNS longer.

clonazepam

The two benzodiazepines that are primarily used as second-line AEDs are clonazepam and clorazepate (see next section). Clonazepam (Klonopin) is the most widely used oral AED of the benzodiazepine family in the United States. It is used to treat a variety of seizure disorders. Its greatest value is in the treatment of generalized seizures, but it is also effective in reducing the frequency of absence, generalized tonic-clonic, and myoclonic seizures. A major factor limiting its use is the high frequency of toxicity associated with its use. The three most common adverse effects are drowsiness, ataxia, and behavioral and personality changes. The behavioral disturbances can be marked and include hyperactivity, irritability, moodiness, and aggressive behavior. Many of these can be reduced or prevented by using the lowest effective dose. A tolerence to the drug develops in approximately one third of the patients who initially respond to clonazepam, and their seizures recur, usually within 1 to 6 months of starting therapy. Some of these patients respond to an increased dose, but others no longer respond to clonazepam at any dose. It is classified as a pregnancy category C drug. Clonazepam is available in 0.5-, 1-, and 2-mg tablets. There is no oral liquid preparation. It is a prescription-only drug. Recommended dosages are given in the table on p. 180.

PHARMACOKINETICS

HALF-LIFE	ONSET	PEAK	DURATION
20-46 hr	20-60 min	1-4 hr	6-12 hr

clorazepate dipotassium

Clorazepate dipotassium (Gen-xene, Tranxene) is a long-acting benzodiazepine anxiolytic used primarily as an add-on drug for patients whose seizures continue despite maximum efforts at treating with a single agent. Clorazepate is a pro-drug that is converted to the active drug N-desmethyldiazepam in the liver. It has been shown to be more effective in the treatment of generalized seizures than in the treatment of other types of seizures. Clorazepate is classified as a pregnancy category D agent. It is available in 3.75-, 7.5-, and 15-mg tablets and in 11.25- and 22.5-mg extended-release tablets. It is a prescription-only drug. Recommended dosages are given in the table on p. 180.

PHARMACOKINETICS

HALF-LIFE	ONSET	PEAK	DURATION
55-100 hr	15 min	1-2 hr	4-6 hr

SUCCINIMIDES

ethosuximide

Ethosuximide (Zarontin) is a very safe and effective first-line AED that is used primarily for the treatment of absence seizures. Such seizures occur primarily in childhood. Occasionally, when valproate is ineffective in controlling primary generalized epilepsy involving seizure types other than absence attacks, the addition of ethosuximide improves seizure control. It is in this setting that ethosuximide is used most in adults. Its common side effects are nausea and abdominal discomfort, drowsiness, anorexia, and headache. In rare cases, behavioral changes may be seen, including psychosis. It is classified as a pregnancy category C agent. Ethosuximide is available in syrup (250 mg/5 ml) and capsule (250 mg) form. It is a prescription-only drug. Recommended dosages are given in the table on p. 180.

PHARMACOKINETICS

HALF-LIFE	ONSET	PEAK	DURATION
24-70 hr	4-7 days*	1-4 hr	12-24 hr

*4-7 days until reaches steady state.

BARBITURATES

phenobarbital

Two of the most commonly used AEDs are the barbiturates phenobarbital (Solfoton) and primidone (Mysoline). Primidone is metabolized in the liver to phenobarbital and phenylethylmalonamide, both of which have anticonvulsant properties. Phenobarbital has been used since 1912, principally for controlling tonic-clonic and partial seizures. Phenobarbital is also a first-line agent for the management of status epilepticus and is an effective prophylactic drug for the control of febrile seizures. By far the most common adverse effect is sedation, but tolerance to this effect usually develops with continued therapy. In pediatric patients the most common adverse effects are irritability, hyperactivity, depression, sleep disorders, and cognitive abnormalities. Therapeutic effects are generally seen at serum drug levels of

15 to 40 μg/ml. It interacts with many drugs because it is a major inducer of hepatic enzymes, causing more rapid clearance of some drugs. Its major advantage is that it has the longest half-life of all the standard AEDs, which allows for once-a-day dosing. This can be a substantial advantage for patients who have a hard time remembering to take their medication or for those who have erratic schedules. A patient may take a dose 12 or even 24 hours too late and may still have therapeutic blood levels at that time. In addition, phenobarbital is the most inexpensive AED, costing only pennies a day compared with several dollars for other AEDs. Phenobarbital is classified as a pregnancy category D agent. It is available for oral administration as capsules (16 mg), tablets (8, 15, 16, 30, 32, 60, 65, 100 mg), and an elixir (15 and 20 mg/5 ml). It also is available as an IV injection (30, 60, 65, and 130 mg/ml). It is a prescription-only drug. Recommended dosages are given in the table on p. 180.

PHARMACOKINETICS*

HALF-LIFE	ONSET	PEAK	DURATION
53-118 hr	20-60 min	8-12 hr	6-12 hr

*For PO therapy.

Activity

HYDANTOINS

phenytoin

Phenytoin (Dilantin) has been used as a first-line AED for many years. It is primarily indicated for the management of tonic-clonic and partial seizures. The most common side effects are lethargy, abnormal movements, mental confusion, and cognitive changes. Therapeutic drug levels are 5 to 20 μg/dl. At toxic levels, phenytoin can cause nystagmus, ataxia, dysarthria, and encephalopathy. Long-term phenytoin therapy can cause gingival hyperplasia, acne, hirsutism, and hypertrophy of subcutaneous facial tissue, resulting in an appearance known as "Dilantin facies." Scrupulous dental care can help prevent gingival hypertrophy. Another long-term consequence of phenytoin therapy is osteoporosis. Vitamin D therapy may be necessary to prevent this, particularly in women. Phenytoin can interact with other medications, and there are two main reasons for this. First, it is highly bound to plasma proteins and competes with other highly protein-bound medications for binding sites. Second, it induces hepatic microsomal enzymes, mainly the cytochrome P-450 system, thereby increasing the metabolism of other drugs and decreasing their levels.

Exaggerated phenytoin effects can be seen in patients with very low serum albumin concentrations. This scenario is most commonly seen in patients who are malnourished or have chronic renal failure. In these patients it may be necessary to maintain phenytoin levels well below 20 μg/ml.

With lower levels of albumin in a patient's body, more free, unbound, pharmacologically active phenytoin will be present. Phenytoin has many advantages from the standpoint of long-term therapy. It is usually well tolerated, highly effective, and relatively inexpensive. It can also be given intravenously if needed. Phenytoin's long half-life allows it to be given only twice a day, and in some cases once a day. As stressed earlier, compliance with AED treatment is very important to seizure control. Therefore if a patient only has to remember to take medication once or twice a day, this will lead to increased compliance and an increased likelihood of therapeutic drug levels being reached, and hence better seizure control. Phenytoin is available in both oral and IV forms. Orally administered phenytoin is available as a suspension (30 and 125 mg/5 ml), chewable tablets (50 mg), regular-release tablets (30 and 100 mg), and extended-release tablets (30 and 100 mg). It also is available as a 50-mg/ml injection. Phenytoin is a pregnancy category D agent and a prescription-only drug. The recommended dosages are given in the table on p. 180.

PHARMACOKINETICS

HALF-LIFE	ONSET	PEAK	DURATION
10-34 hr	2-24 hr	1.5-2.5 hr	6-12 hr

valproic acid

Valproic acid (Depakene, Depakote, Depacon) is used primarily in the treatment of generalized seizures (absence, myoclonic, and tonic-clonic). It has also been shown to be effective for controlling partial seizures. The main side effects are drowsiness; nausea, vomiting, and other gastrointestinal disturbances; tremor; weight gain; and transient hair loss. The most serious ones can be fatal—hepatotoxicity and pancreatitis. Valproic acid can interact with many medications. The main reasons for these interactions are protein binding and liver metabolism. It is highly bound to plasma proteins and competes with other highly protein bound medications for binding sites. It also is highly metabolized by hepatic microsomal enzymes and competes for metabolism. Valproic acid is categorized as a pregnancy category D agent. It is available as valproate sodium syrup (250 mg/5 ml), divalproex sodium capsules with sprinkle particles (250 mg), liquid-filled capsules (250 mg), extended-release divalproex sodium tablets (125, 250, and 500 mg), and valproate sodium injection (100 mg/ml). It is a prescription-only drug. Recommended dosages are given in the table on p. 180.

PHARMACOKINETICS

HALF-LIFE	ONSET	PEAK	DURATION
6-16 hr	15-30 min	1-4 hr	4-6 hr

MISCELLANEOUS AGENTS

carbamazepine

Carbamazepine (Tegretol) is the second most frequently prescribed AED in the United States, after phenytoin. It was marketed in the late 1960s for the treatment of epilepsy in adults after its efficacy and safety for the treatment of trigeminal neuralgia were proved. It was granted approval for use in pediatric patients in 1976. It is chemically related to the tricyclic antidepressants and is considered a first-line AED for the treatment of simple partial, complex partial, and generalized tonic-clonic seizures. It is contraindicated in patients with absence and myoclonic seizures and those who have shown a hypersensitivity reaction to it in the past. Carbamazepine is available as an oral suspension (100 mg/5 ml), a 200-mg tablet, and a 100-mg chewable tablet. There are also extended-release tablets available in 100, 200, and 400 mg. The typical therapeutic serum carbamazepine drug level is 8 to 12 μg/ml, but as with all AEDs, the therapeutic concentrations should be used only as a guideline. Carbamazepine is metabolized to carbamazepine epoxide, which has both anticonvulsant and toxic effects. Carbamazepine undergoes **autoinduction,** the process whereby a drug increases its own metabolism over time, leading to lower-than-expected drug concentrations. With carbamazepine this process usually occurs within the first 2 months after the start of therapy. Carbamazepine is classified as a pregnancy category C drug. It is a prescription-only drug. The recommended dosages are given in the table on p. 180.

PHARMACOKINETICS

HALF-LIFE	ONSET	PEAK	DURATION
14-16 hr	Slow	4-8 hr	12-24 hr

gabapentin

Gabapentin (Neurontin) is an add-on agent for the treatment of partial seizures and partial seizures with secondary generalization in adults. It is also commonly used to treat neuropathic pain. The exact mechanism of action of gabapentin is unknown. Many believe that it works by increasing GABA synthesis, increasing GABA accumulation, or binding to an undefined receptor site in the brain to produce anticonvulsant activity. Abrupt discontinuation of gabapentin can lead to withdrawal seizures. It has no contraindications and is rated a pregnancy category C agent by the FDA. Gabapentin is available as a capsule in 100-, 300-, and 400-mg strengths. The recommended dosage is listed in the table on p. 180.

PHARMACOKINETICS

HALF-LIFE	ONSET	PEAK	DURATION
5-7 hr	Unknown	Unknown	Unknown

Activity

nursing process

It is important for the safe use of the various classes of agents used in the management of seizure disorders to understand the nursing process as it relates to each of these major classes. This discussion focuses on the different groups of the barbiturates, benzodiazepines, hydantoins, and oxazolidinediones. Some of these AEDs, such as the barbiturates and benzodiazepines, are also discussed with the sedative-hypnotic agents (see Chapter 11).

● Assessment

When any AED is to be administered, the nurse should first obtain a thorough health history so that any possible drug interactions (see Table 12-4), drug allergies, and previous unusual or untoward reactions to any of these medications can be known in advance. Drug interactions for fosphenytoin are similar to those of phenytoin. In addition, the nurse needs to gather any information regarding cardiac, respiratory tract, renal, liver, or CNS disorders because of the precautions that may be called for in the use of AEDs. In addition to the traditional AED, it is important to assess liver function studies and complete blood count (CBC) laboratory values with the newer agents gabapentin, lamotrigine (Lamictal), and felbamate because of the adverse effects of aplastic anemia and altered liver function. Fosphenytoin is contraindicated in patients with sinus bradycardia, sinoatrial block, second- and third-degree atrioventricular block, and Adams-Stokes syndrome.

Tiagabine, topiramate, and zonisamide are contraindicated in patients with hypersensitivity to them. They should be used cautiously in patients with renal or liver disease, children under 12 years of age, the elderly, and patients who are pregnant or lactating. The patient's mental status, sensorium, and level of consciousness also need to be assessed and documented before and during therapy. Topiramate is also to be used cautiously in patients with cardiac disease. Drug interactions for topiramate include digoxin, oral contraceptives, CNS depressants, alcohol (increased effects), and decreased levels of topiramate with phenytoin, carbamazepine, and valproic acid. Renal and liver studies and CBC levels should be also be done before initiation of therapy. The newer miscellaneous agents (tiagabine, topiramate, and zonisamide) are indicated for use in partial seizures; therefore documentation of this type of seizure activity is important to initiation of drug treatment.

● Nursing Diagnoses

Nursing diagnoses appropriate to the use of anticonvulsants include, but are not limited to, the following:
- Risk for injury related to decreased sensorium stemming from drug effects.
- Deficient knowledge related to lack of familiarity with and information concerning the use of AEDs.
- Noncompliance (therapeutic regimen) related to patient's misuse of drugs or lack of understanding about the seizure disorder and its treatment.

● Planning

The goals of nursing care in a patient taking AEDs are as follows:
- Patient experiences little or no adverse effects associated with noncompliance and/or with overtreatment or undertreatment.
- Patient can identify therapeutic effects of AEDs.
- Patient remains compliant with therapy and without major harm to self during AED treatment.

Outcome Criteria

Outcome criteria related to the use of AEDs include the following:
- Patient will state the therapeutic drug effects as well as the side effects of the AED such as sedation, confusion, CNS depression.
- Patient (or family members) will state the importance of taking the medication exactly the way it has been prescribed such as the same time every day.
- Patient will state the dangers associated with sudden withdrawal of the medication such as rebound convulsions.
- Patient will maintain a protective environment at home and at work to minimize self-injury.

● Implementation

AEDs, specifically the oral agents, should be taken regularly at the same time of day at the recommended dose and with meals to diminish the gastrointestinal upset often associated with these agents. Oral suspensions should be shaken thoroughly, and capsules should not be crushed, opened, or chewed. Because there are both extended-release and immediate-release forms of oral hydantoins, it is important for the nurse to be sure which agent is being prescribed. Extended-release agents are usually taken once a day. If there are any questions about the medication order or the medication prescribed, the physician should be contacted immediately for clarification.

When administered intramuscularly, parenteral agents should be given deep in muscles, usually in the gluteal muscles, with rotation of the sites when more than one injection is being given. A 23-gauge, 1½-inch needle (as used for most IM injections) is recommended, but the nurse should follow the manufacturer's recommendations as well as make decisions on the basis of each patient's situation.

Parenterally administered AEDs should be given with caution to prevent accidental arterial access and possible cardiac or respiratory arrest. If subcutaneous tissue access does occur as a result of infiltration of the drug at the IV site, ischemia and sloughing may occur because of the high alkalinity of some of these agents, specifically the hydantoins. Any of the intravenously administered AEDs, but especially the hydantoins, specifically phenytoin, should be delivered slowly while any changes in the vital signs—usually a decrease in pulse (<60 beats/min), blood pressure (<120/80 mm Hg), and respiratory rate (<12 breaths/min)—are watched for and monitored. The IV site should

NURSING CARE PLAN Epilepsy

A 68-year-old male patient has developed grand mal seizures post left-sided cerebrovascular accident (LCVA). The physician has placed him on phenytoin (Dilantin) 300 mg/day of the extended-release preparation. His caregiver needs discharge instructions about the medication because the patient has never taken any type of antiepileptic medication. The patient is aphasic and paralyzed on the right side but has no major cognitive impairment.

assessment	*Nursing Diagnosis*	Imbalanced nutrition, less than body requirements, related to side effects of medication therapy
	Subjective Data	Patient unable to communicate verbally because of LCVA
	Objective Data	Patient is post-LCVA
		Never taken antiepileptic drugs
		Resides in residential home
		Caregiver eager for instructions
		Phenytoin ordered for patient
		Problems already with lethargy and decreased appetite
planning and outcome criteria	*Goals*	Patient will maintain drug therapy with antiepileptic medications and recommended therapy while at home and before return appointment in 1 month.
	Outcome Criteria	Patient will show compliance to medication regimen as evidenced by the following: • Seizure control while at home • Decreased side effects from taking medication properly • Lack of complications
implementation		Patient and caregiver instructed on the following: • Purchase an ID card or MedicAlert bracelet stating name, diagnosis, drugs being prescribed, phone number, and allergies. • Patient may be drowsy and somewhat sedated when first placed on phenytoin, but will gradually develop a resistance to these adverse effects. • Drug interactions include alcohol, alcohol-containing products (e.g., OTC cough elixirs), and other CNS depressants such as opioids and sedative hypnotic agents. • Caregiver should be aware that this medication must be taken as prescribed and not omitted or discontinued abruptly; weaning is recommended after long-term use should patient need to discontinue medication. • Medication may turn patient's urine pink, red, or brown; this is a normal reaction. • Antacids should not be taken at the same time but need to be spaced within 2-3 hours of taking phenytoin. • Gingival hyperplasia is a side effect, so the patient needs proper and frequent oral hygiene and regularly-scheduled dental appointments. • Nausea and vomiting and constipation may occur with this medication. • Monitor for nausea and vomiting as a side effect of medication; taking medication with meals may be helpful. • If appetite decreases or nausea and vomiting increase, the patient's health care provider should be contacted as soon as possible.
evaluation		Positive therapeutic outcomes include the following: • Decreased-to-no seizure activity • Tolerance to sedating properties • Therapeutic blood levels of medication • No toxicity Patient should be monitored for common side effects of drowsiness, dizziness, hypotension, nausea and vomiting, gingival hyperplasia, and blood dycrasias.

also be checked for any redness or irritation. When administering phenytoin, always check package inserts or drug handbooks for the number of milligrams per seconds or minutes, and do not mix the agent with any other solution because of the attendant risk of precipitate formation. Only normal saline solutions are to be used with phenytoin.

With the advent of fosphenytoin and its use to overcome some of the physical shortcomings of phenytoin sodium, the nurse is required to be aware of its dosing in phenytoin sodium equivalents (PE). For example, 375 mg of fosphenytoin is equivalent to 250 mg of phenytoin sodium; 375 mg of fosphenytoin would be labeled as fosphenytoin 250 mg PE. Fosphenytoin should not be administered at a rate exceeding 150 mg PE/min. Hypotension and cardiovascular collapse may occur with a too rapid IV infusion of fosphenytoin, and hypotension and ventricular fibrillation may occur with a too rapid IV infusion of phenytoin.

Topiramate should be taken whole and not crushed, broken in half, or chewed. It is also very bitter to the taste and seems to be better tolerated with food. Patients taking tiagabine or topiramate will be prone to sedation and should have assistance with ambulation and activities of daily living. Patients taking either of these agents are encouraged to keep a journal of their response to the agent, seizure description, and any side effects. MedicAlert tags or IDs should be carried by patients taking any AED or if they have seizure disorders. These newer medications, as with any AED, should not be discontinued abruptly. Just as with any of the other AEDs, patients should avoid driving or other activities that require alertness until the medication levels become stable. In addition, with tiagabine, patients should increase fiber, bulk, and fluids in their diet to prevent constipation.

Patient teaching tips for anticonvulsant agents are presented in the previous chapter on sedative-hypnotic agents, with additional points for anticonvulsant therapy presented in the box below. Patients must be told that therapy may last several years or may be lifelong. Support groups may be an option for emotional support for the patient and care giver.

● Evaluation

A therapeutic response to AEDs does not mean the patient has been cured of the seizures but only that seizure activity is decreased or absent. Any response to the medication should be documented in the nurses' notes. In addition, when monitoring and evaluating the effects of AEDs, the nurse needs to constantly assess the patient's mental status, mood and mood changes, sensorium, behavioral changes or changes in the level of consciousness, affect, eye problems or visual disorders, sore throat, or fever (blood dyscrasia is a side effect of the hydantoins). The occurrence of vomiting, diplopia, cardiovascular collapse, and Stevens-Johnson syndrome indicates toxicity of the bone marrow, and the physician should be contacted immediately and no further doses administered should these adverse and toxic effects occur.

---

patient teaching tips

Anticonvulsant Therapy

➤ Patients need to fully understand their seizure disorder and the importance of consistent treatment.

➤ Omissions and any problems with dosing should be reported to the physician immediately!

➤ Patients should carry an ID card or wear a Medic-Alert bracelet or necklace at all times naming the diagnosis, the medications they are taking, and any other pertinent facts.

➤ Patients should avoid driving or engaging in other activities that require alertness when taking any anticonvulsants.

➤ Patients should be encouraged to keep a log or journal recording all seizure activity.

➤ Do not take with alcohol or with other medications without checking with the patient's health care provider.

POINTS TO REMEMBER

Epilepsy, Seizures, and Convulsions
- These three terms have very different meanings.
- They should not be used interchangeably.
- Epilepsy: disorder of brain manifested as a chronic, recurrent pattern of seizures.
- Seizures: abnormal electrical activity in brain.
- Convulsions: a type of seizure (spasmodic contractions of involuntary muscles).

Classification of Seizures
- Partial: short alterations in consciousness, repetitive unusual movements, psychologic changes, and confusion.
- Generalized: most common in childhood; temporary lapses in consciousness (seconds); rhythmic movement

of eyes, head, or hands; does not convulse; and may have several a day.

Status Epilepticus
- Common seizure disorder, life-threatening emergency.
- Characterized by tonic-clonic convulsions.
- Brain damage and death: quick, if not treated.

AEDs
- AEDs include carbamazepine, ethosuximide, phenobarbital, primidone, phenytoin, or valproic acid
- Second-line drugs include clonazepam, clorazepate, methsuximide, and acetazolamide.
- Newer AEDs include gababentin (Neurontin), lamotrigine (Lamictal) and felbamate (Felbamate).

Nursing Considerations

- Nurse must distinguish between focal, primary, secondary, status, tonic-clonic, grand mal, and petit mal seizures.

- Documentation of any seizure activity and the specific characteristics of the movements in the patient is important to a diagnosis and to adequate treatment.
- Noncompliance is the most notable factor leading to treatment failure.

REVIEW QUESTIONS

1. One of your patients with a long history of a seizure disorder is scheduled for surgery at 11:00 AM. He has been taking oral forms of phentyoin (Dilantin) for 6 years and is now NPO preoperatively. What is one of your major concerns for this patient?
   a. Administer IV push Dilantin.
   b. Complete your preoperative instructions, and then contact the physician.
   c. The oral Dilantin should be administered regardless of NPO status to ensure blood levels.
   d. Check with the physician and inquire about another dosage form of Dilantin to give the patient.

2. If a female patient who is planning a pregnancy has been taking Dilantin for her AED therapy, which of the following concerns would dictate that the drug should be changed to another agent? The drug:
   a. Has teratogenic effects.
   b. Often results in preeclampsia.
   c. May cause maternal tachycardia.
   d. Increases fetal weight significantly.

3. What would you expect in a patient with a phenytoin (Dilantin) level of 35 μg/ml?
   a. Ataxia
   b. Polyuria
   c. Seizures
   d. Hypertension

4. Which of the following is the most appropriate and effective method of giving an AED?
   a. Administer every 8 hours.
   b. Give one dose IV followed by oral doses every 2 hours.
   c. Maintain a drug regimen based on the half-life of the AED.
   d. Make sure that oral, IM, and IV routes of any AED are alternated during the first few weeks of therapy.

5. During the assessment of your patient with a history of epilepsy, which of the following questions would be most important to pose to the patient about his or her disease and its treatment?
   a. "Do you take the capsule or tablet form?"
   b. "Do your seizures interfere with your appetite?"
   c. "Do you have severe migraines with the seizure?"
   d. "Do you experience any unusual sensations or perceptions before the seizure occurs?"

For Answers see www.harcourthealth.com/MERLIN/Lilley/.

CRITICAL THINKING Activities

1. What specific nursing intervention may help minimize the ataxia and other side effects associated with the rapid absorption of some of the AEDs such as ethychlorvynol?
2. Why is it critical to effective treatment to assess patients in gathering data to help determine the most appropriate AED?
3. Why is it so important to be aware of concurrent medication administration, including OTC agents, with patients taking AEDs?

4. What would the difference be between an allergic reaction and a toxic reaction in a patient taking phenytoin? What is the appropriate nursing action you should take if either of these occur in your patient?
5. M.M. is a 21-year-old woman who was brought to the emergency room in status epilepticus. The physician has decided to treat the woman with intravenous diazepam and phenytoin. He asks you to give a loading dose of 1.5 g at a rate of 50 mg/min. What rate should you set the pump for (in milliliters per hour)?

For Answers see www.harcourthealth.com/MERLIN/Lilley/.

bibliography

Abramowicz M: Cerivastatin for hypercholesterolemia, *The Medical Letter on Drugs and Therapeutics* 40 (1018):13, 1998.

Albanese J, Nutz P: *Mosby's 2001 nursing drug reference and review cards*, St Louis, 2001, Mobsy.

American Hospital Formulary Service: *AHFS drug information*, Bethesda, Md, 2000, American Society of Health-System Pharmacists.

Anderson PO, Knoben JE, Troutman WG: *Handbook of clinical drug data 1999-2000*, ed 9, New York, 1999, McGraw-Hill.

Cohen MR: New antiseizure medication: tricky dosage method, *Nursing 97* 27(2):14, 1997.

Johns Hopkins Hospital, Department of Pediatrics et al: *The Harriet Lane handbook*, ed 15, St Louis, 2000, Mosby.

Joint National Committee on Detection, Evaluation and Treatment of High Blood Pressure: The Sixth Report of the Joint National Committee on . . . *Arch Intern Med* 157(21), 2413, 1997.

Keen JH: *Critical care and emergency drug reference,* ed 3, St Louis, 1996, Mosby.

McLean MJ: Clinical pharmacokinetics of gabapentin, *Neurology* 44[suppl 5]:S17, 1994.

Medical Letter: tiagabine for epilepsy 40(1024), April 10, 1998.

Medical Letter: topiramode for epilepsy 39(1001):S1, 1997.

Mosby's GenRx: a comprehensive reference for generic and brand drugs, ed 10, St Louis, 2000, Mosby.

Ramsay RE: Clinical efficacy and safety of gabapentin, *Neurology* 44[suppl 5]:S23, 1994.

Skidmore-Roth L: *Mosby's 2001 nursing drug reference,* St Louis, 2001, Mosby.

St. Dennis D, Synoground G: Anticonvulsant medications: new drug update, *J Sch Nurs* 13(1);22, 1997.

Taylor CP: Emerging perspectives on the mechanism of action of gabapentin, *Neurology* 44[suppl 5]:S31, 1994.

United States Pharmacopeia: *USPDI: drug information for the health care provider,* Rockville, Md, 2000, the Author.

Remember to check the **Online Worksheet** for additional learning opportunities: **www.harcourthealth.com/MERLIN/Lilley/**

Activity

Chapter 13

Antiparkinsonian Agents

www.harcourthealth.com/MERLIN/Lilley/

objectives

When you reach the end of this chapter, you should be able to do the following:

1 Identify the different classes of medications used as antiparkinsonian agents.

2 Discuss the mechanisms of action, dosages, indications, contraindications, cautions, side effects, and toxic effects associated with the use of each antiparkinsonian agent.

3 Develop a nursing care plan that includes all phases of the nursing process related to the administration of antiparkinsonian agents.

4 Develop a thorough nursing care plan for the newer catechol-o-methyltransferase (COMT) inhibitors and dopamine agents that includes patient teaching guidelines for the caregiver.

Look for this symbol for topics covered in the **Online Worksheet**

drug profiles

amantadine, p. 195

benztropine mesylate, p. 198

bromocriptine and pergolide, p. 196

entacapone, p. 197

levodopa, p. 194

○━ levodopa-carbidopa, p. 195

ropinirole, p. 196

selegiline, p. 192

trihexyphenidyl, p. 198

○━ Key drug.

glossary

Akinesia (a ki ne′ zhə) Motor and psychic hypoactivity or muscular paralysis. (p. 193)

Chorea (kor e′ ə) A condition characterized by involuntary, purposeless, rapid motions such as flexing and extending the fingers, raising and lowering the shoulders, or grimacing. In some forms the person is also irritable, emotionally unstable, weak, restless, and fretful. (p. 191)

Dyskinesia (dis ki ne′ zhə) An impaired ability to execute voluntary movements. Tardive dyskinesia is one type and is caused by prolonged use of phenothiazine medications in elderly patients or by brain injury. (p. 191)

Dystonia (dis to′ ne ə) Any impairment of muscle tone. The condition commonly involves the head, neck, and tongue and often occurs as an adverse effect of a medication. (p. 191)

Parkinson's disease (pahr′ kin sənz) A slowly progressive, degenerative neurologic disorder characterized by resting tremor, pill-rolling of the fingers, a masklike facies, shuffling gait, forward flexion of the trunk, loss of postural reflexes, and muscle rigidity and weakness. It is usually an idiopathic (of no known cause) disease in people over 60 years of age, although it may occur in younger people, especially after acute encephalitis or carbon monoxide or metallic poisoning. (p. 189)

Presynaptic drugs Drugs that exert their antiparkinson effects before the nerve synapse. (p. 193)

Replacement drugs Drugs that attempt to replace the deficiency of dopamine at the nerve ending. (p. 193)

PARKINSON'S DISEASE

Parkinson's disease (PD) is a chronic, progressive, degenerative disorder affecting the dopamine-producing neurons in the brain. Other chronic central nervous system (CNS) neuromuscular disorders are myasthenia gravis, dementia, and Alzheimer's disease. PD was initially recognized in 1817, at which time it was called "shaking palsy." The symptoms of both the early and advanced stages of the disease along with the treatment options were first described by James Parkinson. It was not until the 1960s, however, that the underlying pathologic defect was discovered. It was postulated then that a dopamine deficit in the area of the brain called the *substantia nigra* was the cause of the disorder.

PD afflicts nearly 1 million Americans. It is primarily a disease of the elderly, rarely developing in people under 40 years of age. However, the number of patients with PD will only continue to increase as our aged population grows. There is a 2% chance of PD developing in a person during his or her lifetime. In most patients the disease becomes apparent between 45 and 65 years of age, with the mean age at onset being 56 years. Men and women are equally affected. Family history does not seem to be a contributing factor. PD is also a prominent cause of disability because of the frequent accompanying motor complications.

The primary cause of PD is an imbalance in two neurotransmitters—dopamine and acetylcholine—in the area

189

of the brain called the *basal ganglia*. This imbalance is caused by failure of the nerve terminals in the substantia nigra to produce the essential neurotransmitter dopamine. This neurotransmitter acts in the basal ganglia to control movements. Destruction of the substantia nigra leads to dopamine depletion. Dopamine is an inhibitory neurotransmitter, and acetylcholine (ACh) is an excitatory neurotransmitter in this area of the brain. A correct balance between these two neurotransmitters is needed for the proper regulation of posture, muscle tone, and voluntary movement. Patients who suffer from PD have an imbalance in these neurotransmitters. Figure 13-1 illustrates the difference in neurotransmitter concentrations in normal people and in patients with PD.

A significant advance in our understanding of the etiology and pathogenesis of PD came in 1983 when the potent neurotoxin 1-methyl-4-phenyl-1,2,3,6-tetrahydropyridine (MPTP) and its metabolic breakdown product 1-methyl-4-phenylpyridine (MPP) were discovered. This illegal substance has been produced in home laboratories and used for recreational purposes. MPTP and MPP selectively destroy the substantia nigra, or that area of the brain that is dysfunctional in PD. It has been shown that a parkinsonian syndrome almost identical to idiopathic PD develops in laboratory animals injected with this neurotoxin. Others theorize that PD is the result of an earlier head injury or of excess iron in the substantia nigra, which undergoes oxidation and causes the generation of toxic free radicals. In still another theory, it is thought that because dopamine levels decrease with age, PD represents a premature aging of the nigrostriatal cells resulting from environmental or intrinsic biochemical factors, or both.

There are no readily available laboratory tests that can detect or confirm PD. Results of computerized tomography (CT), magnetic resonance imaging (MRI), cerebrospinal fluid analysis, and electroencephalography are usually normal and of little diagnostic value. These may be useful tools for ruling out other possible diseases as causes of the symptoms. Therefore the diagnosis of PD is usually made on the basis of the classic symptoms and physical findings. The classic symptoms of PD are listed in Table 13-1.

Symptoms of PD do not appear until approximately 80% of the dopamine store in the substantia nigra of the basal ganglia has been depleted. This means that by the time PD is diagnosed, only approximately 20% or less of the patient's original nigral dopaminergic terminals are functioning normally.

Nerve terminals can take up substances, store them, and release them for use when needed. It is this factor that forms the basis for antiparkinsonian treatment. As long as there are functioning nerve terminals that can take up dopamine, the symptoms of PD can be at least partially controlled. However, the blood-brain barrier does not allow exogenously supplied dopamine to enter the brain. It does, nevertheless, allow levodopa, a naturally occurring dopamine precursor, to do so. After levodopa has been taken up by the dopaminergic terminal, it is converted into dopamine and then released as

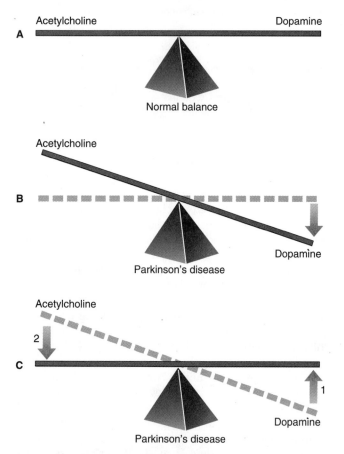

A, Normal balance of acetylcholine and dopamine in the CNS.
B, In Parkinson's disease, a decrease in dopamine results in an imbalance.
C, Drug therapy in Parkinson's disease is aimed at correcting the imbalance between acetylcholine and dopamine. This can be accomplished by either
  1. increasing the supply of dopamine or
  2. blocking or lowering acetylcholine levels.

Fig. 13-1 The neurotransmitter abnormality of Parkinson's disease.

	Classic Parkinsonian Symptoms
13-1	
Symptom	**Description**
Bradykinesia	Slowness of movement
Rigidity	"Cogwheel" rigidity, resistance to passive movement
Tremor	Pill-rolling: tremor of the thumb against the forefinger, seen mostly at rest, is less severe during voluntary activity; starts usually on one side then progresses to the other; is the presenting sign in 70% of the cases
Postural instability	Danger of falling, hesitation in gait as patient starts or stops walking

needed. Levodopa therapy can thus correct the neurotransmitter imbalance in patients with early PD who still have functioning nerve terminals.

Unfortunately, PD is a progressive condition. With time the number of surviving dopaminergic terminals that can take up exogenously administered levodopa and convert it into dopamine decrease. Rapid swings in the response to levodopa (known as the on-off phenomenon) also occur.

The result is worsening PD when too little dopamine is present or dyskinesias when too much is present. **Dyskinesias** is the difficulty in performing voluntary movements that some patients with PD have. The two most commonly associated with antiparkinsonian therapy are **chorea** (irregular, spasmodic, involuntary movements of the limbs or facial muscles) and **dystonia** (abnormal muscle tone in any tissue).

The first step in the treatment of PD is a full explanation of the disease to the patient and his or her family. Physical therapy and speech therapy are almost always needed when the patient is in the later stages of the disease. As previously discussed, drug therapy is aimed at increasing the levels of dopamine as long as there are functioning nerve terminals. It is also aimed at antagonizing or blocking the effects of ACh and slowing the progression of the disease. The agents available for the treatment of PD and their respective categories are listed in Table 13-2.

See the Geriatric Considerations box for antiparkinsonian agents.

NEUROPROTECTIVE THERAPY

In recent years there has been an increasing focus on developing treatment strategies to slow the progression of PD. Selegiline (Eldepryl), a very potent, irreversible monoamine oxidase B (MAO-B) inhibitor derived from amphetamine, has been one means of accomplishing this end.

As early as 1965, nonselective monoamine oxidase inhibitors (MAOIs) were being used to improve the therapeutic effect of levodopa in patients with PD. However, a major adverse effect of MAOIs has been that they interact with tyramine-containing foods (cheese, red wine, beer, and yogurt). This has been termed the *cheese effect,* and the result is severe hypertension. This has considerably restricted the therapeutic use of MAOIs. In 1974 selegiline

was introduced as an investigational option for PD. As an MAO-B inhibitor, selegiline does not elicit the classic cheese effect at doses of 10 mg or less a day. In the years that followed, many investigational studies were conducted, and in October 1989, selegiline received approval by the Food and Drug Administration (FDA) for use in conjunction with levodopa therapy in the treatment of PD. Since then, several small studies and one large study have shown the drug to have a neuroprotective effect. New studies suggest that high doses of the antioxidants vitamin E and vitamin C may be helpful in slowing the progression of PD. A pilot study combining tocopherol (vitamin E) at 3200 IU/day and ascorbate (vitamin C) at 3000 mg/day is showing some promise and may be helpful in treating early PD.

Mechanism of Action

MAO is one of the two major pathways by which dopamine is degraded. Type B accounts for about 70% of all MAO activity in the brain. One of the current theories advanced to explain the etiology of PD is that the neurotoxicity that causes the destruction of the cells of the substantia nigra is accomplished by MPP, the enzymatically active toxin of MPTP. This enzymatic conversion to MPP is accomplished by MAO-B. By blocking this enzyme with the MAO-B inhibitor selegiline, MPP is prevented from being produced and the substantia nigra is spared. Figure 13-2 illustrates this enzymatic inhibition process.

Table 13-2 Antiparkinsonian Agents

Drug Category	Agents
Anticholinergic agents	benztropine, biperiden, diphenhydramine, ethopropazine, procyclidine, trihexyphenidyl
Dopaminergic agents	amantadine, bromocriptine, levodopa, levodopa-carbidopa, pergolide, pramipexole, ropinirole
Neuroprotective agents	selegiline

geriatric considerations

Antiparkinsonian Agents

- Elderly patients taking anticholinergics often used for PD are at risk for the development of health problems associated with the side effects of these medications, such as dry mouth, constipation, impaired thought processes, and urinary retention—especially in men with benign prostatic hypertrophy.
- Anticholinergics are contraindicated in patients with narrow-angle glaucoma or with a history of urinary retention.
- Some aged patients taking anticholinergic agents experience paradoxical reactions, such as excitement, confusion, or irritability.
- Overheating is a problem in patients taking anticholinergics, so the aged should especially avoid excessive exercise during the warm weather and avoid excessive heat exposure.
- Levodopa should be used cautiously, with close monitoring of the aged, especially if there is a history of cardiac, renal, hepatic, endocrine, pulmonary, ulcer, or psychiatric disease.
- The elderly patient taking levodopa is at an increased risk for suffering side effects, especially confusion.
- Levodopa-carbidopa is often started at a low dose because of the increased sensitivity of the aged patient to these medications.

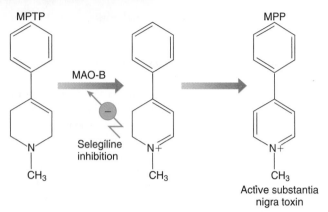

Fig. 13-2 Mechanism of action of selegiline. *MAO-B,* Monoamine oxidase type B; *MPP,* 1-methyl-4 phenylpyridine; *MPTP,* 1-methyl-4-phenyl-1,2,3,6-tetrahydropyridine.

Drug Effects

MAOs are widely distributed throughout the body. The areas where concentrations are high are the liver, kidney, stomach, intestinal wall, and brain. There are two subclasses of MAOs: A and B. Most of MAO-B is in the CNS, primarily in the brain. The primary role of MAOs is the catabolism or breakdown of catecholamines such as dopamine, norepinephrine, and epinephrine, as well as the breakdown of serotonin. Therefore an MAO-B inhibitor like selegiline would cause an increase in the levels of catecholamines and serotonin in the CNS. This can be broadly regarded as stimulation of the sympathetic nervous system (SNS).

Therapeutic Uses

Selegiline is currently approved for use in combination with levodopa or levodopa-carbidopa. It is an adjunctive agent used when a patient's response to levodopa is fluctuating. It allows the dose of levodopa to be decreased. Improvement in functional ability and decreased severity of symptoms are common after selegiline is added. However, only approximately 50% to 60% of patients show a positive response.

Selegiline may be somewhat beneficial as a prophylactic agent. Selegiline administration before exposure to the neurotoxin MPTP has been shown to prevent the onset of a PD-like syndrome in laboratory animals, indicating a possible neuroprotective effect. Several studies have shown that selegiline-treated patients required levodopa therapy approximately 1.8 times later than control patients. One problem that patients with PD experience is that as their disease progresses it becomes more and more difficult to control it with levodopa. Ultimately levodopa no longer controls the PD, and the patient is seriously debilitated. This generally occurs between 5 and 10 years after the start of levodopa therapy. Prophylactic selegiline use may delay the development of serious debilitating PD for 9 to 18 years. Because the average age of patients at the onset of PD is between 55 and 65 years, such a delay would mean most patients will die before the functional disability occurs.

Side Effects and Adverse Effects

The most common adverse effects associated with selegiline use are mild and consist of nausea, lightheadedness,

Selegiline: Adverse Effects

Body System	Side/Adverse Effect
Cardiovascular	Hypotension, dysrhythmia, tachycardia, palpitations, angina, edema
Central nervous system	Altered sensation, pain, dizziness, drowsiness, irritability, anxiety, extrapyramidal side effects
Gastrointestinal	Nausea, vomiting, constipation, diarrhea, anorexia
Respiratory	Asthma, shortness of breath

dizziness, abdominal pain, insomnia, confusion, and dry mouth. The adverse effects seen with selegiline use as they relate to the various body systems are listed in Table 13-3. Reactions seen when the dosage exceeds 10 mg/day include a hypertensive crisis upon the consumption of tyramine-containing food, memory loss, muscular twitches and jerks, and grinding of the teeth.

Interactions

The number of drugs with which selegiline interacts is relatively small, and the degree of interaction is dose dependent. At recommended doses of 10 mg/day, the drug maintains its selective MAO-B inhibition. However, at doses that exceed 10 mg/day, selegiline becomes a nonselective MAOI, contributing to the development of the cheese effect. Meperidine is contraindicated in patients receiving nonselective MAOIs because this has been associated with the occurrence of fatal hypertensive episodes. It is suggested that meperidine as well as other opioids be avoided in patients taking more than 10 mg/day of selegiline.

Dosage

For the recommended dosage of selegiline see the table on p. 193.

drug profiles

selegiline

Selegiline (Eldepryl) is an MAO-B inhibitor used as an adjunctive agent along with levodopa to decrease the amount of levodopa needed. It has also been shown to exert a neuroprotective effect when started early in therapy. It is a prescription-only drug that is available only in an oral form as a 5-mg tablet and a 5-mg capsule. It is classified as a pregnancy category C agent. Selegiline has three active metabolites whose half-lives are listed in the pharmacokinetics table. The recommended dosage for selegiline is given in the dosages table on p. 193.

PHARMACOKINETICS

HALF-LIFE*	ONSET	PEAK	DURATION
2 hr	1 hr	0.5-2 hr	1-3 days

*Selegiline has three active metabolites with long half-lives of 18-21 hours.

agent	pharmacologic class	dosage range	purpose
selegiline (Eldepryl)	Indirect dopaminergic agent/MAOI	*Adult* PO: 5 mg bid with breakfast and lunch in combination with levodopa-carbidopa	Parkinson's disease

MAOI, Monoamine oxidase inhibitor.

DOPAMINERGIC THERAPY

Because in PD little or no dopamine is produced, ACh is left as the predominant neurotransmitter. Dopaminergic agents are used to help replace the lost dopamine or enhance the function of the few neurons that are left to produce their own. Dopaminergic agents can be broken down into three categories based on their underlying mechanisms of action: those that release dopamine (indirect acting), those that increase brain levels of dopamine (replacement), and dopaminergic agonists (direct acting). The ultimate goal is to increase the levels of dopamine in the brain. By doing so and creating a balance with ACh, akinesias, the most detrimental complications of PD, can be reversed. **Akinesias** are symptoms such as a masklike facial expression and impaired postural reflexes. They eventually render the patient unable to care for himself or herself.

Mechanism of Action

Levodopa and the combination product levodopa-carbidopa *directly replace* the deficient neurotransmitter dopamine in the substantia nigra. They are considered the cornerstone of the treatment of PD. Levodopa is the biologic precursor of dopamine required by the brain for dopamine synthesis. These drugs are also referred to as **presynaptic drugs** or **replacement drugs.** This is because they work presynaptically and attempt to increase brain levels of dopamine. Dopamine must be administered in this form because, as mentioned previously, exogenously administered dopamine cannot pass through the blood-brain barrier, whereas levodopa can. Once it does, it is converted directly into dopamine. Traditionally, very large doses of levodopa had to be administered to get enough dopamine to the brain because much of the levodopa administered was broken down outside the CNS by the enzyme dopa decarboxylase. These large doses resulted in high peripheral levels of dopamine and many unwanted side effects such as confusion, involuntary movements, gastrointestinal distress, and hypotension. These problems are avoided when levodopa is given with carbidopa, a peripheral decarboxylase inhibitor that does not cross the blood-brain barrier. Therefore carbidopa prevents levodopa breakdown in the periphery, allowing the levodopa to reach and cross the blood-brain barrier without crossing it itself. Once in the brain, the levodopa is then broken down to dopamine, which can be used directly.

Originally developed and used for the prophylaxis and treatment of viral disorders, amantadine (Symmetrel) has proved to be a valuable adjunct to the traditional antiparkinsonian drugs. Amantadine appears to exert its antiparkinsonian effect by causing the release of dopamine and other catecholamines from their storage sites in the ends of nerves. Amantadine also blocks the reuptake of dopamine into the nerve endings, which allows more dopamine to accumulate both centrally and peripherally. Therefore amantadine's dopaminergic effects are the result of its *indirect actions* on the nerve. Amantadine also has some anticholinergic properties. This may further help with dyskinesias.

Bromocriptine (Parlodel) and pergolide (Permax) are dopaminergic agonists that directly stimulate the dopamine receptors. Chemically, bromocriptine is an ergot alkaloid similar to ergotamine in its chemical structure. Its antiparkinsonian effects are due to its ability to activate dopamine receptors and stimulate the production of more dopamine. This helps correct the imbalance between ACh and dopamine in the CNS. Pergolide, on the other hand, has no effect on dopamine synthesis or dopamine storage sites. It stimulates dopamine receptors in the substantia nigra of the brain, the area believed to be defective in patients with PD. Bromocriptine is a D_2 dopamine agonist, whereas pergolide stimulates D_{1-3} receptors. Another difference between these two postsynaptic drugs is that pergolide is 20 times more potent than bromocriptine and has a half-life that is 3 times longer than that of bromocriptine. Pramipexole (Mirapex) and ropinirole (ReQuip) are two new highly specific D_{2-3} dopamine agonists released in 1997. They are both effective in early and late stages of PD. Two other dopamine agonists are cabergoline and apomorphine. Cabergoline is a D_2 receptor agonist, and apomorphine is an injectable dopamine agonist. Neither is currently available.

Tolcapone (Tasmar) and entacapone (Comtan) are two agents that belong to a totally new class of antiparkinsonian agents. They belong to a class of drugs referred to as catechol-O-methyltransferase (COMT) inhibitors. COMT inhibitors help patients with PD by inhibiting COMT, the enzyme responsible for the breakdown of levodopa. Tolcapone differs slightly from entacapone in that it may act centrally and peripherally. Entacapone cannot cross the blood-brain barrier and therefore only can work peripherally. The main positive effect of these drugs is that they prolong the duration of levodopa benefit. Patients have less "wearing off" and experience prolonged benefits. Along with amantadine, COMT inhibitors are also considered to be indirect acting agents and work as presynaptic agents.

Drug Effects

When broken down in the periphery by dopa decarboxylase, levodopa becomes dopamine. When in the periphery, this dopamine causes involuntary movements, gastrointestinal distress, and orthostatic hypotension. It has even been known to cause dysrhythmias. When levodopa is given with carbidopa, the enzyme inhibitor, much more levodopa then enters the brain, where it can offset the imbalance between dopamine and ACh.

Therapeutic Uses

The therapeutic effects of the replacement drugs levodopa and levodopa-carbidopa are identical. The only difference is that, as already explained, the combination product is more efficient in increasing the dopamine level in the brain.

The therapeutic effects of the indirect-acting dopaminergic agent amantadine are its antidyskinetic effects (its ability to promote voluntary movements) and its antiviral properties (both the prevention and treatment). The direct-acting dopaminergic agents bromocriptine and pergolide also have antidyskinetic effects. In addition they can inhibit lactation, suppress growth hormone production, and inhibit prolactin production. This is because dopamine plays an important role in the regulation of hypothalamic-pituitary function. Dopamine has a direct effect on the adenohypophysis, which is responsible for secretion of growth hormone, prolactin, and other hormones.

Side Effects and Adverse Effects

There are many potential side effects and adverse effects associated with the dopaminergic agents. The most common of these are listed in Table 13-4.

Interactions

The drug interactions involving dopaminergic drugs can cause significant adverse reactions, including a decrease in the efficacy of the dopaminergic drug, a hypertensive crisis, and reversal of the dopaminergic drug's effect. Hydantoins, when given with levodopa, increase the metabolism of levodopa decreasing its effects. Haloperidol or phenothiazines block dopamine receptors in the brain and also result in decreased levodopa effects. MAOIs taken concomitantly with dopaminergic drugs can result in inhibited metabolism, leading to a possible hypertensive crisis. Pyridoxine (vitamin B_6) promotes levodopa breakdown and will reverse levodopa effects. Carbidopa may help prevent this.

Dosages

For the recommended dosages of the dopaminergic agents, see the table on p. 195.

drug profiles

levodopa

As described earlier, the treatment of PD centers around attempts to replace the dopamine deficiency. However, dopamine does not cross the blood-brain barrier, whereas levodopa, a precursor of dopamine, does. However, because levodopa is also converted into dopamine in the rest of the body, the resulting high levels throughout the body cause many unwanted side effects.

Levodopa is a prescription-only drug that is classified as a pregnancy category C medication. It is

Table 13-4 Dopaminergic Agents: Adverse Effects

Body System	Side/Adverse Effects
AMANTADINE	
Central nervous system	Impaired concentration, dizziness, increased irritability, nervousness, blurred vision
Gastrointestinal	Anorexia, nausea, constipation, vomiting
Other	Purple-red skin spots; dryness of mouth, nose, and throat; increased weakness
ENTACAPONE	
Central nervous system	Involuntary movements (dyskinesias)
Gastrointestinal	Nausea, abdominal pain, diarrhea, decreased appetite
Other	Urine discoloration
LEVODOPA AND CARBIDOPA	
Blood	Hemolytic anemia, agranulocytosis
Cardiovascular	Palpitations, orthostatic hypotension
Central nervous system	Agitation; anxiety; psychotic and suicidal episodes; choreiform, dystonic, and other involuntary movements; headache and blurred vision
ROPINIROLE	
Cardiovascular	Syncope sometimes associated with bradycardia, symptomatic orthostatic hypotension
Central nervous system	Hallucinations, somnolence, uncontrolled movement of body, face, tongue, arms, hands, and head
Gastrointestinal	Nausea

contraindicated in patients who have shown a hypersensitivity reaction to it, those with narrow-angle glaucoma or a history of melanoma, and those concurrently taking MAOIs. Levodopa is only available in an oral form as 100-, 250-, and 500-mg capsules and tablets. Recommended dosages are given in the table below.

PHARMACOKINETICS

HALF-LIFE	ONSET	PEAK	DURATION
1-3 hr	2-3 wk*	1-3 hr	<5 hr

*Therapeutic effect.

⊶levodopa-carbidopa

With the addition of the peripheral decarboxylase inhibitor carbidopa, which does not cross the blood-brain barrier, many of the unwanted side effects caused by peripherally broken down levodopa are prevented because more of the levodopa can reach the site of action without being broken down. As a result, much lower daily doses of levodopa are needed. Levodopa-carbidopa (Sinemet, Sinemet CR) has become the cornerstone in the treatment of PD. It also appears to limit the on-off phenomenon that some patients with PD experience. This phenomenon is seen in patients taking levodopa for a long time. Such patients may experience periods when they have good control ("on" time) and periods when they have bad control or break-through PD ("off" time). A variety of studies has shown that Sinemet CR increases "on" time and decreases "off" time. When converting patients from conventional levodopa-carbidopa preparations, the dosage of Sinemet CR should include 10% to 30% more levodopa per day. The interval between dosages of Sinemet CR should be 4 to 8 hours during the waking day. Sinemet CR should not be crushed.

Levodopa-carbidopa is a prescription-only drug that is classified as a pregnancy category C medication. It is contraindicated in patients who have shown a hypersensitivity reaction to it, those with narrow-angle glaucoma or a history of melanoma, and those concurrently taking MAOIs. This combination agent is only available orally as tablets with the following proportions of levodopa to carbidopa, respectively: 100 mg to 10 mg, 100 mg to 25 mg, and 250 mg to 25 mg. There are also controlled-release formulations of this combination product consisting of 100 mg of levodopa and 25 mg of carbidopa or 200 mg of levodopa and 50 mg of carbidopa. Recommended dosages are given in the table below.

Activity

PHARMACOKINETICS

HALF-LIFE	ONSET	PEAK	DURATION
1-3 hr	2-3 wk*	1-3 hr	<5 hr

*Therapeutic effect.

amantadine

Amantadine (Symmetrel) is believed to work in the CNS by eliciting the release of dopamine from nerve endings, causing higher concentrations of dopamine in the CNS. It is most effective in the earlier stages of PD when there are still significant numbers of nerves to act on and dopamine to be

DOSAGES Selected Dopaminergic Agents

agent	pharmacologic class	dosage range	purpose
amantadine (Symmetrel)	Indirect acting	*Adult* PO: 100-400 mg/day divided q12h	Triggers release of dopamine
bromocriptine (Parlodel)	Direct acting	*Adult* PO: 10-40 mg/day	Dopamine agonist
entacapone (Comtan)	Indirect acting	*Adult* PO: 200 mg with each dose of levodopa, up to 10 times/day	Dopamine agonist
⊶**levodopa-carbidopa (Sinemet)**	Replacement	*Adult* PO: 10/100, 1 tablet 3-8 times/day; 25/100, 1 tablet 3-6 times/day; 25/250, 1 tablet 3-4 times/day CR: 1 tablet bid; up to 2-8 tablets at 4- to 8-hr intervals	Replaces dopamine
pergolide (Permax)	Direct acting	*Adult* PO: up to 5 mg/day in combination with levodopa-carbidopa	Dopamine agonist
ropinirole (ReQuip)	Direct acting	*Adult* PO: 0.25 mg 3 times/day slowly titrating to max dose of 24 mg/day	Dopamine agonist

CR, Controlled release.

released. As the disease progresses, however, the population of functioning nerves diminishes, and so does amantadine's effect. Amantadine is usually effective for only 6 to 12 months. After amantadine fails to relieve the hypokinesia and rigidity, a dopamine agonist such as bromocriptine or pergolide is usually tried next.

Amantadine is considered a pregnancy category C medication and is a prescription-only drug. It is contraindicated in patients who have shown a hypersensitivity reaction to it, women who are lactating, and children younger than 1 year of age (remember that amantadine is also an antiviral agent). Amantadine is only available orally as 100-mg tablets and an oral solution that provides 50 mg per 5 ml of syrup. Recommended dosages are given in the table on p. 195.

Activity

PHARMACOKINETICS

HALF-LIFE	ONSET	PEAK	DURATION
11-15 hr	48 hr	2-4 hr	6-12 wk

DOPAMINE AGONISTS

The traditional role of dopamine agonists (bromocriptine, pergolide, pramipexole, ropinirole, and carbergoline) has been as adjuncts to levodopa for management of motor fluctuations only. Recently the agents were evaluated as initial monotherapy or as combination therapy with low-dose levodopa in an attempt to delay levodopa therapy or reduce total exposure to the drug and associated motor complications. The newer agents pramipexole, ropinirole, and carbergoline are more specific for the receptors associated with parkinsonian symptoms, the D_2 family (D_2, D_3, and D_4). This in turn may have more specific antiparkinsonian effects with fewer adverse effects associated with generalized dopaminergic stimulation. These newer dopamine agonists have a promising role in the early treatment of PD. They appear to delay the start of levodopa therapy. Another benefit is that they have less ergot-like effects and dyskinesias. Both bromocriptine and pergolide are structurally similar to ergot derivatives and have some of their unwanted effects. These newer agents have also shown efficacy in patients with advanced PD.

bromocriptine and pergolide

Once amantadine becomes ineffective, a dopamine agonist like pergolide (Permax) or bromocriptine (Parlodel) may be prescribed in its place. Bromocriptine differs from pergolide in that it only stimulates the dopamine-2 receptors and antagonizes or blocks the dopamine-1 receptors. Pergolide stimulates or acts as an agonist at both types of receptors. Eventually levodopa-carbidopa is needed to control the patient's symptoms, but by using amantadine until it

fails then a dopamine agonist until it fails, the need for levodopa therapy may be postponed for up to 3 years. These two agents may also be given with levodopa-carbidopa so that lower doses of the levodopa are needed. This often results in prolonging the "on" periods, when PD is controlled, and decreasing the "off" periods, when PD is not controlled.

Bromocriptine is only available with a prescription and is categorized as a pregnancy category D medication. It is contraindicated in patients who have shown a hypersensitivity reaction to any of the ergot alkaloids, patients with severe ischemic disease, and those with severe peripheral vascular disease. This is primarily because of bromocriptine's ability to stimulate dopamine receptors. Bromocriptine is only available orally as 5-mg capsules and as 2.5-mg tablets. Recommended dosages are given in the table on p. 195.

PHARMACOKINETICS

HALF-LIFE	ONSET	PEAK	DURATION
3-5 hr	0.5-1.5 hr	1-3 hr	4-8 hr

Pergolide is only available with a prescription and is listed as a pregnancy category B medication. It is contraindicated in patients who have shown a hypersensitivity reaction to it or to other ergot alkaloids. It is available only in an oral form as 0.05-, 0.25-, and 1-mg tablets. Recommended dosages are given in the table on p. 195.

PHARMACOKINETICS

HALF-LIFE	ONSET	PEAK	DURATION
27 hr	15-30 min	1-3 hr	1-2 days

ropinirole

Ropinirole (ReQuip) is a new nonergot dopamine agonist indicated for monotherapy for PD and adjunctive therapy with levodopa. It is highly selective for the D_2 family of dopamine receptors. It is categorized as a pregnancy category C medication. It is contraindicated in patients who have shown a hypersensitivity reaction to it. ReQuip is available as 0.25-, 0.5-, 1-, 2-, and 5-mg tablets. Recommended dosages are given in the table on p. 195.

PHARMACOKINETICS

HALF-LIFE	ONSET	PEAK	DURATION
3-5 hr	30 min	1-2 hr	6-10 hr

COMT INHIBITORS

Inhibition of COMT enzyme is a new strategy for prolonging the duration of action of levodopa. Two compounds were developed for this propose, tolcapone (Tasmar) and entacapone (Comtan). Both drugs are reversible inhibitors of COMT. The major difference between them is that tolcapone has a longer duration of action. COMT inhibitors help patients with PD by inhibiting COMT, the enzyme responsible for the breakdown of levodopa. Tolcapone differs slightly from entacapone in that it may act centrally and peripherally. Entacapone cannot cross the blood-brain barrier and therefore can only work peripherally. The main positive effect of these drugs is that they prolong the duration of levodopa benefit. Patients have less "wearing off" and experience prolonged benefits. Along with amantadine the COMT inhibitors are also considered to be indirect acting agents and work presynaptic agents.

entacapone

Entacapone (Comtan) is a new potent COMT inhibitor indicated for the adjunctive treatment of PD. The most recent safety information indicates that entacapone does not appear to be hepatotoxic. Hepatotoxicity was a problem with tolcapone, and no liver tests are required for patients taking entacapone. Entacapone is taken with levodopa and should be effective from the first dose. A patient with PD can feel the benefit of entacapone within a day or two. Entacapone is particularly effective in patients who are experiencing "wearing off" fluctuations. Entacapone, used with levodopa, can reduce the daily "off" and increase the daily "on" time. The levodopa dose and dosing frequency can also be reduced in many cases. It is available in the form of 200-mg film-coated tablets. It is contraindicated in patients who have shown a hypersensitivity reaction to it. Recommended dosages are given in the table on p. 195.

PHARMACOKINETICS

HALF-LIFE	ONSET	PEAK	DURATION
1.5-3.5 hr	1 hr	0.5-1.5 hr	6 hr

ANTICHOLINERGIC THERAPY

Anticholinergics, or drugs that block the effects of ACh, are sometimes useful in treating the muscle tremors and muscle rigidity associated with PD. These two symptoms are caused by excessive cholinergic activity. Anticholinergics do little, however, to relieve the bradykinesia (extremely slow movements) associated with PD. The rationale for the use of anticholinergics is to reduce excessive cholinergic activity in the brain. The first agents in this category to be used were the belladonna alkaloids, atropine and scopolamine. However, because the anticholinergic side effects—dry mouth, urinary retention, blurred vision—can be excessive, new synthetic anticholinergics and antihistamines with better side effect profiles (agents such as benztropine and trihexyphenidyl) were developed.

Mechanism of Action

All anticholinergics work in some way to block ACh (central cholinergic excitatory pathways). Because of the reduced number of dopamine-producing nerves, the ACh-producing nerves are left unchecked and ACh accumulates. This causes an overstimulation of the cholinergic excitatory pathways, resulting in muscle tremors and muscle rigidity. This is sometimes described as *cogwheel rigidity.* The muscle tremors are usually worse while the patient is at rest and consist of a pill-rolling movement and bobbing of the head.

Drug Effects

Anticholinergic drugs have either the opposite effect or oppose the effects of the neurotransmitter ACh, which is responsible for causing increased *s*alivation, *l*acrimation (tearing of the eyes), and *u*rination, as well as *d*iarrhea, increased *g*astrointestinal motility, and possibly *e*mesis (vomiting). The acronym SLUDGE is often used to describe these cholinergic-induced effects. With these in mind, effects of anticholinergics would be the opposite of the SLUDGE symptoms, effects such as antisecretory effects (dry mouth or decreased salivation), urinary retention, decreased gastrointestinal motility (constipation), dilated pupils (mydriasis), and smooth muscle relaxation.

Therapeutic Uses

Anticholinergic agents decrease salivation and relax smooth muscles. They readily cross the blood-brain barrier and therefore can get right to the site of the imbalance in the CNS—the substantia nigra. It is because of their ability to directly relax smooth muscles that the muscle rigidity and akinesia (little or no movement) are reduced. Besides their use as antidyskinetic agents in PD, anticholinergics are also used for the treatment of drug-induced extrapyramidal reactions such as those related to selected antipsychotic agents.

Side Effects and Adverse Effects

The side effects and adverse effects associated with anticholinergic drug use are many, and the most common ones are listed in Table 13-5. They often occur more frequently when the agents are given in high doses. Anticholinergic-induced adverse effects are also more common in the elderly. However, wise and judicious use of such drugs can lead to very effective treatment free of the unwanted side effects.

Table 13-5   Anticholinergic Adverse Effects

Body System	Side/Adverse Effect
Central nervous system	Drowsiness, confusion, disorientation, hallucinations
Gastrointestinal	Constipation, nausea, vomiting
Genitourinary	Urinary retention, pain on urination
Other	Blurred vision, dilated pupils (mydriasis), photophobia, dry skin

Interactions

The interactions that occur between anticholinergic drugs and other drugs and drug classes can be very damaging. Alcohol, CNS depressants, amantadine, phenothiazines, tricyclic antidepressants, and antihistamines can have an additive effect with anticholinergic drugs, resulting in enhanced CNS depressant effects. Antacids, when taken with anticholinergic drugs, alter gastric pH and reduce the absorption and decrease the therapeutic effects of anticholinergic drugs.

Dosages

For information on the dosages of benztropine and trihexyphenidyl in the treatment of PD, see the dosages table below.

drug profiles

Anticholinergics are helpful in alleviating the muscle tremors and rigidity seen in patients with PD. They are not, however, as effective as the other drug classes used in the treatment of PD in correcting the underlying problem. They are very effective for the relief of only minimal symptoms and for the treatment of those patients who cannot tolerate or do not respond to dopamine replacement drugs such as levodopa or the dopaminergics such as amantadine and bromocriptine. Anticholinergics are also useful as adjuncts to these primary drugs. Treatment is usually started with small doses, which are gradually increased until the benefits or side effects appear. Some of the more commonly used agents are trihexyphenidyl (Artane), ethopropazine (Parsidol), diphenhydramine (Benadryl), and benztropine mesylate (Cogentin). They must be used cautiously in the elderly because significant side effects such as confusion, urinary retention, visual blurring, palpitations, and increased intraocular pressure can develop. The most commonly used agents are the synthetic anticholinergics, which are associated with fewer of the side effects commonly seen with the belladonna alkaloid derivatives such as atropine and scopolamine.

benztropine mesylate

Benztropine (Cogentin) is a synthetic anticholinergic agent that resembles both atropine and diphenhydramine (Benadryl) in its chemical structure. Biperiden (Akineton) is also a synthetic anticholinergic agent used in the treatment of PD. They both have anticholinergic, antihistaminic, and local anesthetic properties and are primarily used as adjuncts in the treatment of all forms of PD. They are also useful in the treatment of phenothiazine-induced extrapyramidal reactions. Benztropine is only available with a prescription and comes in an oral form as 0.5-, 1-, and 2-mg tablets and as an IV injection delivering 1 mg/ml. It is rated as a pregnancy category C agent. Its use is contraindicated in patients who have shown a hypersensitivity reaction to it; in those who have narrow-angle glaucoma, myasthenia gravis, urinary retention, a history of peptic ulcer disease, megacolon, or prostate hypertrophy; and in children under 3 years of age. Recommended dosages are given in the dosages table below.

PHARMACOKINETICS

HALF-LIFE	ONSET	PEAK	DURATION
4-8 hr	1 hr	2-4 hr	6-10 hr

trihexyphenidyl

Trihexyphenidyl (Artane) is a synthetic anticholinergic that is used as an adjunctive agent in the treatment of PD. It has weak peripheral anticholinergic effects. It is contraindicated in patients who have shown a hypersensitivity reaction to it and in patients with any of the conditions listed as contraindications to benztropine treatment. It is also considered a pregnancy category C agent. Trihexyphenidyl is only available in oral forms as a 5-mg extended-release capsule, a 2-mg/5 ml elixir, and a 2- and 5-mg tablet. Recommended dosages are given in the dosages table below.

PHARMACOKINETICS

HALF-LIFE	ONSET	PEAK	DURATION
3-4 hr	<1 hr	2-3 hr	6-12 hr

DOSAGES Selected Anticholinergic Agents

agent	pharmacologic class	dosage range	purpose
benztropine (Cogentin)	Anticholinergic	Adult PO: 0.5-6 mg/day 1-4 mg/day	Parkinson's disease Drug-induced extrapyramidal symptoms
trihexyphenidyl (Artane)	Anticholinergic	Adult PO: 6-10 mg/day 5-15 mg/day	Parkinson's disease Drug-induced extrapyramidal symptoms

nursing process

● Assessment

After patients are first confronted with the diagnosis of PD, they soon learn how the disease can affect their every movement and alter activities of daily living (ADL). Before medication is administered, you must perform a thorough assessment and take a thorough nursing history so that the symptoms and the ways in which the disease has affected the patients' ADL are documented and possible contraindications and cautions are identified. The thorough nursing history should include questions about the following activities and body systems:

- CNS: ADL, gait, balance, tremors, weakness, lethargy, and level of consciousness
- Gastrointestinal and genitourinary: appetite, bladder, and bowel patterns
- Psychologic and emotional: mood, affect, depression, and personality changes

Additional signs and symptoms of PD to assess include mask-like expression, speech problems, dysphagia, and rigidity of arms, legs, and neck.

When an anticholinergic agent such as benztropine or trihexyphenidyl is prescribed, you should assess the patient carefully to determine whether he or she has a history of urinary retention, bladder difficulties or obstruction, myasthenia gravis, or acute narrow-angle glaucoma (mydriasis leads to an increase in intraocular pressure), because these are contraindications to the use of these agents. Age is a significant factor as well because of the increased likelihood of side effects or toxicity related to the physiologic changes associated with aging. Other conditions that these agents can exacerbate include tachycardia, benign prostatic hypertrophy (BPH), and peptic ulcer disease, so these patients should be monitored closely. Drugs that interact with these agents include antihistamines, disopyramide, phenothiazines, and tricyclic antidepressants (TCAs) (increase effects). Cholinergic agents decrease the effects of anticholinergics.

When dopaminergic agents such as levodopa, amantadine, or levodopa-carbidopa are prescribed, the patient should be asked whether he or she has a seizure disorder, hypotension, peptic ulcer disease, a renal or hepatic disorder, asthma, a history of myocardial infarction (MI), BPH, or an anemia, or suffers from psychosis or some other affective disorder. These are all contraindications to the use of dopaminergic agents. Drugs that can interact with these agents include MAOIs and furazolidone. Given in combination with the dopaminergic medications, these drugs may result in a hypertensive crisis. Other drug interactions include TCAs, anticholinergics, alcohol, vitamin B_6, and antipsychotic agents.

With the newer agent ropinirole, patients with a history of renal or cardiac disease need to take the drug with caution. Cautious use is also recommended in patients with psychoses, affective disorders, and dysrhythmias. The patient needs to be further assessed for involuntary movements seen in parkinsonism such as akinesia, tremors, staggering gait, rigidity, and drooling. Vital signs should also be assessed during treatment with special attention to blood pressure because of the side effects of hypotension and hypertension. Entacapone is contraindicated in patients with hypersensitivity to the drug. Tolcapone, another newer agent, should not be taken in patients with liver disease. Liver function studies should be taken before treatment. However, entacapone does not have the same effect on the liver, so it may be taken safely by patients with a liver disorder.

Newer dopamine agonists, such as pramipexole, ropinirole, and cabergoline, are contraindicated in patients with sensitivity to these groups of medications.

● Nursing Diagnoses

Nursing diagnoses appropriate to the patient with PD taking antiparkinsonian agents include the following:

- Impaired physical mobility related to the disease process and side effects of medications.
- Disturbed body image related to changes in appearance and mobility due to disease process.
- Urinary retention related to the effects of the disease
- Constipation related to the disease process.
- Risk for injury related to the physical limitations produced by the disease process.
- Imbalanced nutrition, less than body requirements, related to pharmacotherapy and associated side effects.
- Deficient knowledge related to pharmacotherapy and its therapeutic and side effects.

● Planning

Goals of nursing care related to the administration of antiparkinsonian agents include the following:

- Patient remains free of self-injury.
- Patient states the purpose of the specific medications prescribed for the disease.
- Patient states the side effects and toxic effects of medications.
- Patient regains as normal as possible bowel and bladder elimination patterns.
- Patient maintains adequate nutritional status.
- Patient remains as independent as possible.
- Patient is less anxious and fearful.
- Patient regains a positive self-concept.
- Patient remains compliant to therapy.

Outcome Criteria

Outcome criteria related to the administration of antiparkinsonian agents include the following:

- Patient (and significant others) will state ways of preventing self-injury such as use of assistive devices.
- Patient will state purposes, side effects, and toxic effects associated with the specific antiparkinsonian medications such as emesis, nausea, instability, and palpitations.
- Patient will state ways to prevent some of the side effects and toxic effects of antiparkinsonian medications such as frequent mouth care and increased fluids.

- Patient will discuss ways to minimize problems associated with drug-induced alterations in bowel and bladder elimination patterns through changes in diet and fluid intake.
- Patient will discuss measures to ensure an adequate nutritional status with possible antiemetic therapy.
- Patient will begin to perform ADL more independently.
- Patient will openly verbalize fears, anxieties, and changes in self-image with members of the health care team and supportive staff.

● Implementation

Nursing actions related to the administration of the various antiparkinsonian agents focus primarily on safe drug administration and patient education. When patients are receiving anticholinergic agents, you should give oral doses after meals with single daily doses administered at bedtime. Fluid intake and frequent mouth care should be encouraged because of the dryness of the mouth. Any intravenously administered medications, such as benztropine mesylate, should be given slowly, with the patient remaining in bed for an hour afterward. Patients should be informed to not take any other medications without the physician's consent because of many adverse drug interactions with prescription and OTC medications.

During the start of dopaminergic agent therapy, patients should be assisted when walking because of the dizziness caused by these agents. Oral doses should be given with food to help minimize gastrointestinal upset. It is also important to remember that pyridoxine (vitamin B_6) in doses greater than 10 mg will reverse the effects of levodopa. Foods high in vitamin B_6 should therefore also be avoided. Patients should be encouraged to force fluids, unless contraindicated, drinking at least 2000 ml per day, as well as consume an adequate amount of food high in roughage and fiber. A hypertensive crisis may result if levodopa preparations are taken with MAOIs, so these drugs are generally not administered concurrently. At least 2 weeks should be allowed to elapse between the use of these medications. It is also important to remember that dopaminergic agents are generally titrated to the patient's response. Sinemet SR oral form should not be crushed.

Entacapone is generally taken with levodopa and is effective from the first dose. This information about its onset of action should be shared with the patient because often it takes a longer period of time for the other antiparkinsonian agents to have therapeutic effects. It is important to also tell any patient taking antiparkinsonian agents to take them as prescribed and understand their therapeutic onset.

The newer nonergot dopamine agonists have been shown to have more efficacy in patients with advanced forms of PD, and so patient teaching about their effects and their fewer adverse effects is an important part of the patient's care. Patients should be informed about their action but also how they have fewer of the dyskinesia side effects. Entacapone, one of the newer and more potent COMT inhibitors, is generally taken with levodopa and should be effective beginning with the first dose. Patients normally experience the benefit of this agent within a day or two, which is different from the "weeks" for benefits to show with other older agents. Entacapone is also helpful for patients who are experiencing problems with "wearing off" fluctuations. This medication comes in film-coated tablets and should not be crushed.

Patient teaching tips for dopaminergic agents are presented below.

● Evaluation

Monitoring the patient's response to any of the antiparkinsonian medications is crucial to documenting treatment success or failure. Therapeutic responses to the antiparkinsonian agents include an improved sense of well-being; improved mental status; increase in appetite; ability to perform ADL, to concentrate, and to think clearly; and less intense parkinsonism manifestations such as less tremor, shuffling of gait, muscle rigidity, and involuntary movements. In addition to monitoring for therapeutic responses, you must also watch for the occurrence of side effects, such as confusion, anxiety, irritability, depression, paranoia, headache, weakness, lethargy, nausea, vomiting, anorexia, palpitations, postural hypotension, tachycardia, dry mouth, constipation, urinary retention, blurred vision, dark urine, difficulty swallowing, and nightmares. Therapeutic effects of COMT inhibitors may be noticed, as with entacapone, within a few days, whereas with other agents it may take weeks. Side effects for which to monitor with COMT inhibitors include those mentioned previously, but fewer dyskinesias are associated with COMT inhibitors than with dopamine agonists.

---

patient teaching tips

Antiparkinsonian Agents

Dopaminergics

➤ Patients should change positions slowly because of the postural hypotension (drop in blood pressure with position changes) that can occur. Patients should take their time changing positions from lying to sitting and then gradually standing.

➤ Make sure patients know to report to their physician any of the following side effects that may indicate an overdose: excessive twitching, drooling, eye spasms.

➤ Patients should always take their medication exactly as prescribed and should not omit or double a dose. If an omission or error occurs in the administration of these (or any) medications, the physician should be notified immediately.

➤ Avoid sudden withdrawal of medication.

➤ Levodopa preparations may darken the patient's urine and sweat.

➤ Patients should be instructed to avoid taking vitamin B$_6$ supplements and eating vitamin-fortified foods. (Specific food examples [meats, poultry, fish, eggs, sweet potatoes, lima beans, and whole grain cereals] should be given to patients before they undertake home management or are discharged from the hospital.) Vitamin B$_6$ interferes with the action of levodopa. The risk is lower, however, in combination levodopa-carbidopa agents.

➤ These medications should be taken with juice and a low-protein snack or after meals so as to prevent interactions with pyridoxine (vitamin B$_6$) in food.

➤ Encourage patients to keep a journal of their progress and problems.

➤ Sustained release forms should not be crushed.

Anticholinergics

➤ Patients should be instructed to take medication with or after meals to minimize gastrointestinal upset.

➤ Patients should drink lots of fluids, at least 2000 ml per day, unless otherwise instructed by their physician or not allowed this amount of fluid.

➤ Medications should be taken exactly as prescribed and at bedtime to prevent drowsiness during the day.

➤ Patients should understand the importance of not discontinuing medications suddenly.

➤ Patients should avoid taking any OTC medications unless physician has okayed this first.

➤ Patients should avoid operating heavy machinery or driving if they feel sedated or drowsy from the medication.

➤ Patients should be instructed to change positions slowly to prevent falling or fainting because of the postural hypotension (drop in blood pressure with position changes) produced by these agents.

COMT Inhibitors

➤ It is important to tell patients that these newer agents provide a more substantial level of levodopa in the brain, which gives the patient more "good" days.

➤ Often the therapeutic effects are noted in a few days versus several weeks.

➤ Inform patients that these agents are used as an adjunct to levodopa and carbidopa for treatment of PD.

POINTS TO REMEMBER

Neurotransmitter Abnormality in PD

- Chronic, progressive, degenerative disorder of dopamine-producing neurons in brain.
- Normal subject: balance between ACh and dopamine levels in the CNS.
- Patient with PD: raised ACh and lowered dopamine levels.
- Drug therapy: lower ACh level and raise dopamine level.

Classic PD Symptoms

- Bradykinesia (slow movements), rigidity (cogwheel), tremor (pill-rolling), and postural instability.
- Dyskinesias: difficulty performing voluntary movements (two common ones: chorea and dystonias).
- Chorea: irregular, spasmodic, involuntary movements of limbs or facial muscles.
- Dystonias: abnormal muscle tone in any tissue.

Drug therapy for PD

- Neuroprotective, dopaminergic, and anticholinergic.
- Neuroprotective: selegiline—may slow progression of PD.
- Ropinirole (ReQuip) is a new nonergot dopamine agonist indicated for monotherapy for PD and for adjunctive therapy with levodopa.
- COMT inhibitors, such as tolcapone and entacapone, have a longer duration of action and onset that is quicker (i.e., a few days).

- COMT inhibitors are also associated with less "wearing off" effects and prolonged therapeutic benefits.
- Dopaminergic: indirect- and direct-acting and replacement drugs.
- Indirect: release dopamine; direct: stimulate dopamine receptors (agonists); replacement: raise brain dopamine level.

Cornerstone: Levodopa

- Levodopa and levodopa-carbidopa replace deficient dopamine in brain.
- Levodopa: biologic precursor of dopamine.
- Levodopa can pass through blood-brain barrier to get to site of action in the brain; dopamine cannot.

Carbidopa

- Peripheral decarboxylase inhibitor.
- Does not cross blood-brain barrier; prevents levodopa breakdown in periphery.

Patient Considerations

- Require long-term care because of progressive and debilitating nature of illness.
- Require much support and education.
- COMT inhibitors have a quicker onset of a few days versus several days as compared with the traditional agents used for PD.

REVIEW QUESTIONS

1. Which of the following should alert the nurse during the assessment of a patient who is to begin drug treatment with an anticholinergic agent for treatment of his mild Parkinson's disease?
   a. Diarrhea
   b. Drooling
   c. Glaucoma
   d. Irritable bowel syndrome

2. Your patient has recently been ordered amantadine (Symmetrel) for Parkinson's disease. The patient's medication history reveals that she is also on hydrochlorothiazide (HCTZ). Which of the following would be the nurse's most appropriate action?
   a. Do not be concerned because even though there is a drug interaction, the increased effect of the antiparkinsonian agent by the diuretic is a desirable action.
   b. Contact her health care provider about the potential drug interaction with HCTZ leading to toxic effects of amantadine because of its decreased renal excretion.
   c. Encourage the use of both of these agents simultaneously because they are synergistic and result in mood improvement and decrease in gait abnormalities.
   d. Encourage the patient to refuse the medication because research has shown that use of amantadine with diuretics increases the risk of memory impairment.

3. Patient teaching for patients taking antiparkinsonian agents should include all of the following correct information except:
   a. Twitch and eye spasms may indicate overdosage.
   b. Changing of positions should be slow to avoid fainting.

   c. A link exists between antiparkinsonian drug use and Alzheimer's disease.
   d. A link exists between antiparkinsonian drug use and the occurrence of hypotension.

4. If levodopa therapy is not helping a patient with improvement of the effects of Parkinson's disease, the health care provider may consider switching the patient to another antiparkinsonian agent with the corresponding rationale:
   a. Haloperidol (Haldol) with a mechanism of action of dopamine agonism
   b. Methyldopa (Aldomet) with a mechanism of action of antidopaminergism
   c. Amantadine (Symmetrel) with its exclusive mechanism of action of antiviral effects
   d. Levodopa-carbidopa (Sinemet) with its exclusive mechanism of action of inhibition of the decarboxylation of peripheral levodopa

5. Which of the following statements should be emphasized and explained during patient teaching about the use of levodopa?
   a. "There are very few, if any, drug interactions with levodopa."
   b. "Therapeutic effects may take up to several weeks to a few months."
   c. "Make sure that you take a laxative qid with at least 6000 ml of fluids per 8-12 hours."
   d. "Levodopa should be taken as preventive medication to the occurrence of Parkinson's disease."

For Answers see www.harcourthealth.com/MERLIN/Lilley/.

CRITICAL THINKING Activities

1. Mr. P has been diagnosed with Parkinson's disease and is taking levodopa-carbidopa (Sinemet). He also has Alzheimer's disease and is taking tacrine (Cognex). What do you think about the use of these two medications together?

2. You discover that your client who has PD (taking levodopa-carbidopa) is also being given some of his wife's phenothiazine medication to make him "feel even better." Why is this combination unsafe and not rational?

3. Your patient has been placed on a dopaminergic for the management of Parkinson's disease. She also re-

lates to you during the nursing history that she has a diet high in meats, poultry, and whole grain cereals. What would be a concern you may have with this patient's diet and why?

4. How does levodopa help improve the function of the patient diagnosed with Parkinson's disease?

5. After long-term treatment, patients with Parkinson's disease are often placed on a "drug holiday." Explain the rationale for this approach to treatment.

6. Explain the physiology behind the "on-again/off-again" appearance of symptoms that occurs with long-term levodopa treatment.

For Answers see www.harcourthealth.com/MERLIN/Lilley/.

bibliography

Albanese J, Nutz P: *Mosby's 2001 nursing drug reference and review cards*, St Louis, 2001, Mosby.

American Hospital Formulary Service: *AHFS drug information*, Bethesda, Md, 2000. American Society of Health-System Pharmacists.

Anderson PO, Knoben JE, Troutman WG: *Handbook of clinical drug data 1999-2000*, ed 9, New York, 1999, McGraw-Hill.

Berchou RC, Scheife RT, editors: Contemporary issues in the pharmacology of Parkinson's disease, Part 2, *Pharmacotherapy* 20(1):1S, 2000.

Charles PD, Dacis TL: Drug therapy for Parkinson's disease, *South Med J* 89(9):851, 1996.

Johns Hopkins Hospital, Department of Pediatrics et al: *The Harriet Lane handbook*, ed 15, St Louis, 2000, Mosby.

Keen JH: *Critical care and emergency drug reference*, ed 3, St Louis, 1996, Mosby.

Medical Letter: Pramipexole and ropinirole for Parkinson's disease 39(1014), November 21, 1997.

Mosby's GenRx: a comprehensive reference for generic and brand drugs, ed 10, St Louis, 2000, Mosby.

Portyansky E: Parkinsonism patients: when and how should they be treated? *Drug Topics*, p. 66, April 21, 1997.

Pramipexole marketed for Parkinson's disease, *Am J Health Sys Pharm* 54:1925, 1997.

Skidmore-Roth L: *Mosby's 2001 nursing drug reference*, St Louis, 2001, Mosby.

United States Pharmacopeia: *USPDI: drug information for the health care provider*, Rockville, Md, 2000, the Author.

Activity

Chapter 14

Psychotherapeutic Agents

objectives

www.harcourthealth.com/MERLIN/Lilley/

Look for this symbol for topics covered in the **Online Worksheet**

When you reach the end of this chapter, you should be able to do the following:

1 Identify the various drugs in the following classes of psychotherapeutic agents: antianxiety agents, antidepressants, antimanic agents, and antipsychotics.

2 Discuss the mechanisms of action, indications, therapeutic effects, side effects, toxic effects, drug interactions, contraindications, and cautions associated with the various psychotherapeutic agents.

3 Develop a nursing care plan that includes all phases of the nursing process related to the administration of the various psychotherapeutic agents.

4 Develop patient education guidelines for patients receiving psychotherapeutic drugs.

drug profiles

alprazolam, p. 208
o—➤ amitriptyline, p. 213
amoxapine, p. 213
bupropion, p. 218
chlordiazepoxide, p. 208
chlorpromazine, p. 222
o—➤ clozapine, p. 225
diazepam, p. 208
o—➤ fluoxetine, p. 218
fluphenazine, p. 222
o—➤ haloperidol, p. 224
hydroxyzine, p. 210
lithium, p. 219

o—➤ lorazepam, p. 210
loxapine, p. 224
meprobamate, p. 210
molindone, p. 224
nortriptyline, p. 213
paroxetine, p. 218
phenelzine, p. 215
risperidone, p. 225
sertraline, p. 219
thiothixene, p. 223
tranylcypromine, p. 216
trazodone, p. 219

o—➤ Key drug.

glossary

Affective disorders (a fec′ tiv) Emotional disorders that are characterized by changes in mood. (p. 205)

Agoraphobia (a gə rə fo beə) Fear of leaving the familiar setting of home. (p. 205)

Antihistamine (-his tə men) Any substance capable of reducing the physiologic and pharmacologic effects of histamine, including a wide variety of drugs that block histamine receptors. (p. 206)

Antipsychotic (-si ka tik) Of or pertaining to a substance or procedure that counteracts or diminishes symptoms of serious mental illness, such as being out of touch with reality. (p. 219)

Anxiety The unpleasant state of mind in which unreal or imagined dangers are anticipated. (p. 205)

Barbiturates (bar bi chə rət) One of the oldest drug classes used to treat anxiety. (p. 206)

Benzodiazepine (bən zo di a′ zə pen) One of a group of psychotropic agents prescribed to alleviate anxiety. (p. 206)

Biogenic amine hypothesis (BAH) Theory suggesting that depression and mania are due to alterations in neuronal and synaptic catecholamine concentrations. (p. 210)

Bipolar affective disorder (BAD) A major psychologic disorder characterized by episodes of mania, depression, or mixed mood. (p. 205)

Carbamates (kahr bə mat) One of the oldest drug classes used to treat anxiety. (p. 206)

Depression (de presh′ ən) An abnormal emotional state characterized by exaggerated feelings of sadness, melancholy, dejection, worthlessness, emptiness, and hopelessness that are inappropriate and out of proportion to reality. (p. 205)

Dysregulation hypothesis Views depression and affective disorders as not simply decreased or increased catecholamine activity, but as failures of the regulation of these systems. (p. 211)

Gamma-aminobutyric acid (GABA) An inhibitory amino acid in the brain that functions to inhibit nerve transmission in the central nervous system. (p. 206)

Mania (ma ne ə) A state characterized by an expansive emotional state, extreme excitement, excessive elation, hyperactivity, agitation, overtalkativeness, flight of ideas, increased psychomotor activity, fleeting attention, and sometimes violent, destructive, and self-destructive behavior. (p. 205)

Monoamine oxidase inhibitor (MAOI) (mon o′ ə men ok′ si das) Any of a heterogeneous group of drugs used primarily in the treatment of depression. These drugs also exert an antianxiety effect, especially anxiety associated with phobia. (p. 207)

Permissive hypothesis Implicates reduced concentrations of serotonin (5-HT) as the predisposing factor in individuals with affective disorders. (p. 211)

Psychosis (si ko′ sis) Term used to describe a major emotional disorder that impairs the mental function of the affected individual to the point that the individual cannot participate in everyday life. (p. 205)

Psychotherapeutics (si ko ther ə pu' tiks) Refers to the therapy of emotional and mental disorders. (p. 205)

Tetracyclic (tet rə sik' lik) Antidepressant agent used to treat anxiety disorders. (p. 207)

Tricyclic (tri sik' lik) Antidepressant agents, such as amitryptyline and imipramine hydrochloride, that block reuptake of amine neurotransmitters. The exact mechanism of antidepressant action of these drugs is unknown. (p. 207)

The treatment of emotional and mental disorders is called **psychotherapeutics.** When a person's ability to cope with his or her environment—to carry out the activities of daily living and to interact with others—is seriously impaired, a psychotropic drug may be a treatment option. These drugs are among the most commonly prescribed drugs in the United States today. To understand better the nature and goals of this treatment, the types and definitions of these various disorders are presented first.

PSYCHOSIS, AFFECTIVE DISORDERS, AND ANXIETY

Most people experience emotions such as anxiety, depression, and grief. They are normal human emotions. However, the effect of these emotions on one's ability to engage in normal daily activities and to interact with others can vary considerably. The duration and intensity of these emotions can range from occasional depression or anxiety to a state of constant emotional distress that interferes with one's ability to carry on normal activities of daily living.

There are three main emotional and mental disorders: psychoses, affective disorders, and anxiety. A **psychosis** is a major emotional disorder that impairs mental function to the point where the person cannot participate in everyday life. A hallmark of psychosis is a loss of contact with reality. These behavioral problems or psychotic disorders include depressive and drug-induced psychoses, schizophrenia, and autism.

Affective disorders are characterized by changes in mood and range from **mania** (abnormally pronounced emotions) to **depression** (abnormally reduced emotions). Some patients may exhibit both mania and depression, experiencing periodic swings in emotions, from extremely reduced emotions to very intense, hyperactive emotions. This is referred to as a **bipolar affective disorder (BAD).**

Anxiety is the unpleasant state of mind in which unreal or imagined dangers are anticipated. It is divided into several distinct disorders that have been classified by the American Psychiatric Association and the classification published in the fourth edition of the *Diagnostic and Statistical Manual for Mental Disorders,* (DSM-IV). This reference delineates the demographic features and diagnostic criteria for the major psychiatric disorders and has categorized anxiety into the following disorders:
- Obsessive-compulsive disorder (OCD)
- Posttraumatic stress disorder

pediatric considerations

Psychotherapeutic Agents

- Pediatric patients are at a higher risk for suffering side effects from psychotropic agents, especially extrapyramidal symptoms. Always closely monitor pediatric patients taking psychotropic agents!
- The incidence of Reye's syndrome and other adverse reactions is greater in pediatric patients taking psychotropic agents who have had chickenpox, CNS infections, measles, acute illnesses, or dehydration.
- Lithium may lead to decreased bone density or bone formation in children, so children receiving it should be closely monitored for signs and symptoms of lithium toxicity and bone disorders.
- Tricyclic antidepressants (TCAs) are generally not prescribed for patients under 12 years of age. Some antidepressants are used, though, in children with enuresis, attention deficit disorders, and major depressive disorders and may be associated with adverse reactions such as changes in the ECG, nervousness, sleep disorders, fatigue, elevated blood pressure, and gastrointestinal upset. Pediatric patients are generally more sensitive to the effects of most drugs, and this group of agents is no exception. Be aware of the toxicity risk, which can be fatal. Should confusion, lethargy, visual disturbances, insomnia, tremors, palpitations, constipation, or eye pain occur, report this to the physician immediately.

- Generalized anxiety disorder
- Panic disorder
- Social phobia
- Simple phobia

Anxiety is a normal physiologic emotion, but the results of epidemiologic studies show that 2% to 6% of adults suffer from a generalized anxiety disorder, 1% from a panic disorder, and 4% to 5% from **agoraphobia,** the fear of leaving the familiar setting of home. OCD was thought to be rare but is now observed to be twice as common as schizophrenia or panic disorders in the general population. Anxiety may occur as a result of a wide range of medical illnesses (e.g., cardiovascular or pulmonary disease, hypothyroidism, hyperthyroidism, pheochromocytoma, and hypoglycemia). Many of the anxiety disorders are situational. They arise because of a specific event and subside with time. The treatment of these should be limited to psychotherapy. However, when the anxiety disorder markedly affects one's quality of life and relationships or interferes with one's ability to function normally, pharmacotherapy (drug treatment) in conjunction with psychotherapy becomes desirable, and both should be instituted.

The exact causes of mental disorders are not fully understood. Many theories have been advanced in an attempt to explain the causes and pathophysiology of mental dysfunction. In the biochemical imbalance concept, mental disorders are thought to arise as the result of abnormal levels of endogenous chemicals in the brain such as neurotransmitters. There is strong evidence indicating that the brain levels of catecholamines (especially dopamine) and indolamines (serotonin and histamine) play an important role in maintaining mental health. Other biochemicals that seem necessary for the maintenance of normal mental function are **gamma-aminobutyric acid (GABA),** acetylcholine (ACh), and various inorganic ions such as lithium. A knowledge of these various etiologies, especially the biochemical imbalance theory, can aid in an understanding of psychotherapeutic drug action because many of the agents used to treat psychoses, affective disorders, and anxiety block or stimulate the release of these endogenous mediators.

geriatric considerations

Psychotherapeutic Agents

- Elderly patients have higher serum levels of psychotherapeutic agents because of changes in the drug distribution metabolism processes, less serum albumin, decreased lean body mass, less water in tissues, and increased body fat. Because of these changes, elderly patients generally require lower doses of antipsychotic and antidepressant agents.
- Orthostatic hypotension, anticholinergic side effects, sedation, and extrapyramidal symptoms are more common in elderly patients taking psychotherapeutic agents. Careful evaluation and documentation of baseline values and neurologic findings are therefore important to the safe use of these agents.
- Increased anxiety is often associated with the use of tricyclic antidepressants. Patients with a history of cardiac disease may be at a higher risk of experiencing dysrhythmias, tachycardia, stroke, myocardial infarction, or congestive heart failure.
- Lithium is more toxic in elderly patients, and lower doses are often necessary, but close monitoring is important to its safe use in this age group. CNS toxicity, lithium-induced goiter, and hypothyroidism are more frequent in the aged patient.

ANTIANXIETY AGENTS

Medications are only one of the many therapeutic options in people afflicted with the various anxiety disorders. Although benzodiazepines are generally the first-line drug treatment for anxiety disorders, there are other classes of drugs that are also effective. The efficacy of certain classes of medications in the treatment of certain anxiety disorders and their superiority over other drug classes have been documented. These various drug classes are listed in Table 14-1 according to the anxiety disorders they are effective in treating.

Mechanism of Action

Of the several drug classes shown to be effective in the treatment of anxiety disorders, all reduce anxiety by reducing overactivity in the CNS. There are, however, differences among the various drug classes.

Benzodiazepines seem to exert their anxiolytic effects by depressing activity in the areas of the brain called the *brainstem* and the *limbic system.* Benzodiazepines are believed to accomplish this by increasing the action of GABA, an inhibitory amino acid in the brain that functions to inhibit nerve transmission in the CNS. Benzodiazepines have binding sites in the same channels that govern the release of GABA. The binding of benzodiazepines with these sites produces not only an anxiolytic effect but also sedation and muscle relaxation.

There are several other drug classes used for the treatment of anxiety disorders. **Barbiturates** and **carbamates** are probably the oldest such drug classes. Their anxiolytic properties are related to their ability to depress CNS activity and cause sedation. These agents have many undesirable side effects that make them poor drugs for the long-term treatment of anxiety. They are heavily sedating, they interact with many other drugs, and they interfere with normal sleep patterns (suppress rapid eye movement sleep). Meprobamate is one of the more frequently prescribed carbamates used to relieve anxiety.

Antihistamines are also used as anxiolytics because of their ability to depress the CNS by sedating the patient. The antihistamine most commonly used for the relief of anxiety is hydroxyzine. It has few antihistaminic properties but is very sedating. There are two salt forms of hy-

Table 14-1   Various Anxiety Disorders: Drugs of Choice

Disorder	TCA	Benzodiazepine	MAOI	Buspirone	SSRIs
Panic disorder	+++	++++	+++	0	+++
Generalized anxiety disorder	+	++++	?++	+++	
Obsessive-compulsive disorder	+++	?+	?+	0	+++
Posttraumatic stress disorder	+	?+	+	?+	
Simple phobia	0	+	0	0	
Social phobia	+	+	+	0	

TCA, Tricyclic and tetracyclic antidepressants; *MAOI,* monoamine oxidase inhibitors; *SSRI,* selective serotonin reuptake inhibitor; *?,* has shown some efficacy but limited use; +, limited use and efficacy; ++, some use and efficacy; +++, frequent use, good efficacy; ++++, most frequent use, best efficacy; 0, no efficacy or use.

droxyzine: hydroxyzine hydrochloride (Atarax) and hydroxyzine pamoate (Vistaril), both of which are effective anxiolytics.

Monoamine oxidase inhibitors (MAOIs), buspirone (BuSpar), and **tricyclic** antidepressants (TCAs) and **tetracyclic** antidepressants have also been used to treat anxiety disorders. These agents are discussed in greater detail in the section of this chapter, Antidepressant Agents. They relieve anxiety by decreasing overactivity in the CNS.

Drug Effects

Besides their anxiolytic effects just mentioned, antianxiety agents produce several other effects throughout the body. These are sedative, hypnotic, appetite stimulating, analgesic, and anticonvulsant effects. Because of their wide range of effects, they are used for a variety of indications.

Therapeutic Uses

Carbamates such as meprobamate are not only used as anxiolytics but also as sedative-hypnotics. Barbiturates such as phenobarbital are also used in the treatment of seizures, insomnia, hyperbilirubinemia, and chronic cholestasis and for their sedative effects. Antihistamines are used to treat anxiety because of their sedative side effects, but their actual intended therapeutic effect is to block the actions of histamine released in the setting of allergies. TCAs and selective serotonin-reuptake inhibitors (SSRIs) such as fluoxetine are also indicated for the treatment of depression.

However, benzodiazepines are the largest and most commonly prescribed anxiolytic drug class because they offer several advantages over these other drug classes used to treat anxiety. At therapeutic doses they have little effect on consciousness, they are very safe from the standpoint of their side effect profile, and they do not interact with many other drugs. Four very commonly prescribed anxiolytic benzodiazepines are diazepam (Valium), lorazepam (Ativan), alprazolam (Xanax), and midazolam (Versed). They also have a wide variety of therapeutic applications. They are used to relieve anxiety, sedate, produce muscle relaxation, control seizures, treat depression,

and treat alcohol withdrawal. Benzodiazepines commonly used as sedative-hypnotics are described in Chapter 11 and have slightly different therapeutic actions from those of the benzodiazepines used to treat anxiety. The commonly used anxiolytic benzodiazepines and their approved indications are listed in Table 14-2.

Side Effects and Adverse Effects

The most common undesirable effect of the anxiolytic drugs is an overexpression of their therapeutic effects. All these classes of drugs decrease CNS activity, and many of the unwanted effects of these agents are related directly to this action. The most common side effects and adverse effects of benzodiazepines are listed in Table 14-3.

Toxicity and Management of Overdose

There is a potential for benzodiazepines to cause serious life-threatening toxicities, but when taken in normal doses in otherwise healthy patients, they are very safe, effective anxiolytics. When taken with other sedating medications or with alcohol, life-threatening respiratory depression or arrest can occur. This serious consequence can also occur in patients whose metabolism or elimination capabilities are impaired because of liver or kidney dysfunction. In such settings, benzodiazepines can accumulate and not be eliminated. This further accentuates their therapeutic and toxic actions. An overdose of benzodiazepines may result in one or any combination

Table 14-3 Benzodiazepines: Common Adverse Effects

Body System	Side/Adverse Effects
Central nervous system	Drowsiness, sedation, loss of coordination, dizziness, blurred vision, headaches, paradoxical reactions (insomnia, increased excitability, hallucinations)
Gastrointestinal	Nausea, vomiting, constipation, dry mouth, abdominal cramping
Other	Pruritus, skin rash

Table 14-2 Benzodiazepines: Approved Indications

Approved Indications	Benzodiazepines
Alcohol withdrawal	chlordiazepoxide, diazepam, lorazepam, oxazepam
Anxiety	alprazolam, chlordiazepoxide, clorazepate, diazepam, halazepam, lorazepam, oxazepam, prazepam
Depression	alprazolam, oxazepam
Muscle spasm	diazepam
Preoperative sedation	chlordiazepoxide, diazepam, lorazepam
Seizure disorders	clorazepate, diazepam

cultural implications

Psychotherapeutic Agents

Many racial and ethnic groups respond to drugs differently. One example is with benzodiazapines and tricyclic antidepressants. Asians have a lower activity of drug metabolization because of different enzyme deficiencies as compared with Caucasians. Specifically, with the two groups of drugs mentioned, Asians often require lower doses because they have lower levels of metabolizing enzymes (e.g., CY02D6) and are therefore more sensitive to these agents. Beta-blockers, specifically propanolol (Inderal), are also problematic for Asians.

Diazepam (Valium) and Chinese and Japanese Patients

The commonly used antianxiety agent diazepam undergoes different metabolic pathways in the Chinese and Japanese population. These two groups are found to be poor "mephenytoin pathway" metabolizers. Approximately 20% of these individuals metabolize mephenytoin poorly, resulting in rapid drug accumulation. To prevent possible toxicity, lower doses are generally required. As related to nursing implications, nurses may need to watch these individuals more closely for sedation, overdosage, and other adverse reactions to diazepam.

of the following symptoms: somnolence, confusion, coma, or respiratory depression.

The treatment of benzodiazepine intoxication is generally symptomatic and supportive. If ingestion is recent, decontamination of the gastrointestinal system is indicated. As a rule of thumb, gastric decontamination using syrup of ipecac (an agent used to induce vomiting in overdose) is contraindicated in patients who have ingested medications that cause sedation because of the risk of aspiration of the stomach contents. Therefore gastric lavage is generally the best and most effective means of gastric decontamination. Activated charcoal and a salinecathartic may be administered after gastric lavage to remove any remaining drug. Hemodialysis is not useful in the treatment of benzodiazepine overdose.

Many of the therapeutic and toxic effects of benzodiazepines are mediated by receptors in the CNS. Therefore flumazenil (Romazicon), a benzodiazepine receptor blocker (antagonist), is used to reverse the effects of benzodiazepine overdose. It directly opposes the actions of benzodiazepines by directly competing with benzodiazepines for binding at the benzodiazepine receptors in the CNS. It has a stronger affinity for the receptor and thus knocks the benzodiazepine off the receptor, reversing the sedative action of the benzodiazepine. The treatment regimen for the reversal of benzodiazepine overdose is summarized in Table 14-4.

Interactions

There is a wide variety of drug interactions that occur with the use of the anxiolytics, particularly benzodiazepines. Alcohol and CNS depressants, when coadministered with benzodiazepines, can result in additive CNS depression. Cimetidine, disulfiram, MAOIs, and tobacco all can decrease the metabolism of benzodiazepines and result in increased CNS depression.

Dosages

For the recommended dosages of selected antianxiety agents, see the dosages table on p. 209.

Flumazenil Treatment Regimen

Table 14-4

Recommended Regimen	Duration
0.2 mg (2 ml) given IV over 30 sec; wait 30 sec; if still no response, give 0.2 mg (2 ml); may repeat at 60-sec intervals as needed up to four additional times; may be given up to 3 mg in overdose situations	1-4 hr

Important note: Flumazenil has a relatively short half-life and duration of effect of 1 to 4 hr; therefore if the intent is to reverse a long-acting benzodiazepine, the effects of the flumazenil may wear off and the effects of the benzodiazepine may reappear.

drug profiles

BENZODIAZEPINES

Benzodiazepines are contraindicated in patients who have shown a hypersensitivity reaction to them and in patients who have narrow-angle glaucoma. They are all prescription-only drugs and FDA pregnancy category D agents. They are also all scheduled drugs: chlorazepate is a schedule II drug, and the rest are schedule IV drugs.

alprazolam

Alprazolam (Xanax) is most commonly used as an anxiolytic and as an adjunct for the treatment of depression. It is only available for oral administration as a 0.25-, 0.5-, and 1-mg tablet. The 0.25-mg tablet is the dose recommended for the geriatric patient. The commonly recommended dosages are given in the table on p. 209.

PHARMACOKINETICS

HALF-LIFE	ONSET	PEAK	DURATION
11-16 hr	<1 hr	1-2 hr	6-12 hr

chlordiazepoxide

Chlordiazepoxide (Librium) is used for many indications but is most frequently used for the treatment of alcohol withdrawal, for the relief of anxiety, and as a preoperative sedative agent. Chlordiazepoxide combined with the antimuscarinic drug clidinium is Librax, and this is used as an adjunct in the treatment of peptic ulcer disease. It is available orally as a 5-, 10-, and 25-mg capsule and intravenously as a 20-mg/ml injection. The commonly recommended dosages are given in the table on p. 209.

PHARMACOKINETICS

HALF-LIFE	ONSET	PEAK	DURATION
9-34 hr	30-60 min	0.5-4 hr	12-24 hr

diazepam

Diazepam (Valium) is one of the most frequently prescribed benzodiazepines. It is indicated for the

Activity

DOSAGES Selected Antianxiety Agents

agent	pharmacologic class	dosage range	purpose
alprazolam (Xanax)	Benzodiazepine	*Adult* PO: 0.25-0.5 mg tid; do not exceed 4 mg/day	Anxiolytic
		Geriatric PO: 0.25 mg 2-3 times/day	Anxiolytic
chlordiazepoxide (Librium)	Benzodiazepine	*Pediatric* PO: >6 y/o, 5 mg 2-4 times/day *Adult* PO: 5-25 mg 3-4 times/day IM/IV: 50-100 mg; then 25 mg 3-4 times/day for severe anxiety 50-100 mg q2-4h prn for alcoholism	Anxiolytic
		50-100 mg IM before surgery	Preop sedation
diazepam (Valium)	Benzodiazepine	*Pediatric* PO: >6 mo:1.25 mg 3-4 times/day *Adult* PO: 2-10 mg 2-4 times/day *Geriatric* PO: 2-2.5 mg 1-2 times/day	Anxiety, alcoholism, muscle spasm, convulsive disorders
		Pediatric IM/IV: >30 days; 1-2 mg repeated in 3-4 hr prn	Tetanus
		≥5 y/o: 5-10 mg repeated in 3-4 hr prn	Tetanus
		>30 days: 0.2-0.5 mg q2-5 min to a maximum of 5 mg	Status epilepticus
		≥5 y/o: 1 mg q2-5 min to a maximum of 0 mg	Status epilepticus
		Adult IM/IV: 2-10 mg repeated in 3-4 hr prn	Anxiety
		10 mg followed by 5-10 mg in 3-4 hr prn	Alcoholism
		5-10 mg IV w/in 5-20 min before procedure	Cardioversion
		10 mg IM before surgery	Preop sedation
		5-10 mg repeated in 3-4 hr prn	Muscle spasm
		5-10 mg repeated at 10- to 15-min intervals to a maximum of 30 mg; repeat in 3-4 hr prn	Status epilepticus
hydroxyzine (Atarax, Vistaril)	Antihistamine	*Pediatric* <6 y/o PO: 50 mg/day divided ≥ 6 y/o: PO: 50-100 mg/day divided	Anxiolytic/pruritus
		PO: 0.6 mg/kg	Pre/postop sedation
		IM: 1.1 mg/kg	Nausea/vomiting
		Adult PO: 50-100 mg qid	Anxiolytic
		IM: 50-100 mg q4-6h	Anxiolytic
		PO: 25 mg 3-4 times/day	Pruritus
		PO: 50-100 mg	Pre/postpartum sedation
		IM: 25-100 mg	Nausea/vomiting
lorazepam (Ativan)	Benzodiazepine	*Adult* PO: 2-6-mg/day divided	Anxiolytic
		PO: 2-4 mg HS	Hypnotic
		IM: 0.05 mg/kg to a maximum of 4 mg	Preop sedation
		IV: 2-4 mg	Preop sedation
meprobamate (Equanil, Miltown)	Carbamate	*Pediatric* 6-12 y/o PO: 100-200 mg 2-3 times/day	Anxiolytic
		Adult PO: 1.2-1.6 g/day in 3-4 divided doses	Anxiolytic

relief of anxiety, alcohol withdrawal, and seizure disorders (e.g., status epilepticus); for sedation; and as an adjunct for the relief of skeletal muscle spasms. Diazepam has active metabolites that can accumulate in patients who have renal or hepatic dysfunc-

tion. This can result in additive, cumulative effects that may be manifested as prolonged sedation, respiratory depression, or coma. It is available orally as a 2-, 5-, and 10-mg tablet; a 15-mg SR capsule; a 5-mg/5 ml and 5-mg/ml oral solution; and a 2.5-, 10-, and

20-mg rectal gel; and intravenously as a 5-mg/ml injection. The commonly recommended dosages are given in the table on p. 209.

PHARMACOKINETICS

HALF-LIFE	ONSET	PEAK	DURATION
20-50 hr	30-60 min	1-2 hr	12-24 hr

lorazepam

Lorazepam (Ativan) is a widely used benzodiazepine. It is currently approved for use in the management of anxiety disorders, for the short-term relief of anxiety, and as a preoperative medication to provide sedation and light anesthesia and to diminish patient recall (amnesia). It has also shown efficacy in the prevention and treatment of chemotherapy-related nausea and vomiting and of the symptoms of acute alcohol withdrawal. It is available orally as a 0.5-, 1-, and 2-mg tablet and intravenously as a 2- or 4-mg/ml injection. It may also be administered sublingually. When administered in this fashion, its onset of action is similar to that associated with IV administration but without the inconveniences. The commonly recommended dosages are given in the table on p. 209.

PHARMACOKINETICS

HALF-LIFE	ONSET	PEAK	DURATION
IV: 12-16 hr	IV: Rapid	IV: 15-20 min	IV: 4 hr
PO: 12-16 hr	PO: 15-45 min	PO: 2 hr	PO: 12-24 hr

MISCELLANEOUS AGENTS

There are several categories of drugs that can be used in the treatment of anxiety disorders. Although benzodiazepines are by far the most widely prescribed anxiolytics, often drugs in other categories may be prescribed because of certain advantages they offer. Some of the more commonly used drugs are described in the following sections. The efficacy of the carbamates in treating anxiety disorders, with meprobamate the prototype, has been shown. The antihistamine hydroxyzine and the nonbenzodiazepine anxiolytic buspirone are also very effective antianxiety agents.

hydroxyzine

Hydroxyzine is available in two different salt forms: hydrochloride salt (Atarax) and pamoate salt (Vistaril). Both forms are used to treat anxiety disorders. Hydroxyzine is an antihistamine that suppresses activity in the CNS, which makes it useful as both an anxiolytic and antiemetic agent. It is available orally as a 10-mg/5 ml solution; a 25-mg/5 ml suspension; a 10-, 25-, 50-, and 100-mg tablet and capsule; and a 10-, 25-, and 50-mg film-coated tablet. It is also available as a 25- and 50-mg/ml IM injection. The commonly recommended dosages are given in the table on p. 209. Pregnancy category C.

PHARMACOKINETICS

HALF-LIFE	ONSET	PEAK	DURATION
3 hr	15-30 min	30-60 min	4-6 hr

meprobamate

Meprobamate (Equanil, Miltown) is a carbamate-derivative anxiolytic agent. It is the most frequently prescribed carbamate drug for the treatment of anxiety disorders. It is not as frequently prescribed as benzodiazepines because of its high tendency to cause sedation and interfere with motor coordination, and because tolerance rapidly develops in patients taking it. It is contraindicated in patients who have shown a hypersensitivity reaction to carbamates. Meprobamate is similar to the benzodiazepines in that it is also a schedule IV controlled substance and is considered a pregnancy category D drug. It is only available orally as a 200-, 400-, and 600-mg tablet. The commonly recommended dosages are given in the table on p. 209.

PHARMACOKINETICS

HALF-LIFE	ONSET	PEAK	DURATION
PO: 6-16 hr	<1 hr	1-3 hr	6-12 hr
PO-SR: 6-16 hr	Unknown	Unknown	Up to 12 hr

DRUGS USED TO TREAT AFFECTIVE DISORDERS

Several classes of drugs are used in the treatment of the affective disorders. The two main drug categories are antidepressant agents and antimanic agents.

ANTIDEPRESSANT AGENTS

Antidepressants are the pharmacologic treatment of choice for major depressive disorders (see the Research box). Not only are they very effective in treating depression, they are also useful for treating other disorders, such as dysthymia, schizophrenia, eating disorders, and personality disorders. These agents are also commonly used in the treatment of various medical conditions, including migraine headaches, chronic pain syndromes, peptic ulcer disease, and sleep disorders.

Many of the drugs currently used to treat affective disorders increase neurotransmitter concentrations in the CNS. This is based on the belief that alterations in the levels of certain neurotransmitters in the CNS are responsible for causing depression. One of the most widely held hypotheses advanced to explain depression in these terms is the **biogenic amine hypothesis (BAH).** Specifically, it postulates that depression results from a deficiency of neuronal and synaptic catecholamines (primarily norepinephrine) and mania from an excess of amines at the adrenergic receptor sites in the brain. This hypothesis is illustrated in Fig. 14-1.

research

Detecting Depression Among Primary Care Patients

In a study supported in part by the Agency for Health Care Policy and Research (HS06802), 40% of psychiatric patients compared with about 26% of other patients had double depression (a major depression and mild depression and anxiety lasting longer than 2 years), meaning that the most severely depressed patients are treated by psychiatrists, less depressed patients by psychologists or nonphysician therapists, and least depressed patients by primary care physicians in both prepaid and fee-for-service systems of care. Furthermore, patients of primary care physicians were sick enough to warrant treatment and had an average of 13 different symptoms of depression in the year before the study; 75% had recurrent depression. Patients whose depression was diagnosed by general practitioners were only slightly more depressed (characterized by one symptom) than those whose depression was not diagnosed. This study reinforces the importance of improving clinical detection of depressive disorders by general practitioners, especially by primary care providers who serve as referral "gatekeepers" to specialty care in prepaid systems of health care.   ■

Wells M, Burnham A, Camp P: Severity of depression in prepaid and fee-for-service general medical and mental health specialty practices, *Med Care* 33(4): 350, 1995.

Another hypothesis advanced to explain the etiology of affective disorders is the **permissive hypothesis.** It implicates reduced concentrations of serotonin as the predisposing factor in patients with affective disorders. Depression results from decreases in both the serotonin and catecholamine levels, whereas mania results from increased catecholamine but decreased serotonin levels. The permissive hypothesis is illustrated in Fig. 14-2.

A new leading theory attempting to explain the etiology of affective disorders is the **dysregulation hypothesis.** It is essentially a reformulation of the biogenic amine hypothesis. It views depression and affective disorders not simply in terms of decreased or increased catecholamine activity but as a failure of the regulation of these systems.

The drug categories most commonly used in the treatment of affective disorders are TCAs, tetracyclic antidepressants, SSRIs, and MAOIs.

CYCLIC ANTIDEPRESSANTS

Within the cyclic antidepressant drug class there are agents that have a tricyclic chemical structure and those that have a tetracyclic structure. Although they are different structurally, they are similar pharmacologically and therapeutically.

Mechanism of Action

Cyclic antidepressants (tricyclics and tetracyclics) are believed to work by correcting the imbalance in the neurotransmitter concentrations at the nerve endings in the

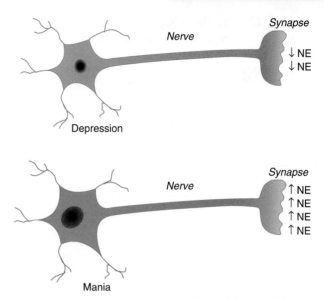

Fig. 14-1 Biogenic amine hypothesis. *NE,* Norepinephrine.

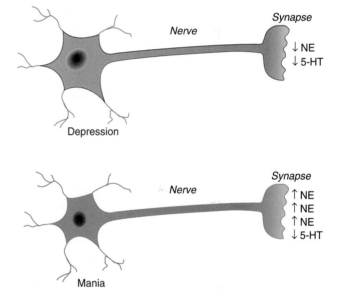

Fig. 14-2 Permissive hypothesis. *NE,* Norepinephrine; *5-HT,* serotonin.

CNS (the biogenic amine hypothesis). This is accomplished by blocking the reuptake of the neurotransmitters and thus causing these neurotransmitters to accumulate at the nerve endings. (It stands to reason that if depression is the result of abnormally low concentrations of these neurotransmitters, then an agent like a cyclic antidepressant that causes the concentrations of neurotransmitters to increase at nerve endings should alleviate the depression.) Some also believe that these agents may help regulate malfunctioning nerves (the dysregulation hypothesis).

Drug Effects

Cyclic antidepressants have several advantageous therapeutic effects, but their use is also associated with many

Table 14-5 Cyclic Antidepressants: Therapeutic and Undesirable Drug Effects by Receptor Site

Blockade of:	Drug Effect*
Andrenergic receptors	Orthostatic hypotension, antihypertensive effects
Dopaminergic receptors	Extrapyramidal and endocrine side effects
Histaminergic receptors	Sedation, weight gain
Muscarinic receptors	Dry mouth, constipation, blurred vision, tachycardia, urinary retention, confusion
Norepinephrine reuptake	*Antidepressant*, tremors, tachycardia, additive pressor effects with sympathomimetic drugs
Serotonergic receptors	*Alleviation of rhinitis*, hypotension
Serotonin reuptake	*Antidepressant*, nausea, headache, anxiety, sexual dysfunction

*Italicized effects are the therapeutic ones.

Table 14-6 Cyclic Antidepressants: Adverse Effects

Body System	Side/Adverse Effects
Cardiovascular	Tremors, tachycardia, orthostatic hypotension, dysrhythmias
Central nervous system	Anxiety, confusion, extrapyramidal effects, sedation
Gastrointestinal	Nausea, constipation, dry mouth
Other	Blurred vision, urinary retention, weight gain, impotence

adverse effects. Both these advantageous and adverse effects can be explained by the functions of the various receptors these agents affect. As previously mentioned, the therapeutic effects of cyclic antidepressants result from their ability to inhibit the reuptake of norepinephrine and serotonin at the nerve endings, but they also block muscarinic, histaminergic, adrenergic, dopaminergic, and serotonergic receptors. This is responsible for their adverse effects. The therapeutic and undesirable effects as they relate to the receptors affected are presented in Table 14-5.

Therapeutic Uses

Cyclic antidepressants are used to treat depression. TCAs have been available for more than 40 years and are widely prescribed. Overall they have demonstrated a remarkable efficacy, and their side effect profiles are well established. They are also considerably less expensive than most of the newer agents, with many of them available in generic formulations. Imipramine and desipramine are probably the most widely prescribed of the TCAs. In addition, imipramine is used as an adjunct in the treatment of childhood enuresis (bed wetting), and clomipramine is useful in the treatment of OCDs. Besides their beneficial antidepressant effects, TCAs are useful as adjunctive analgesics. TCAs have also been used in the treatment of trigeminal neuralgia.

Side Effects and Adverse Effects

The most frequent undesirable effects of cyclic antidepressants are due to their effects on various receptors, mostly the muscarinic receptors. Blockade of these

receptors by TCAs results in many undesirable anticholinergic side effects and adverse effects, the most common being sedation, impotence, and orthostatic hypotension. Older patients have a tendency to suffer more from dizziness, postural hypotension, constipation, delayed micturation, edema, and muscle tremors. The various undesirable effects as they relate to body systems are listed in Table 14-6.

Toxicity and Management of Overdose

TCA overdoses are notoriously lethal. It is estimated that 70% to 80% of patients who die of TCA overdose do so before reaching the hospital. The primary organ systems affected are the CNS and cardiovascular system, and death usually results from either seizures or dysrhythmias. There is no specific antidote for TCA poisoning. Management efforts are aimed at decreasing drug absorption through the administration of multiple doses of activated charcoal. This process speeds up elimination by alkalinizing the urine to a pH of greater than 7.55. It also minimizes damage resulting from CNS and cardiovascular events by giving diazepam for the control seizures or antidysrhythmics for the control of dysrhythmias and provides basic life support.

Interactions

Adrenergics, when coadministered with cyclic antidepressants, may result in increased sympathetic stimulation. Anticholinergics and chlorpromazine taken with cyclic antidepressants may result in increased atropine-like effects. CNS depressants and cyclic antidepressants will have additive CNS depressant effects. MAOIs, when given with cyclic antidepressants, may result in increased therapeutic and toxic effects. Cyclic antidepressants can inhibit the metabolism of warfarin, resulting in increased anticoagulation effects.

Dosages

For the recommended dosages for selected tricyclic antidepressant agents, see the dosages table on p. 213.

DOSAGES Selected Cyclic Antidepressants

agent	pharmacologic class	dosage range	purpose
⊶ amitriptyline (Elavil, Endep)	Tricyclic antidepressant	**Adult** PO: 150-300 mg/day divided **Geriatric** PO: 100-150 mg/day divided	
amoxapine (Asendin)	Tetracyclic antidepressant	**Adolescent/Geriatric** PO: 10 mg tid, 20 mg HS **Adult** PO: 75-300 mg/day divided **Adult** IM: 20-30 mg qid	Depression
nortriptyline (Aventyl, Pamelor)	Tricyclic antidepressant	**Adolescent/Geriatric** PO: 50-150 mg/day divided **Adult** PO: 25-100 mg/day divided	

drug profiles

Cyclic antidepressants are very effective agents in the treatment of various affective disorders, but they are also associated with serious side effects. Therefore patients taking them need to be monitored closely. For this reason all antidepressants are only available with a prescription. Virtually all are rated as pregnancy category C agents, except maprotiline, which is classified as a category B agent.

There are many drugs in the cyclic antidepressant drug class. Within the drug category there are tertiary and secondary TCAs and tetracyclic antidepressants. These are also sometimes referred to as *first-generation antidepressants* because they were the first agents within the cyclic antidepressant drug class to be developed for this purpose. Box 14-1 lists the various cyclic antidepressants according to their respective categories.

⊶amitriptyline

Amitriptyline (Elavil, Endep) is one of the oldest and most widely used of all the TCAs. It is the prototypical tertiary-amine TCA and is also used in the treatment of various pain disorders such as trigeminal neuralgia. It has very potent anticholinergic properties, which can lead to many adverse effects such as dry mouth, constipation, blurred vision, urinary retention, and dysrhythmias. There are two combination products that contain amitriptyline: Limbitrol, which also contains chlordiazepoxide, and Eltrafon or Triavil, which also contains perphenazine. Amitriptyline is available orally as a 10-, 25-, 50-, 75-, 100-, and 150-mg tablet and intravenously as a 10-mg/ml injection. The commonly recommended dosages are given in the table above.

PHARMACOKINETICS

HALF-LIFE	ONSET	PEAK	DURATION
10-50 hr	45 min	2-12 hr	6-12 hr

Activity

amoxapine

Amoxapine (Asendin) is structurally similar to the neuroleptic drug loxapine and is one of the tetracyclic antidepressants. It offers some advantages over older drugs within the cyclic antidepressant class in that it primarily inhibits norepinephrine uptake and is less sedating than other TCAs. Disadvantages to its use are that it causes some of the side effects associated with neuroleptics, such as extrapyramidal side effects, tardive dyskinesia, and neuroleptic malignant syndrome. Amoxapine is only available orally as a 10-, 25-, 50-, 75-, 100-, and 150-mg tablet. The commonly recommended dosages are given in the table above.

PHARMACOKINETICS

HALF-LIFE	ONSET	PEAK	DURATION
8-30 hr	1-2 wk	2-6 wk	6-12 hr

nortriptyline

Nortriptyline (Aventyl, Pamelor) is one of the prototypical secondary-amine TCAs. It is only available orally as either a 10-mg/5 ml solution or as a 10-, 25-, 50-, and 75-mg tablet. The commonly recommended dosages are given in the table above.

PHARMACOKINETICS

HALF-LIFE	ONSET	PEAK	DURATION
18-90 hr	1-2 hr	7-8.5 hr	Variable

Cyclic Antidepressant Categories
BOX 14-1

TERTIARY TCAs
amitriptyline
doxepin
imipramine
trimipramine

SECONDARY TCAs
desipramine
nortriptyline
protriptyline

TETRACYCLIC ANTIDEPRESSANTS
amoxapine
maprotiline
mirtazapine

MONOAMINE OXIDASE INHIBITORS

MAOIs are highly effective antidepressants. They are useful clinically for the treatment of any type of depression but are especially useful for the atypical types such as those characterized by reverse vegetative symptoms (increased sleep and appetite) or by marked panic, phobic, or other anxiety symptoms. In general they are considered second-line agents for the treatment of depression that is not responsive to other pharmacologic therapies such as TCAs. Although MAOIs are effective in the treatment of these disorders, a serious disadvantage to their use is their potential to cause a hypertensive crisis when taken with a substance containing tyramine.

The available MAOI antidepressants phenelzine (Nardil) and tranylcypromine (Parnate) are nonselective inhibitors of both types A and B MAO. Type A is the predominant type of MAO in nerve endings. It preferentially metabolizes serotonin and norepinephrine. On the other hand, type B MAO is the primary type of MAO in the gastrointestinal tract and platelets. It metabolizes phenylethylamine and benzylamine. Dopamine and tyramine are metabolized by both types of MAO.

Mechanism of Action

MAOIs work by inhibiting the enzyme MAO, which is widely distributed in the body, especially in nerves, the liver, and lung tissue. MAO is responsible for inactivating many of the important neurotransmitters in our nervous system, in particular the biogenic amines dopamine, epinephrine, norepinephrine, and serotonin. The antidepressant activity of the MAOIs appears to be related to their inhibition of the MAO system, which in turn results in increased levels of epinephrine, norepinephrine, and serotonin at their storage sites in the nerves. The increased levels of these monoamines in the brain leads to a reduction in depression.

Drug Effects

By inhibiting the MAO enzyme system in the CNS of patients suffering from depression, amines such as dopa-

MAOIs: Adverse Effects
Table 14-7

Body System	Side/Adverse Effects
Cardiovascular	Orthostatic hypotension, tachycardia, palpitations, edema
Central nervous system	Dizziness, drowsiness, restlessness, insomnia, headache
Gastrointestinal	Anorexia, abdominal cramps, nausea
Other	Blurred vision, impotence, skin rashes

mine, serotonin, and norepinephrine are not broken down and therefore higher levels occur. This in turn alleviates the symptoms of depression. The MAOIs were discovered by chance. Research for new chemical derivatives of isoniazid for the treatment of tuberculosis revealed a group of new agents that had antitubercular activity. During clinical trials with these new derivatives, a consistent mood elevation in depressed patients with tuberculosis was noted. So besides their antidepressant effects, some of the older MAOIs have antibacterial effects as well.

Therapeutic Uses

As mentioned previously, MAOIs may be used for the treatment of any type of depression, but they are especially useful for the atypical types including for the treatment of depression that is not responsive to other therapies. However, because of their ability to cause a hypertensive crisis when they are taken with a substance containing tyramine, the MAOIs are generally considered second-line agents. This dangerous and potentially life-threatening condition is discussed with the MAOI interactions.

Side Effects and Adverse Effects

MAOIs are better than the TCAs from the standpoint of undesirable effects in that they produce very few serious effects. The most common cardiovascular effect is orthostatic hypotension. The various side effects and adverse effects that can occur with MAOIs are listed in Table 14-7.

Toxicity and Management of Overdose

Clinical symptoms of MAOI overdose generally do not appear until about 12 hours after ingestion. The primary signs and symptoms are cardiovascular and neurologic in nature. The most serious cardiovascular effects are tachycardia and circulatory collapse, and the neurologic symptoms of major concern are seizures and coma. Hyperthermia and miosis are also generally present in overdose. The recommended treatment is aimed at eliminating the ingested toxin and protecting the organ systems at greatest risk of damage— the brain and heart. Recommended treatments are gastric lavage, urine acidification to a pH of 5, and hemodialysis.

Food and Drink to Avoid When Taking MAOIs

14-8

Food/Drink	Examples
HIGH TYRAMINE CONTENT—NOT PERMITTED	
Aged mature cheeses	Cheddar, blue, Swiss
Smoked/pickled meats, fish, or poultry	Herring, sausage, corned beef, salami, pepperoni
Aged/fermented meats, fish, or poultry	Chicken or beef-liver pate, game
Yeast extracts	Brewer's yeast
Red wines	Chianti, burgundy, sherry, vermouth
Italian broad beans	Fava beans
MODERATE TYRAMINE CONTENT—LIMITED AMOUNTS ALLOWED	
Meat extracts	Bouillon, consomme
Pasteurized light and pale beer	
Ripe avocado	
LOW TYRAMINE CONTENT—PERMISSIBLE	
Distilled spirits (in moderation)	Vodka, gin, rye, scotch
American and mozzarella cheese	Cottage cheese, cream cheese
Chocolate and caffeine beverages	
Fruit	Figs, raisins, grapes, pineapple, oranges
Soy sauce	
Yogurt, sour cream	

Interactions

There is a wide variety of drug interactions that occur with MAOIs.

MAOIs are one of the few drug classes that are capable of interacting with food and leading to a severe reaction. In this case, food containing the amino acid tyramine is the primary culprit, and a hypertensive crisis is the reaction. It is essential for both the patient and the nurse to know the various foods and drinks that should be avoided, and these are listed in Table 14-8. Sympathomimetic agents can also interact with the MAOIs and together cause a hypertensive crisis.

A hypertensive crisis occurs in approximately 8% of patients on MAOIs. It is believed to occur when MAO inactivates gastrointestinal and liver tyramine, which then enters the bloodstream. (Tyramine is normally degraded by MAO in the intestines). The tyramine displaces presynaptic norepinephrine. This norepinephrine, in conjunction with the increase in the norepinephrine stored and released from nerve terminals through the actions of the MAOIs, becomes too much, and hypertension ensues. The chief complaints in such patients are severe occipital headache, stiff neck, flushing, palpitations, diaphoresis, nausea and vomiting, and elevated systolic and diastolic blood pressure. The blood pressure may in-crease abruptly and dramatically, usually within minutes of ingesting the food, beverage, or restricted medication (sympathomimetic agent). This may lead to hyperpyrexia (increased body temperature) and potentially to cerebral hemorrhage, stroke, coma, or death.

Once ingestion occurs, it is considered a medical emergency and immediate treatment should be sought. Patients should be given phentolamine, chlorpromazine, or nifedipine (Procardia), 10 mg sublingually. This is such a sudden and severe reaction that often patients are told they should always have nifedipine available in the event of inadvertent tyramine ingestion. The use of nifedipine sublingually has the potential to cause serious drops in blood pressure and consequently life-threatening adverse effects. Its sublingual use is strongly discouraged.

drug profiles

MAOIs are contraindicated in patients with the following conditions: cerebrovascular or cardiovascular disorders, pheochromocytoma, a known hypersensitivity reaction to them, and liver or renal dysfunction. MAOIs should also not be used in combination with adrenergic agents, tyramine-rich foods, or meperidine. All MAOIs are classified as pregnancy category C agents. Of the agents prescribed for the treatment of depression, phenelzine tends to be prescribed more frequently and tranylcypromine may be more activating (perhaps because of its structural similarity to amphetamine). They are equally effective, although most physicians lean toward a favorite.

Before the start of treatment with MAOIs, it is recommended that the baseline platelet MAO activity be determined. Subsequent measurements obtained after the patient has been started on the MAOI should then be compared with it to determine the change in activity. Measuring the percentage of inhibition during MAOI therapy helps in establishing a therapeutic dose. To achieve maximum benefit, the goal should be 85% to 90% inhibition.

Occasionally a TCA is combined with an MAOI in the treatment of depression refractory to treatment with a TCA alone or with some other agent. Typically this is done by giving an MAOI to a patient already taking a TCA, or the two may be started together at 50% of the usual dose of each. If a patient's depression is stabilized on an MAOI but the physician wishes to add a TCA, then there must be at least a 2-week washout period before the start of TCA treatment. Without this washout period, the patient might experience hyperthermia, delirium, convulsions, and coma.

phenelzine

Phenelzine (Nardil) is an MAOI that has been used for the treatment of affective disorders such as depression. In investigational studies it has also shown some effectiveness in the treatment of panic disorders. It is only available orally as 15-mg tablets. The commonly recommended dosages are given in the table on p. 216.

PHARMACOKINETICS

HALF-LIFE	ONSET	PEAK	DURATION
Variable	2 wk*	<6 wk	2 wk*

*Therapeutic effect.

tranylcypromine

Tranylcypromine (Parnate) is an MAOI used for the treatment of depression. It is structurally similar to amphetamine. It is only available orally as 10-mg tablets. The commonly recommended dosages are given in the table on p. 216.

PHARMACOKINETICS

HALF-LIFE	ONSET	PEAK	DURATION
2-3 hr	<2 hr	1.5-3 hr	3-10 days*

*To reach therapeutic effect.

Dosages

For recommended dosages for selected MAOIs, see the table on p. 216.

SECOND-GENERATION ANTIDEPRESSANTS AND SSRIs

Second-generation antidepressants are a group of newer antidepressant drugs that are generally considered superior to TCAs in terms of their side effect profiles but not from the standpoint of their overall efficacy or onset of action. The individual antidepressants that make up this group of agents are trazodone (Desyrel), bupropion (Wellbutrin), and the SSRIs fluoxetine (Prozac), paroxetine (Paxil), sertraline (Zoloft), fluvoxamine (Luvox), and citalopram (Celexa).

Two new antidepressants venlafaxine (Effexor) and nefazodone (Serzone) also block the reuptake of serotonin but have additive mechanisms of action. Nefazodone is believed to also block the reuptake of norepinephrine. It is unique in that its chemical structure is different than that of the other SSRIs. The chemical structure of venlafaxine is also different than that of the traditional SSRIs. Valafaxine's antidepressant activity is believed to be due to its ability to block the reuptake of serotonin, norepinephrine, and to a lesser degree dopamine. Venlafaxine is currently indicated for the treatment of depression.

The inhibition of serotonin reuptake seems to be the common mechanism of action for trazodone and SSRIs. Bupropion also seems to inhibit reuptake of serotonin and possibly norepinephrine. These newer antidepressants offer several attractive advantages over the traditional TCAs and MAOIs. They are associated with significantly less severe and fewer systemic side effects and adverse effects, especially those to which the elderly have little tolerance—anticholinergic and cardiovascular side effects. They are very safe and have very few drug-drug or drug-food interactions. It does, however, take approximately the same amount of time for them to reach maximum clinical effectiveness, approximately 4 to 6 weeks, as it does for the TCAs and MAOIs.

SSRIs were developed to slow or inhibit the reuptake of serotonin into presynaptic terminals (nerve endings) and thus to increase the levels of serotonin at the nerve endings. Sertraline in the most selective of the three agents in inhibiting serotonin as opposed to norepinephrine reuptake, and fluoxetine is the least selective. Fluoxetine is the only one that has an active metabolite. Fluoxetine along with its active metabolite has an elimination half-life of 2 to 4 days as opposed to a 1-day half-life for sertraline and paroxetine. The individual antidepressants that make up this group of agents are trazodone (Desyrel); bupropion (Wellbutrin and Zyban); and the SSRIs, including fluoxetine (Prozac), paroxetine (Paxil), sertraline (Zoloft), reboxetine (Vestra), fluvoxamine (Luvox), and citalopram (Celexa).

Mechanism of Action

A common feature of second-generation antidepressants is their ability to selectively inhibit serotonin reuptake while having little if any effect on norepinephrine or dopamine reuptake. There are some slight differences between trazodone, bupropion, and SSRIs. Trazodone, marketed in 1982, was the first of these agents to become available. It selectively inhibits serotonin reuptake and has negligible effects on norepinephrine reuptake. Bupropion seems to possess novel pharmacologic actions. It has very weak effects on norepinephrine and serotonin reuptake and also weakly inhibits dopamine reuptake. SSRIs are specific and potent inhibitors of presynaptic serotonin reuptake (reuptake of serotonin into the nerve endings).

DOSAGES MAOIs: Selected Antidepressant Agents

agent	pharmacologic class	dosage range	purpose
phenelzine (Nardil)	Monoamine oxidase inhibitor	*Adult* PO: initial dose, 45-90 mg/day divided, followed by 15 mg/day or qod	Depression
tranylcypromine (Parnate)	Monoamine oxidase inhibitor	*Adult* PO: 30-60 mg/day divided	

Drug Effects

The increase in serotonin reuptake causes increased concentrations of serotonin at nerve endings in the CNS, resulting in numerous functional changes associated with enhanced serotoninergic neurotransmission. This increased serotonin concentration in the CNS seems to lead to a decrease in rapid eye movement (REM) sleep. It also has a potentiating effect when given with opioid analgesics in that the increased serotonin concentration at nerve endings appears to work synergistically with the opioid analgesic in relieving pain.

A primary advantage of SSRIs over TCAs and MAOIs is that SSRIs have little or no effect on the cardiovascular system. The absence of substantial anticholinergic activity, alpha$_1$ adrenergic blocking activity, catecholamine-potentiating effects, and quinidine-like cardiotoxic effects appears to be the principal reason for the general lack of cardiovascular effects associated with SSRIs. They also seem to have very little if any effect on the cardiac conduction system. SSRIs also possess anorectic activity. This appetite-inhibiting action may result from the blocking of serotonin reuptake and the attendant increase in the serotonin concentration at the nerve endings.

Therapeutic Uses

Second-generation agents (trazodone, bupropion, and SSRIs) have been used to treat many affective disorders. Depression, bipolar affective disorder, obesity, eating disorders, OCD, panic attacks or disorders, social anxiety disorders, and myoclonus are only some of the many disorders that this highly effective drug class can be used to treat. Second-generation antidepressants have shown some beneficial effects in the treatment of various substance abuse problems such as alcohol dependence.

Side Effects and Adverse Effects

Second-generation antidepressants offer an advantage over TCAs and MAOIs in that their side effect and adverse effect profiles are very clean. Second-generation antidepressants, especially SSRIs, are associated with very few serious undesirable effects. The various side effects and adverse effects that can occur in patients taking second-generation antidepressants are listed in Table 14-9.

Interactions

Second-generation antidepressants are highly bound to plasma proteins such as albumin. When given with other drugs that are also highly bound to protein (warfarin and dilantin), both compete for binding sites on the surface of albumin. This results in more free, unbound drug and therefore a greater, more pronounced drug effect.

SSRIs have the capacity to inhibit cytochrome P-450. The cytochrome P-450 system is an enzyme system in the liver that is responsible for the metabolism of several drugs. Inhibition of this enzyme system results in higher levels of drugs because they accumulate rather than getting broken down to their inactive metabolites. This also prolongs the action of drugs metabolized by the cytochrome P-450 system. The two SSRIs fluoxetine and paroxetine seem to be more potent inhibitors of this enzyme system than sertraline. There is still controversy over whether the cytochrome P-450 system is inhibited. Many studies have shown that this event is minimal or even nonexistent. The most frequent and significant drug interactions are listed in Table 14-10.

To prevent the potentially fatal pharmacodynamic interactions that can occur between SSRIs and MAOIs, it is recommended that the SSRI be washed out (discontinued) for at least 5 weeks before the start of fluoxetine treatment and for 2 weeks before the start of sertraline or paroxetine treatment.

Dosages

For dosage information for selected second-generation antidepressants, see the dosages table on p. 218.

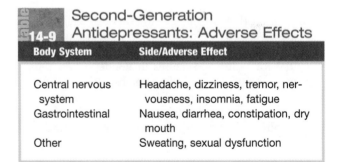

Table 14-9 Second-Generation Antidepressants: Adverse Effects

Body System	Side/Adverse Effect
Central nervous system	Headache, dizziness, tremor, nervousness, insomnia, fatigue
Gastrointestinal	Nausea, diarrhea, constipation, dry mouth
Other	Sweating, sexual dysfunction

Table 14-10 Second-Generation Antidepressants: Drug Interactions

Drug	Mechanism	Result
carbamazepine	Decreases carbamazepine metabolism	Increased carbamazepine levels, carbamazepine toxicity, ocular changes, vertigo, tremor
MAOIs	Enhances serotonin activity	Hyperthermia, diaphoresis, shivering, tremor, seizures, ataxia, autonomic instability
TCAs	Increases TCA toxicity	Sedation, decreased energy, lightheadedness, dry mouth, constipation, elevated TCA levels
warfarin	Warfarin displaced from protein-binding sites	Increased warfarin effects

DOSAGES Selected Second-Generation Antidepressants and SSRIs

agent	pharmacologic class	dosage range	purpose
bupropion (Wellbutrin, Zyban)		*Adult* PO: 200-400 mg/day divided 150 mg/day for 3 days then 150 mg twice a day for 7-12 weeks	Depression Smoking
fluoxetine (Prozac)	Antidepressant	*Adult* PO: 20-80 mg/day divided	
paroxetine (Paxil)		*Adult* PO: 20-50 mg/day divided	Depression
sertraline (Zoloft)		*Adult* PO: 50-200 mg taken once/day	
trazodone (Desyrel)		*Adult* PO: 150-600 mg/day divided	

drug profiles

The second-generation antidepressants trazodone, bupropion, and the SSRIs have proved to be valuable additions to the antidepressant armamentarium. They are highly effective as antidepressants and are associated with very few serious side effects and adverse effects. They are considered first-line agents in the treatment of depression with symptoms of anxiety, depression with suicidal ideations, and patients unable to tolerate adverse reactions to other agents.

bupropion

Bupropion (Wellbutrin, Zyban) was originally approved by the FDA in 1985 but was withdrawn by the manufacturer because of its apparently high potential for inducing seizures in nondepressed patients being treated for bulimia. Subsequent investigations revealed the overall estimated frequency of seizures was approximately 0.4%, and the drug was reintroduced in 1989. Bupropion is a unique antidepressant in terms of both its structure and mechanism of action. It has no appreciable effect either on the uptake of serotonin or norepinephrine or on the activity of MAO. It does, however, have a modest effect on the blockade of dopamine reuptake.

A new sustained-release form of bupropion called Zyban has recently been approved as first-line therapy as an aid in smoking cessation treatment. Zyban is an innovative new treatment because it is the first nocotine-free prescription medicine to treat nicotine dependence.

Bupropion is contraindicated in patients who have shown a hypersensitivity reaction to the drug, those with a seizure disorder or who currently or in the past have suffered from anorexia nervosa or bulimia, and those currently on MAOI treatment. It is considered a pregnancy category B agent. It is avail-

able orally as 75- and 100-mg tablets and as 100- and 150-mg sustained release tablets. The commonly recommended dosages are given in the table above.

PHARMACOKINETICS

HALF-LIFE	ONSET	PEAK	DURATION
10-14 hr	Up to 4 wk*	3 hr	Weeks to months

*Therapeutic effect.

Activity

fluoxetine

Fluoxetine (Prozac) was the first SSRI marketed for the treatment of depression, becoming commercially available in 1988. Since that time, it has become the number one prescribed antidepressant in the United States and one of the most frequently prescribed of all drugs. It is contraindicated in patients who have shown a hypersensitivity reaction to it and in those taking MAOIs. Fluoxetine is available orally as 10-, 20-, and 40-mg capsules, a 10-mg tablet, and a 20-mg/5 ml solution. The commonly recommended dosages are given in the table above. Pregnancy category B.

PHARMACOKINETICS

HALF-LIFE	ONSET	PEAK	DURATION
1-3 days	1-4 wk*	6-8 hr	Unknown

*Therapeutic effect.

paroxetine

Paroxetine (Paxil) is another SSRI antidepressant agent and is the newest of the SSRIs. It is contraindicated in patients who have shown a hypersensitivity reaction to it and those taking MAOIs. Paroxetine is available orally as a 10-, 20-, 30-mg, and 40-mg film-coated tablet. The commonly recommended dosages are given in the table above. Pregnancy category B.

PHARMACOKINETICS

HALF-LIFE	ONSET	PEAK	DURATION
14 hr	1-4 wk*	5-8 hr	Unknown

*Therapeutic effect.

sertraline

Sertraline (Zoloft) is another SSRI antidepressant agent. Of the three SSRIs discussed here, sertraline is the most selective in inhibiting serotonin reuptake and has very little effect on the inhibition of the cytochrome P-450 enzyme system in the liver. It also has no metabolites with clinically significant activity. It is contraindicated in patients who have shown a hypersensitivity to it and those taking MAOIs. Sertraline is available orally as 25-, 50-, and 100-mg tablets. The commonly recommended dosages are given in the table on p. 218. Pregnancy category B.

PHARMACOKINETICS

HALF-LIFE	ONSET	PEAK	DURATION
24 hr	1-8 wk*	6-8 hr	Unknown

*Therapeutic effect.

trazodone

Trazodone (Desyrel) was marketed in the United States in 1982. It was the first of the second-generation antidepressants that could selectively inhibit serotonin reuptake but that negligibly affected norepinephrine reuptake. One advantage of trazodone over TCAs is its minimal adverse effect on the cardiovascular system. It is, however, very sedating. This can be severe and impair cognitive function in the elderly. Trazodone has also rarely been associated with transient nonsexual priapism. This is reportedly the result of alpha-adrenergic blockade.

Trazodone's use is contraindicated in patients who have shown a hypersensitivity reaction to it. It is only available orally as 50-, 100-, 150-, and 300-mg tablets. The commonly recommended dosages are given in the table on p. 218. Pregnancy category C.

PHARMACOKINETICS

HALF-LIFE	ONSET	PEAK	DURATION
6-9 hr	1-2 wk*	2-4 wk*	Weeks*

*Therapeutic effect.

ANTIMANIC AGENTS

Clinical evidence indicates that the catecholamines (dopamine and norepinephrine) play an important pathophysiologic role in the development of mania. Serotonin also appears to be involved. The only drugs currently available that can effectively alleviate the major symptoms of mania are the lithium salts. A variety of medications may be used in conjunction with lithium to regulate mood or stabilize manic patients. Some of these adjunctive medications are benzodiazepines, carbamazepine, clozapine, dopamine receptor agonists, L-tryptophan, calcium channel blockers (CCBs), and valproate.

drug profiles

lithium

The antimanic effect of lithium is not fully understood. Results of studies indicate that lithium ions alter sodium ion transport in nerve cells, resulting in a shift in catecholamine metabolism. The therapeutic levels of lithium that are required are close to the toxic levels, but there is increasingly greater tolerance to these toxic levels during acute manic phases. For the management of acute mania a lithium serum level of 1.0 to 1.5 mEq/L is usually required. Desirable long-term maintenance levels range between 0.6 and 1.2 mEq/L.

Lithium carbonate (Escalith, Lithane, and Lithobid) and lithium citrate (Cibalith-S) are the two currently available salts of lithium. There are no absolute contraindications to lithium therapy, and the side effects and adverse effects are dependent on the serum levels. Levels exceeding 2.0 to 2.5 mEq/L produce moderate to severe toxicity. The most serious adverse effect is cardiac dysrhythmias. Other effects include drowsiness, slurred speech, epileptic-type seizures, choreoathetotic movements, and hypotension. Long-term treatment may cause hypothyroidism.

The concurrent use of thiazides, ACE-inhibitors, and CCBs increase lithium toxicity. Use with haloperidol can result in irreversible brain damage. Lithium is available as 150-, 300-, and 600-mg capsules; 300-mg tablets, 300- and 450-mg slow-release tablets; and a 300-mg/5-ml syrup. Lithium's recommended dosage is 600-1200 mg/day.

PHARMACOKINETICS

HALF-LIFE	ONSET	PEAK	DURATION
18-24 hr	7-14 days*	0.5-2 hr	2-24 hr

*Therapeutic benefit for controlling mania.

Activity

ANTIPSYCHOTIC AGENTS

Antipsychotic agents are used to treat serious mental illness such as bipolar affective disorder, depressive and drug-induced psychoses, schizophrenia, and autism. Antipsychotics are also used to treat extreme mania, certain movement disorders (e.g., Tourette's syndrome), and some medical conditions (nausea and intractable hiccups). Antipsychotics are also referred to as *tranquilizers* or *neuroleptics* because they produce a state of tranquility and work on abnormally functioning nerves.

Constituting about two thirds of all antipsychotics, phenothiazines are the largest group of antipsychotic drugs. However, like many drug discoveries, phenothiazines were discovered by chance, in this case during research for new antihistamines. In 1951 chlorpromazine was the first phenothiazine to be discovered in this way. Phenothiazines are associated with a high incidence of anticholinergic side effects because they are so closely related to antihistamines. Since the early 1950s, therefore, researchers have been working on developing phenothiazines with few side effects. Although phenothiazines can provide much relief to the mentally ill patient, they can also cause many undesirable side effects.

Phenothiazines can be divided into three groups based on structural differences: aliphatic, piperidine, and piperazine phenothiazines. Besides the phenothiazine antipsychotics, there are four other categories of drugs that are commonly used to treat mental illness: thioxanthenes, butyrophenones, dihydroindolones, and dibenzoxazepines. The available neuroleptics or antipsychotics are listed in Table 14-11 according to their respective drug categories and comparative properties. Many of the therapeutic and toxic effects of the antipsychotics are the consequence of their chemical structures.

There is very little difference between traditional antipsychotics in their mechanisms of action; therefore selection of an antipsychotic is based primarily on the least undesirable drug side effect and the patient's type of psy-chosis. Of the currently available antipsychotic agents, no single drug stands out as either more or less effective in the treatment of the symptoms of psychosis. It should also be stressed that antipsychotic drug therapy does not provide a cure for mental illness but is only a way of chemically controlling the symptoms of the illness. These agents represent a significant advance in our treatment of mental illnesses, as borne out by the fact that the early treatment of mental illnesses (before the 1950s) consisted of such extreme measures as isolation, physical restraint, shock therapy, and even lobotomy.

Over the last 2 or 3 years a new class of antipsychotic medications has evolved. They are referred to as *atypical antipsychotics,* and they differ from neuroleptics in both their mechanisms of action and their side effect profiles. Some of these newer atypical antipsychotics include clozopine (Clozaril), risperidone (Risperdal), venlafaxine (Effexor), olanzapine (Zyprexa), and quetiapine (Seroquel). Antipsychotics awaiting approval that show promise include ziprosidone and zotepine.

Mechanism of Action

All antipsychotics are believed to have a common mechanism of action. They are believed to block dopamine receptors in the brain and thus to decrease the dopamine concentration in the CNS. Specifically, phenothiazines block the receptors to which dopamine normally binds postsynaptically in certain areas of the CNS, such as the

Table 14-11 Antipsychotic Agents and Their Comparative Properties

Drug Name	Antipsychotic Potency	MG-MG Ratio*	Sedation	Anticholinergic	Cardiovascular	Extrapyramidal Symptoms
BUTYROPHENONES						
haloperidol	High	1:50	Low	Low	Low	High
DIBENZOXAZEPINE						
loxapine	Inter	1:10	Inter	Inter	Inter	High
DIHYDROINDOLONE						
molindone	Inter	1:100	Inter	Inter	Inter	Inter
PHENOTHIAZINES						
Aliphatic						
chlorpromazine	Low	1:1	High	High	High	Low
triflupromazine	High	1:20	Low	Low	Low	High
Piperidine						
mesoridazine	Low	1:2	High	High	High	Low
thioridazine	Low	1:1	High	High	High	Low
Piperizine						
fluphenazine	High	1:50	Low	Low	Low	High
perphenazine	High	1:15	Low	Low	Low	High
prochlorperazine	High	1:10	Low	Low	Low	High
trifluoperazine	High	1:20	Low	Low	Low	High
THIOXANTHENES						
chlorprothixene	Low	1:2	High	High	High	Low
thiothixene	High	1:50	Low	Low	Low	High

Low, Low incidence; *Inter,* intermediate incidence; *High,* high incidence.
*Compared with chlorpromazine.

limbic system and the basal ganglia. These are the areas associated with emotions, cognitive function, and motor function. This results in a tranquilizing effect in psychotic patients. Both the therapeutic and toxic effects of these agents are the direct result of the dopamine blockade in these areas.

The newer atypical antipsychotics mentioned previously block specific dopamine receptors called *dopamine-2[D2] receptors,* as well as specific serotonin receptors in the brain called *serotonin-2 [5-HT2] receptors.* The different mechanisms of action of the atypical antipsychotics are responsible for their improved efficacy and improved safety profiles.

Drug Effects

Antipsychotics have many effects throughout the body. Besides blocking the dopamine receptors in the CNS, they also block alpha receptors, which results in hypotension and other cardiovascular effects. Many of the adverse effects of these drugs stem from their ability to block histamine receptors (anticholinergic effects). They also block serotonin. This in combination with their ability to block dopamine receptors in the chemoreceptor trigger zone and peripherally, and with their ability to inhibit the vagus nerve in the gastrointestinal tract, accounts for the ability of certain antipsychotics to function as antiemetics. By blocking dopamine receptors in the brainstem reticular system they also have antianxiety effects. Most phenothiazines and haloperidol can also augment prolactin release, which can result in swelling of the breasts and milk secretion in women taking these agents.

Therapeutic Uses

As previously mentioned, the major therapeutic effect of antipsychotic agents is the result of blockade of dopamine receptors in certain areas of the CNS. These are the areas where regulation of dopamine activity tends to be dysfunctional, and this is one possible explanation for mental illness. There are certain areas of the brain where dopamine activity is abnormally increased and others where it is abnormally decreased. The antipsychotics attempt to reestablish dopamine pathways and other neu-rotransmitter systems and restore normal activity. The various areas within the CNS where antipsychotics have a major effect are listed in Table 14-12.

Side Effects and Adverse Effects

The side effects of the individual antipsychotic drugs are many and are important to remember. The antipsychotic agent with the least desirable side effect profile is often the agent that is used. This may vary from patient to patient. The common side effects caused by blockade of the dopamine, muscarinic, histamine, and alpha-adrenergic receptors are listed in Table 14-13.

These undesirable effects can also be classified according to the body system affected. Some of the most significant antipsychotic-induced reactions are agranulocytosis, hemolytic anemia, exfoliative dermatitis, and neuroleptic malignant syndromes. CNS effects include drowsiness, extrapyramidal reactions, and tardive dyskinesia. Ocular adverse effects include blurred vision, corneal lens changes, epithelial keratopathy, and pigmentary retinopathy. Cardiovascular effects include postural hypotension and changes in the electrocardiogram. The common side effects and adverse effects caused by antipsychotic drugs are listed in Table 14-14.

Low-potency antipsychotic agents generally have a low incidence of extrapyramidal symptoms (EPS) and a high incidence of sedation, anticholinergic side effects, and cardiovascular side effects. The opposite is true for high-potency antipsychotic agents. They have a high incidence of EPS and a low incidence of sedation, anticholinergic side effects, and cardiovascular side effects. This is illustrated in Table 14-11.

Interactions

Antacids can decrease antipsychotic absorption when taken together. Antihypertensives may have additive blood-pressure–lowering effects when taken with antipsychotics, and CNS depressants may have additive CNS-depressant effects when taken with antipsychotics.

Dosages

For recommended dosages for selected antipsychotic agents, see the table on p. 223.

Table 14-12 Major Dopamine Systems in the Brain

DA System	DA-Related Function	Effects of DA Receptor Blockade
Hypothalamic-pituitary	Regulates prolactin secretion, temperature, appetite, emesis	Increased prolactin levels resulting in galactorrhea, amenorrhea, and decreased libido; loss of temperature regulation, increased appetite, and antiemetic effects
Mesocortical	Regulates behavior	Therapeutic antipsychotic effects
Mesolimbic	Regulates stereotypical and other behaviors	Therapeutic antipsychotic effects
Nigrostriatal	Mediates function of the extrapyramidal motor system (EPS movement)	*Reversible:* Dystonia, pseudoparkinsonism, akathisia *Irreversible:* Tardive dyskinesia (must catch early to reverse!)

DA, Dopamine; *EPS,* extrapyramidal symptoms.

Antipsychotics: Receptor-Related Side Effects

Table 14-13

Receptor	Side/Adverse Effect	Drug Category
Alpha-adrenergic	Postural hypotension, lightheadedness, reflex tachycardia	Low-potency drugs
Dopamine	Extrapyramidal movement disorders, dystonia, parkinsonism, akathisia, tardive dyskinesia	High-potency drugs
Endocrine	Prolactin secretion (galactorrhea, gynecomastia), menstrual changes, sexual dysfunction	Low-potency drugs
Histamine	Sedation, drowsiness, hypotension, weight gain	Low-potency drugs
Muscarinic	Blurred vision, worsening of narrow-angle glaucoma, dry mouth, tachycardia, constipation, urinary retention, decreased sweating	Low-potency drugs

Antipsychotics: Adverse Effects

Table 14-14

Body System	Side/Adverse Effects
Cardiovascular	Orthostatic hypotension, syncope, dizziness, ECG changes, conduction abnormalities
Central nervous system	Sedation, delirium, neuroleptic malignant syndrome
Dermatologic	Photosensitivity, hyperpigmentation, rash, pruritus
Gastrointestinal	Dry mouth, constipation, paralytic ileus, hepatotoxicity
Genitourinary	Urinary hesitancy, urinary retention, impaired erection, priapism, ejaculatory problems
Hematologic	Leukopenia and agranulocytosis
Metabolic and endocrine	Galactorrhea, irregular menses, amenorrhea, decreased libido, increased appetite, polydipsia, impaired temperature regulation

drug profiles

Antipsychotics, or neuroleptics, are prescription-only medications that are indicated for the treatment of various psychotic disorders. Of the currently available agents, no single drug has stood out as being either more or less effective in the treatment of the symptoms of psychosis. All antipsychotics work through the same mechanism—blocking brain dopamine receptors. Some of the factors that should be considered before selecting an antipsychotic agent are the patient's history of a prior response to an agent and the desired side effect profile. It is also important to start with the lowest possible dose of an orally administered drug. There are many classes of drugs used to treat mental illness; however, as mentioned previously, the largest class and the agents most frequently prescribed are the phenothiazines.

PHENOTHIAZINES

chlorpromazine

Chlorpromazine (Thorazine) has strong anticholinergic and sedative effects and is a strong antiemetic. It is considered a low-potency neuroleptic agent, and therefore the associated incidence of extrapyramidal symptoms is low. The incidence of sedative, anticholinergic, and cardiovascular side effects is high, however. It is indicated for the symptomatic relief of nausea, vomiting, hiccups, and porphyria; for preoperative sedation; and for the treatment of psychotic disorders.

Chlorpromazine is contraindicated in patients who have shown a hypersensitivity reaction to phenothiazines and in those suffering from circulatory collapse, liver dysfunction, blood dyscrasias, coma, bone marrow depression, or alcohol or barbiturate withdrawal. It is classified as a pregnancy category C agent. It is available in oral, rectal, and IV dosage formulations. In the oral form it is available as 30-, 75-, and 150-mg extended-release capsules; 10-, 25-, 50-, 100-, and 200-mg tablets; a 10-mg/5 ml solution; and a 30- and 100-mg/ml concentrated solution. In its rectal formulation it is available as 25- and 100-mg suppositories. The parental form of chlorpromazine is available as a 25-mg/ml injection. The commonly recommended dosages are given in the table on p. 223.

PHARMACOKINETICS

HALF-LIFE	ONSET	PEAK	DURATION
PO: 6 hr	PO: 30-60 min	PO: Unknown	PO: 4-6 hr
PO-ER: 6 hr	PO-ER: 30-60 min	PO-ER: Unknown	PO-ER: 10-12 hr
PR: 6 hr	PR: 1-2 hr	PR: Unknown	PR: 3-4 hr
IM: 6 hr	IM: Unknown	IM: Unknown	IM: 4-8 hr
IV: 6 hr	IV: Rapid	IV: Unknown	IV: Unknown

fluphenazine

Fluphenazine (Prolixin) is available in three different salt forms, which give it varying degrees of antipsychotic potency. The decanoate and enanthate salt forms have the longest durations of action, and the hydrochloride salt form is fairly short in duration. Fluphenazine has the greatest potency of all

DOSAGES Selected Antipsychotic Agents

agent	pharmacologic class	dosage range	purpose
chlorpromazine (Thorazine)	Phenothiazine antipsychotic	*Adult* PO: 30-1000 mg/day divided IM: 25 mg followed by 25-50 mg in 1 hr *Pediatric* PO: 50-200 mg/day divided IM: ≤5 y/o, 40 mg/day divided 5-12 y/o, 75 mg/day divided	Psychotic disorders, mania, schizophrenia
clozapine (Clozaril)	Dibenzodiazepine antipsychotic	*Adult* PO: 330-900 mg/day divided	Management of psychotic symptoms in schizophrenic patients for whom other antipsychotics have failed
fluphenazine (Prolixin)	Phrenothiazine antipsychotic	*Adult* PO: 0.5-20 mg/day divided IM: 2.5-10 mg/day divided *Geriatric* PO: 1-2.5 mg/day divided	Psychotic disorders, schizophrenia
haloperidol (Haldol)	Butyrophenone antipsychotic	*Pediatric* PO: ≥3 y/o, 0.05-0.15 mg/kg/day divided *Adult* PO: 2-100 mg/day divided IM: 2-5 mg for prompt control	Psychotic disorders, control of tics, vocal utterances in Gilles de la Tourette syndrome, short-term treatment of hyperactive children showing excessive motor activity, prolonged parenteral therapy in chronic schizophrenia
loxapine (Loxitane)	Dibenzoxazepine antipsychotic	*Adult* PO: 20-250 mg/day divided	Psychotic disorders
molindone (Moban)	Dihydroindolone antipsychotic	*Adult* PO: 50-225 mg/day divided	Psychotic disorders
risperidone (Risperdal)	Benzisoxazole antipsychotic	*Adult* PO: 2-6 mg/day	Psychotic disorders
thiothixene (Navane)	Thioxanthene antipsychotic	*Adult* PO: 6-30 mg/day divided IM: 4 mg 2-4 times/day	Psychotic disorders, schizophrenia, acute agitation

the phenothiazines: 1 mg of the drug has the antipsychotic potency of 200 mg of chlorphenazine. It is primarily used to treat psychotic disorders and schizophrenia. It is considered a high-potency neuroleptic and is therefore associated with a high incidence of extrapyramidal symptoms; however, the associated incidence of sedative, anticholinergic, and cardiovascular effects is low. It is contraindicated in patients who have shown a hypersensitivity reaction to phenothiazines and in those suffering from circulatory collapse, liver dysfunction, blood dyscrasias, coma, bone marrow depression, or alcohol or barbiturate withdrawal. It is classified as a pregnancy category C agent. The two long-acting salt forms, decanoate and enanthate, are available as 25-mg/ml IM injections. The hydrochloride salt form is available orally as a 2.5-mg/5 ml elixir; a 5-mg/ml solution; and 1-, 2.5-, 5-, and 10-mg tablets. It is also available as a 2.5-mg/ml IM injection. The commonly recommended dosages are given in the table above.

PHARMACOKINETICS

HALF-LIFE	ONSET	PEAK	DURATION
PO: 15-16 hr*	PO (hydrochloride): 1 hr	PO (hydrochloride): 1.5-2 hr	PO (hydrochloride): 6-8 hr
IM: Up to 2 wk†	IM (hydrochloride): 1 hr	IM (hydrochloride): 1.5-2 hr	IM (hydrochloride): 6-8 hr
	IM (enanthate): 24-72 hr	IM (enanthate): Unknown	IM (enanthate): 1-3 wk
	IM (decanoate): 24-72 hr	IM (decanoate): Unknown	IM (decanoate): > or = 4 wk

*Following single dose.
†Following multiple IM injections.

THIOXANTHENES
thiothixene

Thiothixene (Navane) is a high-potency neuroleptic agent. Its use is associated with a high incidence of extrapyramidal symptoms but a low incidence of sedative, anticholinergic, and cardiovascular side effects. Thiothixene is primarily used for the treatment of psychotic disorders, schizophrenia, and acute agitation. It is contraindicated in patients who have shown a hypersensitivity reaction to it and in those suffering from circulatory collapse, liver dysfunction, blood dyscrasias, bone marrow depression, coma, narrow-angle glaucoma, or alcoholism. It is classified as a pregnancy category C agent. Thiothixene is available orally as 1-, 2-, 5-, 10-, and 20-mg capsules and as a 5-mg/ml solution. It is also available as a 10- or 2-mg/ml IM injection. The commonly recommended dosages are given in the table on p. 223.

PHARMACOKINETICS

HALF-LIFE	ONSET	PEAK	DURATION
PO: 34 hr	PO: Days to weeks	PO: Unknown	PO: Unknown
IM: 34 hr	IM: 1-6 hr	IM: Unknown	IM: Unknown

BUTYROPHENONES
haloperidol

Haloperidol (Haldol) is structurally different from the thioxanthenes and the phenothiazines but has similar antipsychotic properties. It is a high-potency neuroleptic agent that has a favorable cardiovascular, anticholinergic, and sedative side effect profile but can often cause extrapyramidal symptoms. Haloperidol is available in three salt forms: the base, decanoate, and lactate salt. Haloperidol decanoate has an extremely long duration of effect. It is used primarily for the long-term treatment of psychosis and is especially useful in patients who are noncompliant with their drug treatment. It is contraindicated in patients who have shown a hypersensitivity reaction to it, those in a comatose state, those taking large amounts of CNS depressants, and those with Parkinson's disease. It is classified as a pregnancy category C agent. It is available in an oral form as 0.5-, 1-, 2-, 5-, 10-, and 20-mg tablets and as a 2-mg/ml solution and an IV form in two injections for IM use: one, the long-acting decanoate salt, comes as a 50- or 100-mg/ml injection; the other, the lactate salt, comes as a 5-mg/ml injection. The commonly recommended dosages are given in the table on p. 223.

PHARMACOKINETICS

HALF-LIFE	ONSET	PEAK	DURATION
PO, IM: 13-35 hr	PO: 2 hr	PO: 2-6 hr	PO: 8-12 hr
x = 21 hr	IM: 20-30 min	IM: 30-45 min	IM: 4-8 hr
IM: 3-9 days*	IM: Unknown	IM: 1 mo	

*Decanoate salt form.

DIHYDROINDOLONES
molindone

Molindone (Moban) is a high-potency neuroleptic agent that is approximately 100 times more potent than chlorpromazine. Molindone, like the phenothiazines, blocks dopamine receptors in the brain. It is primarily used in the treatment of psychotic disorders and schizophrenia. Molindone is only available in an oral form as a 20-mg/ml solution and as 5-, 10-, 25-, 50-, and 100-mg tablets. It is a pregnancy category C drug. Its use is contraindicated in patients who have shown a hypersensitivity reaction to it, those in coma, and children. The commonly recommended dosages are given in the table on p. 223.

PHARMACOKINETICS

HALF-LIFE	ONSET	PEAK	DURATION
Variable	30-60 min	1.5 hr	24-36 hr

DIBENZOXAZEPINES
loxapine

Loxapine (Loxitane) is a tricyclic dibenzoxazepine-derivative antipsychotic agent. Like the phenothiazines, it is indicated for the treatment of psychotic disorders and schizophrenia. Loxapine is available for oral administration as a 25-mg/ml solution and as 5-, 10-, 25-, and 50-mg tablets. It is a pregnancy category C drug. Its use is contraindicated in patients who have shown a hypersensitivity reaction to it and those suffering from circulatory collapse, liver dysfunction, blood dyscrasias, bone marrow depression, coma, narrow-angle glaucoma, or alcoholism. The commonly recommended dosages are given in the table on p. 223.

PHARMACOKINETICS

HALF-LIFE	ONSET	PEAK	DURATION
PO: 4 hr	PO: 30 min	PO: 1.5-3 hr	PO: 12 hr
IM: 12 hr	IM: Unknown	IM: 5 hr	IM: Unknown

ATYPICAL ANTIPSYCHOTICS

There are a number of neuroleptics on the market. All show some efficacy for the positive symptoms of schizophrenia, and over time the improvement may even increase. These so-called *positive symptoms* are hallucinations, delusions, and conceptual disorganization. Unfortunately, neuroleptics are much less effective for negative symptoms. *Negative symptoms* are apathy, social withdrawal, blunted affect, and poverty of speech. It is these negative symptoms that account for most of the social and vocational disability caused by schizophrenia. Another drawback to traditional neuroleptics is that they all cause EPS, including rigidity, tremor, bradykinesia (slow movement), and bradyphrenia (slow thought). To summarize, neuroleptics such as haloperidol are effective for controlling symptoms, but not all symptoms, not in all patients, and not without serious side effects.

Between 1975 and 1990, there was not a single new antipsychotic drug approved in the United

States. Then in 1990 came the approval of clozapine (Clozaril), the first of the atypical antipsychotics. Clozapine was followed in 1995 by risperidone (Risperdal) and in 1996 by olanzapine (Zyprexa). These new agents—plus several more in clinical trials—are in the process of revolutionizing the treatment of psychosis and schizophrenia.

clozapine

Clozapine (Clozaril) is a unique antipsychotic agent. It is similar to loxapine in its chemical structure in that it is a piperazine-substituted tricyclic antipsychotic; however, pharmacologically it is different from all the currently available antipsychotics in terms of its mechanism of action. Because of these pharmacologic differences, clozapine is considered an atypical antipsychotic agent. Clozapine is believed to work on the serotoninergic, adrenergic, and cholinergic neurotransmitter systems in the brain. It also more selectively blocks the dopaminergic receptors in the mesolimbic system. Other antipsychotic agents block dopamine receptors in an area of the brain called the *neostriatum*, but blockade in this area of the brain is believed to give rise to the unwanted extrapyramidal symptoms. Because clozapine has very weak dopamine-blocking abilities in this area, it is associated with minor or no extrapyramidal symptoms.

Clozapine has been extremely useful for the treatment of patients who have failed treatment with other antipsychotic agents, especially those with schizophrenia. Patients taking clozapine must be monitored very closely for the development of agranulocytosis, which is a dangerous drug-induced blood disorder. The risk of agranulocytosis developing as the result of clozapine therapy is 1% to 2% after the first year; this compares with a risk of 0.1% to 1% for phenothiazines. Clozapine is only available in an oral form as 25- and 100-mg tablets. It is a pregnancy category B drug. Its use is contraindicated in patients who have shown a hypersensitivity reaction to it and in those with myeloproliferative disorders, severe granulocytopenia, CNS depression, coma, or narrow-angle glaucoma. The commonly recommended dosages are given in the table on p. 223.

PHARMACOKINETICS

HALF-LIFE	ONSET	PEAK	DURATION
6 hr	PO: 1-6 hr	Weeks	4-12 hr

risperidone

Risperidone (Risperdal) was the second atypical antipsychotic to receive FDA approval. It is even more active than clozapine at the serotonin (5-HT2) receptor. It is effective for refractory schizophrenia, including negative symptoms, and causes minimal EPS at therapeutic dosages (1-6 mg/day). After less

than 2 years, close to one fifth of all new prescriptions for antipsychotics are for risperidone. The FDA classifies risperidone as a pregnancy C agent. It is available as 0.25-, 0.5-, 1-, 2-, 3-, and 4-mg tablets and a 1-mg/1-ml solution. The use of risperidone is contraindicated in patients who have shown a hypersensitivity reaction to it. The commonly recommended dosages are given in the table on p. 223.

PHARMACOKINETICS

HALF-LIFE	ONSET	PEAK	DURATION
20-30 hr	1-2 wk*	Unknown	7 mo

*Therapeutic effects.

Other Atypical Antipsychotics

Olanzapine (Zyprexa) is a recent atypical antipsychotic to receive FDA approval. It too interacts with D2 and 5-HT2A receptors. Like clozapine it also has blocking action on a variety of other receptors such as other dopamine receptors besides D2 receptors, other serotonin receptors, alpha-1 receptors, and histamine receptors. Olanzapine is a thiobenzodiazepine derivative. It was designated 1S (new molecular entity) by the FDA and approved without advisory committee review.

A fourth atypical agent quetiapine (Seroquel) has been approved for the treatment of psychosis. Quetiapine is a dibenzothiazepine antipsychotic like clozapine but seems to be much safer. Quetiapine appears to have affinity for D2 and 5-HT2A receptors and an improved EPS profile. It also blocks histamine and alpha-adrenergic receptors.

All of these agents have a place in the treatment of schizophrenia. The lack of the traditional neurologic side effects is a tremendous benefit. It encourages the early use of antipsychotics when therapy is the most beneficial. Physicians have been very reluctant in the past to prescribe drugs early in therapy. With the evolution of the atypical antipsychotics, early therapy is not only possible but safe and well tolerated.

nursing process

• Assessment

Both the physical and emotional status of patients taking psychotherapeutic drugs need to be assessed. Often patients are so mentally distressed that their physical needs go unmet, resulting in a complexity of problems. Before therapy with any of the psychotherapeutic agents, the baseline values of all vital signs need to be documented. This includes postural (lying and standing) blood pressure readings so that the degree of a drop in blood pressure caused by medication effects can be identified and documented. It is also important to have liver and renal function studies performed before and during psychotropic drug therapy. These are especially important in patients on long-term therapy so that complications and potential toxicity can be prevented or identified early. The patient's level of consciousness (LOC), mental alertness, and potential for injury to self and others also need to be assessed and documented.

With any of these agents, the nurse should always check the patient's mouth to make sure he or she has swallowed oral doses. This can prevent possible hiding or hoarding of medications, which may lead to toxicity, overdose, or noncompliance. Use of liquid preparations, when available, may minimize such problems. Appetite, sleeping patterns, addictive behaviors, elimination difficulties, hypersensitivity, and other conditions and complaints also need to be watched for and documented.

When administering any of the antianxiety agents, first check the patient for the following:
- History of a hypersensitivity reaction to the agent, especially to benzodiazepines
- Chemical abuse
- Pregnancy
- Narrow-angle glaucoma
- Younger than 12 years of age (see Pediatric Considerations box, p. 205).

All of these situations are contraindications to the use of antianxiety agents (see Chapter 11).

Patients receiving these medications who have liver or renal disease or who are aged or in a debilitated state should be observed closely (see Geriatric Considerations box, p. 206). If patients are deemed elderly, weak, or debilitated, it is critical to document these findings and make safety a top priority in their nursing care. Laboratory studies that should be done before the start of anxiolytic therapy include a complete blood count (CBC) and lactate dehydrogenase, creatinine, alkaline phosphatase, and blood urea nitrogen (BUN) measurements. In addition, if you identify a drop in systolic blood pressure of 20 mm Hg or greater, you must inform the physician of this immediately.

The antidepressant agents most commonly used are either TCAs or MAOIs. TCAs are contraindicated in patients who have shown a hypersensitivity reaction to them, who are actively suicidal, or who are recovering from an MI. Cautious administration is recommended for patients with the following characteristics:
- History of benign prostatic hypertrophy
- Urinary retention
- Anemia
- Seizure disorder
- Psychosis
- Suicidal thoughts
- Narrow-angle glaucoma
- Liver dysfunction
- Renal disease
- Thyroid disease
- Heart block
- Elderly
- Children younger than 12 years of age

Patients with cardiac disease and the elderly may be at risk for cardiac disturbances associated with toxicity or overdose.

There are many cautions, contraindications, and interactions pertaining to the use of MAOIs (see Table 14-10 for drug interactions). Contraindications include hypersensitivity reactions, elderly age, and severe cardiac, renal, or hepatic disease. Patients receiving MAOIs who have a history of suicide attempts or suicidal ideations, or who have seizure disorders, hyperactivity, diabetes, or psychosis, should also be closely monitored. This pertains to pregnant women as well. Foods and beverages high in tyramine, such as cheese, beer, wine (especially red wines), soy sauce, meat tenderizer, figs, chicken liver, beef liver, bananas, avocados, yogurt, sour cream, and sherry, should be avoided because sudden and severe hypertension can occur when these are taken with an MAOI (see Table 14-7). Caffeinated beverages should also be avoided because of the hypertension and dysrhythmias that can develop.

With second-generation antidepressants, cautious use with close monitoring is recommended in patients who are pregnant, lactating, or elderly or who have diabetes. These agents should also be used cautiously in children. Drug interactions include the following: (1) MAOIs should *not* be used with these drugs, (2) increased side effects occur with those medications that are highly protein-bound, and (3) toxicity also occurs when these agents are given concurrently with lithium and carbamazepine. Alcohol and other CNS depressants should also be avoided. Some of the other newer second-generation antidepressants also include SSRIs (such as sertraline) and should be used cautiously in the same situations as listed previously with cautious use in patients with epilepsy or renal or hepatic disease. Drug interactions associated with SSRIs include MAOIs, cimetidine, diazepam, tolbutamide, warfarin, lithium, and benzodiazepines. If used with the SSRIs, MAOIs may result in fatal reactions. In addition, the herbal product St. John's Wort should not be used with these SSRIs (see Herbal Interactions box). Newer SSRIs that carry many of the same assessment concerns include reboxetine and citalpram.

Phenothiazines are the major group of antipsychotic agents and differ in their potency and side effects. Haloperidol is similar to other "high-potency" neuroleptics in that its sedating effects are low but the incidence of EPS is high. These include tremors and muscle twitching and result from the blockade of the dopamine receptors, which has an inhibitory effect on specific movements in the musculoskeletal system. Extrapyramidal movement disorders are manifested as parkinsonism-like motor disturbances and are very irritating and uncomfortable for the person experiencing them. Drug interactions for phenothiazines include antacids, antihypertensives, alcohol, and CNS depressants. Contraindications to these agents generally include hypersentitivity to the agent, liver dysfunction, blood dyscrasias, bone marrow suppression, and alcohol or barbiturate withdrawal. For home health and community points see the box on p. 227.

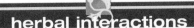

herbal interactions

St. John's Wort

BENEFIT OF HERB

Improves mood, relieves mild or moderate depression

POTENTIAL INTERACTIONS

Can cause confusion, agitation, muscle spasms, twitching; tremors with antidepressant use

CAUTIONS AND NOTES

Side effects include dizziness, increased sensitivity to sun, dry mouth; should be stored in cool, dry place away from light

home health/community points

Phenothiazines

- Tell patients that, if they experience dizziness, lightheadedness, or palpitations, they should inform the physician of this, and the problem should then be assessed. These symptoms may be indicative of postural hypotension and may be prevented by changing positions slowly, especially lying to sitting or standing. Encourage patients to sit on the side of the bed for a few minutes before standing.
- Patients should be informed that it may take up to 3 weeks before a therapeutic response occurs.
- Patients need to protect themselves from exposure to sun and avoid the use of tanning beds. Sunscreen should be used whenever there is a possibility for exposure to the sun, such as when going for a walk outdoors or working in the yard. This is to prevent "solar" erythema.
- Patients need to understand the importance of good and regular dental care to prevent infections and oral candidiasis related to drug-induced dry mouth.
- Patients should avoid temperature extremes such as swimming in cold water, walking in hot weather, and soaking in hot tubs because of the increased risk of hyperthermia leading to heat prostration or of hypothermia.
- Alcohol and alcohol-containing products, such as cough syrups, must be avoided because of the increased risk of CNS depression.
- Follow-up medical visits, therapy sessions, and follow-up laboratory studies to monitor therapeutic drug levels are to be encouraged and patients frequently reminded of this.

Quetiapine, a newer agent used for the treatment of psychosis, is much like the antipsychotic clozapine. Contraindications include hypersensitivity. Cautious use with close monitoring is recommended with children, with the elderly, during pregnancy, and lactation, and in patients with seizure disorders, breast cancer, or hepatic disease. Drug interactions include cimetidine, phenytoin, barbiturates, thioridazine, glucocorticoids, levodopa, and lorazepam. A thorough mental status examination should be performed and documented in the nurse's notes before initiation of the drug. An assessment of musculoskeletal functioning and monitoring for any EPS reactions is also important for safe drug therapy. Laboratory studies to be assessed before and during treatment include bilirubin and other liver function studies, CBC, and a urinalysis. Blood pressures, supine and standing, should also be assessed and documented. A drop of 30 mm Hg or more should be reported to the physician immediately. In addition, with the elderly the health care provider may order reduced doses, and antiparkinsonian agents may be indicated for prevention or treatment of EPS reactions.

Loxapine, molindone, and thiothixene (nonphenothiazine antipsychotic agents) are miscellaneous agents. Each is associated with contraindications, cautions, and drug interactions. Thiothixene is contraindicated in patients who have shown a hypersensitivity reaction to it, in those with blood dyscrasias or bone marrow depression, and in children younger than 2 years of age. It should be used with caution and the effects in patients showing adverse reactions; in women who are pregnant or lactating; and in patients with seizure disorders, high blood pressure, or hepatic or cardiac disease should be closely monitored. It is important to assess the patient's history carefully regarding cardiac disease because of the orthostatic hypotension and tachycardia these agents can induce, which are potentially life-threatening in the elderly patient. The patient's medication history and the current medications being taken should also be carefully noted because of the possible drug interactions that can occur.

There are also several important contraindications to and cautions concerning the use of nonphenothiazine agents. Loxapine and such agents are contraindicated in patients who have shown hypersensitivity reactions to them; in those suffering from blood dyscrasias, brain damage, bone marrow depression, or alcohol or barbiturate withdrawal; and in children. They should be used cautiously in pregnant or lactating women; patients with cardiac, seizure, or liver disorders; men with benign prostatic hypertrophy; and patients younger than 16 years of age.

Besides the same situations cited for loxapine, haloperidol (or butyrophenone) is also contraindicated in patients with Parkinson's disease, angina, urinary retention, or narrow-angle glaucoma. Haloperidol, as a butyrophenone, is also contraindicated in patients who take large doses of CNS depressants.

Drug interactions for which to assess with the use of lithium include thiazides, ACE inhibitors, and CCBs because these agents increase lithium toxicity. Irreversible brain damage is possible when lithium is used with haloperidol.

It takes about 3 weeks before therapeutic blood levels of lithium are reached, so patients should be closely watched before and during this time and given supportive care. Lithium is contraindicated in patients who have shown a hypersensitivity reaction to it; in those with renal disease, liver disease, organic brain syndrome, brain trauma, schizophrenia, severe dehydration, or cardiac disease; in pregnant or lactating women; and in children younger than 12 years of age. Cautious use is recommended in the elderly, in patients with endocrine disorders such as diabetes mellitus and thyroid disorders, and in those with a seizure disorder or urinary retention. Baseline urine laboratory studies should include measurement of the albumin, uric acid, and glucose levels and of the specific gravity. Baseline assessment of sodium intake and skin turgor is important because decreased sodium and fluid intake may lead to lithium toxicity, whereas increased sodium and fluid intake may lead to lithium loss. A baseline assessment of neuromotor functioning is also important because poor coordination, tremors, and weakness that arise after the start of therapy can be symptoms of toxicity.

Clozapine is contraindicated in patients with a hypersensitivity reaction to it, as well as patients with blood dyscrasias, CNS depression, coma, or narrow-angle glaucoma.

● Nursing Diagnoses

Nursing diagnoses appropriate to the nursing care of patients receiving any of the psychotherapeutic agents include the following:

- Disturbed thought processes related to impaired mental state.
- Impaired social interaction related to disease state and isolation from others.
- Risk for injury related to disease state and possible side effects of medications.
- Imbalanced nutrition, less than body requirements, related to influence of mental disorder.
- Disturbed sleep pattern related to mental illness or from drug therapy.
- Situational low self-esteem related to disease process and or side effects of medication.
- Urinary retention related to side effects of psychotherapeutic agents.
- Deficient knowledge related to lack of information about the specific psychotherapeutic drugs and their side effects.

● Planning

Goals related to the administration of psychotherapeutic medications include the following:

- Patient experiences no further deterioration in thought processes.
- Patient does not sustain injury while on medication.
- Patient exhibits improved nutritional status.
- Patient regains normal sleep patterns.
- Patient exhibits (overtly and covertly) a more positive self-image.
- Patient remains free of any alterations in urinary elimination patterns.
- Patient remains compliant with therapy.
- Patient is free of complications associated with the drug and with food and drug interactions.

Outcome Criteria

Outcome criteria related to the aforementioned goals include the following:

- Patient will demonstrate improved or no deterioration in thought processes and will be less hostile, withdrawn, and delusional once medication has reached steady state.
- Patient will demonstrate more open and appropriate behavior and communication with health care team and significant others.
- Patient will be free from falls, dizziness, and fainting attributable to side effects.
- Patient will show healthy nutrition habits with appropriate weight gain and a diet that includes foods from the USDA Food Guide Pyramid.
- Patient will report improved sleep patterns and feeling more rested.
- Patient will openly discuss feelings of poor self-image and self-concept with staff.
- Patient will report any problems with urinary retention.
- Patient will state the importance of taking medications exactly as prescribed at the same time every day and without omissions.
- Patient will state the importance of appointments with the physician or other health care providers to follow improvement and monitor therapy.
- Patient will state the common side effects of the medication as well as those adverse effects (e.g., confusion and changes in LOC) to be reported to the physician.
- Patient will list those medications and foods to be avoided while taking any psychotherapeutic medication.

● Implementation

Regardless of the psychotherapeutic agent prescribed, several general nursing actions are important to the safe administration of these agents. First and foremost is a firm (unless the patient is confrontational or aggressive) but patient attitude. Simple explanations about the drug and its effects as well as the length of time before therapeutic effects can be expected should be given. Vital signs should be monitored during therapy, especially in the elderly and in patients with a history of cardiac disease. The name of the drug, the dosage and route of administration, and more specifically, the patient's response should all be documented. Abrupt withdrawal of any of these medications should be avoided.

More specific nursing actions in patients taking anxiolytics include frequent checks of vital signs because of the orthostatic hypotension that can occur. Patients may be told to wear elastic compression stockings should orthostatic hypotension be problematic. Advise patients to change positions slowly, especially from a sitting or reclining position, and to avoid operating heavy equipment or machinery should sedation or drowsiness occur. The combination of psychotherapy and drug therapy is emphasized because patients need to learn and acquire more effective coping skills. Drug therapy alone is not as effective as it is when combined with psychotherapy. Patients should be reminded to keep anxiolytics and other medications out of the reach of children, and only small amounts of medications should be dispensed at any one time to minimize the risk of suicide attempts. Even though these agents have a wide safety margin, their simultaneous use with alcohol or other CNS depressants can prove fatal. When administering hydroxyzine intramuscularly, it is important to use a Z-track method to prevent tissue injury at the site of injection. Lorazepam is often administered intravenously as an adjunct to anesthesia; in this setting it should be administered with the proper diluent in equal amounts and infused at a rate of 2 mg or less over 1 minute. Lorazepam given intramuscularly should be given deep into a large muscle mass, such as the gluteus maximus.

Antidepressants must be administered carefully per the physician's order, and it is important for patients to realize that it often takes 1 to 3 and often 4 weeks before the therapeutic effects are evident. Careful monitoring of the patient and the provision of supportive care and therapy are important during this time. Make sure the patient understands this and continues to take the medication as prescribed. You may administer the oral forms with meals to prevent gastrointestinal upset. Sedation often occurs in patients taking TCAs. If this lasts more than 2 weeks and interferes with normal activities, the physician should be notified of the problem. When administering an antidepressant for the first time, especially to elderly or weakened patients, assist them with ambulation and other activities during which falls may occur as a result of drowsiness or postural hypotension. Encourage the patient to consume at least 2000 ml of water or other fluids a day and to increase his or her intake of bulk to try to counteract constipation. Sucking on hard candy or chewing gum is helpful for relieving the discomfort of dry mouth.

If a patient who has been taking TCAs is scheduled to undergo a surgical procedure, it is important to wean him or her off the medication a few days beforehand so that an interaction with the anesthesic agents does not occur; however, this is only done with a physician's order. During TCA treatment, it is important to recognize and document the occurrence of blurred vision, excessive drowsiness or sleepiness, urinary retention, or constipation and to consult and discuss this with the physician. It is also important to emphasize the need for the patient on long-term therapy to wear a medication ID bracelet or tag naming the agent being taken.

MAOIs are very potent antidepressants and are reserved for those patients who do not respond to TCA or other modes of therapy. The side effects of these agents are often severe, and these include orthostatic hypotension, dysrhythymias, ataxia, hallucinations, seizures, tremors, dry mouth, and impotence. Patients should be told to contact their physician should any of these occur. In addition, tachycardia, seizures, respiratory depression, mental confusion, and restlessness may occur as a result of overdose and can persist for several weeks. The onset of any of these symptoms should be reported to and discussed immediately with the physician. The desired antidepressant effects of MAOIs do not usually occur before 1 to 4 weeks after the start of therapy. Patients should be weaned carefully from these medications a few weeks before any surgical procedure.

Antipsychotic agents, mainly phenothiazines, can be administered orally or parenterally. The oral forms are well absorbed and will cause less gastrointestinal upset if taken with food or a full glass of water. Hard candy or gum may be used to relieve dry mouth. Perspiration may be increased, so patients should be warned about engaging in excessive activity or being exposed to hot or humid climates. Excessive sweating could lead to dehydration and then drug toxicity. You should contact the physician immediately should the patient exhibit tremors, uncontrollable movements of the tongue, muscle spasms, sore throat, or fever.

With the newer antipsychotic agent, quetiapine, the nurse should assist with ambulation until the patient has been stabilized on the medication. Patients should be taught to change positions slowly to avoid fainting caused by postural hypotension. Increasing fluids may help decrease constipation, and sips of water, candy, and gum may help with dry mouth.

Haloperidol is another antipsychotic agent that may take up to 3 weeks for the full therapeutic effects to occur. It may be given orally or intramuscularly. Its high protein binding characteristic may lead to toxicity as the result of slower metabolism and excretion.

Lithium is used mainly for patients who are in manic states, but its exact mechanism of action is unknown. Crucial to its safe use, however, is keeping the patient adequately hydrated and in a state of electrolyte balance because its excretion is decreased (therefore leading to increased serum levels) in the setting of hyponatremia. Patients who are dehydrated may also experience lithium toxicity.

Clozapine is available in oral forms, and dosages should be carefully checked, as with all medications. In addition, patients must be closely monitored for the development of agranulocytosis.

With all categories of psychotropic medications, patients should be aware of drug interactions and proper dosing. They also need to be receiving psychotherapy or counseling concurrent with the medications as per physician's orders.

Patient teaching tips for these agents are presented on p. 230.

● Evaluation

Both of the therapeutic effects of psychotropic medications and the patient's progress within the treatment regimen must be monitored. Mental alertness, cognition, affect, mood, the ability to carry out activities of daily living, appetite, and sleep patterns are all areas that need to be closely monitored and documented. In concert with the drug therapy, the patient must acquire more effective coping skills. Psychotherapy, relaxation therapy, and an increase in exercise can all help in this regard.

The therapeutic effects of anxiolytics are evidenced by improved mental alertness, cognition, and mood; fewer anxiety and panic attacks; improved sleep patterns and appetite; more interest in self and others; less tension and irritability; and less feeling of fear, impending doom, and stress. Adverse effects to watch for in patients taking anxiolytic agents include hypotension, lethargy, fatigue, drowsiness, confusion, constipation, dry mouth, blood dyscrasias, lightheadedness, and insomnia.

Evidence of the therapeutic effects of antidepressants, which may take 1 to 4 weeks before appearing, include improved sleep patterns and nutrition, increased feelings of self-esteem, less feeling of hopelessness, increased interest in self and appearance, increased interest in daily activities, and less depressive manifestations or suicidal thoughts and ideations. Adverse reactions consist of drowsiness, dry mouth, constipation, dizziness, postural hypotension, sedation, blood dyscrasias, and tremors. Overdose is evidenced by irritability, agitation, CNS irritability, seizures, and then progression to CNS depression with respiratory or cardiac depression.

MAOIs are very potent antidepressants, but therapeutic effects do not occur for up to 4 weeks after the start of therapy. These effects are similar to the ones produced by TCAs. Adverse effects include sedation, dry mouth, constipation, postural hypotension, blurred vision, seizures, and tremors. Toxic reactions are manifested by confusion or hypotension and possibly by respiratory or cardiac distress. The potential for drug-food interactions cannot be overemphasized because of the violent hypertension that can result when these agents are taken with foods and beverages high in tyramine.

The therapeutic effects of antipsychotic drugs (e.g., phenothiazines, nonphenothiazines, and quetiapine) should include improvement in mood and affect and alleviation of the psychotic symptoms and episodes. Emotional instability, hallucinations, paranoia, delusions, garbled speech, and inability to cope should begin to abate once the patient has been on the medication for several weeks. It is also critical to carefully monitor a patient's potential to injure himself or herself or others during the delay between the start of therapy and symptomatic improvement. It is also important to watch the patient for the development of adverse reactions to phenothiazines. These include dizziness and syncope stemming from orthostatic hypotension, tachycardia, confusion, drowsiness, insomnia, hyperglycemia, blood dyscrasias, and dry mouth. Overdose is manifested by excessive CNS depression, severe hypotension, and EPS such as dyskinesias and tremors. These symptoms should be reported immediately to the physician.

The therapeutic effects of haloperidol, another antipsychotic agent, are similar to those of the other agents, but you should monitor your patient for adverse reactions particular to haloperidol. These include sedation; ticlike, trembling movements of the hands, face, neck, and head; hypotension; and dry mouth. Overdose is manifested by severe sedation, hypotension, respiratory depression, and coma. It takes approximately 3 weeks for the therapeutic effects of haloperidol to appear, but it is still important to watch the patient for possible dyskinesia and trembling during this time. Should these occur, the nurse should consult the physician immediately to discuss possible actions.

Lithium's therapeutic effects are characterized by less mania, and it is during the manic phase that lithium is better tolerated by the patient. Therapeutic levels of lithium range from 1.0 to 1.5 mEq/L and should be determined frequently, every few days initially and then at least every few months while the patient is on the drug. You should also monitor the patient's mood, affect, and emotional stability. Adverse reactions to lithium include dysrhythymias, hypotension, sedation, slurred speech, slowed motor abilities, and weight gain. Gastrointestinal symptoms such as diarrhea and vomiting, drowsiness, weakness, and unsteady gait are indicative of overdose. The physician should be consulted immediately if these occur.

Patients taking clozapine should exhibit improvement in their schizophrenic state. In evaluating for adverse effects such as development of agranulocytosis, it is important to remember that it is associated with minor to no EPS.

patient teaching tips

Psychotherapeutic Agents

Anxiolytics and Antidepressants

➤ Patients taking antidepressants should be informed that it may take 2 to 4 weeks to notice the full therapeutic effects of the drug. Therefore some of these drugs remain in the body long after they have been discontinued.

➤ Inform patients to take medications as prescribed and that they are generally weaned off of these drugs.

➤ Take your medication exactly as prescribed by your physician. Do not skip or omit any doses and do not double up on the medication. If you remember you have not taken your medication and it is within an hour or 2 hours of the time you would have taken it, than go ahead and take the dose. If it is more than 2 hours after this time, skip that dose and take the medication at the next scheduled time.

➤ Keep medications out of reach of children.

➤ Change positions slowly to avoid fainting or dizziness. Call your physician immediately should you experience any fainting episodes while taking these medications.

➤ Do not suddenly stop taking this medication.

➤ If you experience drowsiness and sedating effects, do not operate heavy equipment or machinery.

➤ Avoid consuming alcohol and taking other CNS depressants.

➤ Do not take over-the-counter medication or any other medication without checking with your physician first to make sure this is okay.

➤ You may experience more drowsiness during the beginning of treatment. With the TCAs this should decrease after the first few weeks of therapy.

➤ You should contact your physician should you experience sores in the mouth, fever, sore throat, hallucinations, confusion, disorientation, shortness of breath, difficulty in breathing, yellow discoloration of the skin or eyes, or irritability.

➤ Caffeine and caffeinated beverages such as cola, tea, and coffee as well as cigarette smoking decrease the effectiveness of your medication.

➤ Keep all appointments and follow-up visits with your physician and other health care providers.

➤ Always carry or have about you a MedicAlert tag or bracelet naming the medication you are taking.

➤ The therapeutic effects of MAOIs may not occur for up to 4 weeks. Therefore do not alter your dosing if you are not feeling better before this time. Remember a hypertensive crisis may occur if you consume foods high in tyramine, foods such as cheese, beer, wine, avocados, bananas, and liver. Caffeinated beverages should also be avoided. Remember that the drug will remain in the body for up to 2 weeks after discontinuing the medication. Contact your physician should you experience chest pain, a severe throbbing headache, rapid pulse, or nausea.

➤ Avoid abrupt withdrawal.

Phenothiazines and Haloperidol

➤ Take all medications exactly as prescribed. Do not double, omit, or skip doses. Remember, it may be several weeks before an improvement is experienced.

➤ Phenothiazines may cause drowsiness, dizziness, or fainting, so change positions slowly.

➤ You should wear sunscreen when taking phenothiazines because of the photosensitivity they cause.

➤ Avoid taking antacids or antidiarrheal preparations within 1 hour of a dose of a phenothiazine.

➤ Notify your physician immediately should you note fever, sore throat, yellow discoloration of the skin, or uncontrollable movements of the tongue while taking a phenothiazine.

➤ Do not take phenothiazines or haloperidol with alcohol or with any other CNS depressant.

➤ Long-term haloperidol therapy may result in tremors, nausea, vomiting, or uncontrollable shaking of small muscle groups, and any of these symptoms should be reported to your physician.

➤ You may take the oral forms of these medications with meals to decrease GI upset.

➤ Avoid abrupt withdrawal.

Lithium

➤ Take your medication exactly as prescribed. Do not double, skip, or omit doses.

➤ It may take several weeks before you notice any improvement related to the drug therapy.

➤ You may take your medicine with meals to decrease gastrointestinal upset.

➤ If you become ill with vomiting or diarrhea or are unable to eat or drink, it is important that you notify your physician of this immediately. Dehydration of any type, even as the result of excessive sweating, may result in drug toxicity.

➤ Many of the side effects of lithium will disappear with time; however, you should contact your physician should you experience any excessive vomiting, tremors, weakness, or any involuntary movements.

➤ Make sure to keep your appointments, especially ones when blood is drawn to determine the serum lithium levels.

➤ Always wear a MedicAlert tag naming the agent you are taking.

➤ Keep the medication out of the reach of children.

➤ Avoid abrupt withdrawal.

POINTS TO REMEMBER

Psychosis

- Major emotional disorder; impairs mental function; person cannot participate in everyday life.
- Hallmark: loss of contact with reality.

Affective Disorders

- Emotional disorder characterized by changes in mood.
- Range from mania (abnormally elevated emotions) to depression (abnormally reduced emotions).

Anxiety

- A normal physiologic emotion.
- Six main types: obsessive-compulsive disorder, post-traumatic stress disorder, generalized anxiety disorder, panic disorder, social phobia, and simple phobia.

- Situational; arise because of specific events.
- Treat with drugs when markedly affects quality of life, relationships, or normal functioning.

Benzodiazepines

- Drug of choice.
- Most commonly prescribed; several advantages over other categories of drugs.
- Little effect on consciousness; very safe; do not interact with many other drugs.
- Most common ones are diazepam and lorazepam.

Flumazenil: Benzodiazepine Antagonist

- Blocks the benzodiazepine receptor; directly opposes the actions of the benzodiazepines.
- Used to reverse the sedative effects of benzodiazepines.

Selective Serotonin-Reuptake Inhibitors

- Second-generation antidepressants; newer anti-depressants.
- Generally considered superior to TCAs in terms of side effect and safety profiles.
- Specifically and potently inhibit presynaptic serotonin reuptake.

Antipsychotics, Tranquilizers, or Neuroleptics

- All terms used to refer to the drugs commonly used to treat serious mental illness.
- Used for bipolar affective disorder, psychoses, schizophrenia, and autism.

- Called *tranquilizers* because produce a stated of tranquility.
- Called *neuroleptics* because they work on abnormal functioning nerves.

Nursing Considerations

- Assessment of medication and drug history or use is critical to patient safety.
- All medications, including psychotherapeutic agents, must be taken *exactly* as prescribed.
- Avoiding alcohol and other CNS depressants is important to patient safety.
- Patients are to avoid illicit drugs and over-the-counter (OTC) products.

REVIEW QUESTIONS

1. One of your patients has been diagnosed with delusional thoughts and depression and has been placed on thioridazine (Mellaril) 25 mg tid. The physician wants to see how the patient responds to the medication. In assessing the patient for side effects of this medication, what would you mostly likely expect to see?
   a. Polyuria with gross proteinuria
   b. Hypertension with severe emesis
   c. Various anemias accompanied by bradydysrhythmias
   d. Gastrointestinal complaints accompanied by possible photosensitivity

2. A tricyclic antidepressant is sometimes ordered for depression. Patient teaching with these agents would include which of the following important points?
   a. Therapeutic effects may take up to 2 to 3 weeks.
   b. Alcohol is permitted with these agents, unlike other groups of antidepressants.
   c. The medication may be withdrawn without regard to weaning off of the medication.
   d. If a dose is missed, it is important for the patient to double up on the doses to maintain adequate blood levels.

3. Depression is a complex disorder that is manifested by other symptoms besides a change in mood. Tricyclics,

used to treat depression, may also help decrease which of the other manifestations of depression?
   a. Hepatitis
   b. Nephritis
   c. Anorexia
   d. Akathisia

4. Before patients begin taking thioridazine (Mellaril), they should be thoroughly assessed for which of the following drug interactions with associated rationale?
   a. Acetaminophen, because it enhances Mellaril's constriction on vessels
   b. Alcohol, because it vasoconstricts and would increase Mellaril's side effect of hypertension
   c. Beta-blockers because they will exacerbate the orthostatic hypotension associated with Mellaril
   d. Sodium warfarin (Coumadin), because it potentiates Mellaril's common side effect of hemorrhage

5. Which of the following, when administered with lithium, increases the risk of toxicity?
   a. Diuretics
   b. Lomefloxacin
   c. Calcium iodide
   d. Sodium bicarbonate

For Answers see www.harcourthealth.com/MERLIN/Lilley/.

CRITICAL THINKING Activities

1. What conditions would be responsible for decreasing the excretion of lithium from the body? Explain the impact of this decrease on the patient.

2. Mrs. Biggs has inadvertently been given too much lorazepam and is experiencing respiratory arrest. You have identified that use of the benzodiazepine reversal agent flumazenil is indicated. The dose called for is 0.2 mg delivered over 15 seconds, then another 0.2 mg if consciousness does not occur after 45 seconds. This is to be repeated at 60-second intervals as needed up to four additional times for a maximum total dose of 1 mg. Flumazenil (Romazicon) is available as a 0.1-mg/ml vial. What dose should you draw up into the needle to deliver 0.2 mg each time?

3. Mr. Hatchet has a psychotic disorder that has been controlled on chlorpromazine therapy (50 mg q4h) until recently, when severe anticholinergic side effects from the chlorpromazine a low-potency antipsychotic, have necessitated his being switched to haloperidol, a high-potency antipsychotic. The physician would like to know what the equivalent daily dose of haloperidol would be. What is the equivalent daily dose of haloperidol?

4. A 51-year-old patient arrives at the doctor's office for his annual physical. As the "intake" nurse, you do a brief assessment and take a short drug history. You note that he states that he has started taking St. John's Wort for depression and wants to know what the doctor thinks. You document this in the chart and research this information because you are not that familiar with the herbal products. Just what is St. John's Wort? Is it safe for patients to use for depressive symptoms? What information is important to remember about this herbal? What information is really crucial to share with patients in the future if they state that they are taking this supplement?

For Answers see www.harcourthealth.com/MERLIN/Lilley/.

bibliography

Albanese J, Nutz P: *Mosby's 2001 nursing drug reference and review cards,* St Louis, 2001, Mosby.

American Hospital Formulary Service: *AHFS drug information,* Bethesda, Md, 2000, American Society of Health-System Pharmacists.

Anderson PO, Knoben JE, Troutman WG: *Handbook of critical drug data 1999-2000,* ed 9, New York, 1999, McGraw-Hill.

Cooper G: Network briefs, *Family Therapy Networker* 21(5):15, 1997.

Johns Hopkins Hospital, Department of Pediatrics et al: *The Harriet Lane handbook,* ed 15, St Louis, 2000, Mosby.

Keen JH: *Critical care and emergency drug reference,* ed 3, St Louis, 1996, Mosby.

Mental health and pharmacy, *Drug Topics,* 9S-47S, April, 1997.

Mosby's GenRx: a comprehensive reference for generic and brand drugs, ed 10, St Louis, 2000, Mosby.

Preskorn SH: Recent pharmacologic advances in antidepressant therapy for the elderly, *Am J Med* 94(suppl 5A): 2S, 1993.

Skidmore-Roth L: *Mosby's 2001 nursing drug reference,* St Louis, 2001, Mosby.

United States Pharmacopeia: USPDI: *Drug information for the health care provider,* Rockville, Md, 2000, the Author.

Remember to check the **Online Worksheet** for additional learning opportunities: **www.harcourthealth.com/MERLIN/Lilley/**

Activity

Central Nervous System Stimulant Agents

objectives

When you reach the end of this chapter, you should be able to do the following:

1 Identify the various CNS stimulants.

2 Define the following terms: *analeptic, CNS stimulant,* and *methylxanthines.*

3 Discuss the mechanisms of action, indications, contraindications, cautions, side effects, and toxic effects of CNS stimulants.

4 Identify the variety of conditions and disorders being treated with CNS stimulants.

5 Develop a nursing care plan that includes all phases of the nursing process related to the patient receiving CNS stimulants.

www.harcourthealth.com/MERLIN/Lilley/

Look for this symbol for topics covered in the
Online Worksheet
Activity

drug profiles

amphetamine, p. 240
caffeine, p. 238
doxapram, p. 239
methylphenidate hydrochloride, p. 240
modafinil, p. 241
orlistat, p. 239
sibutramine, p. 240
sumatriptan, p. 241

Key drug.

glossary

Amphetamines (am fet' ə menz) CNS stimulants that produce mood elevation or euphoria, increase mental alertness and capacity to work, decrease fatigue and drowsiness, and prolong wakefulness. (p. 235)

Analeptics (an' ə lep tik) CNS stimulants that have generalized effects on the brainstem and spinal cord, which in turn produces an increase in responsiveness to external stimuli and stimulates respiration. (p. 235)

Anorexiants (an' o rek se ənt) Drugs used to control or suppress appetite. These also stimulate the CNS. (p. 235)

Attention-deficit hyperactivity disorder (ADHD) Syndrome affecting children, adolescents, and rarely adults. It is characterized by learning disabilities and behavioral problems. (p. 235)

CNS stimulants Drugs that stimulate a specific area of the brain or spinal cord. (p. 234)

Narcolepsy (nahr' ko lep se) Syndrome characterized by sudden sleep attacks, cataplexy, sleep paralysis, and visual or auditory hallucinations at the onset of sleep. (p. 237)

Serotonin agonists (ser' ə tō nin ag' ə nist) A new class of CNS stimulants used to treat migraines; they work by stimulating 5-HT$_1$ receptors in the brain and are sometimes referred to as *selective serotonin receptor agonists* (SSRAs) or *triptans.* (p. 235)

Sympathomimetic agents (sim' pə tho mi met' ik) Another name for CNS stimulants. (p. 234)

CENTRAL NERVOUS SYSTEM STIMULANTS

CNS stimulants are drugs that stimulate a specific area of the brain or spinal cord. Many of the actions mimic those of the sympathetic nervous system (SNS) neurotransmitters norepinephrine and epinephrine. For this reason they are sometimes referred to as **sympathomimetic agents.** CNS stimulants elevate mood, produce a sense of increased energy and alertness, decrease appetite, and enhance the performance of tasks impaired by fatigue or boredom. Two of the oldest known stimulants are cocaine and amphetamine. These are also the prototypical agents. Cocaine is a natural alkaloid that was first extracted from the plant *Erythroxylon coca* in the mid-nineteenth century but had been used by natives of the Andes for its stimulant effects for centuries before. Caffeine, which is contained in coffee and tea, is another plant-derived CNS stimulant.

CNS activity is regulated by a checks-and-balances system, which consists of both excitatory and inhibitory systems. CNS stimulation can result from either excessive stimulation of the excitatory neurons or blockade of the inhibitory neurons; however, most CNS stimulants act by stimulating the excitatory neurons in the brain. There are many such drugs, but only a few have therapeutic properties.

There are two ways to classify these therapeutic CNS stimulants. The first is according to their location of action in the CNS, and hence the site where they produce their therapeutic effects. The agents are listed in this way in Table 15-1. CNS stimulants may also be classified on the basis of structural similarities and are listed in this way in Table 15-2. However CNS stimulants are classified, their therapeutic applications are limited to five areas. They can be used as analeptics; as appetite suppressants; and for the treatment of **attention-deficit hyperactivity disorder (ADHD),** narcolepsy, and migraine headache.

Amphetamines produce mood elevation or euphoria, increase mental alertness and the capacity for work, decrease fatigue and drowsiness, and prolong wakefulness. They are used to treat narcolepsy and ADHD. Amphetamines produce tolerance and psychologic dependence. They are associated with a high abuse potential and are therefore classified as schedule II drugs under the Controlled Substances Act. Because of this high abuse potential, this class of CNS stimulants is used more frequently for nonmedical (recreational) purposes than for therapeutic ones.

Analeptics were used primarily to stimulate respiration when the natural reflex was lost. However, their use has waned as modern techniques of respiratory therapy have come available that can adequately ventilate a patient by mechanical means. In addition, respiratory paralysis caused by overdoses of opioids, alcohol, barbiturates, and general anesthetics can now be appropriately treated with reversal agents or by more reliable and effective methods of mechanical assistance.

Anorexiants suppress appetite and are used in the treatment of exogenous obesity. According to the National Institutes of Health and the Centers for Disease Control and Prevention (CDC), more than 30% of Americans are 20% or more overweight. At any given time, one third of women and one quarter of men are trying to lose weight. An estimated 60 million Americans are overweight with the incidence higher among women and minorities. Obesity increases the risk for hypertension, coronary artery disease, type 2 diabetes mellitus, gallbladder disease, sleep apnea, gout, and certain types of cancer. Some 300,000 deaths each year are attributed to obesity, making it the second leading cause of preventable deaths in the United States. The cost to society is around $70 billion annually, yet most people who attempt weight loss do so for cosmetic reasons, not for health reasons. Even health care professionals may have a prejudice against overweight people, often believing that the obese do not deserve medical treatment for their condition, and insisting that the patient lose weight before receiving treatment for other medical conditions (e.g., hypertension).

In 2000 the Food and Drug Administration (FDA) took steps to remove a sympathomimetic anorexiant, phenylpropanolamine (PPA), from the market. This action calls for the removal of all forms of PPA alone or in combination with other products. The FDA's Nonprescription Drug Advisory Committee (NDAC) used information from a recently published study as well as other data to support this decision. Their conclusion is that there is an association between the use of PPA and the incidence of hemorrhagic stroke.

Serotonin agonists, also referred to as *selective serotonin receptor agonists* (SSRAs), have made dramatic improvements in the treatment of migraine headaches. They have quickly become a standard for the initial choice of therapy for an acute migraine attack. Migraines, a common type of chronic headache, affect about 6 out of 100 people.

Table 15-1 CNS Stimulants: Site of Action

Site of Action	CNS Stimulant
Brainstem	Serotonin agonist
Cerebral cortex	Amphetamines
Hypothalamic and limbic regions	Anorexiants
Medulla and brainstem	Analeptics

Table 15-2 Structurally Related CNS Stimulants

Chemical Category	CNS Stimulant
Amphetamines	amphetamine, dextroamphetamine, methamphetamine, methylphenidate, pemoline
Serotonin agonists	naratriptan, rizatriptan, sumatriptan, zolmitriptan
Sympathomimetics	phentermine
Xanthines	caffeine, theophylline

legal & ethical principles

Handling of Prescription Drugs

It is important for the nurse to understand the following amendments to the federal laws and apply to the handling of all prescription drugs by the registered nurse (please note that these are summarizing statements and not the law in entirety):

The registered nurse is prohibited from doing the following:
- Compounding or dispensing the designated drugs for legal distribution and administration
- Distributing the drugs to any individuals who are not licensed or authorized by federal or state law to receive the drugs (e.g., those individuals outside the physician-patient relationship); the penalties for such actions are generally severe
- Making, selling, keeping, or concealing any counterfeit drug equipment
- Possession of any type of stimulant or depressant drug as authorized by law (as a patient)

It is important to adhere to these legal guidelines in the practice of drug administration to avoid legal penalties and possible loss of licensure or other staunch penalties. ■

Activity

Migraines most commonly occur in women and usually begin between 10 and 46 years of age. In some cases they appear to be hereditary.

Mechanism of Action

CNS stimulants have varying mechanisms of action and many effects on the CNS. Analeptics (aminophylline, theophylline, caffeine, and doxapram) have generalized effects on the brainstem and spinal cord and, as previously stated, tend to stimulate respiration. Methylxanthine analeptics (caffeine, aminophylline, and theophylline) work by inhibiting the enzyme phosphodiesterase. This enzyme breaks down a substance called *cyclic adenosine monophosphate* (cAMP). When the breakdown of cAMP is blocked, it accumulates. This results in the relaxation of smooth muscle in the respiratory tract, the dilation of pulmonary arterioles, and stimulation of the CNS. Caffeine can stimulate the CNS at almost any level depending on the dose. Its ability to stimulate areas in the CNS is greater than that of the other two methylxanthines. Doxapram's mechanism of action is similar to that of the three methylxanthines, but it has a greater affinity for the area of the brain that senses carbon dioxide content. When the carbon dioxide content of the blood is high, this stimulates the respiratory center in the brain to induce deeper and faster breathing in an attempt to exchange more oxygen for carbon dioxide.

Anorexiants are believed to work by suppressing appetite control centers in the brain, although this has yet to be proved scientifically. There are some minor differences between these agents in terms of their individual actions. Benzphetamine and mazindol resemble the amphetamines from the standpoint of their activity in the CNS, but diethylpropion has little effect on the cardiovascular system. Orlistat works by irreversibly inhibiting the enzyme lipase. This results in decreased amounts of ingested dietary fat absorption and increased fecal fat excretion. Sibutramine works by inhibiting the reuptake of serotonin (enhancing satiety) and norepinephrine (raising metabolic rate) centrally. Phentermine has very little effect on mood but does cause some cardiovascular stimulation.

As previously mentioned, amphetamines are used to treat ADHD and narcolepsy. These are very potent stimulators of the CNS, and therefore the abuse potential associated with their use is very high. Amphetamines increase the amount and the duration of effect of catecholamine neurotransmitters in the CNS responsible for stimulation, mainly norepinephrine and dopamine. The drugs used to treat ADHD and narcolepsy cause an increase in the release of these neurotransmitters and block their reuptake. As a result of this blockade, norepinephrine and dopamine are in contact with their receptors longer, and therefore their duration of action and effectiveness are prolonged. A novel new agent for the treatment of narcolepsy is modafinil. It is a nonamphetamine stimulant that works by decreasing GABA-mediated neurotransmission in the brain.

Drug Effects

Many of the effects of CNS stimulants are dose related. Their pharmacologic actions are similar to the actions of the SNS in that the CNS and the respiratory system are the primary body systems affected. The CNS effects most frequently noted are increased motor activity and mental alertness, diminished sense of fatigue, emotional or mood elevation, and mild euphoria. The respiratory effects most commonly seen are relaxation of bronchial smooth muscle, increased respiration, and dilation of pulmonary arteries. Other body systems can also be affected by CNS stimulants, including the cardiovascular, gastrointestinal, genitourinary, and endocrine systems. Often stimulation of these other body

---

research

OTC Drug for Migraines

In 1999 the FDA expanded the indications for Excedrin Migraine, an over-the-counter (OTC) drug produced by Bristol-Myers Squibb. This product contains 250 mg of acetaminophen, 250 mg of aspirin, and 65 mg of caffeine and has a new indication of "treats migraines." The label states that the drug is "for the temporary relief of mild-to-moderate pain associated with migraine headache." The entire range of symptoms often accompanying migraines is also listed, including severe pain, nausea, and sensitivity to light. Excedrin Migraine is the first FDA-approved OTC drug for migraine and its accompanying symptoms.

Table 15-3 CNS Stimulants: Common Adverse Effects

Body System	Side/Adverse Effects
Cardiovascular	Palpitations, tachycardia, hypertension, angina, dysrhythmias
Central nervous system	Nervousness, restlessness, jitteriness, anxiety, insomnia, headache tremor, blurred vision
Endocrine*	Hypoglycemia, hyperglycemia, increased metabolic rate
Gastrointestinal	Nausea, vomiting, diarrhea, abdominal pain, dry mouth
Genitourinary	Increased urinary frequency, diuresis

*Apply to methylxanthines, such as theophylline, only.

systems results in the unwanted effects, as discussed later.

Therapeutic Uses

The therapeutic effects of CNS stimulants are varied and best discussed from the standpoint of the individual drug category. The therapeutic effects of analeptics are limited to the relaxation of smooth muscle in the respiratory tract, dilation of pulmonary arterioles, and stimulation of areas within the CNS that control respiration, mainly the medulla and spinal cord.

Anorexiants primarily work by broadly stimulating the CNS. As mentioned previously, it is believed that their action specifically targets the appetite control centers in the brain, but this has yet to be proved. Some evidence points toward increased fat mobilization, decreased absorption of dietary fat, and increased cellular glucose uptake as other possible therapeutic effects.

The agents used to treat ADHD stimulate the areas of the brain responsible for mental alertness and attentiveness—the cerebral cortex and subcortical structures such as the thalamus. This results in increased motor activity and mental alertness and a diminished sense of fatigue.

Narcolepsy is a condition in which patients unexpectedly fall asleep in the middle of normal activity. Therefore an agent that can increase mental alertness would be most beneficial in treating a condition such as this, and that is what the amphetamines, the primary agents used to treat narcolepsy, do. The amphetamines' main sites of action in the CNS appear to be the cerebral cortex and possibly the reticular activating system. Stimulation of these areas also results in increased motor activity and a diminished sense of fatigue.

Other therapeutic effects are seen with CNS stimulants such as caffeine. Caffeine may induce diuresis and is a helpful agent in the treatment of migraines when coadministered with other drugs. It does this by increasing blood flow to the kidneys and decreasing the resorption of sodium and water. The constriction of the cerebral blood vessels that caffeine may induce also potentiates the action of the other agents given in combination with it. The constriction of cerebral blood vessels by SSRAs accounts for their beneficial effects in the treatment of migraines as well. However, the mechanism by which SSRAs do this is much different than that of caffeine.

Side Effects and Adverse Effects

CNS stimulants have a wide range of adverse effects that most often arise when these agents are administered at doses higher than the therapeutic doses. These drugs tend to "speed up" body systems. For example, effects on the cardiovascular system include increased heart rate and blood pressure. The most common undesirable effects associated with the administration of CNS stimulants are listed in Table 15-3 according to the body system affected.

Interactions

The drug interactions associated with CNS stimulants vary greatly from class to class. The drug interactions that occur with analeptics and anorexiants differ from those seen for amphetamines. Those drug interactions most commonly encountered for the three classes of CNS stimulants are listed in Table 15-4.

Dosages

The recommended dosages for selected CNS stimulants are given in the table on page 238.

CNS Stimulants: Common Drug Interactions

Drug	Mechanism	Result
AMPHETAMINES		
Beta-blockers	Increase alpha-adrenergic effects	Hypertension, bradycardia, dysrhythmias, heart block
CNS stimulants	Additive toxicities	Cardiovascular adverse effects, nervousness, insomnia, convulsions
Digoxin	Additive toxicity	Increased risk of dysrhythmias
MAOIs	Increase release of catecholamines	Headaches, dysrhythmias, severe hypertension
Tricyclic antidepressants	Additive toxicities	Cardiovascular adverse effects (dysrhythmias, tachycardia, hypertension)
ANOREXIANTS AND ANALEPTICS		
CNS stimulants	Additive toxicities	Nervousness, irritability, insomnia, dysrhythmias, seizures
MAOIs	Increase release of catecholamines	Headaches, dysrhythmias, severe hypertension
Quinolones	Interfere with metabolism	Reduce clearance of caffeine and prolong caffeine's effect
Serotonergic agents	Additive toxicity	Cardiovascular adverse effects, nervousness, insomnia, convulsions

DOSAGES Selected CNS Stimulants

agent	pharmacologic class	dosage range	purpose
amphetamine (Adderall)	CNS stimulant	*Pediatric 3-5 y/o* PO: 2.5 mg/day and increased weekly until desired effect	Attention-deficit hyperactivity disorder
		Pediatric ≥ 6 y/o PO: 5 mg 1-2 times/day and increased weekly until desired effect to a daily maximum of 40 mg	Attention-deficit hyperactivity disorder
		Adult PO: 5-10 mg tid ½-1 hr ac	Appetite control in obesity
caffeine (Nō-Dōz)	Xanthine cerebral stimulant	*Adult* PO: 100-200 mg q3-4h	Aids in staying awake
doxapram (Dopram)	Respiratory stimulant (analeptic)	*Adult/Pediatric > 12 y/o* 0.5-1 mg/kg IV as a single injection note to exceed 1.5 mg/kg, or infusion of 5 mg/min until desired effect, then reduced to 1-3 mg/min	Postanesthetic respiratory depression
		1-2 mg IV given twice at 5-min intervals then repeated at 1-2 hr intervals prn	Drug-induced respiratory depression
		Infusion 1-2 mg/min for up to 2 hr	Acute hypercapnia
methylphenidate (Ritalin)	CNS stimulant	*Pediatric ≥ 6 y/o* PO: 5 mg twice daily before breakfast and lunch and increased weekly until desired effect to a daily maximum of 60 mg	Attention-deficit hyperactivity disorder
		Adult PO: 20-60 mg/day divided in 2-3 doses 30-45 min ac	Narcolepsy
modafinil (Provigil)	CNS stimulant	*Adult* PO: 200 mg daily; up to 400 mg daily	Narcolepsy
orlistat (Xenical)	Lipase inhibitor	*Adult* PO: 120 mg three times a day with each meal containing fat	Appetite control in obesity
sibutramine (Meridia)	CNS stimulant (anorexiant)	*Adult* PO: 10 mg daily; up to max of 15 mg/day	Appetite control in obesity
sumatriptan (Imitrex)	Serotonin agonist	*Adult* PO: 25, 50, or 100 mg orally; can repeat after 2 hr (max 40 mg/daily) SC: 6 mg can repeat in 1 hr (max two injections/daily) IN: 5 or 20 mg, can repeat after 2 hr (max 40 mg/daily)	Migraines

drug profiles

ANALEPTICS

Most analeptic CNS stimulants are highly toxic and have a high abuse potential and are therefore only available with a prescription. Caffeine is the exception. The profiles for aminophylline and theophylline can be found in Part Six on respiratory system drugs.

caffeine

Caffeine (Nō-Dōz) is a CNS stimulant that can be found in OTC drugs and combination-prescription drugs. It is also contained in many beverages and foods. Just a few of the many foods and drugs that contain caffeine are listed in Box 15-1. Caffeine is contraindicated in patients with a known hypersensitivity to the drug and should be used with caution in patients who have a history of peptic ulcers or cardiac dysrhythmias or who have recently suffered an myocardial infarction (MI). Caffeine is available orally as 200- and 250-mg extended-release capsules and as 100-, 150-, and 200-mg regular-release tablets. It is available parenterally as a 250-mg/ml injection. Caffeine is considered a pregnancy category B drug. For the recommended adult and neonate dosages, refer to the table above.

PHARMACOKINETICS

HALF-LIFE	ONSET	PEAK	DURATION
3-4 hr	15-45 min	50-75 min	<6 hr

BOX 15-1 Caffeine-Containing Foods and Drugs

MEDICATIONS
Nonprescription medications
Analgesics
Anacin	32 mg/tablet
Excedrin	65 mg/tablet

Cold medications
Dristan AF	16.2 mg/tablet

Stimulants
NoDoz	100 mg/tablet
Vivarin	200 mg/tablet

Prescription medications (for migraines)
Fioricet	40 mg/tablet
Esgic	40 mg/tablet
Cafergot	100 mg/tablet

BEVERAGES
Coffee (brewed)	80-150 mg/5-oz cup
Coffee (instant)	80-150 mg/5-oz cup
Coffee (decaffeinated)	2-4 mg/5-oz cup
Tea (brewed)	30-75 mg/5-oz cup
Soft drinks	35-60 mg/12-oz cup
Cocoa	5-40 mg/5-oz cup

doxapram

Doxapram (Dopram) is another analeptic that is commonly used in conjunction with supportive measures to hasten arousal and to treat the respiratory depression associated with an overdose of CNS depressants (e.g., barbiturates, opioid analgesics, and general anesthetics), the acute respiratory insufficiency associated with chronic obstructive pulmonary disease (COPD), or respiratory depression in the postoperative recovery period that is not caused by skeletal muscle relaxants.

Doxapram is contraindicated in newborns because of the benzyl alcohol in the injectable formulation of the drug. It is also contraindicated in patients with epilepsy or other convulsive disorders, those who have shown a hypersensitivity reaction to the drug, those showing evidence of head injury, those suffering from cardiovascular impairment or severe hypertension, and patients who have had a cerebrovascular accident. It is only available parenterally as a 20-mg/ml injection. Doxapram is considered a pregnancy category B drug. For the recommended dosages, refer to the table on p. 238.

PHARMACOKINETICS

HALF-LIFE	ONSET	PEAK	DURATION
2-4 hr*	<30 sec	<2 min	5-12 min

*Metabolites: 4-8 hr.

ANOREXIANTS

The majority of anorexiants are CNS stimulants. Benzphetamine (Didrex), diethylpropion (Tenuate), and sibutramine (Meridia) suppress appetite control centers in the brain by elevating levels of neurotransmitters like norepinephrine, serotonin, and dopamine. Until recently the anorexiants were all closely related in chemical structure and mechanism of action. Orlistat is a promising new anorexiant that works by altering fat metabolism. Sibutramine and orlistat are the newest anorexiant agents and appear to offer advantages over older agents with respect to safety and tolerability.

orlistat

Orlistat (Xenical) is one of the newest anorexiants. It is unrelated to any of the other anorexiants in that it works by blocking the absorption of fat from the gastrointestinal tract. Orlistat binds to gastric and pancreatic enzymes called *lipases*. This binding results in inactivation of the enzyme, which prevents absorption of about 30% of dietary fat. Restricting dietary intake of fat to less than 30% of total calories can help reduce some of the gastrointestinal side effects. Flatulence with discharge, oily spotting, and fecal urgency can occur in 20% to 40% of patients. Decreases in serum concentrations of vitamins A, D, and E along with beta-carotene are seen as a result of the blocking of fat absorption. Supplementation with fat-soluble vitamins will correct this deficiency. Orlistat is available in 120-mg capsules. It is classified as a pregnancy category B agent. Recommended dosages are given in the table on p. 238.

PHARMACOKINETICS

HALF-LIFE	ONSET	PEAK	DURATION
16 hr	3 mo*	6-8 hr	Unknown

*Therapeutic effect.

sibutramine

Sibutramine (Meridia) is one of the newest anorexiants and is structurally related to amphetamine. It is approved for treatment of obesity, classified as a schedule IV controlled substance, and classified as a pregnancy category C agent. Sibutramine works by inhibiting primarily the reuptake of norepinephrine and serotonin. These neurotransmitters along with dopamine are elevated in the brain, resulting in decreased appetite.

The most common side effects are dry mouth, headache, insomnia, and constipation. As with the other amphetamines, some concerns exist over increases in blood pressure and heart rate increases. However, to date no heart valve abnormalities have occurred like those that led to removal of fenfluramine and dexfenfluramine (Redux) from the market. Another benefit is that patients taking

Activity

sibutramine have not developed primary pulmonary hypertension, which occurred rarely with some of the other anorexiants.

Sibutramine should not be used with other drugs that elevate serotonin, such as the SSRIs used for depression, SSRAs used for migraines, lithium, meperidine, fentanyl, dextromethorphan, pentazocine, or within 2 weeks of using an MAOI. It is contraindicated in patients who have shown a hypersensitivity reaction to it or in patients receiving MAOIs, patients who have anorexia nervosa, or patients taking other centrally acting appetite-suppressant drugs. Sibutramine is available as 5-, 10-, 15-mg tablets. Recommended dosages are listed in the table on p. 238.

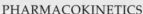

PHARMACOKINETICS

HALF-LIFE	ONSET	PEAK	DURATION
14-16 hr	8 wk	6 mo*	12 mo*

*Therapeutic effects.

AMPHETAMINES

As mentioned previously, the class of CNS stimulants used to treat ADHD and narcolepsy are the amphetamines, and they do so by increasing the amount and duration of effect of the catecholamine neurotransmitters. The overall response is global CNS excitement and stimulation, with improved mental alertness and attentiveness the therapeutic effect.

amphetamine

Amphetamine (Adderall and others) is the prototypical CNS stimulant used to treat ADHD, narcolepsy, and obesity. When used in the treatment of these conditions, it is only as an adjunct to psychologic, educational, and social therapies. Its use is associated with a wide array of CNS effects, many of which are undesirable or unintended. It is for these reasons that many of the other anorexiants and the other drugs used to treat narcolepsy and ADHD were developed. Amphetamine is contraindicated in patients who have shown a hypersensitivity reaction to it as well as those with the contraindications that apply to the other CNS stimulants. It is available orally as 5- and 10-mg capsules and tablets. A mixture of amphetamine salts (dextroamphetamine sulfate, dextroamphetamine saccharate, amphetamine sulfate, and amphetamine aspartate) is known as Adderall. It is available in 5-, 10-, 20-, and 30-mg tablets. It, like many other CNS stimulants, is rated as a pregnancy category X drug; therefore its use should be avoided during pregnancy. It is a C-II controlled substance. For recommended dosages, refer to the table on p. 238.

PHARMACOKINETICS

HALF-LIFE	ONSET	PEAK	DURATION
7-14 hr*	30-60 min	<2 hr	10 hr

*pH <6.6.

methylphenidate hydrochloride

Methylphenidate (Concerta, Ritalin) has become the drug of choice for the treatment of ADHD and narcolepsy. Much attention of late has been focused on this CNS stimulant because of its dramatic effect in the treatment of ADHD, a condition that may affect adults as well as children. However, this heightened interest may have more to do with the better diagnosis and a growing awareness of the disorder than with the drug's particular attributes. Like the other CNS stimulants, its use should be considered adjunctive to psychologic, educational, social, and other remedial measures in the treatment of ADHD, narcolepsy, and weight loss. The side effect profile of methylphenidate is much less unfavorable than that of many other CNS stimulants. As a result of its relative safety, it can be used in more patients without as much concern regarding some of the more severe toxicities seen with other CNS stimulants. Overstimulation of the CNS (severe cardiovascular and nervous system complications) can still occur, but this is a much less common event. Methylphenidate is contraindicated in patients with a history of marked anxiety, tension, and agitation. It is also contraindicated in patients with glaucoma and in those with a known hypersensitivity to it. Methylphenidate is classified as a pregnancy category C drug. It is available orally as 5-, 10-, and 20-mg tablets and 10- and 20-mg extended-release tablets. For recommended dosages, refer to the table on p. 238.

PHARMACOKINETICS

HALF-LIFE	ONSET	PEAK	DURATION
1-3 hr	30-60 min	1-3 hr	4-6 hr

modafinil

Modafinil (Provigil) is indicated to improve wakefulness in patients with excessive daytime sleepiness associated with narcolepsy. It is pharmacologically unrelated to methylphenidate, amphetamine, or pemoline. It has less abuse potential than amphetamine and methylphenidate. Modafinil appears to work indirectly by decreasing GABA-mediated neurotransmission. Some of the most common side effects are headache, nausea, nervousness, anxiety, and insomnia. It is available is 100- and 200-mg tablets. Modafinil is classified as a schedule IV controlled substance and as a pregnancy category C agent. Recommended dosages are given in the table on p. 238.

PHARMACOKINETICS

HALF-LIFE	ONSET	PEAK	DURATION
8-15 hr	1-2 mo*	2-4 hr	Unknown

*Therapeutic effects.

SEROTONIN AGONISTS

The serotonin agonists are a new class of CNS stimulants used to treat migraines. They often can produce relief from moderate to severe migraines within 2 hours in 70% to 80% of patients. They work by stimulating 5-HT$_1$ receptors in the brain and are sometimes referred to as *selective serotonin receptor agonists* (SSRAs) or *triptans*. This stimulation results in constriction of dilated blood vessels in the brain and decreased release of inflammatory neuropeptides. They are available in a variety of formulations from subcutaneous self-injections, oral formulations, and nasal sprays. A common effect of migraines is nausea and vomiting. Orally administered medications often are not tolerated in these individuals. Alternative formulations such as subcutaneous self-injections and nasal sprays are advantageous. They also are typically quicker in onset, producing relief in some patients in 10 to 15 minutes compared with 1 to 2 hours with tablets.

Currently four SSRAs are available: zolmitriptan (Zomig), naratriptan (Amerge), rizatriptan (Maxalt), and sumatriptan (Imitrex). Zolmitriptan, naratriptan, and rizatriptan are also known as *second-generation triptans*. Eletriptan is the next most likely SSRA to come to market, and alnitidan, almotriptan, and frovatriptan are all under development in the United States and in other countries.

Slight differences exist between these products. The most clinical experience has been with sumatriptan since it has been available the longest. Sumatriptan also has the most available dosage forms: subcutaneous injection, tablets, and nasal spray. Of the available oral SSRAs, zolmitriptan and rizatriptan have the most rapid onset of action. Rizatriptan is also available as a wafer that dissolves on the tongue (Maxalt-MLT). This may be advantageous for two reasons: (1) A migraine-related decrease in gastrointestinal motility reduces oral absorption of drugs. In addition, nausea, vomiting, and disabling pain make it difficult for patients to take certain formulations. (2) Sublingual absorption is typically quicker than oral administration. Naratriptan has the longest half-life and therefore may have the longest protection against recurrence of migraines.

sumatriptan

Sumatriptan (Imitrex) is indicated in the acute treatment of migraines. Sumatriptan is contraindicated in patients with ischemic heart disease, signs and symptoms consistent with ischemic heart disease, or Prinzmetal's angina. It is possible to experience a slight increase in blood pressure after administration, so it is also contraindicated in patients with uncontrolled hypertension. It should not be given to patients who may have underlying unrecognized coronary artery disease (CAD) without a thorough cardiac evaluation. It is also contraindicated in patients who are hypersensitive to sumatriptan or any of its active ingredients.

Sumatriptan has some important drug interactions. It should not be taken concurrently with an MAOI or within 2 weeks of discontinuing one. It should not be taken within 24 hours of an ergotamine-containing or ergot-like compound such as DHE or methysergide. Patients should not take other triptans for 24 hours after taking sumatriptan. Sumatriptan is available as 25- and 50-mg tablets, a 12-mg/ml injection, and a 5- and 20-mg nasal spray. It is classified as a pregnancy category C agent. Recommended dosages are given in the table on p. 238.

PHARMACOKINETICS

HALF-LIFE	ONSET	PEAK	DURATION
2.5 hr	0.5-1 hr	2.5 hr	4 hr

For orally administered sumatriptan.

pediatric considerations

Use of Ritalin

Children diagnosed with attention-deficit hyperactivity disorder (ADHD) generally have a variety of symptoms that lead to difficulty in social interactions. Now researchers have found that this disease may persist into adolescence and adulthood and that other disorders seem to correspond with ADHD, such as bipolar disorders. A long-standing controversy exists on the treatment of ADHD in children because the drug of choice, methylphenidate (Ritalin), is a CNS stimulant with concerning side effects. The controversy has been over the possible frequency of diagnosis and whether too many children are receiving the drug who may not need it. However, clinical trials continue to show the effectiveness of CNS stimulants in children with ADHD in reducing hyperactivity, impulsivity, and inattentiveness. The main concern for children with Ritalin is its possible toxicity characterized by agitation, confusion, delirium, seizures, and coma along with dysrhythmias and hypertension. On the other hand, depression, excessive tiredness, weakness, and bizarre behavior may be seen with drug withdrawal. Therefore it is important for caregivers to do the following:

- Always confirm the dosage and frequency.
- Be alert to toxicity.
- Seek medical advice when it appears that the drug is not working or if there are signs of toxicity.
- Always be sure that children or any patient goes through a "weaning" process before the drug is discontinued to prevent withdrawal.

From Goldman LS et al: Diagnosis of attention deficit/hyperactivity disorder in children and adolescents, *JAMA* 279:1100, 1998.

Activity

nursing process

• Assessment

CNS stimulants are most often used for the treatment of drug-induced or postanesthetic respiratory depression. These agents are also used for the treatment of ADHD with hyperactivity, as well as for the treatment of narcolepsy and exogenous obesity. Before administering these agents, you must carefully assess the patient and gather data from his or her nursing history regarding potential contraindications, cautions, and drug interactions. Also assess for the use of any herbal or OTC products that contain ephedra or ginseng. These agents also stimulate the CNS, and many complications may occur, such as seizures, palpitations, and dysrhythmias. Contraindications to the use of these medications include a hypersensitivity to them, seizure disorders, and liver dysfunction. Contraindications to doxapram include all of the foregoing plus hypertension and severe cardiac disorders. Vital signs, especially blood pressure in patients with a history of cardiac disease, should be assessed and the findings recorded for baseline purposes. The height and weight of children who are taking methylphenidate should be measured and recorded before therapy is initiated, and their growth rate should be plotted during therapy because this agent may retard growth. Patients need to be questioned about other medications they are taking, specifically whether they are taking MAOIs or vasopressors, antihypertensive agents, oral anticoagulants, tricyclic antidepressants (TCAs), or anticonvulsants. For patients with ADHD it is particularly important to assess thoroughly their vital signs, blood pressure, and pulse rate and rhythm. Typical behavior, attention span, and history of social problems or problems in school are also important to assess and document.

Sibutramine, a newer anorexiant similar to amphetamines, should not be used with other drugs that elevate serotonin, such as the SSRIs that are used to treat depression. SSRAs, used for migraines, as well as lithium, meperidine, fentanyl, and dextromethorphan are also contraindicated. Sibutramine should also be avoided within 2 weeks of using an MAOI. Sibutramine is also contraindicated in patients who have shown an allergic reaction to MAOIs, have anorexia nervosa, or are taking any other centrally acting appetite suppressant.

Orlistat is another new anorexiant used to treat obesity. It is the first drug in a new class of nonsystemically acting antiobesity agents to be used in patients with a body mass index (BMI) of 30 or more or if the BMI is 27 and the patient is also hypertensive or has high cholesterol or diabetes (a patient who is 5 feet 5 inches and weighs 180 lb has a BMI of about 30). Nutritional assessments and a physician's order would be needed with a concentration on the possibility that this medication may lead to a reduction of some fat-soluble vitamins (A, D, E, K) and beta carotene. Orlistat has become a popular agent for obesity because most anorexiant agents are systemic and increase the risk for addiction, pulmonary hypertension, valvular heart disease, and hypertension. However, this newer drug acts directly at the site of the lumen of the stomach and small intestine, decreasing the incidence of these adverse effects.

The serotonin agonists are a newer class of CNS stimulants and are commonly used in the treatment of migraines but not without concern for possible adverse reactions or for contraindications and drug interactions. Most of these agents are contraindicated in patients with a history of ischemic heart disease or in patients with symptoms consistent with ischemic heart disease or Prinzmetal's angina. Since an elevation in blood pressure may occur, even though usually only a slight elevation, these agents should not be used in patients with uncontrolled hypertension. Patients with CAD should not receive these serotonin agonists unless they have had a thorough cardiac evaluation and their use is approved. Drug interactions include MAOIs (serotonin agonists should not be administered within 2 weeks MAOI use), and these agents should not be taken within 24 hours of use of ergotamine-containing products or even DHE or methysergide. Other triptans should not be taken within 24 hours of taking sumatriptan.

• Nursing Diagnoses

Nursing diagnoses appropriate to patients taking CNS stimulants include the following:
- Imbalanced nutrition, less than body requirements, related to drug effects.
- Disturbed sleep pattern (decreased sleep) related to drug effects.
- Decreased cardiac output related to side effects of palpitations and tachycardia.
- Situational low self-esteem related to possible altered growth in children.
- Anxiety related to drug effects.
- Deficient knowledge related to lack of information about drug regimen.

• Planning

Goals associated with the use of CNS stimulants include the following:
- Patient maintains normal body weight and height.
- Patient continues normal growth and development while on medications.
- Patient experiences minimal sleep deprivation.
- Patient is free of cardiac symptoms and associated complications of drug therapy.
- Patient maintains positive self-esteem.
- Patient appears less anxious.
- Patient remains compliant to drug therapy.
- Patient remains free of complications related to antimigraine treatment.

Outcome Criteria

Outcome criteria related to the nursing care of patients receiving CNS stimulants include the following:

- Patient will maintain normal body weight and height (if pediatric patient, will continue normal growth and development patterns with weight and height falling within normal limits on growth chart) while taking CNS stimulants.
- Patient will show improved sensorium and level of consciousness with increased attentiveness.
- Patient will experience more restful sleep using non-pharmacologic measures.
- Patient's vital signs, specifically blood pressure and pulse, will be within normal limits.
- Patient will communicate feelings of self-image, self-esteem, anxiety, and anger as needed and openly.
- Patient will state symptoms (e.g., palpitations, chest pain) to report to the physician immediately.
- Patient will report a decrease in headaches.

● Implementation

Doxapram is administered intravenously (see the dosages table on p. 238) but at different doses (not to exceed 1.5 mg/kg) depending on the purpose. These infusions should be administered at the rate of approximately 1 to 3 mg/min for the reversal of anesthesia-induced respiratory depression and should not be mixed in alkaline solutions that include theophylline, thiopental sodium, and bicarbonate. 5% dextrose in water (D5W) is usually the diluent used with doxapram, and these solutions should be infused by means of an IV pump. Because patients' sensorium is generally diminished in this situation, placing them in a Sims' or semi-Fowler's position is necessary to prevent possible aspiration. If side effects occur, the infusion should be discontinued immediately and the physician notified.

Methylphenidate should be administered at least 6 hours before bedtime to diminish the insomnia it causes. Methylphenidate should also be given approximately 45 minutes before meals. Because dry mouth is an expected side effect, the patient should perform frequent mouth care, and sucking on hard candy or frequently sipping fluids may provide some relief. If the patient is taking the CNS stimulant for the treatment of obesity, a holistic approach should be used that includes exercise and dietary teaching, all under the supervision of a physician. A journal of responses to the drug therapy at home, play, and school is important in "charting" of the effectiveness of the drug for the child. In addition, counseling is generally a part of the treatment, with the family involved in goal setting for the treatment regimen. A journal to record any side effects—such as weight loss, hypertension, and changes in sensorium or affect—is also important to the progress of the patient.

Phentermine and other cerebral stimulants used for control of appetite should be given at least 6 hours before bedtime to avoid problems with insomnia. Most of these agents are usually given 30 minutes before meals, but the physician's orders should be followed. Gum, hard candy, and frequent sips of water may help decrease dry mouth. Patients should be encouraged to have follow-up visits with their physician since some of the newer agents (anorexiants) are recommended to be taken on a short-term basis.

When taking sibutramine, patients should be instructed about the fact that the therapeutic effects may take up to 8 weeks and peak effects will occur at about 6 months. Strict dietary instructions should supplement use with any anorexiant with special emphasis on the need for exercise with any weight-control program. Patients may also need approval from physicians before beginning exercise, especially if they are not used to a regular exercise program. With orlistat, patients need to be careful of dietary fat intake; restricting the intake of fat to less than 30% of total caloric intake may help in decreasing the occurrence of the gastrointestinal side effects. In addition, orlistat is to be taken with meals that contain fat. Supplementation with fat-soluble vitamins may be indicated.

Serotonin agonists come in a variety of dosage forms. Rizatriptan comes in a wafer that dissolves on the tongue, leading to rapid absorption even if the patient is experiencing nausea and vomiting, making oral administration undersirable. The nasal spray or self-injectable forms of the serotonin agonists are desirable especially in patients experiencing the nausea and vomiting that often occurs with migraine headaches. Oral forms are well tolerated but only if nausea and vomiting are not occurring. Self-injectable forms and nasal sprays also have the benefit of an onset of action of about 10 to 15 minutes as compared with 1 to 2 hours with tablet forms. Patient teaching should include instructions about the dosing. The subcutaneous injection for adults is not to exceed 12 mg/24 hr, the oral form is a maximum of 100 mg, and the nasal spray is one dose in one nostril with repeating of dose in 2 hours at 40 mg/24 hr. Also, foods containing tyramine should be avoided because tyramine is known to precipitate severe headaches. Tyramine-containing foods include beer, wine, aged cheese, food additives, preservatives, artificial sweeteners, chocolate, and caffeine. The patient will often complain of pain at the injection site along with a tingling, hot sensation, and burning at the site. A journal of headaches, precipitating factors, and response to drug therapy is also encouraged to properly follow the patient's progress.

Patient teaching tips for CNS stimulants are presented on p. 244.

● Evaluation

Therapeutic responses to agents used in the management of hyperkinesia include decreased hyperactivity, increased attention span and concentration, and improved behavior. The therapeutic response to agents used for the management of narcolepsy is the ability to remain awake. Anorexiants should cause the patient's appetite to decrease and weight loss to occur. You also need to monitor the patient for the development of adverse effects to these medications; these included mental status changes and changes in sensorium, mood, affect, and sleep patterns; physical dependency; irritability; and withdrawal symptoms such as headache, nausea, and vomiting.

Therapeutic effects of sibutramine include appetite control and weight loss for the treatment of obesity. Adverse effects of sibutramine include dry mouth, headache, insomnia, and constipation. Concerns also exist for increases in blood pressure and heart rate because of the similarity of structure to amphetamines or CNS stimulation. However, less concern exists about heart valve abnormalities, and the same concern does not exist with pulmonary hypertension as with previous anorexiants that were removed from the market (fenfluramine and dexfenfluramine). Therapeutic effects of orlistat, another new anorexiant but one that is a lipase inhibitor instead of a CNS stimulant, includes appetite control in obesity. Adverse effects mainly caused by the drug's action of inhibiting lipase include flatulence with discharge of an oily-type spotting and fecal urgency. The patient also needs to be closely evaluated for decreases in fat-soluble vitamins (A, D, E, and beta carotene) because these vitamins are affected by the decrease in absorption of fats.

Therapeutic responses to modafinil include a decrease in sleepiness associated with narcolepsy. Adverse effects for which to monitor with modafinil include headache, nausea, nervousness, and anxiety.

Therapeutic responses to the serotonin agonists include an improvement in the frequency, duration, and severity of migraine headaches with improved daily functioning and performance because of the decrease in headaches. Adverse effects for which to monitor include pain at the injection site (temporary in nature), flushing, chest tightness or pressure, weakness, sedation, dizziness, sweating, increase in blood pressure and pulse, and bad taste with the nasal spray formulation, which may precipitate nausea.

patient teaching tips

Central Nervous System Stimulants
➤ Patients should avoid other sources of CNS stimulants such as caffeine, which is found in coffee, tea, cola products, and chocolate.
➤ Patients should take their medication exactly as prescribed by their physician. They should not skip, omit, or double-up on doses.
➤ Patients should avoid taking OTC preparations unless they are approved by their physician. Herbal products, such as ephedra and ginseng, should also be avoided.
➤ Patients should not drink alcohol or consume any products that contain alcohol.
➤ Patients should keep a log of their daily activities.
➤ Patients should not stop taking these medications abruptly.
➤ Patients should take medication at least 6 hours before bedtime so as to decrease insomnia.
➤ If taking medication for treatment of obesity, patients should take it 30 to 45 minutes before meals.
➤ Patients should suck on hard candy, chew gum, or sip fluids to minimize dry mouth.

Serotonin Agonists
➤ Tyramine-containing foods should be avoided.
➤ Taking the exact dose and frequency with these medications is critical to their safe use.
➤ Instructions for dosing and dosage forms should accompany instructions to use a journal to record headaches, treatment, and results.

Appetite Suppressants
➤ Caffeine consumption should be decreased to avoid excessive CNS stimulation. Foods and beverages high in caffeine include chocolate, tea, coffee, and cola.
➤ OTC preparations should be avoided, unless physician contacted and patient advised, to avoid serious drug interactions.
➤ Patients should avoid alcohol consumption.
➤ Tapering of doses may be necessary before discontinuing medication to avoid adverse reactions from physical dependency.

POINTS TO REMEMBER

CNS Stimulants
- Drugs that stimulate the brain or spinal cord (e.g., cocaine and caffeine).
- Actions mimic those of the sympathetic nervous system (SNS) neurotransmitters norepinephrine and epinephrine.
- Also called sympathomimetic agents because they mimic the SNS neurotransmitters.

Amphetamines, Analeptics, and Anorexiants
- Family of CNS stimulants.
- Therapeutic uses: analeptics, appetite control, ADHD, and narcolepsy.

Amphetamines
- Elevate mood or produce euphoria; increase mental alertness and capacity for work.
- Decrease fatigue and drowsiness; prolong wakefulness.
- Treat narcolepsy and ADHD.

Analeptics
- Generalized effects on brainstem and spinal cord.
- Increase responsiveness to external stimuli and stimulate respiration.
- Treat respiratory paralysis caused by overdose of opioids, alcohol, barbiturates, and general anesthetic agents.

Anorexiants

- Control or suppress appetite; may also be used to stimulate the CNS.
- Work by suppressing appetite control centers in brain.
- Contraindications to use of CNS stimulants in a patient's history include hypersensitivity, seizure activity, convulsive disorders, and liver dysfunction.

Serotonin Agonists

- A newer class of CNS stimulants generally used to treat migraine headaches.
- Contraindications include CAD, Prinzmetal's angina, and ischemic heart disease.

Nursing Considerations

- Children who take methylphenidate should always have baseline height and weight recorded before initiating drug therapy and should continue to plot their height and weight in a journal during therapy.
- Therapeutic responses to agents used in treatment of hyperkinesia include decreased hyperactivity, increased attention span and concentration, and improved behavior patterns.
- Side effects to monitor for in individuals taking CNS stimulants include changes in mental status or sensorium, mood, affect, and sleep patterns; physical dependency, and irritability.
- Serotonin agonists may be administered subcutaneously, as a nasal spray, and as oral tablets.

REVIEW QUESTIONS

1. A patient with narcolepsy and obesity will probably be ordered to begin treatment with a CNS stimulant. Side effects that the patient may likely encounter include which of the following?
   a. Bradycardia
   b. Nervousness
   c. Mental clouding
   d. Drowsiness at night

2. One of your patients is to begin treatment with an anorexiant. Which side effect may be anticipated with this drug?
   a. Polyuria
   b. Irritability
   c. Bradycardia
   d. Drowsiness at all times

3. Patients being treated with anorexiants are most likely being treated for which of the following nursing diagnoses?
   a. Fluid volume deficit
   b. Fluid volume excess

   c. Altered nutrition: less than body requirements
   d. Altered nutrition: more than body requirements

4. Which of the following drugs cannot be administered with an amphetamine drug?
   a. Caffeine
   b. Estrogen
   c. Morphine
   d. Meperidine

5. Which of the following would alert the nurse to a possible contraindication or caution to the use of an anorexiant?
   a. Fatigue
   b. Overweight
   c. Questionable alcohol abuse
   d. Headaches 1 to 2 times per year

For Answers see www.harcourthealth.com/MERLIN/Lilley/.

CRITICAL THINKING Activities

1. HF is a 67-year-old man who has not resumed spontaneous breathing after surgery despite reversal of the nondepolarizing muscle relaxant given to him for the procedure. The anesthesiologist asks you to administer a 1.5 mg/kg bolus of doxapram followed by an infusion delivered at a rate of 2 mg/min. HF weighs 78 kg. The pharmacist delivers a 20-mg/ml vial of doxapram for injection and a 250-ml bag of doxapram for infusion, the concentration of which is 1 mg/ml.
   a. Calculate how many milliliters of the injection the patient should be given to accomplish the 1.5 mg/kg dose.

   b. What rate (ml/hr) should you set the pump at to deliver the 2-mg/min infusion of doxapram?

2. Narcolepsy has been diagnosed in Ms. Potter, a 68-year-old retired nurse, and she has been on a CNS stimulant for the past 6 months. Formulate a list of questions to ask her caregiver that will help to determine the effectiveness of her drug therapy.

3. Why would you, as a nurse practitioner, recommend or not recommend appetite suppressants for an adult who is obese?

For Answers see www.harcourthealth.com/MERLIN/Lilley/.

bibliography

Albanese J, Nutz P: *Mosby's 2001 nursing drug reference and review cards,* St Louis, 2001, Mosby.

American Hospital Formulary Serivce: *AHFS drug information,* Bethesda, Md, 2000, American Society of Health-System Pharmacists.

Anderson PO, Knoben JE, Troutman WG: *Handbook of critical drug data 1999-2000,* ed 9, New York, 1999, McGraw-Hill.

Facts and comparisons: Fax-stat on drugs 8(45):1, 1999.

FDA approves orlistat for obesity, Rockville, Md, USDHHS. Available at www.fda.gov/bbs/topics.

Johns Hopkins Hospital, Department of Pediatrics et al: *The Harriet Lane handbook,* ed 15, St Louis, 2000, Mosby.

Keen JH: *Critical care and emergency drug reference,* ed 3, St Louis, 1996, Mosby.

Kernan WN et al: Phenylpropanolamine and the risk of hemorrhagic stroke, *N Engl J Med* 343(25):1826, 2000.

Medical Letter: New "triptans" and other drugs for migraine, 40(1037), October 9, 1998.

Medical Letter: Orlistat for obesity, 41(1055), June 18, 1999.

Medical Letter: Sibutramine for obesity, 40(1022), March 13, 1998.

Medical Letter: Zolmitriptan for migraine, 40(1021), February 27, 1998.

Mosby's GenRx: a comprehensive reference for generic and brand drugs, ed 10, St Louis, 2000, Mosby.

Orlistat: A new option in weight loss, Available at www.pharminfo. com/pubs/msb/orlistat250.html.

Riley TN, DeRuiter J: New drugs review, *US Pharmacist,* October 1999, p. 129, 1999.

Sjostrom L et al: Randomized placebo-controlled trial of orlistat for weight loss and prevention of weight regain in obese patients, *Lancet* 352:167, 1998.

Skidmore-Roth L: *Mosby's 2001 nursing drug reference,* St Louis, 2001, Mosby.

Weitzel KW: Migraine: a comprehensive review of new treatment options, *Pharmacotherapy* 19(8):957, 1999.

Remember to check the **Online Worksheet** for additional learning opportunities: **www.harcourthealth.com/MERLIN/Lilley/**

Activity

Drugs Affecting the Autonomic Nervous System: Study Skills Tips

- PURR Application

PURR APPLICATION

Planning for the PART

The basic explanation provided for the PURR model in the Study Skills Tips for Part One demonstrates the application process as it relates to individual chapters. There is another application for the PURR model that can be very useful. This application encourages the learner to take a broader view of the assignment. In the case of this text, you have noticed that the chapters are grouped together into multiple chapter blocks called *parts*. Part organization is not some random process applied by the author to further complicate the subject. Part organization is a carefully thought-out process to put content together in a fashion that is logical and meaningful. Since the author has spent considerable time trying to link the chapters together in the most logical pattern, it is to your advantage as a student to learn to take advantage of the work already done for you.

Part Title

Begin the process of part planning by looking at the Part Three title, "Drugs Affecting the Autonomic Nervous System." Then look at the part structure. There are five chapters contained in Part Three. All these chapters must be concerned with the autonomic nervous system. Even before you have done any reading in any chapter, you are beginning to look for the links that will establish the relationship not only for the ideas in individual chapters, but also the broader link that connects the five chapters in this part with each other and with the ideas that have come in earlier parts and will follow in later parts.

There is a clear example in this part of the way in which parts relate to one another. Look back at Part Two, "Drugs Affecting the Central Nervous System." Clearly that part deals with some aspect of the nervous system as does this part. One learning objective you should establish for yourself is the relationship between these two parts. You must be able to define and explain *central nervous system* and *autonomic nervous system*. However, defining these and going on further limits the learning you can achieve. Ask yourself some additional questions that will help you establish a connection between these parts. "What is the difference in functions of the central and the autonomic nervous systems?" "Are there pharmacologic agents that have application in both the central and autonomic nervous systems?" The principle is to keep stressing the links that must exist throughout all the parts and chapters you are studying. The normal study pattern that most students apply is one that focuses on the individual chapters, but it is essential that the broader scope of chapter and part be maintained.

Part Chapters

After considering the part title and looking for relationships between the new part and past parts studied, the next step in applying the Plan step of PURR to a part is to spend a few minutes studying the chapter title and looking for the relationships that must exist. Part Three has five chapters, and there is a clear pattern in these chapters. Chapters 16 and 17 both contain the term *adrenergic.* Clearly the two chapters are dealing with the same broad topic. However, Chapter 16 covers adrenergic agents and Chapter 17 covers adrenergic-blocking agents. Apply questioning strategies at this point. "What does adrenergic mean?" "What is an adrenergic agent?" These two questions are essential in mastering the content of Chapter 16, and should be questions that you ask yourself almost without thinking. However, the next step is one that can greatly enhance your understanding when you start to read the material. This is a step that is easily overlooked. Notice that Chapter 16 deals with agents and Chapter 17 deals with blocking agents. There must be a difference between an agent and a blocking agent. Focus now with a few questions that will keep you aware that the content in Chapter 16 has a direct relationship to the content in Chapter 17. "What is the difference between an agent and a blocking agent? When is the pharmacologic application of an agent appropriate? Under what conditions should a blocking agent be chosen?" Then ask a question to help maintain the focus on the concept of the entire part. "What aspects of the autonomic nervous system are related to the adrenergic agents and blocking agents?"

Chapters 18 and 19

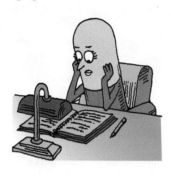

Once you begin to focus on the relationship of chapters within a part, certain things will begin to become apparent. Chapters 18 and 19 cover agents and blocking agents. These two chapters develop the concept as related to cholinergics, rather than adrenergics. But the same questions you used as a focus for Chapters 16 and 17 can be recycled in setting up the study of Chapters 18 and 19. Simply replace the term adrenergic with cholinergic and you are ready to begin reading these two chapters with a clear personal learning objective.

Active Questioning

This is the key concept to master in working through the process for planning your learning for an entire part rather than for single chapters. The idea is to view the part as a whole rather than seeing only the content of individual chapters. In the preceding discussion I have provided a number of sample questions to help you begin the process. These questions should not be seen as the only questions you should ask, but rather as samples to help you develop a questioning process.

Keep in mind that you may ask questions that seem useful and appropriate when you are using only the chapter titles as the question stimulus. Some of the questions will prove to be very useful when reading the chapter. On the other hand, some of the initial questions you generate may have little or no application as you read and understand the content of an individual chapter. Do not worry about the quality of the questions when planning on the part level. Questions can (and sometimes should) be revised or discarded when the details of the chapter become clearer. The important point is that you begin the part with some questions to help you focus your own reading and learning. Also, you will find that the more you apply active questioning as a part of your learning strategy the better your questions will become.

Chapter 16

Adrenergic Agents

www.harcourthealth.com/MERLIN/Lilley/

objectives

When you reach the end of this chapter, you should be able to do the following:

1 Briefly discuss the sympathetic nervous system as related to drug therapy with adrenergic agonists.

2 List the various adrenergic agonists, or sympathomimetics.

3 Discuss the mechanisms of action, therapeutic effects, uses, and adverse and toxic effects of adrenergic agonists, as well as the antidotes to overdose and to the unwanted effects.

4 Develop a nursing care plan that includes all phases of the nursing process related to the administration of the various adrenergic agents and the treatment of side effects and overdose or toxicity stemming from the use of these agents.

Look for this symbol for topics covered in the **Online Worksheet**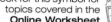

drug profiles

- ☞ **albuterol sulfate**, p. 255
- ☞ **dobutamine**, p. 257
- **dopamine**, p. 257
- ☞ **epinephrine**, p. 256, 258
- **fenoldopam**, p. 259
- **isoproterenol**, p. 259
- **isoproterenol hydrochloride**, p. 256
- **midodrine**, p. 259
- **norepinephrine**, p. 259
- **phenylephrine**, p. 259
- **pseudoephedrine hydrochloride**, p. 256
- **salmeterol**, p. 256
- **tetrahydrozoline**, p. 257

☞ Key drug.

glossary

Adrenergics (ad′ ren ər′ jiks) Drugs that stimulate the sympathetic nervous system. They are also referred to as *adrenergic agonists* or *sympathomimetics* because they mimic the effects of the sympathetic neurotransmitters norepinephrine and epinephrine. (p. 249)

Adrenergic receptors Receptor sites for the sympathetic neurotransmitters norepinephrine and epinephrine. (p. 250)

Alpha-adrenergic receptors Adrenergic receptors that are further divided into alpha₁- and alpha₂-adrenergic receptors and are differentiated by their location on nerves. (p. 250)

Beta-adrenergic receptors Located on postsynaptic effector cells—the cells, muscles, and organs that the nerves stimulate. Beta₁-adrenergic receptors differ from beta₂-adrenergic receptors in that they are primarily in the heart; beta₂-adrenergic receptors are located in the smooth muscle of the bronchioles and arterioles and in visceral organs. (p. 250)

Catecholamines (kat′ ə kol′ ə menz) Substances that can produce a sympathomimetic response. They are either endogenous catecholamines (such as epinephrine, norepi-

nephrine, and dopamine) or synthetic catecholamines (such as isoproterenol and dobutamine). (p. 249)

Dopaminergic receptors (do′ pə men er′ jik) Adrenergic receptors that, when stimulated by dopamine, cause the renal, mesenteric, coronary, and cerebral arteries to dilate and the flow of blood to increase. (p. 250)

Ophthalmics (of thal′ mikz) Topically applied eye medications. (p. 253)

Positive chronotropic effect (kron′ o trop′ ik) Refers to an increased heart rate. (p. 252)

Positive dromotropic effect (drom′ o trop′ ik) Causes an increase in conduction through the atrioventricular node. (p. 252)

Positive inotropic effect (in o trop′ ik) Refers to an increased force of contraction. (p. 252)

Synaptic cleft (si nap′ tik) The space between the nerve ending and the effector organ. (p. 250)

Adrenergics are a large group of both exogenous (synthetic) and endogenous (naturally occurring) substances. They have a wide variety of therapeutic uses depending on their site of action and their effect on receptors. Adrenergics stimulate the sympathetic nervous system (SNS) and are also called adrenergic agonists, or sympathomimetics, because they mimic the effects of the SNS neurotransmitters norepinephrine and epinephrine, which are referred to chemically as **catecholamines**. In describing the adrenergic class of medications, it is helpful to understand how the SNS operates in relation to the rest of the nervous system.

SYMPATHETIC NERVOUS SYSTEM

Figure 16-1 depicts the divisions of the nervous system, showing the relationship of the SNS to the entire nervous system. The SNS is the counterpart to the

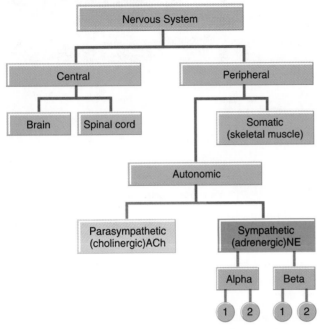

Fig. 16-1 The sympathetic nervous system in relationship to the entire nervous system.

Table 16-1 Adrenergic Receptor Responses to Stimulation

Location	Receptor	Response
CARDIOVASCULAR		
Blood vessels	Alpha$_1$/beta$_2$	Constriction/dilation
Cardiac muscle	Beta$_1$	Increased contractility
Atrioventricular node	Beta$_1$	Increased heart rate
Sinoatrial node	Beta$_1$	Increased heart rate
GASTROINTESTINAL		
Muscle	Beta$_2$	Decreased motility
Sphincters	Alpha$_1$	Constriction
GENITOURINARY		
Bladder sphincter	Alpha$_1$	Constriction
Penis	Alpha$_1$	Ejaculation
Uterus	Alpha$_1$/beta$_2$	Contraction/relaxation
RESPIRATORY		
Bronchial muscles	Beta$_2$	Dilation

parasympathetic nervous system (PSNS); together they make up the autonomic nervous system. They provide a checks-and-balances system for maintaining the normal homeostasis of the autonomic functions of the human body.

Throughout the body there are receptor sites for catecholamines norepinephrine and epinephrine. These are referred to as **adrenergic receptors,** and these are the sites where adrenergic drugs bind and produce their effects. Adrenergic receptors are located at many anatomic sites, and many physiologic responses are produced when they are stimulated or blocked. Adrenergic receptors are further divided into **alpha-adrenergic** and **beta-adrenergic receptors,** depending on whether they respond to norepinephrine or epinephrine, respectively. Both types of adrenergic receptors have subtypes, designated 1 and 2, and these provide a further means of checks and balances that control stimulation and blockade, constriction and dilation, and the increased and decreased production of a substance.

Alpha$_1$- and alpha$_2$-adrenergic receptors are differentiated by their location on nerves. Alpha$_1$-adrenergic receptors are located on postsynaptic effector cells (the cell, muscle, or organ that the nerve stimulates). Alpha$_2$-adrenergic receptors are located on the presynaptic nerve terminals, actually on the nerve that stimulates the effector cells. They control the release of neurotransmitters. The predominant alpha-adrenergic agonist response is vasoconstriction and CNS stimulation.

Beta-adrenergic receptors are all located on postsynaptic effector cells. Beta$_1$-adrenergic receptors are different from beta$_2$-adrenergic receptors in that they are primarily located in the heart; beta$_2$-adrenergic receptors are located in the smooth muscle of the bronchioles, arterioles,

and visceral organs. A beta-adrenergic agonist response results in bronchial, gastrointestinal, and uterine smooth muscle relaxation; glycogenolysis; and cardiac stimulation. Table 16-1 contains a more detailed listing of the adrenergic receptors and the responses elicited when they are stimulated by a neurotransmitter or a drug that acts like a neurotransmitter (see also Fig. 16-2).

There is another adrenergic receptor besides the alpha- and beta-adrenergic receptors called the **dopaminergic receptor.** When stimulated by dopamine, these receptors cause the vessels of the renal, mesenteric, coronary, and cerebral arteries to dilate and the flow of blood to increase. Dopamine is the only substance that can stimulate these receptors.

Catecholamines are produced by the SNS and are stored in vesicles or granules located in the ends of nerves. Here the transmitter waits until the nerve is stimulated, whereupon the vesicles move to the nerve ending and release their contents into the space between the nerve ending and the effector organ called the **synaptic cleft.** The released contents of the vesicle (catecholamines) then have the opportunity to bind to the receptor sites located all along the effector organ. Once the neurotransmitter binds to the receptors, the effector organ responds. Depending on the function of the particular organ, this elicits smooth muscle contraction, an increased heart rate, the increased production of a substance, or contraction of a blood vessel. This process is stopped by the action of enzymes and by reuptake of the neurotransmitter. Catecholamines are specifically metabolized by two enzymes, monoamine oxidase (MAO) and catechol O-methyltransferase (COMT). Each enzyme breaks down the catecholamine but is responsible for doing it in a different area. MAO breaks down the cate-

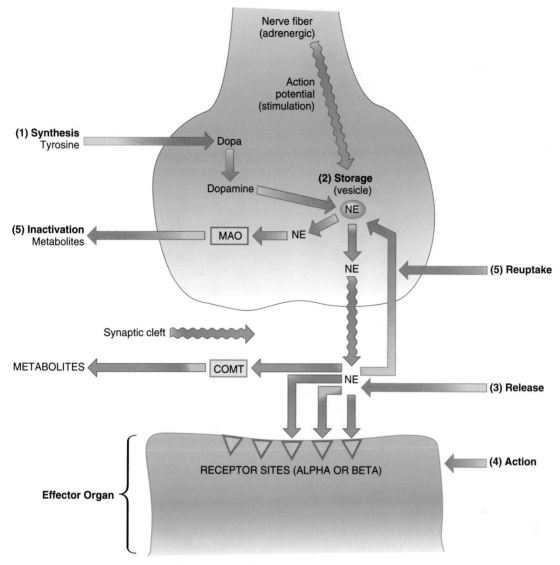

Fig. 16-2 The mechanism by which stimulation of a nerve fiber results in a physiologic process; adrenergic drugs mimic this same process.

cholamines that are in the nerve ending, and COMT breaks down the catecholamines that are outside the nerve ending at the synaptic cleft. The neurotransmitter is also actively taken back up into the nerve ending by a pump. This restores the catecholamine to the vesicle and provides another means of maintaining an adequate supply of the substance. This process is illustrated in Fig. 16-2.

ADRENERGIC DRUGS

Drugs that have effects similar to or that mimic the effects of the SNS neurotransmitters norepinephrine, epinephrine, and dopamine are referred to as adrenergics. As mentioned previously, these neurotransmitters are referred to as *catecholamines*. However, this term refers specifically to an adrenergic drug that has a basic chemical structure similar to that of norepinephrine, epinephrine, or dopamine. Catecholamines produce a sympathomimetic response and are either endogenous substances such as epinephrine, norepinephrine, and dopamine or

synthetic substances such as isoproterenol, dobutamine, and phenylephrine.

Catecholamines that are used therapeutically produce the same result as the endogenous ones but without the need to stimulate the nerve to release the neurotransmitter. Instead, when epinephrine, dobutamine, or any of the adrenergic drugs are given, they bathe the area between the nerve and the effector organ (synaptic cleft). Once there, they have the opportunity to induce a response. This can be accomplished in one of three ways: direct stimulation, indirect stimulation, or a combination of the two.

A direct-acting sympathomimetic binds directly to the receptor and causes a physiologic response (Fig. 16-3). Phenylephrine is an example of such an agent. An indirect-acting sympathomimetic is an adrenergic drug that when given causes the release of the catecholamine from the storage sites (vesicles) in the nerve endings, which then binds to the receptors and causes a physiologic response (Fig. 16-4). Amphetamine and other related anorexiants are

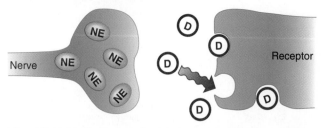

Fig. 16-3 Mechanism of physiologic response by direct-acting sympathomimetics. *D,* Drug; *NE,* norepinephrine.

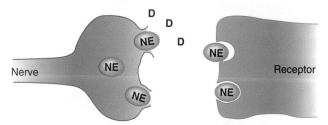

Fig. 16-4 Mechanism of physiologic response by indirect-acting sympathomimetics. *D,* Drug; *NE,* norepinephrine.

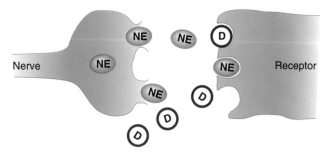

Fig. 16-5 Mechanism of physiologic response by mixed-acting sympathomimetics. *D,* Drug; *NE,* norepinephrine.

examples of such agents. A mixed-acting sympathomimetic both directly stimulates the receptor by binding to it and indirectly stimulates the receptor by causing the release of the neurotransmitter stored in vesicles at the nerve endings (Fig. 16-5). Ephedrine is an example of a mixed-adrenergic drug.

There are also noncatecholamine adrenergic drugs such as phenylephrine, metaproterenol, and albuterol. In general these drugs have a longer duration of action than either the endogenous or synthetic catecholamines.

Catecholamines and noncatecholamines can act at very specific receptors, they can act at different receptors depending on their dose, or they can act at several different receptors all at once. Examples of a few of the catecholamines and the dose-specific selectivity of these agents for various adrenergic receptors are given in Table 16-2.

Although adrenergics work primarily at postganglionic receptors (the receptors that immediately innervate the effector organ, gland, muscle, etc.), certain agents are also capable of working centrally.

The two most common ways of classifying the adrenergics are either by the specific receptors they affect or by the indications for their use.

Mechanism of Action

To fully understand the mechanism of action of adrenergics it is necessary to have a working knowledge of normal adrenergic transmission, which takes place at the junction between the nerve (postganglionic sympathetic neuron) and the innervated organ (effector organ or receptor site). The process of SNS stimulation is illustrated in Fig. 16-2 and discussed earlier in this chapter.

Drug Effects

When adrenergic drugs stimulate alpha-adrenergic receptor sites located on smooth muscles, vasoconstriction

most commonly occurs. A notable exception is adrenergic stimulation of the beta$_2$ receptors on the airways. Many areas of the body are covered by smooth muscles with alpha-adrenergic receptors on them. The binding of adrenergic drugs to these alpha-adrenergic receptors on the smooth muscle of blood vessels, for instance, causes vasoconstriction; at other sites, this causes the relaxation of gastrointestinal smooth muscle, contraction of the uterus and bladder, male ejaculation, decreased insulin release, and contraction of the ciliary muscles of the eye, causing them to dilate.

Activation of beta$_1$-adrenergic receptors by adrenergic drugs produces increased cardiac contractility, increased atrioventricular (AV) nodal conduction, and increased heart rate. Beta$_1$-adrenergic receptor stimulation also causes cardiac stimulation. There are beta$_1$-adrenergic receptors on the myocardium and in the conduction system of the heart, the sinoatrial (SA) node, and the AV node. When these beta$_1$-adrenergic receptors are stimulated by an adrenergic drug, this results in an increased force of contraction, or a **positive inotropic effect;** an increased heart rate, or a **positive chronotropic effect;** and an increase in conduction through the AV node, or a **positive dromotropic effect.** Activation of beta$_2$-adrenergic receptors produces relaxation of the bronchi (bronchodilation) and uterine relaxation. Beta$_2$-adrenergic receptors also cause stimulation in the liver with glycogenolysis and an increase in renin secretion in the kidneys.

Therapeutic Uses

Adrenergics, or sympathomimetics, are employed in the treatment of a wide variety of illnesses and conditions. Their selectivity for either alpha- or beta-adrenergic receptors and their affinity for certain tissues or organs determines the settings in which they are most commonly used. Some adrenergics are used as adjuncts to diet in the short-term treatment of obesity. These drugs are discussed in greater detail in Chapter 15.

Certain adrenergic drugs have an affinity for the adrenergic receptors located in the respiratory system and are classified as bronchodilators. They tend to preferentially stimulate the beta-adrenergic receptors rather than the alpha-adrenergic receptors and cause bronchodilation. These drugs are helpful in treating conditions such as asthma and bronchitis. Of the two subtypes of beta-adrenergic receptors, these adrenergics are more attracted

Table 16-2   Catecholamines and Their Dose-Response Relationship

Drug	Dosage	Receptor
dobutamine (Dobutrex)	Maintenance: 2-10 μg/kg/min High: 40 μg/kg/min	Beta$_1$>>beta$_2$ > alpha$_1$
dopamine (Intropin)	Low: 0.5-2 μg/kg/min Moderate: 2-4 or <10 μg/kg/min High: >10 μg/kg/min	Dopaminergic Beta$_1$ Alpha$_1$
epinephrine (Adrenalin)	Low: 1-4 μg/min High: 4-40 μg/min	Beta$_1$ > beta$_2$>>alpha$_1$ Alpha$_1$ $\geq$ beta$_1$

to the beta$_2$-adrenergic receptors on the bronchial, uterine, and vascular smooth muscles than the beta$_1$-adrenergic receptors on the heart. Following are some common bronchodilators that are beta-adrenergics:

- albuterol
- bitolterol
- ephedrine
- epinephrine
- ethylnorepinephrine
- isoetharine
- isoproterenol
- levalbuterol
- metaproterenol
- salmeterol
- terbutaline

Adrenergics can also be used to reduce intraocular pressure and dilate pupils (mydriasis), properties that make them useful in the treatment of open-angle glaucoma. They accomplish these tasks by stimulating alpha- or beta$_2$-adrenergic receptors or both. The two adrenergics used for this purpose are epinephrine and dipivefrin.

The intranasal application of certain adrenergics can cause the constriction of dilated arterioles and a reduction in nasal blood flow, thus decreasing congestion. These adrenergic drugs work by stimulating alpha-adrenergic receptors and have little or no effect on beta-adrenergic receptors. Following is a list of these nasal decongestants:

- epinephrine
- ephedrine
- naphazoline
- oxymetazoline
- phenylephrine
- tetrahydrolzoline

In another topical application, some adrenergics can be applied to the surface of the eye. These are called **ophthalmics** and work much the same way as nasal decongestants except that they affect the vasculature of the eye. When administered, they stimulate alpha-adrenergic receptors located on small arterioles in the eye and temporarily relieve conjunctival congestion. Following is a list of these ophthalmic adrenergics:

- epinephrine
- naphazoline
- phenylephrine
- tetrahydrozoline

The final group of adrenergics are sometimes referred to as *vasoactive sympathomimetics, pressors, inotropes,* or *cardio-selective sympathomimetics* because they are used to support the heart during cardiac failure or shock. These agents have a variety of effects on the various alpha- and beta-adrenergic receptors, and these effects can also be related to the specific dose of the adrenergic agent. Following is a list of the common vasoactive adrenergic agents:

- dobutamine
- dopamine
- ephedrine
- epinephrine
- fenoldopam
- isoproterenol
- metaraminol
- methoxamine
- norepinephrine
- phenylephrine

Activity

Side Effects and Adverse Effects

Some of the most frequent unwanted CNS effects of the alpha-adrenergic agents include headache, restlessness, excitement, insomnia, and euphoria. The cardiovascular effects of the alpha-adrenergics include palpitations or dysrhythmias, tachycardia, vasoconstriction, and hypertension. Effects on other body systems include anorexia or loss of appetite, dry mouth, nausea, vomiting, and, rarely, taste changes.

Beta-adrenergic agents can adversely affect the CNS, causing mild tremors, headache, nervousness, and dizziness. Beta-adrenergic agents can also have unwanted effects on the cardiovascular system, including increased heart rate (positive chronotrope), palpitations (dysrhythmias), and fluctuations in blood pressure. Other significant effects include sweating, nausea, vomiting, and muscle cramps. See the Pediatric and Geriatric Considerations boxes for additional information.

Toxicity and Management of Overdose

The toxic effects of adrenergic drugs are mainly an extension of their common adverse effects (e.g., seizures, hypotension or hypertension, dysrhythmias, palpitation,

pediatric considerations

Beta-Adrenergic Agonist Administration

- Children are usually more sensitive to most medications; therefore watch children closely for excessive cardiac or CNS stimulations with palpitations, tachycardia, irritability, chest pain, etc.
- Terbutaline is generally not used in children 12 years old and under.
- Other medications, including OTC medications, should not be used unless physician has been notified and approves concurrent use.

geriatric considerations

Beta-Adrenergic Agonist Administration

- Older persons are more sensitive to medications, so monitor for excessive cardiac and CNS stimulation.
- Because of the possible presence of other medical conditions such as hypertension, peripheral vascular disease, and cardiovascular disease, elderly patients need to be monitored carefully before, during, and after the use of these medications.
- Immediately report any chest pain, palpitations, blurred vision, headache, seizures, or hallucinations to the physician.
- Cautions use is recommended with OTC and other medications. Contact the physician for further instructions.
- Monitor vital signs, especially blood pressure and pulse rate with these medications because of their cardiovascular effects.

nervousness, dizziness, fatigue, malaise, insomnia, headache, tremor, dry mouth, and nausea). The two most life-threatening toxic effects involve the CNS and cardiovascular system. In the acute setting, seizures can be effectively managed with diazepam. Intracranial bleeding can also occur, often as a result of extremely elevated blood pressures. These elevated blood pressures not only run the risk of precipitating hemorrhage in the brain but elsewhere in the body as well. The best and most effective treatment in this situation is lowering the blood pressure using a rapid-acting alpha-adrenergic—blocking drug. This can directly reverse the adrenergic-induced state.

Many adrenergic drugs are either synthetic analogues of our own naturally occurring neurotransmitters (norepinephrine, epinephrine, and dopamine) or are the actual endogenous adrenergic compound. Therefore, when these drugs are taken in an overdose or signs and symptoms of toxicity develop, reversing these effects takes a relatively short time. The majority of these compounds have very short half-lives, and therefore their effects are relatively short-lived. Stopping the drug should quickly cause the toxic symptoms to subside. The recommended treatment of overdoses often involves treating the symptoms and supporting the patient. If death occurs, it is usually the result of either respiratory failure or cardiac arrest. The treatment of an overdose should be aimed at the support of these two body systems.

Interactions

The potential drug interactions that can occur with adrenergic agents are significant. Although many of the interactions only result in a diminished adrenergic effect because of direct antagonism at and competition for receptor sites, some reactions can be life-threatening. The following are some of the more serious drug-drug interactions involving adrenergic agents. Alpha- and beta-adrenergic agents, when given with adrenergic agents, directly antagonize each other, resulting in reduced therapeutic effects. Adrenergics, when given with anesthetic agents, can cause increased risk of cardiac dysrhythmias. Tricyclic antidepressants, when given with adrenergics, can cause increased vasopressor effects, acute hypertensive crisis, and possibly respiratory depression. Adrenergics, when given with MAOIs, can lead to hypertensive crisis. Antihistamines and thyroid preparations can increase the adrenergic effects of this class of drugs. Antihypertensives and adrenergics may directly antagonize each other's therapeutic effects. The combination of MAOIs with adrenergic agents can lead to life-threatening hypertensive crisis.

Laboratory Test Interactions

Alpha-adrenergic agents can cause the serum levels of corticosteriods to be increased and the glucose levels to be increased. Therefore interpretations of these laboratory results should be done with caution in patients taking these medications. Alpha-adrenergic agents can cause the plasma cortisol and corticotropin concentrations to be elevated.

Dosages

For the recommended dosages of various adrenergic agents, see the dosages tables on p. 255.

drug profiles

Adrenergics are used in the treatment of a variety of illnesses, and there are many indications for their use. Their selectivity for either alpha- or beta-adrenergic receptors and their affinity for various tissues or organs defines the settings in which they are most commonly used.

BRONCHODILATORS

The bronchodilating adrenergic agents are mostly beta-adrenergic in their actions. They are very effective as antiasthmatic agents and are used in the treatment of acute attacks because of their rapid onset of action and efficacy. Ephedrine, ethylnorepinephrine, and epinephrine also possess alpha-

DOSAGES Selected Bronchodilator Adrenergics

agent	pharmacologic class	dosage range	purpose
albuterol (Proventil, Ventolin, Volmax)	Beta$_2$-adrenergic	*Adult/Pediatric ≥ 4 y/o* Aerosol: 2 inhal. (180 μg) q4-6h *Pediatric 2-6 y/o* PO: 2 mg 3-4 times/day *Adult/Pediatric ≥ 12 y/o* PO: 2-4 mg 3-5 times/day; max 32 mg/day *Adult/Pediatric ≥ 12 y/o* Solution: 2.5 mg 3-4 times/day by nebulization *Adult/Pediatric ≥ 12 y/o* Powder: 200 μg q4-6h by rotohaler device	
epinephrine (Primatene, Bronkaid, others)	Beta-adrenergic	*Adult/Pediatric ≥ 4 y/o* Aerosol: 160-250 μg q3h or more *Adult/Pediatric ≥ 4 y/o* Solution: 8-15 gtt of a 1%, 2%, 2.25% solution by nebulizations q3h or more	

isoetharine (Arm-a-med, Bronkometer, Beta-2, and others)	Beta$_2$-adrenergic	*Adult*
		Aerosol: 1-2 inhal. (340-680 μg) q4h or more
		Adult
		Solution: 0.25-0.5 ml of 1% solution diluted 1:3
		   by oxygen aerosolization or IPPB; or 3-7 inhal.
		   of undiluted 1% solution by hand nebulizer.
		   Consult package insert for % solutions dosages	

isoproterenol (Medihaler-Iso, others)	Beta-adrenergic	*Adult/Pediatric*
		Aerosol: 1-2 inhal. (120-262 μg); do not exceed
		   6 doses in 24 hr
		Pediatric
		SL tablets: 5-10 mg; do not exceed 30 mg/day
		Adult
		SL tablets: 10-20 mg; do not exceed 60 mg/day
		Adult/Pediatric
		Solution: 1:100 solution: 3-7 deep inhal. by
		   hand nebulizer up to 5 times/day
		1:200 solution: 5-15 deep inhal. up to 5 times/day
			Bronchodilation

salmeterol (Serevent)	Beta$_2$-adrenergic	*Adult* Aerosol: one 50-μg inhalation 30-60 min before exercise or one 50-μg inhalation q12h	
terbutaline (Brethine, Brethaire Bricanyl)	Beta$_2$-adrenergic	*Adult/Pediatric ≥ 12 y/o* Aerosol: 2 inhal. (400 μg) q4-6h *Pediatric* SC: 3.5-5 μg/kg *Adult* SC: 0.25 mg; do not exceed 0.5 mg in 4-hr period *Pediatric 12-15 y/o* PO: 2.5 mg tid; do not exceed 7.5 mg/day *Adult* PO: 5 mg q6h 3 times/day; do not exceed 15 mg/day	

IPPB, Intermittent positive-pressure breathing.

adrenergic activity. Although most of these agents are prescription-only drugs, a few are available as OTC medications.

Activation of beta$_2$-adrenergic receptors causes the bronchi to dilate. The beta$_2$-adrenergics are the preferred bronchodilators because they produce fewer cardiac-related side effects than the nonselective beta agents. These drugs are preg-nancy category C agents, except terbutaline, which is listed as a pregnancy category B drug. These drugs are available in oral, aerosol, and injection forms.

Activity

albuterol sulfate

Albuterol (Proventil, Salbutamol, Ventolin, Volmax) is a selective beta$_2$-adrenergic bronchodilator. It is contraindicated in patients with a known hypersensitivity to it. It can be administered by inhalation, orally, and by injection. It is available as an inhaler or as 2- and 4-mg tablets. See the table on p. 255 for dosage information.

PHARMACOKINETICS

HALF-LIFE	ONSET	PEAK	DURATION
PO: 2.5 hr	PO: 30 min	PO: 2.5 hr	PO: 4-6 hr
Inhaler: 4 hr	Inhaler: 5-15 min	Inhaler: 1-1.5 hr	Inhaler: 4-6 hr

epinephrine

Epinephrine (Adrenalin) is a naturally occurring catecholamine produced by the adrenal medulla. It is a very potent alpha-beta–adrenergic agent that produces vasoconstriction, increased blood pressure, cardiac stimulation, and dilatation of the bronchioles. It is the drug of choice for the relief of acute asthma attacks and for the treatment of anaphylaxis. In addition, epinephrine is used to treat open-angle glaucoma, to restore cardiac rhythm in cardiac arrest, and to control bleeding. It is also used as an ophthalmic agent and a nasal decongestant and to prolong the activity of infiltrated local anesthetics. Its use is contraindicated in many settings, including hypersensitivity, narrow-angle glaucoma, shock due to trauma, halogenated general anesthetics, coronary insufficiency, and labor. In addition, its use with local anesthetics administered in the toes or fingers is not recommended because distal circulation may be decreased from its vasoconstricting properties. See the table on p. 255 for dosage information.

PHARMACOKINETICS

HALF-LIFE	ONSET	PEAK	DURATION
Variable (min)	SC: 5-10 min PO inhalation, IV: 1 min	SC: 20 min PO inhalation, IV: <20 min	SC: 20 min PO inhalation, IV: <30 min

isoproterenol hydrochloride

Isoproterenol (Isuprel) is a nonselective beta-sympathomimetic (beta$_1$-beta$_2$) antiasthmatic agent. The beta$_1$-adrenergic activity results in a positive inotropic and chronotropic cardiac effect with a corresponding increase in the stroke volume and oxygen consumption. Beta$_2$-adrenergic activation produces bronchial, gastointestinal tract, and uterine smooth muscle relaxation. Isoproterenol is indicated for the treatment of acute and chronic forms of asthma, bronchitis, and bronchiectasis. Other indications include cardiac arrest, Adams-Stokes syndrome, and ventricular dysrhythmias resulting from AV block.

Isoproterenol is contraindicated in patients with a known hypersensitivity to it and in those suffering from digitalis-induced tachycardia or with pre-existing cardiac dysrhythmias. See the table on p. 255 for dosage information.

PHARMACOKINETICS

HALF-LIFE	ONSET	PEAK	DURATION
IV: 2 min	IV: Immediate	IV: <15 min	IV: <1 hr
Inhalation: 2 min	Inhalation: Immediate	Inhalation: Rapid	Inhalation: 1 hr
SL: 2 min	SL: 30 min	SL: Variable	SL: 2 hr

salmeterol

Salmeterol (Serevent, Serevent Diskus) is a new beta$_2$ agonist indicated for long-term maintenance treatment of asthma, prevention of bronchospasm, and prevention of exercise-induced bronchospasm. It is not indicated for acute exacerbations of asthma or bronchospasms. It is classified as a pregnancy category C agent and is contraindicated in patients with known hypersensitivity to salmeterol. It is available as a 50-μg aerosol inhaler. Recommended dosages are given in the table on p. 255.

PHARMACOKINETICS

HALF-LIFE	ONSET	PEAK	DURATION
5.5 hr	10-20 min	3 hr	12 hr

NASAL DECONGESTANTS

The sympathomimetic agents used as nasal decongestants consist of both alpha- and alpha-beta–adrenergic agents. The alpha-adrenergic activity of these agents is responsible for causing vasoconstriction in the nasal mucosa. This produces shrinkage of the mucosa, which promotes easier nasal breathing. However, excessive use of nasal decongestants can lead to greater congestion because of a rebound phenomenon that occurs when use of the product is stopped. However, this is not seen with the oral agents. The decongestants are administered topically with nasal drops or sprays, which are instilled into each nostril. The ephedrine salts, neosynephrine, phenylephrine hydrochloride, and pseudoephedrine, can produce nasal decongestion when taken, either as sole agents or in combination with allergy, cold, cough, and sinus relief preparations.

The contraindications to the use of the systemically administered nasal decongestants are the same for all of the agents and include hypersensitivity, diabetes, hypertension, thyroid disorders, and enlargement of the prostate gland.

pseudoephedrine hydrochloride

Pseudoephedrine (Sudafed, Afrin) is a natural plant alkaloid that is obtained from the *Ephedra* plant. It is a stereoisomer of ephedrine and is a widely used, orally administered decongestant. See the table on p. 257 for the recommended dosages. Pregnancy category C.

DOSAGES Selected Nasal and Ophthalmic Decongestant Adrenergics

agent	pharmacologic class	dosage range	purpose
pseudoephedrine (Sudafed, Afrin, Pediacare drops, others)	Alpha-, beta-adrenergic	*Pediatric 3-6 mo* PO drops: 1-1.5 gtt q4-6h for 4 doses *Pediatric 1-2 y/o* PO drops: 2 gtt q4-6h for 4 doses *Pediatric 2-5 y/o* PO 15 mg q4-6h. Do not exceed 60 mg/day *Pediatric 6-12 y/o* 30 mg q4-6h. Do not exceed 120 mg/day *Adult/Pediatric ≥ 12 y/o* 60 mg q4-6h. Do not exceed 240 mg/day	Nasal decongestant
tetrahydrozoline (Tyzine Pediatric, Tyzine)	Alpha-adrenergic	*Adult/Pediatric <2 yr* 1-2 gtt bid or tid	Ophthalmic decongestant

PHARMACOKINETICS

HALF-LIFE	ONSET	PEAK	DURATION
Variable (min)*	15-30 min	30-60 min	4-6 hr SR: 8-12 hr

*Half-life is pH-dependent; pH of 5.5-6 = 9-16 hr.

OPHTHALMIC DECONGESTANTS

Ophthalmic decongestants are adrenergics that are applied topically to the eye. When instilled into the eye, they stimulate alpha-adrenergic receptors located on the small arterioles in the eye. This results in constriction and relieves conjunctival congestion, thus decreasing redness in the eye. Although epinephrine, phenylephrine, and naphazoline are all used as ophthalmic decongestants, tetrahydrozoline is the one most widely used.

tetrahydrozoline

Tetrahydrozoline (Murine, Visine, and others) is applied topically to the eye to temporarily relieve congestion, itching, and minor irritation in patients with red and irritated eyes. It causes constriction of the blood vessels of the eye and is sometimes also used during some diagnostic eye procedures. It is the active ingredient in such OTC products as Visine, Soothe, and Murine Plus eyedrops. It is contraindicated in patients with a hypersensitivity reaction to it and in those with narrow-angle glaucoma. The recommended dosages are given in the table above. Pregnancy category C.

PHARMACOKINETICS

HALF-LIFE	ONSET	PEAK	DURATION
Variable (min)	<3 min	Short (min)	4-8 hr

VASOACTIVE ADRENERGICS

Adrenergics that have primarily cardioselective effects are referred to as *vasoactive adrenergics*. They are used to support a failing heart or to treat shock. They may also be used to treat individuals with or-

thostatic hypotension. These agents have a wide range of effects on alpha- and beta-adrenergic receptors, depending on the dose. The vasoactive adrenergics are very potent, quick-acting, injectable drugs. They are listed by the FDA as pregnancy category C agents. Although dosage recommendations are given in the table on p. 258, all of these drugs are titrated to the desired physiologic response. All of the vasoactive adrenergics (with the exception of midodrine) are rapid in onset, and their effects very quickly cease when they are stopped. Therefore careful titration and monitoring of vital signs and electrocardiogram (ECG) are required in patients receiving them.

dobutamine

Dobutamine (Dobutrex) is a beta$_1$-selective vasoactive adrenergic drug that is structurally similar to the naturally occurring catecholamine dopamine. By stimulating the beta$_1$ receptors on the heart (myocardium), it increases cardiac output by increasing contractility (positive inotrope) and increases the stroke volume, especially in patients with congestive heart failure. Dobutamine is available as an IV injected drug. The recommended dosages are listed in the table on p. 258.

PHARMACOKINETICS

HALF-LIFE	ONSET	PEAK	DURATION
2-5 min	<2 min	<10 min	<10 min

dopamine

Dopamine (Intropin) is a naturally occurring catecholamine neurotransmitter in the SNS. It has potent dopaminergic and beta$_1$- and alpha$_1$-adrenergic receptor activity, depending on the dose. Dopamine, when used at low doses, can dilate blood vessels in the brain, heart, kidneys, and mesentery. This increases blood flow to these areas. At higher infusion rates dopamine can improve contractility and

DOSAGES Selected Vasoactive Adrenergics

agent	pharmacologic class	dosage range	purpose
dobutamine (Dobutrex)	Beta$_1$-adrenergic	*Adult* IV infusion: 2.5-40 µg/kg/min	Cardiac decompensation
dopamine (Intropin)	Beta$_1$-adrenergic	*Adult* IV infusion: initiate at 1-5 µg/kg/min and increase if needed; for severe cases, initiate at 5 µg/kg/min and gradually increase in 5-10 µg/min increments to 20-30 µg/kg/min if needed	Shock syndrome
epinephrine (Adrenalin)	Alpha-beta-adrenergic	*Pediatric* SC: 10 µg/kg repeated every 20 min if required *Adult* SC: 0.1-0.5 mg repeated every 10-15 min if required	Anaphylaxis
		Neonatal IV: 10-30 µg/kg every 3-5 min if required *Pediatric* IV: 10 µg/kg every 3-5 min if required *Adult* IV: 0.5-1 mg every 3-5 min if required	Cardiopulmonary resuscitation
fenoldopam (Corlopam)	Dopamine-1 agonist	*Adult* IV: 0.1 to 1.6 µg/kg/min up to 48 hr	Lower blood pressure
isoproterenol (Isuprel)	Beta-adrenergic	*Adult* IV infusion: 0.5-5 µg/min Intracardiac: 0.02 mg IM: 0.2 mg: subsequently 0.02-1 mg IV: 0.02-0.06 mg; subsequently 0.01-0.2 mg Infusion: 5 µg/min range, 2-20 µg/min SC: 0.2 mg; subsequently 0.15-0.2 mg	Heart block/ dysrhythmias
midodrine (ProAmatine)	Alpha$_1$-adrenergic	*Adult* PO 10 mg tid shortly before or upon arising in the morning, midday, and late afternoon (not later than 6 pm)	Orthostatic hypotension
norepinephrine (Levophed)	Alpha-beta adrenergic	*Pediatric* IV infusion: usual rate, 0.1-1 µg/kg/min *Adult* IV infusion: usual rate, 8-12 µg/min	Hypotensive states
phenylephrine (Neosynephrine)	Alpha-adrenergic	*Adult* IM/SC: 1-10 mg; do not exceed initial dose of 5 mg IV infusion: 10 mg/500 ml solution; initial rate, 100-180 µg/min; maintenance dose, 40-60 µg/min	Hypotension
		IV: 0.5 mg in 15-20 sec; subsequent dose, 0.1-0.2 mg	Paroxysmal supraventricular tachycardia

cardiac output. The drug is contraindicated in patients who have a tumor that secretes catecholamines, a pheochromocytoma. It is available as an intravenously injectable drug. The recommended vasoactive dosages are given in the table above.

PHARMACOKINETICS

HALF-LIFE	ONSET	PEAK	DURATION
<2 min	2-5 min	Rapid	10 min

epinephrine

Epinephrine (Adrenalin) is also an endogenous vasoactive catecholamine. It acts directly on both the alpha- and beta-adrenergic receptors of tissues innervated by the SNS. It is used in emergency situations and is one of the primary vasoactive drugs used in many advanced cardiac life support (ACLS) protocols. The physiologic response it elicits is dose related. At low dosages it stimulates mostly beta-adrenergic receptors, increasing the force of contraction and heart rate. At high dosages it stimulates mostly alpha-adrenergic receptors, causing vasoconstriction, which elevates the blood pressure. The dosages recommended for the treatment of various disorders are given in the table above.

PHARMACOKINETICS

HALF-LIFE	ONSET	PEAK	DURATION
<5 min	<2 min	Rapid	5-30 min

fenoldopam

Fenoldopam (Corlopam) is a peripheral dopamine-1 (DA$_1$) agonist indicated for parenteral use in lowering blood pressure. Fenoldopam produces its blood-pressure–lowering effects by inducing arteriolar vasodilation mainly through stimulation of DA$_1$ receptors. It appears to be as effective as sodium nitroprusside for short-term treatment of severe hypertension and may have beneficial effects on renal function. It is available as a 10 mg/ml injection. Recommended dosages are given in the table on p. 258.

PHARMACOKINETICS

HALF-LIFE	ONSET	PEAK	DURATION
5 min	5 min	20 min	10 min

isoproterenol

Isoproterenol (Isuprel) acts directly on the beta-adrenergic receptors. In normal doses it has little or no effect on alpha-adrenergic receptors. The main effects of therapeutic doses of isoproterenol are relaxation of smooth muscle of the bronchial tree, cardiac stimulation, and peripheral vasodilation. It can also relax gastrointestinal and uterine smooth muscle by stimulating the beta$_2$-adrenergic receptors. In addition, isoproterenol inhibits the anaphylaxis-induced release of histamine and may be used to treat patients experiencing an anaphylactic reaction. Common dosages are given in the table on p. 258.

PHARMACOKINETICS

HALF-LIFE	ONSET	PEAK	DURATION
<2 min	Immediate	<15 min	8-50 min

midodrine

Midodrine (ProAmatine) is a prodrug converted to its active form, desglymidodrine, in the liver. It is this active metabolite that accounts for the primary pharmacologic action of midodrine, which is alpha$_1$ adrenergic receptor stimulation. Alpha$_1$ stimulation causes constriction of both arterioles and veins resulting in peripheral vasoconstriction. Midodrine is primarily indicated for the treatment of symptomatic orthostatic hypotension. Midodrine is available as 2.5- and 5-mg tablets. Common dosages are given in the table on p. 258.

PHARMACOKINETICS

HALF-LIFE	ONSET	PEAK	DURATION
3-4 hr	45-90 min	1 hr	6-8 hr

norepinephrine

Norepinephrine (Levophed) acts predominantly by directly stimulating alpha-adrenergic receptors. It also has some direct-stimulating beta-adrenergic effects on the heart (beta$_1$-adrenergic receptors) but none on the lung (beta$_2$-adrenergic receptors). The most evident effects, however, are those on the alpha-adrenergic receptors, which lead to vasoconstriction. Norepinephrine is directly metabolized to dopamine and is primarily used in the treatment of hypotension and shock. Common dosages are given in the table on p. 258.

PHARMACOKINETICS

HALF-LIFE	ONSET	PEAK	DURATION
<5 min	Immediate	1-2 min	1-2 min

phenylephrine

Phenylephrine (Neosynephrine) works almost exclusively on the alpha-adrenergic receptors. It is also believed to act indirectly by causing the release of norepinephrine from its storage sites. It is primarily used as a short-term agent to augment blood pressure in patients in shock, to control some dysrhythmias (supraventricular tachycardias), and to produce vasoconstriction with regional anesthesia. It is also used as an ophthalmic agent and administered topically as a nasal decongestant. Common vasoactive dosages are listed in the table on p. 258.

PHARMACOKINETICS

HALF-LIFE	ONSET	PEAK	DURATION
<5 min*	Immediate*	Rapid*	15-20 min*

*IV use.

nursing process

• Assessment

Adrenergic, or sympathomimetic, drugs have a variety of effects depending on the receptors they stimulate. Stimulation of the alpha-adrenergic receptors results in vasoconstriction, stimulation of beta$_1$-adrenergic receptors produces cardiac stimulation, and stimulation of the beta$_2$-adrenergic receptors results in bronchodilation. Because of these properties, the use of adrenergics requires careful patient assessment to minimize the possible side effects and maximize the therapeutic effects.

In a thorough assessment, the nurse should first gather information about the patient's allergies and past and present medical conditions. A system overview and a thorough medication history should also form part of this assessment. Some pertinent questions to ask the patient include the following:

• Are you allergic to any medication, food, topical products, environmental products, and so on?

- Are you asthmatic, and if so, how frequent and severe are the attacks?
- What are their manifestations and precipitating factors?
- What previous treatment have you received for the asthma, and has it been successful or failed?
- Do you have a history of hypertension, cardiac dysrhythmias, or any other cardiovascular disease?

Assessment of renal and hepatic functioning are also important before initiating treatment. Adrenergic drugs may precipitate tachycardia, hypertension, myocardial infarction (MI), or heart failure. Therefore they should be given cautiously in patients receiving them who have these later disorders, and such patients should be closely monitored. Baseline vital signs and assessment of peripheral pulses, skin color, temperature, and capillary refill should be obtained and documented. In particular for midodrine, postural blood pressures (supine, sitting, and standing—as ordered) and pulses may need to be documented before and during its administration.

In particular with salmeterol, contraindications include a hypersensitivity to it or to adrenergic amines. It should *not* be used within 2 weeks of use of an MAOI, and it is *not* to be used for patients during an acute asthmatic attack. Cautious use is recommended with patients who have a history of cerebrovascular disease, dysrythmias, tachycardia, CNS disorders such as seizures, or diabetes; during pregnancy, and lactation; and in the elderly. Drug interactions include MAOIs, tricyclic antidepressants, and beta-blockers. Assessment of the patient's symptoms and disease progression and manifestations are important to proper treatment. Assess and document lung sounds and any abnormalities, especially for baseline and comparative purposes. Vital signs and a CNS assessment are also important.

Fenoldopam is a peripheral dopamine agonist and an adrenergic agent, but it is used for lowering blood pressure. Assessing and monitoring all vital signs, especially blood pressure and pulse, is important with initiation of the agent and durng its use. Generally this agent is used for short-term treatment and is titrated by IV use, and so careful monitoring during treatment with use of an IV pump and close monitoring of the IV infusion is indicated.

Activity

● Nursing Diagnoses

Nursing diagnoses associated with the use of adrenergic agonists include, but are not limited to, the following:
- Acute pain related to side effects of tachycardia and palpitations.
- Deficient knowledge regarding therapeutic regimen, side effects, drug interactions, and precautions related to use of sympathomimetics.
- Risk for injury related to possible side effects (nervousness, vertigo, hypertension, or tremors) or from potential drug interactions.
- Disturbed sleep pattern related to CNS stimulation caused by adrenergic agents.
- Noncompliance to therapy related to lack of information about the importance of taking the medication as ordered.

- Decreased cardiac output related to cardiovascular side effects consisting of palpitations, hypertension, tachycardia, and anginal pain.

● Planning

Goals for the patient receiving sympathomimetics include the following:
- Patient takes drugs as ordered and follow directions explicitly.
- Patient's symptoms are relieved.
- Patient remains compliant with the drug therapy.
- Patient demonstrates an adequate knowledge about the use of the specific medications.

Outcome Criteria

Outcome criteria related to the administration of adrenergic agonists include the following:
- Patient will state the importance of pharmacologic and nonpharmacologic treatment of the respiratory or other disorder that is present, such as asthma.
- Patient will state the importance of compliance with the therapy and the risks and complications associated with overuse of the medication such as excessive CNS stimulation, insomnia, tachycardia.
- Patient will state conditions and side effects that should be reported to the physician such as chest pain, restlessness, insomnia.
- Patient will state the importance of scheduling and keeping follow-up appointments with the physician to monitor effectiveness of drug therapy.
- Patient will improve in his or her condition once on the medication regimen with decreased signs and symptoms, such as decreased coughing or wheezing.

● Implementation

There are several nursing interventions that can maximize the therapeutic effects of adrenergic agents and minimize the side effects. Always check the packaging inserts concerning dilutional agents and the amount. Use a TB syringe when giving these agents subcutaneously so that accurate, small doses are administered. When these agents are to be administered by an inhaler or nebulizer, teach the patient how to correctly administer the agent and how to properly clean the equipment. Be careful not to administer two adrenergic agents such as epinephrine and isoproterenol at the same time because of the high risk of the precipitating side effects such as tachycardia and hypertension. At least 4 hours should elapse between doses of these medications to prevent serious cardiac dysrhythmias from occurring. Often these medications are used in combination with other agents in the management of asthma because of their synergistic effects.

When administering IV infusions of these agents, check the IV site frequently for patency and to rule out infiltration. Also, with IV infusions, only use clear solutions, mix in 5% dextrose in water, and administer with an infusion device such as an IV pump (all vasoactive substances should be given via IV pump) in conjunction with cardiac monitoring. Infuse the agent slowly so as to not precipitate drastic and possibly dangerous cardiovascular changes, such as in the patient's blood pressure or pulse rate. If giving as an ophthalmic preparation, do not let the eye dropper touch the eye so that the remaining solution in the dropper and container is not contaminated. Drop the solution into the conjunctival sac.

Patients with chronic lung disease who are receiving an adrenergic agent should avoid any of the factors that can exacerbate their condition (e.g., allergens, foods, and cigarette smoking) and implement those measures that can help diminish the risk of respiratory infection. Fluid intake of up to 3000 ml per day should be encouraged to ensure adequate hydration, unless contraindicated. Patients should be encouraged to keep a journal of their symptoms and any improvement or worsening in their condition. Midodrine, which is given orally in patients with orthostatic intolerance (postural hypotension), should be taken as prescribed. Doses are often noted to not be taken after 6 PM.

Salmeterol is indicated for asthma and prevention of bronchospasms in patients over 12 years of age who may need long-term maintenance of their asthma. It is *not* to be used for relief of acute symptoms, and education about its dosing is important. Dosing of salmeterol is usually 2 puffs twice daily 12 hours apart for the maintenance effects. With prevention of exercise-induced asthma, it is recommended to take 2 puffs 1/2 hour to 1 hour before exercise and no additional dosing for 12 hours. The self-administered inhalant form is to be used by the following method: exhale slowly and thoroughly through nose, inhale deeply through mouth while administering the aerosol inhaler, hold breath for at least 3 seconds, and wait 1 minute in between inhalations. If using another type of inhalant, such as a steroid, use the bronchodilator first and wait approximately 5 minutes. All equipment should be rinsed, and the patient should be encouraged to perform mouth care after the use of any inhalant forms of medication.

Patient teaching tips for the adrenergic agents are listed in the box below.

● Evaluation

Therapeutic effects for which to monitor in patients receiving adrenergic agents for the treatment of hypotension, shock, or cardiac arrest include a decrease in edema, increased urinary output, return to normal vital signs (blood pressure, > or = 120/80 mm Hg or increase in blood pressure with each reading; pulse, >60 but <120 beats/min; respiratory rate, >12 but <20 breaths/min), improved skin color (pallor to pink) and temperature (cool to warm), and increased level of consciousness. Improvement in the condition of patients with bronchial asthma would be evidenced by return to a normal respiratory rate (>12 but <20 breaths/min); improved breath sounds throughout the lung fields with less rales; increased air exchange, including that in the lung bases; decreased to no cough; less dyspnea; improved blood gas levels; and increased tolerance of activity. If these agents are used for nasal congestion, the patient should report less congestion and a better ability to breathe. Therapeutic effects of midodrine (an alpha₁ agonist) include less postural intolerance.

Side effects of these medications that your patients should be aware of include, but are not limited to, cardiac dysrhythmias, hypertension, tachycardia, nervousness, anxiety, tremors, insomnia, and restlessness. Rebound nasal congestion, rhinitis, and nasal mucosa ulcerations are possible adverse effects of the nasal decongestants. Side effects related to the use of midodrine include "goose bumps," itchy scalp, and possible hypertension.

Therapeutic response to salmeterol includes an improvement in asthma with improved lung sounds, less wheezing, less respiratory distress, and an overall improved respiratory status. Side effects for which to monitor include CNS stimulation with headache, nervousness, hyperactivity, dizziness, GI upset, tremors, tachycardia, elevated blood pressure, and palpitations.

⚡ patient teaching tips

Adrenergic Agents

➤ Patients should always take medications as prescribed, as excessive dosing may cause CNS and cardiovascular stimulation.

➤ When taking inhaled forms of medication for metered-dose administration, patients should shake the container thoroughly, exhale through nose, and administer medication by aerosol while inhaling or breathing in deeply through mouthpiece of inhaler. Patients should hold their breath for a few seconds and exhale slowly. When using the inhaler for more than one breath application, patients should wait 2 minutes between inhalations of the agent and *only* take amount ordered!

➤ If patients have a history of diabetes mellitus, hypertension, hyperthyroidism, dysrhythmias, chest pain, or seizures, they should make sure their physician knows of these and of any other medications they may be taking for these conditions. Because of the CNS and cardiovascular stimulation produced by adrenergic agents, these medical conditions need to be very closely monitored and the agents must be carefully used to prevent worsening of the preexisting CNS or cardiac disorder.

➤ Patients should not take OTC medication or any other medications without their physician's approval.

➤ If patients' respiratory difficulties increase with use of these medications, they should contact their physician immediately because of the possible tolerance to their actions this may represent.

➤ Patients taking inhaled forms of isoproterenol (Isuprel) should be told not to be alarmed if their sputum or saliva turns pink; this is caused by the medication.

➤ Patients should be informed that sublingual forms of these medications should be held under the tongue, and *not* swallowed until they are completely dissolved. Patients should rinse out their mouths afterward so as to prevent dental problems such as tooth decay.

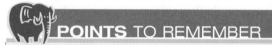

POINTS TO REMEMBER

Adrenergics

- Drugs that stimulate the sympathetic nervous system; also called *adrenergic agonists* and *sympathomimetics.*
- Mimic the CNS neurotransmitters norepinephrine and epinephrine.

Dopaminergic Receptors

- Predominant response when stimulated: vasodilation.
- Located on *postsynaptic* effector cells, blood vessels, and organs.
- Primary site; renal, mesenteric, coronary, and cerebral arteries.

Catecholamines

- Substances that produce a sympathomimetic response (stimulate the SNS).

- Endogenous (natural) catecholamines: epinephrine, norepinephrine, and dopamine.
- Exogenous (synthetic) catecholamines: isoproterenol and dobutamine.

Nursing Considerations

- Patients should avoid respiratory irritants and patients with infections should try to minimize situation that require the use of the adrenergic agonists.
- Patients should avoid any OTC or other prescribed medications because of possible drug interactions.
- With nasal preparations, rebound nasal congestion or ulcerations of the nasal mucosa may occur if drugs are overused. Educate patient to use only as directed.
- Medications should be used only as directed.
- Overuse of inhalant agents can lead to toxicity.

REVIEW QUESTIONS

1. Use of an adrenergic agonist beta$_1$ stimulator agent will result in increased cardiac contractility or a positive:
   a. Inotropic effect
   b. Cholotromic effect
   c. Dromotropic effect
   d. Chronotropic effect

2. Which of the following should the patient expect if he or she is taking an adrenergic agonist?
   a. Increased heart rate
   b. Increased GI peristalsis
   c. Increased bronchial resistance
   d. Vasodilation of only cutaneous vessels

3. Which of the following would be contraindicated in a patient taking epinephrine?
   a. Asthma
   b. Cardiac arrest
   c. Shock from trauma
   d. Acute bronchospasms

4. Your patient is receiving low-dose dobutamine for congestive heart failure and is now complaining of "tightness of the chest" but is feeling better. Heart rate is 110 beats/min, blood pressure is 152/98 mm Hg, and respirations are 20 breaths/min (baseline vital signs were P86, BP 120/82, R18). Which of the following would be your most immediate concern?
   a. The patient is most likely anaphylactic.
   b. These are normal side effects of the drug.
   c. The medication may be worsening a possible pre-existing cardiac disorder.
   d. These vital signs indicate that she is not improving and the dose should increase.

5. Which of the following would occur with an adrenergic beta$_2$-stimulating agent?
   a. Tachycardia
   b. Bronchodilation
   c. Sinus bradycardia
   d. Bronchoconstriction

For Answers see www.harcourthealth.com/MERLIN/Lilley/.

CRITICAL THINKING Activities

1. Why is it important to carefully assess the elderly patient for the presence of medical conditions before administering any beta-adrenergic agonist agents?
2. What is the potential harm to a patient who is about to receive both epinephrine inhalant therapy and isuprel subcutaneous injection for treatment of an acute exacerbation of asthma?
3. Discuss the rationale behind careful titration and monitoring of patients receiving vasoactive adrenergic agents.

For Answers see www.harcourthealth.com/MERLIN/Lilley/.

bibliography

Albanese J, Nutz P: *Mosby's 2001 nursing drug reference and review cards*, St Louis, 2001, Mosby.

American Hospital Formulary Service: *AHFS drug information*, Bethesda, Md, 2000, American Society of Health-System Pharmacists.

Anderson PO, Knoben JE, Troutman WG: *Handbook of clinical drug data 1999-2000*, ed 9, New York, 1999, McGraw-Hill.

Johns Hopkins Hospital, Department of Pediatrics et al: *The Harriet Lane handbook*, ed 15, St Louis, 2000, Mosby.

Keen JH: *Critical care and emergency drug reference*, ed 3, St Louis, 1996, Mosby.

Medical Letter: Fenoldopam: a new drug for parenteral treatment of severe hypertension 40(1027), May 22, 1998.

Mosby's GenRx: a comprehensive reference for generic and brand drugs, ed 10, St Louis, 2000, Mosby.

Skidmore-Roth L: *Mosby's 2001 nursing drug reference*, St Louis, 2001, Mosby.

Remember to check the **Online Worksheet** for additional learning opportunities: **www.harcourthealth.com/MERLIN/Lilley/**

Chapter 17

Adrenergic-Blocking Agents

www.harcourthealth.com/MERLIN/Lilley/

objectives

When you reach the end of this chapter, you should be able to do the following:

Look for this symbol for topics covered in the **Online Worksheet**

1 Discuss the normal anatomy and physiology of the autonomic nervous system as it pertains to adrenergic-blocking agents or sympatholytics.

2 List examples of the various adrenergic antagonists or adrenergic blockers.

3 Discuss the mechanisms of action, therapeutic effects, uses, and adverse and toxic effects of adrenergic antagonists.

4 Identify the antidotes used to treat an adrenergic-blocking agent overdose.

5 Develop a nursing care plan that includes all phases of the nursing process as related to the administration of the various adrenergic antagonists and the treatment of side effects and overdose or toxicity stemming from use of these agents.

drug profiles

acebutolol, p. 271
atenolol, p. 271
carvedilol, p. 271
ergotamine tartrate, p. 267
esmolol, p. 272
labetalol, p. 272
○━ metoprolol, p. 273

phenoxybenzamine hydrochloride, p. 267
phentolamine, p. 267
prazosin, p. 268
○━ propranolol, p. 273
○━ sotalol, p. 273
tolazoline, p. 269

○━ Key drug.

glossary

Agonists (ag′ ə nists) Drugs with a specific cellular affinity that produces a "mimic" response. (p. 264)

Angina (an ji′ nə) Paroxysmal chest pain caused by myocardial ischemia. (p. 270)

Antagonists (an tag′ ə nists) Drugs that bind to adrenergic receptors and inhibit or block neurotransmitters. (p. 264)

Blood-brain barrier Semipermeable membrane that selectively allows substances with specific characteristics to pass into the brain. (p. 270)

Cardioprotective The characteristic of beta-blockers to inhibit stimulation by circulating catecholamines. (p. 270)

Cardioselective beta-blockers Beta-blocking drugs that are selective for beta₁-adrenergic receptors. Also called *beta₁-blocking agents*. (p. 269)

Dysrhythmia (dis rith′ me ah) Irregular heartbeat. (p. 270)

Extravasation (ek strav′ ə sa′ shən) Leaking of fluid from the blood vessel into the tissues. (p. 266)

Glycogenolysis (gli′ ko jə nol′ ə sis) The production of glucose from glycogen in the liver, which is reduced by beta-blockers. (p. 270)

Intrinsic sympathomimetic activity (ISA) (in trin′ zik \ sim′ pə tho′ mi met ik) Action of agents within the beta-blocking class. A drug that mimics the activity of the adrenergic system, such as certain beta-blockers (acebutolol). (p. 269)

Lipophilicity (lip′ o fil is ət e) Attraction to lipid or fat. (p. 270)

Nonspecific beta-blockers Beta-blocking drugs that block both beta₁- and beta₂-adrenergic receptors. (p. 269)

Orthostatic hypotension (or tho′ stat′ ik \ hi′ po ten′ shən) Abnormally low blood pressure occurring when a person assumes the standing position. (p. 268)

Oxytocics (ok′ si to′ sikz) Drugs used to treat postpartum and postabortion bleeding caused by uterine relaxation and enlargement. They stimulate the smooth muscle of the uterus to contract. (p. 265)

Pheochromocytoma (fe′ o kro′ mo si to′ mə) Vascular tumor that secretes norepinephrine and stimulates the CNS. (p. 265)

Sympatholytics Another name for adrenergic antagonists. (p. 264)

Vaughan Williams classification System of classifying antidysrhythmic agents. (p. 270)

The autonomic nervous system consists of the parasympathetic and sympathetic nervous systems. The class of drugs discussed in this chapter works primarily on the sympathetic nervous system (SNS). As discussed in Chapter 16, the adrenergic drugs stimulate the SNS. These drugs are also called **agonists** because they bind to receptors and cause a response. The adrenergic blockers have the opposite effect and are therefore referred to as

antagonists. They also bind to adrenergic receptors but in doing so inhibit or block stimulation of the SNS. They are also referred to as **sympatholytics** because they "lyse," or inhibit, SNS stimulation.

Throughout the body there are receptor sites for the sympathetic neurotransmitters norepinephrine and epinephrine. These are called the *adrenergic receptors,* and there are two basic types—alpha and beta. There are subtypes of both the alpha- and beta-adrenergic receptors, designated 1 and 2. Alpha$_1$- and alpha$_2$-adrenergic receptors are differentiated by their location on nerves. Alpha$_1$-adrenergic receptors are located on the cell, muscle, or organ that the nerve is stimulating (postsynaptic effector cells). The alpha$_2$-adrenergic receptors are located on the actual nerves that stimulate the effector cells. Beta$_1$-adrenergic receptors are located primarily on the heart. Beta$_2$-adrenergic receptors are located primarily on the smooth muscles of the bronchioles and blood vessels. It is at these receptors that adrenergic blockers work, and these agents are classified by the type of adrenergic receptor they block—alpha or beta. Hence they are called *alpha-blockers* and *beta-blockers.*

ALPHA-BLOCKERS

Alpha-adrenergic–blocking agents, or alpha-blockers, interrupt or block the stimulation of the SNS at the alpha-adrenergic receptor. Various physiologic responses occur when the stimulation of the alpha-adrenergic receptors is inhibited. Adrenergic blockade at the alpha-adrenergic receptors leads to vasodilation, decreased blood pressure, miosis or constriction of the pupil, or suppressed ejaculation. The ergot alkaloids dihydroergotamine mesylate, ergoloid mesylate, ergotamine tartrate, and ergonovine maleate are alpha-blockers that are used mainly for their vasoconstrictor properties. The alpha-blockers doxazosin, prazosin, and terazosin are used as antihypertensive agents because they cause vasodilation. Each of these two groups of agents block alpha-adrenergic receptors, but they have an affinity for different sites in the body, and therefore the resultant effects differ. Other alpha-blockers are phenoxybenzamine, phentolamine, and tolazoline.

Mechanism of Action

As previously mentioned, alpha-blockers work by blocking or inhibiting the normal stimulation of the SNS. They do this either by directly competing with the SNS neurotransmitter norepinephrine or by a noncompetitive process. Most alpha-blockers are competitive in their actions. They have a higher affinity for the alpha-adrenergic receptor than norepinephrine and occupy the receptor before the neurotransmitter can do so. Once this competitive alpha-blocker binds to the receptor, it causes the receptor to be less responsive. This blockade is reversible. Noncompetitive alpha-blockers work in a different fashion. They also bind to the alpha-adrenergic receptors, but this type of bond (a covalent bond) is irreversible. An example of an irreversible antagonist is phenoxybenzamine. Regardless of which way the blockade is accom-

plished, the result is a decreased response to stimulation of the SNS. Figure 17-1 illustrates these two mechanisms.

Drug Effects

Alpha-blockers have many effects on the normal physiologic functions of the body. The effects of each agent differ depending on the agent's selectivity for particular tissues or cells in the body. Ergot alkaloids can cause peripheral vasoconstriction as well as the constriction of dilated arteries. Certain alpha-blockers can stimulate uterine contractions. Others can block alpha-adrenergic receptors on both vascular and nonvascular smooth muscle. The vascular smooth muscle for which these alpha-blockers have an affinity is that in the bladder and its sphincters, the gastrointestinal tract and its sphincters, the prostate, and the ureters. The nonvascular smooth muscle for which these agents have an affinity is in the CNS, liver, and kidneys. Unlike ergot alkaloids, some alpha-blockers can induce arterial and venous dilation and thus decrease peripheral vascular resistance and blood pressure. Alpha-blockers can also affect certain concentrations of neurotransmitters, causing a depletion of catecholamines such as norepinephrine and epinephrine. Others can directly block a neurotransmitter such as serotonin (5-hydroxytryptamine) or indirectly cause it to be depleted.

Therapeutic Uses

Alpha-blockers have many therapeutic effects, but these effects differ greatly depending on the particular agent. Ergot alkaloids constrict the dilated arteries going to the brain (carotid arteries) that are often responsible for causing vascular headaches such as migraines. The vasoconstriction of these dilated arteries relieves headache and other symptoms. They are also used as **oxytocics,** agents used to control postpartum and postabortion bleeding caused by uterine relaxation and enlargement. These agents increase the intensity of uterine contractions and induce local vasoconstriction.

Alpha-blockers such as doxazosin, prazosin, terazosin, and tamsulosin cause both arterial and venous dilation. This reduces peripheral vascular resistance and blood pressure; thus these agents are used to treat hypertension. Alpha-adrenergic receptors are also present on the prostate and bladder, and for this reason alpha-blockers are used in patients with benign prostatic hyperplasia (BPH) to decrease resistance to urinary outflow. This reduces urinary obstruction and relieves some of the effects of BPH.

Other alpha-blockers can inhibit excitatory responses to adrenergic stimulation. These agents noncompetitively block alpha-adrenergic receptors on smooth muscle and various exocrine glands. Because of this action, these alpha-blockers are very useful in controlling or preventing hypertension in patients who have a **pheochromocytoma,** a tumor that forms on the adrenal glands on top of the kidneys and secretes norepinephrine, thus causing SNS stimulation. Alpha-blockers are also useful in the treatment of patients who have increased alpha-adrenergic

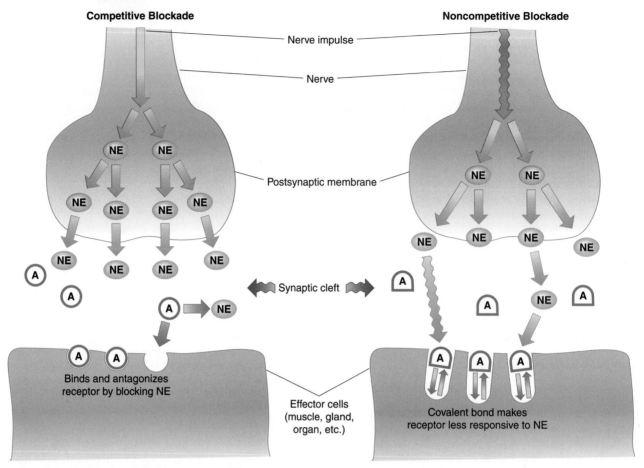

Competitive Blockade

Noncompetitive Blockade

Nerve impulse

Nerve

NE NE

NE NE

Postsynaptic membrane

NE NE NE NE

NE NE NE NE

NE NE

NE NE NE NE

A

A

Synaptic cleft

A

A

A NE

A

NE A

A A

A A A

Binds and antagonizes
receptor by blocking NE

Effector cells
(muscle, gland,
organ, etc.)

Covalent bond makes
receptor less responsive to NE

Fig. 17-1 Alpha-blocker mechanisms for alpha-adrenergic competitive and noncompetitive blockade.

activity. Three such conditions are Raynaud's disease, acrocyanosis, and frostbite. Phenoxybenzamine is an alpha-blocker useful for the treatment of these syndromes.

Other alpha-blockers are effective at antagonizing responses injected catecholamines such as epinephrine and norepinephrine. This causes peripheral vasodilation and decreases peripheral resistance by blocking catecholamine-stimulated vasoconstriction. They can also be used to treat pheochromocytomas. Because of their potent vasodilating properties and their fast onset of action, they are also used to prevent skin necrosis and sloughing after the **extravasation** of vasopressors such as norepinephrine or epinephrine. When these drugs extravasate, or leak out of the blood vessel into the surrounding tissue, this causes vasoconstriction and ultimately tissue death, or necrosis. If the vasoconstriction is not reversed quickly, the whole limb can be lost. Phentolamine, an alpha-blocker, can reverse this potent vasoconstriction and restore blood flow to the ischemic, vasoconstricted area.

Side Effects and Adverse Effects

The primary side effects and adverse effects of alpha-blockers are those related to their effects on the vasculature. The alpha-blockers' primary side effects and adverse effects are listed by body system in Table 17-1.

Toxicity and Management of Overdose

In an acute overdose, the patient's stomach should be emptied immediately either by inducing emesis with syrup of ipecac or by gastric lavage. After this, activated charcoal should be administered to bind to the drug and remove it from the stomach and the circulation. To hasten elimination of the drug bound to the activated charcoal, the first dose should be given with a cathartic such as sorbitol. Symptomatic and supportive measures should be instituted as needed. Blood pressure support with the administration of fluids, volume expanders, and vasopressor agents and the administration of anticonvulsants such as diazepam for the control of seizures are examples of such measures.

Interactions

The most severe of the drug interactions with alpha-blockers are the ones that potentiate the alpha-blockers' effects. Alpha-blockers as a whole are very highly protein bound and compete for binding sites with other drugs that are highly protein bound. With limited sites for binding on protein and increased competition for these sites, the result is that more drug is not bound; therefore more drug circulates freely in the bloodstream. Because drug that is not bound to protein is active, the result is a more pronounced drug effect. Some of the common drugs that

Alpha-Blockers: Adverse Effects

17-1

Body System	Side/Adverse Effects
Cardiovascular	Palpitations, orthostatic, hypotension, tachycardia, edema, dysrhythmias, chest pain
Central nervous system	Dizziness, headache, drowsiness, anxiety, depression, vertigo, weakness, numbness, fatigue
Gastrointestinal	Nausea, vomiting, diarrhea, constipation, abdominal pain
Other	Incontinence, nose bleeding, tinnitus, dry mouth, pharyngitis, rhinitis

Alpha-Blockers: Common Drug Interactions

17-2

Drug	Mechanism	Results
Beta-blockers Calcium channel blockers Diuretics	Additive effects	Profound hypotension
Protein-bound drugs	Compete for binding	Increased effect

interact with alpha-blockers and the results of these interactions are given in Table 17-2.

Dosages

For the recommended dosages of alpha-blockers, see the table on p. 268.

drug profiles

Alpha-blockers are prescription-only drugs that are available in many dosage forms. The oral forms include tablets, capsules, solutions, and sublingual tablets. Parenteral formulations include IV, IM, and SC injections. They are also available as rectal suppositories. Most alpha-blockers are rated as pregnancy category C agents by the FDA. Ergot alkaloids, however, are rated as pregnancy category X drugs.

ergotamine tartrate

Ergotamine (Ergostat) is an ergot alkaloid. All ergot alkaloids are obtained from a fungus called *Claviceps purpurea* that grows on rye. It causes dilated blood vessels in the brain, the carotid arteries, to constrict. These dilated arteries are responsible for causing vascular headaches such as migraines and cluster headaches. Ergotamine is contraindicated in patients with peripheral vascular disease, coronary artery disease, sepsis, impaired hepatic or renal function, and severe hypertension, as well as in pregnant women. It is available as a sublingual 2-mg tablet, an aerosolized inhaler, and as a rectal suppository that contains 2 mg of ergotamine and 100 mg of caffeine. There are also several combination-drug preparations available in oral tablet form. These combinations vary; some of the other agents combined with ergotamine in these preparations are beladonna alkaloids, phenobarbital, and caffeine. The dosages table on page 268 contains the dosing information for the 2-mg sublingual tablets as well as the aerosol preparation.

PHARMACOKINETICS

HALF-LIFE	ONSET	PEAK	DURATION
21 hr	30 min-2 hr	30 min-3 hr	3-4 hr

phenoxybenzamine hydrochloride

Phenoxybenzamine (Dibenzyline) is an alpha-blocker that reduces blood pressure by reducing peripheral vascular resistance. It is used to treat the hypertension caused by pheochromocytoma. Phenoxybenzamine is also useful in the treatment of vascular disorders such as frostbite, Raynaud's disease, and acrocyanosis, which have as an underlying cause increased alpha-adrenergic activity. Phenoxybenzamine directly blocks the alpha-adrenergic receptors and is therefore very useful in the treatment of these vasospastic disorders. The drug is contraindicated in patients who have shown a hypersensitivity reaction to it or who have conditions in which hypotension is undesirable. It is available as a 10-mg capsule. The recommended dosage is given in the table on p. 268.

PHARMACOKINETICS

HALF-LIFE	ONSET	PEAK	DURATION
24 hr	<2 hr	4-6 hr	3-4 days

phentolamine

Phentolamine (Regitine) is an alpha-blocker that reduces peripheral vascular resistance and is also used to treat hypertension. Unlike phenoxybenzamine, it can be used to help establish the diagnosis of pheochromocytoma as well as treat the high blood pressure caused by this catecholamine-secreting tumor. To help establish a diagnosis of pheochromocytoma using phentolamine, a single IV dose of the drug is given to the hypertensive patient who is suspected of having the tumor. If the blood pressure declines rapidly, it is highly likely that the patient has a pheochromocytoma. It is only available as an IV preparation, but this confers some advantages because it can then be used to treat the extravasation of vasoconstricting IV drugs such as norepinephrine, epinephrine, and dopamine, which when given intravenously can leak out of the vein, especially if the

DOSAGES Selected Alpha-Adrenergic–Blocking Agents

agent	pharmacologic class	dosage range	purpose
ergotamine tartrate (Ergostat)	Alpha-blocker	*Adult* Aerosol: one inhalation (0.36 mg) repeated at ≥5-min intervals; do not exceed 6 doses/day or 15/wk SL tablets: 2 mg; repeat at ½-hr intervals; do not exceed 6 mg/day or 5 tablets/week	Vascular headache
phenoxybenzamine hydrochloride (Dibenzyline)	Alpha-blocker	*Adult* PO: initial dose of 10 mg bid; usual range 20-40 mg 2-3 times/day	Hypertension
phentolamine (Regitine)	Alpha-blocker	*Pediatric* IM/IV: 0.05-0.1 mg/kg/dose preop and prn during surgery *Adult* IM/IV: 5 mg 1-2 hr preop and 5 mg prn during surgery	Control/prevention of hypertension during surgery
		Adult IV: 5-15 mg	Hypertensive crises
		Adult 5-10 mg into extravasation site *Pediatric* 0.1-0.2 mg/kg into extravasation site	Treatment of norepinephrine dermal necrosis
prazosin (Minipress)	Alpha₁-blocker	*Adult* PO: 1 mg 2-3/day; maintenance range, 6-15 mg/day divided	Hypertension
tolazoline (Priscoline)	Alpha-blocker	*Neonatal* IV: 1-2 mg/kg via scalp vein, followed by 1-2 mg/kg/hr infusion	Neonatal pulmonary hypertension

IV tube is not correctly positioned. If the drug is allowed to extravasate into the surrounding tissue, this leads to intense vasoconstriction, decreased blood flow, necrosis, and potential loss of the limb. When phentolamine is injected subcutaneously in a circular fashion around the extravasation site, this causes alpha-adrenergic receptor blockade and vasodilation, which in turn increases blood flow to the ischemic tissue, thus preventing permanent damage. It is contraindicated in patients who have shown a hypersensitivity to it, those who have suffered a myocardial infarction (MI), and those with coronary artery disease. The recommended dosages are given in the table above.

PHARMACOKINETICS

HALF-LIFE	ONSET	PEAK	DURATION
19 min	Immediate	2 min	15-30 min

prazosin

Prazosin (Minipress) is an alpha₁-adrenergic-blocking agent primarily used to treat hypertension and to reduce urinary obstruction in men with BPH. Other drugs that are chemically and pharmacologically related to prazosin are doxazosin (Cardura), terazosin (Hytrin), and tamsulosin (Flomax). Its primary antihypertensive effects are related to its selective and competitive inhibition of alpha₁-adrenergic receptors. In men with BPH, prazosin relieves the impaired urinary flow and urinary flow and urinary frequency by relaxing and dilating the vasculature and smooth muscle in the area surrounding the prostate. It also rather dramatically lowers blood pressure. A patient's ability to tolerate this drop in blood pressure must be taken into consideration when prescribing alpha-blockers for the treatment of BPH. Often when patients are first started on the drug, they become very lightheaded and may even pass out when standing up after sitting or lying down. This is referred to as **orthostatic hypotension.** Although it is a fairly common problem specific to the alpha₁-blockers prazosin, doxazosin, terazosin, and tamsalosin, patients quickly acquire a tolerance to it, most after the first dose. Often patients taking their first dose are told to take it at bedtime to circumvent the problem. Prazosin is contraindicated in patients who have shown hypersensitivity reactions to it. It is available as a 1-, 2-, and 5-mg capsule and as a combination product containing the diuretic polythiazide. This preparation is called Minizide. The normally recommended dosages of prazosin are given in the table on p. 268.

PHARMACOKINETICS

HALF-LIFE	ONSET	PEAK	DURATION
2-3 hr	2 hr	1-3 hr	6-12 hr

tolazoline

Tolazoline (Priscoline) is an alpha-blocker that causes peripheral vasodilation and decreases peripheral resistance. It does this primarily by directly relaxing vascular smooth muscle through the competitive blockade of alpha-adrenergic receptors. It is primarily used for the treatment of hypertension in neonates when the hypertension causes the oxygen level in the neonate's blood-stream to decrease and the usual supportive measures are not able to compensate for this. Tolazoline is contraindicated in patients who have had hypersensitivity reactions to it and in patients with known or suspected coronary artery disease. It is also contraindicated in patients who have suffered a cerebrovascular accident. It is available only as a parenteral (IV, IM, or SC) injection. The normal dosages are given in the table on p. 268.

PHARMACOKINETICS

HALF-LIFE	ONSET	PEAK	DURATION
3-10 hr	<30 min	30-60 min	3-4 hr

BETA-BLOCKERS

Beta-adrenergic–blocking agents (beta-blockers) block SNS stimulation of the beta-adrenergic receptors by competing with the endogenous catecholamines norepinephrine and epinephrine. Beta-blockers can be either selective or nonselective, depending on the type of beta-adrenergic receptors they antagonize or block. As mentioned earlier, beta$_1$-adrenergic receptors are located primarily on the heart. Beta-blockers selective for these receptors are sometimes called **cardioselective beta-blockers,** or beta$_1$-blocking agents. Other beta-blockers block both beta$_1$- and beta$_2$-adrenergic receptors, the latter located primarily on the smooth muscles of the bronchioles and blood vessels. Beta-blockers that block both types of beta-adrenergic receptors are referred to as **nonspecific beta-blockers.** The agents within the beta-blocker class can be further categorized according to whether they have **intrinsic sympathomimetic activity (ISA).** Agents with ISA (acebutolol, penbutolol, and timolol) not only block beta-adrenergic receptors but also partially stimulate them. This was initially believed to be an advantageous characteristic, but clinical use has not borne this out. Box 17-1 lists the currently available beta-blockers.

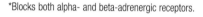

> **BOX 17-1** Currently Available Beta-Blockers
>
> **NONSPECIFIC BETA-BLOCKERS**
> - carteolol (Cartrol)
> - carvedilol (Coreg)
> - labetalol (Normodyne and Trandate)*
> - nadolol (Corgard)
> - penbutolol (Levatol)
> - pindolol (Visken)
> - propranolol (Inderal)
> - sotalol (Betapace)
> - timolol (Blocadren)
>
> **CARDIOSELECTIVE BETA-BLOCKERS**
> - acebutolol (Sectral)
> - atenolol (Tenormin)
> - betaxolol (Kerlone)
> - bisoprolol (Zebeta)
> - esmolol (Brevibloc)
> - metoprolol (Lopressor and Toprol XL)

*Blocks both alpha- and beta-adrenergic receptors.

Activity

Mechanism of Action

Because beta-blockers compete with and block norepinephrine and epinephrine at the beta-adrenergic receptors located throughout the body, the beta-adrenergic receptor sites can then no longer be stimulated by the neurotransmitters and SNS stimulation is blocked. Although beta-adrenergic receptors are located throughout the body, the most important ones in terms of these agents are the ones located on the surface of the heart, the smooth muscle of the bronchi, and the smooth muscle of blood vessels. Cardioselective beta$_1$-blockers block the beta$_1$-adrenergic receptors on the surface of the heart. This decreases heart rate, slows conduction through the atrioventricular (AV) node, prolongs sinoatrial (SA) node recovery, and decreases myocardial oxygen demand by decreasing myocardial contractility. Nonspecific beta-blockers also have this effect on the heart, but they block beta$_2$-adrenergic receptors on the smooth muscle of the bronchioles and blood vessels as well. This can cause the bronchioles to constrict, which in turn leads to narrowing of the airways and shortness of breath. Nonspecific beta-blockers can also constrict blood vessels by blocking beta$_2$-adrenergic receptors on the smooth muscle of blood vessels.

Drug Effects

When the beta-adrenergic receptors of the SNS on the heart are blocked, myocardial stimulation is blocked. This results in both decreased contractile force and decreased myocardial oxygen consumption. The smooth muscle that surrounds blood vessels controls the size of the blood vessels and can cause them to dilate or constrict depending on whether the alpha- or beta-adrenergic receptors are stimulated. When SNS stimulation at these smooth muscles is blocked by a beta-blocker, the muscles are then stimulated by the alpha-adrenergic receptors and contract. This causes increased peripheral vascular resistance.

Beta-blockers also affect the conduction cells in the SA and AV nodes. They tend to slow conduction through these cells and decrease heart rate and contractility. Catecholamines promote **glycogenolysis,** the production of glucose from glycogen, and mobilize glucose in response to hypoglycemia. Nonspecific beta-blockers impair this process. Nonspecific beta-blockers also impair the secretion of insulin from the pancreas, which causes an elevated blood glucose level. Beta-blockers can cause the release of free fatty acids from adipose tissue and moderately elevate blood levels of triglycerides, decreasing levels of good cholesterol, called high-density lipoproteins (HDLs).

Smooth muscle also surrounds the airways in the lungs called *bronchioles*. When beta$_2$-adrenergic receptors are blocked on these, the smooth muscle contracts, causing these airways to narrow.

Many of the beta-blockers that are lipid soluble can cross the **blood-brain barrier,** a semipermeable membrane that selectively allows substances with certain characteristics such as lipid solubility to pass into the brain. Lipid-soluble beta-blockers that can as a result cross into the brain produce weakness, lethargy, and fatigue.

Therapeutic Uses

The drug effects mentioned in the preceding section vary from beta-blocker to beta-blocker depending on the specific chemical characteristics of the agent. Some beta-blockers are used primarily in the treatment of **angina,** or chest pain. These work by decreasing demand for myocardial energy and oxygen consumption, which helps shift the supply-and-demand ratio to the supply side and allows more oxygen to get to the heart muscle. This in turn helps relieve the pain in the heart muscle caused by the lack of oxygen.

Other beta-blockers are considered **cardioprotective** because they inhibit stimulation by the circulating catecholamines. Catecholamines are released during muscle damage such as that caused by a myocardial infarction (MI), or heart attack. When a beta-blocker occupies their receptors, the circulating catecholamines cannot then bind to the receptors. Thus, the beta-blockers "protect" the heart from being stimulated by these catecholamines, which would only further increase the heart rate and the contractile force, thereby increasing myocardial oxygen demand. As a result, beta-blockers are frequently given to patients after they have suffered an MI to protect the heart from the effects of these released catecholamines.

As mentioned previously, beta-blockers also have a profound effect on the conduction system of the heart. The AV node normally receives impulse stimulation from the SA node and slows it down so that the ventricles have time to fill before they are stimulated to contract. Conduction in the SA node, which spontaneously depolarizes at the most frequent rate, is further slowed by beta-blockers, resulting in a decreased heart rate. They also slow conduction

Table 17-3	Beta-Blockers: Common Adverse Effects
Body System	**Side/Adverse Effects**
Blood	Agranulocytosis, thrombocytopenia
Cadiovascular	AV block, bradycardia, congestive heart failure, peripheral vascular insufficiency
Central nervous system	Dizziness, mental depression, lethargy, hallucinations
Gastrointestinal	Nausea, dry mouth, vomiting, diarrhea, cramps, ischemic colitis
Other	Impotence, rash, alopecia, bronchospasms

through the AV node. These effects of beta-blockers on the conduction system of the heart make them useful agents in the treatment of various types of irregular heartbeats called **dysrhythmias.** In the **Vaughan Williams classification** of antidysrhythmic drugs, the beta-blockers are in the class II category.

By blocking peripheral adrenergic receptors and decreasing stimulation from the SNS, beta-blockers are useful in treating hypertension. Traditionally beta-blockers were thought to worsen congestive heart failure (CHF). However, recent studies have shown benefit when using beta-blockers. Certain beta-blockers such as carvedilol and metoprolol have had the best results to date. The form of CHF that has a diastolic dysfunction component responds favorably to beta-blockers.

Because of their **lipophilicity** (attraction to lipid or fat), other beta-blockers can easily gain entry into the CNS and brain. These beta-blockers are used to treat migraine headaches. The topical application of beta-blockers on the eye has also been very effective in treating ocular disorders such as glaucoma.

Side Effects and Adverse Effects

The side effects and adverse effects of beta-blockers are primarily extensions of their pharmacologic activity. Most such effects are mild and diminish with time. Some of the most serious undesirable effects can be caused by acute withdrawal of the drug. This may exacerbate the underlying angina they are being used to treat, or it may precipitate an MI. Beta-blockers may also mask the signs and symptoms of hypoglycemia. Beta-blocker–induced side effects and adverse effects are listed by body site in Table 17-3.

Toxicity and Management of Overdose

After the acute ingestion of an overdose of a beta-blocker, the stomach should be emptied immediately either by inducing emesis or by gastric lavage. Treatment primarily consists of symptomatic and supportive care. Atropine may be given intravenously for the management of bradycardia. If the bradycardia persists despite atropine treatment, isoproterenol may be administered. If

Beta-Blockers: Drug Interactions

Drug	Mechanism	Result
Antacids (aluminum hydroxide type)	Decrease absorption	Decreased beta-blocker activity
Antimuscarinics/anticholinergics	Antagonism	Reduced beta-blocker effects
Diuretics and cardiovascular drugs	Additive effect	Additive hypotensive effects
Neuromuscular blocking agents	Additive effect	Prolonged neuromuscular blockade
Oral hypoglycemic agents	Antagonism	Decreased hypoglycemic effects

the bradycardia still persists, placement of a transvenous cardiac pacemaker should be considered. For the treatment of severe hypotension, vasopressors should be titrated until the desired blood pressure and heart rate are achieved. Intravenously administered diazepam may be useful for the treatment of seizures. Most beta-blockers are dialyzable; therefore hemodialysis may be useful in enhancing elimination in the event of severe overdose.

Interactions

Most of the drug interactions with beta-blockers result from either the additive effects of the coadministered medications, ones with similar mechanisms of action, or the antagonistic effects of the agents. Some of the common drugs that interact with beta-blockers and the results of this are given in Table 17-4.

Dosages

For information on the recommended dosages for selected beta-blockers, see the table on p. 272.

drug profiles

Beta-blockers are prescription-only drugs that are available in oral preparations as tablets and capsules and parenteral forms as intermittent injections or continuous IV infusions. Topically administered forms are also available. Beta-blocker eyedrops are used in the treatment of glaucoma. All beta-blockers except for acebutolol are rated as pregnancy category C agents. Acebutolol is a pregnancy category B agent.

acebutolol

Acebutolol (Sectral) is a cardioselective beta₁-blocker used for the treatment of hypertension, ventricular and supraventricular dysrhythmias, and angina, and in patients in the immediate period after an MI. It is commonly used alone as an antihypertensive agent or in combination with a diuretic for the additive antihypertensive effects. It is one of the few beta-blockers that possess ISA. It is contraindicated in patients who have had a hypersensitivity reaction to it; in those with severe bradycardia, heart block greater than first degree, Raynaud's disease, or malignant hypertension; and in those in cardio-

genic shock or cardiac failure. It is available as 200- and 400-mg capsules. The commonly recommended dosages are given in the table on p. 272.

PHARMACOKINETICS

HALF-LIFE	ONSET	PEAK	DURATION
3-4 hr	1.5-8 hr	3 hr	10-24 hr

atenolol

Atenolol (Tenormin) is a cardioselective beta-blocker that is commonly used to prevent future MIs in patients who have had an MI. It is also used in the treatment of hypertension and angina. It is available as an 0.5-mg/ml injection and as 25-, 50-, and 100-mg tablets. See the table on p. 272 for the recommended dosages.

PHARMACOKINETICS

HALF-LIFE	ONSET	PEAK	DURATION
6-7 hr	IV: Immediate	IV: <5 min	IV: <12 hr
	PO: <30 min	PO: 2-4 hr	PO: 24 hr

carvedilol

Carvedilol (Coreg) is new beta-blocker. It has many actions, including acting as a nonspecific beta-blocker, an alpha₁-blocker, a calcium channel blocker, and possibly an antioxidant. It is primarily used in the treatment of CHF but is also beneficial in hypertension and angina. It has been shown to slow progression of heart failure and decrease the frequency of hospitalization in patients with mild to moderate (class II-III) heart failure. Carvedilol is most commonly added to digoxin, furosemide, and ACE inhibitors when used to treat CHF. It is classified as a pregnancy category C agent. It is contraindicated in patients with class IV decompensated heart failure, asthma, second- or third-degree AV block, cardiogenic shock, and severe bradycardia. It is available as a 3.125-, 6.25-, 12.5-, and 25-mg tablet. Recommended dosages are given in the table on p. 272.

PHARMACOKINETICS

HALF-LIFE	ONSET	PEAK	DURATION
7-10 hr	30 min	1-2 hr	24 hr

DOSAGES Selected Beta-Adrenergic Agents

agent	pharmacologic class	dosage range	purpose
acebutolol (Sectral)	Beta$_1$-blocker	*Adult* PO: 400-800 mg/day divided 600-1200 mg/day divided	Hypertension Premature ventricular beats
atenolol (Tenormin)	Beta$_1$-blocker	*Adult* PO: 50-100 mg/day divided 50-200 mg/day divided IV: 5 mg over 5 min followed by 5 mg over 10 min	Hypertension Angina Acute myocardial infarction
carvedilol (Coreg)	Alpha and beta blocker	*Adult* PO: 3.125 mg twice a day; may double dose every 2 wk to highest tolerated dose	Heart failure, angina, and hypertension
esmolol (Brevibloc)	Beta$_1$-blocker	*Adult* IV: Bolus of 500 μg/kg/min followed by 4 min of 50 μg/kg/min and evaluate IV: 80 mg bolus over 30 min followed by 150 μg/kg/min infusion if needed	Supraventricular tachydysrhythmias Intraoperative-postop/ hypertension
labetalol (Normodyne, Trandate)	Alpha$_1$-beta blocker	*Adult* PO: 200-800 mg/day divided IV: 20 mg with additional doses of 40-80 mg at 10-min intervals until desired effect or a total dose of 300 mg is injected; maintenance infusion of 2 mg/min	Hypertension Severe hypertension
metoprolol (Lopressor, Toprol XL)	Beta$_1$-blocker	*Adult* PO: 100-450 mg/day divided 100 mg bid IV/PO: 3 bolus injections of 5 mg at 2-min intervals followed in 15-min by 50 mg PO q6h for 48-hr; thereafter 100 mg bid	Hypertension Late myocardial infarction Early myocardial infarction
propranolol (Inderal)	Beta-blocker	*Adult* PO: 80-320 mg/day divided 120-240 mg/day divided 10-30 mg 3-4 times/day 180-240 mg/day divided 20-40 mg 3-4 times/day 120-320 mg/day divided 160-240 mg/day divided 60 mg/day divided for 3 days before surgery with an alpha-blocker IV: 1-3 mg	Angina Hypertension Dysrhythmias Post-myocardial infarction Hypertrophic subaortic stenosis Essential tremor Migraine Pheochromocytoma surgery Serious dysrhythmias
sotalol (Betapace)	Beta-blocker	*Adult* PO: 160-320 mg/day divided	Life-threatening ventricular dysrhythmias

esmolol

Esmolol (Brevibloc) is a very potent short-acting beta$_1$-blocker. It is primarily used in acute situations to provide rapid, temporary control of the ventricular rate in patients with supraventricular tachydysrhythmias (SVTs). Because of its very short half-life, it is only given as an IV infusion, and the serum levels are titrated to control the patient's symptoms. It is available as a 250-mg/ml concentrate for injection and as a 10-mg/ml injection. Recommended dosages are given in the table above.

PHARMACOKINETICS

HALF-LIFE	ONSET	PEAK	DURATION
9 min	Immediate	6 min	15-20 min

labetalol

Labetalol (Normodyne, Trandate) is unusual in that it can block both alpha- and beta-adrenergic receptors. It is used in the treatment of severe hypertension and hypertensive emergencies to quickly lower the blood pressure before permanent damage is done. It is available both parenterally as a

5-mg/ml IV injection and in oral forms as 100-, 200-, and 300-mg tablets. The normal dosages are given in the table on p. 272.

PHARMACOKINETICS

HALF-LIFE	ONSET	PEAK	DURATION
6-8 hr	IV: 2-5 min	IV: 5-15 min	IV: 2-4 hr
	PO: 20-120 min	PO: 1-4 hr	PO: 8-24 hr

metoprolol

Metoprolol (Lopressor, Toprol XL) is a beta$_1$-blocker that has become very popular for use in the post-MI patient. Recent studies of metoprolol have shown increased survival in patients given the agent after they have suffered an MI. It is available as 1-mg/ml injection or as 50-, 100-, and 200-mg tablets (Lopressor) and 50-, 100-, and 200-mg extended-release tablets (Toprol XL). It is also available in combination with the diuretic hydrochlorothiazide (Lopressor HCT). Commonly recommended dosages are given in the table on p. 272.

PHARMACOKINETICS

HALF-LIFE	ONSET	PEAK	DURATION
3-4 hr	IV: Immediate	IV: 10 min	IV: 5-8 hr
	PO: 10 min	PO: 1.5-4 hr	PO: 24 hr

propranolol

Propranolol (Inderal) is the prototypical nonspecific beta$_1$- and beta$_2$-blocking agent. It was one of the very first beta-blockers to be used. The lengthy experience with it has yielded many uses for it. Besides the indications mentioned for acebutolol, propranolol has also been used in the treatment of the tachydysrhythmias associated with cardiac glycoside intoxication and for the treatment of hypertrophic subaortic stenosis, pheochromocytoma, thyrotoxicosis, migraine headaches, and essential tremors, as well as many other conditions. The same contraindications that apply to the cardioselective beta-blockers (cited in the discussion on acebutolol) apply to propranolol as well. In addition, it is contraindicated in patients with bronchial asthma. It is available as an IV injection, as 60-, 80-, 120-, and 160-mg oral long-acting capsules, and 10-, 20-, 40-, 60-, and 80-mg tablets. The recommended dosages are given in the table on p. 272.

PHARMACOKINETICS

HALF-LIFE	ONSET	PEAK	DURATION
3-4 hr	30 min	1-1.5 hr	8-12 hr

sotalol

Sotalol (Betapace) is a nonspecific beta-blocker that has very potent antidysrhythmic properties. It is commonly used for the management of difficult-to-treat dysrhythmias. Often these dysrhythmias are life-threatening ventricular dysrhythmias such as sustained ventricular tachycardia. Because it is a nonspecific beta-blocker, it causes some of the unwanted side effects typical of these agents. It is available in oral tablet form in 80-, 160-, and 240-mg amounts. Commonly recommended dosages are given in the table on p. 272.

PHARMACOKINETICS

HALF-LIFE	ONSET	PEAK	DURATION
12 hr	<1 hr	2.5-4 hr	8-12 hr

NEWER BETA-BLOCKERS

Many of the newer beta-blockers are cardioselective beta$_1$-blockers that only need to be taken once a day. The advantage to them is that they do not produce some of the unwanted side effects associated with nonspecific beta-blockers, such as bronchiole constriction and increased peripheral vascular resistance. The once-a-day dosing is another advantage. This helps promote patient compliance, which is very important for the patient taking several other medications to control their hypertension and possibly other diseases as well. Examples of some of these agents are betaxolol and bisoprolol.

nursing process

• Assessment

Adrenergic-blocking agents, or sympatholytics, produce a variety of effects on the patient, depending on the type of receptor blocked. Because of the clinical impact all of these agents have on mainly the cardiac and respiratory systems, their use requires careful assessment of the patient to minimize the side effects and maximize the therapeutic effects. To begin a thorough assessment, information should be gathered about the patient's allergies and past and present medical conditions. A system overview and a thorough medication history should form part of this process. Some pertinent questions to pose to the patient who is to receive an adrenergic blocking agent might include the following:

• Are you allergic to any medications or foods?
• Do you have a history of a chronic obstructive pulmonary disease such as emphysema, asthma, or chronic bronchitis?
• Do you have a history of hypotension, cardiac dysrhythmias, bradycardia, CHF, or any other cardiovascular disease?

These questions are important because alpha-blockers may precipitate hypotension, whereas beta-blockers may precipitate bradycardia, hypotension, heart block, CHF, and bronchoconstriction or increased airway resistance. Any preexisting condition that might be ex-

NURSING CARE PLAN Dysrhythmia

Ms. T.K., a 48-year-old professional journalist, is about to be discharged. The physician has prescribed atenolol (Tenormin) for treatment of cardiac dysrhythmias associated with a moderate mitral valve prolapse. She is asking many questions about the medication since this is a newly diagnosed condition. She is curious about the drug's mechanism of action and side effects as well as how she can minimize the side effects associated with the medication. You are about to begin a teaching session related to the administration of atenolol, and you have decided to give her a printed copy to take home because of her increased level of interest and inquiry about the drug.

assessment	*Nursing Diagnosis*	Risk for injury or fall related to possible postural hypotension or bradycardia as a side effect of atenolol
	Subjective Data	"What type of medication am I going to be on?"
		"Will I have to take this medication forever?"
		"What kind of side effects can I expect, and when is it necessary to see a physician?"
	Objective Data	Recent diagnosis of mitral valve prolapse
		No major complications related to the disease
		Education level of 4 years of college
		Readiness level: asking questions about the medication
planning and outcome criteria	*Goals Outcome Criteria*	Patient will be free of dysrhythmias upon return to physician's office in 1 month. Patient will show compliance to mediation therapy as evidenced by the following:
		• No complaints of palpitations or chest discomfort
		• Normal ECG upon return to physician's office
		• Decrease side effects because of proper home administration of medications
		• Lack of complications of drug therapy
implementation		Inform patient of the following information about atenolol therapy:
		• There are many drug interactions associated with atenolol, including alcohol, epinephrine, hydralazine, indomethacin, insulin, methyldopa, thyroid preparations, prazosin, and verapamil. You should be aware of these interactions so as to prevent side effects, particularly reoccurrence of dysrhythmias, chest pain, and palpitations.
		• These interactions may result in decreased effectiveness, more pronounced action, and other problems that you want to prevent from occurring while taking atenolol.
		• You should not discontinue the medication, your physician will most likely taper your dose over a 2-week period. Stopping this medication abruptly may lead to chest pain.
		• Take the medication as ordered.
		• Do not use OTC products containing alpha-adrenergic stimulants (nasal decongestants, cold preparations); this will help prevent any complications or adverse interactions with the medication.
		• Avoid alcohol and nicotine, since these will adversely affect the action of atenolol.
		• We will instruct you how to monitor your pulse so that you will know when to contact your physician (i.e., pulse <50 beats/min since bradycardia is a side effect).
		• Make sure you comply with all the aspects of your medication regimen, such as adequate exercise, dietary changes, weight control, and any other changes your health care provider has ordered.
		• It is suggested that you purchase a MedicAlert bracelet stating name, diagnosis, drugs being prescribed, phone number, and allergies.
		• Remember that this medication controls symptoms but does not provide a cure.
		• Should you experience shortness of breath, coughing at night, swelling of feet, pulse <50 beats/min, dizziness, fever, or depression, it is important to contact your physician.

NURSING CARE PLAN Dysrhythmia—cont'd

implementation	Inform patient of the following information about atenolol therapy: • Do not skip any doses or double up on this medication. • Blood pressure may be lowered because of medication and should be monitored. • Syncope may occur if postural hypotension occurs. • Change positions slowly to avoid dizziness or syncope.
evaluation	Positive therapeutic outcomes include the following: • Absence or decreased occurrence of dysrhythmia • Absence or decreased occurrence of palpitations • No chest pain Patient is monitored for common side effects of insomnia, fatigue, dizziness, mental changes, nausea, and diarrhea.

acerbated by the use of these agents might be a contraindication to their use.

Patients should be asked whether they are taking any of the drugs that can interact with the adrenergic-blocking agent that has been prescribed for them. These include alpha-blockers (ergotamines); beta-blockers, which could cause vasoconstriction, especially propranolol; and the other agents listed in Table 17-4. The contraindications to the use of these medications are related to their receptor-blocking effects and resulting cardiovascular actions, so these drugs are contraindicated in patients with peripheral vascular disease, CHF, or bradydysrhythmias. With the newer beta-blocker carvedilol, there are similar contraindications such as class IV decompensated heart failure, asthma, severe bradycardia, second- and third-degree heart block, and cardiogenic shock.

● Nursing Diagnoses

Nursing diagnoses related to the use of adrenergic antagonists, or sympatholytics, include, but are not limited to, the following:
• Deficient knowledge related to therapeutic regimen, side effects, drug interactions, and precautions to be taken.
• Risk for injury related to possible side effects of adrenergic antagonistics (e.g., numbness and tingling of fingers and toes).
• Imbalanced nutrition, less than body requirements because of nausea and vomiting, related to use of adrenergic blockers.
• Ineffective tissue perfusion related to cardiovascular side effects of hypertension.
• Disturbed sensory perception related to CNS adverse effects of drug.

● Planning

Goals for the patient receiving sympatholytics include, but are not limited to, the following:
• Patient takes medication exactly as prescribed.
• Patient experiences relief of the symptoms for which the medication was prescribed.

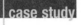 **Nutritional Supplements for Migraine Headaches**

Your 47-year-old patient has a 20-year history of migraine headaches. She has decided to try to treat her headaches, which have improved over the last 2 years, with nutritional supplementation. She is currently in excellent health. She takes one capsule of Fiorinal #3 every 6 hours as needed for headache pain and one 25-mg phenerghan suppository every 6 hours as needed for nausea and vomiting occurring with the headache. In your patient teaching session, you are to inform her of nutritional remedies used to help in migraines.
● *After doing research, what type of supplementation would you recommend (if you were able to prescribe) and why?*
● *What side effects have occurred with the type of supplement that you think is best?*

From Schoenen J, Jacquy J, Lenaerts M: Effectiveness of high-dose riboflavin in migraine prophylaxis, *Neurology* 50(2):466, 1998.

For Answers see www.harcourthealth.com/MERLIN/Lilley/.

• Patient remains compliant with the drug therapy.
• Patient demonstrates an adequate knowledge concerning the use of the specific medications, the side effects, and the appropriate dosing routine to be followed at home.
• Patient is free of injury to self as the result of adverse effects of the medications.

Outcome Criteria

Outcome criteria related to the administration of adrenergic blockers include the following:
• Patient will state the importance of both the pharmacologic and nonpharmacologic treatment of his or her migraine headaches, hypertension, or other reason for drug therapy.
• Patient will state reasons for compliance with the medication therapy and the risks and complications such as syncope, dizziness, and hypotension arising as a result of overuse of the medication.

- Patient will demonstrate the correct method of taking blood pressure with self-taking digital cuff or by using community resources.
- Patient will identify community resources for monitoring blood pressure (e.g., rescue squads, fire departments).
- Patient taking these medications for the treatment of migraine headaches will state the importance of remaining in a quiet, calm, and dark room during a headache.
- Patient will state those conditions that may occur of which the physician should be informed immediately, such as palpitations, chest pain, insomnia, and excessive agitation.
- Patient will keep all follow-up appointments with the physician to maintain safe therapy.
- Patient will follow instructions regarding the avoidance of sudden withdrawal of hypertensive agents to avoid rebound hypertensive crises and will experience minimal complications.

● Implementation

Several nursing interventions can maximize the therapeutic effects of adrenergic-blocking agents and minimize the side effects. Thorough patient education is a must in ensuring good compliance. Patients taking alpha-blockers should be encouraged to change positions slowly so as to prevent or minimize postural hypotension. When using beta-blockers, patients should know to take their apical pulse for one full minute as well as their blood pressure because of the cardiac depression that can occur with these agents. They should be told to contact the physician if the systolic blood pressure decreases to less than 100 mm Hg or the pulse decreases to less than 60 beats/min. The physician should also be notified if the blood pressure continues to decrease, even by a few millimeters of mercury. Patients should also know to report any weight gain, especially more than 2 pounds (1 kg) in a week, weakness, shortness of breath, and edema to their physician immediately. Make sure that patients are weaned off these medications slowly, if this is indicated, because of the possible rebound hypertension or chest pain that rapid withdrawal can precipitate.

Carvedilol, which is a beta-blocker, alpha$_1$-blocker, and calcium channel blocker, is generally given at 3.125 mg bid with possible doubling of dosage every 2 weeks until reaching the highest tolerated dose. Therefore patient education regarding side effects is important to the safe dosing of this agent. Since carvedilol is often used with digoxin, furosemide, and ACE inhibitors, patient teaching about dietary intake of potassium, recording of pulse rates before doses, and reporting of adverse effects (e.g., postural hypotension and bradycardia) is crucial to patient safety. Patients should be encouraged to keep a journal of their responses to the medication regimen and record their daily (or more frequent) blood pressures.

Patient teaching tips for adrenergic-blocking agents are listed below.

● Evaluation

Therapeutic effects for which to monitor in patients receiving adrenergic-blocking agents include, but are not limited to, the following:
- Decrease in blood pressure, pulse rate, and palpitations in patients with a pheochromocytoma
- Alleviation of the symptoms of Raynaud's disease
- Return to normal blood pressure and pulse with lowering of the blood pressure toward 120/80 mm Hg or the pulse to within normal limits (60 beats/min)
- Decrease in chest pain in patients with angina

Patients must also be monitored for the occurrence of the side effects of these medications, which include, but are not limited to, the following:
- Hypotension
- Tachycardia (alpha-blockers)
- Bradycardia
- Heart block
- CHF
- Increased airway resistance
- Fatigue
- Lethargy
- Depression
- Insomnia
- Vivid nightmares

---

patient teaching tips

Adrenergic-Blocking Agents

Alpha-Blockers
➤ Encourage patients to take medication as prescribed and to never abruptly stop taking medication.
➤ Patients should avoid OTC medications because of drug interactions.
➤ Keep these and all other medications out of the reach of children.
➤ Patients should notify their physician if palpitations, dyspnea, nausea, or vomiting occur.
➤ Patients should avoid caffeine because of excessive irritability.

➤ Patients should avoid alcohol ingestion and should not engage in hazardous activities until stable blood levels are achieved.

Beta-Blockers
➤ Encourage patients to always take medication as prescribed, no more and no less.
➤ Tell patients to never abruptly stop taking the medication.
➤ Encourage patients to contact their physician should they become ill and unable to take the prescribed doses. Rebound hypertension or chest pain may occur if this medication is discontinued abruptly.

➤ Patients should report any weight gain of more than 2 pounds (1 kg) within a week as well as any problems with fluid buildup or edema of the feet or ankles, any shortness of breath, or excessive fatigue or weakness.

➤ Patients should notify their physician if they experience any syncope or dizziness.

➤ Inform patients that they may notice a decrease in their tolerance to exercise, and dizziness or fainting may occur with increased activity. Patients should be encouraged to change positions slowly and to contact their physician if any of the above problems occur.

➤ Patients should be warned to not take OTC medications without the approval of their physician!

POINTS TO REMEMBER

Alpha-Blockers

- Block stimulation of the alpha$_1$- and alpha$_2$-adrenergic receptors by norepinephrine or epinephrine.
- Cause a variety of physiologic responses depending on what receptors are blocked.
- Some agents may stimulate the alpha-adrenergic receptors at regular doses and block them at high doses.

Alpha$_1$-Blockers

- Predominant response when blocked: vasodilation and relaxation.
- Block postsynaptic alpha-adrenergic receptors from the stimulatory actions of norepinephrine and epinephrine.
- Drugs such as prazosin, doxazosin, and terazosin.
- Vasodilation: drop in blood pressure; reduces urinary obstruction, which leads to increased urinary flow rates.

Beta-Blockers

- Block stimulation of beta-adrenergic receptors by SNS neurotransmitters norepinephrine and epinephrine as well as dopamine.
- Predominant response when blocked: constriction and cardiac depression.
- Have both selective and nonselective beta-blockers.

- Located on postsynaptic effector cells (cells, muscles, and organs that nerves stimulate).

Cardioselective Beta-Blockers

- Block just beta$_1$-adrenergic receptors on the heart.
- Beneficial effects: decreased heart rate, cardiac conduction, and myocardial contractility.

Nonselective Beta-Blockers

- Block both beta$_1$- and beta$_2$-adrenergic receptors; affect heart and smooth muscle.
- Have beneficial effects of the selective agents.
- Have detrimental effects of nonselective agents (constriction of bronchioles and blood vessels).

Nursing Considerations

- Patients should avoid sudden changes in position because of possible postural hypotension.
- Patients should report constipation or the development of any urinary hesitancy or bladder distention (discomfort over symphisis pubis).
- Confusion, depression, hallucinations, nightmares, palpitations, and dizziness should be reported to the physician.

REVIEW QUESTIONS

1. Atenolol (Tenormin) falls into which category of medications?
   a. Beta-blocker
   b. Alpha-blocker
   c. Sympathomimetic
   d. Parasympatholytic
2. For patients taking atenolol, which of the following statements is correct?
   a. It may be discontinued without any time restraints.
   b. Postural hypotension is not a problem with this agent.
   c. Weaning off the medication is necessary to prevent rebound hypertension.
   d. The patient should stop taking the medication at once should he or she gain 3 to 4 pounds per week.

3. If IV dopamine extravasates, you should do which of the followng?
   a. Apply hot packs to the area.
   b. Apply cold packs to the area and document.
   c. Discontinue the IV medication and administer phentolamine as per protocol.
   d. Discontinue the IV medication and administer SC injections of sodium bicarbonate around the site.
4. Patients taking adrenergic-blockers such as prazosin for hypertension and who have BPH will most likely do which of the following?
   a. Experience major urinary retentive problems
   b. Take the medication SC if the oral forms are not helping

c. Not have any effects on the urinary flow and should not be taking this medication

d. Have some relief of the impaired urinary flow as well as antihypertensive effects

5. Your 62-year-old male patient with a status post MI is ready to be discharged. He complains about being put on metoprolol because he says he does not have high blood pressure. Your best response is:

a. "Alpha-agonists should be used instead."

b. "You are correct. This is not a drug you should be taking."

c. "Beta-blockers are often always used after an MI because they have cardioprotective properties."

d. "Beta-blockers, even though they have cardioprotective properties, may still not be indicated in your case, so let me call the physician."

For Answers see www.harcourthealth.com/MERLIN/Lilley/.

CRITICAL THINKING Activities

1. Essay question: Develop patient teaching plans for the use of the following medications:
   a. ergotamine tartrate (Ergostat)
   b. prazosin (Minipress)
   c. atenolol (Tenormin)

2. One of your patients, a 46-year-old mother of two adolescent children, is now taking propranolol for the control of tachycardia and hypertension. What instructions should you give her if she says: "Well, if if doesn't work after a month or two, I'll just quit taking it!"

3. You have just come on your shift and are taking over for a nurse who already has your patient's heart rate controlled on an esmolol infusion. It is running at a rate of 54 ml/hr. The physician is making rounds and asks you how many μg/kg/min of esmolol the patient is controlled on. The patient weighs 90 kg and the normal concentration of esmolol is 10 mg/ml. How many μg/kg/min of esmolol is the patient receiving?

For Answers see www.harcourthealth.com/MERLIN/Lilley/.

bibliography

Albanese J, Nutz P: *Mosby's 2001 nursing drug reference and review cards*, St Louis, 2001, Mosby.

American Hospital Formulary Service: *AHFS drug information*, Bethesda, Md, 2000, American Society of Health-System Pharmacists.

Anderson PO, Knoben JE, Troutman WG: *Handbook of clinical drug data 1999-2000*, ed 9, New York, 1999, McGraw-Hill.

Johns Hopkins Hospital, Department of Pediatrics et al: *The Harriet Lane handbook*, ed 15, St Louis, 2000, Mosby.

Keen JH: *Critical care and emergency drug reference*, ed 3, St Louis, 1996, Mosby.

Mosby's GenRx: a comprehensive reference for generic and brand drugs, ed 10, St Louis, 2000, Mosby.

Skidmore-Roth L: *Mosby's 2001 nursing drug reference*, St Louis, 2001, Mosby.

United States Pharmacopeial Convention: *USP DI: advice for the patient: drug information in lay language*, vol 11, ed 20, Englewood, Co, 2000, Micromedex.

Activity

Remember to check the **Online Worksheet** for additional learning opportunities: **www.harcourthealth.com/MERLIN/Lilley/**

Chapter 18

Cholinergic Agents

www.harcourthealth.com/MERLIN/Lilley/

objectives

When you reach the end of this chapter, you should be able to do the following:

1 Briefly discuss the normal anatomy and physiology of the autonomic nervous system, including the events that occur during synaptic transmission within the parasympathetic divisions.

2 Cite various examples of the cholinergic drugs.

3 Discuss the mechanisms of action, therapeutic effects, uses, adverse effects, and antidotes to overdose of the cholinergic drugs.

4 Develop a nursing care plan that includes all phases of the nursing process related to the administration of the various cholinergic agents.

Look for this symbol for topics covered in the **Online Worksheet**

drug profiles

bethanechol, p. 283	⊶ **physostigmine**, p. 283
donepezil, p. 283	**pyridostigmine**, p. 284

⊶ Key drug.

glossary

Acetylcholine (ACh) (as′ ə təl ko len) Neurotransmitter responsible for transmission of nerve impulses to effector cells in the parasympathetic nervous system. (p. 279)

Alzheimer's disease A disease that is characterized by progressive mental deterioration manifested by loss of memory, ability to calculate, and visual-spatial orientations; confusion; and disorientation. (p. 281)

Cholinergic agents (ko′ lin ər′ jik) Drugs that stimulate the parasympathetic nervous system. (p. 280)

Cholinesterase (ko′ lin es tər as) Enzyme responsible for the breakdown of acetylcholine. (p. 280)

Direct-acting cholinergic agonists Agents that bind to cholinergic receptors to activate them. (p. 280)

Indirect-acting cholinergic agonists Agents that make more acetylcholine available at the receptor site. (p. 280)

Irreversible cholinesterase inhibitors Agents that form a permanent covalent bond with cholinesterase. (p. 280)

Miosis Contraction of the pupil. (p. 281)

Muscarinic receptors (mus′ kə rin ik) Cholinergic receptors located postsynaptically in the smooth muscle, cardiac muscle, and glands of the parasympathetic fibers and in the effector organs of the cholinergic sympathetic fibers; can be stimulated by the alkaloid muscarine. (p. 279)

Nicotinic receptors (nik′ o tin ik) Cholinergic receptors located in the ganglia of both the parasympathetic and sympathetic nervous systems; can be stimulated by the alkaloid nicotine. (p. 279)

Parasympathomimetics Another name for cholinergic agents that mimic the effects of acetylcholine. (p. 280)

Reversible cholinesterase inhibitors Agents that bind to cholinesterase for minutes to hours but do not form a permanent bond. (p. 280)

Cholinergics, cholinergic agonists, and *parasympathomimetics* are all terms that refer to the class of drugs that stimulate the parasympathetic nervous system (PSNS). To better understand how these agents work, it is helpful to know how the PSNS operates in relation to the rest of the nervous system.

PARASYMPATHETIC NERVOUS SYSTEM

The PSNS is the opposing system to the sympathetic nervous system (SNS) in the autonomic nervous system (Fig. 18-1). The neurotransmitter responsible for the transmission of nerve impulses to effector cells in the PSNS is **acetylcholine (ACh).** The receptor that binds the ACh and mediates its actions is called a *cholinergic receptor.* These cholinergic receptors consist of two types, as determined by their location and their action once stimulated. **Nicotinic receptors** are located in the ganglia of both the PSNS and SNS. They are called *nicotinic* because they can be stimulated by the alkaloid nicotine. The other cholinergic receptors are the **muscarinic receptors.** These receptors are located postsynaptically in the smooth muscle, cardiac muscle, and glands of the parasympathetic fibers and in the effector organs of the cholinergic sympathetic fibers. They are called *muscarinic* because they are stimulated by the alkaloid muscarine, a substance isolated from mushrooms. Figure 18-2 shows how the nicotinic and muscarinic receptors are arranged in the PSNS.

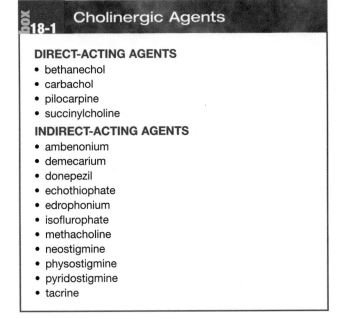

Fig. 18-1 The parasympathetic and sympathetic nervous systems and their relationships to one another.

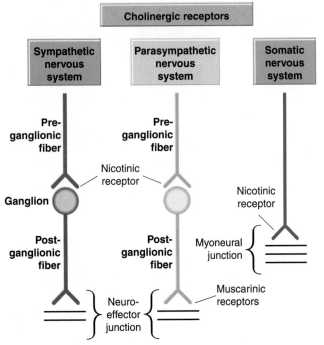

Fig. 18-2 The sympathetic, parasympathetic (PSNS), and somatic nervous systems. Note the location of the nicotinic and muscarinic receptors within the PSNS.

CHOLINERGIC AGENTS

Cholinergic agents mimic the effects of ACh and are therefore sometimes referred to as **parasympathomimetics.** These drugs can stimulate their receptors either directly or indirectly. **Direct-acting cholinergic agonists** bind to cholinergic receptors and activate them. Indirect-

BOX 18-1 Cholinergic Agents

DIRECT-ACTING AGENTS
- bethanechol
- carbachol
- pilocarpine
- succinylcholine

INDIRECT-ACTING AGENTS
- ambenonium
- demecarium
- donepezil
- echothiophate
- edrophonium
- isoflurophate
- methacholine
- neostigmine
- physostigmine
- pyridostigmine
- tacrine

acting cholinergic agonists act by making more ACh available at the receptor site, thereby allowing the ACh to bind to and stimulate the receptor. They do this by inhibiting **cholinesterase,** the enzyme responsible for breaking down ACh. The indirect-acting cholinergic agents bind to the cholinesterase in one of two ways—reversibly or irreversibly. **Reversible cholinesterase inhibitors** bind to cholinesterase for a period of minutes to hours; **irreversible cholinesterase inhibitors** bind to cholinesterase and form a permanent covalent bond. The body must then generate new enzymes to override the ef-

Table 18-1 Cholinergic Agents: Drug Effects

Body Tissue	Response to Stimulation	
	Muscarinic	Nicotinic
Bronchi (lung)	None	Increased secretion, constriction
Cardiovascular		
Blood vessels	Dilation	Constriction
Heart rate	Slowed	Increased
Blood pressure	Decreased	Increased
Eye	Pupil constriction, decreased accommodation	Pupil constriction, decreased accommodation
Gastrointestinal		
Tone	Increased	Increased
Motility	Increased	Increased
Sphincters	Relaxed	None
Genitourinary		
Tone	Increased	Increased
Motility	Increased	Increased
Sphincter	Relaxed	Relaxed
Glandular secretions	Increased intestinal, lacrimal, salivary, and sweat gland secretion	—
Skeletal muscle	—	Increased contraction

fects of the irreversible agents. Box 18-1 lists the direct- and indirect-acting cholinergics.

These agents are used primarily to reduce intraocular pressure in patients with glaucoma or in those undergoing ocular surgery, to treat various gastrointestinal and bladder disorders, and to diagnose and treat myasthenia gravis.

Mechanism of Action

As described, cholinergic drugs all work by stimulating the PSNS. The direct-acting cholinergics act as an agonist at the receptor, directly binding to the ACh receptors and causing stimulation. Indirect-acting agents protect ACh from being broken down by acetylcholinesterase (AChE), making more of this neurotransmitter available to act directly with the receptor. When ACh directly binds to its receptor, stimulation occurs. Once binding occurs on the effector cells (the cell membranes of the target organs), the permeability of the cells changes and calcium and sodium are permitted to flow into the cells. This depolarizes the cell membrane and stimulates the muscle.

Drug Effects

The effects of direct- and indirect-acting cholinergics are those that are generally seen when the PSNS is stimulated. There are many ways to remember these effects. One way is to think of the PSNS as the "rest-and-digest" system. Another way of remembering the effects of cholinergic poisoning is by using the acronym SLUDGE, which stands for salivation, lacrimation, urinary incontinence, diarrhea, gastrointestinal cramps, and emesis.

Cholinergic drugs stimulate the intestine and bladder, resulting in increased gastric secretions, gastrointestinal motility, and increased urinary frequency. They also stimulate the pupil to constrict, causing **miosis.** This helps decrease intraocular pressure. In addition, stimulation of the PSNS by the parasympathomimetics causes increased salivation and sweating. The cardiovascular effects are decreased heart rate and vasodilation. These agents also cause the bronchi of the lungs to constrict and the airways to narrow. ACh is also needed for normal brain function. It is in short supply in patients with **Alzheimer's disease.**

At recommended doses, cholinergics primarily affect the muscarinic receptors, but at high doses the nicotinic receptors can also be stimulated. The desired effects come from muscarinic receptor stimulation; many of the undesirable effects are due to nicotinic receptor stimulation. The various beneficial and undesirable effects of the cholinergic agents are listed in Table 18-1 according to the receptors stimulated.

Therapeutic Uses

Most of the direct-acting agents (ACh, carbachol, and pilocarpine) are used topically to reduce intraocular pressure in patients with glaucoma or in those undergoing ocular surgery. They are poorly absorbed orally because they have large quaternary amines in their chemical structure. This is what limits their use to mostly topical application. One exception is the direct-acting cholinergic drug bethanechol, which can be administered orally or as a SC injection. It primarily affects the detrusor muscle of the urinary bladder and the smooth muscle of the gastrointestinal tract. When given, it causes increased bladder and gastrointestinal tract tone and motility, thereby increasing the movement of contents through these areas. It also causes the sphincters in the bladder and the gastrointestinal tract to relax, allowing them to empty. It is therefore used to treat atony of the bladder and gastrointestinal tract, which sometimes occurs after a surgical procedure.

Indirect-acting agents work by increasing ACh concentrations at the receptor sites stimulating the effector cells. They cause skeletal muscle contraction and are therefore used for the diagnosis and treatment of myasthenia gravis. Their ability to inhibit AChE also makes them useful for the reversal of neuromuscular blockade produced either by neuromuscular blocking agents or by anticholinergic poisoning. For this reason, physostigmine is considered the antidote for anticholinergic poisoning as well as poisoning by irreversible cholinesterase inhibitors such as organophosphates and carbonates, the common insecticides.

In the treatment of Alzheimer's disease, cholinergic agents increase concentrations of ACh in the brain, thereby improving cholinergic function. The ability to increase ACh levels in the brain by inhibiting AChE and preventing the degradation of endogenously released ACh increases or maintains memory and learning capabilities.

Side Effects and Adverse Effects

The primary side effects and adverse effects of cholinergic agents are the consequence of overstimulation of the PSNS. They are extensions of the cholinergic reactions that affect many body functions. The major effects are listed by body system in Table 18-2.

Toxicity and Management of Overdose

There is very little systemic absorption of the typically administered agents and therefore little systemic toxicity. When administered locally in the eye, they can cause temporary ocular changes such as transient blurring and dimming of vision, which can be bothersome to the patient. Systemic toxicity with topically applied cholinergics is seen most commonly when longer-acting agents are given repeatedly for a long time. This can result in overstimulation of the PSNS and in all the attendant responses. Treatment is generally symptomatic and supportive, and the administration of a reversal agent is rarely required.

The likelihood of toxicity is greater for cholinergics that are given orally or intravenously. The most severe consequence of an overdose of a cholinergic agent is a cholinergic crisis. The symptoms of such a reaction may include circulatory collapse, hypotension, bloody diarrhea, shock, and cardiac arrest. Early signs include abdominal cramps, salivation, flushing of the skin, nausea, and vomiting. Transient syncope, transient complete heart block, dyspnea, and orthostatic hypotension may also occur. These can be re-

Table 18-2	Cholinergic Agents: Adverse Effects
Body System	**Side/Adverse Effects**
Cardiovascular	Bradycardia, hypotension, conduction abnormalities (atrioventricular block and cardiac arrest)
Central nervous system	Headache, dizziness, convulsions
Gastrointestinal	Abdominal cramps, increased secretions, nausea, vomiting
Respiratory	Increased bronchial secretions, bronchospasms
Other	Lacrimation, sweating, salivation, loss of binocular accommodation, miosis

DOSAGES Selected Cholinergic Agents

agent	pharmacologic class	dosage range	purpose
bethanechol (Urecholine)	Direct-acting muscarinic	*Adult* PO: 10-50 mg 3-4 times/day SC: 2.5-5 mg every 15-30 min up to max of 4 doses	Postop and postpartum functional urinary retention
donepezil (Aricept)	Anticholinesterase (indirect-acting)	*Adult* PO: 5-10 mg/day as a single dose	Alzheimer's disease
physostigmine (Antilirium)	Anticholinesterase (indirect-acting)	*Pediatric* IM/IV: 0.02 mg/kg repeated at 5-10 min intervals until desired effect or a dose of 2 mg is reached *Adult* IM/IV: 0.5-2 mg repeated every 20 min if needed	Anticholinergic and tricyclic antidepressant antidote
pyridostigmine (Mestinon)	Anticholinesterase (indirect-acting)	*Pediatric* PO: 7 mg/kg/day divided into 5-6 doses *Adult* PO: 60-1500 mg/day divided to provide maximum therapeutic effect IV: 10-20 mg with a suitable anticholinergic	Myasthenia gravis Myasthenia gravis Reversal of nondepolarizing neuromuscular blocking agents

GERD, Gastroesophageal reflux disease.

versed promptly by the administration of atropine. Severe cardiovascular reactions or bronchoconstriction may be alleviated by epinephrine. Janssen Pharmaceutica, the makers of cisapride (Propulsid), stopped marketing the drug on July 14, 2000. As of December 31, 1999, use of cisapride has been associated with 341 reports of heart rhythm abnormalities, including 80 reports of deaths. Most of these events occurred in patients who were taking other medications or suffering from underlying conditions known to increase risk of cardiac dysrhythmia associated with cisapride. Since July 14, cisapride has been available only through an investigational limited access program.

Interactions

The potential drug interactions that can occur with the cholinergics are significant with regard to severity. Anticholinergics, antihistamines, and sympathomimetics may antagonize cholinergic agents, resulting in decreased response to them.

Dosages

For the recommended dosages of the cholinergic agents, see the dosages table on p. 282.

drug profiles

Of the direct-acting cholinergic agents, bethanechol is the only agent that is administered orally. ACh, carbachol, and pilocarpine are applied topically to the eye for the treatment of glaucoma or for a reduction in intraocular pressure during ocular surgery and are discussed in greater detail in Chapter 54, as are the indirect-acting cholinergics echothiophate, demecarium, and isoflurophate, which are used primarily for the treatment of eye disorders or for surgical purposes. The cholinergics are available orally as tablets and syrups, topically as eyedrops, and parenterally as IV and SC injections. The cholinergics are all prescription-only drugs. Most of the cholinergics are rated pregnancy category C agents by the FDA.

bethanechol

Bethanechol (Urecholine) is a direct-acting cholinergic agonist that stimulates the cholinergic receptors located on the smooth muscle of the bladder. This stimulation results in increased bladder tone, increased motility, and relaxation of the sphincter of the bladder. It is used in the treatment of acute postoperative and postpartum nonobstructive urinary retention as well as for the management of neurogenic atony of the bladder with retention. It has also been used to prevent and treat the side effects of other classes of drugs such as phenothiazine- and tricyclic antidepressant (TCA)–induced bladder dysfunction. In addition, it is used in the treatment of postoperative gastrointestinal atony and gastric retention, chronic refractory heartburn, and familial dysautonomia as well as in the diagnostic test for

infantile cystic fibrosis. IM and IV use are contraindicated. It is also contraindicated in patients with hyperthyroidism, peptic ulcer, active bronchial asthma, cardiac disease or coronary artery disease, epilepsy, and parkinsonism. Its use should also be avoided in patients with conditions in which the strength or integrity of the gastrointestinal tract or bladder wall is questionable or with conditions in which increased muscular activity could prove harmful. Bethanechol is available in both oral and parenteral formulations. Oral tablets are available in 5-, 10-, 25-, and 50-mg strengths, and a parenteral formulation is available as a 5-mg/ml SC injection. Commonly recommended dosages are given in the table on p. 282. Pregnancy category C.

PHARMACOKINETICS

HALF-LIFE	ONSET	PEAK	DURATION
Variable	30-90 min	<30 min	1-6 hr

donepezil

Donepezil (Aricept) is an indirect-acting anticholinesterase drug that works centrally in the brain to increase levels of ACh by blocking its breakdown. It is used in the treatment of mild to moderate Alzheimer's disease. Drugs with anticholinergic properties should be avoided in patients on donepezil because they may counteract the effects of donepezil.

Donepezil offers many advantages over tacrine (Cognex), the first agent in this class of indirect-acting anticholinesterase drugs. Donepezil is dosed only once a day compared with four times a day with tacrine. It is more specific for AChE in the CNS, which decreases the incidence of drug interactions currently seen with tacrine. It is classified as a pregnancy category C agent. Donepezil is available as 5- and 10-mg tablets. Recommended dosages are given in the table on p. 282.

PHARMACOKINETICS

HALF-LIFE	ONSET	PEAK	DURATION
72-80 hr	3 wk*	3-4 hr	2 wk*

*Therapeutic effect.

physostigmine

Physostigmine (Antilirium) is a synthetic quaternary ammonium compound that is very similar in structure to edrophonium, pyridostigmine, neostigmine, and ambenonium. It is an indirect-acting cholinergic agent that works indirectly to increase ACh by inhibiting the enzyme that breaks down ACh. It has been shown to improve muscle strength and is therefore used in the symptomatic treatment of myasthenia gravis. Neostigmine, pyridostigmine, and ambenonium are the standard agents used for symptomatic treatment of myasthenia gravis. Endrophonium, another indirect-acting cholinergic agent, is commonly used to diagnose this disorder. It is also useful for reversing the effects of nondepolarizing neuromuscular-blocking agents after surgery. It may also be used in treatment of severe TCA overdoses. It is contraindicated in patients who have shown a hypersensitivity or severe cholinergic reaction to the drug. It should be used with caution in patients with epilepsy, bronchial asthma, bradycardia, recent coronary artery occlusion, hyperthyroidism, cardiac dysrhythmias, or peptic ulcer. It is available parenterally as an intravenously administered injection (1 mg/ml) and topically as an ophthalmic solution and ointment. Recommended dosages are given in the table on p. 282. Pregnancy category C.

PHARMACOKINETICS

HALF-LIFE	ONSET	PEAK	DURATION
15-40 min	<5 min	5 min	30-60 min

pyridostigmine

Pyridostigmine (Mestinon) is also a synthetic quaternary ammonium compound that is very similar structurally to edrophonium, neostigmine, and ambenonium. It is an indirect-acting cholinergic agent and is used in the symptomatic treatment of myasthenia gravis. It is also useful for reversing the effects of nondepolarizing neuromuscular-blocking agents after surgery. It is contraindicated in patients who have shown a hypersensitivity or severe cholinergic reaction to it. It should be used with caution in patients with epilepsy, bronchial asthma, bradycardia, recent coronary artery occlusion, hyperthyroidism, cardiac dysrhythmias, or peptic ulcer. It is available orally as a regular and extended-release tablet and as a solution. The oral solution is 60 mg/ml, the regular-release tablets are 60 mg, and the extended-release tablets are 180 mg. It is also available as a parenteral preparation as a 5 mg/ml injection. Recommended dosages are given in the table on p. 282. Pregnancy category C.

PHARMACOKINETICS

HALF-LIFE	ONSET	PEAK	DURATION
Variable	PO: 30-45 min IV: <5 min	PO: 2-5 min IV: 3-6 hr	PO: <30 min IV: 2-4 hr

nursing process

• Assessment

Cholinergic drugs, or parasympathomimetics, produce a variety of effects stemming from their ability to stimulate the PSNS and mimic the action of ACh. These agents have the following effects:
- Decrease heart rate
- Increase gastrointestinal and genitourinary tone and contractility by stimulating smooth muscle
- Increase the contractility and tone of bronchial smooth muscle
- Increase respiratory secretions
- Produce miosis.

Patients who are to receive a cholinergic agent need to be assessed to determine whether they suffer from gastrointestinal or genitourinary obstruction, asthma, peptic ulcer disease, or coronary artery disease because of the potential for these agents to exacerbate these problems. Information about the patient's allergies and past and present medical conditions should also be gathered. In addition, a system overview and a thorough medication history should form part of this assessment so that possible drug interactions or contraindications to use of the cholinergic agent can be identified in advance.

Before administering donepezil for Alzheimer's disease, the patient needs to be assessed for allergies to this agent or to any piperidine derivative. Cautious use is indicated in patients with sick sinus syndrome, asthma, GI bleeding, liver disease, ulcer disease, GU obstruction, seizure disorders, or COPD; in pediatric patients; and during pregnancy or lactation. Drug interactions include synergistic effects with cholinesterase inhibitors, cholinergic agonists, and succinylcholine. Other drug interactions include NSAIDS and anticholinergics. Also, before initiation of drug therapy with donepezil, it is important to assess and document the patient's vital signs, GI and GU history and status, mental status, mood, affect, changes in behavior, depression, suicidal tendencies, and level of consciousness. Once the patient has begun the medication, it is crucial to assess his or her response to the drug because if no improvement is noted within 6-week period, the health care provider may find it necessary to adjust the dosing.

• Nursing Diagnoses

Nursing diagnoses associated with the use of cholinergics include, but are not limited to, the following:
- Acute pain related to nausea, vomiting, or increased peristalsis.
- Deficient knowledge regarding therapeutic regimen, side effects, drug interactions, and precautions related to the use of cholinergic agents.
- Risk for injury related to possible side effects of cholinergic agents (bradycardia and hypotension).
- Decreased cardiac output related to the cardiovascular side effects of dysrhythmias, hypotension, and bradycardia.
- Disturbed sensory perception related to adverse CNS effects of cholinergic drugs.

• Planning

Goals for the patient receiving cholinergic agents include, but are not limited to, the following:
- Patient receives or takes medications as prescribed.
- Patient experiences relief of the symptoms for which the medication was prescribed.

- Patient remains compliant with the drug therapy regimen.
- Patient demonstrates an adequate knowledge concerning the use of the specific medication, its side effects, and the appropriate dosing at home.
- Patient remains free of self-injury resulting from adverse effects of the medication.

Outcome Criteria

Outcome criteria related to the administration of cholinergic agents include the following:
- Patient will state the importance of both the pharmacologic and nonpharmacologic treatment of their gastrointestinal or genitourinary disorder or glaucoma in achieving good health.
- Patient will state reasons for compliance with the medication therapy and the risks associated with noncompliance as well as the complications associated with overuse of the medication such as bronchospasms, increased abdominal cramping, decreased pulse and blood pressure, etc.
- Patient will state conditions under which to contact the physician such as wheezing, bradycardia, and increased abdominal pain.
- Patient will state the importance of scheduling and keeping follow-up appointments with the physician as related to management of the disorder for which medication has been prescribed.

● Implementation

There are several nursing interventions that can be implemented to maximize the therapeutic effects of cholinergic agents and minimize their side effects. One is to always make sure patients who have undergone an operation ambulate as early as possible as ordered after their procedure to help minimize or prevent gastric and urinary retention and maximize the effects of these medications. Another intervention for drugs use for myasthenia gravis is to give the medication about 30 minutes before meals to allow for onset of action and therapeutic effects (e.g., decreased dysphagia). The packaging inserts should always be checked for instructions concerning dilutional agents and the route of administration (e.g., bethanechol is administered orally or subcutaneously). Atropine is the antidote to the cholinergics, so this medication should be taped to the wall next to the patient's bed or it should be available somewhere in the patient's room.

Donepezil is not a cure for Alzheimer's disease or dementia, so be honest with the patient and caregivers about the fact that this drug is only for symptomatic improvement. While beginning the medication, patients will most likely need continued ADL assistance and help with ambulation because the medication may increase dizziness and cause gait imbalances at the initiation of treatment. Patients and family members or caregivers need to also understand the importance of taking the medication exactly as ordered. In addition, patients should be instructed not to abruptly withdraw themselves off the medication or increase the dosage without physician approval because of the potential of serious complications or overdosage.

Patient teaching tips are presented below.

● Evaluation

Following are some therapeutic effects for which to monitor in patients receiving cholinergic agents. In patients with myasthenia gravis, the signs and symptoms of the disease should be alleviated (see patient teaching tips). In patients suffering a decrease in gastrointestinal peristalsis postoperatively, there should be an increase in bowel sounds, the passage of flatus, and the occurrence of bowel movements that indicate increased gastrointestinal peristalsis. In patients suffering from a hypotonic bladder with urinary retention, micturition should occur within about 60 minutes of the administration of bethanecol.

The nurse must also be alert to the occurrence of the side effects of these medications, including increased respiratory secretions, bronchospasms, difficulty breathing, nausea, vomiting, diarrhea, abdominal cramping, dysrhythmias, hypotension, bradycardia, increased sweating, and an increase in the frequency and urgency of the voiding patterns.

Therapeutic effects of donepezil may not occur for up to 6 weeks but include an improvement of the symptoms of the disease. Adverse effects include hypotension or hypertension, dizziness, insomnia, headache, fatigue, syncope, nausea, vomiting, and anorexia.

---

patient teaching tips

Cholinergic Agents (Parasympathomimetics)

➤ Patients should always take the medication as ordered because an overdose can cause life-threatening problems.

➤ It is often more effective to space the doses of these medications evenly apart to optimize the effects of the medication. Make sure patients understand this before discharge.

➤ Encourage patients to call their physician should they experience increased muscle weakness, abdominal cramps, diarrhea, or difficulty breathing.

➤ Inform patients that if they are taking the medications for the treatment of myasthenia gravis, symptoms associated with the disease should abate; that is, he or she should experience less ptosis (eyelid drooping), less diplopia (double vision), less difficulty swallowing and chewing, and less weakness.

➤ Encourage patients with myasthenia gravis to take medications 30 minutes before meals to help improve swallowing and chewing.

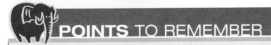

POINTS TO REMEMBER

Cholinergics, Cholinergic Agonists, and Parasympathomimetics

- Names for the class of drugs that stimulate the PSNS.
- PSNS: branch of CNS that opposes the SNS.
- Neurotransmitter of PSNS: acetylcholine.
- Drugs that mimic acetylcholine: parasympathomimetics.

Nicotinic Receptors

- One of the two types of cholinergic receptors.
- Called *nicotinic* because they are stimulated by nicotine.
- Located on preganglionic nerve fibers in the PSNS, SNS, and adrenal medulla.

Muscarinic Receptors

- One of the two types of cholinergic receptors.
- Called *muscarinic* because they are stimulated by muscarine.
- Located on postsynaptic cells, muscles, and glands (not on nerve!).

Cholinesterase

- Enzyme responsible for the breakdown of acetylcholine.
- Indirect-acting cholinergics act by inhibiting this enzyme.
- These agents can either reversibly or irreversibly bind to this enzyme.

Nursing Considerations

- Cholinergics should be given as directed and the patient carefully monitored.
- Bradycardia, hypotension, headache, dizziness, respiratory depression, or bronchospasms occurring in a patient taking cholinergics should be reported immediately to the physician, and the patient monitored carefully.
- Always encourage patients taking cholinergics to change positions slowly to avoid dizziness and fainting resulting from postural hypotension.

REVIEW QUESTIONS

1. What is the rationale for the use of cholinergic agents with patients who have bladder atony?
   a. Blockage of ACh occurs with an increased bladder wall pressure.
   b. The synthetic drugs work predominantly in the muscarinic receptors.
   c. Increased bladder tone and motility occur with increased emptying of the bladder.
   d. Decreased dopamine levels occur with a stimulation of alpha cholinergic receptors.

2. The elderly patient needs to be more cautious when taking bethanechol (Urecholine) because of which side effect?
   a. Dyspnea
   b. Diaphoresis
   c. Hypotension
   d. Hyperthermia

3. With the patient taking the ophthalmic form of physostigmine for glaucoma, it is important to include in patient teaching which of the following statements?
   a. If the solution is yellowish-brown it is still fine to use it.
   b. The applicator tip of the bottle should touch the cornea to ensure contact with the eye.
   c. If a dose has been omitted, do not administer the dose even if within 24 hours because of possible toxicity.

   d. For a brief time the patient may experience blurred vision or there may be a change in his or her near or distant vision.

4. Patient education instructions for use of ophthalmic pilocarpine include all of the following except:
   a. Store medication away from heat, light, and children.
   b. Apply pressure to the inner canthus to prevent systemic absorption.
   c. Open eyelid and pull lower eyelid away from the eye for administration into the conjunctival sac.
   d. Wash your hands, put on sterile gloves, and place the drug in the inner canthus for greater drug distribution.

5. Your patient is taking oral bethanechol (Urecholine) and has been taking it before meals. He has begun to complain of nausea and vomiting. Which of the following statements would *not* be an appropriate response?
   a. "Take with meals if nausea is problematic."
   b. "Urecholine is best tolerated if all doses are taken at bedtime."
   c. "If you take it with at least 180 ml of fluid you may decrease GI upset."
   d. "If nausea and vomiting are severe, contact your health care provider for further instructions."

For Answers see www.harcourthealth.com/MERLIN/Lilley/.

CRITICAL THINKING Activities

1. Your patient underwent a bladder resection 3 days ago and is now experiencing difficulty urinating. The physician orders bethanechol, starting with 10 mg orally, tid. What should you do at this time regarding the use of bethanechol in your patient?

2. Discuss the implications for assessment of patients who may be on either a direct- or an indirect-acting parasympathomimetic.

3. What are the advantages of the synthetic or natural derivatives of belladonna alkaloids?

For Answers see www.harcourthealth.com/MERLIN/Lilley/.

bibliography

Albanese J, Nutz P: *Mosby's 2001 nursing drug reference and review cards,* St Louis, 2001, Mosby.

American Hospital Formulary Service: *AHFS drug information,* Bethesda, Md, 2000, American Society of Health-System Pharmacists.

Anderson PO, Knoben JE, Troutman WG: *Handbook of critical drug data 1999-2000,* ed 9, New York, 1999, McGraw-Hill.

Goldsmith C: Parkinson's disease, *AJN* 99(2):46, 1999.

Hickey J: Myasthenia crisis: your assessment counts, *RN* 54(5):54, 1991.

Johns Hopkins Hospital, Department of Pediatrics et al: *The Harriet Lane handbook,* ed 15, St Louis, 2000, Mosby.

Keen JH: *Critical care and emergency drug reference,* ed 3, St Louis, 1996, Mosby.

Medical Letter: Donepezil (Arecept) for Alzheimer's disease, 39(1002):53, 1997.

Mosby's GenRx: a comprehensive reference for generic and brand drugs, ed 10, St Louis, 2000, Mosby.

Skidmore-Roth, L: *Mosby's 2001 nursing drug reference,* St Louis, 2001, Mosby.

Tatro DS: Keeping up: update-cisapride drug interactions, *Facts and Comparisons Drug Link,* September 1999, Vol. 9, p. 67.

Turkoski BB: *Drug information handbook for nursing 1999-2000: including assessment, administration, monitoring guidelines, and patient education,* ed 2, Cleveland, 1999, Lexi-Comp.

United States Pharmacopeial Convention: *USP DI: drug information for the health care professional, vol. 1,* ed 20, Englewood, Co., 2000, Micromedex.

Remember to check the **Online Worksheet** for additional learning opportunities: **www.harcourthealth.com/MERLIN/Lilley/**

Activity

Chapter 19

Cholinergic-Blocking Agents

www.harcourthealth.com/MERLIN/Lilley/

objectives

When you reach the end of this chapter, you should be able to do the following:

Look for this symbol for topics covered in the **Online Worksheet**

1 Briefly discuss the normal anatomy and physiology of the autonomic nervous system, including the events that are blocked with the use of anticholinergic agents.

2 List examples of the various anticholinergic drugs.

3 Discuss the mechanisms of action, therapeutic effects, uses, and adverse and toxic effects of the anticholinergic drugs and the antidotes to overdose and to the unwanted effects.

4 Develop a nursing care plan that includes all phases of the nursing process related to the administration of the various anticholinergic agents and the treatment of side effects and overdose or toxicity stemming from the use of these various agents.

5 Identify the drug interactions associated with the use of anticholinergics.

6 Evaluate the therapeutic versus side effects of the different anticholinergics.

drug profiles

atropine, p. 291
dicyclomine, p. 291
glycopyrrolate, p. 291
scopolamine, p. 292
tolterodine, p. 293

○—Key drug.

glossary

Anticholinergics (an ti ko lə nər' jik) Another name for a cholinergic-blocking agent. (p. 288)

Cholinergic-blocking agent Any agent that blocks the action of acetylcholine and substances similar to acetylcholine at receptor sites in the synapse. Such agents in effect block the action of cholinergic nerves that transmit impulses through the release of acetylcholine at their synapses. (p. 288)

Competitive antagonist A drug or other substance that is an antagonist or that resembles a normal human metabolite and interferes with its function in the body, usually by competing for the metabolite's receptors or enzymes. Also called an *antimetabolite*. (p. 288)

Mydriasis (mi dri' ə sis) Dilation of the pupil of the eye caused by contraction of the dilator muscle of the iris. (p. 289)

Cholinergic blockers, anticholinergics, parasympatholytics, and *antimuscarinic agents* are all terms for the class of drugs that block or inhibit the actions of acetylcholine (ACh) in the parasympathetic nervous system (PSNS). **Cholinergic-blocking agents** block the action of the neurotransmitter ACh at the muscarinic receptors in the PSNS. ACh released from the stimulated nerve fiber is then unable to bind to the receptor site and fails to produce a cholinergic effect. This is why the cholinergic blockers are also referred to as **anticholinergics.** Blocking the parasympathetic nerves allows the sympathetic (adrenergic) nervous system (SNS) to dominate. Because of this, cholinergic blockers have many of the same effects as the adrenergics. Figure 19-1 illustrates the site of action of the cholinergic blockers within the PSNS.

Cholinergic blockers have many important therapeutic uses and are one of the oldest groups of therapeutic agents. Originally they were derived from various plant sources, but today these naturally occurring substances are only part of a larger group of cholinergic blockers that include both synthetic and semisynthetic agents. Box 19-1 lists the currently available cholinergic blockers grouped according to their chemical class.

Mechanism of Action

Cholinergic blockers are largely **competitive antagonists.** They compete with ACh for binding at the muscarinic receptors of the PSNS. Once they have bound to the receptor, they inhibit nerve transmission at these receptors. This generally occurs at the neuroeffector junction of smooth muscle, cardiac muscle, and exocrine glands. Cholinergic blockers have little effect at the nicotinic receptors, although at high doses they can have partial blocking effects.

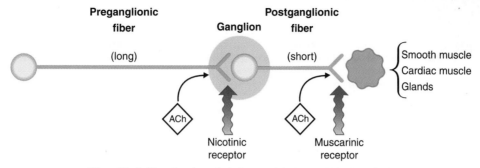

Fig. 19-1 Site of action of cholinergic blockers within the PSNS.

Drug Effects

The major sites of action of the anticholinergics are the heart, respiratory tract, gastrointestinal tract, urinary bladder, eye, and exocrine glands. In general the anticholinergics have effects opposite those of the cholinergics at these sites of action.

The blockade of ACh by cholinergic blockers causes the pupils to dilate and increases intraocular pressure. This can occur because the ciliary muscles and the sphincter muscle of the iris are innervated by cholinergic nerve fibers. Cholinergic blockers can therefore keep the sphincter muscle of the iris from contracting and allow unopposed radial muscle stimulation. This results in a dilated pupil **(mydriasis)** and a relaxed eye (cycloplegia). However, this can be detrimental to patients with glaucoma because it results in increased intraocular pressure.

In the gastrointestinal tract, cholinergic blockers cause a decrease in gastrointestinal motility, gastrointestinal secretions, and salivation. In the cardiovascular system these agents cause an increased heart rate. In the genitourinary system, anticholinergics lead to decreased bladder contraction, which can result in urinary retention. In the skin they reduce sweating, and in the respiratory system they dry mucous membranes and cause bronchial dilation. These effects are listed according to body system in Table 19-1. Many of these cholinergic-blocking agents are available in a variety of forms (IV, IM, PO, SC). Depending upon their route of administration, the same drug could have multiple onsets of action, durations of effect, and peak effects.

Therapeutic Uses

The CNS effects of cholinergic blockers have the therapeutic effect of decreasing muscle rigidity and diminishing tremors. This is of benefit in the treatment of both Parkinson's disease and drug-induced extrapyramidal reactions. The therapeutic cardiovascular effects of anticholinergics are related to their cholinergic-blocking effects on the heart's conduction system. At low doses the anticholinergics slow the heart rate by means of their effects on the cardiac center in the portion of the brain called the *medulla.* At large doses, cholinergic blockers block the inhibitory vagal effects on the pacemaker cells of the sinoatrial (SA) and atrioventricular (AV) nodes and accelerate the heart rate. Atropine is primarily used

BOX 19-1	**Cholinergic Blockers Grouped According to Chemical Class**

NATURAL AGENTS
- atropine
- belladonna
- hyoscyamine
- scopolamine

SYNTHETIC AND SEMISYNTHETIC AGENTS
- anisotropine
- clidinium
- dicyclomine
- glycopyrrolate
- hexocyclium
- homatropine
- ipratropium
- isopropamide
- mepenzolate
- methantheline
- methscopolamine
- oxybutynin
- oxyphencyclimine
- propantheline
- tolterodine
- tridihexethyl

in the setting of cardiovascular disorders, such as for the diagnosis of sinus node dysfunction, the treatment of patients with symptomatic second-degree AV block, and advanced life support in the treatment of sinus bradycardia that is accompanied by hemodynamic compromise.

As previously mentioned, when the cholinergic stimulation of the PSNS is blocked by cholinergic blockers, the SNS effects go unopposed. In the respiratory tract this results in decreased secretions from the nose, mouth, pharynx, and bronchi. It also causes relaxation of the smooth muscles in the bronchi and bronchioles, which results in decreased airway resistance and bronchodilation. Because of this, the cholinergic blockers have proved beneficial in treating exercise-induced bronchospasms, chronic bronchitis, asthma, and chronic obstructive pulmonary disease.

Gastric secretions as well as the smooth muscle responsible for producing gastric motility are both under the control of the PSNS, which is primarily under the

Table 19-1 Cholinergic Blockers: Drug Effects

Body System	Cholinergic Blocker Effects
Cardiovascular	*Small doses:* decrease heart rate *Large doses:* increase heart rate
Central nervous system	*Small doses:* Decrease muscle rigidity and tremors *Large doses:* drowsiness, disorientation, hallucinations
Eye	Dilate pupils (mydriasis), decrease accommodation by paralyzing ciliary muscles (cycloplegia)
Gastrointestinal	Relax smooth muscle tone of gastrointestinal tract, decrease intestinal and gastric secretions, decrease motility and peristalsis
Genitourinary	Relax detrusor muscle of bladder, increase constriction of internal sphincter; these two may result in urinary retention
Glandular	Decrease bronchial secretions, salivation, sweating
Respiratory	Decrease bronchial secretions, dilate bronchial airways

Table 19-2 Cholinergic Blockers: Adverse Effects

Body System	Cholinergic-Blocking Effects
Cardiovascular	Increased heart rate, dysrhythmias
Central nervous system	CNS excitation, restlessness, irritability, disorientation, hallucinations, delirium
Eye	Dilated pupils, decreased visual accommodation, increased intraocular pressure
Gastrointestinal	Decreased salivation, gastric secretions, and motility
Genitourinary	Urinary retention
Glandular	Decreased sweating
Respiratory	Decreased bronchial secretions

control of muscarinic receptors. Cholinergic blockers antagonize these receptors, causing decreased secretions, relaxation of smooth muscle, and decreased gastrointestinal motility and peristalsis. For these reasons cholinergic blockers are commonly used in the treatment of peptic ulcer disease, irritable bowel disease, and gastrointestinal hypersecretory states.

It has been shown that a large number of patients with peptic ulcer disease may be infected with a bacteria known as *Helicobacter pylori.* Treatment with antibiotics can cure peptic ulcer disease. Cholinergic blockers may still be used to decrease symptoms caused by peptic ulcer disease.

The effects that anticholinergics have on the bladder have made them useful in the treatment of such genitourinary tract disorders as reflex neurogenic bladder and incontinence. They relax the detrusor muscles of the bladder and increase constriction of the internal sphincter. The cholinergic blockers' ability to decrease glandular secretions also make them potentially useful agents for reducing gastric and pancreatic secretions in patients with acute pancreatitis.

Side Effects and Adverse Effects

Many body systems are affected adversely by cholinergic blockers. This is a function of the cholinergic blockers' site of action. The muscarinic receptors are located in a variety of tissues, organs, glands, and cells throughout the body. Therefore blockade of these receptors by the anticholinergics produces a wide range of effects, some desirable, as described in the previous section, and some not so desirable. The various side effects and adverse effects of cholinergic blockers are listed by body system in Table 19-2.

Other factors contributing to the wide variety of possible adverse effects of cholinergic blockers are the affinity of the muscarinic receptors for specific drugs and the drug dose. There are also certain patient populations that are more susceptible to the effects of these drugs. These include infants, the elderly, fair-skinned children with Down syndrome, and children with spastic paralysis or brain damage.

Toxicity and Management of Overdose

The dose of cholinergic blockers is particularly important because there is a very narrow difference between therapeutic and toxic doses. This drug characteristic is commonly referred to as a narrow therapeutic index. The treatment of cholinergic blocker overdose consists of symptomatic and supportive therapy. The patient should be hospitalized, and close, continuous monitoring including continuous electrocardiogram (ECG) monitoring should be initiated. The stomach should be emptied by whichever route is most appropriate, inducing emesis with syrup of ipecac if the patient is awake and not convulsing or performing lavage if this not the case. Activated charcoal has proved very effective in removing drug that is already absorbed.

Fluid therapy and other standard measures used for the treatment of shock should be instituted as needed. Delirium, hallucinations, coma, and cardiac dysrhythmias respond favorably to physostigmine treatment. Its routine use as an antidote for cholinergic blocker overdose is controversial, however. It has the potential for producing severe adverse effects such as seizures and asystole and should therefore be reserved for the treatment of patients showing extreme delirium or agitation who could inflict injury on themselves.

Interactions

The potential drug interactions that can occur with cholinergic blockers are significant. Knowledge of the broad categories of drugs that should not be coadministered with cholinergic blockers can help prevent potentially serious consequences. Additive cholinergic effects can be seen when antihistamines, phenothiazines, tricyclic antidepressants (TCAs), and monoamine oxidase inhibitors (MAOIs) are given with cholinergic blockers. Isopropamide can also alter the results of thyroid function tests.

Dosages

For the recommended dosages of selected cholinergic blockers, see the table on p. 292.

drug profiles

All cholinergic blockers are prescription-only drugs. They are available in many dosage formulations: oral, topical, and injectable. Most of the cholinergic blockers are classified as pregnancy category C agents; dicyclomine and mephenzolate are classified as pregnancy category B agents.

Among the oldest and best known naturally occurring cholinergic blockers are the belladonna alkaloids. It is the belladonna alkaloid contained in these agents that is responsible for their therapeutic effects. Of these, atropine is the prototypical agent. It has been in use for hundreds of years and continues to be widely used because of its effectiveness. Besides atropine, scopolamine is the other major naturally occurring drug. These drugs come from a variety of plants within the potato family (Solanaceae). Some examples are *Atropa belladonna* (deadly nightshade), *Hyoscyamus niger* (henbane), and *Datura stramonium* (jimson weed or thorn apple).

Of the semisynthetic and synthetic cholinergic blockers, there are many therapeutically useful agents. These agents are used in the treatment of a variety of illnesses and conditions ranging from peptic ulcer disease and irritable bowel syndrome to the symptoms of the common cold, as well as preoperatively to dry up secretions. They are the synthetic derivatives of the plant-derived belladonna alkaloids and are generally more specific in binding predominantly with muscarinic receptors. They may also be associated with fewer side effects.

atropine

Atropine is a naturally occurring antimuscarinic. It may be prepared synthetically but is usually obtained by extraction from various members of the Solanaceae family of plants (deadly nightshade or jimson weed). In general, atropine is more potent than scopolamine in its cholinergic-blocking effects on the heart and in its effects on the smooth muscles of the bronchi and intestines. Atropine is effective in the treatment of many of the conditions listed in the Therapeutic Uses section. It is contraindicated in patients with angle-closure glaucoma, adhesions between the iris and lens, certain types of asthma

(not cholinergic associated), advanced hepatic and renal dysfunction, hiatal hernia associated with reflux esophagitis, intestinal atony, obstructive gastrointestinal or urinary conditions, and severe ulcerative colitis. It is available as a parenteral injection in several concentrations and strengths, as a solution to be mixed with normal saline solution and inhaled, as a 0.4-mg tablet, or in combination with phenobarbital as an oral solution. The recommended dosages are given in the table on p. 292. Pregnancy category C.

PHARMACOKINETICS

HALF-LIFE	ONSET	PEAK	DURATION
IV: 2.5 hr	Immediate	2-4 min	4-6 hr

dicyclomine

Dicyclomine (Bentyl and others) is a synthetic, antispasmodic cholinergic blocker primarily used in the treatment of functional disturbances of gastrointestinal motility such as irritable bowel syndrome. It has also been used alone and in combination with phenobarbital for the treatment of colic and enterocolitis in infants. It is most commonly administered orally as either a 10-mg capsule or a 20-mg capsule or tablet. It is also available as an orally administered syrup that contains 10 mg/5 ml of the drug. As a parenteral preparation it is available as a 10-mg/ml IM injection. IV administration is not recommended. It is contraindicated in patients who have a known hypersensitivity to anticholinergics and in those with narrow-angle glaucoma, gastrointestinal obstruction, myasthenia gravis, paralytic ileus, gastrointestinal atony, or toxic megacolon. The recommended dosages can be found in the table on p. 292. Pregnancy category B.

PHARMACOKINETICS

HALF-LIFE	ONSET	PEAK	DURATION
9-10 hr	1-2 hr	1-1.5 hr	3-4 hr

glycopyrrolate

Glycopyrrolate (Robinul) is a synthetic antimuscarinic agent that blocks receptor sites in the autonomic nervous system that control the production of secretions and the concentration of free acids in the stomach. It is most commonly used as an adjunct in the treatment of peptic ulcer disease and as a preoperative medication to reduce salivation and excessive secretions in the respiratory and gastrointestinal tracts. It is contraindicated in patients who have a hypersensitivity to it and in those with narrow-angle glaucoma, myasthenia gravis, gastrointestinal or genitourinary obstruction, tachycardia, myocardial ischemia, hepatic disease, ulcerative colitis, and toxic megacolon. It should also not be given to children younger than 3 years of age.

Glycopyrrolate is available orally as a 1- and 2-mg tablet and parenterally as a 0.2-mg/ml IM or IV injection. The normal recommended dosages are given in the table below. Pregnancy category B.

PHARMACOKINETICS

HALF-LIFE	ONSET	PEAK	DURATION
Variable	IV: 1 min	IV: 10-15 min	IV: 4 hr
	PO: <45 min	PO: 1 hr	PO: 6 hr

⊶scopolamine

Scopolamine (Transderm Scop) is another naturally occurring cholinergic blocker and one of the principal belladonna alkaloids. It appears to be the most potent antimuscarinic for the prevention of motion sickness. It seems to accomplish this by correcting the imbalance between ACh and norepinephrine in the higher centers in the brain, particularly in the vomiting center, responsible for the symptoms of motion sickness. Ipratropium, a derivative of scopolamine, has potent effects on the lungs and is discussed in Chapter 34. It is available in several different delivery systems that make it very useful for various indications. For the prevention of motion sickness it is available in a convenient transdermal delivery system, a patch that can be applied just behind the ear 4 to 5 hours before travel. It is also available in several parenteral formulations for injection by various routes: IV, IM, and SC. The transdermal patch Transderm Scop is now available

DOSAGES Selected Cholinergic-Blocking Agents

agent	pharmacologic class	dosage range	purpose
atropine		*Pediatric*	
		PO/IM/IV/SC: 0.01 mg/kg q4-6h	Therapeutic anticholinergic effect
		IM: 3 kg, 0.1 mg; 7-9 kg, 0.2 mg; 12-16 kg, 0.3 mg; 20-27 kg, 0.4 mg; 32 kg, 0.5 mg; 41 kg, 0.6 mg	Preop
		IV: 0.02 mg/kg	Bradycardia
		IV: 0.05 mg/kg repeated every 10-30 min if required	Anticholinesterase (insecticide antidote)
		Adult	
		PO: 0.1-1.2 mg q4-6h	
		IM/IV/SC: 0.3-1.2 mg q4-6h	
		IM: 1 mg	Hypotonic radiography
		IV: 0.5-1 mg	Bradycardia
		1-2 mg followed by 2 mg IM/IV q5-60 min prn	Anticholinesterase (insecticide antidote)
dicyclomine (Bentyl)		*Adult* PO: start with 20 mg qid and slowly increase to the most effective dose, which is 40 mg qid	Irritable bowel syndrome
glycopyrrolate (Robinul)	Anticholinergic	*Pediatric 1 mo-12 y/o* IM/IV: 0.002 mg/kg 30-60 min before surgery; a higher dose of 0.004 mg/kg may be required for children 1 mo-2 y/o	Preanesthetic inhibition of secetions and intraoperatively for control of vagal cardiac irregularities
		Adult IM: 0.1-0.2 mg 3-4 times/day	Peptic ulcer
		IV: 0.1 mg repeated as needed every 2-3 min	Preanesthetic
		Adult/pediatric ≥ 12 y/o PO: 1 mg tid or 2 mg 2-3 times/day	Peptic ulcer
		Adult/pediatric IV: 0.2 mg for each 1 mg of neostigmine or 5 mg of pyridostigmine	Reversal of neuromuscular blockade
⊶ scopolamine (Transderm Scop)		*Pediatric* IM/IV/SC: 0.006 mg/kg	Adjunct to anesthesia
		Adult IM/IV/SC: 0.3-0.65 mg	Adjunct to anesthesia
		Transdermal: 1 patch (1.5 mg) delivers 0.5 mg/day for 3 days	Prevention of motion sickness
tolterodine (Detrol)		*Adult* PO: 1-2 mg twice a day	Overactive bladder

by prescription. It is also available as a topical preparation for ocular indications and as a 0.25-mg capsule. The contraindications that apply to atropine apply to it as well. The recommended dosages for various indications can be found in the table on p. 292. Pregnancy category C.

PHARMACOKINETICS

HALF-LIFE	ONSET	PEAK	DURATION
Variable	IV: 30-60 min	IV: 30-45 min	IV: 4 hr
	Patch: 4-5 hr	Patch: 6 hr	Patch: 72 hr

tolterodine

Tolterodine (Detrol) is new muscarinic receptor blocker now being widely promoted for treatment of urinary frequency, urgency, and urge incontinence caused by bladder (detrusor) overactivity. Another drug that is commonly used to treat these conditions is oxybutynin (Ditropan), which is one of the most commonly prescribed. Other agents also used include propantheline (Pro-Banthine), hyoscyamine (Cystospaz-M and others), flavoxate (Urispas), and the TCA imipramine (Tofranil). These agents are used less frequently because of their antimuscarinic adverse effects, particularly dry mouth. Tolterodine appears to have a much lower incidence of dry mouth in part because of tolterodine's specificity for the bladder as opposed to the salivary glands.

Tolterodine should not be used in patients with narrow-angle glaucoma or urinary retention. For patients with markedly decreased hepatic function or in poor metabolizers taking drugs that inhibit CYP3A4, such as erythromycin or ketoconazole, one should start with 1 mg twice a day instead of the normal recommended dose of 2 mg twice a day. Tolterodine is classified as a pregnancy category C agent. It is available as 1- and 2-mg tablets. Recommended dosages are given in the table on p. 292.

PHARMACOKINETICS

HALF-LIFE	ONSET	PEAK	DURATION
2-4 hr	1 hr	1-2 hr	5 hr

nursing process

● Assessment

Anticholinergic drugs, or parasympatholytics, produce a variety of effects resulting from the blocking of ACh in the PSNS. Because of their various effects at different body sites, such as smooth muscle relaxation, decreased glandular secretion, and mydriasis, the nurse must perform a thorough medical and medication history and a head-to-toe assessment so that any of the following contraindications to the use of cholinergic-blocking agents can be revealed: benign prostatic hypertrophy, glaucoma, tachycardia, myocardial infarction, congestive heart failure, and hiatal hernia. In general the cholinergic blockers should not be used in patients with gastrointestinal or genitourinary obstruction and in children under 3 years of age. Drug interactions are discussed earlier in this chapter. The head-to-toe assessment will also help document baseline findings related to the disease and to assessing drug effectiveness.

Tolterodine, oxybutynin, imipramine, and flavoxate are some of the newer agents being used to treat urinary incontinence. Tolterodine is a muscarinic-receptor–blocking agent that has been most recently introduced for treatment of a variety of urinary symptoms and problems ranging from frequency and urgency to incontinence. Tolterodine and oxybutynin are probably the agents that are most commonly used at this time. Patients who have narrow-angle glaucoma or urinary retention should not take tolterodine. If they have poor renal function or are taking drugs that inhibit CYP3A4, the enzyme for metabolism (such as with erythromycin or ketoconazole), then a lower dosage such as 1 mg bid may be recommended. Cautious use is advised in patients who are pregnant or lactating. Oxybutynin is contraindicated in patients with GI or GU obstruction, GI hemorrhage, glaucoma, colitis, and myasthenia gravis. Cautious use is recommended for patients who are pregnant, lactating, elderly, or under 12 years of age. Drug interactions with oxybutynin include atenolol, digoxin, acetaminophen, haloperidol, levodopa, and phenothiazines. Impramine is contraindicated with an allergy to TCAs, seizure disorders, and benign prostatic hypertrophy (BPH). Cautious use is recommended in patients who are suicidal; have severe depression, narrow-angle glaucoma, urinary retention, cardiac or hepatic disease, or hypothyroidism; and are elderly. Drug interactions are numerous and include many antihypertensive agents, sympathomimetics, alcohol, barbiturates, benzodiazepines, CNS depressants, and MAOIs. Flavoxate is a spasmolytic and is contraindicated in patients with GI or GU obstruction or hemorrhage and used cautiously in patients who are elderly, under 12 years of age, pregnant, lactating, or with a history of glaucoma.

Activity

● Nursing Diagnoses

Nursing diagnoses associated with the use of cholinergic-blocking agents include, but are not limited to, the following:

- Ineffective tissue perfusion related to tachycardia and preexisting cardiac disorders.
- Risk for injury related to possible excessive CNS stimulation that results in tremors, confusion, sedation, and amnesia.
- Acute pain related to side effects of dry mouth.
- Impaired gas exchange related to thickened respiratory secretions from side effects of drug.

- Urinary retention related to loss of bladder tone as a result of side effects of medication.
- Risk for injury (heat stroke) related to decreased sweating and loss of normal heat-regulating mechanisms (especially in the elderly and in those who engage in excessive exercise or who are in high environmental temperatures) and possible heat stroke.
- Risk for injury related to changes in vision related to the mydriatic effects of the medication and from increased sensitivity to the drug in the elderly.
- Deficient knowledge related to the therapeutic regimen, side effects, drug interactions, and precautions related to the use of anticholinergic agents.

● Planning

Goals for the patient receiving cholinergic blockers include, but are not limited to, the following:
- Patient self-administers medications as prescribed.
- Patient experiences relief of symptoms for which the medication was prescribed.
- Patient remains compliant with the drug therapy.
- Patient demonstrates an adequate knowledge about the use of the specific medications, side effects, and the appropriate dosing at home.
- Patient is free of injury to self stemming from adverse effects of the medication.

Outcome Criteria

Outcome criteria include the following:
- Patient will state rationale for the use of cholinergic blockers in preoperative preparation, such as decreasing the risk of complications associated with anesthesia.
- Patient will state importance of compliance with medication regimen, such as avoiding complications of Parkinson's disease.
- Patient will state the importance of taking the medication as prescribed and not suddenly withdrawing the medication because of risk of increasing symptomatology.
- Patient will state those conditions of which the physician should be notified immediately (e.g., palpitations, dysrhythmias, chest pain), if they occur.
- Patient will keep follow-up appointments with the physician to avoid unnecessary adverse effects of complications of treatment or noncompliance.

● Implementation

Preventive nursing care is important to the effective use of cholinergic-blocking agents, especially teaching patients how to decrease their need for these medications, such as those with peptic ulcers. There are several nursing interventions that can also serve to maximize the therapeutic effects of anticholinergics and minimize the side effects. For example, always encourage patients to take the medications as prescribed, especially those with Parkinson's disease or with parkinsonian symptoms produced by certain medications such as phenothiazines and major antipsychotic agents. As another example, patients taking these medications for the treatment of peptic ulcer disease should be told to take the larger doses at bedtime because this often helps decrease the ulcer pain, which can be a source of frequent awakenings during the night.

Because atropine is compatible with some of the other commonly used preoperative medications such as meperidine (Demerol), morphine, and promethazine (Phenergan), it can be combined with these agents in the same syringe for preoperative administration. However, whenever mixing several medications together in one syringe, always calculate the doses very carefully. When administering optical solutions to produce mydriasis, always check the concentration of medication and apply pressure to the inner canthus to prevent more systemic absorption. Remember that the antidote to atropine is physostigmine salicylate (Antilirium) given slowly intravenously.

Tolterodine should be taken as directed and is usually well tolerated when taken with food. Oxybutynin, like flavoxate, should be taken as directed with fluids 1 hour before or 2 hours after meals, if tolerated. With flavoxate and the other drugs in this category, drowsiness may occur, so it is important to inform patients about caution with driving while beginning this medication. Dry mouth associated with these drugs may be handled best with chewing gum, frequent mouth care, and availability of hard candy. As with tolterodine, oxybutynin, flavoxate, and other agents used for urinary incontinence, constipation, and inability to sweat or perspire should be managed with increased fluids and bulk and avoidance of extremes of heat. Patients taking any of these medications for urinary incontinence or other urinary disorders should also be informed to report any unresolved constipation, palpitations, alterations in gait, excessive dizziness, or difficulty in urinating to their health care provider immediately.

Patient teaching tips are presented in the box on p. 295.

● Evaluation

There are some therapeutic effects to look for in patients receiving anticholinergics. Patients with Parkinson's disease should experience fewer problems with tremors, salivation, and drooling. Patients taking these medications for the relief of peptic ulcer disease should experience less abdominal pain. The nurse must also evaluate the patient to determine whether any of the side effects of these medications are occurring, such as constipation, tachycardia, tremors, confusion, hallucinations, CNS depression (which occurs with large doses of atropine), sedation, urinary retention, hot and dry skin, and fever.

patient teaching tips

Anticholinergics

➤ Patients should always take their medication as ordered because a overdose can cause life-threatening problems.

➤ Dry mouth is a common side effect of these medications, so patients taking them on a long-term basis should regularly brush their teeth to combat dental cavities. Patients can chew gum or suck on hard candy to relieve dryness, if these foods are allowed.

➤ Patients should know to be careful when engaging in various activities such as driving a car or operating machinery because of the blurred vision that commonly occurs with these medications.

➤ Patients may experience sensitivity to light and may therefore want to wear dark glasses or sunglasses.

➤ Patients should always get the okay of their physician before taking any other medication, including OTC medications.

➤ If patients are elderly and taking an anticholinergic, they should be reminded that they are at particular risk for suffering heat stroke because of the effects of these agents on the heat-regulating mechanisms in the body. They should therefore avoid exposure to high temperatures as well as strenuous exercise. They should limit physical exertion and always remember the importance of adequate fluid and salt intake, if this is allowed. Also they should use fans, air conditioners, and adequate ventilation to prevent overheating.

➤ Patients should be told to contact their physician should they experience urinary hesitancy and/or retention, constipation, palpitations, tremors, confusion, sedation or amnesia, excessive dry mouth dryness (especially if they have chronic lung infections or chronic lung disease), or fever.

POINTS TO REMEMBER

Cholinergic Blockers, Anticholinergics, Parasympatholytics, Antimuscarinics

- All names for the drugs that block or inhibit the actions of acetylcholine in the PSNS.
- Block the action of acetylcholine at the *muscarinic receptor.*
- Allow the SNS to dominate; therefore these agents have actions similar to those of the adrenergics.

Chemical Classification

- Natural, semisynthetic, and synthetic anticholinergics.

Receptor Action

- Competitive antagonists (blockers).
- Compete with acetylcholine at the muscarinic receptors; high doses: partial blocking actions at nicotinic receptors.
- Bind to and block acetylcholine at muscarinic receptors located on the cells that the nerve stimulates.

- Contraindications to the use of cholinergic blocking agents include patients with a history of benign prostatic hypertrophy, glaucoma, tachycardia, myocardial infarction, congestive heart failure, and hiatal hernia.
- Cautious use of the anticholinergic (cholinergic blocking drugs) include patients with gastrointestinal or genitourinary obstruction or in children under 3 years of age.
- Parkinsonian symptoms may occur with certain medications such as phenothiazines. Anticholinergics help prevent their side effects *but* compliance is key to the therapeutic effect.

Nursing Considerations

- Check compatibility of medication in syringe when administering preoperatively.
- Apply pressure to inner canthus for a few seconds after ophthalmic use for mydriasis.
- The antidote for atropine is physostigmine salicylate.

REVIEW QUESTIONS

1. Elderly patients taking anticholinergics should be reminded to:
   a. Avoid exposure to high temperatures.
   b. Take the drug with antiglaucoma medications.
   c. Participate in exercises and use a hot tub for relaxation.

   d. Not be alarmed if there is constipation, confusion, and palpations.
2. Contraindications to the use of cholinergic blockers include:
   a. Tachycardia.
   b. Peptic ulcer disease.

c. Irritable bowel syndrome.
d. Benign prostatic hypertrophy (BPH).

3. Side effects associated with the use of cholinergic blockers include all of the following except:
a. Mydriasis.
b. Diaphoresis.
c. Tachycardia.
d. CNS excitation.

4. An expected effect from a parasympatholytic includes:
a. Miosis.
b. Increased muscle rigidity.

c. Increased bronchial secretions.
d. Decreased motility and peristalsis.

5. During an assessment of a patient about to receive a cholinergic-blocking agent, you should look for drug interactions such as:
a. Narcotics.
b. Phenothiazines.
c. Meperidine (Demerol).
d. Glycopyrrolate (Robinul).

For Answers see www.harcourthealth.com/MERLIN/Lilley/.

CRITICAL THINKING Activities

1. You are getting ready to administer preoperative medications to a 75-year-old woman undergoing minor surgery. She has a history of smoking, congestive heart failure, and open-angle glaucoma. What is the rationale for why you do not administer the atropine preoperatively to this patient, as ordered? Also, what is your rationale for contacting the physician about this drug interaction and your subsequent action.

2. You are caring for a patient who has just coded in the cardiac care unit. The patient is in second-degree heart block, has sinus bradycardia with a heart rate of 30, and has passed out. You recommend that the cholinergic blocker _____ be given to _____ the heart rate.
   1. belladonna   2. esmolol   3. atropine
   4. increase   5. decrease   6. slow
      a. 1 and 6   b. 2 and 6   c. 3 and 4
      d. 3 and 5

3. You are chaperoning a group of 8 year olds on a deep-sea fishing trip. One of the parents of these children is an anesthesiologist. She has given all the children a medication to take that is supposed to keep them from getting sick while at sea. Three hours into the fishing expedition you notice that your group of 8 year olds are disoriented, hallucinating, irritable, and cannot sit still. You realize the children are suffering from _____ side effects from the cholinergic blocker _____.
   1. central nervous system   2. cardiovascular
   3. respiratory   4. belladonna
   5. pilocarpine   6. scopolamine
      a. 1 and 6   b. 2 and 4   c. 3 and 5
      d. 1 and 5

4. In question number 3 you are asked to give 0.5 mg of atropine to your patient. The vial concentration is 1 mg/ml In the haste of this emergency situation, 5 ml of atropine is given. How many milligrams of atropine was given to your patient?

5. If the sympathetic nervous system is for mobilizing the organism in times of stress or during emergency situations, what is the importance of the parasympathetic nervous system? Why are patients at risk for hyperthermia when taking drugs such as atropine?

For Answers see www.harcourthealth.com/MERLIN/Lilley/.

bibliography

Albanese J, Nutz P: *Mosby's 2001 nursing drug reference and review cards,* St Louis, 2001, Mosby.

American Hospital Formulary Service: *AHFS drug information,* Bethesda, Md, 2000, American Society of Health-System Pharmacists.

Anderson PO, Knoben JE, Troutman WG: *Handbook of clinical drug data 1999-2000,* ed 9, New York, 1999, McGraw-Hill.

Johns Hopkins Hospital, Department of Pediatrics et al: *The Harriet Lane handbook,* ed 15, St Louis, 2000, Mosby.

Keen JH: *Critical care and emergency drug reference,* ed 3, St Louis, 1996, Mosby.

Medical Letter: Tolterodine for overactive bladder 40(1038), October 23, 1998.

Mosby's GenRx: a comprehensive reference for generic and brand drugs, ed 10, St Louis, 2000, Mosby.

Skidmore-Roth L: *Mosby's 2001 nursing drug reference,* St Louis, 2001, Mosby.

Turkoski BB, Lance BR, Bonfiglio MF: *Drug information handbook for nursing,* ed 2, Cleveland, 2000, LexiComp, Inc.

United States Pharmacopeial Convention: *USP DI: advice for the patient: drug information in lay language,* vol. 11, ed 20, Englewood, Colo, 2000, Micromedex.

Activity

Remember to check the **Online Worksheet** for additional learning opportunities: **www.harcourthealth.com/MERLIN/Lilley/**

Drugs Affecting the Cardiovascular and Renal Systems: Study Skills Tips

- Linking Learning
- Text Notation

LINKING LEARNING

The Part Three Study Skills Tips stressed the importance of planning for the part as a whole. With that in mind, what is the focus of Part Four? The part title is "Drugs Affecting the Cardiovascular and Renal Systems." What is the first question you think you should ask about this part? I would begin by asking, "What are the cardiovascular and renal systems?" This is a very obvious question and might seem to be so basic that it need not be asked, but the next six chapters will all develop around this part title. Asking the obvious question sometimes is exactly the thing that should be done to get started.

Chapter Structure

Just as there is a structure to each part in the text, which is constant from one part to the next, there is also a structure in the chapters. This structure is a repeating model that was created by the authors in an attempt to organize the material and present it in the clearest way possible. The chapter structure is a valuable learning asset for those who make use of it.

Chapter Objectives

Each chapter begins with a set of objectives. These are established by the authors and serve to tell you what they expect you will know and be able to do when you have completed the chapter. It is sometimes tempting to ignore the objectives and get right on with the task of reading the chapter. Do not give in to that temptation. Read the objectives and spend some time thinking about what they reveal about the content of the chapter.

Example Based on Chapter 20 Objectives

Objective 1. Define *inotropic*, *chronotropic*, and *dromotropic*.

What can you learn from this objective? First, there is the vocabulary. This objective makes it clear that you have some terms to learn. This means that you may want to have some blank note cards available to start setting up vocabulary cards for this chapter. In fact, you should write each of the terms in objective 1 on a separate card and be ready to complete the card as the terms are introduced and explained in the chapter.

The next thing that stands out in this first objective is that the three terms contain a common element, tropic. This should bring active questioning into play. What does the suffix "tropic" mean? Asking this question now is a way of noting that these three terms do have some common meaning. Also it serves to provide an immediate focus for personal learning when you begin to read the chapter.

Objective 2. Briefly discuss the effect of cardiac glycosides and positive inotropics on a failing heart.

From this comes the potential for a new question relating to the first objective. What do inotropic, chronotropic, and dromotropic have to do with the heart? Just as it is essential to see the relationship between parts and chapters, it is also essential to see relationships within the chapters. These first two objectives should cause you to consider those relationships and make your own learning much more active.

Chapter Headings

The next chapter structure to consider in this process are the chapter headings. Chapter 20 has the major sections:

Cardiac Glycosides and Nursing Process. What is the importance of this heading structure? It tells you that the authors will focus on the pharmacologic aspects first and then

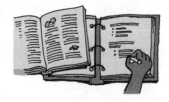

explain how this relates to nursing. This does not tell the learner a great deal about what to anticipate in terms of chapter content, but it does make clear a structure that is consistent in most of the chapters in this text.

Cardiac Glycosides is broken down into subsections in this chapter. Spend several minutes considering the organization of these subsections. The first subtopic to be treated is "Mechanism of Action." What is meant by mechanism of action? How do cardiac glycosides act? On what do they act? It does not matter that you cannot answer these questions at this point. What is important is that you ask them as a means of fostering an active and participatory learning attitude when you begin to read the chapter. Think, question, anticipate, then read. This sequence will enhance your learning.

Continue this process of looking at the subtopics and thinking ahead to what will be explained in the chapter. These subsections are the same in every chapter, and this thinking process should become automatic very quickly.

Glossary

The next chapter structure is one that I have already stressed in previous Study Skills Tips, and it is one that is essential to learning. The glossary is a mini-dictionary for each chapter. Words that have not been introduced earlier in the text and that are central to the content of this chapter are presented here. The listing is in alphabetical order, which means that the glossary terms will not necessarily occur in the same order in the body of the chapter.

As you read terms as presented in the glossary, be aware of the nature of the definition. A glossary definition is specific and brief. It is a very useful place to begin to learn the new terms in the chapter, but the definition presented may not be enough for full understanding. You will find that full understanding will come after reading the chapter and encountering the term within the fuller context of sentences and paragraphs of text that explain not only the term but how it applies in the particular situation.

Glossary and Text Relationship

The term *inotropic agents* is defined in the Chapter 20 glossary. As I read it I understand that inotropic has to do with force or energy of muscle contractions. The glossary states that an inotropic agent is a drug that increases myocardial contractility. Some of this information is clear, and some of it is still somewhat hazy. It should become clearer when connected with the chapter text. The first paragraph of the chapter introduces inotropic agents: "Drugs that increase the force of myocardial contraction are called *positive* **inotropic agents,** and such drugs have a beneficial role in the treatment of a failing heart muscle."

With this sentence I find I have a much clearer understanding of what is meant by inotropic agents, and I have the added benefit of knowing that there are positive inotropic drugs. This is what must happen to fully master the content-specific vocabulary. You must see the core definition as presented in the glossary, but you must also read to determine how that core definition is expanded and exemplified in the body of the text.

When preparing vocabulary cards it is not a good idea to simply copy the definition from the glossary and assume that definition will serve your purpose. Wait to fill out the card until after you encounter the same term in the body of the chapter, and then pick and choose the information from the glossary and the body that will provide you with the clearest understanding of the term. Also, when placing information on vocabulary cards, it is always useful to include chapter number and page numbers so that you can locate the source of your definition quickly should you find it necessary later.

These chapter structures can provide you with a clear picture of what you are expected to learn and the organizational pattern in which the material will be presented. Being aware of the structures and making use of them in this way will improve your concentration when you begin to read the chapter for understanding and memory. The time spent working with chapter structure is not

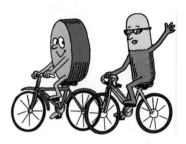

wasted and does not significantly increase the study time of the chapter. In fact, the time you spend working with the objectives, headings, and glossary will generally save time when you are doing intensive reading and study.

TEXT NOTATION

Highlighting or underlining text materials is a tool that can be very helpful when rehearsing and reviewing materials after the study reading. The problem as discussed in the *Study Guide* is that it is often difficult to limit the quantity of material that is marked. Although a good general guideline is to try to limit yourself to marking no more than 20% to 25% of the total, this guideline applies to large blocks of material. However, some paragraphs contain essential information and must be marked extensively, while other paragraphs may need only one or two sentences marked. In this Study Skills Tips section, the object is to look at how the author's structure and language can help you to select what should be marked.

Text Notation Application

Reproduced below are two paragraphs from Chapter 25 with my model underlining completed, followed by a discussion of the reasons for which I made the choices. You should not view the model underlining as a "perfect" example. The decision as to what to mark is very much an individual choice based on a number of factors, including prior experience with the subject matter and awareness of personal learning objectives and needs. These model paragraphs with the accompanying discussion are intended to provide you with a basic model to adapt to your own learning style and needs.

Chapter 25, Paragraphs One and Two

"Fluid and electrolyte management is one of the cornerstones of patient care. Most disease processes, tissue injuries, and surgical procedures greatly influence the physiologic status of fluids and electrolytes in the body. A prerequisite to the understanding of fluid and electrolyte management is knowledge of the extent and composition of the various body fluid compartments.

Sixty percent of the adult human body is water. This is referred to as the *total body water (TBW)*, and it is distributed to the three main compartments in the following proportions: intracellular fluid (ICF) 67%, interstitial fluid (ISF) 25%, and plasma volume (PV) 8%."

Discussion. The first thing you should notice is that the underlining I have done exceeds the 20% to 25% guideline. This is the first paragraph in the chapter. First paragraphs are usually introductions to the topic and may vary a great deal in the quantity of important information. This chapter, in my view, contains a number of key points that must be considered. Because the content seems important, I have chosen to underline more.

Sentence one was chosen because of the word "cornerstones." This word suggests that fluid management is extremely important in patient care and I must be sure to keep that focus throughout the chapter. Paying careful attention to the author's word choices plays a major role in selecting materials for text notation.

Paying attention to language led me to the third sentence, which begins: "A prerequisite to the understanding . . ." That phrase should immediately capture your attention. The phrase says that there is something that must be understood before anything else that follows will make complete sense. The phrase should also serve as an instant cue to generate a question for reading. "What is the prerequisite to understanding fluid and electrolyte management?" This question is answered directly by the sentence containing the phrase. The phrase serves as a language cue that there is something important. This in turn suggests that you probably will want to underline or highlight some information. The question helps you select what should be marked. Everything you do at this point serves as a guide to help you establish clear learning objectives and makes the process of selecting the best information for marking easier to accomplish.

The next segment was chosen because it stands out from the body of the paragraph. *"Total body water (TBW)"* is italicized. This is a print convention used as a means of putting emphasis on something that the author believes to be of special importance. The decision to underline words and phrases that are already emphasized is a personal one. You may feel that, since the author has already marked it, you have no need to add your own marks. I

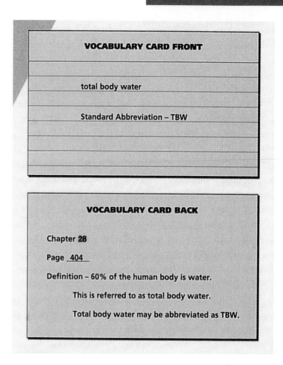

find that my own marking, even of italicized or bold print material, serves as a double reminder of the importance of the information. This is an excellent example of what I mean when I say that text notation is highly personal. Whether you choose to add your own marking or not there is one aspect of this phrase that is essential. "Total body water" is part of the vocabulary of fluids and electrolytes. That means it is time to add to your vocabulary cards.

This term served as a lead-in to the next key point that I have marked. The next sentence is "TBW is distributed to the three main compartments . . ." Whenever you see a phrase with a number and a word such as "main," you should be aware that this is potentially important material. This phrase should generate a new question that will aid in your selection of material to mark. "What are the three main compartments?" You see immediately that the rest of this sentence answers that question, and therefore identifies what needs to be marked. This marking also identifies three additional vocabulary items to be added to your cards for this chapter. As you set up your cards, be careful. One fluid is "intra-," and the second is "inter-." It would be easy to confuse the two, but they have very different meanings. If you are not sure what the difference is between intra- and inter-, make use of a dictionary.

Chapter 25, Paragraph Three

"The TBW can be described as being in or out of the blood vessels, or vasculature. If this terminology is used, then the term **intravascular fluid** (IVF) describes fluid inside the blood vessels, and the term **extravascular fluid** (EVF) describes fluid outside the blood vessels. The term **plasma** is used to describe the fluid that flows through the blood vessels that is intravascular.

Interstitial fluid is the fluid that is in the <u>space between cells, tissues, and organs.</u> Both <u>plasma and interstitial fluid</u> make up <u>extracellular volume.</u> Both <u>interstitial fluid and intracellular fluid make up extravascular volume.</u> These terms are often confused and misused. Table 25-1 lists these definitions for further clarity and understanding."

Discussion. The language conventions and the print conventions, *bold italics,* are the same that I used to help in the previous paragraph. This paragraph also makes a point about the possibility of confusing and/or misusing the terms introduced. Being told that there is confusing material suggests that it is crucial that you be able to identify, define, and explain each of the terms used, and that it will take some careful thought to do so. There is one additional point in this paragraph that is important. The last sentence points you to a table, Table 25-1. There are many tables in this text. Always remember that tables are often used in an effort to simplify complex mate-rial and to clarify the relationships between the items presented in the table. In these opening paragraphs, with the repeated reference to the confusing nature of the descriptions, Table 25-1 will almost certainly be important to your learning.

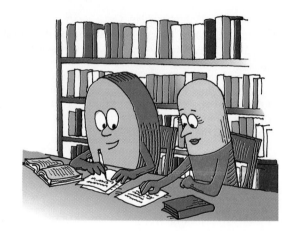

Chapter 20

Positive Inotropic Agents

objectives

www.harcourthealth.com/MERLIN/Lilley/

Look for this symbol for topics covered in the **Online Worksheet** Activity

When you reach the end of the chapter, you should be able to do the following:

1 Define *inotropic, chronotropic,* and *dromotropic.*

2 Briefly discuss the effect of cardiac glycosides and positive inotropics on a failing heart.

3 Explain the digitalizing process, especially the differences between rapid and slow digitalization.

4 Discuss the nursing care required for patients undergoing digitalization and the specific problems associated with rapid and slow digitalization.

5 Discuss the peak onset, duration of action, metabolism, and excretion of positive inotropic agents.

6 Develop a nursing care plan that includes all phases of the nursing process based on actual and potential problems that can occur in the patient receiving positive inotropics.

7 Identify significant drugs, laboratory tests, and food interactions associated with positive inotropic agents.

8 Explain why specific diseases, conditions, and drugs are considered interactions, cautions, or contraindications to the use of a digoxin and other positive inotropic agents.

9 Discuss the nurse's responsibility in patients experiencing digoxin toxicity and to patients receiving digoxin immune FAB (Digibind).

drug profiles

⚷ **digoxin,** p. 305   **milrinone,** p. 307

digoxin immune FAB, p. 305

⚷ Key drug.

glossary

Automaticity (aw to mə tis i te) A property of specialized excitable tissue that allows self-activation through the spontaneous development of an action potential, as in the pacemaker cells of the heart. (p. 302)

Cardiac glycoside (gli′ ko sid) A glycoside is any of several carbohydrates that yield a sugar and a nonsugar as the result of hydrolysis. The plant *Digitalis purpurea* yields a glycoside used in the treatment of heart disease; these glycosides are called *cardiac glycosides.* (p. 302)

Chronotropic agent (kron′ o tropik) An agent that influences the rate of the heartbeat. A positive chronotropic agent increases the heart rate. (p. 302)

Congestive heart failure (CHF) An abnormal condition in which cardiac pumping is impaired as the result of myocardial infarction, ischemic heart disease, or cardiomyopathy. Failure of the ventricle to eject blood efficiently results in volume overload, chamber dilatation, and elevated intracardiac pressure. The retrograde transmission of increased hydro-static pressure from the left ventricle leads to pulmonary congestion; elevated right ventricular pressure leads to systemic venous congestion and peripheral edema. (p. 302)

Dromotropic agent (drom′ o trop′ ik) An agent that influences the conduction of electrical impulses. A positive dromotropic agent enhances the conduction of electrical impulses in the heart. (p. 302)

Ejection fraction The proportion of blood that is ejected during each ventricular contraction compared with the total ventricular filling volume. It is an index of left ventricular function, and the normal fraction is 65% (0.65). (p. 302)

Inotropic agents (in′ o trop′ ik) *Inotropic* refers to the force or energy of muscular contractions, particularly contraction of the heart muscle. Positive inotropic agents are drugs that increase myocardial contractility. (p. 302)

Left ventricular end-diastolic volume (ven trik′ u lər \ di′ ə stol′ ik) Ventricular diastole begins with the onset of the second heart sound and ends with the first heart sound. The *left ventricular end-diastolic volume* is the total amount of blood in the ventricle before it contracts, or the preload. (p. 302)

Lusitropic Heart muscle and blood vessel relaxation caused by quick reuptake of calcium back into sarcoplasmic reticulum storage sites. (p. 307)

Refractory period The period during which a pulse generator (e.g., the heart) is unresponsive to an input signal of specified amplitude and during which it is impossible for the myocardium to respond. This is the period when the cardiac cell is readjusting its sodium and potassium levels and the cardiac cell cannot be depolarized again. (p. 302)

Therapeutic window The drug level range in the blood that is considered beneficial, as opposed to toxic. (p. 304)

Drugs that increase the force of myocardial contraction are called *positive* **inotropic agents,** and such drugs have a beneficial role in the treatment of a failing heart muscle. A drug that increases the rate at which the heart beats is called a positive **chronotropic agent.** Drugs may also affect how quickly electrical impulses travel through the conduction system of the heart (the sinoatrial [SA] node, atrioventricular [AV] node, bundle of His, and Purkinje fibers). Drugs that accelerate conduction are referred to as positive **dromotropic agents.** This chapter focuses on two of the main classes of positive inotropic agents: **cardiac glycosides** and *phosphodiesterase inhibitors.*

It has been estimated that close to 2 million office and 1.5 million hospital visits a year are necessitated by exacerbations of congestive heart failure (CHF). Findings yielded by one of the largest and most frequently cited studies involving patients with CHF, the Framingham study, show that the 5-year survival rate in patients with CHF is approximately 50%. Therefore any drug that could lengthen survival in affected patients or help the failing heart perform its essential duties would be extremely valuable. The glycosides are a prime example. Data contrary to this were recently released. Digoxin's use as a first-line treatment for CHF did not improve mortality rates. Angiotensin-converting enzyme (ACE) inhibitors and diuretics were recommended as the mainstays; however, digoxin may still offer benefit in some patients.

CONGESTIVE HEART FAILURE AND CARDIAC DYSRHYTHMIAS

Heart failure is a pathologic state in which the heart is unable to pump blood in sufficient amounts from the ventricles (i.e., cardiac output) to meet the body's metabolic needs. The signs and symptoms typically associated with heart failure constitute the syndrome of **congestive heart failure (CHF).** This syndrome can be limited to the left ventricle (producing pulmonary edema and symptoms of dyspnea or cough) or the right ventricle (producing symptoms such as pedal edema, jugular venous distention, ascites, and hepatic congestion), or it may affect both ventricles.

In patients with CHF, the overworked, failing heart cannot meet the demands placed on it and blood is not ejected efficiently from the ventricles. This occurs because the **ejection fraction** (the amount of blood ejected with each contraction) compared with the total amount of blood in the ventricle just before contraction **(left ventricular end-diastolic volume)** is decreased. (Normally the ejection fraction is approximately 65% [0.65] of the total volume in the ventricle.) As more blood accumulates in the right and left ventricles, more pressure builds up in the blood vessels leading to the heart. The retrograde transmission of this increased hydrostatic pressure from the left ventricle leads to pulmonary congestion, whereas elevated right ventricular pressure causes systemic venous congestion and peripheral edema.

Because the heart cannot then meet the increased demands placed on it, the blood supply to certain organs is reduced. The organs most dependent on blood supply, the brain and heart, are the last to be deprived of blood. As an organ that is relatively less dependent on blood supply, the kidney has its blood supply shunted away. Therefore the filtration of fluids and removal of waste products is impaired. When these fluids and waste products accumulate, the patient experiences such symptoms as pulmonary edema and shortness of breath, resulting in kidney failure.

The physical defects producing CHF are of two types: (1) a cardiac defect (myocardial deficiency such as myocardial infarction [MI] or valve insufficiency), which leads to inadequate cardiac contractility and filling, and (2) a defect outside the heart (systemic defect such as coronary artery disease, pulmonary hypertension, or diabetes), which results in an overload on an otherwise normal heart. Either or both of these defects may be present in the same patient. Common causes of myocardial deficiency and systemic defects are listed in Box 20-1.

In patients with supraventricular dysrhythmias, atrial fibrillation, or atrial flutter, the top aspects of the heart (atria) are contracting several hundred times a minute. Not only are the atria contracting frequently, but several areas in the atria besides the SA node are then acting as the pacemaker of the heart. Normally the AV node controls how slowly or quickly impulses arrive in the ventricles, and it also has the ability to receive all these depolarizations and to allow only a certain number to pass through the ventricles. This keeps the patient from going into ventricular fibrillation, which is fatal. It also gives the ventricles time to fill with blood, an equally important aspect. However, during atrial fibrillation or flutter, patients may show symptoms such as CHF.

All cells in the heart can depolarize spontaneously, a property called **automaticity.** The **refractory period** is the time when the cardiac cells are readjusting their sodium and potassium levels. During this time the cardiac cells cannot depolarize again. It is the sodium-potassium ATPase pump that is responsible for the movement of potassium ions in and sodium ions out of the cardiac cells after they have depolarized, an action potential has been generated, and the electrical impulse has been generated. In patients with either atrial fibrillation or flutter, the AV node is circumvented and the impulses arrive in the ventricle before the refractory period is over. The resultant slow spread of impulses from the atrium through refractory muscle results in continuous atrial excitation—atrial fibrillation or flutter. (The cardiac conduction system and the abnormalities responsible for causing dysrhythmias are described in greater detail in Chapter 21.)

CARDIAC GLYCOSIDES

According to the survival statistics cited earlier, any drug that can lengthen survival in patients with CHF by helping the failing heart perform its essential duties would be extremely valuable. Glycosides may be able to do this in certain patients. They are one of the oldest and most ef-

Myocardial Deficiency and Increased Work Load: Common Causes

BOX 20-1

MYOCARDIAL DEFICIENCY
Inadequate contractility
Myocardial infarction
Coronary artery disease
Cardiomyopathy
Infection

Inadequate filling
Atrial fibrillation
Infection
Tamponade
Ischemia

INCREASED WORK LOAD
Pressure overload
Hypertension
Outflow obstruction

Volume overload
Hypervolemia
Congenital abnormalities
Anemia
Thyroid disease

---

pediatric considerations

Cardiac Glycosides

- Digoxin should be given according to a regular time schedule 1 hour before or 2 hours after the child's or infant's feeding.
- Make sure that the dosing of these agents is accompanied by close monitoring and individualized dosing and nursing care. Calculating dosages is of great importance to safe and cautious nursing care—caution, caution, and more caution is needed, as a one-decimal-point placement error may result in a tenfold dosage error, which would be fatal! All medication calculations should be double-checked by another registered nurse or by a pharmacist or physician because of this narrow margin of error.
- Toxicity is manifested in children by nausea, vomiting, bradycardia, anorexia, and dysrhythmias.
- The physician should be notified immediately should the following symptoms indicative of CHF develop: increased fatigue, sudden weight gain (2 lb or greater in 1 week), respiratory distress, or profuse scalp sweating. ■

---

fective groups of drugs. Not only do they have beneficial effects in the failing heart but they also help control the ventricular response to atrial fibrillation or flutter. They were originally obtained from either the *Digitalis purpurea* or the *Digitalis lanata* plant, both commonly referred to as *foxglove*. Cardiac glycosides have been the mainstay of therapy for CHF for more than 200 years, and they continue to be one of the most frequently used positive inotropic agents. Digoxin is the most commonly prescribed digitalis preparation. The widespread and enduring popularity of digitalis is the result of several years of clinical use. Critically ill patients can be restored to near-normal states within hours after digitalization.

Mechanism of Action

The primary beneficial effect of a cardiac glycoside (e.g., digoxin) is thought to be an increase in myocardial contractility. This occurs secondarily to the inhibition of the sodium pump. By inhibiting this enzyme complex, the cellular sodium concentration and subsequently calcium concentration increase. The overall result is enhanced myocardial contraction. Digoxin also augments vagal tone, resulting in increased diastolic filling.

Cardiac glycosides also change the electrical conduction properties of the heart, and this markedly affects the conduction system and cardiac automaticity. Glycosides decrease the velocity (rate) of electrical conduction and prolong the refractory period in the conduction system. The particular area of the conduction system where this occurs is between the atria and the ventricles (SA node to AV node through the ventricles). The cardiac cell remains in a state of depolarization and is unable to start another electrical impulse.

Drug Effects

Cardiac glycosides, especially digitoxin and digoxin, are almost identical in their ability to treat CHF and dysrhythmias. The two glycosides vary, however, in terms of their water solubility, half-life, and excretion, and the clinical profile of the patient determines which glycoside is selected. All cardiac glycosides produce dramatic inotropic, chronotropic, and dromotropic cardiac effects. (*Inotropic* refers to the force or energy of muscular contractions; *chronotropic* refers to the rate of the heart beat; and *dromotropic* refers to the conduction of electrical impulses.) These effects include the following:

- A *positive inotropic* effect resulting in an increase in the force and velocity of myocardial contraction without a corresponding increase in oxygen consumption
- A *negative chronotropic* effect producing a reduced heart rate
- A *negative dromotropic* effect that decreases automaticity at the SA node, decreases AV nodal conduction, reduces conductivity at the bundle of His, and prolongs the atrial and ventricular refractory periods
- An increase in stroke volume
- A reduction in heart size during diastole
- A decrease in venous blood pressure and vein engorgement
- An increase in coronary circulation
- Promotion of diuresis as the result of improved blood circulation
- Palliation of exertional and paroxysmal nocturnal dyspnea, cough, and cyanosis

Therapeutic Uses

Cardiac glycosides are primarily used in the treatment of CHF and supraventricular dysrhythmias. In CHF the therapeutic effects of digoxin are secondary to its ability to increase the force of contraction, its positive inotropic action. There are many therapeutic benefits to this. Increasing the force of contraction increases the ejection fraction compared with the left ventricular end-diastolic volume, or preload. As more blood is ejected with each contraction of the heart, there is less blood remaining in the ventricle and thus less pressure that builds up. With this the symptoms of pulmonary edema, pulmonary hypertension, and right-sided ventricular failure subside.

Another benefit of this positive inotropic action is that it promotes diuresis by ensuring that adequate blood is supplied to the kidneys. As a result, fluids are filtered and waste products removed, resulting in the relief of shortness of breath and pulmonary edema.

Cardiac glycosides are also effective in the treatment of dysrhythmias such as atrial fibrillation and atrial flutter because of their negative chronotropic (decreased heart rate) and negative dromotropic (slowed conduction velocity) actions. Automaticity, conduction velocity, and the refractory period are all affected. Digoxin can slow the depolarization of the SA node and other areas of the atria that may be acting as pacemakers. Thus the glycosides such as digoxin directly slow conduction through the AV node (decreasing the ventricular rate) and increase the vagal action on the heart. In addition, the cardiac glycosides lengthen the refractory period, which allows the correct levels of sodium and potassium ions to be reached before depolarization.

Side Effects and Adverse Effects

The side effects and adverse effects associated with cardiac glycoside use can be very serious. The primary cardiac glycoside in use today is digoxin, and close monitoring of patients' clinical response to it and the possible development of toxic symptoms is essential. Digoxin has a very narrow **therapeutic window,** meaning there is a small range of the drug level in the blood that is considered therapeutic. Monitoring of digoxin levels after the drug reaches steady state is only necessary if there is suspicion of toxicity noncompliance, or deteriorating renal

function. Low potassium levels increase its toxicity, so frequent serum electrolyte level checks are also important. It has been estimated that as many as 20% of patients taking digoxin exhibit toxic symptoms. The common undesirable effects associated with cardiac glycoside use are listed in Table 20-1.

Toxicity and Management of Overdose

The treatment strategies for digoxin toxicity depend on the severity of the symptoms. These strategies can range from simply withholding the next dose to instituting aggressive therapies. The steps usually taken in the management of cardiac glycoside toxicity are listed in Table 20-2.

When significant toxicity develops as a result of cardiac glycoside therapy, the administration of Digibind (digoxin immune FAB) may be indicated. Digibind is an antibody that recognizes digoxin as an antigen and forms an antibody-antigen complex thus inactivating the free digoxin. Digibind therapy is not indicated in every patient who is showing signs of digoxin toxicity. Following are the clinical settings in which its use may be indicated:

- Hyperkalemia (serum potassium level >5 mEq/L) in a digitalis-toxic patient
- Life-threatening cardiac dysrhythmias, sustained ventricular tachycardia or fibrillation, and severe sinus bradycardia or heart block unresponsive to atropine treatment or cardiac pacing
- Life-threatening digoxin or digitoxin overdose: >10 mg of digoxin in adults; >4 mg of digoxin in children

Interactions

There are a number of significant drug interactions that are possible with cardiac glycosides. The common ones are listed in Table 20-3. One food interaction, bran in large amounts, may decrease the absorption of oral digitalis drugs.

Dosages

For dosage information on the cardiac glycosides, see the table on p. 305.

Table 20-1	Cardiac Glycosides: Common Adverse Effects	
Body System	**Side/Adverse Effect**
Cardiovascular	Any type of dysrhythmia including bradycardia or tachycardia
Central nervous system	Headache, fatigue, malaise, confusion, convulsions
Gastrointestinal	Anorexia, nausea, vomiting, diarrhea
Visual	Colored vision (i.e., green, yellow, or purple), halo vision, or flickering lights

Table 20-2	Digoxin Toxicity: Step Management	
Step	**Management**
1	Discontinue drug.
2	Determine digoxin and electrolyte levels.
3	Administer potassium supplements for hypokalemia
4	Institute supportive therapy for gastrointestinal symptoms (nausea, vomiting, or diarrhea)
5	Start electrocardiographic monitoring for cardiac arrhythmias; administer appropriate antidysrhythmic drugs (lidocaine or phenytoin).
6	Administer digibind for severe overdose.

drug profiles

Cardiac glycosides get their name from their chemical structures. Glycosides are complex, steroidlike structures linked to sugar molecules. Because the particular drugs derived from the *Digitalis* plant have potent actions on the heart, they are referred to as *cardiac glycosides,* with digoxin by far the most commonly prescribed digitalis preparation. Deslanoside and digitoxin are other less commonly prescribed preparations. The widespread and long-standing popularity of cardiac glycosides such as digoxin is the result of their unequaled efficacy in the treatment of CHF. Cardiac glycosides are prescription-only drugs and are classified as pregnancy category C agents.

◦━digoxin

Digoxin (Lanoxin, LanoxiCaps) is by far the most commonly prescribed digitalis glycoside. It is a highly effective agent for the treatment of both CHF and atrial fibrillation and flutter. It may also be used clinically to improve myocardial contractility and thus reverse cardiogenic shock or other low cardiac output states. Digoxin is contraindicated in patients who have shown a hypersensitivity to it, and in those with ventricular tachycardia and fibrillation, beriberi heart disease, or hypersensitive carotid sinus syndrome. Normal therapeutic drug levels of digoxin should be between 0.5 and 2 ng/ml. Higher levels than 2 ng/ml are typically desirable for the treatment of atrial fibrillation. Orally, digoxin is available as a 50-μg/ml elixir, a 50-, 100-, and 200-μg liquid-filled capsule, and a 125-, 250-, and 500-μg tablet. Parenterally it comes as a 100- and 250-μg/ml IV injection. Because of digoxin's fairly long duration of action and half-life, a loading, or "digitalizing," dose is often given to bring serum levels of the drug up to a desirable therapeutic level more quickly. See the table on p. 306 for the recommended digitalizing doses and the daily oral and IV adult and pediatric dosages.

PHARMACOKINETICS

HALF-LIFE	ONSET	PEAK	DURATION
33-44 hr	30-120 min	2-6 hr	2-4 days

digoxin immune FAB

Digoxin immune FAB (Digibind) is the antidote for severe digoxin overdose and is indicated for the reversal of such life-threatening cardiotoxic effects as severe bradycardia, advanced heart block,

---

Table 20-3

Cardiac Glycosides: Drug Interactions

Drug	Mechanism	Result
Adrenergics reserpine succinylcholine	Increase cardiac irritability	Increased digoxin toxicity
amphotericin-B chlorthalidone ethoxzolamine Loop diuretics Laxatives Steroids (adrenal) Thiazide diuretics	Hypokalemia	Increased digoxin toxicity
Antacids Antidiarrheals cholestyramine colistipol	Decrease PO absorption	Reduced therapeutic effect
Anticholinergics	Increase PO absorption	Increased therapeutic effect
Barbiturates oxyphenobutazone phenylbutazone	Enzyme inducer	Reduced therapeutic effect
quinidine verapamil amiodarone	Decrease clearance	Increased digoxin levels (2×); digoxin dose should be reduced 50%

A digoxin preparation can also interfere with the results of several laboratory tests. It can cause the plasma levels of estrone to be raised and the levels of lactate dehydrogenase and testosterone to be lowered. It can also cause the erythrocyte sodium concentration to be increased and the erythrocyte potassium concentration to be reduced.

In addition to the drug and laboratory test interactions, digoxin can also interact with certain foods. The consumption of excessive amounts of potassium-rich food can decrease its therapeutic effect, whereas the consumption of excessive amounts of licorice can increase digoxin toxicity as the result of the hypokalemia produced.

DOSAGES Selected Digitalis Cardiac Glycosides and Phosphodiesterase Inhibitors

agent	pharmacologic class	dosage range	purpose

digoxin (Lanoxin, LanoxiCaps)	Digitalis cardiac glycoside	*Pediatric*
		Digitalizing dose
		IV: Premature: 0.015-0.025 mg/kg
		     Newborn: 0.020-0.030 mg/kg
		     1 mo-2 y/o: 0.030-0.050 mg/kg
		     2-5 y/o 0.025-0.035 mg/kg
		     5-10 y/o: 0.015-0.030 mg/kg
		     >10 y/o: 0.008-0.012 mg/kg
		PO: Premature: 0.020-0.030 mg/kg
		     Newborn: 0.025-0.035 mg/kg
		     1 mo-2 y/o: 0.035-0.060 mg/kg
		     2-5 y/o: 0.030-0.040 mg/kg
		     5-10 y/o: 0.020-0.035 mg/kg
		     >10 y/o: 0.010-0.015 mg/kg
		Usual maintenance dose, 20%-35% of digitalizing dose
		Adult
		PO/IV: usual digitalizing dose, 1-1.5 mg/day; usual maintenance dose, 0.125-0.5 mg/day
			Congestive heart failure; supraventricular dysrhythmias

milrinone (Primacor)	Phosphodiesterase inhibitor	*Adult* IV loading dose: 50 μg/kg IV continuous infusion dose: 0.375-0.75 μg/kg/min	Congestive heart failure

ventricular tachycardia or fibrillation, and severe hyperkalemia. It has a unique mechanism of action. As previously mentioned, it is believed to work by binding to free (unbound) digoxin, which then blocks or reverses all the drug effects and symptoms of toxicity. Digibind is contraindicated in patients who have shown a hypersensitivity to it. It is only available parenterally as a 40-mg vial. Digibind is dosed either in milligrams or by the number of vials, depending on the dose calculation method or the reference chart used. It is commonly dosed based on the patient's serum digoxin level in conjunction with his or her weight. The recommended dosages vary according to the amount of cardiac glycoside ingested. Each milligram can neutralize 15 μg of digoxin or digitoxin. For recommended dosages consult the manufacturer's latest dosage table recommendations. It is important to bear in mind that after Digibind is given, all subsequent digoxin serum levels will be elevated for days to weeks because of the presence of both the free (unbound) digoxin (toxic digoxin) and the digoxin that has been bound by the Digibind (nontoxic digoxin). Therefore, at this point, the clinical signs and symptoms of digoxin toxicity rather than the digoxin serum levels should be used to monitor the effectiveness of reversal therapy.

PHARMACOKINETICS

HALF-LIFE	ONSET	PEAK	DURATION
14-20 hr	Immediate	Immediate	Days to weeks

PHOSPHODIESTERASE INHIBITORS

As the name implies, phosphodiesterase inhibitors are a group of inotropic agents that work by inhibiting an enzyme called *phosphodiesterase.* The inhibition of his enzyme results in two very beneficial effects in an individual with heart failure: a positive inotropic response and vasodilation. For this reason this class of drugs may also be referred to as *inodilators* (inotropes and dilators). These agents were discovered in the search for positive inotropic drugs with a better therapeutic window than digoxin. There are presently only two agents in this category: amrinone and milrinone. These inodilators share a similar pharmacologic action with methylxanthines such as theophylline. They both inhibit phosphodiesterase resulting in an increase in intracellular cyclic adenosine monophosphate (cAMP). However, the inodilators are more specific for phosphodiesterase type III in the heart and vascular smooth muscles.

Mechanism of Action

The mechanism of action of phosphodiesterase inhibitors differs from other inotropic agents such as cardiac glycosides and catecholamines. The beneficial effects of phosphodiesterase inhibitors come from cAMP, the build-up of a substance that the phosphodiesterase enzyme normally breaks down. Amrinone and milrinone, the two currently available phosphodiesterase inhibitors, work by selectively inhibiting phosphodiesterase type III, which is in high concentrations in the heart and vascular smooth muscle. Inhibition of phosphodiesterase results in more calcium being available for the heart to use in muscle contraction. It also results in dilation of blood vessels, which in turn decreases the work load of the heart.

Drug Effects

Amrinone and milrinone have specificity for phosphodiesterase type III, which is located in heart and blood vessel muscle. The effects on heart muscle result in an increase in the force of contraction, positive inotropic action. The effects on the smooth muscle that surrounds blood vessels results in relaxation of smooth muscle and therefore causes dilation of blood vessels. The increase in calcium present in heart muscle is also taken back up into its storage sites in the sarcoplasmic reticulum at a much faster rate than normal. This results in the heart muscle relaxing more than normal as well as being more compliant. This effect is known as a **lusitropic** effect. In summary, phosphodiesterase inhibitors have positive inotropic and lusitropic effects. They may also increase heart rate in some instances and therefore may also have positive chronotropic effects.

Therapeutic Uses

Phosphodiesterase inhibitors are primarily used for the short-term management of CHF. In CHF the therapeutic benefits of the inodilators are secondary to their ability to increase the force of contraction (inotropic effects) and to relax blood vessels (lusitropic effects). The inodilators have 10 to 100 times greater affinity for smooth muscle surrounding blood vessels than they do for heart muscle. This suggest that the primary beneficial effects of inodilators are due to their ability to dilate blood vessels. This causes a reduction in afterload or the force that the heart has to pump against to eject its volume.

Traditionally, phosphodiesterase inhibitors are given to patients who can be closely monitored and who have not responded adequately to digoxin, diuretics, and/or vasodilators. Phosphodiesterase inhibitors do not require a receptor-mediated effect to increase contraction. Other positive inotropic agents, such as beta-agonists (e.g., dobutamine, dopamine) require stimulation of a receptor to increase contraction. The repetitive stimulation of these receptors can cause the body to become less sensitive to stimulation over time. In patients with end-stage heart failure who require positive inotropic support, a continual dosage increase would be needed to maintain positive results. As these drug dosages are increased they produce more unwanted cardiac effects. Because phosphodiesterase inhibitors do not use receptors to increase force of contraction, they do not have this unwanted problem. Many hospitals that treat large numbers of patients with heart failure now treat these end-stage heart failure patients with weekly 6-hour infusions of phosphodiesterase inhibitors. This has been shown to increase the quality of life and decrease the number of readmissions to the hospital for exacerbations of heart failure.

Side Effects and Adverse Effects

Although amrinone and milrinone are both phosphodiesterase inhibitors, they have very different side effect profiles. The side effect that is most worrisome with amrinone is thrombocytopenia. Amrinone-induced thrombocytopenia occurs at a rate of about 2.4% and is more frequent in high doses given over long periods of time. The other side effects associated with amrinone therapy are primarily related to the gastrointestinal tract. They are dysarhythmia (3%), nausea (1.7%), and hypotension (1.3%). With long-term use, increased liver enzymes may be noticed.

The primary side effect seen with milrinone therapy is dysrhythmia. These dysrhythmias are mainly ventricular in nature. Ventricular dysrhythmias occur in approximately 12% of patients treated with milrinone. Some other side effects seen with milrinone therapy are hypotension (2.9%), angina (chest pain) (1.2%), hypokalemia (0.6%), tremor (0.4%), and thrombocytopenia (0.4%).

Toxicity and Management of Overdose

No specific antidote exists for an overdose of either amrinone or milrinone. Hypotension is the primary effect seen with excessive doses of these two phosphodiesterase inhibitors. This hypotension is due the drug's ability to cause vasodilation. It is recommended to reduce or temporarily discontinue the phosphodiesterase inhibitor if excessive hypotension occurs. This should be done until the patient's condition is stabilized. General measures for circulatory support are also recommended.

Interactions

There are limited data available regarding potential drug interactions with phosphodiesterase inhibitors. They are given concurrently with a wide variety of cardiovascular medications in intensive care settings without interactions. What little data that is present states safe concurrent administration with the following: digoxin, lidocaine, quinidine, hydralazine, prazosin, isosorbide dinitrate, nitroglycerin, chlorthalidone, furosemde, hydrochlorothiazide, spironolactone, captopril, heparin, warfarin, diazepam, insulin, and potassium supplements. Do not inject furosemide in IV lines of amrinone or milrinone because it will precipitate immediately. Glucose-containing solutions should not be used when mixing amrinone. This will cause a 11% to 13% loss in amrinone's activity over 24 hours because of a slow chemical interaction.

Dosages

For dosage information on the phosphodiesterase inhibitors, see the dosages table on p. 306.

drug profiles

milrinone

Milrinone (Primacor) is one of the two presently available phosphodiesterase inhibitors. Amrinone was the first of the two phosphodiesterase inhibitors to be used clinically for the short-term treatment of CHF. Milrinone and amrinone are referred to as *inodilators* because they exert both a positive inotropic effect and a vasodilatory effect. Both of these agents are contraindicated in patients who have shown a hypersensitivity to them. Milrinone is only available as an IV product and is available in a 5-mg (1-mg/ml) Carpuject sterile cartridge unit and a 100-ml (200 μg/ml) in 5% dextrose injection. It is classified as a pregnancy category C agent. Recommended dosages are given in the table on p. 306.

PHARMACOKINETICS

HALF-LIFE	ONSET	PEAK	DURATION
2.3 hr	5-15 min	6-12 hr	8-10 hr

nursing process

Because of the high incidence of CHF, an understanding of the nursing implications associated with its medical treatment is critical to the safe and effective care of patients receiving cardiac glycosides as the mainstay of treatment. Owing to the narrow therapeutic index of cardiac glycosides, the nurse needs to constantly assess the patient, update the plans of care, intervene appropriately, and evaluate or monitor the therapeutic and adverse effects of the drug.

NURSING CARE PLAN Congestive Heart Failure

Mr. E.D. a 72-year-old man admitted with CHF, has been started on digoxin 0.125 mg for maintenance doses. He will be on your nursing unit for the next 1 to 2 days and will require frequent monitoring of the effects of the cardiac glycoside. Vital parameters are as follows upon admission to your unit: confused in early PM, UO about 240 cc/shift, P110, RR 33, BP 100/56, 1+ pitting pedal edema, SOB, DOE, < energy levels, unable to dress self, and skin intact. Lab studies show normal H&H, BUN, urinalysis, but K+ at 3.4.

assessment	**Nursing Diagnosis**	Impaired tissue perfusion related to tachycardia from CHF
	Subjective Data	Complaints of SOB, DOE, pedal edema
	Objective Data	Rales lower bases; weight >2 lb in 5 days; RR 32, P 102, BP 100/60
planning and outcome criteria	**Goals**	Patient will show improved tissue perfusion within 48 hours of treatment
	Outcome Criteria	Patient will have increased tissue perfusion, cardiopulmonary within 8 hours as evidenced by the following: • Urinary output >30 ml/hr • Decreased weight resulting from fluid loss • Rales • P <60 <100 • RR 16-20 • Decreased pedal edema
implementation		• Take patient's vital signs q4h and prn, including apical pulse • I&O q8h • Daily weights • Monitor digitalis levels as ordered • Monitor serum electrolytes • Take apical pulse for 1 full minute and notify physician if P <60; hold drug until further orders • Breath sounds q4h and prn • Elevate head of bed • Keep feet elevated at all times • Passive ROM
evaluation		Patient will show the following therapeutic responses to digitalis treatment: • Decreased weight • Ease of breathing • Increased UO • Decreased edema • Decreased SOB/DOE • Increased ability to perform ADL • Vital signs within normal limits Patient will be monitored for (and experience minimal) side effects associated with digitalis therapy such as bradycardia, headache, gastrointestinal symptoms, blurred vision, anorexia.

H&H, Hematocrit and hemoglobin; *SOB*, shortness of breath; *DOE*, dyspnea on exertion; *UO*, urinary output; *ROM*, range of motion; *ADL*, activities of daily living; *RR*, respiratory rate; *P*, pulse; *BP*, blood pressure.

Assessment

Before the administration of a cardiac glycoside, data must be collected concerning the patient's medication history (past and present over-the-counter [OTC], herbal [see Herbal Interactions box], prescription, or illegal drugs used) and any drug allergies he or she may have. An assessment of the patient's medical history, including both diseases and conditions, is also crucial and may yield findings that dictate either very cautious use of the agent or even contraindicate its use (Table 20-4).

Before initiating digoxin therapy, and even during maintenance therapy, several clinical parameters need to be assessed. These include the following:
- Blood pressure
- Apical pulse for 1 full minute
- Heart sounds
- Breath sounds
- Weight
- Intake and output amounts
- Electrocardiograms
- Renal function laboratory values (blood urea nitrogen [BUN] and creatinine)
- Liver function values (AST, ALT, creatine phosphokinase, lactate dehydrogenase, and alkaline phosphatase).

The baseline status of any edema, confusion, nausea, vomiting, anorexia, or diarrhea also needs to be documented. In addition, to assess for possible drug or food interactions, the patient's medication record or a list of the current medications being taken by the patient and his or dietary habits needs to be compiled and recorded. The use of thyroid preparations may result in decreased digoxin levels. One important food interaction for which to assess is whether the patient consumes large amounts of bran, which will decrease the absorption of oral digitalis drugs.

Contraindications to the use of amrinone lactate include hypersensitivity to amrinone or bisulfites, acute MI, dehydration, and severe aortic or pulmonic disease. Cautious use is recommended in patients with decreased renal and hepatic disease.

The newer agent milrinone is used for the short-term IV therapy of CHF. Before its use patients should be assessed for any allergy to it or to amrinone, and it should be used cautiously with patients with COPD, aortic or pulmonary valvular diseases, ventricular dysrhythmias, atrial fibrillation or flutter, or renal dysfunction. It is also used cautiously in pregnancy. The patient's vital signs and ECG should be monitored during infusion of the drug.

Nursing Diagnoses

Appropriate diagnoses in patients who are to receive positive inotropic agents include, but are not limited to, the following:
- Ineffective tissue perfusion related to pathophysiologic influence of CHF.
- Deficient knowledge related to first-time use of a cardiac glycoside and lack of information on CHF and its treatment.
- Risk for injury related to pathologic impact of CHF and potential side effects of medication therapy.
- Imbalanced nutritional status, less than body requirements, related to gastrointestinal side effects and potential digoxin toxicity.

Table 20-4 Conditions Predisposing to Digitalis Toxicity

Condition/Disease	Significance
Cardiac pacemakers	Patients with these devices may exhibit digitalis toxicity at lower-than-usual doses.
Hepatic dysfunction	Decreased hepatic elimination of digitoxin necessitating a reduction of digitoxin.
Hypokalemia	Increases a patient's risk of serious dysrhythmias and renders him or her more predisposed to digitalis toxcity.
Hypercalcemia	Places the patient at higher risk of suffering sinus bradycardia, dysrhythmias, and heart block.
Atrioventricular block	Heart block may worsen with increasing levels or digitalis.
Dysrhythmias	Dysrhythmias may occur that did not exist before digitalis use, and thus could be related to digitalis toxicity.
Hypothyroid, respiratory, or renal disease	Patients with these disorders require lower doses because of the renal disease resultant delayed drug excretion they cause.
Elderly age	Because of decreased renal function and the resultant diminished drug excretion along with decreased body mass in this patient population, a lower-than-usual dose is needed to prevent toxicity. The practice of polypharmacy may also lead to toxicity.
Ventricular fibrillation	Ventricular rate may actually increase with digitalis use.

- Ineffective tissue perfusion related to digoxin-related dysrhythmias.
- Noncompliance to therapy related to lack of information about the drug effects and adverse effects.

● Planning

Goals of care related to the administration of positive inotropic agents include the following:

- Patient exhibits improved cardiac output once therapy is initiated.
- Patient states use, action, side effects, and toxic effects of therapy.
- Patient is free from injury related to medication therapy.
- Patient's appetite is improved or he or she is free of anorexia while on positive inotropic agents.

In planning for the administration of these preparations, it important to check the dosage when administering either digoxin or digitoxin because of the difference in the pharmacokinetic properties of these drugs; for example, 80% of digoxin is excreted by the kidneys and 90% of digitoxin is first metabolized by the liver. These differences, in conjunction with the patient's particular medical history, often determine whether the physician prescribes digoxin (preferred in patients with impaired liver function) or digitoxin (preferred in patients with impaired renal function).

Outcome Criteria

Outcome criteria in patients receiving a positive inotropic agent include the following:

- Patient will have improved to strong peripheral pulses, increased endurance for activity, decreased fatigue, and pink, warm extremities.
- Patient will have increased urinary output resulting from therapeutic effects of the drug.
- Patient will have improved heart and lung sounds with decreased dysrythmias and rales.
- Patient will lose appropriate weight and have less edema from the therapeutic effects of the drug (increased urinary output due to increased cardiac output).
- Patient's skin and mucous membranes (color and temperature) will be improved to pink and warm.
- Patient will maintain appetite while on therapy and report anorexia, nausea, and vomiting immediately to physician.
- Patient will be free of toxicity as evidenced by no bradycardia or complaints of anorexia, nausea, or vomiting.
- Patient will demonstrate proper technique for taking radial pulse for 1 full minute before taking medication.
- Patient will be able to cite drug-related problems to report to the physician, such as palpitations, dysrhythmias, chest pain, and pulse less than 60 beats/min.

● Implementation

Before administering any dose of a cardiac glycoside, the nurse should count the patient's apical pulse and auscultate the heart beat for 1 full minute. If the pulse is 60 beats/min or less or greater than 120 beats/min, then the dose should be withheld and the physician notified of the problem. In addition, the physician should be contacted if the patient experiences any of the following manifestations of toxicity: anorexia, nausea, vomiting or diarrhea, and visual disturbances such as blurred vision or the perception of green or yellow halos around objects.

Other nursing interventions include checking the dosage form and amounts *carefully* as well as the physician's order to make sure the specific drug ordered has been dispensed (such as digitoxin versus digoxin). Digoxin may be administered with meals but not with foods high in fiber because the fiber will bind to the digitalis, which will make less drug available for absorption. If the medication is to be given intravenously, the following interventions are critical: administer undiluted IV forms at around 0.25 mg/min or over more than 5 minutes. The administration of IM forms of cardiac glycosides is extremely painful and is not indicated or recommended because of tissue necrosis and erratic absorption that may ensue. Digoxin and digitoxin are incompatible with any other medication in solution or syringe. It is important to remember that, regardless of the dosage form, if the patient's apical pulse is less than 60 or more than 120 beats/min, the dose should be withheld, the physician notified of the problem, the vital signs monitored, and all interventions documented. Should toxicity become life-threatening, Digibind, the antidote to digoxin or digitoxin toxicity, should be administered over 30 minutes or given as an IV bolus if cardiac arrest is imminent. See the Home Health/Community Points box on p. 311.

The nursing interventions for patients undergoing digitalization need to be considered separately. Although not commonly used in contemporary practice, digitalization may still be done in some areas of practice for the management of CHF. Rapid digitalization (to get faster action) is generally reserved for patients with CHF who are in acute distress. Such patients are hospitalized because digitalis toxicities can appear quickly in this setting and are directly correlated to the high drug concentrations used. Should the patient undergoing rapid digitalization exhibit *any* of the manifestations of toxicity, the physician should be contacted immediately. Such patients should be observed constantly and serum digoxin or digitoxin levels measured frequently. Slow digitalization is generally performed on an outpatient basis in patients with CHF who are not in such acute distress. In this context it takes longer for toxic effects to appear (depending on the specific drug's half-life) than it does for the toxic effects stemming from rapid digitalization. The main advantages of slow digitalization are that it can be done on an outpatient basis and with oral dosage forms and it is safer than rapid digitalization. Disadvantages are that it takes longer for the therapeutic effects to occur and the symptoms of toxicity are more gradual, and

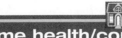

home health/community points

Digoxin

- Patients should be instructed on how to take radial pulse before each dose of digoxin. For the elderly and physically or mentally challenged it is important to have home health care personnel supervise the medication regimen, because these individuals will be at risk for possible interactions with other medications or for possible toxicity.
- Patients should keep a journal at home in reference to the following: date, day, time of dose, amount of medication taken, dietary intake, any unusual side effects or changes in conditions, and pulse rate. The following is an example of a chart-type journal, which may help to identify therapeutic as well as side effects and toxicity associated with the medication administration at home (see below):

- Patients should be encouraged to contact the physician or health care provider with any unusual complaints or if the pulse is *below* 60 beats/min or erratic, or if they are experiencing anorexia, nausea, or vomiting. Any changes in visual acuity should also be reported to their health care provider or home health care nurse.
- Patients taking digoxin should be encouraged to wear a MedicAlert ID band, and have one ordered before discharge from the hospital.
- A weight gain of 1 or 2 lb a day or 5 lb or more in a week should be reported to the health care provider or to the home health care nurse.

Drug dose	Date and time	Apical pulse rate	Weight	Side effects	Diet intake	Any changes or unusual complaints	Misc.

---

therefore more insidious, in onset. With amrinone, IV forms should not be mixed with dextrose and it should be kept in mind that the true color of IV amrinone is clear yellow. Intake and output, heart rate, blood pressure, daily weight, and respiration should be monitored during amrinone or milrinone therapy. Amrinone administration (IV) with any evidence of hypokalemia should be noted and reported to the physician. All vital signs should be closely monitored during milrinone therapy as well.

Milrinone should only be infused using an infusion pump. During treatment, the patient should be encouraged and monitored for any discomfort at the IV site, numbness, tingling of the extremities, or difficulty breathing.

Patient teaching tips for patients on digoxin are listed on p. 312.

Evaluation

Monitoring patients after the administration of positive inotropic agents is crucial for identifying therapeutic effects as opposed to side effects. Because positive inotropic agents increase the force of myocardial contractility (positive inotropic effect), alter electrophysiologic properties (decrease rate negative chronotropic effect), and decrease AV node conduction (negative dromotropic effect), the therapeutic effects include the following:

- Increased urinary output
- Decreased edema

- Decreased shortness of breath, dyspnea, and rales
- Decreased fatigue
- Resolving of paroxysmal nocturnal dyspnea
- Improved peripheral pulses, skin color, and temperature

While monitoring for the therapeutic effects, it is essential (because of the low therapeutic index of digitalis preparations) to assess patients for the development of side effects such as anorexia, nausea, vomiting, diarrhea, ventricular dysrhythmias, heart block, bradycardia, and confusion. Monitoring laboratory values such as the serum creatinine, potassium, calcium, sodium, and chloride levels as well as the digoxin (0.5-2 ng/ml) and digitoxin (13-25 ng/ml) therapeutic levels will also help ensure the delivery of safe and efficacious treatment. For patients receiving amrinone, all vital signs and hemodynamic parameters (cardiac output, central venous pressure) must be constantly evaluated. Therapeutic effects of milrinone include an improvement in cardiac function with an improvement noted in the patient's CHF. Side effects for which to monitor include hypotension, dysrhythmias, headache, ventricular fibrillation, chest pain, and hypokalemia. Patients on milrinone should be evaluated for significant hypotension, and the drug should be discontinued or the infusion rate decreased per physician's orders.

patient teaching tips

Positive Inotropic Agents

➤ Patients should be told to take medication at the same time every day and exactly as ordered.

➤ Patients should be warned to never double up on a dose and never skip a dose unless told to do so by physician.

➤ Patients should use only the dropper supplied with the elixir form to administer the medication.

➤ Patients should be warned to not change brands when refilling prescriptions.

➤ Patients should be told to check with their physician before taking any other medication with the digoxin, whether prescribed or OTC medication or herbal.

➤ Patients should know to notify their physician if their radial pulse is less than 60 or more than 120 beats/min or if it is erratic and also if they are experiencing anorexia, nausea, vomiting, diarrhea, or blurred vision, or seeing green or yellow halos around objects. In the event of any of these problems, patients should withhold the dose.

➤ Patients should inform the physician if they experience a weight gain of 2 lb or greater (about 1 kg) per day.

➤ It is important for patients to wear a MedicAlert bracelet or necklace naming the medication, or medications, they are taking and their cardiac condition as well as to carry an alert card on their person. Patients should be told to contact their local emergency medical services department to find out how to post or supply information in their home regarding their cardiac condition and the medications they are taking.

➤ Patients taking antacids or eating ice cream, milk products, yogurt, or cheeses should be told to take their dose 2 hours before or after they take these medications or foods.

➤ Family members must also be taught the side effects and the importance of taking the patient's pulse before giving the drug as well as the signs and symptoms of toxicity.

➤ Patients should be encouraged to consume foods high in potassium, especially if they are also taking a potassium-depleting diuretic. They should report any signs and symptoms of weakness, fatigue, or lethargy.

➤ Patients should know that anorexia is an early manifestation of toxicity.

➤ Patients should weigh themselves daily before breakfast to check for possible weight loss or gain resulting from fluid overload or loss and report immediately 1- to 2-lb weight increase that occurs within 1 day.

➤ Patients should be told to never withdraw or discontinue the drug abruptly.

POINTS TO REMEMBER

Inotropic

- Refers to the force of myocardial contraction.
- Positive inotropic agents increase the force of contractions (e.g., digoxin).
- Negative inotropic agents decrease force of contraction (e.g., beta-blockers, calcium channel blockers).

Chronotropic

- Refers to the rate at which the heart beats (beats/min).
- Positive chronotropic agents increase the heart rate (e.g., epinephrine, atropine).

Dromotropic

- Refers to the conduction of electrical impulses through the heart.
- Positive dromotropic agents increase the speed of the electrical impulse through the heart.
- Cardiac conduction: start in SA node and goes to AV node, then down bundle to His to Purkinje fibers.

Cardiac Glycosides

- One of the oldest and most effective group of drugs obtained from a plant source.
- Originally obtained from *Digitalis* plant, commonly referred to as *foxglove.*
- Mainstay of CHF treatment for over 200 years.

Ejection Fraction

- Amount of blood ejected at each contraction over amount of blood in heart before contraction.
- Normally around 65% (0.65).
- Patients with CHF have low ejection fractions because their hearts are failing as pumps.

Nursing Considerations

- Contraindications to the use of digoxin include patients with a history of allergy to the medications, ventricular tachycardia and fibrillations, beriberi heart disease, AV block, and hypersensitive carotid sinus syndrome.
- Predisposers to digitalis toxicity include hypokalemia, hypercalcemia, hypothyroid states, renal dysfunction, and elderly.
- Taking an apical pulse for 1 full minute is a standard of care expected when administering digoxin.
- A physician should be notified at the first signs of anorexia, nausea, vomiting, or for bradycardia with a pulse below 60 beats per minute for a patient receiving digoxin.
- Hypotension, dysrhythmias, and thrombocytopenia are major adverse effects of amrinone and milrinone.

REVIEW QUESTIONS

1. Which is the correct order of steps in treatment of digoxin toxicity?
   1) Discontinue the drug.
   2) Administer digibind for severe doses.
   3) Determine digoxin and electrolyte levels.
   4) Give potassium supplements for hypokalemia.
   5) Start ECG monitoring for any cardiac dysrhythmias.
   a. 1, 3, 4, 5, 2.
   b. 1, 4, 3, 5, 2.
   c. 3, 1, 4, 2, 5.
   d. 3, 5, 2, 1, 4.

2. Digibind therapy is indicated in which of the following situations?
   a. Severe sinus tachycardia
   b. Digoxin level of 5 mg in adults
   c. Serum potassium level <5 mEq/L
   d. Life-threatening cardiac dysrhythmias

3. An added benefit to the positive inotropic action of digoxin is that it promotes:
   a. Diuresis.
   b. Proteinuria.
   c. Bradycardia.
   d. Chronotropy.

4. Bradycardia, as a side effect of digoxin, is related to which of the following effects?
   a. Positive chronotropic
   b. Negative chronotroic
   c. Positive chromotropic
   d. Negative chromotropic

5. Which of the following medications would be safe to administer concurrently with digoxin?
   a. Verapamil
   b. Anticholinergics
   c. Benzodiazepines
   d. Steroids (adrenal)

For Answers see www.harcourthealth.com/MERLIN/Lilley/.

CRITICAL THINKING Activities

1. Atrial fibrillation develops in the patient for whom you are caring. The patient is not currently on any agent to treat this and is becoming quite symptomatic. The physician prescribes digoxin at a dosage of 0.5 mg IV stat, followed by 0.25 mg IV every 6 hours for two doses. On hand is a vial of digoxin with the following strength: 250 mcg/ml. How much digoxin (in milliliters) should you give each time?

2. Your patient, a 78-year-old-man, has a potassium level of 3.0 mEq/L. He states that he has been nauseous and without an appetite and has experienced some diarrhea. He has been taking digoxin for the past few weeks for the treatment of recently diagnosed CHF. Discuss the implication of hypokalemia in a patient who is on digoxin.

3. Explain why the elderly patient with hypothyroid dis-

For Answers see www.harcourthealth.com/MERLIN/Lilley/.

bibliography

Albanese J, Nutz P: *Mosby's 2001 nursing drug reference and review cards*, St Louis, 2001, Mosby.

American Hospital Formulary Service: *AHFS drug information*, Bethesda, Md, 2000, American Society of Health-System Pharmacists.

Anderson PO, Knoben JE, Troutman WG: *Handbook of clinical drug data 1999-2000*, ed 9, New York, 1999, McGraw-Hill.

Clayton BD, Stock YN: *Basic pharmacology for nurses*, ed 12, St Louis, 2001, Mosby.

Digitalis Investigation Group: The effect of digoxin on mortality and morbidity in patients with heart failure, *N Engl J Med* 336:525, 1997.

Johns Hopkins Hospital, Department of Pediatrics et al: *The Harriet Lane handbook*, ed 15, St Louis, 2000, Mosby.

Keen JH: *Critical care and emergency drug reference*, ed 3, St Louis, 1996, Mosby.

Mosby's GenRx: a comprehensive reference for generic and brand drugs, ed 10, St Louis, 2000, Mosby.

Skidmore-Roth L: *Mosby's 2001 nursing drug reference*, St Louis, 2001, Mosby.

Turkoski BB: *Drug information handbook for nursing 1999-2000: including assessment, administration, monitoring guidelines, and patient education*, ed 2, Cleveland, 1999, Lexi-Comp.

Remember to check the **Online Worksheet** for additional learning opportunities: **www.harcourthealth.com/MERLIN/Lilley/**

Activity

Chapter 21

Antidysrhythmic Agents

objectives

When you reach the end of this chapter, you should be able to do the following:

1 Define the most commonly encountered dysrhythmias.

2 Describe normal cardiac function.

3 Identify the various classes of antidysrhythmic agents as determined by their mechanism of action.

4 Provide examples of specific drugs within each class of antidysrhythmic agents.

5 Discuss the mechanisms of action, therapeutic effects, and adverse effects of the various antidysrhythmics and the various uses for these agents.

6 Develop a nursing care plan that includes all phases of the nursing process related to the administration of the various antidysrhythmics and the treatment of overdose or toxicity.

www.harcourthealth.com/MERLIN/Lilley/

Look for this symbol for topics covered in the **Online Worksheet**

drug profiles

adenosine, p. 329
⚬━ amiodarone, p. 327
atenolol, p. 326
bretylium, p. 328
diltiazem, p. 329
disopyramide, p. 320
encainide and flecainide, p. 324
⚬━ esmolol, p. 326
ibutilide, p. 328

⚬━ lidocaine, p. 321
metoprolol, p. 326
mexiletine, p. 324
procainamide, p. 320
propafenone, p. 325
propranolol, p. 326
⚬━ quinidine, p. 321
sotalol, p. 327
tocainide, p. 324
⚬━ verapamil, p. 329

⚬━Key drug.

glossary

Action potential An electrical impulse consisting of a self-propagating series of polarizations and depolarizations that is transmitted across the cell membranes of a nerve fiber during the transmission of a nerve impulse and across the cell membranes of a muscle cell during contraction or other activity of the cell. (p. 315)

Action potential duration The interval during which a cell is repolarizing to its baseline membrane potential. (p. 316)

Arrhythmia (ə rith′ me ə) In the most literal sense, the absence of a rhythmic pattern. A term also commonly used to refer to any deviation from the normal pattern of the heartbeat, or dysrhythmia. (p. 315)

Cardiac Arrhythmia Suppression Trial The name of the major research study conducted by the National Heart, Lung, and Blood Institute to investigate the possibility of eliminating sudden cardiac death in patients with asymptomatic, non–life-threatening ectopy that has arisen after a myocardial infarction. (p. 324)

Dysrhythmia (dis rith′ me ə) Any disturbance or abnormality in a normal rhythmic pattern. (p. 315)

Effective refractory period The period after the firing of an impulse during which a cell may respond to a stimulus but the response will not be passed along or continued. (p. 316)

Fast channels, sodium channels Other terms for *fast-response channels.* These cells can rapidly conduct electrical impulses. (p. 315)

Internodal pathways, Bachmann's bundle Special pathways in the atria that carry electrical impulses that are spontaneously generated by the sinoatrial node. These impulses cause the heart to beat. (p. 317)

Relative refractory period The time during which a depressed response to a strong stimulus is possible. (p. 316)

Resting membrane potential The transmembrane voltage that exists when the heart muscle is at rest. (p. 315)

Sodium-potassium ATPase pump A mechanism for transporting sodium and potassium ions across cell membranes against an opposing concentration gradient. Energy for this transport system is obtained from the hydrolysis of adenosine triphosphate by means of an enzyme called *adenosine triphosphatase* (ATPase). (p. 315)

Sudden cardiac death Unexplained cessation, or death, of cardiac function. (p. 324)

Threshold potential The spontaneous depolarization of cells after a critical state of electrical tension is reached. (p. 317)

Vaughan Williams classification The most commonly used system used to classify antidysrhythmic drugs. (p. 317; see also Table 21-2, p. 318)

DYSRHYTHMIAS AND NORMAL CARDIAC ELECTROPHYSIOLOGY

A **dysrhythmia** is any deviation from the normal rhythm of the heart. The term **arrhythmia,** which is also used to refer to these deviations, literally means "no rhythm," which implies asystole or no heartbeat at all. Thus the more accurate term for an irregular heart rhythm is *dysrhythmia* because a patient who has no cardiac rhythm is in asystole, or dead. There are many conditions in which dysrhythmias can develop. Some of the more common arise after a myocardial infarction (MI) or cardiac surgery or as the result of coronary artery disease. These dysrhythmias are usually serious and require treatment with an antidysrhythmic agent, though not all have to be treated.

Disturbances in cardiac rhythm are the result of abnormally functioning cardiac cells. Therefore, to help understand the pathologic mechanism responsible for dysrhythmias, it is first necessary to review the electrical properties of cardiac cells. Figure 21-1 illustrates the process from the standpoint of a single cardiac cell. Inside a cardiac cell there exists a net negative charge relative to the outside of the cell. This difference in the electronegative charge exists in all types of cardiac cells and is referred to as the **resting membrane potential** (RMP). The RMP results from an uneven distribution of ions (sodium, potassium, and calcium) across the cell membrane. To maintain this uneven distribution of ions requires the **sodium-potassium ATPase pump,** an energy-requiring ionic pump. Cardiac cells become excited when there is a change in this distribution of ions across its membrane, and this movement of ions across the cardiac cell's membrane results in the propagation of an electrical impulse and the subsequent contraction of the myocardial muscle. This is called an **action potential** and consists of four phases. Phase 1 of the action potential starts when the fast sodium channel closes and a period of rapid repolarization begins. During phase 2, calcium ion influx occurs through the slow channels. This causes a plateau phase during which the membrane potential changes only slightly. Over time, potassium ions flow outward and the

cell is repolarized to its baseline level (phase 3). To restore the cell to its original state, the energy-dependent, sodium-potassium ATPase pump, or sodium pump, moves sodium ions out and potassium ions into the cell. Phase 4 is the RMP.

The movement of ions across the cardiac cell's membranes (action potential) varies in speed from one area to another in the heart's conduction system. Figure 21-2 illustrates the action potentials in two different types of cells found in the conduction system of the heart. The action potential of the specialized electrical conducting cells in the sinoatrial (SA) node is shown in Fig. 21-2, *A,* and the action potential of a Purkinje cell (fiber) located in the specialized electrical conducting system is depicted in Fig. 21-2, *B.* Figure 21-3 also illustrates the movement of sodium, potassium, and calcium ions into and out of a Purkinje cell during the four phases of the action potential. There are several important differences in the action potentials of the SA node and Purkinje cell. The RMP in the Purkinje cell is approximately -80 to -90 mV compared with -50 to -60 mV in the SA nodal cell. The level of the RMP (phase 4) is an important determinant of the rate of impulse conduction to other cells. The less negative the RMP at the onset of phase 0, the slower the upstroke velocity of phase 0. The slope or rate of rise of phase 0 is directly related to the impulse conduction velocity or speed. If the slope of phase 0 is steep such as it is in the Purkinje cells, this means that electrical conduction through these cells is fast.

The action potential of the Purkinje cells illustrated in Fig. 21-2, *B,* has a rapid rate of rise of phase 0, and therefore electrical impulses are conducted quickly. These cells are referred to as *fast-response cells,* or *fast-channel cells.* During this phase, channels open, permitting a rapid influx of sodium ions into the cell. The terms **fast channels** and **sodium channels** both refer to these fast-response channels. Many antidysrhythmic agents affect the RMP and sodium channels, which in turn affects the rate of impulse conduction.

Because the cells of the SA or atrioventricular (AV) nodes have RMPs of -50 to -60 mV, they have a much

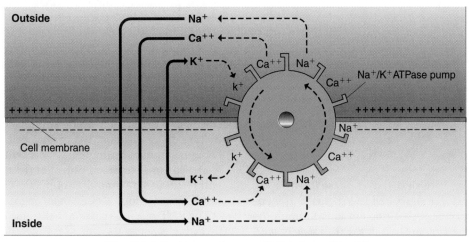

Fig. 21-1 Resting membrane potential of a cardiac cell.

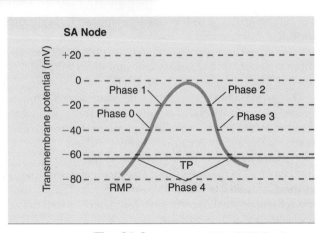

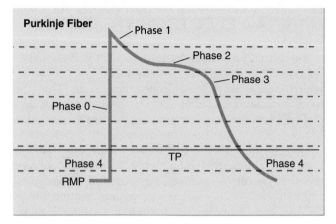

Fig. 21-2 Action potentials. *RMP*, Resting membrane potential; *SA*, sinoatrial; *TP*, threshold potential.

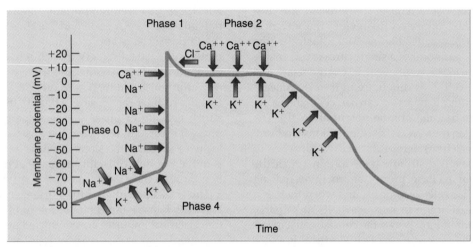

Fig. 21-3 Purkinje fiber action potential.

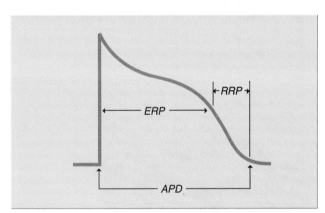

Fig. 21-4 Aspects of an action potential. *APD*, Action potential duration; *ERP*, effective refractory period; *RRP*, relative refractory period.

slower upstroke velocity, or a slower phase 0. This slow rate of rise in phase 0 of the SA and AV nodes is primarily dependent on the entry of calcium ions through the slow channel. These cells are therefore called *slow-channel tissue*, or *calcium channels*, and conduction in these cells is

slower than that in the myocardial or other electrical conduction tissue. Drugs that affect calcium ion movement into or out of these cells tend to have significant effects on the SA and AV nodal conduction rates.

The interval between phase 0 and phase 4 when the cell is repolarizing and returning to its RMP is called the **action potential duration** (APD). The period between phase 0 and midway through phase 3 is called the absolute or **effective refractory period** (ERP). During the ERP the cardiac cell cannot be stimulated to depolarize and conduct electricity. During the remainder of phase 3 until the return to the RMP (phase 4), the cardiac cell is vulnerable to depolarization if it receives an impulse. This period is referred to as the **relative refractory period** (RRP), and during it a strong stimulus can initiate a premature depolarization. If a cardiac cell receives a strong enough stimulus during the RRP, it will be when the cell is at a lower membrane potential (less negative), which will result in slow impulse conduction. Figure 21-4 illustrates these various aspects of an action potential.

The RMP of certain cardiac cells gradually and spontaneously decreases (becomes less negative) over time, and this is probably secondary to small changes in the flux of

Table 21-1 Comparison of Action Potentials in Different Cardiac Tissue

Tissue	Action Potential Wave	Speed of Response	Threshold Potential (m V)	Conduction Velocity (m/sec)
SA node	⟋⟍	Slow	−60	<0.05
Atrium	⅃⟍	Fast	−90	−1
AV node	⟋⟍	Slow	−60	<0.05
His-Purkinje	⅃⟍	Fast	−95	3
Ventricle	⅃⟍	Fast	−90	1

sodium and potassium ions. Depolarization eventually occurs when a certain critical voltage is reached (**threshold potential** [TP]). This process of spontaneous depolarization is referred to as *automaticity,* or *pacemaker activity.* It is normal when it occurs in the SA node, AV node, and His-Purkinje system. When tissues besides these assume the property of spontaneous depolarization, dysrhythmias occur.

The SA node, AV node, and His-Purkinje cells all possess automaticity, but the SA node is the pacemaker of the heart because it spontaneously depolarizes the fastest. The SA node has an intrinsic rate of 60 to 100 depolarizations, or beats per minute; that of the AV node is 40 to 60 beats per minute; and that of the ventricular Purkinje fibers is 40 or less beats per minute. The action potentials in different areas of the heart along with other characteristics of the cells in these different areas are compared in Table 21-1.

As the pacemaker of the heart, the SA node, which is located near the top of the right atrium, generates the electrical impulse needed to produce the heartbeat. This impulse then travels through the atria via specialized pathways called the **internodal pathways** and **Bachmann's bundle.** While the impulse is traveling through these specialized pathways, it is causing the myocardial muscle in the atria to contract. This impulse is then received by the AV node, which is located near the bottom of the right atrium. The AV node slows this very fast-moving electrical impulse just long enough to allow the ventricles to accept the blood that the atria have just squeezed into them. If the AV node did not slow the impulse, the ventricles would contract almost at the same time as the atria, resulting in a smaller volume of blood being injected (decreased cardiac output).

Upon stimulation, the AV node generates an electrical impulse that passes into the bundle of His, a band of cardiac muscle fibers located between both the right and left ventricles in what is called the *ventricular septum.* The bundle of His distributes the impulse into both ventricles via the right and left bundle branch. Each branch terminates in the Purkinje fibers that are located in the myocardium of the ventricles. The stimulation of the Purkinje fibers causes ventricular contraction and blood to leave the ventricles, going to the lungs from the right ventricle and to the rest of the body from the left ventricle.

Any abnormality in cardiac automaticity or impulse conduction will result in some type of dysrhythmia.

ANTIDYSRHYTHMIC AGENTS

There are numerous drugs available to treat dysrhythmias, and these are classified based on where and how they affect cardiac cells. The most commonly used system is the **Vaughan Williams classification,** which uses as its basis the effect produced by the particular agent on the action potential. This approach has yielded four major groups of agents. Class I antidysrhythmics are considered membrane-stabilizing agents, but they are further divided into Ia, Ib, and Ic agents, depending on the magnitude of their effects on phase 0, the APD, and the ERP. Class II drugs are beta-blockers that depress phase 4 depolarization. Class III drugs primarily prolong repolarization during phase 3. Class IV drugs depress phase 4 depolarization and prolong repolarization during phases 1 and 2. Calcium channel blockers (CCBs) (slow channel blockers) like verapamil belong to class IV. The various agents in these four classes are listed in Table 21-2. Several antidysrhythmics exert more than one type of effect on the action potential. Moricizine is such an agent, but it is classified most commonly by itself in class I because it exhibits the properties of class Ia, Ib, and Ic agents.

Mechanism of Action

Antidysrhythmic drugs can correct abnormal cardiac electrophysiologic function by various mechanisms of action. As the membrane-stabilizing agents, class I drugs exert their actions on the sodium (fast) channels; however, as already noted, there are some slight differences in the actions of the agents within this class, resulting in three subgroups of agents. Class Ia agents (quinidine, procainamide, and disopyramide) block sodium channels; more specifically they delay repolarization and increase the APD. Class Ib agents (tocainide, mexiletine, phenytoin, and lidocaine) block the sodium channels, but unlike class Ia agents, they accelerate repolarization and decrease the APD. Class Ic agents (flecainide, encainide, and propafenone) have a more pronounced effect on the blockade of sodium channels but have little effect on repolarization or the APD. As previously mentioned, moricizine is most frequently classified simply as a class I drug with no subclass specifications because it has characteristics of all three subclasses.

Table 21-2 Vaughan Williams Classification of Antidysrhythmic Drugs

Functional Class	Drugs
Class I: Membrane-stabilizing agents; fast sodium channel blockers	moricizine
Ia: ↑ blockade of sodium channel, delay repolarization, ↑ APD	quinidine, disopyramide, procainamide
Ib: ↑ blockade of sodium channel, accelerate repolarization, ↓ APD	tocainide, mexiletine, phenytoin, lidocaine
Ic: ↑ ↑ ↑ blockade of sodium channel ± on repolarization	flecainide, encainide, propafenone
Class II: Beta-blocking agents	All beta-blockers
Class III: Principal effect on cardiac tissue is to ↑ APD	amiodarone, bretylium, sotalol, ibutalide
Class IV: Calcium channel blockers	verapamil, diltiazem
Other: Antidysrhythmic drugs that have the properties of several classes and therefore cannot be placed in one particular class	digoxin, adenosine

APD, Action potential duration; ↑, increase ↓, decrease; ±, increase or decrease.

Table 21-3 Antidysrhythmics: Mechanisms of Action

Vaughan Williams class	I	II	III	IV
Action	Blocks sodium channels, affects phase 0	Decreases spontaneous depolarization, affects phase 4	Prolongs APD	Blocks slow calcium channels
Tissue	Fast	Slow	Fast	Slow
Effect on action potential				

APD, Action potential duration.

Class II agents are beta-blockers. They work by reducing or blocking sympathetic nervous system stimulation to the heart and, as a result, the transmission of impulses in the heart's conduction system. This results in depression of phase 4 depolarization. These drugs mostly affect slow tissue.

Class III agents (amiodarone, bretylium, ibutilide, and sotalol) increase the APD by prolonging repolarization in phase 3. They affect fast tissue and are most commonly used to manage dysrhythmias that are difficult to treat.

Class IV agents are CCBs. As their name implies, they work by inhibiting the slow-channel pathways, or the calcium-dependent channels. By doing this, they depress phase 4 depolarization. Diltiazem and verapamil are by far the most commonly used CCBs for cardiac rhythm disturbances.

The mechanisms of action of the major classes of antidysrhythmics are summarized in Table 21-3.

Drug Effects

Antidysrhythmic drugs primarily alter cardiac electrophysiology. These effects include changes in the SA node and ectopic pacemakers, AV node, conduction velocity, autonomic nervous system innervation, ERPs, and various segments of the electrocardiogram (ECG).

The effects for the various classes of agents are summarized in Box 21-1.

Therapeutic Uses

Antidysrhythmic agents are effective in treating a variety of cardiac dysrhythmias. The antidysrhythmic drugs and the most common indications for their use are listed in Table 21-4.

Side Effects and Adverse Effects

Side effects and adverse effects common to most antidysrhythmics include hypersensitivity reactions, nausea, vomiting, and diarrhea. Other common effects include dizziness, headache, and blurred vision. In addition, any antidysrhythmic is capable of producing a proarrhythmic (dysrhythmic) effect. This occurs most frequently in association with quinidine, amiodarone, moricizine, or propafenone therapy.

Toxicity and Management of Overdose

The main toxic effects of the antidysrhythmics involve the heart, circulation, and CNS. Specific antidotes are not available, and the management of an overdose involves maintaining adequate circulation and respiration using general support measures and any required symptomatic treatment (Table 21-5).

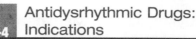

Box 21-1 Drug Effects of Antidysrhythmic Drugs

CLASS I: MORICIZINE
- Prolongs AV node conduction velocity
- Prolongs bundle of His and Purkinje cell conduction velocity
- Prolongs the PR and QRS complex intervals of the ECG
- Eliminates or reduces ectopic foci stimulation
- Minimal effect on the SA node and automaticity

CLASS IA: DISOPYRAMIDE, PROCAINAMIDE, QUINIDINE
- Depress myocardial excitability
- Prolong the ERP
- Eliminate or reduce ectopic foci stimulation
- Decrease inotropic effect
- Anticholinergic (vagolytic)

CLASS IB: LIDOCAINE, MEXILETINE, PHENYTOIN, TOCAINIDE
- Decrease myocardial excitability in the ventricles
- Eliminate or reduce ectopic foci stimulation in the ventricles
- Minimal effect on the SA node and automaticity
- Minimal effect on the AV node and conduction
- Minimal anticholinergic (vagolytic) activity

CLASS IC: FLECAINIDE, PROPAFENONE, ENCAINIDE
- Dose-related depression of cardiac conduction, especially in the bundle of His-Purkinje system
- Minimal effect on atrial conduction
- Eliminate or reduce ectopic foci stimulation in the ventricles
- Minimal anticholinergic (vagolytic) activity

CLASS II: ACEBUTOLOL, ESMOLOL, PROPRANOLOL
- Block beta-adrenergic cardiac stimulation
- Reduce SA node activity
- Eliminate or reduce atrial ectopic foci stimulation
- Reduce ventricular contraction rate
- Reduce cardiac output and blood pressure

CLASS III: AMIODARONE, BRETYLIUM, SOTALOL, IBUTILIDE
- Prolong the ERP
- Prolong myocardial action potential
- Block both alpha- and beta-adrenergic cardiac stimulation

CLASS IV: VERAPAMIL, DILTIAZEM
- Prolong AV node ERP
- Reduce AV node conduction
- Reduce rapid ventricular conduction caused by atrial flutter

Table 21-4 Antidysrhythmic Drugs: Indications

Drug	Indications
CLASS IA disopyramide procainamide quinidine	Atrial fibrillation, premature atrial contractions, premature ventricular contractions, ventricular tachycardia, Wolff-Parkinson-White syndrome
CLASS IB lidocaine mexiletine tocainide	Ventricular dysrhythmias only (premature ventricular contractions, ventricular tachycardia, ventricular fibrillation)
CLASS IC encainide flecainide propafenone	Severe ventricular dysrhythmias only May use in atrial fibrillation/flutter
CLASS I moricizine	Symptomatic ventricular and life-threatening dysrhythmias
CLASS II Beta-blockers atenolol esmolol metaprolol propranolol	General myocardial depressants for both supraventricular and ventricular dysrhythmias
CLASS III amiodarone bretylium ibutalide sotalol	Life-threatening ventricular tachycardia or fibrillation, atrial fibrillation or flutter; resistant to other drugs; also sustained ventricular tachycardia Ventricular tachycardia or fibrillation Same as amiodarone's
CLASS IV Calcium channel blockers diltiazem verapamil	Paroxysmal supraventricular tachycardia; rate control for atrial fibrillation and flutter

ther the therapeutic or toxic effects. See Table 21-6 for a summary of the drug interactions.

Dosages

For information on the dosages of the various antidysrhythmics see the dosages table on p. 322.

Interactions

Antidysrhythmics can interact with many different categories of drugs. The most serious drug interactions are the ones that can result in dysrhythmias, hypotension or hypertension, respiratory distress, or a summation of ei-

drug profiles

CLASS Ia DRUGS

Class Ia drugs are considered membrane-stabilizing drugs because they possess local anesthetic properties. They stabilize the membrane and have depressant effects on phase 0 of the action potential.

Antidysrhythmics: Management of Overdose

Table 21-5

Drug	Toxic Effect	Management
acebutolol	Bradycardia	1-3 mg IV atropine divided
	Bronchospasm	Beta$_2$-adrenergic or theophylline
	Cardiac failure	Digitalization
	Hypotension	Vasopressor
adenosine	Usually self-limiting due to very short half-life	Competitive antagonists caffeine or theophylline
amiodarone	Bradycardia	Beta-adrenergic agent
	Hypotension	Positive inotropic agent or vasopressor
bretylium	Hypertension	Nitroprusside
	Hypotension	Dopamine or norepinephrine and fluid therapy
digoxin	Decrease clearance	Quinidine, verapamil, and amiodarone; increase digoxin levels
disopyramide	Loss of consciousness, cardiac and respiratory arrest	Neostigmine for anticholinergic effects, induced emesis, activated charcoal, and hemodialysis
esmolol	Same as acebutolol's	Same as acebutolol's
flecainide	Reduced heart rate	Dopamine or dobutamine; acidify very alkaline urine
lidocaine	Convulsions	Diazepam or thiopental
mexiletine	Bradycardia, hypotension	Atropine; acidify urine to promote excretion
moricizine	Hypotension, CHF, and MI	Gastric evacuation and advanced life support systems
phenytoin	Circulatory and respiratory arrest, convulsions	Life support systems when required
procainamide	Cardiac depression	IVpressor agents and supportive measures
propafenone	Convulsions	Diazepam and mechanical assisted respiration
propranolol	Same as acebutolol's	Same as acebutolol's
quinidine	Cardiac dysrhythmias	Sodium lactate reduces toxicity except in alkalosis; lidocaine
sotalol	Same as acebutolol's	Same as acebutolol's
tocainide	Convulsions	Diazepam or short-acting barbiturate
verapamil	Bradycardia	Atropine
	Cardiac failure	Dopamine or dobutamine
	Conduction problems	Cardiac pacing
	Hypotension	Vasopressors, 10% calcium chloride solution

All class Ia agents are classified as pregnancy category C agents.

disopyramide

Disopyramide (Norpace, Norpace CR) is used primarily for the treatment of ventricular dysrhythmias. Its therapeutic efficacy is comparable to that of quinidine and procainamide, but it can produce significant side effects, including anticholinergic effects, ventricular dysrhythmias, and particularly cardiovascular depression. For these reasons its use is limited, especially in patients with poor left ventricular (LV) function.

Significant adverse reactions from disopyramide are hypotension and widening of the QRS interval on the ECG, as well as those mentioned for quinidine and procainamide. The incidence of systemic lupus erythematosus associated with its use is less than that associated with the use of procainamide. Contraindications to its use are similar to those of quinidine and procainamide. Disopyramide is only available orally as 100- and 150-mg regular-release and extended-release capsules. Common dosages are listed in the dosages table on p. 322. Pregnancy category C.

PHARMACOKINETICS

HALF-LIFE	ONSET	PEAK	DURATION
PO: 4-10 hr	PO: 30 min-3.5 hr	PO: 30 min-3 hr	PO: 6-12 hr
		x̄: 2.5 hr	

procainamide

The electrophysiologic effect of procainamide (Pronestyl, Procanbid, Pronestyl-SR, Procan SR) is similar to that of quinidine, but it differs from quinidine in that its indirect effect (anticholinergic action) is weaker. Procainamide is useful in the management of atrial and ventricular tachydysrhythmias. It is reported to be more effective in the treatment of ventricular disturbances, especially in suppressing premature ventricular contractions and preventing the recurrence of ventricular tachy-

Activity

Table 21-6 Antidysrhythmics: Drug Interactions

Drug	Mechanism	Result
Anticoagulants	Anticoagulant displaced from protein-binding sites	More pronounced anticoagulant effects
Antidysrhythmics	Additive	Proarrhythmic, may cause dysrhythmias
Phenytoin	Phenytoin displaced from protein-binding sites	More pronounced phenytoin effects
Sulfonylurea compounds	Sulfonylurea displaced from protein-binding sites	More pronounced sulfonylurea effects

cardia. The IV form of procainamide is generally preferred over that of quinidine. Procainamide is chemically related to the local anesthetic procaine. Significant adverse effects of the agent include ventricular dysrhythmias and blood disorders. It can cause a lupus erythematosus–like syndrome, which occurs in about 30% of patients on long-term therapy. It can also cause gastrointestinal effects such as nausea, vomiting, and diarrhea, but these are less intense than those of quinidine. Other side effects include fever, leukopenia, maculopapular rash, urticaria, pruritus, flushing, and torsades de pointes resulting from prolongation of the QT interval.

Procainamide is contraindicated in patients who have shown hypersensitivity reactions to it and in those with complete heart block, lupus erythematosus, and second- or third-degree heart block. It is available in four different oral forms: 250-, 375-, and 500-mg capsules; 250-500-, 750-, and 1000-mg extended-release, film-coated tablets; 250-, 375-, and 500-mg film-coated tablets; and 500- and 1000-mg T-kote, controlled-release tablets. Parenterally procainamide comes as a 100- and 500-mg/ml injection. Common dosages are listed in the dosages table on p. 323. Pregnancy category C.

PHARMACOKINETICS

HALF-LIFE	ONSET	PEAK	DURATION
IV/IM: 3 hr	IV/IM: 10-30 min	IV/IM: 10-60 min	IV/IM: 3 hr
PO: 3 hr	PO: 0.5-1 hr	PO: 1-2 hr	PO: 3 hr*

*8-hr extended release.

∘ฺquinidine

Quinidine (Quinidex, Cardioquin, Quinaglute, DuraTab) has both a direct action on the electrical activity of the heart and an indirect (anticholinergic) effect. Its anticholinergic action results in inhibition of the parasympathetic nervous system (PSNS) and allows sympathetic nervous system (SNS) activity to go unopposed. This accelerates the rate of electrical impulse formation and conduction. Significant adverse effects of the agent include cardiac asystole and ventricular ectopic beats. Like other cinchona alkaloids and the salicylates, quinidine can cause cinchonism. Symptoms of mild cinchonism include tinnitus, loss of hearing, slight blurring of vision, and gastrointestinal upset. Contraindications to the use of the drug include hypersensitivity to it, thrombocytopenic purpura resulting from previous therapy, AV block, intraventricular conduction defects, and abnormal rhythms (proarrhythmic effects such as torsades de pointes). Quinidine is available both orally and parenterally and in three different salt forms. The oral preparations consist of 324-mg extended-release quinidine gluconate tablets, 275-mg quinidine polygalacturonate tablets, and 200- and 300-mg regular-release and 300-mg extended-release quinidine sulfate tablets. Parenterally, quinidine gluconate comes as an 80-mg/ml injection. Common dosages are listed in the dosages table on p. 323. Pregnancy category C.

PHARMACOKINETICS

HALF-LIFE	ONSET	PEAK	DURATION
PO: 6-7 hr	1-3 hr	PO: 0.5-6 hr	PO: 6-8 hr*

*12-hr sustained-release.

CLASS Ib DRUGS

Class Ib drugs share many characteristics with class Ia agents but are grouped together because they act preferentially on ischemic myocardial tissue. They have little effect on conduction velocity in normal tissue. Class Ib agents have a weak depressive effect on phase 0 depolarization, the APD, and the ERP. They include lidocaine, tocainide, and mexiletine. Mexiletine and tocainide are classified as pregnancy category C agents, and lidocaine is classified as a pregnancy category B agent.

∘ฺlidocaine

Lidocaine (Xylocaine) is the prototypical Ib agent. It is one of the most effective drugs for the treatment of ventricular dysrhythmias, but it can only be administered intravenously because it has an extensive first-pass effect (i.e., when taken orally, the liver metabolizes most of it to inactive metabolites).

Lidocaine exerts its effects on the conduction system of the heart by making it difficult for the ventricles to develop a dysrhythmia, an action called *raising the ventricular fibrillation threshold*. It does this by decreasing the sensitivity of the cardiac cell membrane to impulses and decreasing the cell's

DOSAGES Selected Antidysrhythmic Agents

agent	pharmacologic class	dosage range	purpose
adenosine (Adenocard)	Unclassified antidysrhythmic	**Adult** IV: 6-mg bolus over 1-2 sec. If needed, a second rapid bolus of 12 mg, which may be repeated a second time if required	Supraventricular tachycardia, conversion to normal sinus rhythm
amiodarone (Cordarone)	Class III antidysrhythmic	**Adult** IV: 150 mg over 10 min, then 60 mg/hr for 6 hr, then 30 mg/hr as maintenance dose PO: 800-1600 mg/day for 1-3 wk and reduced to 600-800 mg/day for 5 wk: usual maintenance dose, 400 mg/day PO: 200-400 mg/day	Ventricular dysrhythmias Atrial dysrhythmias
atenolol (Tenormin)	Beta₁-blocker (class II antidysrhythmic)	**Adult** IV: 5 mg over 5 min followed by 5 mg over 10 min followed by 50 mg PO 10 min after last IV injection and another 50 mg 12 hr later, then 100 mg/day for a further 6-9 days	Acute MI
bretylium (Bretylol)	Class III antidysrhythmic	**Adult** IM/IV: 5-10 mg/kg repeated at 5-30 min intervals if needed to a total dose of 30-35 mg/kg	Ventricular dysrhythmias
diltiazem (Cardizem)	Calcium channel blocker	**Adult** IV: bolus dose, 0.25 mg/kg over 2 min; second dose, 0.35 mg/kg over 2 min after 15 min prn; then 5-10 mg/hr or higher by continuous infusion	Supraventricular dysrhythmias
disopyramide (Norpace, Norpace CR)	Class Ia antidysrhythmic	**Adult** PO: 150 mg q6h; CR: 300 mg q12h with a daily range of 400-800 mg divided	Ventricular dysrhythmias
encainide (Enkaid)	Class Ic antidysrhythmic	**Adult** PO: Start with 25 mg q8h. If required, raise dosage to 35 mg q8h after 3-5 days. Some patients may require 50 mg q6h or 75 mg q6h. Dose increment requires an interval of 3-5 days and 75 mg is the maximum single dose	Life-threatening dysrhythmias
esmolol (Brevibloc)	Beta₁-blocker (class II antidysrhythmic)	**Adult** IV: bolus dose of 500 μg/kg/min followed by 4 min of 50 μg/kg/min and evaluate	Supraventricular tachyarrhythmias
flecainide (Tambocor)	Class Ic antidysrhythmic	**Adult** PO: 50 mg q12h can be increased by 50 mg bid every 4 days until desired effect with a daily maximum of 300 mg for PSVT. 100 mg q12h with increment of 50 mg bid every 4 days if needed; usual dose, 150 mg q12h with daily maximum of 400 mg	Paroxysmal supraventricular tachycardia-paroxysmal atrial flutter/fibrillation Sustained ventricular tachycardia
ibutalide (Corvert)	Class III antidysrhythmic	**Adult** IV: 1 mg infusion over 10 min (*if <60 kg then 0.1 ml/kg)	Atrial fibrillation/flutter
lidocaine (Xylocaine)	Class Ib antidysrhythmic	**Pediatric** IV: suggested bolus dose, 1 mg kg; usual maintenance infusion rate, 20-50 μg/kg/min **Adult** IM: 4-3 mg/kg; may be repeated after 60-90 min IV: bolus dose, 50-100 mg; may be repeated in 5 min. Do not exceed 200-300 mg over 1 hr. Usual maintenance infusion rate, 1-4 mg/min	Ventricular dysrhythmias

DOSAGES Selected Antidysrhythmic Agents—cont'd

agent	pharmacologic class	dosage range	purpose
metoprolol (Lopressor)	Beta₁-blocker	*Adult* IV/PO: 3 bolus injections of 5 mg at 2-min intervals followed by 50 mg PO every 6 hr for 48 hr, thereafter 100 mg bid PO: 100 mg bid	Early MI Late MI
mexiletine (Mexitil)	Class Ib antidysrhythmic	*Adult* PO: start with 200 mg q8h. A minimum of 2-3 days is required between dosage adjustments, which are 50- or 100-mg increments up or down. For rapid control, 400 mg followed by 200 mg in 8 hr. Stabilized patients may be put on a 12-hr schedule with a maximum dose of 450 mg q12h	Ventricular dysrhythmias
procainamide (Pronestyl, Pronestyl-SR, Procan SR, Procanbid)	Class Ia antidysrhythmic	*Adult* PO: 250-500 mg q3-6h; 0.5-1 g q6h (sustained release); or 0.5-1 g q12h (Procanbid) IM: 50 mg/kg/day divided into fractional doses of 1/4-1/8 q3-6h IV: 50-100 mg every 5 min up to 500 mg with a maintenance infusion of 1-6 mg/min	Atrial dysrhythmias Ventricular dysrhythmias Alternate PO dosage Dysrhythmias during surgery Rapid dysrhythmia control
propafenone (Rythmol)	Class Ic antidysrhythmic)	*Adult* PO: start with 150 mg q8h and increase every 3-4 days; usual range, 450-900 mg/day divided	Ventricular dysrhythmias
propranolol (Inderal)	Beta-blocker (class II antidysrhythmic)	*Adult* IV: 1-3 mg; if needed, repeated in 2 min and additional doses if needed q ≥ 4h. Switch to PO as soon as possible PO: 80-320 mg/day divided 2-4 times/day	Serious dysrhythmias Angina
quinidine (Quinidex [sulfate], Cardioquin [polygalacturonate], Quinaglute DuraTab [gluconate])	Class Ia antidysrhythmic	*Adult* Gluconate PO: 324-648 mg q8-12h IM: 600 mg followed by 400 mg q2h or more if needed IV: 330-750 mg Polygalacturonate: PO: 275 mg 3-4 times/day Sulfate PO: 200 mg q2-3h for 5-8 doses with daily increases until sinus rhythm is restored or toxic effects occur 200-300 mg 3-4 times/day	Atrial dysrhythmias Ventricular dysrhythmias Atrial dysrhythmias Conversion of atrial fibrillation Atrial dysrhythmias
sotalol (Betapace)	Class II antidysrhythmic	*Adult* PO: 160-320 mg/day divided into 2-3 doses	Life-threatening dysrhythmias
tocainide (Tonocard)	Class Ib antidysrhythmic	*Adult* PO: initial dose, 400 mg q8h with a daily range of 1200-1800 mg in 3 doses with a maximum of ≤2400 mg/day	Ventricular dysrhythmias
verapamil (Calan, Isoptin, Verelan)	Calcium channel blocker (class IV antidysrhythmic)	*Pediatric* IV: ≤1 y/o: 0.1-0.2 mg/kg bolus over 2 min; repeat dose after 30 min IV: 1-15 y/o: 0.1-0.3 mg/kg bolus over 2 min. Do not exceed 5-mg dose. Repeat dose not exceeding 10 mg may be given after 30 min. *Adult* PO: Start with 80 mg 3-4 times/day; daily range, 240-480 mg IV: 5-10 mg bolus over 2 min; repeat dose of ≤10 mg may be given after 30 min.	Supraventricular tachyarrhythmias

ability to depolarize on its own (decreasing automaticity). Many of these effects are accomplished by blockade of fast sodium channels.

Lidocaine is the drug of choice for treating the acute ventricular dysrhythmias associated with MI. Significant adverse effects include CNS toxicities such as twitching, convulsions, and confusion; respiratory depression or arrest; and the cardiovascular effects of hypotension, bradycardia, and dysrhythmias. It is contraindicated in patients who are hypersensitive to its use, have severe SA or AV intraventricular block, or have Stokes-Adams or Wolff-Parkinson-White syndrome. Lidocaine is only available parenterally for IM or IV administration. It comes as a 100-mg/ml IM injection and as a 10-, 20-, 40-, 100-, and 200-mg/ml IV injection. Common dosages are listed in the dosages table on p. 322. Pregnancy category B.

PHARMACOKINETICS

HALF-LIFE	ONSET	PEAK	DURATION
IV/IM: 8 min, 1-2 hr (terminal)	IV/IM: 2-15 min	IV/IM: 5-10 min	IV/IM: 20 min-1.5 hr

Activity

mexiletine

Mexiletine (Mexitil) is structurally and pharmacologically similar to lidocaine, and its effects on the conduction system of the heart are also very similar. As with tocainide, a response to parenteral lidocaine does not predict a response to mexiletine. Mexiletine effectively suppresses PVCs in patients suffering from an acute MI, chronic coronary artery disease, or digitalis toxicity, and in those undergoing cardiac surgery. It has proved particularly useful when taken in combination with selected class Ia or Ic agents or with beta-blockers.

The most frequent adverse effects are nausea, vomiting, dizziness, and tremor. These reactions are usually not serious, however, and are dose related and minimized by taking the drug with food or an antacid. Contraindications to its use include hypersensitivity, cardiogenic shock, and second- or third-degree AV block. It is available orally only as 150-, 200-, and 250-mg capsules. Common dosages are listed in the dosages table. Pregnancy category C.

PHARMACOKINETICS

HALF-LIFE	ONSET	PEAK	DURATION
PO: 12 hr	0.5-2 hr	PO: 2-3 hr	Unknown

tocainide

Tocainide (Tonocard) is an orally active chemical derivative of lidocaine. However, in only about 60% of those patients whose dysrhythmia is stabilized on lidocaine will tocainide have the same success. Conversely, if lidocaine does not control the dys-

rhythmia, it is unlikely tocainide will do so. Tocainide does not undergo extensive first-pass metabolism, so it can be administered orally. It is useful for the treatment of various ventricular dysrhythmias. Its efficacy is probably due to its relatively long half-life of approximately 15 hours. It effectively suppresses the frequency of premature ventricular contractions (PVCs) but is less effective than the other class I agents in preventing chronic, recurrent ventricular tachycardia or fibrillation.

The most frequent side effects include dizziness, paresthesias (tingling), and tremor. Other complaints include nausea and vomiting, which can be minimized by taking the medication with food or an antacid. The most serious side effects are hematologic in nature and include agranulocytosis, leukopenia, and thrombocytopenia. Pulmonary disorders such as pulmonary fibrosis, interstitial pneumonitis, pulmonary edema, and pneumonia may also occur.

Tocainide is contraindicated in patients with a known hypersensitivity to it and in those with second- or third-degree heart block. It is available orally as 400- and 600-mg film-coated tablets. Common dosages are listed in the dosages table on p. 323. Pregnancy category C.

PHARMACOKINETICS

HALF-LIFE	ONSET	PEAK	DURATION
PO: 10-17 hr	Unknown	PO: 0.5-3 hr	8 hr

CLASS Ic DRUGS

Class Ic drugs (flecainide, encainide, and propafenone) have a more pronounced effect on sodium channel blockade than the Ia and Ib agents but have little effect on repolarization or the APD. These drugs markedly slow conduction in the atria, AV node, and ventricles. Because of their marked effect on conduction, these drugs strongly suppress PVCs, reducing or eliminating them in a large number of patients. All class Ic drugs are classified as pregnancy category C agents except for encainide.

encainide and flecainide

Encainide (Enkaid) and flecainide (Tambocor) have many similar characteristics. They are both chemical analogues of procainamide, with flecainide a fluorinated local anesthetic analogue of procainamide. Encainide decreases cardiac contractility and cardiac output less than does flecainide. A large, multicenter, double-blind, placebo-controlled study called the **Cardiac Arrhythmia Suppression Trial** was conducted by the National Heart, Lung, and Blood Institute to determine whether the incidence of **sudden cardiac death** rate could be reduced in post-MI patients with asymptomatic non life-threatening ectopy through the use of either encainide or flecainide. The findings showed that the excessive mortality and nonfatal cardiac arrest rates in patients treated with flecainide or encainide were actually comparable with or worse than those seen in patients who received placebo. Because of these findings, the FDA required that the labeling for flecainide and encainide be revised to indicate that their use should be limited to the treatment of documented, life-threatening, ventricular dysrhythmias such as sustained ventricular tachycardia. Treatment with either agent should be initiated in the hospital. These drugs are not indicated for the management of less severe dysrhythmias such as nonsustained ventricular tachycardia or frequent PVCs.

Although flecainide and encainide are better tolerated than quinidine or procainamide and more effective than mexiletine or tocainide, they are more proarrhythmic. It is this proarrhythmic potential that limits their use to the management of life-threatening dysrhythmias. Flecainide has a negative inotropic effect and depresses LV function. Unlike flecainide, encainide is less likely to significantly depress LV function. Less serious but more frequent noncardiac adverse effects include dizziness, visual disturbances, and dyspnea. Contraindications to their use include hypersensitivity, cardiogenic shock, second- or third-degree AV block, and non life-threatening dysrhythmias.

Encainide and flecainide are both available as oral preparations. Encainide is available as 25-, 35-, and 50-mg capsules and flecainide as 50-, 100-, and 150-mg tablets. Common dosages are listed in the dosages table. Encainide is a pregnancy category B agent. Flecainide is a pregnancy category C agent. Encainide was voluntarily withdrawn from the market by the manufacturer. The drug may still be obtained outside the United States. It is rare to encounter a patient who is still taking it.

PHARMACOKINETICS

HALF-LIFE	ONSET	PEAK	DURATION
Encainide 1-2 hr	Unknown	0.5-1.5 hr	Unknown
Flecainide PO: 12-27 hr	Unknown	PO: 3 hr	Unknown

propafenone

Propafenone (Rythmol) is similar in action to flecainide and encainide. It reduces the fast inward sodium current in Purkinje fibers and to a lesser extent in myocardial fibers. Unlike other class I drugs, propafenone has mild beta-blocking effects. This may contribute to its overall effects on the conduction system. It is also believed to have calcium channel blocking effects, which may contribute to propafenone's mild negative inotropic effects.

Until recently propafenone's use has been limited to the treatment of documented, life-threatening, ventricular dysrhythmias such as sustained ventricular tachycardia. Recent findings suggest that at low doses it has benefit in the treatment of atrial fibrillation as well. Treatment should also be started while the patient is in the hospital. Unlike encainide and flecainide, however, propafenone can be used in patients with depressed LV function. It may be a better antidysrhythmic agent than disopyramide, procainamide, and quinidine in these patients. However, it should be used with caution in patients with congestive heart failure (CHF) because it has some beta-blocking properties and dose-dependent negative inotropic effects.

Propafenone is generally well tolerated. The most frequently reported adverse reaction is dizziness. Patients may also complain of a metallic taste, constipation, and headache, along with nausea and vomiting. These gastrointestinal side effects may be reduced by taking propafenone with food. Propafenone is contraindicated in patients with a known hypersensitivity to it, and in those with bradycardia, bronchial asthma, significant hypotension, uncontrolled CHF, cardiogenic shock, or various conduction disorders. It is available orally as 150- and 300-mg film-coated tablets. Common dosages are listed in the dosages table on p. 323. Pregnancy category C.

PHARMACOKINETICS

HALF-LIFE	ONSET	PEAK	DURATION
2-10 hr	Unknown	3-5 hr	Unknown

CLASS II DRUGS

Class II antidysrhythmics are also known as beta-blockers. These agents work by reducing or blocking SNS stimulation to the heart and the heart's conduction system. By doing this, beta-blockers prevent catecholamine-mediated actions on the heart. The resulting cardiovascular effects include a reduced heart rate, delayed AV node conduction, reduced myocardial contractility, and decreased myocardial automaticity. The pharmacologically induced effects of the beta-blockers are especially beneficial after an MI because of the many catecholamines released at this time, making the heart hyperirritable and predisposed to many types of dysrhythmias. Beta-blockers offer protection from these potentially very dangerous complications. Several studies have demonstrated a significant reduction in the incidence of sudden cardiac death after MI in patients treated with beta-blockers on an ongoing basis. This reduction is on the average of 25%.

Although there are several beta-blockers, only a handful are commonly used as antidysrhythmic drugs. These FDA-approved, antidysrhythmic, class

Activity

II agents are described in the following drug profiles. The class II agents are classified as pregnancy category C agents except acebutolol, pindolol, and sotalol, which are all category B agents.

atenolol

Atenolol (Tenormin) is a cardioselective beta-blocker, which means that it preferentially blocks the beta$_1$-adrenergic receptors that are primarily located on the heart. Noncardioselective beta blockers not only block the beta$_1$-adrenergic receptors on the heart but also the beta$_2$-adrenergic receptors in the lungs, and could therefore exacerbate a preexisting case of asthma or chronic obstructive pulmonary disease. Besides atenolol's class II antidysrhythmic properties, it is also useful in the treatment of hypertension and angina.

Atenolol is contraindicated in patients with severe bradycardia, second- or third-degree heart block, CHF, cardiogenic shock, or a known hypersensitivity to it. Orally atenolol comes as 25-, 50-, and 100-mg tablets. Parenterally it comes as 0.5-mg/ml IV injections. Common dosages are listed in the dosages table on p. 322. Pregnancy category C.

PHARMACOKINETICS

HALF-LIFE	ONSET	PEAK	DURATION
PO: 6-7 hr	PO: 1 hr	PO: 2-4 hr	PO: > or = 24 hr

esmolol

Esmolol (Brevibloc) is a short-acting beta-blocker with pharmacologic and electrophysiologic effects on the heart's conduction system similar to those of atenolol. Esmolol is also a cardioselective beta-blocker that primarily and preferentially blocks the beta$_1$-adrenergic receptors on the heart. It is used in the acute treatment of supraventricular tachyarrhythmias or dysrhythmias that originate above the ventricles and are fast instead of slow. It is also used to control hypertension and tachyarrhythmias that develop after an acute MI.

Esmolol is contraindicated in patients with severe bradycardia, second- or third-degree heart block, CHF, cardiogenic shock, severe asthma, or a known hypersensitivity to it. Esmolol is only available parenterally as a concentrated 250-mg/ml injection for IV infusion and a 10-mg/ml IV injection. Common dosages are listed in the dosages table on p. 322. Pregnancy category C.

PHARMACOKINETICS

HALF-LIFE	ONSET	PEAK	DURATION
IV: 9 min	IV: Very rapid	IV: Rapid	IV: Short

metoprolol

Metoprolol (Lopressor) is another cardioselective beta-blocker commonly given after an MI to reduce the risk of sudden cardiac death. It is also used in the treatment of hypertension and angina. It is available orally as 50-, 100-, and 200-mg extended-release tablets; and as 50- and 100-mg regular-release tablets. Parenterally it comes as a 1-mg/ml IV injection. In the treatment of hypertension it is combined with the thiazide diuretic hydrochlorothiazide in a product called *Lopressor HCT*. The contraindications to metoprolol use are the same as those of both atenolol and esmolol. Common dosages are listed in the dosages table on p. 323. Pregnancy category C.

PHARMACOKINETICS

HALF-LIFE	ONSET	PEAK	DURATION
PO: 3-4 hr	PO: 1 hr	PO: 2-4 hr	PO: 13-19 hr

propranolol

Propranolol (Inderal) was one of the first beta-blockers introduced into clinical practice, which occurred in 1967. It was then primarily used in the treatment of dysrhythmias. Propranolol is a nonspecific beta-blocker that blocks both beta$_1$- and beta$_2$-adrenergic receptors on the heart and lungs. Its primary effect on the conduction system of the heart is the blockade of cardiac beta$_1$-adrenergic receptors, thereby preventing catecholamine-mediated stimulation of the heart. The resulting cardiovascular effects are a reduced heart rate, delayed AV node conduction, reduced myocardial contractility, and decreased myocardial automaticity. Propranolol is also believed to have membrane-stabilizing properties that may play a small role in its overall antidysrhythmic effect.

Because propranolol is the oldest of this class of drugs, there are now many indications for its use. Hypertension, angina, supraventricular dysrhythmias, ventricular tachycardia, the tachyarrhythmias associated with cardiac glycoside toxicity, hypertrophic subaortic stenosis, pheochromocytoma, thyrotoxicosis, migraines, post-MI, and essential tremor are just some of these. The contraindications to propranolol use are the same as for atenolol. It is available in both oral and parenteral dosage forms. Orally it is available as 60-, 80-, 120-, and 160-mg extended-release capsules; 10-, 20-, 40-, 60-, 80-, and 90-mg tablets; and a 20-mg/5 ml and a 40-mg/5 ml oral solution and an 80-mg/ml concentrated oral solution. Parenterally propranolol comes as a 1-mg/ml injection. Common dosages are listed in the dosages table on p. 323. Pregnancy category C.

PHARMACOKINETICS

HALF-LIFE	ONSET	PEAK	DURATION
3-5 hr	IV: 2 min	IV: 15 min	IV: 3-6 hr
	PO: 30 min	PO: 1-1.5 hr	PO: 8-11 hr

sotalol

Sotalol (Betapace) is another nonselective beta-blocker that is used to treat dysrhythmias. It is unique in that it possesses antidysrhythmic properties similar to those of the class III agents (such as amiodarone) while simultaneously exerting beta-blocker or class II effects on the conduction system of the heart. In addition, sotalol has proarrhythmic properties similar to those of the class Ic agents. This means that while patients are taking sotalol, it can cause serious dysrhythmias such as torsades de pointes or a new ventricular tachycardia or fibrillation. For this reason, sotalol is usually reserved for the treatment of documented, life-threatening, ventricular dysrhythmias such as sustained ventricular tachycardia.

Contraindications to sotalol use include hypersensitivity to it, bronchial asthma, cardiogenic shock, and sinus bradycardia. Sotalol is available only orally as 80-, 120-, 160-, 240-, and 320-mg tablets. Common dosages are listed in the dosages table on p. 323. Pregnancy category C.

PHARMACOKINETICS

HALF-LIFE	ONSET	PEAK	DURATION
PO: 12 hr	PO: 1-2 hr	PO: 2-4 hr	PO: 12-24 hr

CLASS III DRUGS

Class III agents consist of amiodarone, ibutilide, and bretylium. Amiodarone and bretylium control dysrhythmias by inhibiting repolarization and markedly prolonging refractoriness and the APD. Ibutilide is indicated for conversion of atrial fibrillation/flutter to a normal sinus rhythm. Amiodarone and bretylium are indicated for the management of life-threatening ventricular tachycardia or ventricular fibrillation that is resistant to other drug therapy. Amiodarone and bretylium have also been very effective in the treatment of sustained ventricular tachycardias. Amiodarone has recently been used more frequently to treat atrial dysrhythmias as well. These agents are classified as pregnancy category C agents.

⌐amiodarone

Amiodarone (Cordarone and Pacerone) markedly prolongs the APD and the ERP in all cardiac tissues. Besides these dramatic effects it is also known to block both the alpha- and beta-adrenergic receptors of the SNS. Clinically it is one of the most effective antidysrhythmic agents for controlling supraventricular and ventricular dysrhythmias. It is indicated for the management of sustained ventricular tachycardia, ventricular fibrillation, and nonsustained ventricular tachycardia. It is reported to be effective in 40% to 60% of all patients with ventricular tachycardia. Recently it has shown promise in the management of atrial dysrhythmias that are difficult to treat or resistant.

Amiodarone has many unwanted adverse effects, and many of these can be attributed to its chemical properties. Amiodarone is very lipophilic, or "fat loving." Therefore it can penetrate and concentrate in the adipose tissue of any organ in the body, where it may cause unwanted effects. It also has iodine in its chemical structure. One organ that sequesters iodine from our diets is the thyroid gland. As a result, amiodarone can cause either hypothyroidism or hyperthyroidism. Adverse reactions occur in approximately 75% of the patients treated with the agent, but the incidence and severity of these are more common in association with higher doses (those exceeding 400 mg/day) and prolonged therapy. The most common reaction is corneal microdeposits, which may cause visual halos, photophobia, and dry eyes. This occurs in virtually all adults who take the drug for more than 6 months.

The most serious adverse effect is pulmonary toxicity, which is fatal in about 10% of patients and involves a clinical syndrome of progressive dyspnea and cough accompanied by damage to the alveoli. The result can be pulmonary fibrosis. Another serious complication of amiodarone therapy is that it too may not only treat the dysrhythmias but may also provoke them.

Amiodarone has an exceptionally long half-life, approaching many days. As a result, the therapeutic as well as any adverse effects of amiodarone may linger long after the drug has been discontinued. In fact, it may take as long as 2 to 3 months after the drug has been discontinued for some side effects to subside. For all these reasons, although very effective, amiodarone is typically considered a drug of last resort. Therapy is typically started in the hospital and closely monitored until the serum levels are within a therapeutic range.

Amiodarone is contraindicated in patients who have a known hypersensitivity to it, as well as in those with severe sinus bradycardia or second- or third-degree heart block. Amiodarone is available orally as 200-mg tablets and as a parenteral formulation in ampules containing 3 ml of a 50 mg/ml solution. Common dosages are listed in the dosages table. Amiodarone is classified as a pregnancy category C agent.

If it is indicated to maintain a patient on long-term, orally administered amiodarone after intravenously administered amiodarone, then there are recommended conversions. When transition of a patient on IV amiodarone to oral amiodarone is feasible, the recommendations in Table 21-7 are helpful.

<table>
<tr><td>Table
21-7</td><td colspan="2">Recommendations for Oral
Dosage After IV Infusion</td></tr>
</table>

Duration of Amiodarone IV Infusion	Initial Daily Dose of Oral Amiodarone
<1 wk	800-1600 mg
1-3 wk	600-800 mg
>3 wk	400 mg

PHARMACOKINETICS

HALF-LIFE	ONSET	PEAK	DURATION
PO: 15-100 days	PO: 1-3 wk	PO: 2-10 hr	PO: 10-150 days

bretylium

Bretylium (Bretylol) was initially marketed as an antihypertensive agent, but not much later its effects on the conduction system were noted. It has both a direct and an indirect effect on cardiac conduction. The direct effect prolongs the APD of the Purkinje fibers and ventricular myocardium and the ERP. The indirect effect is due to an adrenergic-blocking effect, in that bretylium accumulates in the nerve endings of the SNS, where it displaces norepinephrine. This results in a short-term rise in blood pressure; however, after this, the further release of norepinephrine is blocked and ultimately the reuptake of norepinephrine is inhibited.

Bretylium is only available parenterally. It is used for the treatment of serious dysrhythmias such as life-threatening ventricular tachycardia or fibrillation. Therefore bretylium is most commonly used in intensive care unit settings and cardiac codes in patients who do not respond to lidocaine, quinidine, procainamide, or disopyramide treatment. The major adverse effect associated with its use is postural hypotension, occurring in about 50% of patients. Other common side effects include nausea and vomiting. However, all of these side effects can be reduced by administering it by slow IV infusion. Bretylium is contraindicated in patients with a known hypersensitivity to it. It is only available parenterally as a 2- and 4-mg/ml injection for IV infusions and as a 50-mg/ml bolus injection. Common dosages are listed in the dosages table on p. 322. Pregnancy category C.

PHARMACOKINETICS

HALF-LIFE	ONSET	PEAK	DURATION
4-17 hr	6-20 min	IV: Rapid (<1 hr)	IV: 6-24 hr

ibutilide

Ibutilide (Corvert) is a class III antiarrhythmic agent. Unlike the other two agents in the class III group of antiarrhythmics, ibutilide is indicated for

atrial dysrhythmias. Atrial fibrillation and atrial flutter cause irregular contractions of the heart and can lead to serious conditions such as decreased cardiac output, congestive heart failure, low blood pressure, and stroke. Although other pharmacologic therapies are used to treat atrial fibrillation and flutter, ibutilide is the only drug therapy available for rapid conversion of these two conditions to normal sinus rhythm. The only other treatment available for rapid conversion is electrical cardioversion. Although it is effective, electrical cardioversion carries the risk, expense, and inconvenience of both the procedure itself and the anesthesia it requires.

Ibutilide is only available parenterally as a single-dose, 10-ml vial in a 0.1 mg/ml concentration. It is dosed based on patient weight. Ibutilide is contraindicated in patients who have previously demonstrated hypersensitivity to it. As with other antidysrhythmic agents, ibutilide should be used with caution because it can have a prodysrhythmic effect, most significantly ventricular tachycardia and torsades de pointes. Class Ia antidysrhythmic drugs (e.g., disopyramide, quinidine, and procainamide) and other class III drugs (e.g., amiodarone and sotalol) should not be given concomitantly with ibutilide. They should not be given within 4 hours after infusion of ibutilide either because of their potential to prolong refractoriness. Common dosages are listed in the dosages table on p. 322.

PHARMACOKINETICS

HALF-LIFE	ONSET	PEAK	DURATION
6 hr	10 min	30 min	4 hr

CLASS IV DRUGS

Class IV antidysrhythmic drugs are CCBs. Although there are more than nine such agents currently available, only a few are commonly used as antidysrhythmics. Besides their effectiveness as antidysrhythmics, CCBs are effective in the treatment of hypertension and angina.

Verapamil and diltiazem are the two CCBs most commonly used for the following:

- Treating dysrhythmias, specifically those that arise above the ventricles (paroxysmal supraventricular tachycardia [PSVT])
- Controlling the ventricular response to atrial fibrillation and flutter by slowing conduction and prolonging refractoriness of the AV node (i.e., not allowing the ventricles to beat as fast). These agents block the slow inward flow of calcium ions into the slow (calcium) channels in cardiac conduction tissue. The conduction effects of these agents are limited to the atria and the AV node, where conduction is prolonged and the tis-

sues are made more refractory to stimulation. These agents have little effect on the ventricular tissues.

diltiazem

Diltiazem (Cardizem) is primarily indicated for the temporary control of a rapid ventricular response in a patient with atrial fibrillation or flutter and PSVT. Its use is contraindicated in the settings of hypersensitivity, acute MI, pulmonary congestion, Wolff-Parkinson-White syndrome, severe hypotension, cardiogenic shock, sick sinus syndrome, or second- or third-degree AV block. Diltiazem is available both orally and parenterally. Orally diltiazem is available as 30-, 60-, 90-, and 120-mg tablets; 60-, 90-, and 120-mg sustained-release, twice-a-day capsules; and 120-, 180-, 240-, 300-, and 360-mg controlled-delivery, once-a-day capsules. Parenterally diltiazem is available as a 5-mg/ml injection. Common dosages are listed in the dosages table on p. 322. Pregnancy category C.

PHARMACOKINETICS

HALF-LIFE	ONSET	PEAK	DURATION
PO: 3.5-9 hr	PO: 0.5-1 hr	2-3 hr	PO: 4-8 hr 12 hr*

*For extended-release product.

verapamil

Verapamil (Calan, Isoptin, Verelan) has actions similar to those of diltiazem in that it also inhibits calcium ion influx across the slow calcium channels in cardiac conduction tissue. This results in dramatic effects on the AV node. Verapamil is used to prevent and convert recurrent PSVT and to control ventricular response in atrial flutter or fibrillation. It can also temporarily control a rapid ventricular response to these frequent atrial stimulations, usually decreasing the heart rate by at least 20%. Besides its use for the management of various dysrhythmias, verapamil is also used to treat angina, hypertension, and hypertrophic cardiomyopathy.

The contraindications that apply to diltiazem apply to verapamil as well, and it is also available both orally and parenterally. Orally it as 40-, 80-, and 120-mg film-coated tablets and 120-, 180-, and 240-mg extended-release tablets and capsules. Parenterally it is available as a 2.5-mg/ml injection for IV administration. Common dosages are listed in the dosages table on p. 323. Pregnancy category C.

PHARMACOKINETICS

HALF-LIFE	ONSET	PEAK	DURATION
PO: 2.8-7.4 hr	PO: 30 min	PO: 1-2 hr	PO: 6-8 hr
IV: 2-5 hr	IV: 1-2 min	IV: 3-5 min	IV: 10-60 min

UNCLASSIFIED ANTIDYSRHYTHMICS

adenosine

Adenosine (Adenocard) is an unclassified antidysrhythmic agent. It is a naturally occurring nucleoside that slows the electrical conduction time through the AV node and is indicated for the conversion of PSVT to sinus rhythm. It is particularly useful for the treatment of PSVT that has failed to respond to verapamil or when a patient has coexisting conditions such as CHF, hypotension, or LV dysfunction that limit the use of verapamil. It is contraindicated in patients with second- or third-degree heart block, sick sinus syndrome, atrial flutter or fibrillation, or ventricular tachycardia, as well as in those with a known hypersensitivity to it. It has an extremely short half-life of less than 10 seconds. For this reason, it is only administered intravenously and only as a fast IV push. It will frequently cause asystole for a period of seconds. All other side effects are minimal because of its very short duration of action. It is only available parenterally as a 3-mg/ml injection. Common dosages are listed in the dosages table on p. 322. Pregnancy category C.

PHARMACOKINETICS

HALF-LIFE	ONSET	PEAK	DURATION
<10 sec	1 min	Immediate	1-2 min

nursing process

Because the four classes of antidysrhythmics produce a variety of effects on the action potential of the cardiac cell, they exert a major effect on cardiac electrophysiologic function. This diversity of therapeutic effect and the attendant side effects pose a special challenge to the nurse, who is responsible for ensuring the safe and efficacious use of these agents. Because the nursing process that applies to the administration of these agents varies for each of the four classes of agents, each group is discussed.

● Assessment

Before administering any class I antidysrhythmics to a patient, the nurse must obtain a thorough drug and medical history. Contraindications to the administration of these drugs include the following:

- Known hypersensitivity to them
- CHF
- Complete heart block
- Hypotension
- Myasthenia gravis
- Urinary retention
- Hepatic or renal insufficiency
- Congenitally prolonged QT interval (class Ia agents)

home health/community points

Antidysrhythmics

- Patients taking antidysrhthmics at home need to be closely monitored by the home health care nurse or by the physician or other health care provider. This should include frequent measurements of the blood levels of the medication as well as frequent monitoring of the blood pressure and pulse. These measures are important, especially in the elderly, because of the toxic effects these agents can have.
- Patient education using pamphlets, posters, journals, and other printed, video, or audio (often available free of charge from pharmaceutical companies) material is encouraged. The patient should be given as much reference material as possible. It is important to provide education and supportive material and resources because of the toxic effects of the medicines, the often seriousness of the disease, and the polypharmacy that is frequently a part of the clinical picture in these patients.
- Make sure patients know to notify the physician or other health care provider of any worsening of their dysrhythmia, as well as any shortness of breath, edema, chest pain, dizziness, or syncope. They should also know to report any of the adverse reactions or possible signs of toxicity of the particular agent they are taking.

- Second- or third-degree heart block
- Hypersensitivity to the local anesthetics lidocaine and tocainide
- Cardiogenic shock
- Hypokalemia (class Ic agent).

Class Ia agents should be administered cautiously in patients with electrolyte imbalances, especially hypokalemia. Class Ib agents should be administered cautiously in patients with hepatic or renal disease, CHF, bradycardia, a markedly altered urinary pH (affects excretion), and weights of less than 50 kg (111 lb), as well as in the elderly. The cautious administration of class Ic agents is required in patients with severe renal or liver disease, CHF, prolonged QT intervals, and blood dyscrasias.

Drugs that interact with class I antidysrhythmics include the following:
- Neuromuscular blockers, which interact with quinidine, procainamide, and disopyramide, resulting in increased skeletal muscle relaxation
- Anticholinergic drugs, which results in an enhanced anticholinergic effect
- Coumarin anticoagulants, which interact with quinidine, resulting in hypothrombinemia
- Digoxin and quinidine, which results in increased serum digoxin levels
- Nifedipine, which interacts with quinidine, resulting in decreased serum quinidine levels

- Cimetidine, which interacts with quinidine, resulting in increased serum quinidine
- Anticonvulsants, which interact with quinidine or disopyramide, resulting in increased metabolism of these antidysrhythmics
- Cimetidine, which interacts with procainamide, resulting in increased levels of the procainamide.

In addition, an increased urinary pH will cause the serum levels of quinidine to be elevated.

Class Ib antidysrhythmic drugs interact with other antidysrhythmics and with lidocaine. Lidocaine toxicity may result from the concurrent administration of propranolol or cimetidine.

Class Ic agents interact with digoxin (which leads to an increase in the serum digoxin levels and digoxin toxicity) and with flecainide and alkalinizing drugs (which leads to a decrease in the urinary excretion of flecainide). (See Table 21-6 for a summary of the drug interactions that occur with the antidysrhythmics.)

Before administering any class II antidysrhythmics, the nurse needs to obtain a thorough drug and medical history. Contraindications to the administration of these drugs include a known hypersensitivity to them, asthma and other forms of chronic obstructive pulmonary disease, sinus bradycardia, second- or third-degree heart block, diabetes mellitus, and peripheral vascular disease. Drugs that interact with the class II agents propranolol and acebutolol hydrochloride include phenothiazines and antihypertensive agents, with hypotension the effect. Propranolol also interacts with cimetidine, resulting in decreased metabolism of the propranolol.

Before administering either of the class III antidysrhythmic agents, bretylium and amiodarone, the nurse should collect data regarding the patient's medication history, present and past medical history, drug allergies, and specific laboratory test results. A very thorough assessment is crucial to the safe use of these antidysrhythmics because of the adverse reactions patients can have to them. In fact, it is because of these severe adverse reactions that they are not the first choice for antidysrhythmic therapy. Amiodarone must be administered cautiously in patients who have preexisting bradycardia, conduction or sinus node disorders, severely depressed or compromised ventricular function, or marked cardiomegaly. Bretylium must be administered cautiously in patients with aortic stenosis, pulmonary hypertension, or digitalis-induced dysrhythmias. Drugs they can interact with include digoxin, which results in increased digoxin levels, and warfarin, which results in increased clotting times with hypoprothrombinemia. Remember that ibutilide is for treatment of atrial dysrhythmias.

With class IV antidysrhythmic agents such as verapamil and diltiazem, the nurse should collect data on the patient's medication history, present and past medical history, drug allergies, and specific laboratory results. Cautious administration of this agent is warranted in patients with hypotension, CHF, sick sinus syndrome, AV conduction disturbances, or hepatic impairment. Indications for its use include PSVT with rapid ventricular response rates. Drugs that interact with it include other antidysrhythmics and antihypertensive agents, which enhance the risk of hypotension and heart failure; digoxin, which increases the digoxin levels and causes digitalis toxicity; and highly protein bound drugs such as hydantoin, aspirin, sulfonamide antibiotics, and sulfonylureas, which result in the adverse effects of either verapamil, diltiazem, or the other medication.

● Nursing Diagnoses

Nursing diagnoses related to the administration of antidysrhythmics include the following:
- Decreased tissue perfusion related to the impact of the dysrhythmia.
- Risk for injury related to side effects of the medications.
- Deficient knowledge related to disease and medication therapy.
- Impaired gaseous exchange (decreased) related to adverse reaction to the medications.
- Diarrhea related to adverse reaction to the medications.
- Disturbed body image related to changes in lifestyle and sexual functioning due to side effects of the medications and impact of the disease process.

● Planning

Therapeutic goals appropriate for patients receiving antidysrhythmic agents include the following:
- Patient is free of further symptoms related to cardiac dysrythmias once therapy is initiated.
- Patient has improved tolerance to activity and improved general sense of well-being.
- Patient is free of complications associated with noncompliance or with sudden withdrawal of medication.
- Patient reports any increase in the symptoms of the dysrhythmia.
- Patient demonstrates adequate knowledge of drug therapy and its side effects.

Outcome Criteria

Outcome criteria for patients receiving antidysrhythmics include the following:
- Patient's dysrhythmia symptoms such as shortness of breath and chest pain will be alleviated by the medication therapy.
- Patient will exhibit signs and symptoms of improved cardiac output, as evidenced by regular apical and radial pulses; vital signs within normal limits; and a decrease in weight, edema, crackles, and shortness of breath attributable to compliance with therapy.
- Patient will state the importance of complying with the medication regimen and of coming in for follow-up visits with the physician (i.e., decreasing complications and manifestations of dysrhythmias).
- Patient will state the common side effects of the medication such as constipation and dry mouth.

● Implementation

The administration of class I antidysrhythmics requires some very specific nursing interventions. Initially the

ECG and vital signs must be monitored closely in patients who are receiving these medications because, if the QT interval is prolonged by more than 50%, this may precipitate a variety of conduction disturbances. An IV pump is needed when administering procainamide intravenously. When switching from IV to oral forms, the infusion should be continued for 2 hours after the start of the oral agent, or as prescribed. Solutions of lidocaine containing epinephrine should not be used except as a local anesthetic.

The administration of any of the class II antidysrhythmics requires some very specific nursing interventions. Initially the ECG and vital signs must be closely monitored in patients receiving these medications because of the cardiovascular adverse effects they can precipitate, such as hypotension, bradycardia, and AV blocks. These problems usually occur when the drug is first given. Patients taking propranolol should be cautioned to report the appearance of any shortness of breath or skin rash. Should the parenteral solution of any of these drugs appear discolored or contain particulate matter, it should be discarded. IV solutions should be administered over a 3-minute period, especially in elderly patients, so as to minimize the risk of adverse effects. Patients should also be cautioned not to skip doses.

As with the other classes of antidysrhythmics, there are some very specific nursing interventions called for in patients receiving a class IV antidysrhythmic. Patients who are receiving such an agent initially or having their doses altered must be monitored by ECG. In addition, blood pressure and other vital signs need to be monitored frequently. IV bolus doses should be administered over a 2-minute period, but this should be done over 3 minutes in elderly patients to minimize the adverse effects that can arise in these patients. It is crucial to remember that verapamil and beta-blockers cannot be administered intravenously at the same time or within a few hours of each other.

See p. 332 for patient teaching tips for antidysrhythmic agents.

● Evaluation

Monitoring patients receiving class I antidysrhythmics is important in identifying the therapeutic as opposed to the adverse and toxic effects. Therapeutic effects include improved cardiac output, decreased chest discomfort, decreased fatigue; improved vital signs, skin color, and urinary output; and improvement in irregularities to normal rhythm. Adverse effects include bradycardia, dizziness, headache, cinchonism, chest pain, CHF, and peripheral edema. Toxic effects range from cardiac failure and bradycardia to CNS-related effects such as confusion or convulsions.

The monitoring of patients receiving any of the class II antidysrhythmics is important in identifying both the therapeutic effects and the adverse and toxic effects. Therapeutic effects include improved cardiac output, decreased chest discomfort, decreased fatigue, regular pulse rate or improvement in irregularities, and improved vital signs, skin color, and urinary output. Adverse effects include bradycardia, dizziness, headache, and peripheral edema. Toxic effects consist of cardiac failure, bradycardia, bronchospasms, hypotension, and conduction problems.

Monitoring patients receiving class III antidysrhythmics is important for identifying both the therapeutic effects and the side and toxic effects. Therapeutic effects include improved cardiac output, more regular rhythm, decreased chest discomfort, decreased fatigue, and improved vital signs, skin color, and urinary output. Adverse effects include peripheral neuropathies, extrapyramidal symptoms, headache, fatigue, lethargy, dizziness (bretylium use only), bradycardia, hypotension, dysrhythmias, severe orthostatic hypotension (bretylium use only), microdeposits on the cornea with visual disturbances, hypothyroidism or hyperthyroidism, nausea, vomiting, constipation, hepatic dysfunction with abnormal liver enzyme activity, electrolyte imbalances, photo-

sensitivity, blue-gray skin color changes, severe pulmonary changes with development of pneumonitis, alveolitis with high doses, pulmonary fibrosis, and pulmonary muscle weakness. The patient's thyroid function should be monitored carefully during therapy so that abnormal function can be identified before any further adverse effects appear. Toxic effects include hypotension or hypertension and bradycardia.

It is important to monitor patients receiving a class IV antidysrhythmic to identify both the therapeutic effects and the side and toxic effects. Therapeutic effects include improved cardiac output, decreased chest discomfort, decreased fatigue, and improved vital signs, skin color, and urinary output. Adverse effects include bradycardia, CHF, hypotension, AV conduction disorders, ventricular asystole, peripheral edema, and constipation. Toxic effects include hypotension, bradycardia, heart failure, and conduction disorders.

✍ patient teaching tips

Antidysrhythmic Agents

Class I Antidysrhythmics

➤ Patients should be told to take medication without omissions but not to double up on doses to make up for missed doses. Patients should contact their physician if uncertain about what to do in the event of any missed or skipped doses. This is true for classes I-IV.

➤ Patients should not crush or chew any of the oral sustained-release preparations (with any class of agent).

➤ If patients should notice a tablet or capsule in their stool, they should know that this is usually just the wax matrix of the preparation that has not been absorbed and that the medication has been extracted in the intestines.

➤ Adverse reactions associated with the class la antidysrhythmics that patients should be aware of include ringing of the ears, anticholinergic effects such as dryness of the mouth and constipation, GI upset, headache, fever, light-headedness, blurred vision, and cinchonism. which results from a reaction to the source of quinidine, *Cinchona*, and includes headache, fever, and light-headedness. Class la antidysrhythmic toxicity is manifested by cardiac or respiratory arrest or by loss of consciousness, so careful administration at home is important and should be monitored with a calendar or some other means of dose identification.

➤ Adverse reactions associated with class lb agents include confusion, tremors (shakiness), convulsions, light-headedness, hypotension, dizziness, tinnitus, double vision, lethargy, and sensations of cold. Class lb toxicity is manifested by confusion or convulsions.

➤ Adverse reactions associated with class lc agents include dizziness, headaches, fatigue, shakiness, CHF (shortness of breath, lethargy, decreased urine output,

swelling of feet, and weight gain of 2 lbs [1 kg] or more in a week), GI upset, edema, and chest pain. Class lc toxicity is manifested by bradycardia.

Class II Antidysrhythmics

➤ Propranolol toxicity is manifested by bradycardia, bronchospasms, heart failure, and hypotension, and patients should report increased lethargy and shortness of breath, edema, a weight gain of 2 lbs or more in a week, cough, decreased urinary output, dizziness, syncopal (fainting) spells, or heart palpitations to their physician.

➤ Oral forms of propranolol hydrochloride should be taken before meals and at bedtime, as ordered by the physician (i.e., if taken 3-4 times a day).

➤ Patients should always take the drug after counting their radial pulse for 1 full minute. If the pulse is less than 60 beats/min, they should notify their physician.

Class III Antidysrhythmics

➤ Patients should use sunscreen products when out in the sun because of the photosensitivity (increased risk of sunburn with minimal exposure) these agents cause. They should report any unusual tingling of the skin that is followed by blistering or erythematous (reddening) reactions.

➤ Patients should contact their physician should they exhibit any of the following signs and symptoms while receiving amiodarone: lethargy, weight gain, cool and dry skin, bradycardia, hypotension, or intolerance to cold (indicative of hypothyroidism associated with the therapy); or nervousness, palpitations, weight loss, warm and moist skin, and tachycardia (indicative of the hyperthyroidism associated with the therapy).

➤ Side effects of these drugs include numbness and tingling of the extremities, uncontrolled shaking of the head and hands, headache, weakness, fatigue and loss of energy, dizziness, fainting spells (especially with changes of position from lying to standing or sitting to standing or sudden position changes such as stooping over), visual problems, nausea, vomiting, constipation, sunburn (even with very limited sun exposure), blue-gray skin discoloration, or cough.

Class IV Antidysrhythmics

➤ Patients should know the various drugs that interact with class IV agents: digoxin, antihypertensives, other antidysrhythmics, sulfonamides (i.e., Septra, Bactrim),

sulfonylureas (oral antidiabetic agents), aspirin-containing drugs or aspirin products, phenytoin, coumarin.

➤ Patients should be aware of the adverse effects of diltiazem: dizziness, fatigue, headache, transient hypotension, heart failure (edema or swelling, shortness of breath, cough, palpitations, decreased urine output, and lethargy), and constipation. Signs and symptoms of toxicity include bradycardia (pulse <60 beats min), heart failure, palpitations and skipped heartbeats, and hypotension.

POINTS TO REMEMBER

Dysrhythmias and Dysrhythmic Agents

• Any disturbance or abnormality in a normal pattern of the heartbeat.
• Antidysrhythmic drugs are used to correct dysrhythmias.
• Antidysrhythmics may cause dysrhythmias and for this reason are called *prodysrhythmic.*

Mechanisms of Antidysrhythmic Agents

• *Class I:* Membrane-stabilizing agents.
• *Class II:* Beta-adrenergic blockers; depress phase 4 depolarization.
• *Class III:* Prolong repolarization in phase 3.
• *Class IV:* Depress phase 4 depolarization and prolong repolarization of phases 1 and 2.

Vaughan Williams Classification

• Most commonly used system to classify antidysrhythmic drugs.
• Groups drugs according to where and how they affect cardiac cells.
• Broken down into four main classes:class Ia (quinidine), Ib (lidocaine), and Ic (flecainide); class II (beta-blockers); class III (bretylium, amiodarone, and sotalol), and class IV (calcium channel blockers).

Sodium-Potassium ATPase Pump

• Mechanism for transporting sodium and potassium ions across cell membranes against an opposing concentration gradient.
• Energy for this transport system is obtained from the hydrolysis of adenosine triphosphate by means of an enzyme called *adenosine triphosphatase* (ATPase).
• Cardiac glycosides (digoxin) work by inhibiting this pump.

Conduction System of the Heart

• SA (sinoatrial) node → AV (atrioventricular) node → His-Purkinje cells.
• All cells in these areas have what is known as *automaticity* (they can depolarize spontaneously).

• The SA node is the pacemaker because it can spontaneously depolarize easier and faster than the others.

Action Potential

• An electrical impulse consisting of a self-propagating series of polarizations and depolarizations.
• Caused by ions (sodium and potassium) leaking into or out of a cardiac cell.
• Responsible for the release of calcium into the myocardial actin and myosin.
• Therefore responsible for coupling excitation with contraction.
• An electrical phenomenon (depolarization) coupled with a physiologic phenomenon (heart muscle contraction).

Nursing Consideration

• Some of the classes of antidysrhythmics are more toxic than others, but astute nursing assessment and close monitoring are required for all.
• Close monitoring requires ECGs, but heart rate, blood pressure, heart rhythms, general well-being, skin color, temperature, and heart and breath sounds are also important factors.
• It is important to assess the plasma drug levels and to check for possible drug interactions and certain medical conditions before the use of antidysrhythmics.
• Serum potassium levels should be measured before the initiation of therapy.
• Blood pressure, pulse rate, and intake and output amounts should all be measured and documented before the initiation of therapy.
• The therapeutic response to antidysrhythmics includes a decrease in blood pressure in hypertensive patients, a decrease in edema, and a regular pulse rate or pulse rate without major irregularities or improved regularity as opposed to the irregularity that existed before therapy.
• Patient education about the dosage schedule and the side effects to report to the physician is important to safe and effective therapy.

REVIEW QUESTIONS

1. Which of the following symptoms should the patient report to the physician immediately when taking amiodarone?
   a. Dyspnea
   b. Photosensitivity
   c. Muscle weakness
   d. Capillary refill less than 5 seconds.
2. Adverse reactions associated with Class 1a antidysrhthmics include which of the following:
   a. Glycosuria.
   b. Crystalluria.
   c. Cinchonism.
   d. Dysphagia.
3. Side effects associated with the use of procainamide include all of the following except:
   a. Diarrhea.
   b. Ventricular dysrhythmias.
   c. Systemic lupus erythematous.
   d. Photosensitivity

4. Which of the following nursing diagnoses is most appropriate for patients taking antidysrhythmics?
   a. Risk for infection related to adverse effects
   b. Fluid volume excess related to pulmonary edema as a side effect
   c. Risk for self-injury related to side effect of orthostatic hypotension
   d. Disturbed body image related to changes in sexual functioning due to adverse effects of the medication.
5. Your patient has suffered an acute myocardial infarction. Which of the following drugs would most likely be ordered to prevent acute ventricular dysrhythmias?
   a. Digitalis
   b. Lidocaine
   c. Adenosine
   d. Furosemide

For Answers see www.harcourthealth.com/MERLIN/Lilley/.

CRITICAL THINKING Activities

1. J.K. is a 68-year-old man who has undergone coronary artery bypass grafting 1 day before. Some irregular heartbeats (dysrhythmias) have developed, and he has been put on procainamide, infused at a rate of 4 mg/min. The nephrologist is concerned about the total volume your patient is receiving because his urine output is very low and asks you to determine how much fluid the patient is receiving a day from his procainamide infusion. The standard procainamide concentration at your hospital is 1 mg/ml.
   a. How many milliliters of fluid is J.K. receiving from his procainamide infusion per day?
   b. The nephrologist would like to keep J.K.'s fluid intake to less than 1000 ml/day. What concentration will accomplish this: 1, 2, 4, or 8 mg/ml.

2. What is the nature of the therapeutic response you would expect in a patient prescribed a diuretic and antidysrhythmic to treat CHF? Explain your answer.
3. Mrs. T.L. has been discharged to home on quinidine for the treatment of ventricular ectopy. What instructions are crucial for her to understand before her discharge?
4. Amiodarone (Cordarone) has many precautions associated with its use. Discuss problems that you would warn your patient about, especially since summer is around the corner.

For Answers see www.harcourthealth.com/MERLIN/Lilley/.

bibliography

Albanese J, Nutz P: *Mosby's 2001 nursing drug reference and review cards*, St Louis, 2001, Mosby.

American Hospital Formulary Service: *AHFS drug information*, Bethesda, Md, 2000, American Society of Health-System Pharmacists.

Anderson PO, Knoben JE, Troutman WG: *Handbook of clinical drug data 1999-2000*, ed 9, New York, 1999, McGraw-Hill.

Chase S, Cerrato PL: Pharmacology in practice: antiarrhythmics, *RN* 60(5):41, 1997.

Hayes DD: Bradycardia: keeping the current flowing, *Nursing 97* 27(6):50, 1997.

Johns Hopkins Hospital, Department of Pediatrics et al: *The Harriet Lane handbook*, ed 15, St Louis, 2000, Mosby.

Keen JH: *Critical care and emergency drug reference*, ed 3, St Louis, 1996, Mosby.

Lazzara D: Dealing confidently with deadly arrhythmias, *Nursing 98* 28(1):41, 1998.

Mancini ME, Kaye W: AEDs: changing the way you respond to cardiac arrest, *AJN* 99(5):26, 1999.

Mosby's GenRx: a comprehensive reference for generic and brand drugs, ed 10, St Louis, 2000, Mosby.

Skidmore-Roth L: *Mosby's 2001 nursing drug reference,* St Louis, 2001, Mosby.

Turkoski BB: *Drug information handbook for nursing 1999-2000: including assessment, administration, monitoring guidelines, and patient education,* ed 2, Cleveland, 1999, Lexi-Comp.

United States Pharmacopeial Convention: *USP DI: drug information for the health care professional, vol. 1,* ed 20, Englewood, Colo, 2000, Micromedex.

Activity

Remember to check the **Online Worksheet** for additional learning opportunities: **www.harcourthealth.com/MERLIN/Lilley/**

Chapter 22

Antianginal Agents

objectives

www.harcourthealth.com/MERLIN/Lilley/

When you reach the end of this chapter, you should be able to do the following:

Look for this symbol for topics covered in the **Online Worksheet** Activity

1 Define *angina*.

2 Explain how cellular ischemia is responsible for causing angina.

3 Discuss how antianginal agents such as nitrates, beta-blockers, and calcium channel blockers decrease anginal pain.

4 Identify the various dosage forms of nitrates, beta-blockers, and calcium channel blockers, along with their indications, advantages, and cautions.

5 Develop a nursing care plan that includes all phases of the nursing process related to the administration and treatment of angina with nitrates, nitrites, beta-blockers, and calcium channel blockers.

6 Evaluate the therapeutic versus the adverse and toxic effects of the different antianginal agents.

drug profiles

○━**atenolol,** p. 342
diltiazem, p. 344
isosorbide dinitrate, p. 339
isosorbide mononitrate, p. 339

○━**metoprolol,** p. 343
○━**nifedipine,** p. 345
○━**nitroglycerin,** p. 339
pentaerythrital tetranitrate, p. 340
verapamil, p. 345

○━Key drug.

glossary

Angina pectoris (an ji′ nə, an′ jə nə\ pek to′ ris) Chest pain occurring when the level of oxygen and energy-rich nutrients in the blood is insufficient to meet the demands of the heart. (p. 336)

Chronic stable angina Chest pain that has atherosclerosis as its primary cause. (p. 337)

Coronary arteries Arteries that deliver oxygen to the heart muscle. (p. 336)

Coronary artery disease Any one of the abnormal conditions that can affect the arteries of the heart and produce various pathologic effects, especially a reduced supply of oxygen and nutrients to the myocardium. (p. 336)

Ischemia (is ke′ me ə) Poor blood supply to an organ. (p. 336)

Ischemic heart disease Poor blood supply to the heart. (p. 336)

Reflex tachycardia (tak′ i kahr′ de ə) A rapid heart sinus rhythm caused by a variety of autonomic nervous system effects, such as blood pressure changes, fever, or emotional stress. (p. 338)

Unstable angina Early stage of progressive coronary artery disease. (p. 337)

Vasospastic angina (vas′ o spas′ tik) Ischemia-induced myocardial chest pain caused by spasms of the coronary arteries. (p. 337)

ANGINA AND CORONARY ARTERY DISEASE

The heart is a very efficient organ, but it is very demanding in an aerobic sense because it requires a large supply of oxygen to meet the incredible demand placed on it. Pumping blood to all the tissues and organs of the body is a difficult job. The heart's much-needed oxygen supply is delivered to the heart muscle by means of the **coronary arteries.** However, when the supply of oxygen and energy-rich nutrients in blood is insufficient to meet the demands of the heart, the heart muscle (or myocardium) aches. This is called **angina pectoris,** or chest pain. Poor blood supply to an organ is referred to as **ischemia.** When the organ involved is the heart, the condition is called **ischemic heart disease.**

Ischemic heart disease is the number one killer in the United States today, and the primary cause is disease of the coronary arteries resulting from atherosclerosis. When atherosclerotic plaques form in the lumens (channels) of these vessels, they become narrow. The supply of oxygen and energy-rich nutrients needed for the heart to meet the demands placed on it is then decreased. This disorder is called **coronary artery disease**

(CAD). The result of CAD and of ischemic heart disease is a myocardial infarction (MI), or heart attack. It occurs when blood flow through the coronary arteries to the myocardium is completely blocked, so that the heart muscle cannot receive any of the substances necessary for normal function. If this process is not reversed immediately, that area of the heart will die and become necrotic and nonfunctioning.

The rate at which the heart pumps and the strength of each heart beat (contractility) also place oxygen demands on this organ. There are many substances and situations that can increase heart rate and contractility and thus increase oxygen demand. Some of these substances are caffeine, exercise, and stress. These substances or situations result in stimulation of the sympathetic nervous system (SNS), which results in increased heart rate and contractility. In an already overburdened heart such as one in a patient with CAD, this can worsen the balance between myocardial oxygen supply and demand and result in angina. Some drugs that are used to treat angina are aimed at correcting the imbalance between myocardial oxygen supply and demand by decreasing heart rate and contractility. Beta-blockers and calcium channel blockers (CCBs) are two examples.

The pain of angina results from the following process: Under ischemic conditions when the myocardium is deprived of oxygen, the heart shifts to anaerobic metabolism to meet its energy needs. One of the by-products of anaerobic metabolism is lactic acid. The accumulation of lactic acid and other metabolic by-products causes the pain receptors surrounding the heart to be stimulated, producing the heart pain known as angina. It is the same pathophysiologic mechanism responsible for causing the soreness in skeletal muscles after vigorous exercise.

There are three classic types of chest pain, or angina pectoris. **Chronic stable angina** has atherosclerosis as its primary cause. *Classic angina* and *effort angina* are other names for it. Chronic stable angina can be triggered by either exertion or stress (cold, fear, or emotions). Smoking or the consumption of alcohol, coffee, or drugs that stimulate the SNS can exacerbate it. The pain of chronic stable angina is commonly intense but subsides within 15 minutes with either rest or drug therapy. **Unstable angina** is usually the early stage of progressive CAD. It often culminates in MI in subsequent years. For this reason, unstable angina is also called *preinfarction angina*. Another term for this type of angina is *crescendo angina* because the pain increases in severity and in the frequency of attacks. In the later stages, pain may even occur while the patient is at rest. **Vasospastic angina** results from spasms of the layer of smooth muscle that surrounds the atherosclerotic coronary arteries. This pain often happens at rest and without any precipitating cause. It does, however, seem to follow a regular pattern, usually occurring at the same time of day. This type of angina is also called *Prinzmetal's angina* or *variant angina*. Dysrhythmias and electrocardiogram (ECG) changes often accompany these anginal attacks.

ANTIANGINAL DRUGS

Recent advances in pharmacotherapy have resulted in the development of a host of new antianginal agents that have been approved for clinical use. The three main classes of drugs used to treat angina pectoris are the nitrates/nitrites, beta-blockers, CCBs. Their various therapeutic effects are summarized in Table 22-1. There are three main therapeutic objectives of antianginal drug therapy. It must (1) minimize the frequency of attacks and decrease the duration and intensity of the anginal pain; (2) improve the patient's functional capacity with as few side effects as possible; and (3) prevent or delay the worst possible outcome, MI. The object of antianginal drug therapy is to increase blood flow to ischemic myocardium, decrease myocardial oxygen demand, or accomplish both. Figure 22-1 illustrates how drug therapy works to alleviate angina.

Table 22-1   Antianginal Agents: Therapeutic Effects

Therapeutic Effect	Nitrates	Beta-Blockers*	Calcium Channel Blockers		
			Nifedipine	**Verapamil**	**Diltiazem**
SUPPLY					
Blood flow	↑↑	↑	↑↑↑	↑↑↑	↑↑↑
Duration of diastole	0	↑↑↑	0/↑	↑↑↑	↑↑
DEMAND					
Preload†	↓↓↓	↑	↓/0	0	0/↓
Afterload	↓	0/↓	↓↓↓	↓↓	↓↓
Contractility	0	↓↓↓	↓	↓↓↓	↓↓
Heart rate	0/↑	↓↓↓	0/↑	↓↓	↓↓

↓ = Decrease ↑ = increase; 0 = little or no effect.
*In particular those that are cardioselective and do not have intrinsic sympathomimetic activity (ISA).
†*Preload* is pressure in the heart caused by blood volume. The nitrates effectively move part of this blood out of the heart and into blood vessels thereby decreasing preload or filling pressure.

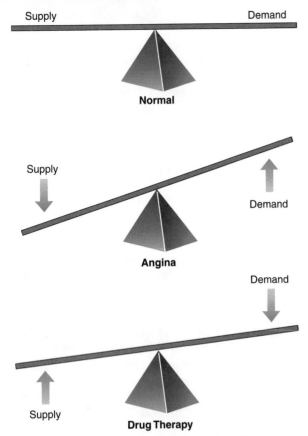

Fig. 22-1 Benefit of drug therapy for angina with increasing oxygen supply and decreasing oxygen demands.

NITRATES/NITRITES

Nitrates, and in particular nitroglycerin, have long been the mainstay of both the prophylaxis and treatment for angina and other cardiac problems. This class of antianginal agents was first discovered by Sir Thomas Lauder Brunton in England, who noted that amyl nitrite was just as effective as venesection in the management of angina. A few years later, a chemically related substance, glyceryl trinitrate (nitroglycerin), was successfully isolated and used for this purpose. Today there are several chemical derivatives of these early precursors, all of which are organic nitrate esters. They are available in a wide variety of preparations, including sublingual, buccal, chewable, and oral tablets; capsules; ointments; patches; inhalable sprays; and IV solutions. Following is a list of the rapid- and long-acting nitrates available for clinical use:

- Rapid-acting agents
  - amyl nitrite
  - nitroglycerin
- Long-acting agents
  - isosorbide dinitrate
  - isosorbide mononitrate

Mechanism of Action

Nitrates dilate all blood vessels, but they primarily affect the blood vessels of the venous circulation. However, at low doses they do have slight arterial vasodilator properties. This venodilation is the result of relaxation of the smooth muscle that surrounds veins. Nitrates also have a potent dilating effect on the coronary arteries.

Drug Effects

If the nitrate-induced venodilation just described occurs rapidly, this causes the cardiovascular system to overcompensate and increase its heart rate, a condition referred to as **reflex tachycardia.** This occurs because the venodilation causes most of the blood to be in the venous circulation and out of the heart. The heart then falsely senses that there has been a dramatic loss of blood volume. If this were true, it would be appropriate for the heart to accelerate its rate to move the smaller volume of blood more quickly throughout the body. The heart soon realizes, however, that there has not been a loss of blood volume but that the volume of blood missing in the heart is now in the periphery (e.g., venous system) and slows its rate back to normal.

Therapeutic Uses

Nitrate-induced vasodilation has many therapeutic effects (see Table 22-1). By causing venodilation, the nitrates bring about a decrease in venous return and in turn a lower left ventricular, end-diastolic volume (preload) and pressure. Left ventricular systolic wall tension is also reduced, and myocardial oxygen demand is thereby lowered.

The nitrates cause both large and small coronary vessels to dilate. Often this causes blood to be redistributed and therefore oxygen to be delivered to previously ischemic tissue (myocardium). The nitrates also alleviate coronary artery spasms (vasospastic angina). In addition, coronary arteries that are diseased and have been narrowed by atherosclerosis can also be dilated as long as there is smooth muscle surrounding the coronary artery. Exercise-induced constriction or spasms of atherosclerotic coronary arteries can be reversed or even prevented by nitrates.

Side Effects and Adverse Effects

Nitrates are well tolerated, and most side effects are usually transient and involve the cardiovascular system. The most frequent undesirable effect is headache, which usually diminishes in intensity and frequency soon after the start of therapy. Other cardiovascular effects include tachycardia and postural hypotension. Methemoglobinemia is an extremely rare adverse effect and usually occurs in patients with an inherited genetic propensity for the condition. Topical nitrate dosage forms can produce various contact dermatitides, but these are actually reactions to the dosage delivery system and not to the drug (nitroglycerin).

Tolerance to the nitrates' antianginal effects can occur in some patients, especially those on long-acting formulations or taking nitrates around the clock. To prevent this, a regular nitrate-free period allows certain enzymatic pathways to replenish themselves. A common reg-

DOSAGES Selected Antianginal Nitrate Coronary Vasodilators

agent	pharmacologic class	dosage range	purpose
isosorbide dinitrate (Isordil, Sorbitrate, Dilatrate SR)		*Adult* Chewable/sublingual: 2.5-10 mg prn PO: 5-30 mg 2-3/day and 40-80 mg q8-12h for sustained-release formulations	
isosorbide mononitrate (Imdur, Monoket, ISMO)	Antianginal nitrate coronary vasodilator	*Adult* PO: 20 mg bid given 7 hr apart and 60-120 mg once daily for sustained-release formulations	Angina
nitroglycerin (Nitro-Bid, Nitrostat, Nitrol, others)		*Adult* Ointment: 1-2 inch ribbon q8h, up to 4-5 inch ribbon q4h PO: 2.5-6.5 mg 2-3 times daily (during the day) Spray: 0.4-0.8 mg onto or under the tongue prn Buccal: 1 mg q3-5h prn place tablet between lip and gum	

imen with transdermal patches is to remove them at night for 8 hours and apply a new patch in the morning. This has been shown to prevent tolerance to the beneficial effects of nitrates.

Interactions

Nitrate antianginal drugs can produce additive hypotensive effects when taken in combination with alcohol, beta-blockers, CCBs, or phenothiazines.

Dosages

The organic nitrates are available in an array of forms and doses. See the dosages table above for more information.

drug profiles

isosorbide dinitrate

Isosorbide dinitrate (Isordil, Sorbitrate, Dilatrate-SR) is an organic nitrate and therefore a powerful explosive. It exerts the same effects as the other nitrates. When isosorbide dinitrate is metabolized in the liver, it is broken down into two active metabolites, both of which have the same therapeutic actions as isosorbide dinitrate itself. Isosorbide dinitrate is used for the acute relief of angina pectoris, for prophylaxis in situations likely to provoke angina attacks (e.g., exercise), and for the long-term prophylaxis of angina pectoris. The contraindications to isosorbide dinitrate use are the same as those of nitroglycerin, and it is also a pregnancy category C agent. Isosorbide dinitrate is only available orally as 40-mg extended-release capsules and tablets; 5-, 10-, 20-, 30-, and 40-mg tablets; 5- and 10-mg chewable tablets; and 2.5-, 5-, and 10-mg sublingual tablets. Refer to the dosages table above for the recommended dosages.

PHARMACOKINETICS

HALF-LIFE	ONSET	PEAK	DURATION
Variable	1 hr	Unknown	4-6 hr

isosorbide mononitrate

Isosorbide mononitrate (Imdur, Monoket, ISMO) is one of the two active metabolites of isosorbide dinitrate, but it has no active metabolites. As a result of these qualities, it produces a more consistent, steady therapeutic response, with less variation in the response within the same patient and between patients. Its contraindications are the same as those of nitroglycerin, and it is also a pregnancy category C agent. It is only available in oral formulations: two regular-release products, ISMO and Monoket, and a sustained-release form, Indur. The ISMO and Monoket are taken twice a day, with 7 hours the recommended interval between the first and second dose. This 7-hour interval is believed to delay the development of nitrate tolerance, a limitation to long-term nitrate therapy. ISMO is available as 20-mg tablets and Monoket as 10- and 20-mg tablets. Imdur is available as a 30-, 60-, and 120-mg tablets and is taken only once a day. Refer to the dosages table above for dosage recommendations.

PHARMACOKINETICS

HALF-LIFE	ONSET	PEAK	DURATION
5 hr	15-30 min	0.5-1 hr	5-12 hr

nitroglycerin

Nitroglycerin is the prototypical nitrate and is made by many pharmaceutical companies, so it goes by many trade names (e.g., Nitro-Bid, Nitrostat, and Nitrong). It has traditionally been the most important drug used in the symptomatic treatment of ischemic heart conditions such as angina. Nitroglycerin is contraindicated in patients with a known hypersensitivity to it, and in those suffering from increased intracranial pressure, inadequate cerebral perfusion, constrictive pericarditis, pericardial tamponade, severe hypotension, or severe anemia. It is classified as a pregnancy category C agent.

When given orally, nitroglycerin goes to the liver to be metabolized before it can be active in the body. During this process a very large amount of the nitroglycerin is removed from the circulation. This is called a *large first-pass effect*. For this reason, nitroglycerin is administered by many other routes to bypass the first-pass effect. It also is available in many formulations and has proved useful for the treatment of a variety of cardiovascular conditions. The sublingual and buccal routes of administration are employed for the treatment of chest pain or angina of acute onset, or for the prevention of angina when patients find themselves in situations likely to provoke an attack. These routes are advantageous for ameliorating these acute conditions because the area under the tongue and inside the cheek is highly vascular. This means that the nitroglycerin is absorbed quickly and directly into the bloodstream and hence its therapeutic effects occur rapidly.

Sublingual nitroglycerin is available as 0.15-, 0.3-, 0.4-, 0.6-mg tablets. Buccal extended-release tablets are available in 1-, 2-, and 3-mg doses. Nitroglycerin also comes as a 0.4-mg/per metered dose aerosol that is sprayed under the tongue. Nitroglycerin is available in an IV form that is used for blood pressure control in the perioperative hypertensive patient as well as for the treatment of ischemic pain, congestive heart failure (CHF), or the pulmonary edema associated with acute MI. These IV infusions are available in concentrations of 0.5 or 5 mg/ml. Oral and topical dosage formulations are used for the long-term prophylactic management of angina pectoris. The oral forms are available as 2.5-, 6.5-, 9-, and 13-mg extended-release capsules and as 2.6- and 6.5-mg extended-release tablets. Topical formulations offer the same advantages as the sublingual and buccal formulations in that they also bypass the liver and the first-pass effect. They also allow for the continuous slow delivery of nitroglycerin, which supplies a steady dose of nitroglycerin to the patient. The topical delivery forms are available as a 2% ointment or as 0.1-, 0.2-, 0.3-, 0.4-, 0.6, and 0.8-mg/hr patches that supply 24 hours' worth of nitroglycerin. See the dosages table on p. 339 for the recommended dosages.

PHARMACOKINETICS

HALF-LIFE	ONSET	PEAK	DURATION
1-4 min	SL: 2-3 min	Unknown	0.5-1 hr*

*For short-acting oral preparations.

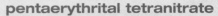

pentaerythrital tetranitrate

Pentaerythrital tetranitrate (Peritrate) is metabolized to several active metabolites and is recommended only for the long-term prophylactic management of angina. It is not effective for the acute treatment of anginal attacks. It must be taken three to four times a day, and patient response varies considerably. For these reasons, pentaerythrital tetranitrate and erythrityl tetranitrate are seldom used. They offer few benefits compared with the newer nitrate formulations, which have comparatively reliable pharmacodynamic characteristics and only need to be taken once or twice a day. Extended-release formulations of pentaerythrital tetranitrate are available, but these still do not confer the pharmacodynamic advantages of mononitrates. Contraindications to its use are similar to those of the other nitrates, and it is also a pregnancy category C agent. It is available in oral forms as 10-, 20-, and 40-mg regular-release tablets; 30-, 45-, and 80-mg extended-release capsules; and 80-mg extended release tablets.

PHARMACOKINETICS

HALF-LIFE	ONSET	PEAK	DURATION
Unknown	30 min	Unknown	4-5 hr

BETA-BLOCKERS

Beta-adrenergic blockers, more commonly referred to as beta-blockers, have become the mainstay in the treatment of a wide range of cardiovascular diseases. Most available beta-blockers demonstrate antianginal efficacy, although not all have been approved for this use. Those beta-blockers approved as antianginal agents are atenolol, metoprolol, nadolol, and propranolol.

The main beneficial effect of beta-blockers in the treatment of angina is slowing the heart rate and decreasing contractility. These two effects have two favorable physiologic results. First, decreasing the heart rate decreases myocardial oxygen demand, because a rapidly beating heart requires more energy and oxygen than a slowly or normally beating heart. In addition, this increases oxygen delivery to the myocardium. Second, by decreasing contractility, the beta-blockers help conserve energy, or decrease demand. As mentioned in previous chapters, beta-blockers bind to and thus block the beta-adrenergic receptors, which would otherwise bind to the SNS neurotransmitters epinephrine and norepinephrine. These catecholamines would ordinarily be released in greater quantities in the setting of exercise or stress to stimulate the heart muscle to contract further, and the physiologic act of contractility requires energy in the form of adenosine triphosphate (ATP), oxygen, and many other vital substances. Therefore any decrease in the energy demands on the heart would be beneficial in alleviating conditions such as angina, in which the supply of these substances is already deficient because of the ischemia.

Beta-blockers are most effective in the treatment of typical exertional angina. This is because the usual physiologic increase in the heart rate and systolic blood pressure that occurs during exercise or stress is blunted, thereby decreasing the myocardial oxygen demand.

One drawback to the use of beta-blockers is their negative effect on physical performance. Fatigue and lethargy are the most common patient complaints and may be due to either a decreased cardiac output or a direct CNS effect.

There are a number of contraindications to the use of beta-blockers, including bronchial asthma and serious conduction disturbances. They should be used with caution in patients with systolic CHF. Additionally, several common yet sometimes subtle conditions in elderly patients may be exacerbated by beta-blockers. These include mental depression and peripheral vascular disease. The decision to initiate antiischemic therapy with a beta-blocker in any patient should therefore be made carefully, weighing both the risks and the benefits.

Mechanism of Action

As previously mentioned, beta-blockers are effective in the treatment of angina because they slow the heart rate and decrease contractility by binding to and blocking the beta-adrenergic receptors located on the heart's conduction system and throughout the myocardium. This has the ultimate effect of decreasing the work load of the heart.

Slowing the heart rate is very beneficial in a patient with ischemic heart disease because the coronary arteries have more time to fill with oxygen-rich and nutrient-rich blood when the heart is relaxed during diastole and to deliver these vital substances to the myocardium. At a normal heart rate of 60 to 80 beats/min, the heart spends 60% to 70% of the time in diastole. As the heart rate increases in the setting of stress or exercise, however, the heart spends more and more time in systole and less and less time in diastole. The physiologic consequence is that the coronary arteries receive increasingly less blood and eventually the myocardium becomes ischemic.

In an ischemic heart the increased demand of increasing contractility also leads to more ischemia and chest pain. By blocking this mechanism, a beta-blocker causes contractility and hence the energy needs to be decreased. This shifts the supply-and-demand back toward a more balanced ratio.

Drug Effects

The primary drug effects of the beta-blockers are related to the cardiovascular system. As covered in previous chapters, the predominant beta-adrenergic receptors in the heart are the beta$_1$-adrenergic receptors. They are responsible for the conduction effects of the conduction system. When they are blocked by beta-blockers, the rate at which the pacemaker (sinoatrial [SA] node) fires decreases, and the time it takes for the node to recover increases. The re-

research

More Consultation Enhances Care for Heart Attack Patients

Research is supporting consultations with cardiologists for patients who are being treated for heart attacks. Consultation by a generalist to a cardiologist may improve the quality of care for patients who suffer or are suffering from an acute myocardial infarction (AMI) because the cardiologist is more likely than the generalist to order the "life-saving" medications. This study comes at a time when there are many "cost-containing" measures, including less focus on the "more expensive specialist" versus the generalist physician. It shows that the debate on "cost-efficiency" should not overlook results from research conducted several years ago. Chart reviews of 1716 AMI patients at 22 Minnesota hospitals between 1992 and 1993 showed that patients treated by a cardiologist or a generalist who consulted regularly with a cardiologist were more likely to receive life-saving medications such as thrombolytics, aspirin, beta-blockers, and lidocaine. In addition, there was no variation in the "care" practiced with patients by a generalist consulting with a cardiologist and those cared for by a cardiologist. Money should not be the issue when it comes to saving lives, but the issue should be with the use of the more appropriate physicians and modes of care. ■

Data from Willison DJ et al: Consultation between cardiologists and generalists in the management of acute myocardial infarction: implications for quality of care, *Arch Intern Med* 158(16):1778, 1998.

sult is a decrease in heart rate. Beta-blockers slow conduction through the atrioventricular (AV) node as well, which contributes to slowing the heart rate.

Beta-blockers may also suppress renin activity and the renin-aldosterone-angiotensin system. Renin is a potent vasoconstrictor that the kidneys release when they sense they are not being adequately perfused and receiving enough blood. When beta-blockers inhibit its release, the blood vessels to and in the kidney dilate, which decreases blood pressure.

Therapeutic Uses

The primary therapeutic effects of the beta-blockers are their antihypertensive, antianginal, and cardioprotective effects, the latter of value after an MI.

Beta-blockers produce their antihypertensive effects either by blocking both peripheral and cardiac beta-adrenergic receptors, by decreasing sympathetic outflow from the CNS, by suppressing renal renin release, or by a combination of these processes.

The antianginal effects of the beta-blockers are related to the supply-and-demand imbalance present in the setting of ischemic heart disease and angina. In this condition blood supply is decreased because the blood vessels have been narrowed by atherosclerosis or vasospasm. This has the overall effect of increasing the work load of the heart (increased demand). The two alone or together cause an imbalance between the needed oxygen supply and demand, which the beta-blockers rectify by slowing the heart rate and decreasing contractility.

There are many therapeutic effects of beta-blockers after an MI. After a patient has suffered an MI, there is a high level of circulating catecholamines (norepinephrine and epinephrine), the release of which has been triggered by the myocardial damage resulting from the infarction. These catecholamines will produce several harmful consequences if their actions go unopposed. They essentially irritate the heart. They cause the heart rate to increase, causing a further imbalance in the supply-and-demand ratio, and they irritate the conduction system of the heart to the point where dysrhythmias may ensue that can be fatal. The beta-blockers block all these harmful effects and have been shown to improve the chances for survival in such patients. They should be given to all patients in the acute stages after an MI, unless contraindicated.

Side Effects and Adverse Effects

The side effects of the beta-blockers are related to their ability to block beta-adrenergic receptors in areas where they are not intended to. For example, the smooth muscle that surrounds many blood vessels throughout the circulation as well as the airways in the lungs has beta$_2$-adrenergic receptors on its surface. When these beta$_2$-adrenergic receptors are stimulated, they cause the smooth muscle to relax. When this occurs in blood vessels, they dilate and blood pressure decreases. When this occurs in the airways of the lungs, they dilate and oxygen delivery increases. A beta-blocker that blocks beta$_2$-adrenergic receptors thus causes the opposite of these physiologic actions, such that blood vessels constrict and hypertension occurs or the airways constrict and the delivery of oxygen decreases. This may in turn exacerbate a patient's underlying asthma or chronic obstructive pulmonary disease (COPD). The most common beta-blocker related side effects and adverse effects are listed in Table 22-2.

Interactions

There are many important drug interactions that involve the beta-blockers. The more common and important of these are listed in Table 22-3.

Table 22-2 Beta-Blockers: Adverse Effects

Body System	Side/Adverse Effects
Cardiovascular	Bradycardia, hypotension, second- or third-degree heart block, heart failure
Central nervous system	Dizziness, fatigue, mental depression, lethargy, drowsiness, unusual dreams
Metabolic	Alter glucose and lipid metabolism
Other	Wheezing, dyspnea, impotence

Dosages

For information on the dosages of selected beta-blockers used for the treatment of angina, see the dosages table on p. 343.

drug profiles

As pointed out earlier, beta-blockers are the mainstay in the treatment of a wide range of cardiovascular diseases, mainly hypertension, angina, and the acute stages of myocardial infarction. The beta-blockers are all classified as pregnancy category C agents except acebutolol, pindolol, and sotalol. Contraindications to their use include hypersensitivity to the particular agent, cardiac failure or shock, second- or third-degree heart block, bronchospastic disease (primarily pertains to use of nonspecific beta-blockers), and hypotension. Beta-blockers can be used in the treatment of CHF. The three most commonly used are carvedilol, metoprolol, and bisoprolol. The drug profile for carvedilol is in Chapter 17 on p. 271.

⚬═atenolol

Atenolol (Tenormin) is a cardioselective beta$_1$-adrenergic receptor blocker and is indicated for the prophylactic treatment of angina pectoris. Atenolol's use after an MI has been shown to lead to a decrease in mortality. It is available in a parenteral form, which is an advantage because often during and immediately after an MI, blood flow to the gastrointestinal tract is poor and patients may be intubated. This rules out enteral administration of an agent. In its parenteral form atenolol is available as a 0.5-mg/ml injection. It is also available orally as 25-, 50-, and 100-mg tablets. Re-

Table 22-3 Beta-Blockers: Drug Interactions

Drug	Mechanism	Result
Anticholinergics	Antagonize	Decrease beta-blocker
cimetidine	Decreases metabolism	Increases propranolol and metoprolol levels and pharmacodynamic effects
Diuretics and antihypertensives	Additive	Hypotension
phenothiazine	Additive hypotensive effects	Hypotension and cardiac arrest

fer to the dosages table on p. 343 for the recommended dosages. Pregnancy category C.

PHARMACOKINETICS

HALF-LIFE	ONSET	PEAK	DURATION
6-7 hr	1 hr	2-4 hr	24 hr

*All values are for PO atenolol.

metoprolol

Metoprolol (Lopressor) is also a cardioselective beta$_1$-adrenergic receptor blocker that is used for the prophylactic treatment of angina and has many of the same characteristics as atenolol. It has shown similar efficacy in reducing mortality in the victims of MI and in treating angina. It is available both orally and parenterally. Orally it is available as 50- and 100-mg tablets and as 50-, 100-, and 200-mg extended-release tablets. Parenterally it is available as a 1-mg/ml injection. Refer to the dosages table below for recommended dosages. Pregnancy category C.

PHARMACOKINETICS

HALF-LIFE	ONSET	PEAK	DURATION
3-7 hr	1 hr	2-4 hr	13-19 hr

CALCIUM CHANNEL BLOCKERS

CCBs are the most recent antianginal drugs to come available. The three main classes are phenylalkylamine, benzothiazepine, and dihydropyridine, traditionally represented by verapamil, diltiazem, and nifedipine, respectively. Although they all block calcium channels, their chemical structures and therefore their mechanisms of action differ slightly. There are more than nine CCBs available today, with more on the way. Those that are used for the treatment of chronic stable angina are amlodipine, diltiazem, nicardipine, nifedipine, verapamil, and bepridil.

CCBs affect both myocardial oxygen demand and supply. They decrease myocardial oxygen demand by causing peripheral arterial vasodilation and by a negative inotropic action (i.e., reduced myocardial contractility). CCBs may be particularly effective for the treatment of coronary artery spasms secondary to the relaxation of the smooth muscles in the vessel walls. However, they may not be as effective as beta-blockers in blunting exercise-induced elevations in heart rate and blood pressure.

Mechanism of Action

The cardiovascular effects of CCBs include depressing the automaticity of and conduction through the SA and AV nodes, decreasing myocardial contractility, and decreasing peripheral and coronary artery tone. Verapamil and diltiazem will also decrease heart rate. Their most dramatic antianginal effects, however, are secondary to their effects on myocardial contractility and the smooth muscle tone of peripheral and coronary arteries.

Calcium plays an important role in the excitation-contraction coupling process that occurs in the heart and vascular smooth muscle cells. It is a vital component in the contraction of any muscle, whether it is smooth muscle or skeletal muscle. Preventing calcium from entering into and interacting in the contraction process therefore prevents muscle contraction, and the result is relaxation. Relaxation of the smooth muscles that surround the coronary arteries cause them to dilate. This increases blood flow to the heart, which in turn increases the oxygen supply and helps shift the supply-and-demand ratio back to normal. This also occurs in the arteries throughout the body, resulting in a decrease in the force (systemic vascular resistance) that the heart has to exert itself against when delivering blood to the body (afterload). Decreasing afterload reduces the work load of the heart and therefore reduces myocardial oxygen demand. This is the primary beneficial antianginal effect of the dihydropyridine CCBs, and of nifedipine in particular.

Both diltiazem and verapamil have dramatic effects on the cells of the cardiac conduction system, or calcium channels, which are discussed in depth in Chapter 21. It is these channels that are blocked when these CCBs are given. The electrophysiologic effect of this blockade is a slowing of AV node conduction and a prolonging of the

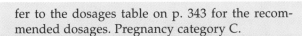

agent	pharmacologic class	dosage range		purpose
atenolol (Tenormin)	Beta$_1$-blocker	*Adult* PO: 50-200 mg/day as a single dose		Angina
metoprolol (Lopressor)	Beta$_1$-blocker	*Adult* PO: 100-400 mg/day in 2 divided doses		Angina

DOSAGES Selected Beta-Adrenergic Agents

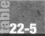

Body System	Side/Adverse Effect
Cardiovascular	Hypotension, palpitations, tachycardia or bradycardia, heart failure
Gastrointestinal	Constipation, nausea
Other	Dermatitis, dyspnea, rash, flushing, peripheral edema, wheezing

TABLE 22-4 Calcium Channel Blockers: Adverse Effects

TABLE 22-5 Calcium Channel Blockers: Drug Interactions

Drug	Mechanism	Result
Beta-blockers	Additive effects	Bradycardia and AV block
Digoxin	Interferes with elimination of digoxin	Can increase digoxin levels
H$_2$ blockers	Decrease clearance	Elevated levels of calcium channel blockers

refractory period, also discussed in Chapter 21. This is very beneficial, especially in the setting of atrial fibrillation or flutter, because if these rapidly firing impulses are allowed to pass unhindered to the ventricles, the result could be life-threatening ventricular fibrillation or tachycardia.

Drug Effects

The effects of CCBs are mostly limited to the cardiovascular system. They are a very safe and effective class of drugs with little if any extracardiovascular effects. As previously mentioned, by relaxing vascular smooth muscle, they cause a decrease in systemic vascular resistance and in turn a decrease in afterload. They also affect the cardiac conduction system by slowing AV node conduction and prolonging the effective refractory period. This helps the AV node function better as a filter that catches all the electrical impulses from the atria and slows them down.

Therapeutic Uses

The therapeutic benefits of the CCBs are numerous. Because of their very acceptable side effect and safety profile, they are considered first-line agents for the treatment of such conditions as angina, hypertension, and supraventricular tachycardia. They are also used for the short-term management of atrial fibrillation and flutter, migraines, Raynaud's disease, and subarachnoid hemorrhage. (Their use in these other conditions is described in the appropriate chapters.)

Side Effects and Adverse Effects

The side effects of the CCBs are very limited and primarily related to overexpression of their therapeutic effects. The most common of the CCB related adverse effects are listed in Table 22-4.

Interactions

The drug interactions that can occur with CCBs vary with the particular agent, although there are not actually many such interactions. One of particular note because of its beneficial effect is the interaction that occurs between cyclosporin and diltiazem. Because diltiazem interferes with the metabolism and elimination of cyclosporin (and thus cyclosporin is not broken down as quickly), smaller doses of the cyclosporin are needed. This is advantageous because one of cyclosporin's most frequent and devastat-

ing effects is that it can destroy the kidney and cause renal failure. Other important drug interactions that involve CCBs are listed in Table 22-5.

Dosages

For information on the dosages of selected CCBs, see the dosages table on p. 345.

Activity

drug profiles

CCBs are beneficial, highly effective agents used to treat angina. Because they have a greater affinity for peripheral vascular smooth muscle, the dihydropyridines are therefore more suited for the treatment of the hypertension that occurs in the setting of exertional angina. This class of CCBs has grown enormously. As a class they are very safe and effective. However, because of their potent peripheral vasodilating properties, they have a greater propensity to cause peripheral edema and reflex tachycardia. They are effective in the treatment of angina because they are potent decreasers of afterload. The benzothiazepines and phenylalkylamines have a greater affinity for the cells of the conduction system and the coronary arteries, making them more suited for the management of dysrhythmias and for the dilation of atherosclerotic coronary arteries. The various agents are listed in Table 22-6 according to their respective chemical category, although not all of the agents are used as antianginal drugs even though they all have antianginal effects.

CCBs are very safe and effective drugs with few contraindications. Some of the contraindications are hypersensitivity to them, second- or third-degree AV block, hypotension, acute MI, and cardiogenic shock. They are all classified as pregnancy category C agents.

diltiazem

Diltiazem (Cardizem, Dilacor, Tiazac) is the only benzothiazepine CCB. It has a particular affinity for the cardiac conduction system and is very ef-

DOSAGES Selected Calcium Channel-Blocking Antianginal Agents

agent	pharmacologic class	dosage range	purpose
diltiazem (Cardizem, Dilacor, Tiazac)		*Adult* PO: initial dose, 30 mg qid ac and hs; range 180-360 mg divided in 3-4 doses; or 1 daily for the CD (extended-release) capsule. Dosages of 480 mg/day may be needed.	
nifedipine (Adalat, Procardia)	Calcium channel blocker	*Adult* PO: 30-120 mg XL qd	Angina
verapamil (Calan, Covera HS,* Isoptin, Verelan)		*Adult* PO: initial dose, 80-120 mg tid; range 240-480 mg/day divided. Do not exceed 480 mg/day. *PO: 180 mg daily at bedtime; max 480 mg/day.	

fective for the oral treatment of angina pectoris resulting from coronary insufficiency and hypertension. It is one of the few CCBs that is also available parenterally, for which it is used for the treatment of atrial fibrillation and flutter along with paroxysmal supraventricular tachycardia. There are two sustained-delivery formulations of Cardizem, which can be confused with each other. There is a Cardizem SR, which is taken twice a day, and Cardizem CD, which is taken once a day. Two competing pharmaceutical companies make once-a-day diltiazem preparations called Dilacor XR and Tiazac. Oral forms of diltiazem are available as 30-, 60-, 90-, and 120-mg tablets; 60-, 90-, and 120-mg extended-release capsules; and 120-, 180-, 240-, and 300-mg dual-release capsules and tablets. Tiazac is available in 120-, 180-, 240-, 300-, 360-, and 420-mg extended-release capsules. Refer to the dosages table above for recommended dosages. Pregnancy category C.

PHARMACOKINETICS

HALF-LIFE	ONSET	PEAK	DURATION
3.5-9 hr	30 min	2-3 hr	Up to 24 hr*

*With extended dosage forms.

nifedipine

Nifedipine (Adalat, Adalat CC, Procardia, Procardia XL) was the first dihydropyridine CCB to be developed and introduced into clinical use. In the past, the liquid-filled nifedipine capsules have been squeezed to release their liquid contents under the tongue. This practice is no longer recommended because of several studies showing that it increases the mortality rate. Nifedipine is only available orally as 10- and 20-mg liquid-filled capsules and as 30-, 60-, and 90-mg extended-release, film-coated tablets. Refer to the dosages table above for recommended dosages. Pregnancy category C.

Classification of Calcium Channel Blockers

22-6

Generic Name	Trade Name	Available Routes
BENZOTHIAZEPINES		
diltiazem	Cardizem, Dilacor, Tiazac	PO/IV
DIHYDROPYRIDINES		
amlodipine	Norvasc	PO
bepridil	Vascor	PO
felodipine	Plendil	PO
isradipine	DynaCirc	PO
nicardipine	Cardene	PO/IV
nifedipine	Adalat, Procardia	PO
nimodipine	Nimotop	PO
PHENYLALKYLAMINES		
verapamil	Calan, Isoptin, Verelan	PO/IV

PHARMACOKINETICS

HALF-LIFE	ONSET	PEAK	DURATION
2-5 hr	20 min	30-60 min	IR: 6 hr XL: 24 hr

verapamil

Verapamil (Calan, Isoptin, Verelan, Covera HS) is the only phenylalkylamine CCB. Like diltiazem, it has a greater affinity for the conduction system of the heart than dihydropyridine CCBs such as nifedipine and is therefore effective in treating such rhythm disturbances as paroxysmal supraventricular tachycardias. Verapamil is also used for the treatment of angina, hypertension, and hypertrophic cardiomyopathy. The most common side effect of verapamil is constipation, occurring in less than 9% of patients. Verapamil is available in many oral dosage formulations and is also available in a parenteral preparation. Verapamil is available as a 40-, 80-, and 120-mg film-coated tablet and as a 120-, 180-, 240-mg extended-release capsule and film-coated, extended-release tablet. Parenterally verapamil is available as a 2.5-mg/ml injection. Refer to the dosages table on p. 345 for recommended dosages. Pregnancy category C.

PHARMACOKINETICS

HALF-LIFE	ONSET	PEAK	DURATION
4.5-12 hr	0.5-2 hr	1-2 hr	Unknown

nursing process

In patients with coronary artery disease, the clinical symptoms result from a lack or inadequate delivery of blood and the attendant oxygen and nutrients to the heart, which results in ischemic heart disease. Antianginal agents such as nitrates, nitrites, beta-blockers, and CCBs are used to reduce ischemia by increasing the delivery of oxygen- and nutrient-rich blood to cardiac tissues or by reducing oxygen consumption by the coronary vessels. Either of these mechanisms can reduce ischemia and lead to a decrease in anginal pain. Nitrates and nitrites work mainly by decreasing venous return to the heart (preload) and decreasing systemic vascular resistance (afterload). CCBs decrease calcium influx into the smooth muscle causing vascular relaxation. This either reverses or prevents the spasms of coronary vessels that cause the anginal pain associated with Prinzmetal's or vasospastic angina and with chronic anginal pain. Beta-blockers help by slowing the heart rate and decreasing contractility thereby decreasing oxygen demands. Even though these groups of drugs have similar clinical effects, the nursing process required for each is somewhat specific in terms of the characteristics and effects of the agents and the indications for and contraindications to their use.

● Assessment

Before administering any nitrates or nitrites, a complete health history must be obtained to determine whether the patient has any past or present medical conditions or diseases that would either be a contraindication to the use of these agents or call for cautious use. Other drugs being taken by the patient should also be documented. Patients should be encouraged to describe their anginal attacks because this will help in the selection of the appropriate therapy. Contraindications to the use of nitrates and nitrites include hypersensitivity to these agents, severe anemia, acute MI, increased intracranial pressure, hypertension, and cerebral hemorrhage. Cautious use is called for in patients suffering from head injuries or postural hypotension as well as in women who are pregnant or lactating. It is also necessary to assess a patient's vital signs, including respiratory patterns and rate, before and during therapy. Drugs that interact with these agents include beta-blockers, narcotics, diuretics, antihypertensives, anticoagulants, alcohol (results in increased hypotension and even cardiovascular collapse), sympathomimetics (may antagonize the effects of nitrates and nitrites), and tricyclic antidepressants (their effect is enhanced when they are taken with nitrates). Cold temperature and tobacco use can reduce the effectiveness of nitrates. Nitrates also interact with sildenafil (Viagra) (discussed in Chapter 33). It is also important to remember that cross-tolerance may develop when nitrates and nitrites are taken together.

Before administering a CCB as an antianginal agent, the nurse should check to make sure the patient has no conditions that are contraindications, such as sick sinus syndrome, second- or third-degree heart block, hypotension with a systolic blood pressure of less than 90 mm Hg, or cardiogenic shock. Cautious use is called for in pregnant or lactating women, children, and patients with renal or liver disease, hypotension, or CHF. Drugs that interact with CCBs include theophylline, beta-blockers, antihypertensives, digitalis, cimetidine, lithium, and quinidine. These drugs should be used cautiously in conjunction with CCB. Contraindications to the use of beta-blockers include patients with asthma, CHF, or serious conduction disturbances. Cautious use is recommended in the elderly.

Amlodipine, a commonly used calcium channel blocker for treatment of angina, should be used with caution in patients with bradycardia or CHF. It is also used with caution in patients who have a decreased renal and hepatic functioning, which would have an influence on the excretion and metabolism of the drug. Drug interactions for which to assess include beta-blockers, digitalis glycosides, and other antidysrhythmic agents.

● Nursing Diagnoses

Nursing diagnoses related to the administration of antianginal agents include the following:
- Acute pain related to pathologic impact of tissue ischemia.
- Impaired physical mobility related to the ischemia angina.
- Deficient knowledge related to first-time use of antianginals.
- Risk for injury related to side effects of antianginals.

● Planning

Goals of nursing care related to the administration of antianginals include the following:
- Patient experiences fewer episodes of chest pain with appropriate use of antianginals.
- Patient is able to perform activities of daily living with increasing comfort and less chest pain.
- Patient tolerates moderate, supervised exercise.
- Patient states actions to take when chest pain is unrelieved.
- Patient states side effects of therapy to report.

NURSING CARE PLAN Chest Pain

Mr. L.L., a 59-year-old high school principal, was admitted to the ER with complaints of chest pain after a high school basketball game, which he attended after a 12-hour day at work. He experienced chest pain and was taken by ambulance to a local chest pain center where the following were completed: 12 lead ECG and serum enzyme studies to rule out possible MI. Over the next 24 hours he was observed and monitored in the chest pain unit. All studies were negative, and there were no further complaints of chest pain. He was discharged on SL nitroglycerin and is scheduled for an ultrasound and stress test with thallium scan in 1 week.

assessment	*Nursing Diagnosis*	Deficient knowledge related to lack of knowledge and experience with treatment of chest pain
	Subjective Data	Complaints of chest pain and palpitations
	Objective Data	• Smoker × 20 yr of 2 packs/day • Occasional wine drinker • Principal of high school • Family history of MI • History of hypertension × 2 yr • Minimal exercise and does not watch diet for fat intake
planning and outcome criteria	*Goals*	Patient will verbalize dosing, importance of compliance, side effects, and drug interactions to nitroglycerin, before discharge
	Outcome Criteria	Patient will be able to demonstrate understanding of medication regimen by being able to accurately verbalize the following: • Use of nitroglycerin • Side effects of medication • Drug interactions • Symptoms and side effects to report to the physician immediately • When to call 911 • How to minimize side effects
implementation		SL nitroglycerin is taken to abort acute attacks of angina with an onset of action in 1-3 min, and lasts only 30 min; therefore, it is important to follow these guidelines: • Place SL tab under the tongue, DO NOT CHEW, let dissolve, and DO NOT SWALLOW until dissolved; take SL tabs at ONE tab every 5 min until chest pain relieved, but no more than 3 tabs with 15 min, and if chest pain unrelieved then activate EMS by calling 911!! These instructions are very important to the effectiveness of the drug. • Avoid alcohol and OTC drugs with this medication. • A headache may occur with the dose of drug, and you may develop tolerance to the headache as time goes on; however, a nonnarcotic analgesic is recommended. • If the drug stings when in contact with the mucous membranes, it is still potent. • The drug loses potency in about 6 months; always have fresh refills available. • Keep the SL nitroglycerin container away from light, heat, and moisture because these decrease the drug's effectiveness. • Once you take the nitroglycerin, lie down and be sure to change positions slowly to avoid falling or fainting. • You may be instructed by the physician to take this medication prior to stressful activities such as exercise or sexual activity to prevent angina. • Be sure to take the medication exactly as prescribed.
evaluation		Patient shows therapeutic response to nitroglycerin therapy as evidenced by decreased occurrence of chest pain Patient is monitored for and reports minimal side effects such as: • Headache • Dizziness

NURSING CARE PLAN Chest Pain—cont'd

evaluation	
	• Nausea
	• Vomiting
	• Pallor
	• Sweating
	• Hypotension
	• Tachycardia
	• Fainting
	• Flushing of the face

Outcome Criteria

Outcome criteria related to the administration of antianginals include the following:

- Patient will have increased comfort related to therapeutic effects of antianginals with fewer precipitating events and episodes.
- Patient will experience increased tolerance for activity while on antianginals with less chest pain with increasing exercise.
- Patient will state those symptoms to report to the physician, such as syncope, excessive dizziness, severe headache, or chest pain.

• Implementation

When patients first begin antianginal therapy, it is crucial for the nurse to review the patient's baseline vital signs as well as any documentation of their anginal pain and precipitating factors. If the patient is taking sublingual forms, he or she should be told to take nitroglycerin at the first sign of angina. The patient should be lying down to prevent or decrease dizziness and fainting resulting from drug-induced hypotension, which may last for up to a half hour. When administering nitroglycerin intravenously, it must be diluted in 5% dextrose in water or 0.9% sodium chloride and must not be given with any other drugs or solutions. Intravenously administered nitroglycerin must be contained in glass IV bottles, with the rate of administration set at the one specified by the manufacturer. Because IV filters or volume-control chambers will absorb the drug, these should not be used for its administration. In addition, IV forms of nitroglycerin are only stable for 96 hours after preparation.

Infusion pumps must be used, and aluminum foil should be wrapped around the bottle and tubing (unless packaging inserts instruct otherwise), or use special IV tubing provided, usually non-PVC tubing. Any parenteral solution that is discolored blue, green, or dark red should be discarded. If the patient is on long-term treatment with sodium nitroprusside (only administered intravenously and in a hypertensive crisis), his or her thiocyanate levels should be monitored daily. In addition, it is important to remember that amyl nitrite is highly flammable and should be kept away from flames or smoking materials. Because the active ingredient in nitroglycerin is

easily destroyed, nitrates and nitrites should be stored in an airtight, cotton filler—free, dark glass bottle with a metal cap.

The rapid-acting agents (amyl nitrite, sublingual nitroglycerin, and sublingual or chewable isosorbide dinitrate) are indicated for the relief of acute angina attacks. The longer-acting nitrates, along with the topical, transdermal, transmucosal, and oral sustained-release forms, are used prophylactically to prevent anginal attacks or decrease their frequency and severity as well as to prevent predictable anginal episodes. Skin exposure to ointment forms of nitrates should be avoided because of possible absorption of the drug.

When administering oral CCBs, the agents should be taken before meals and as ordered. Some of the agents, such as diltiazem, must be stored in a tight container and at room temperature. See the patient teaching tips box for CCBs and beta blockers. Beta-blockers should be given or taken as ordered. Measures to decrease constipation include a high-fiber diet and forcing fluids.

Patient and family instructions for antianginal agents are included in the patient teaching tips on p. 349.

• Evaluation

Patients taking antianginal agents must be monitored carefully for the occurrence of an allergic reaction, which may be manifested by dyspnea, swelling of the face, or hives. In addition, the patient needs to be monitored for adverse reactions such as headache, light-headedness, decreased blood pressure, or dizziness, which may indicate the need for a decreased dose. The patient's journal on his or her angina (duration, time of onset, activity being performed, and the character) should be reviewed continuously. If the patient is receiving IV nitrates, it is important to look for the development of pedal edema, skin turgor, nausea, vomiting, rales, dyspnea, or orthopnea. Vital signs should be monitored frequently during acute exacerbations of the angina and during IV administration.

In addition, patients should be monitored for the therapeutic effects of the agents, such as relief of the angina, decreased blood pressure, or both. If the patient is experiencing blurred vision or dry mouth, the drug should be discontinued and the physician notified. If patients report that parts of the sustained-release forms of antianginal medication are appearing in their stool, then the medication is possibly moving too fast through the gastrointestinal tract and patients may need to be switched to another dosage form. It is important to monitor the blood levels of CCBs to make sure they are therapeutic (e.g., diltiazem; 0.025-0.1 μg/ml). Patients taking beta-blockers should monitor pulse rate daily and report any rate lower than 60 beats per minute. Dizziness or fainting should also be reported.

---

patient teaching tips

Antianginal Agents

Nitrate Antianginal Agents

➤ When suffering from an acute anginal attack, patients should know to take one (sublingual) SL tablet as soon as possible after the pain begins, then to lie down and rest. If there is no relief after three SL nitrates taken every 5 minutes for 15 minutes, then 911 should be called and emergency rescue personnel told to respond.

➤ Patients should never chew or swallow the SL forms, because this will interfere with the action and effectiveness of the nitrate. SL forms should be placed under the tongue and allowed to dissolve before swallowing it. If they cause a burning sensation under the tongue, the patients should know this shows the drug is still potent.

➤ Transmucosal nitroglycerin tablets should also not be chewed, crushed, or swallowed and should be placed inside the cheek or under the lip and allowed to dissolve slowly.

➤ Patients should be instructed to always keep a fresh supply of nitroglycerin on hand, because even under the best circumstances it loses its strength in about 3 months after the bottle has been opened.

➤ Patients should be aware of the adverse effects of nitrates: flushing of the face, dizziness, fainting, brief throbbing headache, increase in heart rate, and lightheadedness. The headaches usually last no longer than 20 minutes and are usually relieved with analgesics.

➤ Medications should be kept out of the reach of children.

➤ Patients should keep a record of the frequency and the characteristics of their anginal attacks, any precipitating factors, the number of pills taken, and adverse effects. Any therapeutic response to any of the antianginal agents should also be recorded in this journal, as well as a description of any symptoms of the medications.

➤ Remember that in addition to certain medications, patients should know to avoid those activities or factors that precipitate angina, such as stress, loss of sleep, overeating, heavy exercise, or the excessive intake of stimulants such as those contained in coffee, tea, chocolate, soft drinks, and cigarettes or other tobacco products.

➤ Alcohol consumption and hot baths plus spending time in jacuzzis, hot tubs, or saunas will result in vessel dilation, with a resultant increase in the chance of hypotension, and thus fainting.

➤ Nitrate topical ointments should be spread in a thin layer on the applicator paper provided with the product. Patients should always use the appropriate applicator paper because the various ointment preparations and applicator papers are not interchangeable. Ointments should not be rubbed or massaged into the skin. Any residue from the old site should be washed off before new ointment is applied. Ointments can be applied to any nonhairy site on the patient's body, not necessarily on the chest or over the heart. The ointment should be covered with either plastic wrap or the application papers to prevent staining or inadvertent removal of the medication.

➤ Rotation of sites is encouraged, and the old ointment or patch should be removed before another application.

➤ Transdermal patches should be applied to a hairless part of the body only after the old patch has been removed and the old site cleansed. These patches can be worn while swimming or bathing, but if one does come off, patient should cleanse the old site and apply a new patch.

➤ Resistance or tolerance to the nitrates may occur, so the patients should contact the physician if anginal symptoms recur.

➤ In general nitrates should be taken at the first hint of anginal pain.

➤ Patients should be encouraged to change positions slowly at all times to prevent a further drop in their blood pressure or fainting.

➤ The physician should be notified if the patient experiences blurred vision, a persistent headache, or dry mouth.

➤ Caution is encouraged whenever the patient engages in hazardous activities because of the dizziness that can occur.

Calcium Channel Blockers

➤ Patients need to take their calcium channel blocker the same time every day and to be careful to take it as prescribed.

➤ Patients should avoid hazardous activities until the drug effects have stabilized and dizziness is no longer a problem.

➤ Patients need to know how to monitor their pulse rate before taking each dose and to record pulse rates and a description of any anginal pain.

➤ Patients should be encouraged to limit their caffeine intake (coffee, caffeinated soft drinks, tea, excess chocolate).

➤ Patients should be instructed to not take OTC medications unless otherwise instructed by their physician.

➤ Patients should be instructed about the various drug interactions of agents such as Norvasc with other prescribed agents and OTC products and herbals.

➤ Patients should be instructed about the possibility of hypotension and to change positions slowly to avoid falling or fainting.

➤ Patients should be instructed about the side effects of calcium channel blockers, including headache, dizziness, edema, and hypotension.

➤ Patients should be encouraged to keep a daily journal of symptoms, relief of symptoms, precipitating events, and control of symptoms, depending on what the physician has suggested or encouraged them to do.

➤ Patients should report to their health care provider an increase of 2 pounds of weight in 1 day or 5 or more pounds in 1 week.

Beta-Blockers

➤ Beta-blockers are used for long-term prevention of angina, and patients should be aware that they are not for immediate relief or to abort an attack.

➤ Constipation is a common problem with beta blockers. Forcing fluids and eating a diet high in fiber (fresh figs, prunes, raisins, bran, wheat germ) is recommended unless contraindicated.

➤ These medications should never be discontinued abruptly due to risk of a rebound hypertensive crisis.

➤ Patients should take this medication exactly as prescribed.

➤ Alcohol intake, heat, hot baths, and spending time in jacuzzis, hot tubs, or saunas will result in vasodilation and resultant hypotension and risk for fainting and injury.

➤ Patients should report chest pain, palpitations, excessive dizziness, fainting episodes, pulse rates under 60 bpm, edema, and any dyspnea to their physician.

POINTS TO REMEMBER

Angina

- Angina pectoris or chest pain occurs because of a mismatch between the oxygen supply and oxygen demand.
- Either too much oxygen demand or too little oxygen delivery.
- The heart is a very aerobic or oxygen-requiring muscle.
- When it does not receive enough oxygen, it becomes ischemic; this produces pain.
- Coronary arteries deliver oxygen to the heart muscle; they can become blocked: heart attack.

Coronary Artery Disease

- Abnormal condition of the arteries (blood vessels) that deliver oxygen to the heart muscle.
- Become narrowed, resulting in reduced flow of oxygen and nutrients to the myocardium.
- Nitrates, calcium channel blockers, and beta-blockers may be used to treat the symptoms.

Nitrates

- Nitroglycerin is the prototypical nitrate.
- Dilate constricted coronary arteries, helping to increase oxygen and nutrient supply to the heart muscle.
- Isosorbide dinitrates were the first group of oral agents used for angina.
- Isosorbide mononitrates are the new and improved nitrates for angina.
- Nitroglycerin is the main intravenous nitrate used for angina.

- Dilate coronary arteries, and thus *increase oxygen supply.*

Calcium Channel Blockers

- Relieve angina by reducing afterload (the force the ventricles must push against to eject their blood).
- By reducing afterload they reduce the work load of the heart and therefore the oxygen demand on the heart. These drugs *reduce oxygen demand.*
- Relax the smooth muscle surrounding the blood vessels, causing them to dilate and blood pressure to drop.
- Some may dilate coronary arteries and therefore *increase oxygen supply* as well.

Beta-Blockers

- Relieve angina by slowing the heart rate.
- Slowing the heart rate reduces the work load of the heart.
- This *decreases oxygen demand* on the heart.

Nursing Considerations

- Contraindications to the use of antianginals include allergies, severe anemia, increased intracranial pressure, hypertension, and cerebral hemorrhage.
- Cautious use is called for in patients with head injuries or postural hypotension, and in pregnant or lactating women.
- Calcium channel blockers are often used as antianginals and are contraindicated in patients who have sick sinus syndrome, second- or third-degree heart block, hypotension, or cardiogenic shock.

- The IV administration of nitrates should be done in accordance with manufacturer guidelines and institutional policies.
- The various dosage forms of nitrates cannot be used interchangeably.
- Beta-blockers are contraindicated in patients with CHF or second- or third-degree heart block.

- Beta-blockers may exacerbate conditions in patients with respiratory disease such as chronic obstructive pulmonary disease.
- Norvasc and other calcium channel blockers may be ordered for angina and are associated with side effects of hypotension, headache, dizziness, and edema.

REVIEW QUESTIONS

1. When applying topical nitroglycerin ointment, which of the following reflects the *most appropriate* nursing intervention or nursing decision about its use?
   a. Only apply the ointment when trying to abort an attack of angina.
   b. Only apply the ointment to an area directly over the ventricular area.
   c. Do not leave the previous ointment dose in place; remove it and apply new ointment.
   d. Vigorously apply using your ungloved fingers and rub until all ointment is absorbed into the skin.
2. Which of the following statements is *incorrect* regarding the administration of IV nitroglycerin?
   a. IV nitroglycerin is only stable for 18 to 24 hours.
   b. IV filters will absorb the drug and should not be used.
   c. The IV tubing and bag should be a non-PVC type material.
   d. Nitroglycerin is generally incompatible with other IV medications.
3. Which of the following statements from your patient reflect that he needs *more* patient teaching about his SL nitroglycerin?
   a. Let the tablet dissolve completely before swallowing.
   b. Once you take a dose, lie down and change positions very slowly to avoid fainting.

   c. Take up to five doses at 15-minute intervals, and call 911 if you experience no relief after the five doses or a 1 hour and 15 minute time period.
   d. The SL nitroglycerin is no longer potent if you don't experience burning under the tongue with its administration.
4. Which of the following situations or conditions would cause a cautious use of nitrates and nitrites?
   a. History of CHF
   b. History of liver dysfunction
   c. Blood pressure of 120/80 mm Hg
   d. Smoking history of two packs per day
5. Your patient is going to begin taking a beta-blocker for part of his treatment regimen for a myocardial infarction. Which of the following would you need to include in his patient teaching?
   a. Chew any extended-release preparations thoroughly.
   b. Report tachycardia, a common side effect, to your health care provider.
   c. Do not be concerned with abrupt withdrawing or discontinuation of the medication.
   d. If you have chest pain, fainting, fluid retention or swelling, or shortness of breath, contact your health care provider immediately.

For Answers see www.harcourthealth.com/MERLIN/Lilley/.

CRITICAL THINKING Activities

1. M.J. is a 45-year-old man with stable angina who has recently been prescribed sublingual nitroglycerin tablets for the relief of his anginal attacks. He asks you how many milligrams of nitroglycerin are in his tablets. All the bottle says is "1/150 gr tablets." How many milligrams of nitroglycerin are in M.J.'s 1/150 gr tablets?
2. Your patient has been switched from sublingual nitroglycerin to a transdermal form. What instructions do

   you need to give him regarding the difference in his therapeutic regimen?
3. You are caring for a patient who has just suffered a myocardial infarction, for which he has received a thrombolytic agent, aspirin, heparin, oxygen, and now a nitroglycerin infusion. The infusion is running at a rate of 33 μg/min, and the concentration of the infusion is 200 μg/ml. At what rate should the infusion pump be set in milliliters per hour?

For Answers see www.harcourthealth.com/MERLIN/Lilley/.

bibliography

Albanese J, Nutz P: *Mosby's 2001 nursing drug reference and review cards,* St Louis, 2001, Mosby.

American Hospital Formulary Service: *AHFS drug information,* Bethesda, Md, 2000, American Society of Health-System Pharmacists.

Anderson KA: A practical guide to nitrate use, *Postgrad Med* 89(1):67, 1991.

Anderson PO, Knoben JE, Troutman WG: *Handbook of clinical drug data 1999-2000,* ed 9, New York, 1999, McGraw-Hill.

Davis L, Stecy P: Pharmacologic management of cardiovascular problems in women, *J Nurse Midwife* 42(3):176, 1997.

Johns Hopkins Hospital, Department of Pediatrics et al: *The Harriet Lane handbook,* ed 15, St Louis, 2000, Mosby.

Keen JH: *Critical care and emergency drug reference,* ed 3, St Louis, 1996, Mosby.

Medical Letter: Drugs for chronic heart failure 41(1045), January 29, 1999.

Mosby's GenRx: a comprehensive reference for generic and brand drugs, ed 10, St Louis, 2000, Mosby.

Skidmore-Roth L: *Mosby's 2001 nursing drug reference,* St Louis, 2001, Mosby.

Turkoski BB: *Drug information handbook for nursing 1999-2000: including assessment, administration, monitoring guidelines, and patient education,* ed 2, Cleveland, 1999, Lexi-Comp.

United States Pharmacopeial Convention: *USP DI: advise for the patient: drug information in lay language, vol. 1I,* ed 20, Englewood, Colo, 2000, Micromedex.

Willison DJ et al: Consultation between cardiologists and generalists in the management of acute myocardial infarction: implications for quality of care, *Arch Intern Med* 158(16):1778, 1998.

Activity

Chapter 23

Antihypertensive Agents

objectives

When you reach the end of this chapter, you should be able to do the following:

1 Briefly discuss the normal anatomy and physiology of the autonomic nervous system, including the events that take place during synaptic transmission within the sympathetic and parasympathetic division.

2 Define *hypertension.*

3 Describe the different forms of hypertension.

4 Discuss the rationale for using a stepped-care approach in the management of hypertension.

5 Identify the various classes of drugs used in the treatment of hypertension.

6 Describe the actions of the different classes of drugs used to treat hypertension.

7 Identify the contraindications to and cautions pertaining to the various antihypertensive agents, as well as their side effects and toxic effects.

8 Develop a nursing care plan that includes all phases of the nursing process for patients receiving antihypertensive agents.

drug profiles

- **captopril**, p. 363
- **clonidine**, p. 360
- **diazoxide**, p. 367
- **enalapril**, p. 364
- **guanadrel and guanethidine**, p. 360
- **hydralazine hydrochloride**, p. 367
- **losartan**, p. 364
- **minoxidil**, p. 367
- **prazosin**, p. 359
- **reserpine**, p. 360
- **sodium nitroprusside**, p. 367
- **valsartan**, p. 364

○━ Key drug.

glossary

Adrenergic neuronal blockers Drugs that modify the function of the sympathetic nervous system depleting the stores of norepinephrine. (p. 357)

Alpha₁-blockers Drugs that primarily cause arterial and venous dilation. (p. 357)

Antihypertensives Medications used to treat hypertension. (p. 354)

Cardiac output Amount of blood ejected from the left ventricle and measured in liters per minute. (p. 355)

Centrally acting adrenergic agents Drugs that modify the function of the sympathetic nervous system by stimulating alpha₂-receptors, causing decreased blood pressure. (p. 356)

Essential (idiopathic or primary) hypertension An elevated systemic arterial pressure for which no cause can be found and that is often the only significant clinical finding. (p. 355)

Ganglionic-blocking agents (gang gle on ik) Agents that prevent nerves from responding to the action of acetylcholine by occupying the receptor sites for acetylcholine (i.e., nicotinic receptors) on sympathetic and parasympathetic nerve endings. (p. 354)

Hypertension A common, often asymptomatic disorder in which blood pressure persistently exceeds 140/90 mm Hg. (p. 354)

Idiopathic hypertension (id′ e o path′ ik) High blood pressure that develops without an apparent or known cause. (p. 355)

Nicotinic receptor (nik o tin ik) The receptor and site of action for acetylcholine in both the parasympathetic and sympathetic nervous systems. (p. 356)

Orthostatic hypotension (or tho stat′ ik) Common side effect of adrenergic drugs involving a sudden drop in blood pressure when patients change position. (p. 358)

Primary hypertension Elevated systemic arterial pressure for which no cause can be found and that is often the only significant finding. (p. 355)

Prodrug Drug that is inactive in its present form and must be biotransformed in the liver to its active form. (p. 361)

Rauwolfia alkaloid (rou wool′ fi ə al′ kə loid) Any one of more than 20 alkaloids derived from the root of a climbing shrub, *Rauwolfia serpentina;* used in the treatment of hypertension. (p. 361)

Secondary hypertension High blood pressure associated with several primary diseases, such as renal, pulmonary, endocrine, and vascular diseases. (p. 355)

Step-care approach Antihypertensive treatment program sponsored by National High Blood Pressure Coordinating Committee (NHBPCC) and established to encourage health professionals to use combinations of medications in a systematic fashion with a scientific basis. (p. 354)

Significant advancements have been made in the detection, evaluation, and treatment of high blood pressure, or **hypertension.** Over the past 40 years the development of new medications to treat hypertension **(antihypertensives)** has had an enormous impact on the quality of life of affected persons by reducing the incidence of the various complications associated with hypertension as well as improvements in drug therapy such as drugs with few side effects. Drug therapy for hypertension first became available in the early 1950s with the introduction of **ganglionic-blocking agents.** However, side effects and inconsistent effects were common problems with these agents. Then in 1953 the vasodilator hydralazine was introduced and in 1958 the thiazide diuretics. These agents offered important advantages over the existing antihypertensive drug therapies. In addition, with the discovery of these newer drugs came a better understanding of the disease process itself. Now a myriad of antihypertensive drugs are available, the newer ones commonly being more effective, more versatile, and better tolerated than the older agents. These agents can be used either alone or in combination with other antihypertensive agents. The classes of drugs that can be employed are diuretics, beta-blockers, angiotensin-converting enzyme (ACE) inhibitors, alpha$_1$ antagonists, alpha$_2$ antagonists, angiotension II blockers, and calcium channel blockers (CCBs).

HYPERTENSION

As many as 50 million people in the United States have some form of hypertension, making it the most common disease in the population of the western hemisphere. Not only does hypertension affect a large portion of our society, it has many severe consequences if left untreated because hypertension is a major risk factor for coronary artery disease, cardiovascular disease, and death resulting from cardiovascular causes. It is the most important risk factor for stroke and congestive heart failure (CHF), and it is also a major risk factor for renal failure and peripheral vascular disease.

The diagnosis and treatment of hypertension have varied considerably over the years, which has resulted in a great deal of misunderstanding. The National High Blood Pressure Coordinating Committee (NHBPCC), which is associated with the National Institutes of Health, is a leading group that reviews data on hypertension and makes recommendations concerning its diagnosis and treatment. The original mission of the NHBPCC was to foster nationwide efforts to detect, treat, and control hypertension through the education of both health care professionals and the general public to its existence and dire consequences if left untreated. As part of the treatment efforts, practicing health care professionals were encouraged to use medication combinations in a systematic fashion with a scientific basis, or the **step-care approach.** In this regimen the patient was started on a small dose of an antihypertensive drug, then the dose was increased. Drugs from different classes, or "steps," were added sequentially as needed to achieve and maintain the blood pressure at less than 140/90 mm Hg. Included in this approach were definitions of mild, moderate, and severe hypertension.

There were many misconceptions inherent in this system, however, the most damaging of which was that a person with mild hypertension was only mildly sick and therefore did not need close monitoring or therapy. However, experience showed that there is no such thing as mild hypertension and that it is actually a serious risk factor for cardiovascular disease and death. A new, stricter definition of hypertension was therefore called for because of the overwhelming evidence that raised blood

research

High Blood Pressure

The Joint National Committee on the Detection, Evaluation, and Treatment of High Blood Pressure (Sixth report, 1997) introduced changes that directly affect the way we detect, evaluate, and treat hypertension. One change was the introduction of a more "individualized" therapy, as compared with the traditional stepped-care approach, because it could address specific patient considerations, including pharmacologic alternatives. Health care providers are therefore encouraged to adopt an individualized approach to the planning of drug therapy for hypertension that considers quality of life, use of concurrent therapies, demographic concerns, and presence of concomitant diseases. ∎

Table 23-1 Classification of Blood Pressure

Category*	Systolic Blood Pressure (mm Hg)	Diastolic Blood Pressure (mm Hg)
Normal	<130	<85
High normal	130-139	85-89
Hypertension		
Stage 1	140-159	90-99
Stage 2	160-179	100-109
Stage 3	180-209	110-119
Stage 4	≥210	≥120

*When systolic and diastolic blood pressures fall into different categories, the blood pressure should be classified according to the higher category. For example, a diastolic blood pressure of <90 mm Hg and a systolic blood pressure of >140 mm Hg are classified as isolated systolic hypertension. A blood pressure of 186/70 mm Hg would be stage 3 isolated systolic hypertension.

pressure, especially the diastolic pressure, represents a significant risk regardless of the degree and should be actively treated.

The NHBPCC has now been in existence for more than 20 years. During this period the NHBPCC has developed numerous programs and educational materials for the use of health care professionals and the public. One of the most prominent features of the program has been the consensus reports issued every 4 years by the Joint National Committee on the Detection, Evaluation, and Treatment of High Blood Pressure. In its sixth report released in November 1997, several important changes were introduced that directly affect the way we detect, evaluate, and treat hypertension (see Research box on p. 361).

One of the major changes was a new classification system for blood pressure because of the realization that the term *mild hypertension* did not adequately reflect the serious nature of this condition. This became evident when it was found that even though the vast majority of the 50 million Americans with hypertension have so-called mild hypertension, most of the morbidity and mortality actually occurs in this group. In addition, many practitioners thought that the stepped-care approach to the treatment of hypertension no longer adequately reflected the current scope of pharmacologic alternatives or furnished the type of care dictated by the then thorough scientific understanding of the disorder. In this report, individualized therapy was proposed as a more appropriate treatment strategy than stepped care because it could address specific patient circumstances, including pharmacologic alternatives. Health care providers are therefore now encouraged to adopt an individualized approach to the planning of drug therapy that takes into consideration the demographic concerns of their patient, the presence of concomitant diseases, the use of concurrent therapies, and the patient's quality of life.

The new classification scheme categorizes the degrees of blood pressure according to four stages, rather than as "mild," "moderate," and "severe," which can be misleading. This classification scheme is presented in Table 23-1.

Hypertension can also be defined by its cause. When the specific cause for hypertension is unknown, it may be called **essential, idiopathic,** or **primary hypertension.** About 90% of the cases of hypertension are of this type. **Secondary hypertension** makes up the other 10%. It is most commonly the result of another disease such as pheochromocytoma, the eclampsia of pregnancy, or renal artery disease. It may also result from the use of certain medications. If the cause of secondary hypertension is eliminated, the blood pressure usually returns to normal.

Blood pressure is determined by the product of cardiac output and systemic vascular resistance (SVR). **Cardiac output** is the amount of blood that is ejected from the left ventricle and is measured in liters per minute. Normal cardiac output is 4 to 8 L/min. SVR is the force (resistance) the left ventricle has to overcome to eject its volume of blood. Numerous factors interact to regulate these two major variables and keep the blood pressure within normal limits, and these are illustrated in Fig. 23-1. These are the same factors that can be responsible for causing high blood pressure and are the sites of action of many of the antihypertensive drugs.

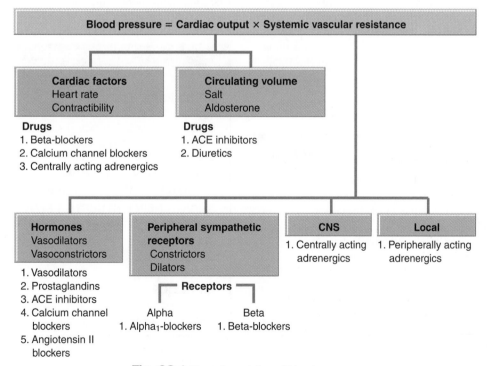

Fig. 23-1 Normal regulation of blood pressure.

ANTIHYPERTENSIVE AGENTS

As previously mentioned, the drug therapy for hypertension should be individualized to accommodate or complement the specific needs or concerns of the patient. Important considerations in planning drug therapy are whether the patient has concomitant medical problems and what the impact of drug therapy on the patient's quality of life will be. Demographic factors, cultural implications (see the Cultural Implications box below), the ease of medication administration (e.g., a once-a-day dosing schedule and transdermal administration), and cost are other important considerations.

There are essentially six main categories of pharmacologic agents: diuretics, adrenergic agents, vasodilators, ACE inhibitors, angiotensin II receptor blockers, and CCBs. These may be used either alone or in combination, and the various antihypertensive agents in each category are listed in Box 23-1. The diuretics are discussed in detail in Chapter 24, and therefore are not discussed here.

NICOTINIC RECEPTOR

The stimulation of the two divisions of the autonomic nervous system, the parasympathetic (PSNS) and sympathetic (SNS) nervous systems, is controlled by the neurotransmitter acetylcholine (ACh). The receptor for ACh in both systems is the **nicotinic receptor.** It gets its name from the fact that it was the administration of the ganglionic stimulant nicotine that first revealed its existence.

In the SNS this receptor is located between the preganglionic and postganglionic fibers. In the PSNS the nicotinic receptor is located between the preganglionic and postganglionic fibers. The receptor located between the postganglionic fiber and the effector cells is called the *muscarinic receptor.* Like the PSNS nicotinic receptor, it is also stimulated by ACh. Figure 23-2 shows how these nicotinic receptors are arranged in both the PSNS and SNS.

GANGLIONIC BLOCKERS

The ganglionic blockers, mecamylamine and trimethaphan, have few uses. They work by blocking the actions of ACh at the nicotinic receptors. They have been primarily used to lower blood pressure in emergency situations. One reason they are seldom used is that tachyphylaxis develops in 24 to 72 hours. They have been replaced with other classes of antihypertensives that are generally more effective and safer.

ADRENERGIC AGENTS

Adrenergic agents are a large group of antihypertensive agents, as shown in Box 23-1. The beta-blockers and combined alpha-beta blockers have been discussed in detail in Chapter 17. The adrenergic agents discussed here have different sites where they exert their antihypertensive action. The centrally and peripherally acting adrenergic agents, which are older agents, are not used as frequently now as the newer alpha$_1$-blockers because of the intolerable side effects they produce.

Mechanism of Action

The **centrally acting adrenergic agents** clonidine, guanabenz, guanfacine, and methyldopa all act by modifying the function of the SNS. Because SNS stimulation leads to an increased heart rate and force of contraction, the constriction of blood vessels, and the release of renin from the kidney, the result is hypertension.

SNS stimulation is increased when its alpha$_1$-adrenergic receptors are stimulated and is decreased when its alpha$_2$-adrenergic receptors are stimulated. Therefore there are two ways to decrease SNS stimulation by means of these receptors and ultimately to decrease blood pressure. The first is by stimulating the alpha$_2$-adrenergic receptors in

---

BOX 23-1 Categories and Subcategories of Antihypertensive Drugs

ADRENERGIC AGENTS
Alpha$_1$-blockers
Beta-blockers (cardioselective and nonselective)
Centrally acting alpha-blockers
Combined alpha-beta blockers
Peripheral acting adrenergic agents

ANGIOTENSIN-CONVERTING ENZYME INHIBITORS

ANGIOTENSIN II RECEPTOR BLOCKERS

CALCIUM CHANNEL BLOCKERS
Benzothiazepines
Dihydropyridines
Phenylalkylamines

DIURETICS
Loop diuretics
Potassium-sparing diuretics
Thiazides

VASODILATORS

the CNS, and the second is by blocking alpha$_1$-adrenergic receptors in the periphery. The centrally acting adrenergic agents decrease blood pressure by stimulating the alpha$_2$-adrenergic receptors, which results in a decreased sympathetic outflow from the CNS.

The **adrenergic neuronal blockers** guanadrel, guanethidine, and reserpine also act by modifying the function of the SNS, but they do so by depleting the stores of norepinephrine, the neurotransmitter of the SNS. Without it the SNS cannot stimulate certain organs such as the heart. The overall result is a decrease in blood pressure.

The peripheral-acting **alpha$_1$-blockers** doxazosin, prazosin, and terazosin have a similar mechanism of action to that of the centrally acting adrenergic agents and the adrenergic neuronal blockers in that they also modify the function of the SNS. However, they do so by blocking the alpha$_1$-adrenergic receptors, which when stimulated produce increased blood pressure. Thus when these receptors are blocked, blood pressure is decreased.

Figure 23-3 illustrates the site and mechanism of action for the various antihypertensive agents.

Drug Effects

The drug effects of the centrally acting adrenergic agents are many and varied. The cardiovascular effects are decreased blood pressure and heart rate. The stimulation of the alpha$_2$-adrenergic receptors by the centrally acting alpha adrenergics also affects the kidneys by reducing the activity of renin, a potent vasoconstrictor. Renovascular resistance is decreased without affecting renal blood flow or the glomerular filtration rate. Growth hormone release is also stimulated by alpha-agonists in both adults and children, but the effects are short-lived. The centrally act-

ing adrenergics are also known to decrease gastrointestinal motility and increase the absorption of sodium and water. In addition, they decrease the production of aqueous humor, which results in decreased intraocular pressure.

The drug effects of the adrenergic neuronal blockers are primarily cardiovascular. These agents cause a decrease in blood pressure and the heart rate. Venous dilation and the peripheral pooling of blood may also occur, and slight decreases in SVR usually occur. Postural and postexercise hypotension are common. In addition, adrenergic neuronal blockers cause the retention of sodium and water and expansion of blood volume, which may result in tolerance to their hypotensive effect during prolonged therapy, especially if a diuretic is not administered concurrently.

The drug effects of the alpha$_1$-blockers are primarily related to their ability to dilate arteries and veins, with reduced peripheral vascular resistance and subsequent decrease in blood pressure. This produces a marked decrease in the systemic and pulmonary venous pressures and an increase in cardiac output. Alpha$_1$-blockers increase urinary flow rates and decrease outflow obstruction by preventing smooth muscle contractions in the bladder neck and urethra.

Therapeutic Uses

The centrally acting adrenergic agents clonidine, guanabenz, guanfacine, and methyldopa are mainly used for the treatment of hypertension, either alone or in combination with other antihypertensive agents. Particular centrally acting adrenergics may also be used prophylactically to prevent migraine headaches and for the treatment of severe dysmenorrhea or menopausal flushing.

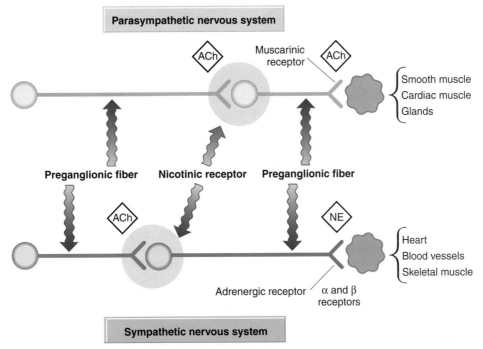

Fig. 23-2 Location of the nicotinic receptors within the parasympathetic and sympathetic nervous systems.

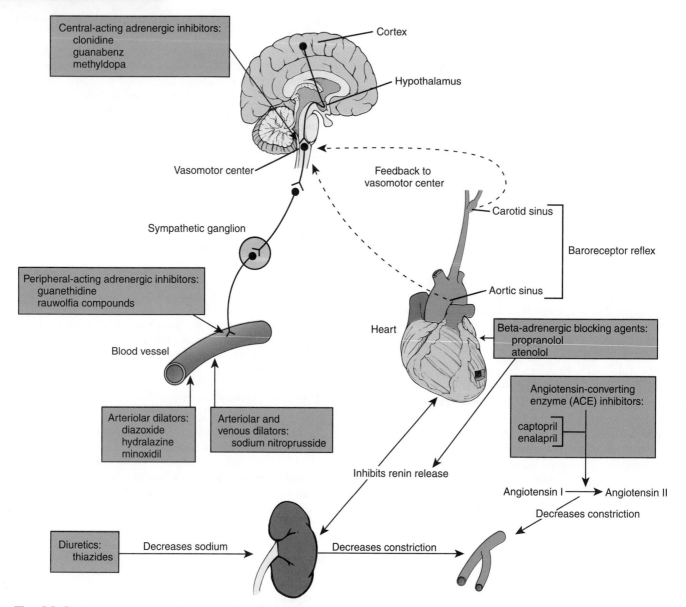

Fig. 23-3 Site and mechanism of action for the various antihypertensive agents. (From Lewis SM, Heitkemper MM, Dirksen SR: *Medical-surgical nursing: assessment and management of clinical problems,* ed 5, St Louis, 2000, Mosby.)

Clonidine is also useful in the management of withdrawal symptoms in opioid- or nicotine-dependent persons. Various forms of glaucoma may also respond to treatment with certain centrally acting adrenergics.

The adrenergic neuronal blockers guanadrel, guanethidine, and reserpine used in the treatment of hypertension are commonly administered along with other agents such as diuretics to increase their effectiveness and prevent resistance to their antihypertensive effects. Various forms of glaucoma may also respond to treatment with certain adrenergic neuronal blockers.

The therapeutic effects of the alpha$_1$-blockers doxazosin, prazosin, and terazosin are related to their ability to dilate arteries and veins. They have been used to treat hypertension and relieve the symptoms associated with BPH. They have also proved effective in the management of severe CHF when used with cardiac glycosides and diuretics.

Side Effects and Adverse Effects

As with all drug classes, adrenergic drugs can cause side effects and adverse effects. The most common side effects of these agents are dry mouth, drowsiness, sedation, and constipation. Other effects include headaches, sleep disturbances, nausea, rash, and cardiac disturbances such as palpitations. There is also a high incidence of **orthostatic hypotension** in patients taking them, a condition in which there is a sudden drop in blood pressure during changes in position.

Interactions

Adrenergic agents interact primarily with CNS depressants such as alcohol, barbiturates, and opioids. The additive effects of these combinations of agents increase CNS depression. Otherwise they are relatively free of drug and laboratory test interactions, although their co-

Adrenergics: Drug Interactions

23-2

Drug	Interacts With	Mechanism	Result
clonidine	Opioids Sedatives Hypnotics Anesthetics Alcohol	Additive	Increased CNS depression
	Tricyclic antidepressants MAOIs Appetite suppressants Amphetamines	Opposing actions	Decreased hypotensive effects
	Diuretics Nitrates Other antihypertensive agents	Additive	Increased hypotensive effects
	Beta-blockers	Additive	May potentiate bradycardia and increase the rebound hypertension in clonidine withdrawal
guanadrel	Diuretics Other antihypertensives	Additive	Increased hypotension
	Tricyclic antidepressants Phenothiazines ephedrine phenylpropanolamine	Opposing effects	Decreased hypotensive effect
prazosin	Diuretics, other hypotensive agents	Additive	Increased hypotension
	indomethacin	Opposing effects	Decreased hypotensive effect
	verapamil	Increased serum prazosin levels	Increased hypotension
reserpine	Diuretics, beta-blockers, other antihypertensives	Additive	Increased hypotension
	quinidine procainaminde	Additive	Increased cardiac depression
	Barbiturates Alcohol	Additive	CNS depression
	MAOIs	Additive	Excitation and hypertension
	Tricyclic antidepressants	Opposing effects	Decreased hypotensive effect

administration with beta-blockers as well as the combination of phenoxybenzamine with epinephrine can both have additive effects and increase hypotension. Terazosin can produce a reduced hematocrit reading. The drug interactions that can occur with certain adrenergic agents are summarized in Table 23-2.

Dosages

For information on the dosages of selected adrenergic antihypertensive agents, see the dosages table on p. 360.

drug profiles

ALPHA₁-BLOCKERS

The alpha₁-blockers are doxazosin, prazosin, tamsulosin, and terazosin. They are the newest of the adrenergics and have the best safety and efficacy profiles, but they are not free of adverse effects.

They are contraindicated in patients who have shown a hypersensitivity to them and are classified as pregnancy category C agents. They are only available in oral preparations.

prazosin

Prazosin (Minipress) is the oldest of the alpha₁-blockers and the prototype. It reduces both peripheral vascular resistance and blood pressure by dilating both arterial and venous blood vessels. It has been shown beneficial in the treatment of hypertension, the relief of the symptoms of obstructive BPH, and as an adjunct to cardiac glycosides and diuretics in the treatment of severe CHF. Prazosin is available as 1-, 2-, and 5-mg capsules and is also available in combination with the diuretic polythiazide (Minizide). Recommended dosages are given in the dosages table on p. 360.

DOSAGES Selected Antihypertensive Agents: Adrenergic/Antiadrenergic Agents

agent	pharmacologic class	dosage range	purpose
clonidine (Catapres)	Alpha$_2$-adrenergic	*Adult* PO: 0.2-0.8 mg/day divided, to a maximum of 2.4 mg/day	
guanadrel (Hylorel)	Peripherally acting sympatholytic (antiadrenergic)	*Adult* PO: 20-75 mg/day divided in 2 doses	Hypertension
prazosin (Minipress)	Alpha$_1$-blocker	*Adult* PO: 1-20 mg in 2 to 3 doses	
reserpine (Novoreserpine, Serpalan)	Peripherally acting sympatholytic (antiadrenergic)	*Adult* PO: 0.1-0.25 mg/day divided or as a single daily dose	

PHARMACOKINETICS

HALF-LIFE	ONSET	PEAK	DURATION
2-4 hr	2 hr	2-4 hr	<24 hr

CENTRALLY ACTING AGENTS (ALPHA$_2$-ADRENERGIC RECEPTOR STIMULATORS)

Of the four centrally acting adrenergics (clonidine, guanabenz, guanfacine, and methyldopa), clonidine is by far the most commonly used and the prototype. Methyldopa is also widely used in the treatment of hypertension and is the drug of choice for treating hypertension in pregnancy. However, these agents are not typically prescribed as first-line antihypertensive agents because their use is associated with a high incidence of unwanted side effects such as orthostatic hypotension, fatigue, and dizziness. They may be used as adjunct agents in the therapy for hypertension after other agents have failed or may be used in conjunction with other antihypertensives such as diuretics.

clonidine

Clonidine (Catapres, Duraclon) is primarily used for its ability to decrease blood pressure. As previously noted, clonidine is also useful in the management of opioid withdrawal.

It has a better safety profile than the other centrally acting adrenergics and has the advantage of being available in several dosage formulations, both topical and oral preparations. Topically clonidine is available as a patch that administers a dose of 0.1, 0.2, and 0.3 mg/24 hours. Orally, clonidine is available as 0.1, 0.2-, and 0.3-mg tablets. Clonidine is also available as a 100 μg/ml, preservative-free, epidural infusion. Epidural infusion of clonidine is indicated for treatment of severe pain in cancer patients. Clonidine should not be abruptly discontinued because of severe rebound hypertension. Its use is contraindicated in patients who have shown hypersensitivity reactions to it and is classified as a pregnancy category C agent. See the dosages table above for recommended dosages.

PHARMACOKINETICS

HALF-LIFE	ONSET	PEAK	DURATION
6-20 hr	30-60 min	3-5 hr	8 hr

PERIPHERALLY ACTING AGENTS (ADRENERGIC NEURONAL BLOCKERS)

The adrenergic neuronal blockers are guanadrel, guanethidine, and reserpine. These agents, like the centrally acting adrenergics, are seldom used because of their frequent side effects and limited effectiveness. Reserpine does have the advantage, however, of being very inexpensive and has a very long half-life and duration of action, but its antihypertensive effects are diminished at high doses, and mental depression develops in many patients taking it.

guanadrel and guanethidine

Guanadrel (Hylorel) is very similar in many aspects to guanethidine (Ismelin). They are both very old antihypertensive agents and their clinical use is limited today. They are now primarily used as adjunctive antihypertensive agents when single-drug therapy has failed to produce a response. They are both only available as oral preparations and are both classified as pregnancy category B agents. Contraindications to their use include hypersensitivity to them, pheochromocytoma, recent myocardial infarction (MI), CHF, cardiac failure, sinus bradycardia, and concurrent use with MAOIs. Guanadrel is available as 10- and 25-mg oral tablets. For the recommended dosages of guanadrel, see the dosages table above.

PHARMACOKINETICS

HALF-LIFE	ONSET	PEAK	DURATION
10-12 hr	0.5-2 hr	4-6 hr	4-14 hr

reserpine

Reserpine (Novoreserpine, Serpalan) is slightly different from guanadrel and guanethidine in that it is one of the **rauwolfia alkaloids.** Others of these plant-derived alkaloids are *Rauwolfia serpentina,* alseroxylon, and deserpidine, but reserpine is the most commonly used of the four. Because these alkaloids promote sodium and water resorption, their antihypertensive effects may diminish with continued use. These drugs are often combined with diuretics in an attempt to offset this effect.

Reserpine is classified as a pregnancy category D drug and is contraindicated in patients suffering from mental depression, active peptic ulcers, or ulcerative colitis, and in those who have shown a hypersensitivity to it. It is only available in oral forms as 0.1- and 0.25-mg tablets. There are many combination products containing reserpine and various diuretics. Recommended dosages are given in the dosages table on p. 360.

PHARMACOKINETICS

HALF-LIFE	ONSET	PEAK	DURATION
4-5 hr -12 days	Very slow	2-3 wk	Unknown

ANGIOTENSIN-CONVERTING ENZYME (ACE) INHIBITORS

The ACE inhibitors represent a large group of antihypertensive agents. There are currently more than 13 agents available for clinical use and many more combination agents in which a thiazide diuretic or a CCB is combined with the parent ACE inhibitor. Some of the newer ACE inhibitors are cilazapril (Inhibace), moexipril (Univasc), perindopril (Aceon), spirapril (Renormax), trandolapril (Mavik), and zofenopril. These agents are very safe and efficacious and are often utilized as the first-line agents in the treatment of both CHF and hypertension. Some of the distinguishing characteristics of the various agents that make up this large class of antihypertensives are summarized in Table 23-3. The ACE inhibitors as a class are very similar and only differ in a few of their chemical properties, but there are some significant differences between them in terms of their clinical properties. Knowing these differences can be helpful in selecting the proper agent for a particular patient.

Captopril has the shortest half-life and therefore must be dosed more frequently than any of the other ACE inhibitors. This may be an important drawback to its use in a patient who has a history of being noncompliant with his or her medication therapy. On the other hand, it may be best to start with a drug that has a short half-life in a patient who is still very critically ill and may not tolerate medications well, so if problems arise, they will be short-lived. Both captopril and enalapril can be dosed multiple times a day.

Captopril and lisinopril are the only two ACE inhibitors that are not prodrugs. A **prodrug** is a drug that is inactive in its present form and must be biotransformed in the liver to its active form to be effective. This is an important advantage in a patient with liver dysfunction,

since all the other ACE inhibitors are prodrugs and their transformation to active forms in such patients would be hindered.

Enalapril is the only ACE inhibitor that is available in a parenteral preparation. All other agents are only available in oral formulations. All the newer ACE inhibitors, such as benazepril, fosinopril, lisinopril, quinapril, and ramipril, have long half-lives and durations of action allowing them to be given only once a day. This is particularly beneficial in a patient who is taking many other medications and may have difficulty keeping track of the various dosing schedules for each. A once-a-day medication regimen promotes excellent patient compliance.

All ACE inhibitors have detrimental effects on the unborn fetus and neonate. They are classified as pregnancy category C agents for women in their first trimester and as pregnancy category D agents for women in their second or third trimester. ACE inhibitors should be used in pregnant women only if there are no safer alternatives. Fetal and neonatal morbidity and mortality have been reported to have occurred in at least 50 women who were receiving ACE inhibitors during their pregnancies. All ACE inhibitors are contraindicated in patients with a known hypersensitivity to them, lactating women, children, and patients with bilateral renal artery stenosis.

Many of the ACE inhibitors are combined with either a diuretic or a CCB. The advantage of such combination products is convenience. Often an individual with hypertension or CHF must take many medications including an ACE inhibitor to control high blood pressure. Combination products are beneficial in that they result in increased patient compliance and a decreased number of medications. Examples of new combination ACE inhibitor/CCB products are benazapril and amlodipine (Lotrel), enalapril and diltiazem (Teczem), and trandolapril and verapamil (Tarka).

Mechanism of Action

As is often the case with pharmaceutical discoveries, the development of the ACE inhibitors was spurred by the discovery of an animal substance found to have beneficial effects in human beings. This particular animal substance was the venom of the South American viper, which was found to inhibit kininase activity. Kininase is an enzyme that normally breaks down bradykinin, a potent vasodilator in the human body.

Table 23-3 · ACE Inhibitors: Distinguishing Characteristics

Generic Name	Trade Name	Combination with Hydrochlorothiazide	Interval	Route	Prodrug
benazepril	Lotensin	Lotensin HCT	Once a day		Yes
captopril	Capoten	Capozide 25/15 and 25/25, Capozide 50/15 and 50/25	Multiple	PO	No
cilazapril	Inhibace	None	Once a day	PO	Yes
enalapril	Vasotec	Vaseretic	Multiple	PO & IV	Yes
fosinopril	Monopril	None		PO	Yes
lisinopril	Prinivil	Prinizide 12.5 and 25			No
	Zestril	Zestoretic 12.5 and 25	Once a day		No
moexipril	Univasc	None		PO	Yes
perindopril	Aceon	None			Yes
quinapril	Accupril	None			Yes
ramipril	Altace	None			Yes
spirapril	Renormax	None	Once a day	PO	Yes
trandolapril	Mavrik	None			Yes

The ACE inhibitors have several beneficial cardiovascular effects. As their name implies, they inhibit the angiotensin-converting enzyme, which is responsible for converting angiotensin I to angiotensin II, the latter a potent vasoconstrictor and stimulator of aldosterone. Aldosterone stimulates sodium and water resorption. This whole system is referred to as the *renin angiotensin–aldosterone system (RAAS)*.

Drug Effects

The primary effects of the ACE inhibitors are cardiovascular and renal. Their cardiovascular effects are due to their ability to reduce blood pressure by decreasing SVR. They do this by preventing the breakdown of the vasodilating substance bradykinin and the formation of angiotensin II. These combined effects decrease afterload, or the resistance against which the left ventricle must eject its volume of blood during contraction. The ACE inhibitors are beneficial in the treatment of CHF because they prevent sodium and water resorption by inhibiting aldosterone secretion. This causes diuresis, which decreases blood volume and return to the heart. This in turn decreases preload, or the left ventricular end-diastolic volume, and the work on the heart.

Although ACE inhibitors prevent sodium and water resorption in the kidney, potassium is resorbed. Therefore its levels may need to be monitored, especially in patients taking potassium-sparing diuretics, because hyperkalemia could develop and cause severe cardiac effects such as dysrhythmias.

Therapeutic Uses

The therapeutic effects of the ACE inhibitors are related to their potent cardiovascular effects. They are excellent antihypertensives and adjunctive agents for the treatment of CHF. They may be used alone or in combination with other agents such as diuretics in the treatment of hypertension or CHF.

The beneficial hemodynamic effects of the ACE inhibitors have been studied extensively. Because of their ability to decrease SVR (a measure of afterload) and preload, ACE inhibitors can stop the progression of left ventricular hypertrophy, which is sometimes seen after an MI. The various therapeutic effects of the ACE inhibitors are listed in Table 23-4, which shows the body substances that ACE inhibitors act on and the resulting beneficial hemodynamic effect.

ACE inhibitors have been shown to decrease morbidity and mortality rates in patients with CHF. They should be considered the drugs of choice for hypertensive patients with CHF. They have also shown to have renal protective effects in patients with diabetes.

Side Effects and Adverse Effects

Major CNS effects of the ACE inhibitors include fatigue, dizziness, mood changes, and headaches. A characteristic dry, nonproductive cough is reversible upon discontinuation of the therapy. A first-dose hypotensive effect can cause a significant decline in blood pressure. Other side effects include loss of taste, proteinuria, hyperkalemia, rash, pruritus, anemia, neutropenia, thrombocytosis, and agranulocytosis. In patients with severe CHF whose renal function may depend on the activity of the RAAS, treatment with ACE inhibitors may cause acute renal failure (ARF).

Toxicity and Management of Overdose

The most pronounced symptom of an overdose of an ACE inhibitor is hypotension. Treatment is symptomatic and supportive, and includes the administration of IV fluids to expand the blood volume. Hemodialysis is effective for the removal of captopril and lisinopril.

ACE Inhibitors: Therapeutic Effects

23-4

Body Substance	Effect In Body	ACE Inhibitor Action	Resulting Hemodynamic Effect
Aldosterone	Causes sodium and water retention	Prevents its formation	Diuretics = ↓ plasma volume = ↓ filling pressures or ↓ preload
Angiotensin II	Potent vasoconstrictor	Prevents its formation	↓ SVR = ↓ afterload
Bradykinin	Potent vasodilator	Prevents its breakdown	↓ SVR = ↓ afterload

*SVR, Systemic vascular resistance; ↓, decreased.

home health/community points

Antihypertensive Agents

One of the major side effects of antihypertensive agent is orthostatic hypotension. One of your patients has been discharged after a 6-day hospitalization for hypertensive crises and to rule out a CVA. At 78 years of age, she is somewhat fragile and weakened, lives alone, and has an order for a home health nurse to visit twice weekly to monitor her blood pressure and the success of the prescribed antihypertensive regimen. On one of your first visits, she complains of light-headedness and dizziness. After doing a complete head-to-toe assessment and taking supine and standing blood pressure measurements, it is clear that she is most likely suffering from postural hypotension. You report the symptoms to the physician and make the patient aware of the problem, its signs and symptoms, contributing factors, and other educational information for safe medication use at home. Patient teaching in the home in this situation should include the following information:

- The blood pressure drops because of the medication when the patient moves from sitting or lying to standing. This is characterized by dizziness, light-headedness, lethargy, weakness, and even syncope (fainting).

- Contributing factors include hot climates, saunas, hot showers or baths, alcohol, exercise, hot weather, and dehydration.
- The patient can do several things at home to help this problem, including the following:
  - Keep a consistent and adequate input of fluids (as determined by the physician) at all times, especially during the summer or hot temperatures or when perspiring profusely.
  - Move from one position to another very slowly, and always hold on to a railing or bar when moving from lying to standing or sitting to standing.
  - Take cooler showers or baths.
  - Do not drink alcohol.
  - Support stockings may be beneficial, and calf muscle exercises may also help.
  - Keep a journal of any symptoms and precipitating events, as well as lying, sitting, and standing blood pressure measurements, several times a week.

Interactions

ACE inhibitors can interact with nonsteroidal antiinflammatory drugs (NSAIDs) and potassium-sparing diuretics. ACE inhibitors, when given with other antihypertensives or diuretics, will have additive effects, resulting in increased therapeutic effects. Aspirin and other NSAIDs can have antagonistic effects with ACE inhibitors, resulting in reduced therapeutic effects. Lithium and ACE inhibitors, when given together, can result in lithium toxicity. Potassium supplementation and potassium-sparing diuretics, when given with ACE inhibitors, may result in hyperkalemia.

Acetone may be falsely detected in the urine of patients taking captopril.

Dosages

For information on the dosages for selected ACE inhibitors, see the dosages table on p. 364.

drug profiles

○━captopril

Captopril (Capoten, Capozide) was the first ACE inhibitor to become available and is considered the prototypical agent for the class. Several large multicenter studies have shown its clinical efficacy in minimizing or preventing the left ventricular dilation and dysfunction (also called *ventricular remodeling*) that can arise in the acute period after an MI, thereby improving the patient's chances of survival. It can also reduce the risk of heart failure in these patients and thus the need for subsequent hospitalizations for the treatment of CHF. Because it has the shortest half-life of all the currently available ACE inhibitors, captopril is an excellent agent to give to hospitalized patients who are in a fragile condition

DOSAGES Selected Antihypertensive Agents: ACE Inhibitors and Angiotensin II Receptor Blockers

agent	pharmacologic class	dosage range	purpose
captopril (Capoten) (Capozide)*		*Adult* PO: 25-150 mg 2-3 times/day	Hypertension and heart failure
		PO: Usual dose, 1-2 tablet/day or higher based on the ratio of the two drugs*	Hypertension
enalapril (Vasotec) (Vaseretic)*	ACE inhibitor	*Adult* PO: 10-40 mg/day as a single dose or in 2 equal doses	Hypertension
		PO: 20-50 mg/day as a single dose with digoxin and diuretic	Congestive heart failure
		IV: 1.25 mg q6h over a 5-min period	Hypertension
		PO: Usual dose, 1-2 tablet/day	
losartan (Cozaar)	Angiotensin receptor blocker	*Adult* PO: 25-100 mg in 1 to 2 doses	Hypertension and congestive heart failure
valsartan (Diovan)	Angiotensin receptor blocker	*Adult* PO: 80-320 mg in 1 dose	Hypertension and congestive heart failure

*Fixed-combination tablet with hydrochlorothiazide.

but need afterload and preload reduction. Such a reduction will decrease the work load of a failing heart such as that which exists in the setting of CHF. A very long-acting agent may reduce these hemodynamic variables too much and have lingering effects that may be difficult to compensate for acutely. Captopril is only available orally as 12.5-, 25-, 50-, and 100-mg tablets and as a combination product that includes hydrochlorothiazide. Recommended dosages are given in the dosages table above.

PHARMACOKINETICS

HALF-LIFE	ONSET	PEAK	DURATION
<2 hr	15 min	1-2 hr	2-6 hr

enalapril

Enalapril (Vasotec, Vaseretic) is the only currently available ACE inhibitor that is available in both oral and parenteral preparations. The parenteral formulation (enalaprilat) is an active drug. It offers the hemodynamic benefit of inhibiting ACE activity in an acutely ill patient who cannot tolerate oral medications. Although its half-life is slightly longer than that of captopril, it may in some instances still have to be given twice a day. Enalapril differs from captopril in that it is a prodrug and relies on a functioning liver to be converted to its active form. Like captopril, it too has been shown in many large studies to improve a patient's chances of survival after an MI and to reduce the incidence of heart failure and the need for subsequent hospitalizations for the treatment of CHF in these patients. The oral formulation are available as 2.5-, 5-, 10-, and 20-mg tablets. The parenteral form is

available as a 1.25-mg/ml injection. Recommended dosages are given in the dosages table above.

PHARMACOKINETICS*

HALF-LIFE	ONSET	PEAK	DURATION
<2 hr	1 hr	4-6 hr	12-24 hr

*For oral enalapril.

ANGIOTENSIN II RECEPTOR BLOCKERS

Angiotensin II receptor blockers, also known as AII blockers or ARBs, are one of the newest classes of antihypertensives. Losartan (Cozaar), eposartan (Teveten), valsartan (Diovan), irbesartan (Avapro), candesartan (Atacand), and telmisartan (Micardis) are all ARBs. They work by interfering with the binding of AII to AT_1 receptors and are effective in lowering blood pressure.

Clinically, ACE inhibitors and ARBs appear to be equally effective for treatment of hypertension. Both are well tolerated, but ARBs do not cause cough. It is not clear whether ARBs will be as effective as ACE inhibitors in decreasing mortality rates after a myocardial infarction, in treating CHF, or in their renal-protective effects. Both types of drugs are contraindicated for use in the second or third trimester of pregnancy. Whether one or more of these drugs, particularly newer drugs, could prove to have unique adverse effects with long-term use is unknown.

Mechanism of Action

ARBs block the binding of AII to type I AII receptors. ACE inhibitors such as enalapril block conversion of angiotensin I to AII, but AII may also be formed by other enzymes that are not blocked by ACE inhibitors. In addition, ACE inhibitors block breakdown of bradykinins and substance P, which accumulate and may cause adverse effects such as cough but might also contribute to the drugs' antihypertensive and cardiac- and renal-protective effects. Bradykinins are potent vasodilators and help reduce blood pressure by dilating arteries and decreasing systemic vascular resistance.

Drug Effects

The most prominent effects of ARBs are their effects on the cardiovascular system. AII is a potent vasoconstrictor. It is the primary vasoactive hormone of the renin-angiotensin system and an important component in the pathophysiology of hypertension. AII also stimulates aldosterone secretion by the adrenal cortex. The drug effects of ARBs are primarily seen on vascular smooth muscle and the adrenal gland. By selectively blocking the binding of AII to the AT_1 receptor, ARBs block vasoconstriction and the secretion of aldosterone. AII receptors have been found in other tissues throughout the body, but the effects of blocking these with an ARB are unknown.

Therapeutic Uses

The therapeutic effects of ARBs are related to their potent vasodilating properties. They are excellent antihypertensives and adjunctive agents for the treatment of CHF. They may be used alone or in combination with other agents such as diuretics in the treatment of hypertension or CHF. The beneficial hemodynamic effects of ARBs are their ability to decrease SVR (a measure of afterload). Their use is rapidly growing, and more and more studies are verifying their beneficial effects. Currently they should not be used for patients with diabetes, heart failure, or renal dysfunction except for those who cannot tolerate an ACE inhibitor.

Side Effects and Adverse Effects

The most common side effects of ARBs are upper respiratory infections and headache. Occasionally dizziness, inability to sleep, diarrhea, dyspnea, heartburn, nasal congestion, back pain, and fatigue can occur. Rarely anxiety, muscle pain, sinusitis, cough, and insomnia can also occur.

Toxicity and Management of Overdose

Overdose may manifest as hypotension and tachycardia; bradycardia occurs less often. Treatment is symptomatic and supportive and includes the administration of IV fluids to expand the blood volume.

Interactions

ARBs can interact with cimetidine, phenobarbital, and rifampin. The drugs that interact with these agents, the mechanism responsible, and the result of the interaction are summarized in Table 23-5.

Dosages

For information on the dosages for selected ARBs, see the dosages table on p. 364.

Angiotensin II Receptor Blockers: Drug Interactions

Table 23-5

Drug	Mechanism	Result
cimetidine	Competes with metabolism	Increased ARB effect
lithium	Inhibits lithium elimination	Increased lithium concentrations
phenobarbital, rifampin	Increase metabolism	Decreased ARB effect

drug profiles

losartan

Losartan (Cozaar, Hyzaar) is classified as an ARB. Losartan has been shown to be beneficial in patients with hypertension and congestive heart failure. More and more studies are showing the beneficial effects of ARBs, including losartan, in the treatment of CHF. These studies are showing ARBs to be better tolerating and producing a marginally lower mortality rate than treatment with an ACE inhibitor.

Losartan is classified as a pregnancy category C agent during the first trimester of pregnancy and a pregnancy category D agent during the second and third trimesters. Its use is contraindicated in patients who are hypersensitive to any component of this product. It should be used with caution in patients with renal or hepatic dysfunction and patients with renal artery stenosis. One should avoid breastfeeding while on losartan because it can cause serious adverse effects on the nursing infant. Losartan is available as a 25- and a 50-mg tablet and as a combination product that has 12.5 mg of hydrochlorothiazide and 50 mg of losartan or 25 mg of hydrochlorothiazide and 100 mg of lozartan. Recommended dosages are given in the dosages table on p. 364.

PHARMACOKINETICS

HALF-LIFE	ONSET	PEAK	DURATION
6-9 hr	Unknown	3-4 hr	24 hr

valsartan

Valsartan (Diovan and Diovan HCT) is an ARB. Valsartan is indicated for the treatment of hypertension. It has been shown to be effective in the treatment of CHF. It may be used alone or in combination with other antihypertensive agents. It is generally well tolerated with little side effects.

As with losartan, valsartan is classified as a pregnancy category C agent during the first trimester of pregnancy and a pregnancy category D agent during the second and third trimesters. It has contraindications and precautions similar to those of losartan. Valsartan is available as an 80- and a 160-mg capsule and as a combination product that has 12.5 mg of hydrochlorothiazide and either 80 or 160 mg of valsartan. The two combination products with valsartan are tablets. Recommended dosages are given in the dosages table on p. 364.

PHARMACOKINETICS			
HALF-LIFE	ONSET	PEAK	DURATION
6 hr	Unknown	2-4 hr	24 hr

CALCIUM CHANNEL BLOCKERS

CCBs have been discussed in some detail in the two previous chapters on antidysrhythmic agents (Chapter 21) and antianginal agents (Chapter 22). As a class of medications they are used for several indications and have many beneficial effects and few side effects. CCBs are primarily used for the treatment of hypertension and angina. Their effectiveness in treating hypertension is related to their ability to cause smooth muscle relaxation by blocking the binding of calcium to its receptors, thereby preventing contraction. Because of their effectiveness and safety, they have been added to the list of first-line agents for the treatment of hypertension. CCBs are used for many other indications as well. They are effective antidysrhythmics and migraine medications, they can prevent the cerebral artery spasms that can occur after a subarachnoid hemorrhage, and they are effective in the treatment of Raynaud's disease.

DIURETICS

The diuretics are a highly effective class of antihypertensive agents. Their primary therapeutic effect is decreasing the plasma and extracellular fluid volumes, which results in decreased preload. This leads to a decrease in cardiac output and total peripheral resistance, all of which decrease the work load of the heart. This large group of antihypertensives is discussed in detail in Chapter 24 on diuretics.

VASODILATORS

Vasodilators act directly on arteriolar smooth muscle to cause relaxation. Some vasodilators (diazoxide IV and sodium nitroprusside) are particularly useful in the management of hypertensive emergencies when the blood pressure is severely, or even only moderately, elevated. However, there is a threat of impending end-organ damage, particularly of the brain, heart, or eyes.

Mechanism of Action

The particular mechanism of action of the direct-acting vasodilators that makes them useful as antihypertensive agents is their ability to directly elicit peripheral vasodilation. This results in a reduction in systemic vascular resistance.

Drug Effects

In general the most notable effect of the vasodilators is their hypotensive effect. However, in recent years minoxidil (in its topical form) has received increasing attention because of its effectiveness in restoring hair growth. Oral diazoxide has also proved to have significant antihypoglycemic effects.

Therapeutic Uses

All the vasodilators can be used to treat hypertension, either alone or in combination with other antihypertensives. Diazoxide is also an antihypoglycemic when administered orally. Sodium nitroprusside and diazoxide IV are reserved for the management of hypertensive emergencies. Minoxidil in its topical form is used to restore hair growth.

Side Effects and Adverse Effects

Undesirable effects of diazoxide include dizziness, headache, orthostatic hypotension, dysrhythmias, sodium and water retention, nausea, vomiting, rarely acute pancreatitis, and hyperglycemia in diabetic patients.

The adverse effects of hydralazine include dizziness, headache, anxiety, tachycardia, edema, nasal congestion, dyspnea, anorexia, nausea, vomiting, diarrhea, anemia, agranulocytosis, hepatitis, peripheral neuritis, lupus erythematosus, and rash.

Minoxidil effects include T-wave ECG change, pericardial effusion or tamponade, angina, breast tenderness, rash, and thrombocytopenia.

Sodium nitroprusside effects include bradycardia, decreased platelet aggregation, rash, hypothyroidism, hypotension, and possible cyanide toxicity.

Toxicity and Management of Overdose

The main symptom of diazoxide overdose or toxicity is hypotension, which can usually be controlled by having the patient assume the Trendelenburg position. Sympathomimetics such as dopamine or norepinephrine may also be required. Hydralazine toxicity or overdose produces hypotension, tachycardia, headache, and generalized skin flushing. Treatment is supportive and symptomatic and includes the administration of IV fluids, digitalization, if needed, and the administration of beta-blockers for the control of tachycardia.

Minoxidil overdose or toxicity can precipitate excessive hypotension. Treatment is supportive and symptomatic and includes the administration of IV fluids. Norepinephrine and epinephrine should not be used to reverse the hypotension because of the possibility of causing excessive cardiac stimulation.

The main symptoms of sodium nitroprusside overdose or toxicity are excessive hypotension and cyanide toxicity. Treatment for the hypotension is supportive and symptomatic, and cyanide toxicity can be treated using a standard antidote kit.

23-6 Direct-Acting Vasodilators: Drug Interactions

Drug	Mechanism	Result
DIAZOXIDE		
Antihypertensives/thiazides	Additive effects	Increased hypotensive/hyperglycemic effect
hydralazine	Additive effects	Increased hypotensive effect
PO anticoagulants	Protein storage displacement	Increased anticoagulant effect
Sulfonylureas	Hyperglycemic effect	Decreased hypoglycemic effect of sulfonylureas
HYDRALAZINE		
Adrenergics	Antagonism	Decreased hypotensive effect
Antihypertensives	Additive effects	Increased hypotensive effect
Monoamine oxidase inhibitors	Alters biotransformation	Increased hypotensive effect
MINOXIDIL		
Antihypertensives/thiazides	Additive effects	Increased hypotensive effect
guanethidine	Additive effects	Significant hypotensive effect
SODIUM NITROPRUSSIDE		
Ganglionic-blocking agents	Additive effects	Increased hypotensive effect

Interactions

Although the incidence of drug interactions with the direct-acting vasodilators (especially sodium nitroprusside) is low, as a class of agents they are associated with a variety of drug interactions. These are summarized in Table 23-6.

Dosages

For dosage information for selected vasodilator agents, see the dosages table on p. 368.

drug profiles

diazoxide

Diazoxide (Hyperstat) is contraindicated in patients who have shown a hypersensitivity to it and in those with functional hypoglycemia or the compensatory hypertension associated with coarctation or arteriovenous shunt. Its use as an antihypertensive agent is limited to the management of hypertensive emergencies. Oral agents can control hypoglycemia. See the dosages table on p. 368 for dosage information. Pregnancy category C.

PHARMACOKINETICS

HALF-LIFE	ONSET	PEAK	DURATION
30-36 hr	<1 min	2-5 min	3-12 hr

hydralazine hydrochloride

Hydralazine hydrochloride (Apresoline) is contraindicated in patients with a known hypersensitivity to it as well as in those with coronary artery disease or mitral valvular or rheumatic heart dis-

ease. See the dosages table on p. 368 for dosage information. Pregnancy category C.

PHARMACOKINETICS

HALF-LIFE	ONSET	PEAK	DURATION
3-7 hr	IV: 5-20 min PO: 20-30 min	IV: 30-45 min PO: 1-2 hr	IV: 2-4 hr PO: 6-12 hr

minoxidil

Minoxidil (Loniten, Rogaine) is contraindicated in patients with a known hypersensitivity to it and in those with pheochromocytoma. A topical 2% and 5% minoxidil solution is used to treat hair loss, and a 2.5- and 10-mg tablet is used to treat hypertension. See the dosages table above for dosage information. Pregnancy category C.

PHARMACOKINETICS

HALF-LIFE	ONSET	PEAK	DURATION
4.2 hr	30 min	2-8 hr	2-5 days

sodium nitroprusside

Sodium nitroprusside (Nipride, Nitropress) is contraindicated in patients with a known hypersensitivity to it, as well as in those with the compensatory hypertension associated with coarctation or arteriovenous shunt, congenital Leber's optic atrophy, tobacco amblyopia, or inadequate cerebral circulation. This drug's use is limited to the management of hypertensive emergencies. See the dosages table on p. 368 for dosage information. Pregnancy category C.

PHARMACOKINETICS

HALF-LIFE	ONSET	PEAK	DURATION
2 min	<2 min	2-5 min	1-10 min

Activity

DOSAGES Selected Antihypertensive Agents: Vasodilators

agent	pharmacologic class	dosage range	purpose
diazoxide (Hyperstat)		*Pediatric/Adult* IV: 1-3 mg/kg repeated at 5-15 min intervals; mainte-nance doses can be given at 4-24 hr intervals if required (max of 150 mg/dose)	Acute hypertension
hydralazine hydrochloride (Alazine, Apresoline)	Direct-acting peripheral vasodilator	*Pediatric* PO: 0.75-7.5 mg/kg/day to a max of 200 mg/day *Adult* PO: 10 mg qid for 2-4 days followed by 25 mg qid for balance of week. Second and subsequent weeks, 50 mg qid, then adjust to lowest effective dose for maintenance. IV: 20-40 mg prn	Hypertension
minoxidil (Loniten)		*Pediatric <12 y/o* PO: 0.25-1 mg/kg/day usually as a single dose; do not exceed 50 mg/day. *Pediatric >12 y/o/Adult* PO: 10-40 mg/day as a single dose or divided; do not exceed 100 mg/day	Hypertension
sodium nitroprusside (Nipride, Nitropress)		*Pediatric/Adult* IV: 0.3-10 μg/kg/min	

nursing process

As previously discussed, there are a variety of agents used to treat hypertension. Although much of the nursing process related to their use is similar for the agents as a whole, there are some considerations very specific to the use of the particular classes of agents. Therefore the overall nursing process called for in patients receiving any of the antihypertensive agents is described here (also see Box 23-2), with the patient teaching tips giving details on the nursing process necessary for the individual classes of antihypertensives.

● **Assessment**

Before administering any antihypertensive agent to a patient, the nurse should obtain a thorough health history and perform a head-to-toe physical examination, since this is crucial to ensuring safe drug therapy. During the nursing assessment, it is important to look for underlying causes of the hypertension such as the following:
• Renal or liver dysfunction
• Stressful lifestyle
• Cushing's disease
• Addison's disease
• Renal artery stenosis
• Coarctation of the aorta
• Peripheral vascular disease
• Pheochromocytoma

Many of these diseases demand cautious administration of the antihypertensive agent or may even constitute a contraindication to its use. In addition, if it is primary (idiopathic) hypertension that is being treated, the identification of an underlying cause of what would then be secondary hypertension means that eradication of the primary disease could alleviate the high blood pressure, ruling out the need for antihypertensive therapy. Cautious use of antihypertensives is called for in elderly patients and patients who have chronic illnesses. Specifically, diuretics should be used cautiously in elderly patients and patients with hypotension suffering from fluid and electrolyte disturbances.

Beta-blockers should be used cautiously in patients with chronic obstructive pulmonary disease (COPD), diabetes mellitus, or hyperlipidemia. The adrenergic inhibitor clonidine should be used cautiously in patients suffering from coronary insufficiency, those with Raynaud's disease or a history of mental depression, and recent victims of MI. In addition to cautions listed for clonidine therapy, methyldopa, another adrenergic inhibitor, should not be used in patients with active liver disease and should be used cautiously in patients with hemolytic anemia.

Contraindications to ARBs include pregnancy, hyperaldosteronism, and renal artery stenosis. Caution should be taken with patients who are in volume depletion, renal dysfunction, and renal insufficiency. Drug interactions include potassium salts or supplements, cimetidine, phenobarbital, rifampin, and lithium. Any over-the-counter medications should also be avoided unless advised by the physician. Before beginning treatment the health care provider must monitor and document baseline vital signs, including pulse and blood pressure (standing and sitting), cardiac rate and rhythm, weight, and input and output.

Contraindications to the use of the adrenergic neuronal blockers include COPD, peptic ulcer disease or colitis,

NURSING CARE PLAN Hypertension

Mr. J.C., a 58-year-old African-American male, reports to the doctor's office today and is newly diagnosed as hypertensive. He has never taken any medications for any disorder and has been extremely healthy until this recent bout with headaches and chest pain. His blood pressure at the office today is 172/98, P92, R22, and he is somewhat anxious about his blood pressure and taking any medication. His wife of 25 years is very supportive and has attended each visit with him to the doctor's office. He is a executive vice-president for a local computer company and is a hard-driving, hard-working individual. He denies smoking and drinking, and his weight and height are within normal limits. Nursing assessment is negative for any edema, chest pain, distress, dyspnea, palpitations, or other problems. He exercises regularly and will be instructed on a low-fat diet and be supervised at a local cardiac rehab center for appropriate exercising and stress management. The main concern today is education about his medication, enalapril maleate.

assessment	*Nursing Diagnosis*	Deficient knowledge related to lack of information and experience with medications
	Subjective Data	"I really am not sure about how to take this new blood pressure medicine or anything about its side effects"
		"Are there any medications I can't take when I'm taking this blood pressure medicine"
	Objective Data	• New diagnosis of hypertension
		• Addition of enalapril maleate to regimen
		• BP 168/106
		• P88
		• RR 22
		• SMA6 within normal limits
		• Renal and liver function studies within normal limits
planning and outcome criteria	*Goals*	Patient will remain compliant and with minimal side effects to enalapril maleate therapy within 1 mo
	Outcome Criteria	Patient will repeat the following instructions:
		• How to take the medication
		• How not to skip or double up on doses missed or forgotten
		• How to measure and record BPs with pulse
		• Side effects associated with therapy
		• Ways to maximize the effects of the medication
		• Side effects to report to the physician immediately
		• Importance of compliance to therapy
		• Drug interactions and importance of a holistic approach to therapy such as with exercise and diet
implementation		Patient education focused on the following instructions:
		• Take medication at least 1 hr before meals as ordered.
		• Avoid OTC preparations that are used for colds due to their vasoconstricting properties, which in turn elevate blood pressure.
		• It is important that you take this medication exactly as prescribed and without missing any doses or doubling up on doses; if stopped abruptly it may lead to a "rebound" hypertensive problem in which your blood pressure could elevate at high and dangerous levels.
		• Light-headedness occurs for the first few days of therapy and usually subsides after this time; however, you should always rise slowly to sitting or standing position to avoid postural hypotension and fainting.
		• Make sure you always comply with dosage schedule even if you are feeling better.
		• Photosensitivity may occur, so avoid sunlight or wear sunscreen if outdoors.
		• Contact your physician if you have problems with mouth sores, fever, swelling of hands or feet, palpitations, or irregular heartbeats and chest pain.
		• If you perspire heavily or suffer from dehydration, vomiting, diarrhea, you could have a fall in blood pressure with resulting fainting, dizziness or falling; contact physician should this occur.
		• Take and record in a journal your blood pressures at least 3 times per week or have a local rescue/fire squad member take it for you. They often will provide this service for you if you go by their station.

NURSING CARE PLAN Hypertension—cont'd

evaluation

Patient will display therapeutic response to medication as a result of compliance to drug therapy as evidenced by:
- Taking medications as prescribed
- Blood pressures within normal limits with diastolic consistently <90 mm Hg
- Avoiding interacting medications
- Contacting physician appropriately with problems or concerns
- Positioning self slowly from sitting or standing without fainting or falls
- Taking meds before meals
- Reporting improved health and sense of well being
- Normal appetite
- Without weight gain, edema, dyspnea, wet rales, and signs and symptoms of CHF
- Wearing sunscreen when outdoors
- Suffering minimal side effects and without mouth sores, edema, or irregular heartbeats or chest pain
- Contacting physician when ill and possibly dehydrated
- Patient monitored for side effects but experiences minimal problems
- Recording blood pressures in a journal and sharing them with the physician at appointments; gradual decline in elevated blood pressure to within normal limits

BOX 23-2 Tips for Nurses Caring for Antihypertensive Patients

- Nurses need to be proactive in screening patients for hypertension and take every opportunity to provide patients with both verbal and written information about the disease and the lifestyle changes needed. Information about medications is also important!
- Home health care nurses should take every opportunity to participate in blood pressure screenings in their community and seek occasions to answer patients' questions about hypertension—its causes, risks, complications, and treatment.
- Whenever a nurse identifies a patient with a diastolic blood pressure that exceeds 120 mm Hg, because this is a hypertensive crisis, he or she should make sure the patient gets immediate medical attention.

hypersensitivity to them, and frank CHF not related to hypertension. Cautious use of these agents is called for in the settings of severe renal disease, recent MI, cerebrovascular disease, CHF, sinus bradycardia, diabetes mellitus, impaired liver function, and fever. Rauwolfia alkaloids such as reserpine should be used cautiously in patients with a history of mental depression, gallstones, renal insufficiency, cerebral hemorrhage, epilepsy, cardiac damage, COPD, or parkinsonism. Contraindications to their use include mental depression, ulcerative colitis, and acute peptic ulcers.

Cautious use of the alpha$_1$-blockers is warranted in patients with angina or severe cardiac disease and in the elderly. Vasodilators should be used cautiously in patients with impaired cerebral or cardiac circulation. Arterial and venous dilator drugs should not be used in patients with inadequate cerebral circulation and should be used cautiously in patients suffering from impaired renal or hepatic function or vitamin B$_{12}$ deficiency. ACE inhibitors should not be used as first-line agents because of their potentially serious side effects, and they should be used cautiously in patients with hyperkalemia or reduced renal function. Newer agents, such as Losartan (an ARB), should be used very cautiously with the elderly, in patients with hepatic function impairment or renal impairment, and in patients who are sodium- or fluid-depleted. Patients who are hypokalemic or hypovolemic may show even more dramatic drops in blood pressure. Losartan, in particular, interacts with NSAIDs, diuretics, K-containing medications, and sympathomimetics and results in clinical problems (either decreased or increased blood pressure [sympathomimetics causing increased blood pressure]).

CCBs should be used cautiously in patients suffering from severe aortic stenosis, bradycardia, heart failure, or cardiogenic shock. Their cautious use is recommended in elderly patients as well as in those with impaired renal or liver function.

Nursing Diagnoses

Nursing diagnoses appropriate to patients receiving antihypertensive agents include, but are not limited to, the following:
- Deficient knowledge about medications and treatment protocol related to a newly prescribed treatment with medications and lifestyle changes.
- Noncompliance with the therapy related to lack of familiarity with or acceptance of the disease process.
- Sexual dysfunction related to the sexual dysfunction as a side effect of some antihypertensive drugs.

Hypertension

Hypertension was diagnosed in G.S. when she was 33 years old. Both her mother and sister suffer from hypertension, and both were also in their 30s when it was diagnosed. G.S.'s most current blood pressure is 150/96 mm Hg, and for this reason, the nurse practitioner has recommended she see her primary care provider. After examining her, the physician prescribes hydrochlorothiazide and puts her on a diet low in table salt. After 14 days of this therapy; G.S.'s blood pressure is found to be 145/86 mm Hg. Stress reduction has been the biggest obstacle in her treatment. She is a lawyer in a prominent law firm and has found that her blood pressure is consistently elevated (diastolic readings >100 but <110 mm Hg) whenever she measures it at work.

● *What should G.S. know about her antihypertensive medication therapy?*

● *What lifestyle changes would you, as her nurse, recommend she make, and even more importantly, what information would you give her to help her change her lifestyle and more effectively reduce the stress in her life?*

● *What questions would you ask G.S. to find out more about her stress level and the lifestyle changes she should make?*

For Answers see www.harcourthealth.com/MERLIN/Lilley/.

● Risk for injury related to side effects of the antihypertensive agent such as dizziness, orthostatic hypotension, and syncope.

● Acute pain related to headache as a side effect of some antihypertensive agents.

● Ineffective tissue perfusion related to the influence of the disease process.

● Excess fluid volume related to side effects of some of the antihypertensive agents and treatment protocol.

● Imbalanced nutrition, less than body requirements, related to side effects of the agent.

● Constipation related to the side effects of antihypertensive agents.

● Risk for injury related to possible excessive CNS effects such as paresthesias, sedation, tremors, weakness, and seizures.

● Risk for injury to mucous membranes related to dry mouth effects of drug.

● Disturbed body image related to side effects of hypertension medication (e.g., impotence, sexual dysfunction, weight gain, and fatigue).

● **Planning**

Nursing goals of antihypertensive therapy should focus on educating the patient and his or her family to the need for adequate management to prevent end-organ damage. These goals include making sure the patient understands the nature of the disease, its symptoms and treatment, and the importance of complying with

the treatment regimen. The patient must also come to terms with the diagnosis as well as with the fact that there is no cure for the disease and treatment will be lifelong. The influence of chronic illness as well as the importance of nonpharmacologic therapy, stress reduction, and follow-up care must also be underscored. The nurse needs to plan for ongoing assessment of blood pressure, weight, diet, exercise, smoking habits, alcohol intake, compliance with therapy, and sexual function in such patients.

Specific patient goals include the following:
● Patient takes the drug exactly as prescribed.
● Patient experiences relief of symptoms for which the medication was prescribed.
● Patient demonstrates an adequate knowledge about the use of the specific medications, its side effects, and the appropriate dosing at home.
● Patient is free of self-injury resulting from adverse effects of the medications.
● Patient states the rationale and importance of medication therapy.
● Patient maintains record of medication administration and of any associated side effects that occur.
● Patient reports any change in sexual patterns and function, bowel pattern changes, or activity intolerance.
● Patient implements measures to take to decrease the occurrence of side effects.
● Patient remains compliant to therapy.

Outcome Criteria

Outcome criteria related to the use of antihypertensive agents are as follows:
● Patient will state the risks and complications of potent antihypertensive agents such as tremors, decreased sweating, tachycardia, and hypotension.
● Patient will state conditions that may occur that the physician should be notified of such as syncope and chest pain.
● Patient will state importance of lifelong compliance to the pharmacologic treatment of hypertension to decrease end-organ damage and complications to every organ system.
● Patient will follow instructions to change position slowly, monitor blood pressure, keep follow-up appointments with the physician, and keep a journal to help decrease injury from side effects of drugs.
● Patient will communicate openly with nurses and other members of the health care team regarding the disease and the treatment prescribed and any concerns related to changes in body image or function.
● Patient will report to the physician immediately any edema or weight gain of more than 2 lb in 1 week.
● Patient will maintain normal nutritional status through adherence to a prescribed diet high in fiber and fluids and avoidance of alcohol.

● **Implementation**

Nursing interventions generally can help the patient achieve stable blood pressures and can minimize adverse effects. Many patients have problems complying with treatment because the disease itself is silent whereas the medications often have very altering effects on self-concept and sexual function. Any symptoms patients experience may well be side effects of the medication.

When taking ARBs, the health care provider must emphasize to patients to take these medications exactly as ordered and not to change the dosage or discontinue unless prescribed by the physician. Instructions should be given to the patient about how to change positions slowly to avoid syncope from postural hypotension. These agents are often tolerated better with meals. Patients should report any unusual shortness of breath; difficulty breathing; swelling of the feet, ankles, face, or around the eyes; weight gain or loss; chest pain; palpitations; or excessive fatigue.

Besides monitoring vital signs and educating patients, the nurse should encourage patients to do the following:
- Lose weight
- Avoid stress
- Engage in supervised exercise
- Pay attention to their skin condition, including skin turgor
- Note any leg cramps or general muscle weakness (hypokalemia)
- Watch for interactions with over-the-counter or other drugs
- Monitor for signs of depression such as nightmares, poor appetite, and insomnia
- Change positions slowly
- Avoid straining
- Avoid smoking and consuming alcohol
- Watch their blood glucose levels if they are diabetic
- Inform all health care personnel of medications they are currently taking
- Stay hydrated
- Take caution in hot weather and with exercising
- Protect their extremities from the cold and from possible injury from falls as the result of side effects such as orthostatic hypotension.

Other nursing considerations for all of these agents include education about the importance of not missing a dose and proper dosing. It is important to remember that these drugs should not be withdrawn abruptly because this may trigger a rebound hypertensive crisis that could precipitate a cerebrovascular accident. Oral forms should be given with meals so that absorption of the drug is more gradual and effective. Intravenous forms should be given with extreme caution using an IV pump. Regular blood pressure checks are necessary while the patient is on this medication, and a patient journal should be suggested. Although the restriction of sodium intake has always been a standard aspect of the nonpharmacologic therapy for hypertension, the actual need for it is now being debated. Treatment of hypertension should be managed holistically, and it should be emphasized that the medication therapy is only part of the overall treatment.

See the Herbal Interactions box for goldenseal, an herb commonly taken to prevent colds or flu and to relieve diarrhea and GI inflammation.

Patient teaching tips for antihypertensive agents are listed on p. 373.

● Evaluation

Because patients with hypertension are at high risk for incurring cardiovascular injury, it is critical for them to be compliant with both their pharmacologic and nonpharmacologic treatment. Monitoring patients for the adverse effects (e.g., orthostatic hypotension, dizziness, fatigue) and toxic effects of the various types of antihypertensive agents is important to the identification of potentially life-threatening complications. The most important aspect of the evaluation process is collecting data and monitoring patients for evidence of controlled blood pressure. Blood pressure should be maintained at less than 140/90 mm Hg. Blood pressure monitoring should be at periodic intervals, and education about self-monitoring is very important to the safe use of these drugs. The physician also needs to examine the fundus of patients' eyes, because this is a more reliable indicator of the long-term effectiveness of treatment than blood pressure readings. The patient must constantly be monitored for the development of end-organ damage as well as for specific problems that the medication can cause. Men receiving an antihypertensive agent should be questioned about impotence because they often are not aware that this is an expected side effect of most antihypertensive agents. Follow-up visits to the physician are important for monitoring patient compliance, the effectiveness of or problems with treatment, and complications of the hypertension.

Therapeutic effects of ARBs include an improvement in hypertensive states and in patients with CHF. Patients should report a return to a normal baseline of blood pressure with improved energy levels and improvement in the signs and symptoms of hypertension, such as less edema, improved breath sounds, no abnormal heart sounds, capillary refill <5 seconds, less shortness of breath, or dyspnea. Side effects for which to monitor during the use of ARBs include upper respiratory infections, headache, dizziness, insomnia, GI disturbances (diarrhea, heartburn), fatigue, and cough.

patient teaching tips

Antihypertensive Agents

All Antihypertensives

➤ Patients should be encouraged to take their medication exactly as prescribed by the physician because an overdose can cause life-threatening problems. Taking medications as prescribed is very important in controlling hypertension and preventing complications.

➤ If a dose is missed, patients should check with their physician for instructions on what to do. They should never double up on doses.

➤ Patients should know they must never stop taking their medications on their own without their physician's approval, because this may lead to a very dangerous increase in blood pressure and life-threatening problems.

➤ Medication should be taken with a full glass of fluid, preferably orange juice (unless this is not allowed) because it is high in potassium. Other foods high in potassium are citrus fruits, dried fruits, apricots, bananas, nuts, cantaloupe, watermelon, beef, and fowl.

➤ Remember that medication is only part of a treatment program. Patients need to watch their diet, stress level, weight, and alcohol intake. They should avoid smoking and eating foods high in sodium such as lunch meats, canned soups, processed cheese, snack foods, and Chinese food. They should engage only in supervised exercise.

➤ Keep all medications out of the reach of children.

➤ Patients should wear a MedicAlert tag or bracelet and a medical ID card specifying their condition and the medications they are taking.

Adrenergic Agents

➤ Follow-up visits to the physician are very important so that patients' blood pressure and medication levels can be monitored closely.

➤ As with other antihypertensive agents, patients should not miss doses or stop taking their medication abruptly without a physician's order, because this could precipitate a considerable increase in their blood pressure (rebound hypertension), which could lead to life-threatening problems. These serious problems could occur within 8 to 24 hours after the drug is discontinued.

➤ If patients are experiencing serious side effects or believe that they should stop taking their medication or have their dose changed, they should contact their physician immediately.

➤ The symptoms of a hypertensive crisis or of blood pressure that is elevated such that stroke or other life-threatening problems may ensue include anxiety, sweating, increased pulse, salivation, muscle pain, and stomach pain.

➤ Patients should always keep an adequate supply of these medications on hand, especially while traveling.

➤ Patients should have periodic (every 6 months) eye examinations.

➤ The use of clonidine with other CNS depressants can cause severe drowsiness.

Adrenergic Neuronal Blockers

➤ Dizziness, light-headedness, and fainting occur frequently in patients taking these medications, especially when patients change positions suddenly.

➤ Hot tubs, showers, or baths; hot weather; prolonged sitting or standing; physical exercise; and alcohol ingestion are all conditions that can aggravate low blood pressure, and this may lead to fainting and possible injury. If patients experience dizziness, they should sit or lay down until the symptoms subside.

➤ Patients should inform any other health care personnel who may be treating them (e.g., dentist, surgeon) that they are taking antihypertensives.

➤ Patients should be warned to not take any other medications or OTC drugs that might contain a sympathomimetic that can precipitate high blood pressure.

➤ Follow-up care with the physician is very important to the patient's health and overall well-being.

Rauwolfia Alkaloids

➤ Patients should change positions slowly to prevent possible dizziness and fainting.

➤ These medications have a sedating effect, so patients should be careful about operating hazardous machinery.

➤ Patients should not take other CNS depressants.

➤ Patients should report any awareness of mental depression to their physician.

➤ Sugarless hard candy or gum and/or saliva substitutes may help to relieve the dry mouth that is a side effect of these agents.

➤ Patients should understand the importance of follow-up care with their physician.

Alpha$_1$-Adrenergic Blockers

➤ There is a first-dose effect with prazosin. This means that patients will experience a considerable drop in their blood pressure after they take their first dose, so they should take it while lying down or before bedtime and arise slowly. This first-dose effect decreases with time or with a reduction in the dose, as ordered by the physician.

➤ It often takes 4 to 6 weeks for this drug to be working at its full potential.

➤ Patients should weigh themselves daily and report any increase to their physician.

➤ Patients should not take any other medications, including OTC drugs, without first getting the approval of their physician.

➤ Patients should take their blood pressure frequently and keep a record of the readings.

ACE Inhibitors

➤ It may take several weeks before patients experience the benefits of this medication.

➤ Patients should report any signs of infection and easy bruising or bleeding.

➤ Patients should report any weight gain or loss.

➤ The impaired taste associated with these medications usually goes away in 2 to 3 months.

➤ Patients should be encouraged not to take potassium supplements or increase potassium intake because this may be harmful.

A-II Blockers

➤ Losartan should be taken the same time everyday; do not omit a dose and do not double up on doses.
➤ Take caution when exercising, in hot weather, and with any condition leading to fluid or sodium loss.
➤ Monitor and record blood pressures a few times each week.
➤ Take care when using OTC medications because of interactions.

Calcium Channel Blockers

➤ Patients should always keep a record of their medications. Patients should be encouraged to always keep a record of any chest pain that occurs and note its pattern, duration, and severity. Blood pressure readings should also be recorded.
➤ Encourage patients to change position slowly.
➤ It is important for patients to see their physician regularly.
➤ Patients should monitor their blood pressure and pulse regularly and keep a record of the values. They should report to their physician a pulse of less than 50 beats/minute, headaches, nausea, rashes, vomiting, edema, or a weight gain.
➤ Patients should get the okay of their physician before taking any OTC or other medication.

Diuretics

➤ If patients are diabetic or have gout, they must monitor their condition carefully, because diuretics may cause an increase in uric acid levels as well as hyperglycemia.
➤ Encourage patients to always be cautious about their potassium levels and report any leg cramping, weakness, and muscle cramps.

➤ Encourage patients to increase their intake of potassium-rich foods such as bananas, apricots, and citrus fruits.
➤ Patients should take their diuretic ("fluid pill") early in the day so they won't be up all night voiding.
➤ Patients should be encouraged to check their blood pressure at least three times a week, unless otherwise specified by the physician, and to keep a record of the readings.
➤ If patients are also taking digitalis products, they must be careful to report any of the following symptoms to their physician immediately: very slow pulse (<50 beats/minute), nausea, vomiting, loss of appetite, or visual disorders.
➤ Alcohol, barbiturates, and opioids react with any of these medications and cause the patient's blood pressure to decrease further, which may cause dizziness or fainting.

Vasodilators (Arteriolar)

➤ Patients should be encouraged to take their pulse and blood pressure frequently and report any changes to the physician.
➤ Patients should weigh themselves daily and report any increase to their physician.
➤ Patients should report any shortness of breath, chest pain, cough, or fatigue to their physician.
➤ Systemic lupus may occur in patients taking more than 200 mg of oral hydralazine per day, so they should report any fever, sore throat, joint pain, chest pain, or fatigue to their physician.
➤ Hypertrichosis occurs in about 80% of patients taking minoxidil and involves thickening and increased pigmentation of the fine body hair over the face, shoulders, back, legs, and forearms. It is reversible within 2 to 6 months after the drug is discontinued. Patients should report any problems with hair overgrowth to their physician.

POINTS TO REMEMBER

Blood Pressure

• BP is the product of cardiac output (CO) times the systemic vascular resistance (SVR).
• All antihypertensives in some way affect CO and/or SVR.
• CO: amount of blood ejected from left ventricle measured in liters per minute.
• SVR: force the left ventricle must overcome to eject its end-diastolic volume.
• Four main categories of antihypertensives: diuretics, adrenergics, ACE inhibitors, and calcium channel blockers.

Angiotensin-Converting Enzyme Inhibitors

• Work by blocking a critical enzyme system responsible for the production of angiotensin II (a potent vasoconstrictor).
• By blocking angiotensin converting enzyme, ACE inhibitors prevent vasoconstriction caused by angiotensin II.

• They also prevent aldosterone secretion and therefore sodium and water resorption.
• They also prevent bradykinin (a potent vasodilator) from being broken down by angiotensin II.

Calcium Channel Blockers

• May be used to treat angina, dysryhthmias, and hypertension.
• Relieve high blood pressure by causing smooth muscle relaxation and dilation of blood vessels.
• If calcium not present smooth muscle cannot contract.
• Three chemical categories of calcium channel blockers; the dihydropyridines have the greatest affinity for the peripheral blood vessels.

Nursing Considerations

• A thorough nursing assessment should include finding out whether the patient has any underlying causes of

hypertension, such as renal or liver dysfunction, a stressful lifestyle, Cushing's disease, Addison's disease, renal artery stenosis, peripheral vascular disease, or pheochromocytoma.
- Always check for the existence of contraindications, cautions, and drug interactions before administering any of the antihypertensive agents.
- Patients should be managed not only by pharmacologic means but should also be encouraged to consume a diet low in fat, to make any other modifications in their diet, to engage in regular, supervised exercise, and to reduce stress in their life.

- Contraindications include patients with a history of myocardial infarction, chronic renal disease.
- Cautious use is recommended in patients with renal insufficiency and glaucoma.
- Drug interactions include other antihypertensive agents, anesthetics, and diuretics.
- Therapeutic effects include less hypertensive-related symptoms such as chest pain, severe headaches, and increased BP readings.
- Side effects to constantly monitor for in patients on these medications include tachycardia, confusion, hallucinations, CNS depression, and constipation.

REVIEW QUESTIONS

1. The physician is performing an ophthalmic examination on your patient who has a history of hypertension. What is the rationale for this type of examination?
   a. To assess for end-of-life type of situations.
   b. Visual acuity decreases sometimes rapidly with antihypertensive treatment.
   c. The retina may show signs of bulging, indicating drug toxicity and possible hypotension.
   d. The fundus of the patient's eye is often a more reliable indicator of long-term effectiveness of treatment as compared with blood pressure readings.
2. Which of the following common side effects is usually a major concern for male patients taking antihypertensive agents?
   a. Impotence
   b. Increased libido
   c. Increased weight
   d. Decreased sensorium

3. Your female patient has just begun treatment of hypertension with minoxidil. You have explained to her that she may experience hypertrichosis, which is also:
   a. Increased breast size.
   b. Increased weight gain.
   c. Increased skin discoloration.
   d. Increased pigmentation of fine body hair.
4. Which of the following agents would require the patient to lie down during the first dose of medication to avoid the severe syncope associated with mainly the first dose?
   a. Potassium chloride
   b. Furosemide (Lasix)
   c. Prazosin (Minipress)
   d. Digitalis preparations
5. In general, most antihypertensive agents may cause all of the following side effects except for:
   a. Dry mouth.
   b. Tachycardia.
   c. Profound sedation.
   d. Postural hypotension.

For Answers see www.harcourthealth.com/MERLIN/Lilley/.

CRITICAL THINKING Activities

1. Primary hypertension has been diagnosed in J.M., a 53-year-old woman, and reserpine (0.1 mg PO qd) has been prescribed. Before initiating reserpine therapy, what past medical conditions should the nurse inquire about during the nursing assessment?
2. B.T. is a 78-year-old woman who has been admitted to the emergency room for the treatment of a possible acute myocardial infarction. One of your standing orders is to start a nitroglycerin infusion at a rate of 33 μg/min. The concentration of nitroglycerin in a standard, premixed nitroglycerin infusion bag is 200 μg/ml. What rate in milliliters per hour should you set the infusion pump at to deliver the prescribed dose?

3. You are caring for a patient who needs rapid reduction of blood pressure and is in a hypertensive crisis. The patient cannot tolerate sodium nitroprusside, the preferred agent in this situation. Instead trimethaphan (Arfonad) is ordered. You are to start your patient on a 1-mg/min infusion and titrate to maintain a systolic blood pressure between 100–120 mm Hg. Assuming 1 mg/min achieves your desired endpoint, how long will a 500 mg/250 ml bag of Arfonad last?
4. During the administration of trimethaphan for the treatment of a hypertensive emergency, what is important to do while the patient is receiving the medication? Explain your answer.

For Answers see www.harcourthealth.com/MERLIN/Lilley/.

bibliography

Albanese J, Nutz P: *Mosby's 2001 nursing drug reference and review cards*, St Louis, 2001, Mosby.

American Hospital Formulary Service: *AHFS drug information*, Bethesda, Md, 2000, American Society of Health-System Pharmacists.

Anderson PO, Knoben JE, Troutman WG: *Handbook of clinical drug data 1999-2000*, ed 9, New York, 1999, McGraw-Hill.

Davis L, Stecy P: Pharmacologic management of cardiovascular problems in women, *J Nurse Midwife* 42(3):176, 1997.

Johns Hopkins Hospital, Department of Pediatrics et al: *The Harriet Lane handbook*, ed 15, St Louis, 2000, Mosby.

Joint National Committee on Detection, Evaluation, and Treatment of High Blood Pressure: The sixth report of the Joint National Committee on Detection, Evaluation, and Treatment of High Blood Pressure, *Arch Intern Med* 157(1):2413, 1997.

Keen JH: *Critical care and emergency drug reference*, ed 3, St Louis, 1996, Mosby.

Kuncl N, Nelson KM: Antihypertensive drugs, *Nursing* 27(8):46, 1997.

Loggie JH, Sardegna KM: Latest standards for hypertension in teens, *Patient Care* 15:121, 1997.

Medical Letter: Candesartan for hypertension 40(1040):109, November 20, 1998.

Medical Letter: Drugs for hypertension 41(1048):23, March 12, 1999.

Medical Letter: A new ACE inhibitor and two new angiotensin receptor blockers for hypertension 41(1065):105, November 5, 1999.

Mosby's GenRx: a comprehensive reference for generic and brand drugs, ed 10, St Louis, 2000, Mosby.

Reynolds E, Baron RB: Hypertension in women and the elderly, *Postgrad Med* 100(4):58, 1996.

Skidmore-Roth L: *Mosby's 2001 nursing drug reference*, St Louis, 2001, Mosby.

Turkoski BB: *Drug information handbook for nursing 1999-2000: including assessment, administration, monitoring guidelines, and patient education*, ed 2, Cleveland, 1999, Lexi-Comp.

United States Pharmacopeial Convention: *USP DI: drug information for the health care professional*, vol. 1, ed 20, Englewood, Colo, 2000, Micromedex.

Activity

Remember to check the **Online Worksheet** for additional learning opportunities: **www.harcourthealth.com/MERLIN/Lilley/**

Chapter 24

Diuretic Agents

www.harcourthealth.com/MERLIN/Lilley/

Look for this symbol for
topics covered in the
Online Worksheet

objectives

When you reach the end of this chapter, you should be able to do the following:

1 Discuss the indications for diuretics.

2 Discuss the different types of diuretics and their mechanisms of action as they relate to the various indications.

3 List the commonly used diuretics and the different classes of agents.

4 Describe the rationale for diuretic treatment, the dosages of the agents, their side effects, and the cautions, contraindications, and drug interactions.

5 Develop a nursing care plan that includes all phases of the nursing process for the patient receiving diuretics.

6 Summarize the therapeutic effects anticipated in patients receiving diuretics.

---

drug profiles

acetazolamide, p. 380

amiloride, p. 385

○━**furosemide,** p. 382

hydrochlorothiazide,
p. 387

mannitol, p. 383

metolazone, p. 388

spironolactone, p. 385

triamterene, p.385

○━Key drug.

---

glossary

Afferent arterioles The small blood vessels leading to the glomerulus. (p. 378)

Aldosterone (al′ dos tər on) A mineralocorticoid steroid hormone produced by the adrenal cortex that mediates the actions of the renal tubule in the regulation of sodium and potassium balance in the blood. (p. 379)

Ascites (ə si′ tez) An abnormal intraperitoneal accumulation of fluid containing large amounts of protein and electrolytes. Ascites may be detected when more than 500 ml of fluid has accumulated. (p. 382)

Collecting duct The final common pathway for filtered fluid that starts in the glomerulus. (p. 379)

Distal tubule The structure that anatomically follows the ascending loop of Henle. (p. 379)

Diuretics (di′ u ret′ ik) Drug or other substance that tends to promote the formation and excretion of urine. (p. 377)

Diuretic ceiling effect Daily doses of more than 50 mg of diuretic drugs in a 1-day period rarely produce additional clinical results but do increase drug toxicity. (p. 387)

Efferent arterioles The small blood vessels leaving the glomerulus. (p. 378)

Glomerular filtration rate (glo mer′ u lər) The amount of ultrafiltrate formed per unit of time by the plasma flowing through the glomeruli of the kidney. (p. 378)

Glomerulus (glo mer′ u ləs) Cluster of capillaries that surround each nephron. (p. 378)

Kaliuretic diuretics (ka le u ret′ ik) Agents that induce potassium loss in the urine. (p. 384)

Nephron (nef′ ron) A microscopic structural and functional unit of the kidney that resembles a funnel and consists of a long stem and two convoluted sections. (p. 378)

Open-angle glaucoma (glaw′ ko mə) Elevated pressure in an eye because of obstruction of the outflow of aqueous humor. (p. 379)

Proximal tubule Structure that anatomically follows the glomerulus. (p. 378)

The drugs that accelerate the rate of urine formation are termed **diuretics,** and they accomplish this through a variety of mechanisms. The result is that they remove sodium and water from the body.

Diuretics were discovered by accident when it was noticed that a mercury-based antibiotic had a very potent diuretic effect. Thus began the early developmental stages of diuretics. All the major classes of diuretic drugs in use today were developed between 1950 and 1970, and they remain among the most commonly prescribed drugs in the world. The sixth Joint National Committee on the Detection, Evaluation, and Treatment of Hypertension recently reaffirmed the role of diuretics as the first-line agents in the treatment of hypertension. The hypotensive activity of diuretics may be due to many different mechanisms. They cause direct arteriolar dilation, decreasing peripheral vascular resistance. They also decrease extracellular fluid volume, plasma volume, and cardiac output, which may account for the decrease in blood pressure. They have long been the mainstay of therapy not only for hypertension but also for congestive heart failure (CHF). In fact, diuretics are so potent, safe, and inexpensive that they are almost universally the drug of choice in the treatment of many clinical conditions. The main problem with their use is their metabolic side effects, which are dose related.

This chapter reviews the essential properties and actions of the following important classes of diuretic agents: carbonic anhydrase inhibitors (CAIs), loop diuretics, osmotic diuretics, potassium-sparing diuretics, and thiazide and thiazide-like diuretics. However, before these are discussed in detail, it is first important to quickly review kidney function, because this is the key to understanding the therapeutic effects of these agents.

KIDNEY FUNCTION

The kidney serves a very important role in the day-to-day functioning of our bodies. It filters out toxic waste products from the blood while simultaneously saving essen-

tial ones. This delicate balance between toxins and essential chemicals is maintained by the **nephron.** This is the main structural element in the kidney, and each kidney contains approximately one million of them. It is in the nephron where diuretic agents exert their effect. The actual filtering takes place in the **glomerulus,** a cluster of capillaries surrounded by the glomerular capsule. The rate at which this occurs is referred to as the **glomerular filtration rate** (GFR), and it is used as a gauge of how well the kidneys are functioning as filters. Normally about 180 liters of blood is filtered through them per day. The GFR, which can also be thought of as the rate at which blood flows into and out of the glomerulus, is regulated by the small blood vessels leading to the glomerulus **(afferent arterioles)** and the small blood vessels leaving the glomerulus **(efferent arterioles).** Alterations in blood flow such as occurs in a patient in shock would therefore have a dramatic effect on kidney (renal) function. In low blood flow situations the kidney receives less blood, and therefore less diuretic gets to its site of action. For this reason diuretics may have diminished effects.

The **proximal tubule,** which anatomically follows the glomerulus, resorbs 60% to 70% of the sodium from the filtered fluid (filtrate) back into the bloodstream. Blood vessels surround the nephrons and allow substances to

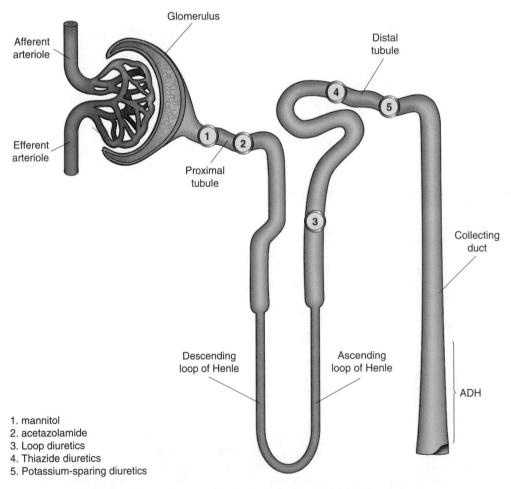

1. mannitol
2. acetazolamide
3. Loop diuretics
4. Thiazide diuretics
5. Potassium-sparing diuretics

Fig. 24-1 The nephron and diuretic sites of action. *ADH,* Antidiuretic hormone.

be directly absorbed from or secreted into the bloodstream. This process is an active one that requires energy. A sodium ion is actively transported back into the blood, this causes the passive resorption of chloride and water. The chloride and water simply follow the sodium. Another 20% to 25% of sodium is resorbed back into the bloodstream in the ascending loop of Henle. This is a passive process that does not require energy because here it is the chloride that is actively resorbed and the sodium that passively follows it.

The remaining 5% to 10% of sodium resorption takes place in the **distal tubule,** which anatomically follows the ascending loop of Henle. Here sodium is actively filtered in exchange for potassium or hydrogen ions, a process regulated by the hormone **aldosterone.** The **collecting duct** is the final common pathway for the filtrate that started in the glomerulus. It is here that antidiuretic hormone acts to increase the absorption of water back into the bloodstream, thereby preventing it from being lost in the urine. This entire process, along with the sites of action of the different classes of diuretics are shown in Fig. 24-1.

DIURETIC AGENTS

The various diuretics are classified according to their sites of action, chemical structure, and diuretic potency. The sites of action of the various diuretics are determined by the way in which they inhibit the sodium and other electrolyte transport systems located along the nephron (see Fig. 24-1). The commonly used classes of agents and the individual drugs in these classes are listed in Table 24-1. The most potent diuretics are the loop diuretics, followed by metolazone (a thiazide-like diuretic), the thiazides, and the potassium-sparing diuretics. Their potency is a function of where they work in the nephron to inhibit sodium and water resorption. The more sodium and water they inhibit from resorption the greater the amount of diuresis and therefore the greater the potency.

CARBONIC ANHYDRASE INHIBITORS

CAIs are chemical derivatives of sulfonamide antibiotics. As their name implies, CAIs inhibit the enzyme carbonic anhydrase, which exists in the kidneys, eyes, and other parts of the body. The site of action of the CAIs depends on the distribution of carbonic anhydrase along the nephron. For instance, acetazolamide acts principally in the proximal tubule, which as previously described is directly behind the glomerulus. Today CAIs are mainly used for the adjunct treatment of chronic simple glaucoma, sometimes referred to as **open-angle glaucoma.** CAIs, and particularly acetazolamide, can also be extremely helpful in the management of patients with CHF who have become resistant to their present diuretic regimens. Acetazolamide can also be useful in prevention or amelioration of symptoms associated with high altitude sickness.

Mechanism of Action

As previously noted, the carbonic anhydrase system in the kidney is located just behind the glomerulus in the proximal tubules, where almost two thirds of all sodium and water is resorbed back into the blood. Here a specific transport system operates that exchanges sodium for hydrogen ions. For sodium and thus water to be resorbed back into the blood, hydrogen must be exchanged for it. Without the hydrogen, this cannot occur, and the sodium and water are eliminated with the urine. The carbonic anhydrase helps make the hydrogen ions available for this exchange. When its actions are inhibited with a CAI such as acetazolamide, little sodium and water can be resorbed into the blood and they are eliminated with the urine. The CAIs reduce the formation of hydrogen (H^+) and bicarbonate (HCO_3^-) ions from carbon dioxide and water by the noncompetitive, reversible inhibition of carbonic anhydrase. This results in a reduction in the availability of these ions, mainly hydrogen, for active transport systems.

Drug Effects

As previously mentioned, the inhibition of carbonic anhydrase causes the hydrogen ion concentration in the renal tubules to be reduced, resulting in an increased excretion of bicarbonate, sodium, water, and potassium. Because the resorption of water is decreased, the urine volume is increased and the urine becomes alkaline. This accounts for the diuretic effects of CAIs. Orally or parenterally administered CAIs can also decrease the formation of aqueous humor in the eye. This has the benefit of lowering intraocular pressure in patients who suffer from glaucoma. However, this effect of CAIs seems to be independent of its diuretic action.

Table 24-1 Classification of Diuretics

Class	Drugs
Carbonic anhydrase inhibitors	dichlorphenamide, acetazolamide, methzolamide
Loop diuretics	furosemide, ethacrynic acid, bumetanide, torsemide
Osmotic diuretics	mannitol
Potassium-sparing diuretics	amiloride, spironolactone, triameterene
Thiazide and thiazide-like diuretics	chlorothiazide, hydrochlorothiazide, bendroflumethiazide, methyclothiazide, quinethazone, metolazone, chlorthalidone, indapamide

CAIs bring about an inhibited formation of bicarbonate and hydrogen ions that has many effects on other parts of the body. The metabolic acidosis induced by CAIs is also beneficial in the prevention of seizures. In addition, CAIs may induce respiratory and metabolic acidosis, which may in turn increase oxygenation during hypoxia by increasing ventilation, cerebral blood flow, and the dissociation of oxygen from oxyhemoglobin. An undesirable effect of CAIs is that they elevate the blood glucose level and cause glycosuria in diabetic patients. This may be due to the decline in the potassium level that CAIs may induce.

Therapeutic Uses

The therapeutic applications of CAIs are wide and varied. They are commonly used in the treatment of glaucoma, edema, epilepsy, and high-altitude sickness.

CAIs are used principally as adjunct agents in the long-term management of open-angle glaucoma that cannot be controlled by topical miotic agents or epinephrine derivatives alone. These agents together can increase the outflow of aqueous humor, the obstruction of which is responsible for the glaucoma. They are also used short term in conjunction with miotics to lower intraocular pressure in preparation for ocular surgery in patients with acute ocular disorders or narrow-angle glaucoma and as an adjunct in the treatment of secondary glaucoma.

CAIs, particularly acetazolamide, are used to manage the edema secondary to CHF that has become resistant to other diuretics. However, as a class, CAIs are much less potent diuretics than loop diuretics or thiazides, and the metabolic acidosis they induce diminishes their diuretic effect in 2 to 4 days.

Acetazolamide may be a useful adjunct to other anticonvulsants in the prophylactic management of various forms of epilepsy. However, tolerance to the anticonvulsant effects of CAIs develops quickly, and they may be ineffective for prolonged therapy. Acetazolamide is also effective in both the prevention and treatment of the symptoms of high-altitude sickness. These symptoms include headache, nausea, shortness of breath, dizziness, drowsiness, and fatigue.

Side Effects and Adverse Effects

The more common undesirable effects of CAIs are metabolic abnormalities such as acidosis. They may also cause drowsiness, anorexia, paresthesias, hematuria, urticaria, photosensitivity, and melena.

Interactions

Significant drug interactions that occur with CAIs include an increase in digitalis toxicity stemming from the hypokalemia that CAIs may induce. Their concomitant use with corticosteroids may cause hypokalemia, and their use with oral hypoglycemic agents and quinidine will induce greater activity or toxicity of the latter agents.

Dosages

For information on the dosages of acetazolamide, see the following drug profile.

drug profiles

Although there are three CAIs (see Table 24-1), by far the most widely prescribed one is acetazolamide, and it is thus the only one profiled here.

acetazolamide

Acetazolamide (Diamox, Diamox Sequels) is classified as a pregnancy category C agent and is contraindicated in patients who have shown a hypersensitivity to it or sulfonamides, as well as in those with significant liver or kidney dysfunction, low serum potassium or sodium levels, acidosis, and adrenal gland failure. Acetazolamide is available both orally and parenterally. Orally it is available as 500-mg extended-release capsules and 125- and 250-mg tablets. Parenterally, acetazolamide is available as a 500-mg injection. A recommended dosages for pediatric patients is oral administration of 5 mg/kg/day. A common oral dosage for adults is 250 to 375 mg/day given on alternate days.

PHARMACOKINETICS			
HALF-LIFE	ONSET	PEAK	DURATION
10-15 hr	1 hr	2-4 hr	8-12 hr

LOOP DIURETICS

Loop diuretics (bumetanide, ethacrynic acid, furosemide, and torsemide) are very potent diuretics that act primarily along the thick ascending limb of the loop of Henle, blocking chloride and secondarily sodium resorption. They are also believed to activate the renal prostaglandins, resulting in dilation of the blood vessels of the kidneys, lungs, and the rest of the body (systemic and pulmonary vascular resistance). The beneficial hemodynamic effects of loop diuretics are a reduction in both the preload and central venous pressures, which are the filling pressures of the ventricles. These actions make them very useful in the treatment of the edema associated with CHF, hepatic cirrhosis, and renal disease.

Loop diuretics are particularly useful when rapid diuresis is desired because their onset of action is rapid. In addition, the diuretic effect lasts at least 2 hours. A distinct advantage they have over thiazide diuretics is that their diuretic action continues even when the creatinine clearance decreases below 25 ml/min. This means that even when the function of the kidney diminishes, loop diuretics can still work. Their combined use with a thiazide (especially metolazone) increases their effectiveness because this results in the blockade of sodium and water resorption at multiple sites in the nephron, a property referred to as *sequential nephron blockade*. Because of their potent diuretic effect and the duration of this effect, loop diuretics are effective as single-dose therapy. This allows the renal tubule time to partially compensate for the potassium depletion and other electrolyte derangements

Table 24-2 Loop Diuretics: Common Adverse Effects

Body System	Side/Adverse Effect
Central nervous system	Dizziness, headache, tinnitus, blurred vision
Gastrointestinal	Nausea, vomiting, diarrhea
Hematologic	Agranulocytosis, thrombocytopenia, neutropenia
Metabolic	Hypokalemia, hyperglycemia, hyperuricemia

that often accompany around-the-clock diuretic therapy. Despite this, the major side effect of loop diuretics is electrolyte disturbances. Though rare, prolonged high doses can also result in hearing loss stemming from ototoxicity. Bumetanide, furosemide, and torsemide are chemically related to the sulfonamides.

Mechanism of Action

Loop diuretics act directly on the ascending limb of the loop of Henle to inhibit sodium and chloride resorption. They have also been shown to inhibit electrolyte resorption in the proximal renal tubule and to increase the concentrations of renal prostaglandins, resulting in the dilation of blood vessels in the kidney, lungs, and possibly the entire body. This reduction in peripheral vascular resistance may account for their antihypertensive effects. However, this effect is reversed when nonsteroidal antiinflammatory drugs (NSAIDs) are given with them.

Drug Effects

Loop diuretics have renal, cardiovascular, and metabolic effects. The renal effects just discussed constitute the loop diuretics' major mechanism of action.

As previously noted, loop diuretics produce a potent diuresis and subsequent loss of fluid. The resulting decreased fluid volume leads to a decreased return of blood to the heart, or decreased filling pressures. This has the following cardiovascular effects:

- Reduces blood pressure
- Reduces pulmonary vascular resistance
- Reduces systemic vascular resistance
- Reduces central venous pressure
- Reduces left ventricular end-diastolic pressure

The metabolic effects of the loop diuretics are secondary to the electrolyte losses, specifically potassium depletion, produced by the potent diuresis. Changes in the plasma insulin, glucagon, and growth hormone levels have been seen as a result in patients taking loop diuretics.

Therapeutic Uses

Loop diuretics are used to manage the edema associated with CHF and hepatic or renal disease, to control hyper-

tension, and to increase the renal excretion of calcium in patients with hypercalcemia.

Side Effects and Adverse Effects

Common undesirable effects of the loop diuretics are listed in Table 24-2. Those commonly associated with bumetanide therapy are muscle cramps, dry mouth, arthritic pain, and encephalopathy. These are especially common in patients with preexisting liver disease. Ethacrynic acid may cause neutropenia and rare episodes of Henoch-Schönlein purpura. Furosemide can produce erythema multiforme, exfoliative dermatitis, photosensitivity, and rare cases of aplastic anemia. Torsemide may rarely cause thrombocytopenia, agranulocytosis, leukopenia, and neutropenia. It may also cause a severe skin disorder called *Stevens-Johnson syndrome.*

Toxicity and Management of Overdose

Electrolyte loss and dehydration, which can result in circulatory failure, are the main toxic effects of loop diuretics that require attention. Treatment involves electrolyte and fluid replacement.

Interactions

Loop diuretics exhibit both neurotoxic and nephrotoxic properties, and they produce additive effects when given in combination with drugs that have similar toxicities. The drug interactions are summarized in Table 24-3.

Loop diuretics also affect certain laboratory results. They cause increases in the serum levels of uric acid, glucose, alanine aminotransferase (ALT), and aspartate aminotransferase (AST).

Dosages

For the recommended dosages of loop diuretics, see the dosages table on p. 382.

Activity

drug profiles

The currently available loop diuretics are bumetanide, ethacrynic acid, furosemide, and torsemide. As a class they are very potent diuretics, but this

Loop Diuretics: Drug Interactions

Table 24-3

Drug	Mechanism	Result
Aminoglycosides capreomycin chloroquine phenylbutazone vancomycin	Additive effect	Increased neurotoxicity, especially ototoxicity
Corticosteroids digitalis	Hypokalemia	Additive hypokalemia Increased digitalis toxicity
lithium	Decreases renal excretion	Increased lithium toxicity
NSAIDs	Inhibit renal prostaglandins	Decreased diuretic activity
Sulfonylureas	Decrease glucose tolerance	Hyperglycemia

DOSAGES Selected Loop Diuretics

agent	pharmacologic class	dosage range	purpose
bumetanide (Bumex)		*Adult* PO: 0.5-2 mg/day as a single dose IM/IV: 0.5-1 mg; may be repeated at intervals of 2-3 hr but not to exceed a total dose of 10 mg/day	Edema
ethacrynic acid (Edecrin)		*Pediatric* IV: 1 mg/kg/dose; max 3 mg/kg/day PO: initial dose 25 mg/day; max 3 mg/kg/day *Adult* IV: 0.5-1 mg/kg; max 200 mg/day	CHF, hypertension, renal failure, pulmonary edema, cirrhosis
furosemide (Lasix)	Loop diuretic	*Pediatric* IM/IV: 1 mg/kg/dose; not to exceed 6 mg/kg/dose PO: 2 mg/kg as a single dose; not to exceed 6 mg/kg/day *Adult* IM/IV: 20-40 mg/dose; max 600 mg/day; administer high dose IV therapy as a controlled infusion at a rate ≤4 mg/ml PO: 20-80 mg/day as a single dose	CHF, hypertension, renal failure, pulmonary edema, cirrhosis
torsemide (Demadex)		*Adult* PO/IV: 20-200 mg once daily	Edema

potency varies between the various agents. The equipotent doses for these various agents are as follows:

BUMETANIDE	TORSEMIDE	FUROSEMIDE	ETHACRYNIC ACID
1 mg	10 mg	40 mg	50 mg

furosemide

Furosemide (Lasix) is by far the loop diuretic most commonly used in clinical practice and the prototype agent in this class. Structurally it is related to the sulfonamides. It has all the therapeutic and adverse characteristics of the loop diuretics mentioned earlier. It is primarily used in the management of pulmonary edema and the edema associated with CHF, liver disease, nephrotic syndrome, and **ascites** (the accumulation of fluid in the peritoneal area). It has also been used in the treatment of hypertension, usually that caused by CHF.

Furosemide is classified as a pregnancy category C agent and is contraindicated in patients who have shown a hypersensitivity to sulfonamides, in infants and lactating women, and in patients suffering from anuria, hypovolemia, and electrolyte depletion. It is available orally as a 40-mg/5 ml and a 10-mg/ml oral solution. It is also available as 20-, 40-, and 80-mg tablets. Parenterally it is available as a 10-mg/ml injection. Recommended dosages are given in the dosages table above.

PHARMACOKINETICS

HALF-LIFE	ONSET	PEAK	DURATION
1-2 hr	1 hr	1-2 hr	6-8 hr

Activit

OSMOTIC DIURETICS

The osmotic diuretics are mannitol, urea, organic acids, and glucose. Mannitol, a nonabsorbable, solute that works along the entire nephron, is the most commonly used of these agents. Its major site of action, however, is the proximal tubule. Because it is nonabsorbable, it produces an osmotic effect, that is, it pulls fluid, or water, into the blood vessels and nephrons from the surrounding tissues. Ultimately this reduces cellular edema and increases urine production, causing diuresis. However, it produces only a slight loss of electrolytes, especially sodium. Because of this, mannitol is not indicated for patients in an edematous state because it does not promote sufficient sodium excretion.

Mannitol may induce vasodilation and in doing so increase both glomerular filtration and renal plasma flow. This makes it an excellent agent for preventing kidney damage during acute renal failure (ARF). It has also been shown to reduce intracranial pressure and cerebral edema resulting from head trauma. In addition, mannitol treatment may be tried when elevated intraocular pressure is unresponsive to other drug therapies.

Mannitol may crystallize when exposed to low temperatures. This is more likely to occur when concentrations exceed 15%. Because of this, mannitol should always be administered intravenously through a filter.

Mechanism of Action

Mannitol and the other osmotic diuretics induce diuresis mainly by increasing the osmotic pressure of the glomerular filtrate, which in turn inhibits the tubular resorption of water and solutes, producing a rapid diuresis. The resulting osmotic effect pulls fluid from the extravascular spaces intravascularly into the tubules or into the blood vessels from the surrounding tissue.

Drug Effects

Besides increasing the osmotic pressure of the glomerular filtrate, mannitol can also induce the rapid excretion of water, sodium, and other electrolytes as well as the rapid excretion of toxic substances from the kidney. This drug also reduces excessive intraocular pressure.

Therapeutic Uses

Mannitol is the osmotic diuretic of choice. It is commonly used in the treatment of patients in the early, oliguric phase of ARF. However, for it to be effective in this setting, enough renal blood flow and glomerular filtration must exist to enable the drug to reach the tubules. Increased renal blood flow resulting from the dilation of blood vessels supplying blood to the kidneys is another therapeutic benefit of mannitol therapy in such patients. It can also be used to promote the excretion of toxic substances, reduce intracranial pressure, and treat cerebral edema. In addition, it can be used as a genitourinary irrigant in the preparation of patients for transurethral surgical procedures and as supportive treatment in patients with edema induced by other conditions.

geriatric considerations

Diuretic Therapy

- Always obtain baseline measurements of the patient's height, weight, intake and output amounts, and serum sodium, potassium, and chloride levels.
- Diuretics should be taken early in the day to prevent nocturia, or voiding at night, which could lead to lack of sleep and possible injury because of the need to get out of bed during the night.
- If the elderly patient is living alone and has no assistance or minimal assistance with his or her medication regimen, visits from a home health or public health professional may help ensure the safety of the therapy and compliance with therapy and diet.
- Caution should be taken with the use of diuretics in the elderly since these patients are more sensitive to the therapeutic effects of diuretics and more likely to experience dehydration, electrolyte loss, dizziness, and syncope.
- Encourage elderly patients to change positions slowly because of the risk of orthostatic hypotension and high risk for falls.

Side Effects and Adverse Effects

Significant undesirable effects of mannitol include convulsions, thrombophlebitis, and pulmonary congestion. Other less significant effects are headaches, chest pains, tachycardia, blurred vision, chills, and fever.

Interactions

There are no drugs that interact significantly with mannitol.

Dosages

For the recommended dosages of mannitol, see the dosages table on p. 384.

drug profiles

mannitol

Mannitol (Resectial, Osmitrol) is the prototypical osmotic diuretic. It is rated as a pregnancy category C agent and is contraindicated in patients with a hypersensitivity to it as well as in those suffering from anuria, severe dehydration, pulmonary congestion, or cerebral hemorrhage. Treatment should be terminated if severe cardiac or renal impairment develops after the initiation of therapy. It is only available parenterally as a 5%, 10%, 15%, 20%, and 25% solution for intravenous injection. Recommended dosages are given in the dosages table on p. 384.

PHARMACOKINETICS

HALF-LIFE	ONSET	PEAK	DURATION
1.5 hr	0.5-1 hr	0.25-2 hr	6-8 hr

DOSAGES Mannitol

agent	pharmacologic class	dosage range	purpose
mannitol (Resectial, Osmitrol)	Osmotic diuretic	*Adult* IV infusion: 50-200 g/day, 1.5-2 g/kg over 30-60 min Suggested loading dose of 25 g, followed by an infusion rate to produce a urine flow of at least 100 ml/hr	Renal failure Reduction of intraocular and intracranial pressure Diuresis for drug intoxication

Table 24-4 Potassium-Sparing Diuretics: Common Adverse Effects

Body System	Side/Adverse Effect
Central nervous system	Dizziness, headache
Gastrointestinal	Cramps, nausea, vomiting, diarrhea
Other	Urinary frequency, weakness, hyperkalemia

POTASSIUM-SPARING DIURETICS

The most commonly prescribed potassium-sparing diuretics are amiloride, spironolactone, and triamterene. These diuretics are also referred to as *aldosterone-inhibiting diuretics* because they block the aldosterone receptors. These agents work in the collecting ducts and distal convoluted tubules, where they interfere with sodium-potassium exchange. They also competitively bind to aldosterone receptors and therefore block the resorption of sodium and water that is induced by aldosterone secretion. They are often prescribed in children with CHF because the cardiac disorder in this setting is often accompanied by an excess secretion of aldosterone and the loop and thiazide diuretics are frequently ineffective in its management.

Because little more than 3% of the total filtered load reaches the collecting ducts, the potassium-sparing diuretics are weak as diuretics. When diuresis is needed, they are generally used as adjuncts to thiazide treatment. This combination is beneficial in two aspects. First, it has synergistic diuretic effects, and second, the two agents counteract the adverse metabolic effects of each other: The thiazide diuretics cause potassium, magnesium, and chloride to be lost in the urine, and the potassium-sparing diuretics counteract this by elevating the potassium and chloride levels.

Mechanism of Action

The diuretic action of potassium-sparing diuretics varies for the different drugs in the class. Amiloride and triamterene, which have similar pharmacologic properties, act directly on the distal renal tubule, which is under the control of mineralocorticoids, especially aldosterone, to inhibit the resorption of sodium ions in exchange for potassium and hydrogen ions. This results in the diuresis of water and sodium and the retention of potassium.

Spironolactone is a competitive antagonist of aldosterone, and for this reason causes sodium and water to be excreted and potassium to be retained.

Drug Effects

As their name implies, potassium-sparing diuretics prevent potassium from being pumped into the tubule, so it is not secreted. They do this by competitively blocking the aldosterone receptors and inhibiting the action of this mineralocorticoid. The excretion of sodium and water is promoted, however. In addition, with the exception of triamterene, these drugs have an antihypertensive effect.

Therapeutic Uses

The therapeutic applications of the potassium-sparing diuretics vary depending on the particular agent. Spironolactone and triamterene are used in the treatment of hyperaldosteronism and hypertension and for reversing the potassium loss caused by the **kaliuretic diuretics** or other potassium-losing drugs. The uses for amiloride are similar to those of spironolactone and triamterene, but it is less effective in the long term. It may be more effective than spironolactone or triamterene in the treatment of metabolic alkalosis, however. It is typically used in the treatment of CHF.

Side Effects and Adverse Effects

Potassium-sparing diuretics have several common undesirable effects. These are listed in Table 24-4. There are also some significant adverse effects that are specific to the individual agents. Spironolactone can cause gynecomastia, amenorrhea, irregular menses, and postmenopausal bleeding. Triamterene may reduce folic acid levels and cause the formation of kidney stones and urinary casts. It may also precipitate megaloblastic anemia. Hyperkalemia also may occur when triamterene is used alone or in combination with other diuretics. Side effects from triamterene use are rare.

Interactions

The concomitant use of these potassium-sparing diuretics with lithium, angiotensin-converting enzyme (ACE) inhibitors, or potassium supplements can result in significant drug interactions. The combined use of ACE inhibitors or potassium supplements with potassium-

DOSAGES Selected Potassium-Sparing Diuretics Agents

agent	pharmacologic class	dosage range	purpose
amiloride (Midamor)		*Adult* PO: 5-20 mg/day	Edema and as an adjunct to kaliuretic diuretics
spironolactone (Aldactone)	Potassium-sparing diuretics	*Pediatric* PO: 3.3 mg/kg/day single or divided *Adult* PO: 25-200 mg/day	Edema
triameterene (Dyrenium)		*Adult* PO: 100 mg bid; do not exceed 300 mg/day	Edema

sparing diuretics can result in hyperkalemia. When given together, lithium and potassium-sparing diuretics can result in lithium toxicity. NSAIDs can inhibit renal protaglandins, decreasing blood flow to the kidneys and therefore decreasing the delivery of diuretic drugs to this site of action. This in turn can lead to a diminished diuretic response.

Dosages

For recommended dosages of potassium-sparing diuretics, see the dosages table above.

drug profiles

amiloride

Amiloride (Midamor) is generally used in combination with a thiazide or loop diuretic in the therapy for CHF. Hyperkalemia may occur in as many as 10% of the patients who are taking amiloride alone. It should be used with caution in patients suffering from renal impairment or diabetes mellitus and in elderly patients. Amiloride is contraindicated in the settings of hypersensitivity, hyperkalemia, and impaired renal function. It has only weak antihypertensive properties. It is a pregnancy category B agent and is only available orally as a 5-mg tablet. It also is available in combination with hydrochlorothiazide in a product called Moduretic. Recommended dosages are given in the dosages table above.

PHARMACOKINETICS

HALF-LIFE	ONSET	PEAK	DURATION
6-9 hr	2 hr	6-10 hr	24 hr

spironolactone

Structurally, spironolactone (Aldactone) is a synthetic steroid that blocks aldosterone receptors. It is used in high doses for the treatment of ascites. This condition is commonly associated with cirrhosis of the liver. The serum potassium level should be monitored frequently in patients taking it who have impaired renal function or who are currently taking

potassium supplements, because hyperkalemia is a frequent complication of spironolactone therapy. It is the potassium-sparing diuretic most frequently prescribed for children who have CHF because this form of CHF frequently causes excess aldosterone to be secreted, which in turn causes increased sodium and water resorption. Recently spironolactone has been shown to reduce morbidity and mortality rates in patients with severe CHF when added to standard therapy. It is contraindicated in patients who have a hypersensitivity to it and those suffering from anuria, significant renal impairment, or hyperkalemia. Of the three commonly used potassium-sparing diuretics, spironolactone has the greatest antihypertensive activity. It is a pregnancy category D agent and is only available orally as 25-mg tablets and as 25-, 50-, and 100-mg film-coated tablets. It also is available in combination with hydrochlorothiazide in a product called Spironazide or Aldactazide. Recommended dosages are given in the dosages table above.

PHARMACOKINETICS

HALF-LIFE	ONSET	PEAK	DURATION
13-24 hr	1-3 days	2-3 days	2-3 days

triamterene

As previously mentioned, the pharmacologic properties of triamterene (Dyrenium) are similar to those of amiloride. Therefore, like amiloride, triamterene acts directly on the distal renal tubule of the nephron to depress the resorption of sodium and the excretion of potassium and hydrogen, processes otherwise stimulated at that site by aldosterone. However, unlike spironolactone, which induces diuresis by directly inhibiting aldosterone, triamterene does so independent of aldosterone. Triamterene is contraindicated in the settings of hypersensitivity, anuria, significant renal or hepatic insufficiency, and hyperkalemia. It has little or no antihypertensive effect. It is a pregnancy category D agent and is only available orally as 50- and 100-mg capsules. It also is available in combination with hydrochlorothiazide in a product called Dyazide or Maxzide. Recommended dosages are given in the dosages table on p. 385.

PHARMACOKINETICS			
HALF-LIFE	ONSET	PEAK	DURATION
2-3 hr	2-4 hr	6-8 hr	12-16 hr

THIAZIDES AND THIAZIDE-LIKE DIURETICS

Thiazide and thiazide-like diuretics are all generally considered equivalent in their effects. However, chlorthalidone is somewhat different because of its long duration of action. Metolazone, which is also frequently prescribed, and quinethazone may be more effective than other agents in the class in the treatment of patients with renal dysfunction. Hydrochlorothiazide is one of the most commonly used and the least expensive of the generic preparations. The thiazide diuretics consist of bendroflumethiazide, benzthiazide, chlorothiazide, polythiazide, and trichlormethiazide. The thiazide-like diuretics are very similar in action to the thiazides and include chlorthalidone, indapamide, metolazone, and quinethazone.

Thiazides are used as adjunct agents in the management of CHF, hepatic cirrhosis, and edema of various origins. The primary site of action of thiazides and thiazide-like diuretics is the distal convoluted tubule, where they inhibit sodium and chloride resorption. Thiazides also cause direct relaxation of the arterioles (small blood vessels). Decreased preload (filling pressures) and decreased afterload (the force the ventricles must overcome to eject the volume of blood they contain) are the beneficial he-

modynamic effects. This makes them very effective for the treatment of both CHF and hypertension.

As renal function decreases, the efficacy of thiazides diminishes, probably because delivery of the drug to the active site is impaired. Thiazides generally should not be used if the creatinine clearance is less than 30 to 50 ml/min. Normal creatinine clearance is 125 ml/min. The only exception is metolazone, which remains effective to a creatinine clearance of 10 ml/min. Major side effects of the agents stem from the electrolyte disturbances they produce. They are noted for precipitating hypokalemia and hypercalcemia as well as metabolic disturbances such as hyperlipidemia, hyperglycemia, and hyperuricemia.

Mechanism of Action

Thiazide diuretics are chemical derivatives (benzothiadiazines) of sulfonamides. Their diuretic effect stems from their ability to inhibit the tubular resorption of sodium and chloride ions, primarily in the ascending loop of Henle and in the early distal tubule of the nephron. As a result, water, sodium, and chloride (and to a lesser extent potassium) are excreted.

Drug Effects

Thiazides and related diuretics cause water, sodium, chloride, and potassium ions to be excreted without altering the pH of the urine. By dilating the arterioles these drugs also lower peripheral vascular resistance.

The antihypertensive effect of the thiazides is the result of sodium depletion and lowered peripheral vascular resistance. They are one of the most prescribed group of agents for the treatment of hypertension.

Therapeutic Uses

In addition to hypertension, the thiazide and thiazide-like diuretics are used in the treatment of edematous states, idiopathic hypercalciuria, and diabetes insipidus. Any of these drugs can be used either as a sole agent or

pediatric considerations

Thiazide Diuretics

- Pediatric dosages of these medications should be calculated carefully. Admission and daily weights should be measured and recorded so that a possible overdose can be identified. Fluid volume and electrolyte loss, hypotension, shock, and possibly death are the consequences of overdose.
- Weights, intake and output amounts, and vital signs, including the rate, depth, and rhythm of respirations, should be checked daily to make sure the child is responding appropriately and to help identify possible adverse reactions to or complications of the therapy.
- The oral forms may be taken with food or milk and should be taken early in the day.
- Sunscreen containing PABA should be avoided, and clothing worn to protect the child from the sun during even brief exposure. Lengthy exposure to either heat or sun should be avoided because of the heat stroke, exhaustion, and fluid volume loss this may precipitate.

	Thiazide and Thiazide-Like Diuretics: Common 24-5 Adverse Effects	
Body System/Process	**Side/Adverse Effect**
Central nervous system	Dizziness, headache, blurred vision, paresthesia, decreased libido
Gastrointestinal	Anorexia, nausea, vomiting, diarrhea, pancreatitis, cholecystitis
Genitourinary	Impotence
Hematologic	Jaundice, leukopenia, purpura, agranulocytosis, aplastic anemia, thrombocytopenia
Integumentary	Urticaria, photosensitivity
Metabolic	Hypokalemia, glycosuria, hyperglycemia, hyperuricemia, hypochloremic alkalosis

in combination with other agents. This group of diuretics may also be useful as adjunct agents in the treatment of edema related to CHF, hepatic cirrhosis, and corticosteroid or estrogen therapy.

Side Effects and Adverse Effects

As previously mentioned, major side effects of the thiazide and thiazide-like diuretics relate to the electrolyte disturbances they cause. These mainly comprise reduced potassium levels and elevated levels of calcium, lipids, glucose, and uric acid. Other effects, such as gastrointestinal disturbances, skin rashes, photosensitivity, thrombocytopenia, pancreatitis, and cholecystitis, are less common. Dizziness and vertigo are common side effects of metolazone therapy and are attributed to sudden shifts in the plasma volume brought about by the agent. Headache, impotence, and decreased libido are other important side effects of these agents. Many of these side effects are dose related and are seen at higher doses, especially above 25 mg. The more common side effects of the thiazide and thiazide-like diuretics are listed in Table 24-5.

Toxicity and Management of Overdose

An overdose of these drugs can lead to an electrolyte imbalance resulting from hypokalemia. Symptoms include anorexia, nausea, lethargy, muscle weakness, mental confusion, and hypotension. Treatment involves electrolyte replacement.

Interactions

Thiazides and related agents interact with corticosteroids, diazoxide, digitalis, and oral hypoglycemics. The mechanisms and results of these interactions are summarized in Table 24-6.

Besides the drug interactions, these agents can increase the serum levels of SGOT and SGPT and alter the glucose levels in urine. In addition, the excessive consumption of licorice can lead to an additive hypokalemia in patients taking them.

Dosages

For information on the dosages for thiazide and thiazide-like diuretics, see the dosages table below.

drug profiles

Thiazide and thiazide-like diuretics are listed in Box 24-1. These drugs fall into several pregnancy categories. Chlorothiazide, hydrochlorothiazide, indapamide, methyclothiazide, and metolazone are category B agents. Benzthiazide, polythiazide, and trichloromethiazide are category C agents, and hydroflumethiazide is the only category D agent in this class. Bendroflumethiazide, chlorthalidone, and quinethazone are not classified in any pregnancy category.

hydrochlorothiazide

Hydrochlorothiazide (Esidrix, HydroDiuril), which is considered the prototypical thiazide diuretic, is a very commonly prescribed and inexpensive thiazide diuretic. It is also a very safe and effective diuretic. There are many combination-drug products that contain hydrochlorothiazide, the other agent being methyldopa, propranolol, spironolactone, triamterene, hydralazine, ACE inhibitors, beta-blockers, or labetalol. Daily doses exceeding 50 mg/day rarely produce additional clinical results and may only increase drug toxicity. This property is known as the **diuretic ceiling effect.**

Table 24-6 Thiazide and Thiazide-like Diuretics: Drug Interactions

Drug	Mechanism	Results
Corticosteroids	Additive effect	Hypokalemia
diazoxide	Additive effect	Hyperkalemia
digitalis	Hypokalemia	Increased digitalis toxicity
lithium	Decrease clearance	Increased lithium toxicity
NSAIDs	Inhibit renal prostaglandins	Decreased diuretic activity
Oral hypo-glycemics	Antagonism	Reduced therapeutic effect

DOSAGES Thiazide and Selected Thiazide-like Diuretic Agents

agent	pharmacologic class	dosage range	purpose
hydrochlorothiazide (Esidrix, HydroDiuril)	Thiazide diuretic	*Pediatric* PO: <6 mo, 3.3 mg/kg/day; 6 mo-2 y/o 12.5-37.5 mg/day in 2 doses; 2-12 y/o, 37.5-100 mg day in 2 doses *Adult* PO: 25-200 mg/day usually divided PO: 25-100 mg/day *Elderly* 12.5-25 mg/day	Edema
metolazone (Mykrox, Diulo, Zaroxolyn)	Thiazide-like diuretic	*Adult* PO: 2.5-20 mg/day	Edema

Hydrochlorothiazide is a pregnancy category B agent and is contraindicated in patients with a known hypersensitivity to thiazides or sulfonamides, and in those suffering from anuria, renal decompensation, or hypomagnesemia. It is only available orally as a 50-mg/5 ml solution and as 25-, 50-, and 100-mg tablets. Recommended dosages are given in the dosages table on p. 387.

PHARMACOKINETICS

HALF-LIFE	ONSET	PEAK	DURATION
5.6-14.8 hr	2 hr	4 hr	6-12 hr

metolazone

Metolazone (Mykrox, Diulo, Zaroxolyn) is a thiazide-like diuretic that appears to be more potent than the thiazide diuretics. This is most visible in patients with renal dysfunction. One striking advantage of metolazone is that it remains effective to a creatinine clearance as low as 10 ml/min. It may also be given in combination with loop diuretics to obtain a potent diuresis in patients with severe symptoms of CHF.

Metolazone is classified as a pregnancy B agent and is contraindicated in patients with a known hypersensitivity to thiazides or sulfonamides, in those with anuria, and in pregnant or lactating women. It is only available orally as 0.5-, 2.5-, 5-, and 10-mg tablets. Do not interchange brands because their bioavailabilities are different. Recommended dosages are given in the dosages table on p. 387.

PHARMACOKINETICS

HALF-LIFE	ONSET	PEAK	DURATION
6-20 hr	1 hr	1-2 hr	Up to 24 hr

BOX 24-1 Thiazide and Thiazide-like Diuretics

THIAZIDE DIURETICS
bendroflumethiazide (Naturetin)
benzthiazide (ExNa)
chlorothiazide (Diuril)
cyclothiazide (Anhydron)
hydrochlorothiazide (Esidrix, Hydro-Diuril)
hydroflumethiazide (Saluron, Diucardin)
methyclothiazide (Enduron, Aquatensen)
polythiazide (Renese)
trichloromethiazide (Metahydrin, Naqua)

THIAZIDE-LIKE DIURETICS
chlorthalidone (Hygroton)
indapamide (Lozol)
metolazone (Mykrox, Zaroxolyn)
quinethazone (Hydromox)

nursing process

● Assessment

Before administering any type of diuretic, the nurse should obtain a thorough patient history. A physical examination must also be completed and the findings documented. Because fluid volume levels and electrolyte concentrations are affected by diuretics, the patient's baseline fluid volume status, intake and output measurements, serum electrolyte values, weight, and vital signs should be documented. Skin turgor, the serum creatinine level, arterial blood gas values, blood pH, and the uric acid level should also be documented before the start of diuretic therapy. Often it is necessary to measure postural blood pressures (lying and standing) in patients who are to receive these agents because they cause fluid to be lost from the intravascular spaces first, and this may precipitate blood pressure changes (both a decrease and postural changes).

Cautious use of diuretics, with close monitoring of fluid volume status, electrolytes, and vital signs, is recommended in patients with the following disorders or conditions: hypokalemia, hypovolemia, renal disease, liver disease, lupus, diabetes, chronic obstructive pulmonary disease (COPD), and gout. Potassium-sparing diuretics should be used cautiously in patients who are dehydrated, those with renal disease, and lactating women. Cautious use of osmotic diuretics is recommended in patients with severe renal disease or CHF, those who are dehydrated, and pregnant or lactating women.

Contraindications to the use of diuretics include allergies to the specific medication, or to sulfonamides in the case of furosemide and thiazide diuretic treatment; anuria; dehydration; hypovolemia; hypotension; and

case study Diuretic Therapy

Primary hypertension has been diagnosed in S.G., a 47-year-old woman. Her blood pressures have been ranging between 158 and 172 mm Hg systolic and 94 and 110 mm Hg diastolic. Her average blood pressure over the past month has been 156/98 mm Hg. She has a strong family history of hypertension and is a single parent of two adolescents. She is also trying to keep up with her responsibilities as a full-time assistant professor of education at a local urban university. There is no evidence of renal insufficiency or cardiac damage at this time nor is there evidence of retinopathy or other signs and symptoms of end-organ disease. No other problems are reported, and S.G. is begun on 50 mg of hydrochlorothiazide daily.

● *Discuss the antihypertensive effects of hydrochlorothiazide.*
● *What sort of guidelines must you give this patient so that she does not have adverse reactions to the diuretic therapy?*
● *What nonpharmacologic measures should the nurse tell the patient about that can help control her blood pressure?*

For Answers see www.harcourthealth.com/MERLIN/Lilley/.

NURSING CARE PLAN Diuretic Therapy

Mr. L.P. is a 59-year-old attorney who is a partner in a local prestigious law firm. His typical work day begins at 7:30 AM and lasts till about 8 PM. He exercises two to three times a week but not regularly. However, he is in good health and cholesterol and lipid profiles are within normal limits. He has been diagnosed with hypertension and needs to lost about 22 pounds per physician's orders. He is to begin taking chlorothiazide (Diuril) at a dosage of 500 mg twice daily and is to follow up in 1 week with the physician and dietician (for further consultation). He has been asked to have his blood pressure taken three times a week and to keep a daily journal of any symptoms as well as record blood-pressure readings.

assessment	*Nursing Diagnosis*	Deficient knowledge related to new treatment of hypertension and lack of experience with medication
	Subjective Data	Complaint of severe headaches
	Objective Data	• Attorney × 24 yr
		• History of stress ulcers
		• Family history of hypertension
		• Blood pressure at physician's office was 180/98 mm Hg

planning and outcome criteria	*Goals*	Patient will remain compliant to diuretic therapy within 1 mo
	Outcome Criteria	Patient will verbalize safe and accurate means of taking diuretic medication as evidenced by:
		• Fewer side effects and
		• Increased therapeutic effects within 1 mo of therapy

implementation		Patient education should include the following statements:
		• Chlorothiazide, a diuretic that will help eliminate water to help decrease your blood pressure. It also eliminates, through urine, sodium, chloride, potassium, and magnesium, which means we monitor electrolytes frequently, along with BPs.
		• Weigh yourself weekly and report a gain in weight of 2 lb or more in 1 wk.
		• Take plenty of fluids, up to 2-3L/day or as per physician's advice.
		• Change positions slowly when you rise from sitting or standing to avoid fainting and dizziness.
		• Take your medication with food.
		• Take this medication early in the morning to prevent urination at nighttime.
		• Eat a diet high in potassium with foods such as strawberries, orange juice, apricots, and bananas to help counter the potassium lost in the urine.
		• Contact physician should you experience muscle cramps, dizziness, nausea, and muscle weakness.
		• Record and monitor your BPs at least 3×/wk for now.
		• Often when patient is taking a diuretic in addition to digoxin or if the patient has dysrhythmias, the physician may add potassium supplementation.
		• Follow up with the physician in 1 wk or as per physician's advice.

evaluation		Patient shows a therapeutic response to diuretic therapy as evidenced by:
		• Improved blood pressure
		• Less edema in feet and hands
		• Improved energy levels
		Patient is monitored for side effects such as:
		• Dizziness
		• Drowsiness
		• Postural hypotension nausea, vomiting, anorexia
		• Muscle cramps
		• Fatigue
		• Headache
		• Hyperglycemia
		• Polyuria
		• Blurred vision

electrolyte disturbances. Their use is also contraindicated in infants and in breast-feeding women. Thiazide diuretics are contraindicated in patients suffering from altered renal function or hypomagnesemia. Potassium-sparing diuretics are contraindicated in patients suffering from hyperkalemia and in pregnant women. Osmotic diuretics are contraindicated in patients with severe pulmonary edema, severe edema, active intracranial bleeding, and severe dehydration.

● Nursing Diagnoses

Nursing diagnoses associated with the use of diuretics include the following:
- Decreased cardiac output related to adverse effects of diuretics.
- Deficient fluid volume related to drug effects of diuretics.
- Risk for injury related to postural hypotension and dizziness.
- Deficient knowledge related to new use of diuretic therapy.
- Acute pain related to occurrence of headache from adverse effects of diuretics.
- Noncompliance to treatment related to lack of information about side effects of medications.

● Planning

Goals related to the administration of diuretics include the following:
- Patient regains fluid and electrolyte balance.
- Patient remains free of the complications associated with diuretic use.
- Patient remains free of injury to self while on diuretics.
- Patient remains compliant with therapy.

Outcome Criteria

The outcome criteria in patients receiving diuretics are as follows:
- Patient will maintain normal electrolyte values (sodium, potassium, and chloride values) while on diuretics.

- Patient will continue to show or regain normal cardiac output while on diuretic therapy as evidenced by vital signs, adequate intake and output within normal limits (pulse <100, >60; BP 120/80; urine output > or = 30 ml/hr).
- Patient's skin turgor will be pliable and without edema or dryness.
- Patient will rise slowly and change positions slowly and cautiously while receiving diuretics.
- Patient will state importance and rationale for follow-up visits with the physician such as monitoring for adverse effects, dehydration, fluid and electrolyte imbalances.
- Patient will report dizziness, fainting, palpitations, tingling, confusion, or disorientation to physician immediately.

● Implementation

Diuretics, including patient education guidelines, were discussed in Chapter 23 on antihypertensive agents. As a reminder, however, diuretics should be taken in the morning as much as possible to avoid their interference with sleep patterns. Potassium supplements are generally not recommended when potassium levels exceed 3.0 mEq/L or unless per physician's advice.

Additional patient teaching tips for diuretic therapy are presented below.

● Evaluation

The therapeutic effects of diuretics include the resolution of or a reduction in the edema, fluid volume overload, CHF, or hypertension or a return to normal intraocular pressures. The patient must also be monitored for the occurrence of adverse reactions such as metabolic alkalosis (monitor arterial blood gas values), drowsiness, lethargy, hypokalemia, tachycardia, hypotension, leg cramps, restlessness, and a decrease in mental alertness.

✎ patient teaching tips

Diuretic Therapy

➤ The patient should be told to always maintain proper nutritional and fluid volume status and to eat more potassium-rich foods when taking *any but the potassium-sparing diuretics*. Foods high in potassium include bananas, oranges, dates, raisins, plums, fresh vegetables, potatoes (especially potato skins), meat, and fish.

➤ If patients are taking a diuretic along with a digitalis preparation, they and/or their family members should be shown how to monitor the pulse rate and know to call the physician at the first signs of toxicity. The symptoms of this consist of anorexia, nausea, vomiting, and bradycardia, or a pulse of less than 60 beats/min.

➤ Diabetic patients who are taking thiazide and/or loop diuretics should be told to closely monitor their blood sugar levels because these drugs can raise them.

➤ Patients taking diuretics should be told to change positions slowly and rise slowly after sitting or lying to prevent dizziness and possible fainting (syncope) related to the orthostatic hypotension resulting from the diuretic therapy.

➤ Encourage patients to return to their physician for follow-up visits and especially for laboratory workups.

➤ Patients taking diuretics should keep a journal or log of their daily weights.

➤ Patients who have been ill and experienced nausea, vomiting, and/or diarrhea should notify their physician

of this because of the electrolyte and fluid loss this may have precipitated. Patients should ask whether to institute fluid volume replacement to prevent any excess fluid or electrolyte loss.
➤ Signs and symptoms of hypokalemia include muscle weakness, constipation, irregular pulse rate, and an overall feeling of lethargy.

➤ Patients should be encouraged to notify the physician immediately should they experience rapid heart rates or syncope, as this may be a result of hypotension or fluid volume loss.
➤ Any weight gain of 2 or more pounds (1 kg) a day or 5 or more pounds (2.25 kg) in a week should be reported to the physician immediately.

POINTS TO REMEMBER

Types of Diuretics
- Five main types of diuretics: carbonic anhydrase inhibitors and loop, osmotic, potassium-sparing, and thiazide and thiazide-like diuretics.
- The loop, potassium-sparing, and thiazide and thiazide-like diuretics are the most commonly used.
- All increase the rate of urine formation.
- Their purpose is to cause a net loss of water from the body and to increase urine output.

Nephron
- The main structural element in the kidney.
- The site where diuretics work.
- Composed of the glomerulus, afferent and efferent arterioles, proximal and distal tubules, loop of Henle, and collecting ducts.

Loop Diuretics
- Very potent diuretics that work in the loop of Henle, where the most of the sodium is resorbed.
- Three main ones currently used: furosemide, bumetanide, and torsemide.
- Ethacrynic acid seldomly used.
- Potency differences: 1 mg of bumetanide = 10 mg of torsemide = 40 mg of furosemide = 50 mg of ethacrynic acid.

Thiazide and Thiazide-Like Diuretics
- Frequently used and least expensive because several generic preparations are available.
- Hydrochlorothiazide is considered the prototypical thiazide diuretic.
- Used as adjunctive therapy to manage hepatic cirrhosis, edema, and CHF.
- May cause adverse metabolic effects: hypokalemia, hypercalcemia, hyperlipidemia, hyperglycemia, hyperuricemia.

Nursing Considerations
- Fluid volume status should be monitored in patients receiving diuretics because of the serious excess and deficit states they can cause.
- Skin and mucous membrane status and sodium, potassium, and chloride levels are ways of monitoring for excess and deficit states.
- Intake and output amounts should be monitored in patients receiving diuretics.
- Elderly patients are very susceptible to the effects of diuretics.
- Adverse reactions to diuretics include metabolic alkalosis, drowsiness, lethargy, hypokalemia, tachycardia, hypotension, leg cramps, restlessness, and decreased mental alertness.

REVIEW QUESTIONS

1. Which of the following is a drug interaction and should be taken with caution with thiazide diuretics?
   a. Potassium salts
   b. Antacid formulas
   c. Digitalis preparations
   d. Over-the-counter aspirin products
2. Patients taking carbonic anyhydrase inhibitors, such as Diamox, experience glycosuria because these agents result in:
   a. Increased blood levels of calcium with resultant diuresis.
   b. Increased levels of mannitol from the nephron and resultant oliguria or polyuria.
   c. Increased serum glucose levels with glycosuria and osmotic diuresis in the patient.
   d. Decreased levels of sodium, inactivation of sodium-potassium pump, and polyuria.
3. Patients taking spironolactone are at risk for developing:
   a. Hypokalemia.
   b. Hyperkalemia.
   c. Hypernatremia.
   d. Hypercalcemia.
4. Which of the following statements should be included in patient education for a patient taking furosemide (Lasix)?
   a. Check weight monthly and report it to the physician.

b. Avoid foods such as oranges and bananas that are high in potassium.

c. Change positions slowly because you may experience dizziness and possible fainting as a result of postural hypotension.

d. If you have a weight gain of more than 5 to 8 pounds per week, you should tell your physician at your next office visit.

5. One of your patients who is taking HCTZ is experiencing moderate light-headedness. He tells you that he is taking the medication exactly as prescribed and drinking many fluids. In your nursing assessment and dietary/drug history, you also discover that he is eating licorice almost on a daily basis. Which of the following side effects will be enhanced in this patient who is eating licorice every day and taking a thiazide diuretic?

a. Hypokalemia

b. Hyponatremia

c. Hypochloremia

d. Hypomagnesemia

For Answers see www.harcourthealth.com/MERLIN/Lilley/.

CRITICAL THINKING Activities

1. G.G. is a 64-year-old man who has been admitted to the coronary care unit because he is suffering from heart failure. He has been given 80 mg of furosemide every 6 hours, but with no relief of his pulmonary and peripheral edema. The physician would like to change him to bumetanide. What would be the equivalent daily dose of bumetanide?

2. What type of caution would you give a patient who is beginning treatment with a potassium-sparing diuretic?

3. Describe the antihypertensive effects of loop diuretics in the treatment of hypertension.

For Answers see www.harcourthealth.com/MERLIN/Lilley/.

bibliography

Albanese J, Nutz P: *Mosby's 2001 nursing drug reference and review cards*, St Louis, 2001, Mosby.

American Hospital Formulary Service: *AHFS drug information*, Bethesda, Md, 2000, American Society of Health-System Pharmacists.

Anderson PO, Knoben JE, Troutman WG: *Handbook of clinical drug data 1999-2000*, ed 9, New York, 1999, McGraw-Hill.

Holcomb SS: Understanding the ins and outs of diuretic therapy, *Nursing* 27(2):34, 1997.

Johns Hopkins Hospital, Department of Pediatrics et al: *The Harriet Lane handbook*, ed 15, St Louis, 2000, Mosby.

Keen JH: *Critical care and emergency drug reference*, ed 3, St Louis, 1996, Mosby.

Medical Letter: Spironolactone for heart failure 41(1061):81, September 10, 1999.

Morrison RT: Edema and principles of diuretic use, *Med Clin North Am* 81(3):689, 1997.

Mosby's GenRx: a comprehensive reference for generic and brand drugs, ed 10, St Louis, 2000, Mosby.

Perez A: Restoring electrolyte balance: hypokalemia, *RN* 58(12):33, 1997.

Skidmore-Roth L: *Mosby's 2001 nursing drug reference*, St Louis, 2001, Mosby.

Turkoski BB: *Drug information handbook for nursing 1999-2000: including assessment, administration, monitoring guidelines, and patient education*, ed 2, Cleveland, 1999, Lexi-Comp.

United States Pharmacopeial Convention: *USP DI: advice for the patient: drug information in lay language*, vol. 1I, ed 20, Englewood, Colo, 2000, Micromedex.

Activity

Remember to check the **Online Worksheet** for additional learning opportunities: **www.harcourthealth.com/MERLIN/Lilley/**

Chapter 25

Fluids and Electrolytes

www.harcourthealth.com/MERLIN/Lilley/

objectives

When you reach the end of this chapter, you should be able to do the following:

Look for this symbol for topics covered in the **Online Worksheet**

1 Identify the various fluid and electrolyte solutions commonly used in the management of fluid and electrolyte disorders.

2 Discuss the mechanisms of action, indications for use, dosages, contraindications and cautions to use, and side effects for patients receiving fluid and electrolyte solutions.

3 Develop a nursing care plan that includes all phases of the nursing process for the patient receiving fluid and electrolyte solutions.

4 Discuss patient education guidelines related to fluid and electrolyte management.

---

drug profiles

albumin, p. 398	**hetastarch,** p. 398
dextran, p. 398	**sodium chloride,** p. 397

○━ Key drug.

---

glossary

Colloid (kol′ oid) A state of matter in which large molecules or aggregates of molecules that do not precipitate and that measure between 1 and 100 nm are dispersed in another medium. (p. 394)

Colloid oncotic pressure (ong kot′ ik) The osmotic pressure exerted by a colloid in solution, such as that produced when the concentration of protein in the plasma on one side of a cell membrane is higher than that in the neighboring interstitial fluid. (p. 394)

Crystalloids (kris′ tə loid) A substance in a solution that diffuses through a semipermeable membrane. (p. 395)

Dehydration (de′ hi dra′ shən) Excessive loss of water from the body tissues. It is accompanied by an imbalance in the essential electrolyte concentrations, particularly sodium, potassium, and chloride. (p. 395)

Edema (ə de mə) The abnormal accumulation of fluid in interstitial spaces, such as in the pericardial sac, intrapleural space, peritoneal cavity, and joint capsules. (p. 395)

Extracellular fluid (eks′ trə sel′ u lər) That portion of the body fluid comprising the interstitial fluid and blood plasma. The adult body contains about 11.2 liters of interstitial fluid, constituting about 16% of the body weight, and about 2.8 liters of plasma, constituting about 4% of the body weight. (p. 394)

Extravascular fluid (eks′ trə vas′ ku lər) Fluids in the body that are outside the blood vessels. Examples include lymph and cerebrospinal fluid. (p. 394)

Hydrostatic pressure (hi′ dro stat′ ik) The pressure exerted by a liquid. (p. 394)

Hypokalemia (hi′ po kə le′ me ə) A condition in which there is an inadequate amount of potassium, the major intracellular cation, in the bloodstream. (p. 401)

Hyponatremia (hi′ po nə tre′ me ə) A condition in which there is an inadequate amount of sodium in the blood, caused either by inadequate excretion of water or by excessive water in the bloodstream. (p. 402)

Interstitial fluid (in′ tər stish′ əl) Extracellular fluid that fills in the spaces between most of the cells of the body and provides a substantial portion of the liquid environment of the body. (p. 394)

Intracellular fluid Fluid located within cell membranes throughout most of the body. It contains dissolved solutes that are essential to maintaining electrolyte balance and healthy metabolism. (p. 394)

Intravascular fluid The fluid inside blood vessels. (p. 394)

Isotonic (i′ so ton′ ik) Having the same concentration of a solute as another solution, hence exerting the same osmotic pressure as that solution, such as an isotonic saline solution that contains an amount of salt equal to that found in the intracellular and extracellular fluid. (p. 394)

Osmotic pressure The pressure exerted on a semipermeable membrane separating a solution from a solvent; the membrane being impermeable to the solutes in the solution and permeable only to the solvent. (p. 394)

Plasma (plaz′ mə) The watery, straw-colored fluid component of lymph and blood in which the leukocytes, erythrocytes, and platelets are suspended. (p. 394)

Fluid and electrolyte management is one of the cornerstones of patient care. Most disease processes, tissue injuries, and surgical procedures greatly influence the physiologic status of fluids and electrolytes in the body. A prerequisite to the understanding of fluid and electrolyte management is knowledge of the extent and composition of the various body fluid compartments.

PHYSIOLOGY OF FLUID BALANCE

About 60% of the adult human body is water. This is referred to as the *total body water* (TBW), and it is distributed to the three main compartments in the following proportions: **intracellular fluid** (ICF), 67%; interstitial fluid (ISF), 25%; and plasma volume (PV), 8%. This distribution is illustrated in Figure 25-1. The actual volume of fluid that would normally be in each compartment in an average 70-kg man with a TBW content of 60% of his total body weight is shown in Table 25-1.

The terms used to identify the various spaces within which the TBW is distributed can be quite confusing, and there are two basic approaches to distinguishing among the locations of the fluid. The TBW can be described as being in or out of the blood vessels, or vasculature. If this terminology is used, then the term **intravascular fluid** (IVF) describes fluid inside the blood vessels, and the term **extravascular fluid** (EVF) describes the fluid outside the blood vessels. The term **plasma** is used to describe the fluid that flows through the blood vessels that is intravascular. **Interstitial fluid** is the fluid that is in the space between cells, tissues, and organs. Both plasma and interstitial fluid make up extracellular volume. Both interstitial fluid and intracellular fluid make up extravascular volume. These terms are often confused and misused. Table 25-1 lists these definitions for further clarity and understanding.

What then keeps fluid inside the blood vessels? All the fluid outside the cells, the **extracellular fluid** (ECF), which consists of both the plasma and the ISF, has about the same concentration of electrolytes. However, there is one big difference between the plasma and the ISF. The plasma has a protein concentration, primarily consisting of albumin but also including globulin and fibrinogen, four times greater than that of the ISF. The reason for this higher concentration of protein is that these solutes (proteins) have a molecular weight that exceeds 69,000 daltons, and this makes them too large to pass through the walls of the blood vessels. Because of the difference in this concentration of plasma proteins (also known as **colloids**), fluid flows from the area of low protein concentration in the interstitial compartment to the area of high concentration inside the blood vessel in order to try to create an isotonic environment. (**Isotonic** means an equal concentration of solutes.) The protein in the blood vessels therefore exerts a constant **osmotic pressure** that prevents the leakage of too much plasma through the capillaries into the tissues. This pressure is called **colloid oncotic pressure** (COP), and normally it is 24 mm Hg. The opposing pressure, that exerted by the ISF, is called **hydrostatic pressure** (HP), and normally it is 17 mm Hg, which, of course, is less than the COP. The phenomenon of COP is illustrated in Figure 25-2.

The regulation of the volume and composition of body water is essential for life because it is the medium in which all metabolic reactions occur. The body maintains

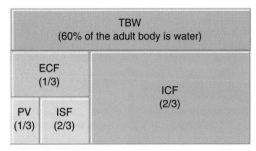

Fig. 25-1 Distribution of total body water (TBW). *ECF,* Extracellular fluid; *ICF,* intracellular fluid; *ISF,* interstitial fluid; *PV,* plasma volume.

Fluid Location: Descriptive Terms and Actual Volumes

Table 25-1

Name	Location	Actual Volumes
		(in a 70-kg man with a TBW content of 60% of his total body weight)
IF THE POINT OF REFERENCE IS THE CELLS, THEN THESE TERMS ARE USED:		
Intracellular fluid (ICF)	Inside of cells	28,000 ml
Extracellular fluid (ECF)	Outside of cells	14,000 ml (composed of both intravascular plasma and interstitial fluid)
IF THE POINT OF REFERENCE IS THE BLOOD VESSELS, THEN THESE TERMS ARE USED:		
Intravascular fluid or plasma volume (PV)	In blood vessels	3500 ml
Extravascular fluid (EVF)	Out of blood vessels	38,500 ml
IF THE POINT OF REFERENCE IS THE TISSUES THEN THESE TERMS ARE USED:		
Interstitial fluid (ISF)	In the spaces between cells, tissues, and organs but not in the plasma or the cells	10,500 ml

the volume and composition remarkably constant by maintaining a balance between intake and excretion. The amount of water gained each day is kept equal to the amount of water lost. When for some reason the body cannot maintain this equilibrium, therapy with various agents becomes necessary. If the amount of water gained exceeds the amount of water lost, a water excess or overhydration occurs. This is referred to as **edema.** If the quantity of water lost exceeds that gained, a water deficit, or **dehydration,** occurs. It has been estimated that death usually occurs when 20% to 25% of the TBW is lost.

Dehydration leads to a disturbance in the balance between the amount of fluid in the extracellular compartment and that in the intracellular compartment. In the initial stages of dehydration, water is lost first from the extracellular compartments. The nature of further fluid losses, COP changes, or both depends on the type of clinical dehydration (see Box 25-1). Clinical conditions that can result in dehydration and fluid loss as well as the symptoms of dehydration and fluid loss are listed in Box 25-2.

When fluid that has been lost must be replaced, there are three categories of agents that can be used to accomplish this: crystalloids, colloids, and blood products. The clinical situation dictates which category of agents is most appropriate.

CRYSTALLOIDS

Crystalloids are fluids that supply water and sodium to maintain the osmotic gradient between the extravascular and intravascular compartments. Their PV-expanding capacity is related to the sodium concentration. They are generally used as maintenance fluids to compensate for insensible fluid losses, as replacement fluids to correct body fluid deficits, and for special purposes (i.e., the treatment of specific fluid and electrolyte disturbances). The different crystalloids are listed in Table 25-2.

Mechanism of Action

As previously mentioned, crystalloids supply sodium and water to maintain the osmotic gradient between the fluid outside the blood vessels (EVF) and the fluid inside

the blood vessels (IVF). This capacity to expand the PV is related to the sodium content. Therefore hypertonic saline (3% sodium chloride) is more efficient than normal saline (0.9% sodium chloride) for expanding the PV.

Drug Effects

Crystalloid solutions contain fluids and electrolytes that are normally found in the body. They do not contain proteins (colloids), which are necessary to maintain the COP and prevent water from leaving the plasma compartment. In fact, the administration of large quantities of crystalloid solutions for fluid resuscitation decreases the COP. Compared with the distribution of colloids, crystalloids are also distributed faster into the interstitial and intracellular compartments, which makes them better for treating dehydration than for expanding the PV, such as in the setting of hypovolemic shock. That is to say, crystalloids cannot expand the PV as well as colloids, and besides this, much larger quantities are initially required to accomplish this.

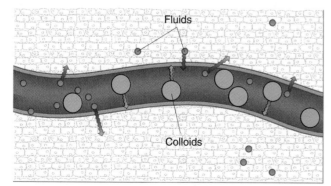

Fig. 25-2 Colloid osmotic pressure. As shown, the colloids inside the blood vessel are too large to pass through the vessel wall. The resulting oncotic pressure exerted by the colloids draws fluid from the surrounding tissues and other extravascular spaces into the blood vessels and also keeps fluid inside the blood vessel.

BOX 25-1 Types of Dehydration

Type of Dehydration	Characteristics
Hypertonic	Caused when water loss is greater than sodium loss, resulting in a concentration of solutes outside the cells and causing the fluid inside the cells to move to the extracellular space, thus dehydrating the cells. *Example:* elevated temperature resulting in perspiration.
Hypotonic	Caused when sodium loss is greater than water loss, resulting in higher concentrations of solute inside the cells, thus pulling fluid from outside the cells (plasma and interstitial spaces) into the cells. *Examples:* renal insufficiency and inadequate aldosterone secretion.
Isotonic	Caused by a loss of sodium and water from the body, resulting in a decrease in the volume of extracellular fluid. *Examples:* diarrhea and vomiting.

BOX 25-2 Dehydration and Fluid Loss: Conditions and Symptoms

Conditions	Symptoms
Bleeding	Increased bleeding and pulse rate
Bowel obstruction	Decreased perspiration and mucous secretions
Diarrhea	Decreased urine output
Fever	Dry skin and mucous membranes
Vomiting	Decreased tears and saliva

Table 25-2 Crystalloids

Product	Composition (mEq/L)						Volume (ml)	Cost*
	Na	**Cl**	**K**	**Ca**	**Mg**	**Lactate**		
Normal saline	154	154	0	0	0	0	1000	1
Hypertonic saline	513	513	0	0	0	0	500	1
Lactated Ringer's	130	109	4	3	0	28	1000	2.5×
5% Dextrose (D5W)	0	0	0	0	0	0	1000	2×
Plasmalyte	140	103	10	5	3	8	1000	5×

Na, Sodium; *Cl*, chloride; *K*, potassium; *Ca*, calcium; *Mg*, magnesium.
*Relative cost; example: D5W is two times the cost of hypertonic saline.

Table 25-3 Crystalloids and Colloids: Dosing Guidelines

	Crystalloids and Colloids			
	0.9% NS	**3% NS**	**5% Colloid***	**25% Colloid†**
To raise plasma volume by 1 liter, administer:	5–6 L	1.5–2 L	1 L	0.5 L
Fluid compartment distributed to:				
Plasma	25%	25%	100%	200–300%
Interstitial space	75%	75%	0	Decreased fluid levels
Intracellular space	0	0	0	Decreased fluid levels

NS, Normal saline.
*Isooncotic solutions such as 5% albumin, dextran 70, and hetastarch.
†Hyperoncotic solutions such as 25% albumin.

Therapeutic Uses

Crystalloid solutions are most commonly used as maintenance fluids. They are used to compensate for insensible fluid losses, to replace fluids when there are body fluid deficits, and to manage specific fluid and electrolyte disturbances. Crystalloids also promote urinary flow. They are much less expensive than colloids and blood products. In addition, there is no risk of viral transmission or anaphylaxis and no alteration in the coagulation profile associated with their use. The choice whether to use a crystalloid or colloid in these situations depends on the severity of the condition. Following are the common indications for either crystalloid or colloid replacement therapy:

- Shock
- Adult respiratory distress syndrome
- Acute nephrosis
- Burns
- Cardiopulmonary bypass
- Renal dialysis
- Hypoproteinemia
- Acute liver failure
- Reduction of the risk of deep vein thrombosis

Side Effects and Adverse Effects

Crystalloids are a very safe and effective means of replacing needed fluid. They do, however, have some unwanted effects. Because they contain no large particles such as proteins, they do not stay within the blood vessels and can leak out of the plasma into the tissues and cells. This may result in edema anywhere in the body. Peripheral edema and pulmonary edema are two common examples. Crystalloids also dilute the proteins that are in the plasma, further reducing the COP. Because crystalloids cannot carry oxygen as the blood products do, their use may result in decreased oxygen tension. Typically, large volumes are required for them to be effective (liters of fluid). As a result, large or prolonged infusions may worsen tissue acidosis or adversely affect CNS function in patients suffering from hepatic insufficiency, renal failure, or hypovolemic shock. Another disadvantage of crystalloids is that their effects are short-lived (transient).

Interactions

Interactions with crystalloid solutions are rare because they are very similar if not identical to normal physiologic substances. Certain electrolytes contained in lactated Ringer's solution may interact with other electrolytes, forming a complex that results in the formation of a precipitate. However, this would be an incompatibility rather than a true interaction.

Dosages

For the recommended dosages of crystalloids, see Table 25-3.

Activity

drug profiles

The most commonly used crystalloid solutions are normal saline (0.9% sodium chloride) and lactated Ringer's solution. The available crystalloid solutions and their compositions are summarized in Table 25-2.

sodium chloride

Sodium chloride (salt, NaCl) is available in several concentrations, the most common being 0.9%. This is the normal concentration of sodium chloride, and for this reason, it is referred to as *normal saline.* Other commonly used concentrations are 0.45% (half-normal saline) and 3% (hypertonic saline). These solutions have different indications, and they are used in different situations depending on how urgently fluid volume restoration is needed and/or the extent of the sodium loss.

Sodium chloride is a physiologic fluid that is present throughout the body. For this reason there are no hypersensitivity reactions to it. It is safe to administer it during any stage of pregnancy, but it is contraindicated in patients with conditions in which the administration of sodium and chloride would be detrimental. Hypertonic saline injections (3% and 5%) are contraindicated in the presence of increased, normal, or only slightly decreased serum electrolyte concentrations. Sodium chloride is available as a 650-mg tablet and as 0.45%, 0.9%, 3%, and 5% solutions.

PHARMACODYNAMICS

PLASMA VOLUME EXPANSION	COLLOID ONCOTIC PRESSURE	DURATION OF EXPANSION
60-70 ml*	30 mm Hg	Few Hours

*500 ml of normal saline will expand the plasma volume by 60 to 70 ml.

The dose of sodium chloride administered depends on the clinical situation. As a general rule, 20% or less of blood is lost more slowly then sodium chloride is required. The amounts of crystalloid or colloid needed to expand the PV by 1 liter, or 1000 milliliters, are given in Table 25-3, and this can be used as a general guide to dosing.

COLLOIDS

Colloids are substances that increase the COP and effectively move fluid from the interstitial compartment to the plasma compartment by pulling the fluid into the blood vessels. Normally this task is performed by the three blood proteins, albumin, globulin, and fibrinogen. However, for them to be effective, the total protein level must be in the range of 7.4 g/dl. If this level drops below 5.3 g/dl, the COP then becomes less than the HP (hydrostatic pressure) and fluid shifts into the tissues. When this happens, colloid replacement therapy is required to reverse this process by increasing the COP. The COP de-

creases with age and also in the settings of hypotension and malnutrition. The commonly used colloids are listed in Table 25-4.

Mechanism of Action

The mechanism of action of colloids is related to their ability to increase the COP. As previously explained, because the colloids cannot pass into the extravascular space, there is ordinarily a higher concentration of solutes (solid particles) inside the blood vessels (intravascular space) than outside the blood vessels. Fluid thus moves toward this hypertonic area in an attempt to make it isotonic. The result is that fluid is pulled from the extravascular space to the intravascular space, thereby increasing the blood volume. Because colloids increase the blood volume, they are sometimes called *plasma expanders.* They also make up part of the total PV.

Drug Effects

Colloids increase the COP and move fluid from outside the blood vessels to inside the blood vessels. They can maintain the COP for several hours. They are naturally occurring products and consist of proteins (albumin), carbohydrates (dextrans or starches), and animal collagen (gelatin). Usually they contain a combination of both small and large particles. The small particles are eliminated quickly and promote diuresis and perfusion of the kidneys; the larger particles maintain the PV. Albumin is the one exception in that it contains particles that are all the same size.

Therapeutic Uses

Colloids are used to treat a wide variety of conditions (see list on p. 396). Clinically colloids are superior to crystalloids in their ability to expand the PV. However, crystalloids are less expensive and are less likely to promote bleeding. On the other hand, crystalloids are more likely to cause edema because of the larger volumes needed to achieve the desired clinical effect.

Side Effects and Adverse Effects

Colloids are relatively safe agents, although there are some disadvantages to their use. They can alter the coagulation system, resulting in impaired coagulation and possibly bleeding. They have no oxygen-carrying ability and contain no clotting factors. They may also dilute the plasma protein concentration, which may impair the function of platelets. Rarely, dextran therapy precipitates anaphylaxis or renal failure. All these undesirable effects should be closely monitored for.

Interactions

Because colloid solutions are so compatible with drugs, they are sometimes used as the medium for delivering them. The drug propofol (Diprivan) is such an example. It is delivered in a 10% lipid emulsion.

Dosages

For the recommended dosages of colloids, see Table 25-3.

Commonly Used Colloids

Table 25-4

Product	Composition (mEq/L)		Volume (ml)	Cost*
	Na	**Cl**		
Dextran 70†	154	154	500	1
Dextran 40†	154	154	500	2×
Hetastarch	154	154	500	5×
5% Albumin	145	145	500	10
25% Albumin	145	145	100	10

*Using the cost of dextran 70 as the means of comparison.
†Dextran is available in NaCl, which has 154 mEq/L of both Na and Cl. It is also available in D5W, which contains no Na or Cl.

drug profiles

The specific colloid used for replacement therapy varies from institution to institution. The three most commonly used are dextran 40, hetastarch, and 5% albumin. They are all very quick in onset and have a long duration of action. They are metabolized in the liver and excreted by the kidneys, with albumin the one exception. It is metabolized by the reticuloendothelial system and excreted by the kidneys and the intestines.

albumin

Albumin (Albuminar, Albutein, Buminate, Plasbumin) is a natural protein that is normally produced by the liver. It is responsible for generating about 70% of the COP. Human albumin is a sterile solution of serum albumin prepared from pooled blood, plasma serum, or placentas obtained from healthy human donors. It is pasteurized (heated at 60° C for 10 hours) to destroy any contaminants.

Albumin is classified as a pregnancy category C agent and is contraindicated in patients with a known hypersensitivity to it and in those with congestive heart failure, severe anemia, or renal insufficiency. Albumin is only available in a parenteral form in concentrations of 5% and 25%. See Table 25-3 for the dosing guidelines.

PHARMACOKINETICS

HALF-LIFE	ONSET	PEAK	DURATION
16 hr	<1 min	Unknown	<24 hr

dextran

Dextran (Gentran, LMD, Rheomacrodex) is a solution of glucose. It is available in two concentrations, dextran 40 and the more concentrated dextran 70, and it has a molecular weight similar to that of albumin. Dextran 40 is the more commonly utilized of the two and is a low-molecular-weight polymer of glucose. It is a derivative of sugar that has actions similar to those of human albumin in that it expands the PV by drawing fluid from the interstitial space to the intravascular space.

Dextran is classified as a pregnancy category C agent and is contraindicated in the settings of hypersensitivity, congestive heart failure, renal insufficiency, and extreme dehydration. It is only available in a parenteral form in either a 5% dextrose solution or a 0.9% sodium chloride solution. See Table 25-3 for the dosing guidelines.

PHARMACOKINETICS

HALF-LIFE	ONSET	PEAK	DURATION
2-6 hr (D-40)	<5 min	Unknown	4-6 hr
12 hr (D-70)	1 hr	Unknown	12 hr

hetastarch

Hetastarch (Hespan) is a synthetic colloid derived from cornstarch. Its molecular weight is similar to that of albumin, and the colloidal properties of the 6% hetastarch solution resemble those of human albumin and dextran. It is similar to dextran in that it is a synthetic colloid and has no protein-binding properties.

Hetastarch is classified as a pregnancy category C agent and is contraindicated in patients who have shown a hypersensitivity to it and in those with severe bleeding disorders, congestive heart failure, or renal insufficiency. Hetastarch is only available in a parenteral form as a 6% concentration in a 0.9% sodium chloride solution. See Table 25-3 for dosing guidelines.

PHARMACOKINETICS

HALF-LIFE	ONSET	PEAK	DURATION
17-48 days	<1 min	Unknown	24-36 hr

BLOOD PRODUCTS

Blood products are also known as *oxygen-carrying resuscitation fluids*. They are the only class of fluids that are able to carry oxygen because they are the only fluid that contains hemoglobin. They not only can increase the PV but

Table 25-5 Blood Products

Product	Dosage	Cost*
Cryoprecipitate		1
Fresh frozen plasma (FFP)		1.7×
Packed RBCs	1 unit	2.2×
Plasma protein fractions (PPF)		1
Whole blood		3.3×

*Using the cost of cryoprecipitate as the means of comparison.

also can improve tissue oxygenation. They are also the most expensive and least available of the three types of fluids (crystalloids, colloids, and blood products) because they are natural products and require human donors. The available blood products are listed in Table 25-5. Their use is called for when a patient has lost more than 25% of his or her blood volume.

Mechanism of Action

The mechanism of action of blood products is related to their ability to increase the COP, and hence the PV. They do so in the same manner as colloids and crystalloids, by pulling fluid from the extravascular space to the intravascular space. Because of this they are also considered plasma expanders. Some also have the ability to carry oxygen. These are the oxygen-carrying resuscitation fluids, and they consist of packed red blood cells (PRBCs) and whole blood.

Drug Effects

Blood products increase COP and move fluid from outside the blood vessels to inside the blood vessels. They can maintain the COP for several hours to days, and because they come from human donors, they have all the effects that our own blood products have. They are administered when our own body is deficient in these products.

Therapeutic Uses

Blood products are used to treat a wide variety of clinical conditions, and the blood product used depends on the specific indication. The available blood products and specific conditions they are used to treat are listed in Box 25-3.

Side Effects and Adverse Effects

There are several undesirable effects of the blood products, some potentially serious. Because these products come from other humans, they can be incompatible with the recipient's immune system. These incompatibilities are tested for before the administration of the particular blood product by determining the respective blood types of the donor and recipient and by doing cross-matching tests. This helps reduce the likelihood of the recipient rejecting the blood products, which would in turn precipitate transfusion reactions and anaphylaxis. These prod-

Box 25-3 Blood Products: Indications

Blood Product	Indication
Cryoprecipitate and PPF	To manage acute bleeding (>50% blood loss slowly or 20% acutely)
FFP	To increase clotting factor levels in patients with a demonstrated deficiency
PRBCs	To increase oxygen-carrying capacity in patients with anemia, in patients with substantial hemoglobin deficits, and in patients who have lost >25% of their total blood volume
Whole blood	Same as for PRBCs

PPF, Plasma protein fraction; *FFP,* fresh frozen plasma; *PRBCs,* packed red blood cells.

Table 25-6 Suggested Guidelines for Blood Products: Management of Bleeding

Amount of Blood Loss	Fluid of Choice
20% or less (slow loss)	Crystalloids
20%–50% (slow loss)	Nonprotein plasma expanders (dextran and hetastarch)
>50% (slow loss) or 20% (acutely)	Whole blood or PPF and FFP
80% or more lost	As above, but for every 5 units of blood given, administer 1–2 units of FFP and 1–2 units of platelets to prevent the hemodilution of clotting factors and bleeding.

ucts can also transmit pathogens from the donor to the recipient. Examples of such pathogens are hepatitis and human immunodeficiency virus (HIV). Various preparation techniques are now utilized to reduce this risk of pathogen transmission, resulting in a drastic reduction in the incidence of such problems.

Interactions

As with crystalloids and colloids, blood products are very similar if not identical to normal physiologic substances, so they interact with very few substances. Calcium and drugs such as aspirin, which normally affect coagulation, may interact with these substances when infused in the body in much the same way they interact with the body's own blood products.

Dosages

For the dosage guidelines pertaining to blood products, see Table 25-6.

Whole blood and PRBCs are currently the most commonly used oxygen-carrying resuscitation fluids. They should be used in patients who have lost more than 25% of their total blood volume. All the blood products are derived from pooled human blood donors. For this reason they can do all of the following: carry oxygen, increase the PV, and improve tissue oxygenation.

PLASMA PROTEIN FRACTION (PPF)

PPF is obtained using a process very similar to the one used to obtain albumin. It involves the fractionation of human plasma with ethanol and its pasteurization at 60° C for 10 hours. More than 83% of PPF is albumin and more than 1% is gamma-globulin. PPF and albumin are similar in that both have similar colloidal properties. The primary advantages to the use of PPF are that it is simpler to manufacture, and greater amounts of protein per unit of plasma are yielded. The disadvantage to its use is that it is more antigenic than albumin. The suggested guidelines are given in Table 25-6.

FRESH FROZEN PLASMA (FFP)

FFP is obtained by centrifuging whole blood and thereby removing the cellular elements. The resulting plasma is then frozen at −18° C. FFP is not recommended for routine fluid resuscitation but may be used as an adjunct to massive blood transfusion in the treatment of patients with underlying coagulation disorders. The plasma-expanding capability of FFP is similar to that of dextran but slightly less than that of hetastarch. The disadvantage to FFP use is that it can transmit pathogens. The suggested guidelines are given in Table 25-6.

PACKED RED BLOOD CELLS

PRBCs are obtained by the centrifugation of whole blood, and their separation from plasma and the other cellular elements. The advantage to PRBC use is that their oxygen-carrying capacity is better than that of the other blood products, and they are less likely to cause cardiac fluid overload. They are small, compact oxygen carriers. The disadvantages are that they have a poor shelf life, their availability fluctuates, they can transmit viruses, they can cause allergic reactions, they can precipitate bleeding abnormalities, and they are expensive. The suggested guidelines are given in Table 25-6.

WHOLE BLOOD

Whole blood is a complete and physiologic volume expander. One unit provides hemoglobin, protein, and water that not only restores lost oxygen-carrying capacity but also expands the PV. The advantages and disadvantages of whole blood transfusion are the same as those associated with PRBC use. The suggested guidelines are given in Table 25-6.

PHYSIOLOGY OF ELECTROLYTE BALANCE

The chemical composition of the fluid compartments varies from compartment to compartment. The principal electrolytes in the ECF are sodium cations (Na^+) and chloride anions (Cl^-); the major electrolyte of the ICF is the potassium cation (K^+). Other important electrolytes are calcium, magnesium, and phosphorus. These different chemical compositions are vital to the normal function of all systems in the body, and they are controlled by the renin-angiotensin-aldosterone system, antidiuretic hormone system, and sympathetic nervous system (SNS). When these compositions are imbalanced, adverse consequences occur.

POTASSIUM

Potassium is the most abundant cationic (positively charged) electrolyte inside cells (the intracellular space), where the normal concentration is approximately 150 mEq/L. Approximately 95% of the potassium in the body is intracellular. In contrast, the potassium content outside the cells in the plasma ranges from 3.5 to 5.0 mEq/L. These plasma levels are critical to normal body function and are maintained by the adrenal gland hormone aldosterone.

Potassium is obtained from a variety of foods, the most common being fruit and juices, fish, vegetables, poultry, meats, and dairy products. It has been estimated that for normal body functions to be maintained, a person must consume 5 to 10 mEq of potassium per day. Fortunately the average daily diet usually provides 35 to 100 mEq of potassium, which is well above the required daily amount. Excess dietary potassium is usually excreted by the kidneys in the urine. However, if the kidneys lose their ability to filter and secrete waste products, potassium can accumulate, leading to toxic levels, and these in turn can precipitate ventricular fibriliation and cardiac arrest. Hyperaldosteronism and potassium-sparing diuretics can alter normal potassium balance as well. *Hyperkalemia* is the term for an excessive serum potassium level, and it is defined as a serum potassium level exceeding 5 mEq/L. There are several causes of hyperkalemia. One, renal failure, was just mentioned. Others are as follows:
- Burns
- Hyperaldosteronism
- Trauma
- Infections

- Metabolic acidosis
- Excessive loss from cells
- Potassium supplements
- Potassium-sparing diuretics

The opposite of hyperkalemia is **hypokalemia,** or a deficiency of potassium. This condition is more a result of excessive potassium loss than of poor dietary intake, however. As with hyperkalemia, there are a multitude of clinical conditions that can cause it. These include the following:

- Malabsorption
- Diarrhea
- Burns*
- Thiazide-like diuretics
- Corticosteroids
- Alkalosis
- Vomiting
- Crash diets
- Loop diuretics
- Ketoacidosis
- An increased secretion of mineralocorticoids (hormones of the adrenal cortex)
- Large amounts of licorice
- Thiazide diuretics
- Prolonged laxative misuse

Too little serum potassium can also greatly increase the toxicity associated with digitalis preparations, and this can precipitate serious ventricular dysrhythmias.

The early detection of hypokalemia is important in the prevention of the serious, life-threatening consequences of this metabolic disturbance if it goes undetected. The key to early detection is knowing its early symptoms, which are generally mild and can easily go undetected. Both the early (mild) symptoms and late (severe) symptoms of hypokalemia are listed in Box 25-4. The treatment of hypokalemia involves both identifying and treating the cause and restoring the serum potassium levels to normal (>3.5 mEq/L). The consumption of potassium-rich foods can usually correct mild hypokalemia, but clinically significant hypokalemia requires the oral or parenteral administration of a potassium supplement, which usually contains potassium chloride.

Mechanism of Action

Potassium's importance as the primarily intracellular electrolyte is highlighted by the enormous number of life-sustaining reactions and everyday physiologic functions that require it, functions that we take for granted and that would not be possible without it. Muscle contraction, the transmission of nerve impulses, and the regulation of heartbeats (the pacemaker function of the heart) are just a few of these functions.

Potassium is also essential for the maintenance of acid-base balance, isotonicity, and the electrodynamic characteristics of the cell. It plays a role in many enzymatic reactions, and it is an essential component of gastric secretion, renal function, tissue synthesis, and carbohydrate metabolism.

*Burn patients can exhibit either hyperkalemia or hypokalemia.

Drug Effects

The drug effects of potassium are numerous, as evidenced by the enormous number of physiologic functions and reactions throughout the body it is involved in. As mentioned previously, it is the major cation inside cells.

Therapeutic Uses

Potassium replacement therapy is called for in the treatment or prevention of potassium depletion in patients whenever dietary measures prove inadequate. The potassium salt used for this purpose is potassium chloride. The chloride is required to correct the hypochloremia (low chloride) that frequently accompanies potassium deficiency.

Other therapeutic effects of potassium are related to its role in the contraction of muscles and the maintenance of the electrical characteristics of cells. Potassium salts may be used to stop irregular heartbeats (dysrhythmias) and to manage the tachyarrhythmias that can occur after cardiac surgery. Potassium may also be used to treat thallium poisoning and to help increase muscular strength in some patients with myasthenia gravis.

Side Effects and Adverse Effects

The adverse effects of potassium therapy are primarily limited to the gastrointestinal tract and occur with the oral administration of potassium preparations. These gastrointestinal effects include diarrhea, nausea, and vomiting. More significant ones include gastrointestinal bleeding and ulceration. The parenteral administration of potassium usually produces pain at the injection site. Cases of phlebitis have been associated with IV administration, and the excessive administration of potassium salts can lead to hyperkalemia and toxic effects.

Toxicity and Management of Overdose

The toxic effects of potassium are the result of hyperkalemia. Symptoms include muscle weakness, paresthesia, paralysis, cardiac rhythm irregularities that can result in ventricular fibrillation, and cardiac arrest. The treatment instituted depends on the degree of the hyperkalemia and ranges from regimens for reversing life-threatening

BOX 25-4 Symptoms of Hypokalemia
EARLY
Anorexia
Hypotension
Lethargy
Mental confusion
Muscle weakness
Nausea
LATE
Cardiac dysrhythmias
Neuropathy
Paralytic ileus
Secondary alkalosis

problems to simple dietary restrictions. In the event of severe hyperkalemia, the IV administration of sodium bicarbonate, calcium gluconate or other calcium salt, and dextrose solution with insulin is required. This should be followed up with sodium polystyrene or hemodialysis to eliminate the extra potassium from the body. Less critical levels can be reduced with ion-exchange resins and by means of dietary restrictions.

Interactions

The use of potassium-sparing diuretics and ACE inhibitors can produce a hyperkalemic state. The use of diuretics, amphotericin B, and mineralosteroids can produce a hypokalemic state.

Dosages

Fluid and electrolyte therapy involves replacing any deficit losses and/or providing maintenance levels for specific patient requirements. Accordingly, specific dosage amounts of fluids or electrolytes depend on several clinical factors that include the following:

- Specific patient losses
- Efficacy of patient physiologic systems involved in fluid and electrolyte metabolism, especially adrenal, cardiovascular, and kidney functions
- Current drug therapy for pathologic conditions that complicate the amount and duration of replacement
- Selection of oral or parenteral replacement formulations

Suggested dosage guidelines with subsequent adjustments for potassium are 10 to 20 mEq administered orally several times a day or parenteral administration of 30 to 60 mEq every 24 hours.

Activity

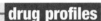

POTASSIUM SUPPLEMENTS

Potassium supplements are administered to either prevent or treat potassium depletion. The acetate, bicarbonate, chloride, citrate, and gluconate salts of potassium are available for oral administration. The parenteral salt forms of potassium for IV administration are acetate, chloride, and phosphate.

The dosage of potassium supplements is usually expressed in milliequivalents of potassium and depends on the requirements of the individual patient. The different salt forms of potassium deliver varying milliequivalent amounts of potassium. These various salt forms and how many grams of each are needed to yield 40 mEq are given in Box 25-5.

Potassium is classified as a pregnancy category A agent and is contraindicated in patients with severe renal disease, severe hemolytic disease, or Addison's disease, and in those suffering from hyperkalemia, acute dehydration, or extensive tissue breakdown stemming from multiple trauma. Potassium is available in many different oral and IV for-

mulations. It is available as a tablet and powder for solution, an extended-release capsule and tablet, and an elixir and oral solution. It is also available as an injection for IV use.

PHARMACOKINETICS

HALF-LIFE	ONSET	PEAK	DURATION
IV: Variable	IV: Immediate	IV: Rapid	IV: Variable
PO: Variable	PO: <30 min	PO: 30 min	PO: Variable

SODIUM

Sodium is the counterpart to potassium in that potassium is the principal cation (positively charged substance) inside cells and sodium is the principal cation outside cells. The normal concentration of sodium outside cells is 135 to 145 mEq/L, and it is maintained through the dietary intake of sodium in the form of sodium chloride, which is obtained from salt, fish, meats, and other foods flavored, seasoned, or preserved with salt.

Hyponatremia is the condition of sodium loss or deficiency and occurs when the serum levels decrease below 135 mEq/L. It is manifested by lethargy, hypotension, stomach cramps, vomiting, diarrhea, and seizures. Some of the same conditions that cause hypokalemia can also cause hyponatremia, and these are listed on p. 401. Other causes of hyponatremia are excessive perspiration, occurring during hot weather or physical work; prolonged diarrhea or vomiting, especially in young children; renal disorders; and adrenocortical impairment.

Hypernatremia is the condition of sodium excess and occurs when the serum levels of sodium exceed 145 mEq/L. Some of the symptoms are water retention (edema) and hypertension. The most common cause, however, is poor renal excretion stemming from kidney malfunction. Inadequate water consumption and dehydration are other causes. Symptoms of hypernatremia include red, flushed skin; dry, sticky mucous membranes; increased thirst; temperature elevation; and decreased or absent urination.

Mechanism of Action

As one of the body's electrolytes, sodium performs many physiologic roles necessary for the normal function of the body. It is the major cation in ECF and is principally involved in the control of water distribution, fluid and electrolyte balance, and osmotic pressure of body fluids. Sodium also participates along with both chloride and bicarbonate in the regulation of acid-base balance. Chloride, the major extracellular anion (negatively charged substance), closely complements the physiologic action of sodium. Sodium is also capable of causing diuresis.

Drug Effects

The drug effects of sodium are numerous. Because it is the major cation, it is involved in an enormous number of physiologic functions and reactions throughout the body.

Potassium: Various Salt Forms

Salt Form	Amount (in grams) Needed to Yield 40 mEq of Potassium
Acetate	3.9
Bicarbonate	4.0
Chloride	3.0
Citrate	4.3
Dibasic phosphate	3.5
Gluconate	9.4
Monobasic phosphate	5.4

Therapeutic Uses

Sodium is primarily administered in the treatment or prevention of sodium depletion when dietary measures have proved inadequate. Sodium chloride is the primary salt used for this purpose. Mild hyponatremia is usually treated with the oral administration of sodium chloride tablets and/or fluid restriction. Pronounced sodium depletion is treated with normal saline or lactated Ringer's solution administered intravenously. These agents have been discussed earlier in this chapter.

Side Effects and Adverse Effects

The oral administration of sodium chloride can cause gastric upset consisting of nausea, vomiting, and cramps. Venous phlebitis can be a consequence of its parenteral administration.

Toxicity and Management of Overdose

Hypernatremia leads to hypertension, edema, thirst, tachycardia, weakness, convulsions, and possibly coma. Treatment consists of increased fluid intake and dietary restrictions. The IV administration of dextrose solution may be required in more serious cases to help promote renal excretion.

Interactions

Sodium is not known to interact significantly with any drugs.

Dosages

Fluid and electrolyte therapy involves replacing any deficit losses and/or providing maintenance levels for specific patient requirements. Accordingly, specific dosage amounts of fluids or electrolytes depend on several clinical factors that include the following:
- Specific patient losses
- Efficacy of patient physiologic systems involved in fluid and electrolyte metabolism, especially adrenal, cardiovascular, and kidney functions
- Current drug therapy for pathologic conditions that complicate the amount and duration of replacement
- Selection of oral or parenteral replacement formulations

Suggested dosage guidelines with subsequent adjustments for sodium chloride are 1 to 2 g administered orally several times a day or parenteral administration of 1 liter of sodium chloride injection (normal saline).

drug profiles

sodium chloride

Sodium chloride is primarily used as a replacement electrolyte for either the prevention or treatment of sodium loss. It is also used as a diluent for the infusion of compatible drugs and in the assessment of kidney function after a fluid challenge. Sodium chloride is classified as a pregnancy category C agent and is contraindicated in patients who are hypersensitive to it. It is available in many IV preparations and orally as a 650-mg tablet and a 1-g and 2.25-g tablet.

PHARMACOKINETICS

HALF-LIFE	ONSET	PEAK	DURATION
Unknown	Immediate	Rapid	Variable

nursing process

• Assessment

Parenterally administered hydrating solutions such as 5% dextrose are used mainly for the prevention of dehydration. Isotonic solutions such as normal saline are customarily used to augment extracellular volumes diminished as the result of blood loss, severe vomiting, or any condition that leads to a chloride loss equal to or greater than the sodium loss. Normal saline is also used as the medium for blood transfusions because 5% dextrose in water results in the hemolysis of RBCs. Hypertonic solutions such as 3.5% sodium chloride are used to treat hypotonic expansion, such as that resulting from water intoxication. Plasmalyte 56 or Plasmalyte 148 are maintenance solutions used to replace electrolytes and water lost as the result of severe diarrhea or vomiting.

Although the physician selects which solution is to be administered, the nurse, by monitoring and assessing the patient, diagnoses the problem and the complications of the therapy and determines the effectiveness or ineffectiveness of the therapy. Today many patients needing replacement therapy are in home care settings, making the nurse even more responsible for ensuring their adequate and proper assessment.

The assessment of a patient who is to receive any parenteral replacement solutions should focus on the patient's past and present medical history, including diseases and gastrointestinal, renal, cardiac, or hepatic dysfunction or disorders. The nurse should question patients about prescription and over-the-counter (OTC) medications they are taking and their dietary habits. Patients' fluid volume and electrolyte status and baseline vital signs should be determined and laboratory studies performed. The skin, mucous membranes, daily weights, and intake and output measurement should also be assessed and any skin turgor noted in patients being treated for a fluid or electrolyte disorder. Pediatric and geriatric patients may be more sensitive to the effects of potassium chloride.

Before administering potassium to patients, it is important to assess the ECG for the presence of peaking T waves, depressed R waves, a prolonged Q-R interval, or a widening QRS complex, as well as the potassium levels and intake and output amounts. Contraindications to the use of potassium include renal disease, severe hemolytic disease, hyperkalemia, Addison's disease, acute dehydration, and multiple trauma that involves severe tissue breakdown. Potassium supplementation should be avoided or used with extreme caution in patients taking angiotensin-converting enzyme (ACE) inhibitors. Cautious use is recommended in patients suffering from cardiac disease or systemic acidosis and those taking potassium-sparing diuretics. The patient's pulse rate, blood pressure, and evidence of edema also need to be reported and documented.

Albumin and other colloids are contraindicated in patients with congestive heart failure or severe anemia and in those who have shown a hypersensitivity to it. Cautious use is called for in the settings of decreased salt intake, decreased cardiac reserve, hepatic disease, and pregnancy, as well as in the absence of an albumin-deficient state. The hematocrit, hemoglobin levels, and serum protein levels should also be noted and documented. Baseline assessment of patients' blood pressure, pulse rate, respiratory status, and intake and output amounts should also be performed and documented and any dyspnea or hypoxia noted.

Before administering blood or blood components, the nurse should obtain a thorough history regarding transfusions patients have received and their response to them. If the patient has any history of adverse reactions, this should be reported to the physician and blood bank or laboratory and the nature of them documented. It is also important to assess venous access as well as to check the patient's laboratory values (e.g., hematocrit [Hct], hemoglobin [Hgb], white blood cells [WBCs], RBCs, clotting factors) and baseline vital signs before infusing the blood or blood product. Even the general appearance of the patient and his or her affect can be a source of early evidence of adverse reactions to a transfusion or infusion of blood components.

• Nursing Diagnoses

Nursing diagnoses relevant to the patient who is to receive blood products, blood components, or related agents include the following:
- Risk for injury (falls) related to transfusion reaction or fluid and electrolyte imbalances.

- Risk for imbalanced fluid volume related to influence of fluid and electrolyte disorders.
- Risk for injury (skin trauma or abnormal clotting) related to altered blood component levels.
- Deficient knowledge about treatment regimen related to lack of patient education about the influence of fluid and electrolyte disturbances on the body and influence of treatment.
- Risk for injury related to complications of the transfusion or infusion of blood products, blood components, or related agents.

• Planning

Following are the goals related to the administration of fluids and electrolytes and blood components:
- Patient has minimal problems with volume overload related to the transfusion or infusion.
- Patient begins minimal exercise and shows increased tolerance daily.
- Patient participates in activities as he or she can tolerate them.
- Patient states measures to implement to minimize self-injury related to altered blood component levels or altered fluid and electrolytes.
- Patient states rationale for treatment and the side effects of replacement agents.
- Patient states symptoms and problems to report to physician.

Outcome Criteria

Following are the outcome criteria for patients receiving fluid, electrolytes, or blood components:
- Patient will remain free of self-injury as the result of adverse reactions (dizziness, volume overload, hypersensitivity) to the transfusion or infusion or of an allergic reaction.
- Patient will regain ability to engage in normal or near-normal exercise showing increased tolerance daily as evidenced by walking small distances and increasing to regular supervised exercise.
- Patient will participate in activities according to his or her ability to tolerate them without dyspnea or chest pain.
- Patient will demonstrate return to normal or near-normal values of blood components or fluid and electrolyte levels.
- Patient will see physician for follow-up as ordered to monitor laboratory values pertinent to treatment.

• Implementation

Continued reassessment of the patient during therapy is crucial in ensuring safe and effective treatment and also important in preventing the complications of overtreatment and undertreatment, which may be life-threatening. Serum electrolyte levels should not exceed normal ranges (sodium, 135-145 mEq/L; chloride, 95-108 mEq/L; potassium, 3.5-5.0 mEq/L; calcium, 4.5-5.8 mEq/L; magnesium, 1.5-2.5 mEq/L) and should be watched carefully after the conclusion of treatment as well. It is important to document all changes in the patient and any changes in assessment findings. Besides monitoring the infusion rate, the appearance of the fluid or solution, and the infusion site, the nurse must also constantly watch for infiltration of the solution, thrombosis, thrombophlebitis, pain at the IV site, pulmonary edema, fever, and air emboli.

With the administration of any fluid and electrolyte solution, a steady and even flow rate must be maintained to prevent complications. If for some reason the nurse cannot administer the solution ordered or in the amount or at the rate specified, this must be dealt with immediately, the situation resolved, the physician notified, an incident report filed, and the matter documented. The nurse must always perform in an especially prudent, safe, and thorough manner when administering fluids to elderly or pediatric patients because they are more sensitive to changes in fluid and electrolyte levels.

When administering potassium replacements parenterally, the nurse should carefully monitor the dosage during infusion. When given intravenously, potassium *must always be given in diluted form* and administered slowly and only to patients with a documented urine output. It is generally recommended that IV solutions should not contain more than 40 mEq/L of potassium and the rate should not exceed 20 mEq/hr. When IV potassium chloride is ordered for a patient, the nurse must remember the danger associated with potassium infusions. Potassium chloride should never be given as an IV bolus or given undiluted since cardiac arrest may occur. When adding potassium chloride to a liter bag of IV solution, it is necessary to mix the bag thoroughly to prevent concentration of potassium chloride in the solution. Oral preparations of potassium should be prescribed whenever possible and in conjunction with a high potassium diet so as to avoid the need for IV administration. Potassium chloride is the salt customarily used for IV infusions.

Oral forms of potassium are usually prepared in doses of 10, 20, or 40 mEq/15 ml and must be diluted in water or fruit juice to minimize gastrointestinal distress or irritation. Powder or effervescent forms should be prepared according to the package guidelines. Both enteric-coated and uncoated forms can cause gastrointestinal ulcers with bleeding, so their use should always be closely monitored. Any complaints of nausea, vomiting, gastrointestinal pain, or gastrointestinal bleeding should be assessed, noted, and reported to the physician immediately and all doses withheld until further orders are received.

Symptoms of hyponatremia include lethargy, hypotension, stomach cramps, vomiting, diarrhea, and seizures. Treatment with Ringer's solution or normal saline is usually helpful in alleviating them, but sodium can also be taken in by consuming a diet high in salt, obtained from such sources as catsup, mustard, cured meats, cheeses, potato chips, peanut butter, popcorn, and table salt. Careful administration with constant monitoring of the IV solution and the rate and site of administration is recommended in any patient undergoing electrolyte replacement therapy.

The IV infusion of albumin and other colloids should always be done slowly and cautiously, with careful monitoring, to prevent fluid overload and possible congestive heart failure, especially in those patients at particular risk for this. The hematocrit and hemoglobin values should also be determined in advance so that any anemia can be detected and care taken not to overload the heart pump with an increased volume. Albumin and any blood products should be infused at room temperature.

legal & ethical principles

Infiltrating IV

Nurses often encounter an infiltrating IV in the routine care of many of their patients. Every action taken is very important to the standard of care of the patient and in ensuring that the nurse has acted as any prudent nurse would. The assessment and action taken by the nurse can be important for the patient as in the case of **Macon-Bibb Hosp. Authority vs. Ross** (335 S.E. 2d 633-GA).

SITUATION

Ms. Ross was brought to the emergency room of the hospital with dyspnea, bradycardia, and a blood pressure of 250/150 mm Hg. She went into respiratory arrest at 2:55 PM; she was intubated with an endotracheal tube, and nitroprusside was administered intravenously to decrease her blood pressure. Because of the rapid drop in blood pressure, an IV administration of dopamine was started at 3:28 PM in her right wrist to increase her blood pressure. When her BP was stable, she was transferred to the cardiac care unit at 4:30 PM. At midnight, a nurse noted that the IV site had a "bruise bluish in color." The next notation was at 11:00 AM the following day, in which it was recorded that the patient's right arm was swollen and painful with a large blistered area around the IV site. The same notation was made at 4:00 PM. It was not until 6:50 PM that a note indicated that a physician was informed of the infiltration. As a result of the extravasation of dopamine, the patient's lower right arm was permanently scarred. On a jury verdict, the court entered judgment for the patient. The hospital appealed.

The court of appeals affirmed the judgment of the lower court. It was noted that, although an infiltration may result from an improper technique, it may also be due to the size of the needle, the status of the patient's veins, or specific intolerance to an IV. However, according to the expert nurse's testimony, supported by suitable references, dopamine should be infused into a "large vein," such as in the antecubital fossa, to minimize the risk of extravasation. In addition, dopamine should be monitored continuously for free flow. If extravasation of dopamine occurs, the recommended treatment of the site is infiltration with a saline solution of phentolamine (Regitine) within 12 hours.

The nurses were criticized for not being sufficiently knowledgeable regarding dopamine, which resulted in their failure to notify a physician of the patient's impaired tissue integrity.

From McKenry LM, Salerno E: *Mosby's pharmacology in nursing,* ed 21, St Louis, 2001, Mosby.

The patient should be carefully assessed and all findings documented at the start of the administration of a blood product or component (e.g., PPF, platelets, and FFP). The patient should then be assessed and the findings documented every 15 minutes, or more frequently if needed, thereafter. At this point the product should be infused at a rate of about 20 drops per minute. Vital signs should be checked and recorded every 15 minutes, or more frequently if possible. Should a reaction occur, the transfusion should be stopped immediately; appropriate nursing measures implemented; the physician notified; and the nature of the event, the corresponding measures taken, and the patient's response documented. Apprehension, restlessness, flushed skin, increased pulse and respirations, dyspnea, rash, swelling, fever and chills (a febrile reaction beginning 1 hour after the start of administration and lasting up to 10 hours), nausea, weakness, and jaundice need to be reported to the physician immediately. The expiration date of blood components should be checked to make sure they are fresh. No outdated blood or blood components should be used.

See the box below for patient teaching tips for these agents.

● Evaluation

The therapeutic response to fluid, electrolyte, and blood or blood component therapy includes the normalization of the following laboratory values: RBCs, WBCs, Hgb, Hct, sodium, potassium, and calcium. In addition, the fluid levels, volume status, and cardiac function should return to normal, and the patient should be able to resume his or her normal or near-normal activities. The patient should also show an increased tolerance to activity, improved skin color, and minimal to no dyspnea, chest pain, weakness, or fatigue. The therapeutic response to albumin therapy includes increased blood pressure, decreased edema, and increased serum albumin levels. Monitoring for the side effects of any of these products as well as for conditions stemming from either an excess or deficit of the particular product is also part of the evaluation process, and any such findings should be reported to the physician, if necessary, and documented. Adverse reactions to albumin include distended neck veins; shortness of breath; anxiety; insomnia; expiratory rales; frothy, blood-tinged sputum; and cyanosis.

---

patient teaching tips

Fluids and Electrolytes

➤ Patients should consume foods high in potassium in order to take in the recommended daily allowance, which is between 40 and 50 mEq for adults and 2 to 3 mEq/kg of body weight for infants. Two medium-sized bananas or an 8-oz glass of orange juice contains 45 mEq; 20 large dried apricots contain 40 mEq; and a level teaspoon of salt substitute (KCl) contains 60 mEq of potassium. Oral doses are usually increased gradually over about 1 week to prevent hyperkalemia.

➤ Sodium may be lost as the result of major tissue or body trauma, vomiting, the syndrome of inadequate antidiuretic hormone secretion, diuretic use, tap water enemas, wound drainage, loss of gastrointestinal fluids, and excessive perspiration. Patients should follow replacement instructions carefully and as the physician prescribed.

➤ Encourage patients taking any type of fluid or electrolyte substance, colloid, or blood component to report any unusual side effects immediately to their physician. Such complaints include chest pain, dizziness, weakness, shortness of breath, or any unusual symptom.

➤ Water intake is important in all patients, especially the elderly and anyone in a hot, humid environment or losing fluids as the result of perspiration, drainage, and the like. Patients should understand that water is important because it is the medium in which all metabolic reactions occur and it is needed for the precise regulation of the volume and composition of body fluid, both of which are essential for life.

POINTS TO REMEMBER

Total Body Water
- Broken down into intracellular (inside the cell) and extracellular (outside the cell) volume.
- The fluid that is outside the cells is either in the plasma (intravascular volume) or between the tissues, cells, or organs (interstitial fluid).

Colloid Oncotic Pressure
- The concentration of colloids such as albumin is four times greater inside blood vessels than outside them.

- Colloids are large protein particles that cannot leak out of the blood vessels.
- Because of their greater concentration inside blood vessels, fluid is pulled into the blood vessels.
- Albumin, hetastarch, and dextran are examples of colloids.

Crystalloids
- Fluids that supply water and sodium to maintain the osmotic gradient between extravascular and intravascular compartments.

- Their PV-expanding capacity is related to the sodium concentration.
- They contain fluids and electrolytes that are normally found in the body.

Blood Products

- Also known as *oxygen-carrying resuscitation fluids.*
- Only class of fluids able to carry oxygen because they are the only fluids that contain hemoglobin.
- They not only increase the oxygen-carrying capabilities but also the COP.

Nursing Considerations—Hydration

- Hydrating solutions include 0.45%, 0.9%, or higher saline in water (hypertonic solutions: 3% and 5%); these are used to hydrate patients and prevent dehydration. Hypertonic solutions should be given slowly (<100 ml/hr).
- Dehydration may be hypotonic, resulting from the loss of salt; hypertonic, resulting from fever with perspiration; or isotonic, resulting from diarrhea or vomiting.
- Each form of dehydration is treated differently.

Nursing Considerations—Potassium Therapy

- Symptoms of hypokalemia include lethargy, weakness, fatigue, respiratory difficulty, paralysis, and ileus.
- IV potassium should always be given slowly and only in appropriate concentrations.

- Hyperkalemia may lead to ventricular fibrillation and cardiac arrest.

Nursing Considerations—Sodium Therapy

- Hyponatremia is manifested by lethargy, hypotension, stomach cramps, vomiting, diarrhea, and possibly seizures.
- Hypernatremia is manifested by red, flushed skin; dry, sticky mucous membranes; increased thirst; temperature elevation; and a decrease in or absence of urination.

Nursing Considerations—Blood Products

- Blood products may cause hemolysis of RBCs, and so adverse reactions such as fever, chills, and back pain should be watched for. If noted, the physician should be notified immediately, the IV infusion discontinued, and the nature of the reactions and all actions taken documented.

Albumin

- During the infusion of albumin and like products, the patient should be constantly monitored for the development of increased central venous pressure, as manifested by the occurrence of distended neck veins; shortness of breath; expiratory rales; anxiety; and frothy, blood-tinged sputum.

REVIEW QUESTIONS

1. Which of the following statements is true about administration of KCl?
   a. IV rates of KCl solutions may safely exceed 20 mEq KCl/hr.
   b. When giving IV KCl it is crucial to *always* give it in diluted form.
   c. IV solutions of KCl should not contain more than 20 mEq KCl.
   d. Oral forms of KCl may be given safely and effectively on an empty stomach.
2. KCl would most likely be contraindicated in patients with which of the following?
   a. Burns
   b. Diarrhea
   c. Multitrauma
   d. Renal disease

3. Mild hyponatremia is most likely to be treated by:
   a. Oral NaCl tablets.
   b. Forcing of fluids only.
   c. IV bolus of KCl and NaCl.
   d. Wide open IV infusion of NS.
4. Blood products should be administered with what type of IV fluids?
   a. NS
   b. D5W
   c. D10W
   d. D5 RL
5. Hypernatremia may result in which of the following conditions?
   a. Diaphoresis
   b. Hypertension
   c. Decreased turgor
   d. Severe bradycardia

For Answers see www.harcourthealth.com/MERLIN/Lilley/.

CRITICAL THINKING Activities

1. Your patient is receiving heparin therapy and warfarin sodium (Coumadin) has also been prescribed. What is the rationale for beginning Coumadin treatment while the patient is already on an anticoagulant?

2. Ms. Wall takes 2500 mg of calcium carbonate daily in the form of an OTC calcium supplement. How much elemental calcium is she actually taking?

3. Contrast the three types of dehydration. List an example of each type.
4. Discuss the importance of crystalloids and their therapeutic effectiveness. Provide examples of crystalloids and the conditions for which they would be ordered.
5. Compare the use of crystalloids with that of colloids.

For Answers see www.harcourthealth.com/MERLIN/Lilley/.

bibliography

Albanese J, Nutz P: *Mosby's 2001 nursing drug reference and review cards,* St Louis, 2001, Mosby.

American Hospital Formulary Service: *AHFS drug information,* Bethesda, Md, 2000, American Society of Health-System Pharmacists.

Anderson PO, Knoben JE, Troutman WG: *Handbook of clinical drug data 1999-2000,* ed 9, New York, 1999, McGraw-Hill.

Johns Hopkins Hospital, Department of Pediatrics et al: *The Harriet Lane handbook,* ed 15, St Louis, 2000, Mosby.

Keen JH: *Critical care and emergency drug reference,* ed 3, St Louis, 1996, Mosby.

McKenry LM, Salerno E: *Mosby's pharmacology in nursing,* ed 21, St Louis, 2001, Mosby.

Mosby's GenRx: a comprehensive reference for generic and brand drugs, ed 10, St Louis, 2000, Mosby.

Skidmore-Roth L: *Mosby's 2001 nursing drug reference,* St. Louis, 2001, Mosby.

Turkoski BB: *Drug information handbook for nursing 1999-2000: including assessment, administration, monitoring guidelines, and patient education,* ed 2, Cleveland, 1999, Lexi-Comp.

United States Pharmacopeial Convention: *USP DI drug information for the health care professional,* vol. 1, ed 20, Englewood, Colo, 2000, Micromedex.

Activity

Remember to check the **Online Worksheet** for additional learning opportunities: **www.harcourthealth.com/MERLIN/Lilley/**

Chapter 26

Coagulation Modifier Agents

objectives

When you reach the end of this chapter, you should be able to do the following:

1 Discuss the mechanisms of action of coagulation modifiers such as anticoagulants, antiplatelet agents, antifibrinolytics, and thrombolytics.

2 Identify the indications for and contraindications to the use of coagulation modifiers.

3 Discuss the administration procedures for these medications.

4 Identify the drug interactions associated with the use of coagulation modifiers, specific observations related to their use, and the antidotes for an overdose.

5 Develop a nursing care plan that includes all phases of the nursing process for patients receiving anticoagulants, antiplatelet agents, antifibrinolytics, and thrombolytics.

drug profiles

alteplase, p. 423
aminocaproic acid, p. 421
anisindione and warfarin sodium, p. 414
○━ aspirin, p. 418
clopidogrel, p. 419

desmopressin, p. 421
enoxaparin, p. 415
○━ heparin, p. 415
pentoxifylline, p. 419
○━ streptokinase, p. 424
urokinase, p. 424

○━ Key drug.

glossary

Anisolated plasminogen streptokinase activator complex A plasminogen-streptokinase complex that has been chemically modified by acylation, allowing a prolonged half-life. (p. 422)

Anticoagulants (an′ ti ko ag′ u lənt) A substance that prevents or delays coagulation of the blood. (p. 410)

Antifibrinolytic (an′ ti fi′ bri no lit ik) Drug that prevents the lysis of fibrin and in doing so promotes clot formation. (p. 420)

Antiplatelet drug (an′ ti plat′ lət) Substance that prevents platelet plugs from forming, which can be beneficial in defending the body against heart attacks and strokes. (p. 410)

Antithrombin III (an′ ti throm′ bin) Substance that turns off the three main activating factors: activated II (thrombin), activated X, and activated IX. (p. 410)

Beta-hemolytic streptococci (group A) The pyogenic streptococci of group A that cause hemolysis of red blood cells in blood agar in laboratory setting. These organisms cause most of the acute streptococcal infections seen in human beings. (p. 422)

Clot specific Refers to whether a thrombolytic agent will lyse clots only in coronary arteries or throughout the body. (p. 422)

Deep vein thrombosis (throm bo′ sis) The formation of a thrombus in one of the deep veins of the body. The deep veins most commonly affected are the iliac and femoral veins. (p. 412)

Embolus (em′ bo ləs) A blood clot that has been dislodged from the wall of a blood vessel and is traveling throughout the bloodstream. (p. 412)

Fibrin (fi′ brin) A stringy, insoluble protein produced by the action of thrombin on fibrinogen during the clotting process. (p. 410)

Fibrinogen A plasma protein that is converted into fibrin by thrombin in the presence of calcium ions. (p. 423)

Fibrinolysis (fi′ bri nol′ ə sis) The continual process of fibrin decomposition produced by the actions of fibrinolysin. It is the normal mechanism for removing small fibrin clots. It is stimulated by anoxia, inflammatory reactions, and other kinds of stress. (p. 412)

Fibrinolytic system A system undergoing fibrinolysis. (p. 412)

Hemorrheologic drugs (he′ mo re′ ol aj ik) Drug that alters platelet function without preventing them from working. (p. 410)

Hemostasis (he′ mo sta′ sis) The termination of bleeding by mechanical or chemical means or by the complex coagulation process of the body, consisting of vasoconstriction, platelet aggregation, and thrombin and fibrin synthesis. (p. 410)

Hemostatic agent A procedure, device, or substance that arrests the flow of blood. (p. 410)

Plasmin (plaz′ min) The enzyme that breaks down fibrin into fibrin degradation products. (p. 412)

Plasminogen (plaz min′ ə jən) A plasma protein that is converted to plasmin and promotes fibrinolysis. (p. 412)

Pulmonary emboli (pool′ mo nar e) The blockage of a pulmonary artery by foreign matter such as fat, air, tumor, or a thrombus that usually arises from a peripheral vein. (p. 412)

Streptokinase (strep' to ki' nase) A fibrinolytic activator that enhances the conversion of plasminogen to the fibrinolytic enzyme plasmin. It is used in the treatment of certain cases of pulmonary and coronary embolism. (p. 422)

Stroke Occlusion of the blood vessels of the brain by an embolus, thrombus, or cerebrovascular hemorrhage, resulting in ischemia of the brain tissue normally perfused by the damaged blood vessels. (p. 412)

Thromboembolic event An event in which a blood vessel is blocked by an embolus carried in the bloodstream from the site of its formation. The area supplied by an obstructed artery may tingle and become cold, numb, and cyanotic. (p. 412)

Thrombolytic drug (throm bo' lit ik) A drug or other agent that dissolves thrombi. (p. 410)

Thrombus (throm' bəs) An aggregation of platelets, fibrin, clotting factors, and the cellular elements of the blood that is attached to the interior wall of a vein or artery, sometimes occluding the lumen of the vessel. (p. 412)

Tissue plasminogen activator A naturally occurring plasminogen activator secreted by vascular endothelial cells (the walls of the blood vessels). (p. 410)

The process that halts bleeding after injury to a blood vessel is called **hemostasis.** Normal hemostasis involves the complex interaction of substances that promote clot formation and substances that either inhibit coagulation or dissolve the formed clot. The drugs discussed in this chapter aid the body in achieving hemostasis, and they can be broken down into several main categories based on their actions. **Anticoagulants** inhibit the action or formation of clotting factors and therefore prevent clots from forming. **Antiplatelet drugs** prevent platelet plugs from forming by inhibiting platelet aggregation, which can be beneficial in preventing heart attacks and strokes. Other agents alter platelet function without preventing them from working. These are sometimes referred to as **hemorrheologic drugs.** Sometimes clots may form and totally block a blood vessel. When this happens in one of the coronary arteries, a heart attack occurs, and the clot blocking the blood vessel must be lysed to prevent or minimize damage to the myocardial muscle. The **thrombolytic drugs** lyse or break down such preformed clots.

This is a unique difference between thrombolytics and the anticoagulants, which can only prevent the formation of a clot. **Hemostatic agents** have the opposite effect of these other classes of agents; they promote blood coagulation and are helpful in the management of conditions in which excessive bleeding would be harmful. The various agents in each category of coagulation modifiers are listed in Table 26-1. Understanding the individual coagulation modifiers and their mechanisms of action requires a basic working knowledge of the coagulation pathway and coagulation factors, which is provided in the next section.

HEMOSTASIS

As previously mentioned, normal hemostasis involves a complex relationship between substances that promote clot formation (platelets, von Willebrand factor, activated clotting factors, and tissue thromboplastin) and substances that either inhibit coagulation (prostacyclin, **antithrombin III,** protein C and S) or dissolve a formed clot **(tissue plasminogen activator).** Each of these systems is discussed along with the description of the actions of the various classes of coagulation modifiers.

The coagulation system is called a cascade because each activated factor serves as a catalyst that amplifies the next reaction. The result is a large concentration of a clot-forming substance called **fibrin.** The coagulation cascade is typically divided into the intrinsic and extrinsic pathways, and these pathways are activated by different types of injury. When blood vessels are damaged, thromboplastin, a substance contained in the walls of blood vessels, is released. This activates the extrinsic pathway by activating factors VII and X. All the components of this intrinsic pathway are present in the blood in their inactive forms. This pathway is activated when factor XII comes in contact with exposed collagen in damaged blood vessels. Figures 26-1 and 26-2 illustrate the steps that occur in the extrinsic and intrinsic pathways, respectively, and the

Table 26-1 Coagulation Modifiers: Categories and Agents

Type of Coagulation Modifier	Drug Class	Individual Agents
PREVENT CLOT FORMATION		
Inhibit certain clotting factors	Anticoagulants	anagrelide, anisindione, ardeparin, dalteparin, enoxaparin, heparin, warfarin
Prevent platelets from working	Antiplatelet drugs	abciximab, aspirin, clopidogrel, dipyridamole, eptifibatide, pentoxifylline, ticlopidine, tirofiban
PROMOTE CLOT FORMATION		
Prevent lysis of fibrin	Antifibrinolytics	aminocaproic acid, tranexamic acid, aprotinin
LYSE A PREFORMED CLOT		
Directly lyse the clot	Thrombolytics	alteplase, anistreplase, reteplase, streptokinase, urokinase
REVERSAL AGENTS	Heparin antagonist	protamine
	Warfarin sodium antagonist	vitamin K

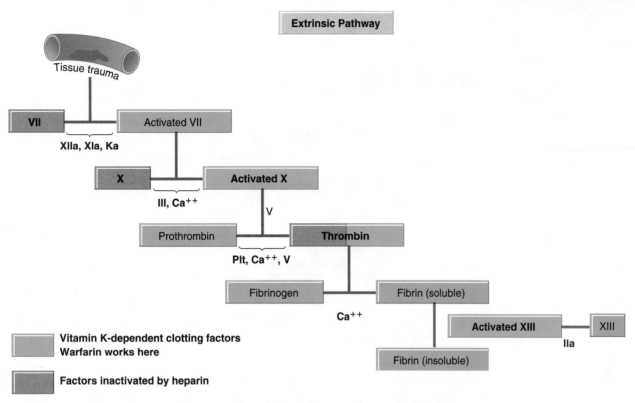

Fig. 26-1 Coagulation pathway and factors. *Plt,* Platelets.

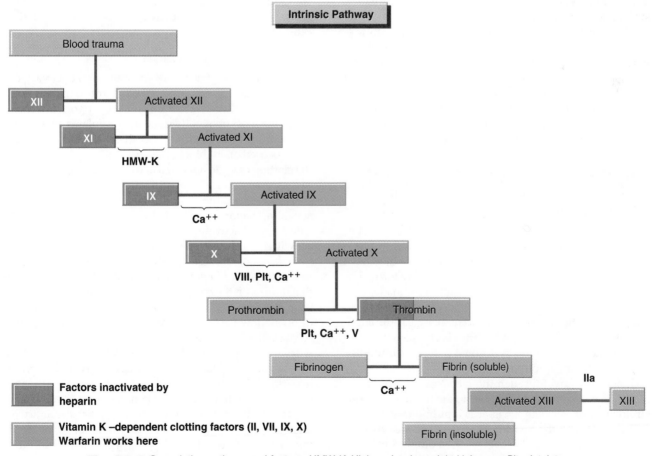

Fig. 26-2 Coagulation pathway and factors. *HMW-K,* High-molecular weight kininogen; *Plt,* platelets.

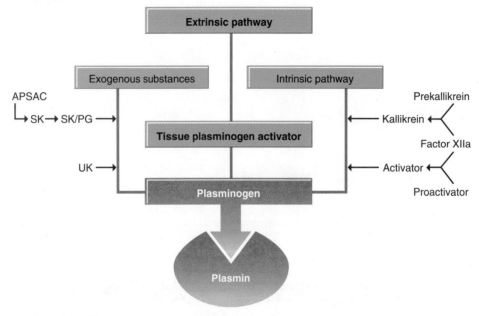

Fig. 26-3 The fibrinolytic system. *APSAC,* Anisolyated plasminogen streptokinase activator complex; *PG,* plasminogen; *SK,* streptokinase; *UK,* urokinase.

factors involved. They also show where in these pathways the various coagulation modifiers work.

Once a clot is formed and fibrin is present, the **fibrinolytic system** is activated. This is the system that regulates the breakdown of clots and keeps the coagulation system from going out of control. **Fibrinolysis** is the mechanism by which formed thrombi are lysed to prevent excessive clot formation and blood vessel blockage. **Plasmin** is the enzyme that eventually breaks fibrin down into the fibrin degradation products, although it must first be activated by **plasminogen.** It is the fibrin in the clot that binds to circulating plasminogen, which in turn activates plasmin and keeps the clot localized. Figure 26-3 illustrates the fibrinolytic system.

COAGULATION MODIFIERS

ANTICOAGULANTS

Drugs that prevent the formation of a clot by inhibiting certain clotting factors are called *anticoagulants.* These agents are only given prophylactically because they have no direct effect on a blood clot that has already formed or on ischemic tissue injured as the result of an inadequate blood supply caused by the clot. By decreasing blood coagulability, anticoagulants prevent intravascular thrombosis. Their uses vary from preventing clot formation to preventing the extension of a preformed clot, or a **thrombus.**

Once a clot forms on the wall of a blood vessel, it may dislodge and travel through the bloodstream. This is referred to as an **embolus.** If it goes to the brain, it causes a **stroke;** if it goes to the lungs, it is a **pulmonary emboli;** and if it goes to the veins in the legs, it is a **deep vein thrombosis (DVT).** Collectively these complications are called **thromboembolic events** because they involve a

thrombus becoming an embolus and causing an "event." Anticoagulants can prevent all of these from occurring if used in the correct manner. There are both orally and parenterally administered anticoagulants, and each agent has a slightly different mechanism of action and indications. All of them have their own risks, mainly that of causing bleeding.

Mechanism of Action

The mechanisms of action of the anticoagulants vary depending on the agent. Although other anticoagulants exist such as anisindione (Miradon) and enoxaparin (Lovenox), by far the most frequently used anticoagulants are heparin and warfarin (Coumadin), and these are the anticoagulants focused on in this chapter. All anticoagulants work in the clotting cascade but do so at different points. As shown in Figs. 26-1 and 26-2, heparin works by binding to a substance called antithrombin III, which turns off three main activating factors: activated II (also called *thrombin*), activated X, and activated IX. (Factors XI and XII are also inactivated but do not play as important a role as the other three factors.) Of these, the thrombin is the most sensitive to the actions of heparin. The overall effect of heparin is that it turns off the coagulation pathway and prevents clots from forming. As previously noted, however, it cannot lyse or break down a clot. The low molecular weight heparins (LMWHs) such as enoxaparin and dalteparin (Fragmin) work similar to the way heparin works. Heparin primarily binds to activated factors II, X, and IX, LMWHs differ from heparin in that they are much more specific for activated factor X (Xa) than for activated factor II (IIa). Unlike heparin, LMWHs have a much more predictable anticoagulant response. Frequent laboratory monitoring of bleeding times such as activated partial thromboplastin times (APTTs) are not required with LMWHs.

Warfarin also works by inhibiting certain clotting factors, in particular clotting factors II, VII, IX, and X. These factors rely heavily on vitamin K for their synthesis, a process that takes place in the liver. Warfarin and the indanedione derivatives (anisindione and dicumarol) specifically work by interfering with the proper production of vitamin K. The result is that the vitamin K needed for the production of clotting factors II, VII, IX, and X is dysfunctional, causing the clotting factors to be dysfunctional. As with heparin, the final effect is the prevention of clot formation. Figures 26-1 and 26-2 show where in the clotting cascade this occurs.

Drug Effects

The primary drug effects of the anticoagulants are confined to the coagulation system and bleeding. Besides preventing the formation of clots, heparin can also reduce the plasma lipid levels. Once the heparin therapy is stopped, a rebound increase in the lipid levels may occur.

Therapeutic Uses

The ability of anticoagulants to prevent clot formation is of benefit in certain settings in which there is a high likelihood of clot formation. These include a myocardial infarction (MI), unstable angina, atrial fibrillation, indwelling devices such as mechanical heart valves, and conditions in which blood flow may be slowed and blood may pool, such as major orthopedic surgery. As previously mentioned, the ultimate consequence of a clot can be a stroke or a heart attack, a DVT, or a pulmonary embolism (PE), so the prevention of these serious events is the ultimate benefit of these agents.

Side Effects and Adverse Effects

Bleeding is the main complication of anticoagulation therapy, and the risk increases with increasing dosages. It also depends on the nature of the patient's underlying clinical disorder and is increased in patients also taking high doses of aspirin or other drugs that impair platelet function. Some of the possible side effects of anticoagulant therapy are listed in Table 26-2.

Toxicity and Management of Overdose

Treatment of the toxic effects of anticoagulants is aimed at reversing the underlying cause. Although the toxic effects of heparin, LMWHs, and warfarin are hemorrhagic in nature, the management of each is different. Symptoms that may be attributed to toxicity or an overdose of anticoagulants are hematuria, melena, petechiae, ecchymoses, and gum or mucous membrane bleeding. In the event of either heparin or warfarin toxicity, the anticoagulant should be discontinued. In the case of heparin, this may be enough to reverse the toxic effects because of the short half-life of the drug (1 to 2 hours). In severe cases or when large doses have been given intentionally (i.e., during cardiopulmonary bypass for heart surgery), a reversal agent may need to be given. If large amounts of blood have been lost, replacement with packed red blood cells (PRBCs) may be necessary. The anticoagulant effects of heparin can be reversed with protamine sulfate. The protamine does

Table 26-2	Anticoagulants: Adverse Effects	
Body System	**Side/Adverse Effects**
Blood	Bleeding, thrombocytopenia, thrombosis
Gastrointestinal	Nausea, vomiting, abdominal cramps, ulcerations, bleeding
Other	Osteoporosis, skin necrosis, hypoaldosteronism, anaphylactic reactions

this by forming a complex with heparin, and this has the effect of completely reversing the heparin's anticoagulant properties. This takes place in as fast as 5 minutes. As a rule of thumb, 1 mg of protamine can reverse the effects of 100 units of heparin. Heparin comes from three different sources and each source has a different anticoagulant potency. In theory, however, the protamine dosing should vary depending on the type of heparin given (1 mg of protamine for 90 units of heparin-sodium from bovine lung tissue, 100 units of heparin calcium from porcine intestinal mucosa, and 115 units of heparin sodium from porcine intestinal mucosa). Protamine may also be used to reverse the effects of LMWHs. A dose of protamine equal to the dose of the LMWH should be used (e.g., 1 mg of protamine/1 mg of enoxaparin).

In the event of warfarin sodium toxicity or overdose (as previously mentioned), the first step is to discontinue the anticoagulant. However, the reversal agent and the therapy after discontinuation differs from those of heparin. As with heparin, the toxicity associated with sodium warfarin use is an extension of its therapeutic effects on the clotting cascade. However, because sodium warfarin functionally inactivates the vitamin K dependent clotting factors and because these clotting factors are synthesized in the liver, it may take 36 to 42 hours before the liver can resynthesize enough clotting factors to reverse the warfarin effects. Treatment with warfarin's reversal agent, vitamin K (phytonadione), can hasten the return to normal coagulation. The dose and route of administration of the vitamin K depend on the clinical situation and its acuity (i.e., how quickly the sodium warfarin induced effects must be reversed). High doses of vitamin K (10 to 15 mg) given intravenously should reverse the anticoagulation within 6 hours. If the warfarin therapy must be reinstated, resistance to its effect will be encountered because the large dose of vitamin K will maintain its reversal effects for up to 1 week. Low doses of vitamin K may minimize the resistance to warfarin therapy when warfarin must be restarted. In acute situations in which bleeding is severe and the time it would take for the vitamin K to take effect is not rapid enough, it may be necessary to administer plasma or factor concentrates.

Interactions

The drug interactions involving the oral anticoagulants are profound and complicated, and the drugs and the result of an interaction are given in Table 26-3. The main interaction mechanisms responsible for increasing anticoagulant activity include the following:

- Enzyme inhibition of biotransformation
- Displacement of the agent from inactive protein-binding sites
- Decrease in vitamin K absorption or synthesis by the bacterial flora of the large intestines
- Alteration in the platelet count or activity

Drugs that can increase the activity of heparin include aspirin, IV ethacrynic acid, and the oral anticoagulants. Antihistamines, digitalis, and the tetracyclines may partially antagonize the anticoagulant effects of heparin.

The main interaction mechanism responsible for decreasing anticoagulant activity is an increase in the biotransformation of the oral agents (enzyme inducers). The drugs that cause this are listed in Table 26-3.

Heparin can alter the serum levels of lipids, glucose, thyroxine, AST, ALT, and also affect T_3 uptake.

Dosages

For the dosages of anticoagulants, see the dosages table on p. 415.

drug profiles

All three anticoagulants discussed here (anisindione, heparin sodium, and warfarin sodium) are prescription medications. Anisindione is available in tablets, warfarin is available in tablets and an injection, and heparin can be given only by SC or IV injection. Several new LMWHs are currently available. These products are made by taking heparin and enzymatically removing part of the heparin molecule making a smaller, more accurate heparin. They are presently used for preventing and treating various thromboembolic events in patients who are at high risk for such events. Some of these high-risk patients undergo surgeries such as total hip or knee surgeries and high-risk general surgery. Some of the currently available LMWHs are enoxaprin and dalteprin. There are occasions when it is appropriate to use an oral anticoagulant like warfarin with an IV anticoagulant like heparin (e.g., while waiting for the full anticoagulant effect of warfarin to take place).

Table 26-3 Anticoagulants: Drug Interactions

Drug	Mechanism	Result
ANISINDIONE/WARFARIN SODIUM		
acetaminophen (high doses) amiodarone bumetanide furosemide	Displaces from inactive protein-binding sites	Increased anticoagulant effect
aspirin/other NSAIDs Broad-spectrum antibiotics cephalosporin	Decreases platelet activity	Increased anticoagulant effect
Mineral oil Vitamin E	Interferes with vitamin K	Increased anticoagulant effect
aminoglutethimide Barbiturates carbamazepine glutethimide rifampin	Enzyme inducer	Decreased anticoagulant effect
amiodarone cimetidine ciprofloxacin erythromycin ketoconazole metronidazole omeprazole Sulfonamides	Enzyme inhibitor	Increased anticoagulant effect
cholestyramine sucralfate	Impairs absorption of warfarin	Decreased anticoagulant effect
HEPARIN		
aspirin/other NSAIDs	Decrease platelet activity	Increased anticoagulant effect
ethacrynic acid	Additive	
Oral anticoagulants	Additive	
Thrombolytics Cephalosporins Penicillins	Additive	Increased anticoagulant effect

anisindione and warfarin sodium

Anisindione (Miradon) is an indanedione derivative. Warfarin sodium (Coumadin, Panwarfin) is a coumarin derivative. Warfarin is one of the most commonly prescribed oral anticoagulants. Both drugs are contraindicated in patients who have shown a hypersensitivity to them and in those with subacute bacterial endocarditis or any type of potential or actual bleeding condition. Because both drugs can also pass the placental barrier, they are also contraindicated in pregnant women. Both are noted as pregnancy category X agents. Anisindione is available as 50-mg tablets. Warfarin sodium is available as an injection (5 mg per vial) and as 1-, 2-, 2.5-, 3-, 4-, 5-, 6-, 7.5-, and 10-mg tablets. See the dosages table below for dosage information on both agents.

PHARMACOKINETICS

HALF-LIFE	ONSET	PEAK	DURATION
Anisindione: 3-5 days	Unknown	1-3 days	1-6 days
Warfarin: 0.5-3 days	12-24 hr	3-4 days	2-5 days

Activity

heparin

Heparin (Hep-Lock) is a natural mucopolysaccharide anticoagulant obtained from the lungs, intestinal mucosa, or other suitable tissues of primarily sheep and cows. It is contraindicated in the settings of hypersensitivity and any potential or actual bleeding condition. Heparin is considered a pregnancy category C agent. It is available in a multitude of concentrations and strengths. Heparin comes as a 10-, 100-, 1000-, 2500-, 5000-, 7500-, 10,000-, 20,000-, and 40,000- U/ml injection as well as a 25,000-U/500 ml infusion. Heparin can be given either subcutaneously or intravenously. See the dosages table below for dosage recommenda-

tions. Note that most institutions have adopted heparin nomograms for the dosing of heparin.

PHARMACOKINETICS

HALF-LIFE	ONSET	PEAK	DURATION
1-2 hr	SC: 20-60 min IV: Immediate	SC: 2-4 hr	Dose-dependent

enoxaparin

Enoxaparin (Lovenox) is an LMWH obtained by enzymatically cleaving large unfractionated heparin molecules into small fragments. These smaller fragments of heparin have a greater affinity for factor Xa than factor IIa, have a higher degree of bioavailability, and longer elimination half-lives than unfractionated heparin. Laboratory monitoring, as done for heparin, is not necessay with enoxaparin because of its high bioavailability and greater affinity for factor Xa. Lovenox is currently indicated for the prevention and treatment of deep vein thrombsis, which may lead to pulmonary embolism after knee or hip replacement surgery. There is new evidence that the agents within this therapeutic class of agents (LMWHs) are also effective for prevention of thromboembolic events in high-risk general surgery patients as well as patients with unstable angina.

Enoxaparin is contraindicated in patients with active major bleeding; thrombocytopenia associated with enoxaparin; or hypersensitivity to enoxaparin, heparin, or other porcine products. Enoxaparin is available in parenteral form only as a 30-, 40-, 80-, 90-, and 100-mg prefilled syringe. Enoxaparin is rated as a pregnancy category B agent. See the dosages table below for dosage information.

PHARMACOKINETICS

HALF-LIFE	ONSET	PEAK	DURATION
4.5 hr	3-5 hr	4-5 hr	12 hr

Activity

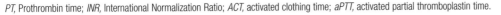

DOSAGES Selected Anticoagulant Agents

agent	pharmacologic class	dosage range	purpose
anisindione (Miradon)	Indanedione anticoagulant	*Adult* PO: First dose, 300 mg, followed by 200 mg on second day and 100 mg on third day; maintenance dose, 25-250 mg/day	
enoxaparin (Lovenox)	Low-molecular-weight heparin (LMWH)	*Adult* SC: 15 mg bid or 30 mg qd for DVT prophylaxis; 1 mg/kg bid or 1.5 mg/kg qd for treatment of DVT; or 1 mg/kg bid for unstable angina and non–Q-wave MI	Anticoagulant
heparin (Hep-Lock)	Natural anticoagulant	*Pediatric* IV: initial 50 U/kg, then 12-25 U/kg/hr increased by 2-4 U/kg/hr q6-8h prn *Adult* SC: 10,000-20,000 U followed by 8,000-10,000 U tid IV: 10,000 U followed by 5,000-10,000 U 4-6 times/day Infusion: 20,000-40,000 U/day ACT *or* aPTT determines maintenance dose	
warfarin sodium (Coumadin)	Coumarin anticoagulant	PT or INR determines maintenance dose, usually 2-10 mg/day	Anticoagulant

PT, Prothrombin time; *INR*, International Normalization Ratio; *ACT*, activated clothing time; *aPTT*, activated partial thromboplastin time.

ANTIPLATELET AGENTS

Another class of coagulation modifiers that prevent clot formation are the antiplatelet drugs, but they accomplish this in an entirely different manner. The anticoagulants work in the clotting cascade, whereas the antiplatelet drugs work at the initial step of the coagulation process, preventing platelet adhesion. As with anticoagulants, an understanding of the role of platelets in the clotting process is essential to understanding how antiplatelet drugs work.

research

Some Fats are Protective!

The American Heart Association has recently recommended replacement of saturated fats with monounsaturated or polyunsaturated fats. Monounsaturated fats are found in olive or canola oil, and polyunsaturated fats are found in corn and soybean oil. Studies have shown that diets high in olive oil are associated with lower risks of heart disease. Many Americans have replaced certain fats with diets high in grains, fruits, and vegetables. These foods associated with reducing LDLs are also associated with reducing HDLs (the "healthy" cholesterols) and need to be increased to be preventive.

©1999 by Facts and Comparisons. Reprinted with permission from *Drug Facts and Comparisons*. 1999 loose leaf edition. St. Louis, MO: Facts and Comparisons, a Wolters Kluwer Company.

Platelets normally flow through blood vessels without adhering to their surfaces. When blood vessels are injured by a disruption to blood flow, trauma, or the rupture of plaque from the vessel wall, substances such as collagen and fibronectin are present in the walls of blood vessels and are exposed. Collagen is a potent stimulator of platelet adhesion. Once platelet adhesion occurs, stimulators (adenosine diphosphate [ADP], thrombin, thromboxane A_2 [TXA_2], and prostaglandin H_2) are released from the damaged blood vessels. These cause the platelets to aggregate at the site of injury. Once there, they change shape and release their contents, which include ADP, serotonin, and platelet factor 4 (PF4). The hemostatic function of these substances is twofold. First, they attract platelets to the site of injury (platelet recruiters); second, they are potent vasoconstrictors. Vasoconstriction limits blood flow to the damaged blood vessel, thus also decreasing blood loss.

A platelet plug that has formed at a site of injury to plug the damaged blood vessel is not stable and can be dislodged. The clotting system is therefore stimulated to form a more permanent fibrin plug. The role of the platelet and the relationship between platelets and the clotting cascade in the generation of a stabilized fibrin clot are illustrated in Fig. 26-4.

Mechanism of Action

The mechanisms of action of the antiplatelet drugs vary depending on the agent. Aspirin, clopidogrel, dipyridam-

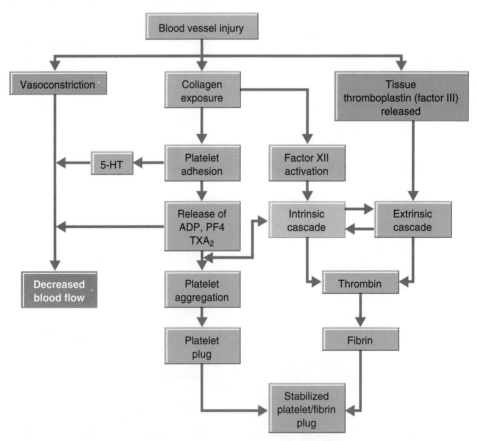

Fig. 26-4 Relationship between platelets and clotting cascade. *ADP,* Adenosine diphosphate; *5-HT,* serotonin; *PF4,* platelet factor 4; *TXA₂,* thromboxane A₂.

ole, pentoxifylline, and ticlopidine all affect the normal function of platelets. Many of the antiplatelet drugs affect the cyclooxygenase pathway, which is one of the common final enzymatic pathways in the complex arachidonic acid pathway that operates in platelets and on blood vessel walls. This pathway as it functions in both platelets and blood vessel walls is illustrated in Fig. 26-5.

Aspirin (acetylsalicylic acid) acetylates and inhibits cyclooxygenase in the platelet irreversibly such that the platelet cannot regenerate this enzyme. Therefore the effects of aspirin last the life span of a platelet, or 7 days. This irreversible inhibition of cyclooxygenase in the platelet prevents the formation of thromboxane (TX), a substance that causes blood vessels to constrict and platelets to aggregate. Thus by preventing TX formation, aspirin prevents these actions, resulting in dilation of the blood vessels and prevention of platelets from aggregating or forming a clot. This system also exists in the blood vessel. However, much higher doses of aspirin (>80 mg per day) are needed to inhibit the cyclooxygenase pathway in the blood vessels. This has the drawback of not only inhibiting the cyclooxygenase but also preventing the formation of prostacyclin, a beneficial substance that causes blood vessel dilation and inhibits platelet aggregation. If prostacylin is prevented from forming, vasoconstriction and platelet aggregation occur. By interfering with the function of the coagulation pathway, aspirin may also have a hematologic action. This is believed to consist in altering the hepatic synthesis of blood coagulation factors VII, IX, and X. Aspirin accomplishes this in much the same way that warfarin does, by interfering with the action of vitamin K.

Dipyridamole, another antiplatelet agent, also works by inhibiting platelet aggregation, which it does by preventing the release of ADP, PF4, and TXA_2, substances that stimulate platelets to aggregate or form a clot. Figure 26-4 shows how these substances accomplish this. Dipyridamole may also directly stimulate the release of prostacyclin and inhibit the formation of TXA_2 (see Fig. 26-5).

Clopidogrel and ticlopidine are two antiplatelet drugs that belong to one of the newest class of antiplatelet drugs called the *ADP inhibitors.* Their mechanism of action is entirely different from that of aspirin in that it inhibits platelet aggregation by altering the platelet membrane so that it can no longer receive the signal to aggregate and form a clot. This signal is usually sent by fibrinogen, which attaches to a glycoprotein receptor (GP IIb-IIIa) on the surface of the platelet. Ticlopidine and clopidogrel inhibit the activation of this receptor. It may take 24 to 48 hours for this action to take effect, which suggests that these therapeutic effects may be produced by ticlopidine metabolites rather than by the ticlopidine itself. Clopidogrel is a new antiplatelet drug, similar to ticlopidine in its actions, that has shown much promise. It has been shown to be significantly better than aspirin at reducing the number of heart attacks, strokes, and vascular deaths in at-risk patients.

Pentoxifylline, another antiplatelet agent, is a methylxanthine derivative with properties similar to those of theobromine, caffeine, theophylline, and other methylxanthines, but in contrast to other methylxanthines, it has little cardiac effects. It has many effects on blood. It can both increase the flexibility of RBCs and reduce the aggregation of platelets. It is sometimes referred to as a hemorrheologic agent, or a drug that alters the normal function of the blood. It affects the RBCs by increasing the flexibility (deformability) of the cells and reducing the

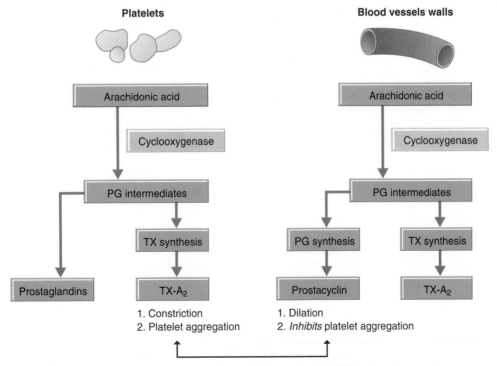

Fig. 26-5 Cyclooxygenase pathway. *PG*, Prostaglandin; *TX-A₂*, thromboxane A₂.

viscosity of whole blood, which it appears to do by facilitating the ability of the RBCs to maintain their integrity. The antiplatelet effects of pentoxifylline are that it inhibits platelet aggregation, which it does by inhibiting ADP, serotonin, and platelet factor 3 (see Fig. 26-4). Pentoxifylline also stimulates the synthesis and release of prostacyclin from blood vessels (see Fig. 26-5). In addition, it may have effects on the system that is responsible for lysing or breaking down clots, the fibrinolytic system. This may involve its increasing the breakdown of fibrin by raising the plasma concentrations of the tissue plasminogen activator (see Fig. 26-3).

Drug Effects

The drug effects of the antiplatelet drugs are multiple, but their primary ones are on the blood and the various mechanisms that maintain hemostasis. Although they have multiple effects on various components of the blood, they primarily inhibit the actions of platelets.

Therapeutic Uses

The therapeutic effects of the antiplatelet drugs depend on the particular agent. Aspirin has multiple therapeutic effects, but many of them vary depending on the dose. Aspirin has analgesic, antiinflammatory, and antipyretic properties. It also has potent antithrombotic and hematologic effects. Dipyridamole is used as an adjunct to warfarin in the prevention of postoperative thromboembolic complications. It is also used to decrease platelet aggregation in the setting of a number of other thromboembolic disorders. Ticlopidine's therapeutic effects are similar to a few of the therapeutic effects of aspirin. It has antithrombotic effects and is useful for reducing the risk of fatal and nonfatal thrombotic stroke.

Side Effects and Adverse Effects

The potential adverse effects of the various antiplatelet drugs can be serious. The most common ones are listed in Table 26-4.

Interactions

There are some potentially dangerous drug interactions that can occur with antiplatelet agents. Coadministration of ticlopidine with antacids results in its decreased absorption. Its use with digoxin causes the plasma levels of the digoxin to be decreased. Concurrent use with aspirin is not recommended. The concurrent use of both dipyridamole and aspirin produces additive antiplatelet activity. Aspirin, when given with NSAIDs, can potentiate bleeding. Also a patient who is allergic to aspirin may also be allergic to NSAIDs. When aspirin is given with oral antidiabetic agents, one can experience a loss of diabetic control. The combined use of steroids or NSAIDs with aspirin can increase the ulcerogenic effects of aspirin.

Ticlopidine can produce elevations in alkaline phosphatase activity, bilirubin level, and transaminase activity.

Dosages

For information on the dosages of selected antiplatelet agents, see the dosages table on p. 419.

see the dosages table on p. 419.

drug profiles

Antiplatelet drugs are extremely useful in the management of thromboembolic disorders. Each has unique pharmacologic properties that make them all somewhat different from one another.

∞ aspirin

Aspirin is available in many combinations with other prescription and nonprescription drugs and goes by many product names. It is classified as a pregnancy category D agent. Aspirin is contraindicated in patients with a known hypersensitivity to salicylates, those with asthma, those with

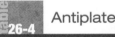

Antiplatelet Drugs: Adverse Effects

Table 26-4

Body System	Side/Adverse Effect
ASPIRIN	
Central nervous system	Stimulation, drowsiness, dizziness, confusion, flushing
Gastrointestinal	Nausea, vomiting, gastrointestinal bleeding, diarrhea, heartburn
Hematologic	Thrombocytopenia, agranulocytosis, leukopenia, neutropenia, hemolytic anemia, bleeding
CLOPIDOGREL	
Cardiovascular	Chest pain, hypertension
Central nervous system	Flu-like symptoms, headache, dizziness, fatigue
Gastrointestinal	Abdominal pain, dyspepsia, diarrhea, nausea
Miscellaneous	Skin disorders, edema, epistaxis, rash
PENTOXIFYLLINE	
Cardiovascular	Angina, dysrhythmias, palpitation, hypotension, chest pain, dyspnea
Central nervous system	Headache, anxiety, tremors, confusion, dizziness
Gastrointestinal	Nausea, vomiting, bloating, constipation, dry mouth, thirst, bad taste

gastrointestinal bleeding or bleeding disorders, children under 12 years of age or with flulike symptoms, lactating women, and patients with vitamin K deficiency or peptic ulcer disease. It is available orally and rectally. Orally it is available in many doses and dosage forms. It is available as chewing gum containing 227 mg per stick; tablets of numerous strengths: 324, 325, 500, and 650 mg; 75- and 81-mg chewable tablets; 165-, 324-, 325-, 500-, 650-, and 975-mg delayed-release tablets; 650- and 800-mg extended-release tablets; and 325- and 500-mg film-coated tablets. For commonly recommended dosages, see the dosages table below.

PHARMACOKINETICS

HALF-LIFE	ONSET	PEAK	DURATION
2-3 hr	15-30 min	0.25-2 hr	4-6 hr

clopidogrel

Clopidogrel (Plavix) and ticlopidine (Ticlid) are the only two ADP inhibitors on the market. They are potent antiplatelet agents. Ticlopidine is primarily used to reduce the risk of fatal and nonfatal thrombotic stroke in patients who have suffered either a completed thrombotic stroke or stroke precursors (e.g., transient ischemic attacks, reversible ischemic neurologic deficit, or minor stroke). Clopidogrel is indicated for the reduction of MI, stroke, vascular death in patients with atherosclerosis documented by recent stroke, or established peripheral arterial disease. They are also used after intracoronary stent implantation to reduce the risk of stent thrombosis.

Ticlopidine's use should be reserved for patients unable to tolerate aspirin therapy because of the life-threatening neutropenia and agranulocytosis that it can precipitate. Clopidogrel has not been shown to cause this side effect to the degree that ticlopidine has, and clopidogrel can be dosed once a day compared with ticlopidine, which must be dosed twice a day. Clopidogrel is classified as a pregnancy category B agent. It is contraindicated in patient with a known hypersensitivity to it and in those with active pathological bleeding such as peptic ulcer or intracranial hemorrhage. Clopidogrel is available as a 75-mg tablet. Recommended dosages are given in the dosages table below.

PHARMACOKINETICS

HALF-LIFE	ONSET	PEAK	DURATION
8 hr	1-2 hr*	1 hr*	7-10 days

*Onset and peak values can be reduced by giving a loading dose of 300-375 mg.

pentoxifylline

Two agents are currently approved for treatment of intermittent claudication caused by occlusive peripheral arterial disease: pentoxifylline (Trental) and cilostazol (Pletal). Pentoxifylline improves erythrocyte flexibility, microcirculatory flow, and tissue oxygenation concentration and reduces blood viscosity. Cilostazol is a phosphodiesterase III inhibitor that is supposed to improve capillary blood flow by increasing the deformability of erythrocytes and decrease blood viscosity.

Pentoxifylline and cilostazol are prescription-only medications. Pentoxifylline is contraindicated in patients with a known hypersensitivity to it or any methylxanthine. It is classified as a pregnancy category C agent and is only available orally as a 400-mg film-coated, extended-release tablet. For commonly recommended dosages see the dosages table below.

PHARMACOKINETICS

HALF-LIFE	ONSET	PEAK	DURATION
0.5-1 hr	Unknown	2-4 hr	Unknown

DOSAGES Selected Antiplatelet Agents

agent	pharmacologic class	dosage range	purpose
aspirin	Salicylate antiplatelet	*Adult* PO: 81-325 mg qd 325-1300 mg/day	MI prophylaxis TIA prophylaxis
clopidogrel (Plavix)	Antiplatelet	*Adult* PO: 75 mg qd; 300-375 mg may be given as a one-time loading dose after coronary stent implantation	Reduction of atherosclerotic events
pentoxifylline (Trental)	Antiplatelet/ hemorrheologic	*Adult* PO: 400 mg tid with meals	Claudication associated with peripheral arterial disease

MI, Myocardial infarction; *TIA*, transient ischemic attack.

ANTIFIBRINOLYTICS

The individual antifibrinolytic agents have varying mechanisms of action, but all prevent the lysis of fibrin, the substance that helps make the platelet plug insoluble and anchors the clot to the damaged blood vessel (see Figs. 26-1 and 26-2). The term **antifibrinolytic** refers to what these drugs do, which is to prevent the lysis of fibrin; in doing so, they promote clot formation. They have the opposite effects of anticoagulant and antiplatelet agents, which prevent clot formation. There are two synthetic antifibrinolytics, aminocaproic acid and tranexamic acid; one natural antifibrinolytic agent, aprotinin; and another antifibrinolytic with a different mechanism of action, desmopressin. Other drugs used to stop excessive bleeding are referred to as hemostatic agents, and these comprise thrombin, microfibrillar collagen, absorbable gelatin, and oxidized cellulose. These agents are not discussed here.

Mechanism of Action

Antifibrinolytics vary in several ways, depending on the particular agent. The various antifibrinolytic agents and their proposed mechanisms of action are described in Table 26-5.

Drug Effects

The drug effects of the antifibrinolytics are very specific and limited. They do not have many effects outside of their hematologic ones. Aminocaproic acid, tranexamic acid, and aprotinin prevent the breakdown of fibrin, which prevents the destruction of the formed platelet clot. Desmopressin increases the resorption of water by the collecting ducts in the kidneys, resulting in increased urine osmolality and a decreased urinary flow rate. It also causes a dose-dependent increase in the concentration of plasma factor VIII (von Willebrand factor) along with an increase in the plasma concentration of tissue plasminogen activator. The overall effect of this is increased platelet aggregation and clot formation.

Therapeutic Uses

Antifibrinolytics are useful in both the prevention and treatment of excessive bleeding resulting from systemic hyperfibrinolysis or surgical complications. They have also proved successful in arresting excessive oozing from surgical sites such as chest tubes, as well as in reducing the total blood loss and the duration of bleeding in the postoperative period.

Desmopressin's therapeutic effects exceed those of the antifibrinolytics. It can be given either intranasally or parenterally to prevent or control polydipsia, polyuria, and dehydration in patients with diabetes insipidus caused by a deficiency of endogenous posterior pituitary vasopressin and in patients with polyuria and polydipsia stemming from trauma or surgery in the pituitary region. It may also be used in patients who have hemophilia A or type I von Willebrand's disease. Desmopressin increases the levels of clotting factors in which these patients are deficient.

Side Effects and Adverse Effects

The adverse effects of antifibrinolytic drugs are infrequent and mild. There have been rare reports of these agents causing thrombotic events such as acute cerebrovascular thrombosis and acute MI. The common side effects of antifibrinolytics are listed in Table 26-6.

Interactions

The concurrent use of drugs such as estrogens or oral contraceptives with aminocaproic acid, tranexamic acid, and aprotinin may have an additive effect, resulting in increased coagulation. Few specific interactions have been reported for desmopressin, although it should be given cautiously in patients receiving lithium, large doses of epinephrine, demeclocycline, heparin, or alcohol because this may lead to a reduced antidiuretic response to the desmopressin. Drugs such as chlorpropamide and fludrocortisone may potentiate the antidiuretic response. The concurrent administration of clofibrate and desmopressin may prolong the antidiuretic effect of desmopressin.

Table 26-5 Antifibrinolytics: Mechanisms of Action

Antifibrinolytic Agent	Mechanism of Action
Synthetic agents: aminocaproic acid and tranexamic acid	Forms a reversible complex with plasminogen and plasmin. By binding to the lysine-binding site of plasminogen, it displaces plasminogen from the surface of fibrin. This prevents plasmin from lysing the fibrin clot. Therefore these drugs can only work if a clot has formed.
Natural agent: aprotinin	Inhibits the proteolytic enzymes trypsin, plasmin, and kallikrein, which lyse proteins that destroy fibrin clots. By inhibiting these enzymes, aprotinin prevents the degradation of the fibrin clot. It is also thought to inhibit the action of the complement system.
Other: desmopressin (DDAVP)	Works by increasing factor VIII (von Willebrand factor), which anchors platelets to damaged vessels via the glycoprotein Ib platelet receptor. It appears that desmopressin acts as a general endothelial stimulant, stimulating factor VIII, prostaglandin I_2, and plasminogen-activated release.

Dosages

For information on the dosages for aminocaproic acid and desmopressin, see the dosages table below.

---

drug profiles

Antifibrinolytics have a very limited use in preventing the lysis of fibrin, which promotes clot formation. The prototypical antifibrinolytic is aminocaproic acid. The effects of tranexamic acid and aprotinin are similar to those of aminocaproic acid, but desmopressin's effects are totally different from those of the other three agents.

aminocaproic acid

Aminocaproic acid (Amicar) is a synthetic antifibrinolytic agent used to prevent and control the excessive bleeding that can result from surgery or overactivity of the fibrinolytic system. Its use is contraindicated in patients who have had a hypersensitivity to it, as well as in the settings of postpartum bleeding, disseminated intravascular coagulation, upper urinary tract bleeding, and new burns. It is considered a pregnancy category C drug. It is available in both oral and parenteral preparations. Orally it is available as a 250-mg/ml syrup and a 500-mg tablet. Parenterally it is available as a 250-mg/ml injection for IV infusion. For commonly recommended dosages, see the dosages table below.

PHARMACOKINETICS

HALF-LIFE	ONSET	PEAK	DURATION
2 hr	Unknown	1.2 hr	<3 hr*

*For IV formulaion.

desmopressin

Desmopressin (DDAVP) is a synthetic polypeptide. It is structurally very similar to vasopressin, which is antidiuretic hormone, the natural human posterior pituitary hormone. Because of these physical characteristics, it is often used to increase the resorption of water by the collecting ducts in the kidneys to prevent or control polydipsia, polyuria, and dehydration in patients with diabetes insipidus caused by a deficiency of endogenous posterior pituitary vasopressin or in patients with polyuria and polydipsia resulting from trauma or surgery in the pituitary region.

Desmopressin also causes a dose-dependent increase in plasma factor VIII (von Willebrand factor) along with an increase in tissue plasminogen activator, resulting in increased platelet aggregation and clot formation. Desmopressin is classified as a pregnancy B agent and is contraindicated in patients with a known hypersensitivity to it and in those with nephrogenic diabetes insipidus. It is available as a 10-mg/0.1 ml intranasal solution and a 4-μg/ml parenteral injection. Desmopressin nasal spray is used for primary nocturnal enuresis. For commonly recommended dosages, see the dosages table below.

PHARMACOKINETICS

HALF-LIFE	ONSET	PEAK	DURATION
<2 hr	15-30 min	1.1-2 hr	Unknown

THROMBOLYTICS

Thrombolytics are coagulation modifiers that break down, or lyse, preformed clots (thrombi) in the blood vessels that supply the heart with blood, the coronary arteries. This reestablishes blood flow to the blood-starved heart muscle. If the blood flow is reestablished soon, the heart

Table 26-6 Antifibrinolytics: Adverse Effects

Body System	Side/Adverse Effects
Cardiovascular	Dysrhythmias, orthostatic hypotension, bradycardia
Central nervous system	Headache, dizziness, fatigue, hallucinations, psychosis, convulsions
Gastrointestinal	Nausea, vomiting, abdominal cramps, diarrhea

DOSAGES Selected Aminocaproic Acid and Desmopressin

agent	pharmacologic class	dosage range	purpose
aminocaproic acid (Amicar)	Hemostatic	*Adult* IV infusion: 4-5 g during first hour, then 1-1.25 g at 1-hr intervals up to a daily max of 30 g	Excessive bleeding caused by systemic hyperfibrinolysis or urinary fibrinolysis
desmopressin (DDAVP)	Synthetic posterior pituitary hormone	*Adult* IV: 0.3 μg/kg infused over 15-30 min. Preop use: agent is administered 30 min before surgery	Surgical and postop hemostasis and management of bleeding in patients with hemophilia A or type I von Willebrand's disease

muscle and left ventricular function can be saved. If blood flow is not reestablished early, the heart muscle becomes ischemic, then necrotic, and eventually nonfunctional.

Thrombolytic therapy made its debut in 1933 when a substance that would break down fibrin clots was isolated from a patient's blood. This substance was observed to be produced by a bacteria growing in the patient. The bacteria was found to be group A **beta-hemolytic streptococci,** and the substance was eventually called **streptokinase** (SK). SK was first used in a patient in 1947 to dissolve a clotted hemothorax, but it was not until 1958 when the first patient with an acute myocardial infarction (AMI) received it. In 1960 a naturally occurring human plasminogen activator called urokinase came available that was found to exert fibrinolytic effects on pulmonary emboli (clots in the lungs). However, the results of the early thrombolytic trials conducted during the 1960s and 1970s and made up of patients who had had an AMI were not taken seriously by the medical community. It was not until the 1980s, when DeWood and colleagues demonstrated that the underlying cause of AMIs was a coronary artery occlusion, that the use of thrombolytics for the early treatment of AMIs took off.

During the past decade, new thrombolytics have been developed and launched. Tissue plasminogen activator and **anisolated plasminogen streptokinase activator complex** (APSAC) are two of these agents. With the advent of these new thrombolytics came the performance of several large landmark thrombolytic research studies, which showed that early thrombolytic therapy could bring about a 50% reduction in mortality, a reduction in the infarct size, an improvement in left ventricular function, and a reduction in the incidence and severity of congestive heart failure. These findings and developments along with a better understanding of the pathogenesis of AMIs have led the way in the advancements made in the treatment of AMIs.

Mechanism of Action

There is a fine balance between the formation and dissolution of a clot. The coagulation system is responsible for clot formation, whereas the fibrinolytic system is responsible for dissolving the clot. The natural fibrinolytic system within blood takes days to break down a clot, and this is of little value in the case of a clotted blood vessel supplying blood to the heart muscle. Necrosis of the myocardium would not be prevented by these natural means, but thrombolytic therapy can activate the fibrinolytic system to break down the clot (thrombus) in the blood vessel quickly so that the delivery of blood to the heart muscle via the coronary arteries is quickly reestablished. This prevents myocardial tissue (heart muscle) and heart function from being destroyed. Thrombolytics accomplish this by activating the conversion of plasminogen to plasmin, which breaks down, or lyses, the thrombus (see Fig. 26-3). Plasmin is a proteolytic enzyme, which means that it breaks down proteins. It is a relatively nonspecific serine protease that is capable of degrading such proteins as fibrin, fibrinogen,

and other procoagulant proteins such as factors V, VIII, and XII. In other words, the substances that form clots are destroyed by plasmin. Essentially, these drugs work by mimicking the body's own process of clot destruction. Although the individual thrombolytic agents are somewhat diverse in their actions, they all have this common result.

SK binds with plasminogen to form an SK-plasminogen complex, which then acts on other plasminogen molecules to form plasmin. The plasmin formed then lyses the clots. SK is not **clot specific,** since it not only does it break down the thrombus in the coronary artery but it also breaks down clots anywhere in the body. It activates fibrinolysis throughout the body. Tissue plasminogen activator (t-PA) is a naturally occurring plasminogen activator secreted by vascular endothelial cells (the walls of blood vessels). However, the amount secreted naturally is not sufficient to dissolve a coronary thrombus quickly enough to restore circulation to the heart and save the heart muscle. t-PA is now made through recombinant DNA techniques and can thus be administered in quantities sufficient enough to dissolve a coronary thrombus quickly. It is fibrin specific and also clot specific, meaning that only the fibrin clot stimulates t-PA to convert plasminogen to plasmin. Therefore it does not induce a systemic lytic state. The APSAC is an SK-plasminogen complex that has been chemically modified by acylation, allowing a prolonged half-life. It, like SK, is not clot specific, so systemic fibrinolysis is induced with its use.

Drug Effects

The drug effects of the thrombolytics are primarily related to their action on the fibrinolytic system. They stimulate the fibrinolytic system to lyse preformed clots, and their action is limited solely to the fibrinolytic system.

Therapeutic Uses

The purpose of all the thrombolytic agents is to activate the conversion of plasminogen to plasmin, the enzyme that breaks down a thrombus. The presence of a thrombus that interferes significantly with normal blood flow on either the venous or the arterial side of the circulation is an indication for the use of thrombolytic therapy. An exception to this may be a thrombus that has formed in blood vessels that directly connects with the CNS. The indications for thrombolytic therapy include AMI, arterial thrombosis, DVT, occlusion of shunts or catheters, and PE. Its use for other thrombotic disorders is currently being evaluated.

Side Effects and Adverse Effects

The most frequent undesirable effect of thrombolytic therapy is internal, intracranial, and superficial bleeding. Other problems include hypersensitivity, anaphylactoid reactions, nausea, vomiting, and hypotension. These drugs can also induce dysrhythmias, and urokinase therapy has been associated with the development of a Guillain-Barré type syndrome.

Toxicity and Management of Overdose

Acute toxicity primarily causes an extension of the side effects of the thrombolytic agent, and treatment is symptomatic and supportive.

Interactions

The most common effect of drug interactions is an increased bleeding tendency resulting from the concurrent use of anticoagulants and antiplatelets or drugs that affect platelet function.

A laboratory test interaction that can occur with thrombolytic agents is a reduction in the plasminogen and fibrinogen levels.

Dosages

For information on the dosages for SK, alteplase, and urokinase, see the dosages table below.

drug profiles

All thrombolytic agents exert their effects by activating plasminogen and converting it to plasmin, which is capable of digesting **fibrinogen,** a major component of clots. The four thrombolytic agents currently approved for IV use in the management of AMIs are SK, APSAC, t-PA, and r-PA. The fifth thrombolytic agent available is urokinase. However, it is administered to lyse peripheral vascular thrombi and is seldom used to treat AMIs.

alteplase

Alteplase (Activase) is a naturally occurring t-PA secreted by vascular endothelial cells. The pharmaceutically available t-PA is made through recombinant DNA techniques, and modified mammalian hamster ovary cells produce the substance. It is clot (fibrin) specific, and thus it does not produce a systemic lytic state. In addition, because it is present in our bodies in a natural state, its administration for therapeutic use does not induce an antigen-antibody reaction. It can therefore be readministered immediately in the event of reinfarction. t-PA has a very short half-life of 5 minutes. It is believed to open the clogged artery faster, but its action is short-lived. Therefore it is given concomitantly with heparin to prevent reocclusion of the infarcted blood vessel.

The contraindications to alteplase use and its pregnancy rating are the same as those for SK. Alteplase is also only available parenterally as 20-, 50-, and 100-mg injections for IV infusion. For the

DOSAGES   Selected Thrombolytic Agents

agent	pharmacologic class	dosage range	purpose
alteplase (Activase; tissue plasminogen activator)	Thrombolytic enzyme	*Adult* IV: 100 mg over 90 min given as a 15-mg IV bolus, then 50 mg over 30 min, and then 35 mg over 60 min	Acute MI
		100 mg over 2 hr or 30-50 mg over 1.5-2 hr via pulmonary artery	Pulmonary embolism
		0.9 mg/kg (total dose not to exceed 90 mg); given as an IV bolus over 1 min	Acute ischemic stroke
streptokinase (Streptase, Kabikinase)	Thrombolytic enzyme	*Adult* IV: 1.5 million IU infused over 60 min or intracoronary infusion initiated with a bolus of 20,000 IU followed by 2000 IU/min for 1 hr	Acute MI
		IV: loading dose of 250,000 IU over 30 min followed by a maintenance infusion of 100,000 IU/hr for 24-72 hr	Deep vein thrombosis, arterial thrombosis and embolism, pulmonary embolism
		IV: 250,000 IU into each occluded limb of the cannula over 25-35 min and clamped for 2 hr followed by aspiration of the infusion cannula with saline and reconnection of the cannula	Arteriovenous cannula occlusion
urokinase (Abbokinase)	Thrombolytic enzyme	*Adult* IV: initial dose of 2000 IU/lb given over 100 min followed by a continuous infusion of 2000 IU/lb/hr for up to 12 hr	Pulmonary embolism
		Infuse into occluded artery at 6000 IU/min for up to 12 hr following an initial bolus dose of 2,5000-10,000 U of heparin	Coronary artery thrombi
		1 ml or 5000 IU for each catheter clearance	Occluded IV catheters
		0.9 mg/kg (total dose not to exceed 90 mg); given as an IV bolus over 1 minute (10% of total calculated dose) followed by an IV infusion of the remainder of total dose over next 60 minutes	Acute ischemic stroke

commonly recommended dosages, see the dosages table on p. 423. Pregnancy category C.

PHARMACOKINETICS

HALF-LIFE	ONSET	PEAK	DURATION
5 min	Unknown	Varies with dose	Unknown

streptokinase

SK (Streptase, Kabikinase) is the oldest thrombolytic agent, the one produced from beta-hemolytic streptococci. It binds with plasminogen, and this SK-plasminogen complex then acts on other plasminogen molecules to form plasmin. As pointed out previously, SK is not clot specific. Because it is made from a nonhuman source, it is antigenic and may provoke allergic reactions. This happens because the body's immune system recognizes it as a foreign substance (an antigen) and launches an antibody against it, resulting in an antigen-antibody reaction. These antibodies develop approximately 5 days after SK therapy and persist for 6 months to 1 year afterwards. It is therefore recommended that patients not be retreated with SK or APSAC during that time. Hypotension secondary to vasodilation occurs in approximately 10% to 15% of patients given SK.

SK is a pregnancy category C agent and is contraindicated in patients with a known hypersensitivity to it, as well as in the settings of active internal bleeding, an aneurysm, uncontrolled hypotension, an intracranial or intraspinal neoplasm, surgery, and trauma. It is only available parenterally in doses of 250,000, 750,000, and 1,500,000 IU per vial. For the commonly recommended dosages, see the dosages table on p. 423.

PHARMACOKINETICS

HALF-LIFE	ONSET	PEAK	DURATION
18 min, then 83 min	1 hr	Varies with dose	24-36 hr

urokinase

Human urokinase (Abbokinase) was the first t-PA. It was initially purified from human urine but in North America is currently prepared from transformed fetal renal parenchymal cells in tissue culture. Urokinase is occasionally used as a thrombolytic agent in the treatment of AMIs, but clinical experience with this use is considerably more limited than that with the other thrombolytics. It is primarily used for the treatment of pulmonary embolism and occluded IV catheters. Its contraindications are the same as those of the other thrombolytics, but it is a pregnancy category B agent. Urokinase is only available in a parenteral preparation and in doses of 250,000, 5000, and 9000 per vial for IV injection. Recent FDA warnings have limited

the use of urokinase products because of the risk of contamination. A synthetic formulation of urokinase has been in development and may replace the current urokinase product that is derived from fetal renal parenchymal cells. For now the current formulation is unavailable. For commonly recommended dosages, see the dosages table on p. 423.

PHARMACOKINETICS

HALF-LIFE	ONSET	PEAK	DURATION
10-20 min	Unknown	Unknown	<3 hr

nursing process

A variety of conditions warrant the use of coagulation modifiers. These conditions range from venous or arterial thromboembolism to vessel injury, and any of the coagulation modifiers such as heparin, warfarin, aspirin, dipyridamole, SK, and urokinase may be required for treatment. These agents with their different mechanisms of action and indications require some very specific nursing processes, and each is discussed under each category of coagulation modifier.

ANTICOAGULANTS

• Assessment

The nursing assessment of patients receiving the anticoagulants heparin or warfarin sodium is very important to the safe care of these patients with some very life-threatening conditions. It is important to obtain a medical and medication history on the patient as well as information on any hypersensitivity reactions to medications before initiating treatment with an anticoagulant. Contraindications to the use of these agents include any condition in which there is a risk of hemorrhage, such as severe hypertension, ulcer disease, ulcerative colitis, aneurysms, malignant hypertension, alcoholism, and head injuries. Women who are pregnant or breast feeding should also not be given warfarin sodium or indanedione derivatives. Extreme caution is necessary when heparin is used in patients undergoing major surgery or in patients receiving any other agents that may precipitate bleeding, agents such as those listed in Table 26-1. Patients with a history of congestive heart failure may also show an increased sensitivity to warfarin sodium and the indanedione derivatives. See also the Herbal Interactions boxes on ginko and ginseng, which can affect blood coagulation.

• Nursing Diagnoses

Nursing diagnoses that pertain to patients receiving anticoagulants include the following:
• Acute pain related to symptoms of underlying disorder or ischemia.

case study | Heparin Therapy

In the past 2 years, Mr. L.L., a 56-year-old attorney, has suffered three episodes of deep vein thrombosis. All occurred without complications and all were treated successfully with anticoagulant therapy and bed rest. He now presents to the urgent care center because of increased pain and swelling in his left calf that has lasted for the past 3 days. Initially he is given 5000 U of heparin. At admission to the hospital for anticoagulant therapy he is started on a continuous infusion of 25,000 U of heparin in 1000 ml of 0.9% sodium chloride.

- *What nursing actions should be implemented to ensure the accuracy and safety of the continuous heparin infusion?*
- *What patient findings would indicate a therapeutic response to the heparin therapy?*
- *If Mr. L.L. suddenly complains of numbness and tingling in his lower extremities with accompanying changes in muscle strength and sensation 12 hours after the initiation and continuation of heparin therapy, what would be the most appropriate nursing action(s) to implement?*

For Answers see www.harcourthealth.com/MERLIN/Lilley/.

- Deficient knowledge related to new medication regimen and need for altered lifestyle.
- Activity intolerance related to underlying tissue disorder or ischemia.
- Risk for injury (bruising or tissue injury) related to side effects of anticoagulants.
- Ineffective tissue perfusion related to underlying disorder or ischemia.

● Planning

Goals for the patient receiving anticoagulants include the following:
- Patient experiences increased comfort and relief of pain.
- Patient exhibits improved blood flow as the result of the therapeutic effects of the anticoagulants.
- Patient remains free from injury stemming from either the disease or the medication being taken.
- Patient is compliant with the lifestyle changes required and with the medication therapy.
- Patient demonstrates adequate knowledge regarding medication therapy and its potential side effects.

Outcome Criteria

Outcome criteria pertaining to the use of anticoagulants include the following:
- Patient will experience relief of symptoms such as decreased pain, swelling, and edema once tissue perfusion is regained as the result of medication therapy.
- Patient will show improved circulation with warm extremities or strong pedal pulses or experience a return to his or her predisease state of tissue perfusion.
- Patient will be free of bruising, bleeding problems, or any other adverse reaction to the medication.

herbal interactions

Ginko

BENEFIT OF HERB
Improves memory, sharpens concentration

POTENTIAL INTERACTIONS
May increase bleeding times with aspirin, dipyridamole, or warfarin

CAUTIONS AND NOTES
Contraindicated in patients taking blood thinners; adverse effects can include GI discomfort, dizziness, or headache

herbal interactions

Ginseng

BENEFIT OF HERB
Relieves stress and the effects of aging; increases energy

POTENTIAL INTERACTIONS
Can affect blood coagulation or platelet adhesion; can increase hypoglycemia with insulin use

CAUTIONS AND NOTES
Used cautiously in patients taking anticoagulants; may cause breast tenderness, headache, nervousness, or increased blood pressure

- Patient will state the rationale for the use of the medication regimen such as decreased clotting or clot formation.
- Patient will state the nature of and rationale for the lifestyle changes needed, such as improved diet, exercise, and no smoking.
- Patient will state side effects, how to monitor for complications of the anticoagulants, the importance of coming in for follow-up appointments with the physician and of frequent laboratory studies, and when to contact the physician so as to prevent complications such as hemorrhage.

● Implementation

Vital signs are routinely monitored in all patients initially taking an anticoagulant as well as during therapy. Various laboratory values should also be monitored in patients receiving an anticoagulant. Any change in pulse rate or rhythm, blood pressure, or level of consciousness, and the occurrence of unexplained restlessness are significant because they are possible indications of bleeding problems related to the anticoagulant. The physician should be notified immediately of the occurrence of any of these problems.

Safe and effective treatment with anticoagulants requires that the nurse have an adequate knowledge about the similarities of and differences between the various anticoagulants. Knowledge of the proper techniques of administration is also crucial for their safe use. For example, it is important to remember that heparin should only be given subcutaneously or intravenously, not intramuscularly. To prevent inadvertent IM injection during SC injection, a ⅝-inch (1.5 cm) needle should be used. Sites of injection include areas of deep subcutaneous fat such as the fatty layer of the abdomen 2 inches (5 cm) away from the umbilicus or the area near the iliac crest. Incisional areas or wounds should be avoided by at least 2 inches. See Box 26-1 for the procedure to follow for subcutaneous heparin administration.

When rapid anticoagulation is needed, the physician will generally order heparin to be given intravenously, either by continuous or intermittent infusion. During continuous IV heparin infusion, blood levels can be maintained and the effects can be easily reversed with the IV administration of protamine sulfate. The effects of SC heparin can also be reversed with protamine sulfate, but it often takes several doses to produce this effect because of the variable rates of absorption of the SC forms. See Box 26-2 for the procedure for the intermittent or continuous IV administration of heparin. LMWHs are presently used in high-risk patients (thromboembolic events). These new agents, such as enoxaparin, have a more predictable anticoagulant response.

When oral anticoagulants such as warfarin sodium and the indanedione derivatives are prescribed, therapy is often initiated with heparin until the prothrombin times indicate an adequate therapeutic response. This is necessary because the action of oral anticoagulants does not appear until about 12 to 24 hours after the first dose, by which time the normal removal of circulating clotting fac-

---

BOX 26-1 Subcutaneous Heparin Administration

- After thoroughly checking the physician's order, assess the patient for the existence of any allergies, contraindications, or cautions.
- Wash your hands thoroughly. Check the heparin bottle for the proper dilution of the agent, the expiration date, and the clarity of the solution. Using a tuberculin syringe, especially for small doses, draw up the exact dose of heparin. Always double-check with another registered nurse to make sure of the right dose. Replace the needle with a new sterile 5/8-in (1.5-cm), 26- to 28-gauge needle so that there is no residual on the needle and to ensure adequate sharpness of the needle for injection.
- Check the patient's identification band to make sure you have the correct patient.
- Put on disposable gloves and select the injection site outside a 2-in (5-cm) area around the umbilicus. Although the abdominal area or the area around the iliac crest is the preferred site of injection, any of the subcutaneous sites may be used. Always check where previous injections have been administered so that you can rotate the sites appropriately.
- Cleanse the site thoroughly with antiseptic but be careful not to massage or rub the site before or after the injection. Let the antiseptic dry before giving the injection.
- Grasp the subcutaneous tissue firmly so as to form a fat pad, then quickly insert the needle at a 90-degree angle. *Do not aspirate,* and be careful not to pinch the skin. Release the skin gently, and slowly inject the heparin. Count for 10 seconds, then withdraw the needle without changing its angle. Press a sterile 2 × 2-in (5 × 5 − cm) gauze pad or sponge over the area and maintain gentle but firm pressure for 10 sec. *Be careful not to massage, rub, or traumatize the skin.*
- Check the site for bleeding or bruising and document the site, time, dose, and any other pertinent information in the appropriate places in the patient's chart and/or medication record. Make sure your patient is comfortable, then remove your gloves and wash your hands.

BOX 26-2 Intravenous Heparin Administration

- For the continuous IV administration of heparin, an IV pump must be used to ensure a steady and precise rate of infusion.
- Always double-check the physician's order for the dose, rate, time, and route before initiating therapy. Generally, about a 6- to 12-hr supply is ordered.
- No other medication should be administered with the heparin or through the heparin line.
- For intermittent infusions, a heparin lock was used in years past. Now in most institutions, heparin locks are called *intermittent infusion locks* and they are generally flushed with normal saline. Some institutions still use heparin locks and administer 10 to 100 USP units of heparin per milliliter of a flushing solution.
- Intermittent infusions of heparin are usually ordered to be given every 4 to 6 hr because of heparin's short half-life. The drug should be infused slowly and given either undiluted or diluted with 50 to 100 ml of isotonic saline solution, though the latter practice is preferred.
- Guidelines for intermittent infusions include injection through the lock after cleansing the diaphragm with 70% alcohol and using a 25- to 27-gauge needle, which helps the diaphragm to reseal after repeated injections.
- Regardless of whether the injection is given through an IV pump or by intermittent or continuous IV infusion, it is crucial to always check the site to determine whether infiltration has occurred, so as to prevent a hematoma from forming there. Should this occur, the lock should be removed and replaced in a new site before the next scheduled infusion. Document your actions appropriately in the nurse's notes.

tors has occurred. The administration procedures for the oral anticoagulants are outlined in Box 26-3.

Patient education is a vital part of the nursing care plan for patients receiving anticoagulants. Not only do patients need to understand the reason why they are receiving anticoagulants, but they also need to understand the importance of laboratory testing to monitor the therapeutic, side, and toxic effects of these drugs.

Should uncontrolled bleeding occur, the nurse must institute emergency measures to stabilize the patient's condition. Laboratory values should be reported to the physician. The antidote to hemorrhage or uncontrolled bleeding resulting from heparin therapy is protamine sulfate and that to oral anticoagulant therapy is vitamin K, which can be administered intravenously, intramuscularly, or orally. However, this may precipate resistance to future use of the oral anticoagulant that may last for some time. Protamine may also be used to reverse effects of LMWHs.

Patient teaching tips for the anticoagulant agents are listed in the box on p. 430.

● Evaluation

Monitoring for the therapeutic and adverse effects of anticoagulants is crucial for their safe use. Adverse effects of heparin therapy include elevated blood pressure, headache, hematoma formation, irritation and pain at the injection site, hemorrhage, thrombocytopenia, shortness of breath, chills, and fever. Early signs of an overdose of anticoagulants include bleeding of the gums while brushing teeth, unexplained nosebleeds or bruising, and heavier-than-usual menstrual bleeding. Abdominal pain, back pain, bloody or tarry stools, bloody urine, constipation, blood in the sputum, severe or continuous headaches, and the vomiting of frank red blood or a

"coffee ground" substance (old blood) are all indications of internal bleeding. Warfarin sodium and the indanedione derivatives can also cause hair loss, rash, abdominal pain, diarrhea, nausea, vomiting, and leukopenia.

Therapeutic levels of anticoagulants can be monitored by laboratory tests. The standard tests for determining the effects of heparin therapy are the clotting times, and these consist of the Lee-White whole blood clotting time, the whole blood activated partial thromboplastin time (WBAPTT), and the APTT, the latter being the test most commonly used. A whole blood clotting time of 2½ to 3 times the control value indicates therapeutic levels have been reached. With IV heparin administrations, especially continuous IV infusions, coagulation studies should be performed every 4 hours. Prothrombin times are used to determine the dose of warfarin sodium. Prothrombin times are determined daily in patients just starting warfarin sodium therapy until a time of 1½ to 2½ times the normal control value is reached, which indicates a therapeutic effect. Once the level of the particular agent stabilizes, the times may be determined at 1- to 4-week intervals depending on the patient's response and physical condition.

Should a heparin overdose occur, the antidote is protamine sulfate, given intravenously over 1 to 3 minutes. Vitamin K, or phytonadione, is the antidote to oral anticoagulant overdose and can be given intramuscularly, subcutaneously, intravenously, or orally, depending on the patient's condition.

Because of the complexity and life-threatening nature of the conditions for which anticoagulants are used, the nurse must continually reassess and monitor the patient's response to the treatment and document the response accordingly. The continuous monitoring of the patient for the signs and symptoms of internal or external bleeding is crucial during both the initiation and maintenance of therapy.

Activity

ANTIPLATELET AGENTS

Another group of agents used to alter coagulation are the antiplatelet agents. Aspirin, dipyridamole, and ticlopidine are the most commonly used drugs in this category.

● Assessment

The nursing assessment of patients receiving any of these agents should begin with the taking of a medication and medical history. Specific contraindications to the use of these agents include hypersensitivity, hypotension, and pregnancy. Aspirin is contraindicated in patients with any bleeding disorder, in children younger than 16 years of age, in children with flulike symptoms, in pregnant or lactating women, and in patients with a vitamin K deficiency or peptic ulcer disease. Clopidogrel is contraindicated in patients with any active bleeding states, coagulation disorders, and liver disease. Cautious use with close monitoring is recommended with patients who are hypertensive, have renal or hepatic disease, and are about to have surgery.

BOX 26-3 Oral Anticoagulant Administration

- It is important to recheck the physician's orders and the patient's medication and medical history before administering the agent. Always check to make sure the patient has no known hypersensitivity to the agent.
- There are many more drugs that can interact with oral anticoagulants than with heparin, especially those that are highly protein bound such as the ones listed in Table 26-3. Always check the patient's medication list before initiating therapy with warfarin sodium or indanedione.
- The dose of the medication is calculated on the basis of the patient's clotting values.
- Oral anticoagulants should be administered at the same time every day to maintain steady blood levels.
- Document the dose, time of administration, and any other pertinent facts.

Drug interactions include warfarin, tamoxifen, tolbutamide, aspirin or aspirin-containing products, and some NSAIDs. Additive antiplatelet effects occur when these agents are coadministered with other aspirin products or with any of the nonsteroidal antiinflammatory agents (NSAIDs). Increased bleeding would occur in conjunction with the use of warfarin sodium. There are several drugs that interact with aspirin, and these are listed in Table 26-6.

Baseline vital signs also need to be determined in all patients. Lying and standing blood pressures are important to monitor because of the orthostatic hypotension these agents can precipitate. Before aspirin therapy is initiated, the patient's renal function, the complete blood count, hematocrit, hemoglobin level, and prothrombin time should all be assessed.

● Nursing Diagnoses

Nursing diagnoses relevant to the patient receiving antiplatelet agents include the following:
- Ineffective tissue perfusion related to the clotting disorder or thrombus formation.
- Impaired physical mobility related to tissue injury or decreased tissue perfusion from coagulation disorders.
- Risk for injury related to possible adverse reactions to antiplatelet therapy.
- Deficient knowledge related to medication treatment regimen due to lack of information.

● Planning

Goals for patients receiving antiplatelet agents include the following:
- Patient regains normal or near-normal tissue perfusion.
- Patient resumes normal daily activities.
- Patient remains free from injury related to medication therapy.
- Patient remains compliant with therapy.

Outcome Criteria

Outcome criteria pertaining to the patient receiving antiplatelet agents include the following:
- Patient will show signs of improved blood flow and tissue perfusion once therapy is initiated, such as improved distal pulses and color and temperature of distal areas.
- Patient will increase mobility gradually every day, as ordered, such as from walking to doorway to walking down hallway.
- Patient will protect self from skin injuries such as abrasions or bruising and avoid contact sports.
- Patient will take medication as prescribed and report any unusual side effects or adverse reactions such as bleeding, easy bruising, or palpitations to the physician immediately.

● Implementation

Safe and effective treatment with antiplatelet agents requires that the nurse have an adequate knowledge about these agents, including knowledge of the drug interactions that can occur and the life-style changes the patient must make. Dipyridamole should be taken on an empty stomach or either 1 hour before or 2 hours after meals so that maximal absorption can take place, whereas aspirin should be taken 30 minutes before or 2 hours after meals to minimize gastrointestinal upset. Patients taking either of these agents should quit smoking because of the vasoconstriction induced by the nicotine. It is important to remember that aspirin will interfere with the results of certain laboratory tests, such as coagulation studies, liver function tests, serum uric acid levels, and serum potassium and cholesterol levels. With clopidogrel, patients need to be aware of the signs and symptoms that need to be reported immediately to their health care provider, such as respiratory difficulty, back pain, skin rash, GI bleeding, bleeding disorders, diarrhea, acute severe headache, or change in vision (blurred vision or loss of vision).

● Evaluation

Monitoring for both the therapeutic and adverse effects of antiplatelet agents is crucial to their safe use. The therapeutic effects include decreased chest pain, dizziness and other neurologic symptoms, and platelet adhesion. Adverse effects of aspirin use include gastrointestinal upset or bleeding, heartburn, headache, hepatitis, thrombocytopenia, agranulocytosis, leukopenia, neutropenia, hemolytic anemia, prolonged prothrombin time, tinnitus, hearing loss, rapid pulse, wheezing, hypoglycemia, hyponatremia, and hypokalemia. Adverse effects of dipyridamole use include postural hypotension, headache, weakness, syncope, gastrointestinal upset, rash, flushing of the face, and dizziness. It is necessary to continually monitor liver, renal, and clotting function with laboratory studies in patients on long-term aspirin therapy. It is also critical to the safe care of patients receiving these medications that the nurse reassess and monitor the patient's response to the treatment and document the response accordingly. Continuous monitoring of the patient for signs of internal or external bleeding is of utmost importance both during the initiation of therapy and during ongoing therapy. Therapeutic effects of clopidogrel and ticlopidine include a decrease in the occurrence of clotting events such as TIAs and CVAs. Side effects for which to monitor with these agents include increased bleeding tendencies, flu-like symptoms, headache, fatigue, chest pain, and epistaxis.

ANTIFIBRINOLYTICS

● Assessment

Nursing assessment of patients receiving these agents should begin with the taking of medication and medical history. Baseline vital signs should also be obtained and recorded as well as blood clotting studies performed.

Drug interactions to assess for include concurrent use of oral contraceptives. Cautious use of desmopressin is recommended in patients receiving lithium, large doses of epinephrine, heparin, or alcohol. Aminocaproic acid is contraindicated in hypersensitivity, postpartum bleeding, disseminated intravascular coagulation, new burns, and upper urinary tract bleeding. Desmopressin is contraindicated in patients with hypersensitivity and nephrogenic diabetes insipidus.

● Nursing Diagnoses

Nursing diagnoses pertaining to the patient receiving antifibrinolytics include the following:
- Ineffective tissue perfusion related to excessive bleeding.
- Risk for injury or shock related to excessive bleeding.
- Risk for injury related to side effects of antifibrinolytics.

● Planning

Goals pertaining to patients receiving antifibrinolytics include the following:
- Patient maintains or regains normal to near normal tissue perfussion.
- Patient has improved hemostasis with drug therapy and supportive treatment.
- Patient experiences minimal adverse or toxic effects of antifibrinolytic agents.

Outcome Criteria

Outcome criteria pertaining to patients receiving antifibrinolytics include the following:
- Patient will experience increased strength of pulses and increased to normal skin temperature and color.
- Patient will exhibit a return to normal vital signs with improved blood pressure (120/80 mm Hg), pulse (>60 but <100 beats/min), and respiration (>16 but <20 respirations/min).
- Patient will be free of signs and symptoms of acute cerebrovascular thrombosis (cerebrovascular accident, or stroke) or acute MI.

● Implementation

Before administering intravenously, check the rate of infusion and dilutional factor for aminocaproic acid because infusion that is too rapid may result in bradycardia or hypotension. Desmopressin should be infused intravenously over 15 to 30 minutes for doses of 0.3 μg/kg. Intranasal dosage form should be administered exactly as ordered.

● Evaluation

Therapeutic effects of antifibrinolytics include arrest of oozing of blood from surgical site or decrease in blood loss. In addition, desmopressin may result in control or prevention of polyuria, polydypsia, and dehydration in patients with diabetes insipidus.

THROMBOLYTICS

Another group of agents used to alter clotting mechanisms are the enzymes used as thrombolytics. These agents are used in patients who are in very acute situations, such as those suffering acute MIs.

● Assessment

A nursing assessment should be performed before initiation of therapy. Possible drug interactions include concurrent use with anticoagulants and antiplatelet agents or any agent altering platelet function. Contraindications and cautions for the use of these drugs are similar to those in previous discussions on coagulation modifiers. However, thrombolytics are contraindicated with active internal bleeding, severe uncontrolled hypertension, and recent CVA. Baseline vital signs as well as related clotting laboratory studies (thrombin time, PT, APTT, Hct, and platelet counts) are also important to obtain and monitor.

● Nursing Diagnoses

Nursing diagnoses appropriate to the use of these agents are similar to the ones discussed in the previous sections on anticoagulants and antiplatelets.

● Planning

Goals and outcome criteria are also similar to the two previously discussed groups of coagulation modifiers.

● Implementation

Nursing considerations related to thrombolytics are similar for these agents. Specifically, their IV administration should be prepared per manufacturer guidelines and per protocol. IV sites should be monitored frequently for bleeding, redness, and pain. IM injections are also contraindicated with the use of these agents. Any bleeding from gums, mucus membranes, or occurrence of epistaxis and increased pulse (>100 beats/min) should be reported to the physician immediately. All vital signs should be monitored frequently as well. Other nursing considerations include monitoring for decreased blood pressure and restlessness, which should be reported to the physician immediately. Patients should be instructed to report pink, red, or cloudy urine; black, tarry stools or frank red blood in the stools; abdominal or chest pain; dizziness; or severe headache.

Reconstitution of IV streptokinase should be done slowly with 5 ml NaCl or D_5W. Roll gently and do not shake. Urokinase is reconstituted with sterile water for injection and then further diluted with 0.9% NaCl or D_5W.

● Evaluation

The therapeutic effects of thrombolytics include improved tissue perfusion, decreased chest pain, decreased leg pain, improved shunt performance, and prevention of further myocardial damage. Adverse effects to monitor for include hypersensitivity, nausea, vomiting, hypotension, dysrhythmias, excessive bleeding, and chest pain.

patient teaching tips

Coagulation Modifiers

Anticoagulants

➤ Patients should be told to report any abnormal bleeding that occurs, such as excessive bleeding from cuts or wounds or any unusual bleeding from anywhere on their body, or any of the symptoms of possible bleeding, such as severe headache; blurred vision; blood-tinged urine, emesis, or sputum; red or dark brown or dark black stools; dizziness; fever; muscular or limb weakness; rash; nose bleeds, or any excessive vaginal or menstrual bleeding.

➤ Patients should be encouraged to avoid having IM injections, brushing with a hard-bristled toothbrush, shaving with a straight razor, and engaging in any activity that would increase his or her risk of tissue injury. They should also avoid or be careful (as per physician's orders) shaving, trimming their nails, and gardening, and should avoid or be careful when participating in rough or contact sports.

➤ Patients should take oral medications only as directed.

➤ Tell patients not to make up for any missed doses and not to double-up on doses. Patients should call their physician if unsure what to do in the event of a missed dose.

➤ Tell patients to wear a MedicAlert bracelet or necklace and to carry a tag in their wallet naming the specific medication and their disorder.

➤ Patients should be encouraged to inform other physicians they are seeing and their dentist of the type of medication they are taking and why.

➤ Patients should know to contact their physician immediately should any bleeding occur that lasts more than 10 minutes after pressure has been applied to the site.

➤ Patients should be taught to avoid eating foods high in vitamin K, foods such as tomatoes, dark leafy vegetables, bananas, and fish.

➤ Patients should be instructed to avoid consuming alcohol.

➤ Patients should be instructed to check the labels of any OTC medications carefully to make sure it is okay to take them with an anticoagulant.

Antiplatelet Agents

➤ Patients taking aspirin or aspirin products should know to report any of the following symptoms to their physician: decrease in urine output; constant ringing of the ears; swelling of the feet, ankles, or legs; dark urine; clay-colored stools; abdominal pain; rash (discontinue use if rash occurs); and blurred vision or the perception of halos around objects.

➤ Make sure patients know to keep these products out of the reach of children.

➤ Patients should be told about not consuming alcohol or smoking.

➤ Patients should understand that these medications are not cures and often need to be taken long term.

➤ Patients should be told to avoid hazardous activities until they are stabilized on dipyridamole therapy because of the dizziness the drug can cause.

➤ Patients should report any unusual symptoms to their physician immediately.

➤ Patients should avoid taking ticlopidine with aspirin or dipyridamole, unless ordered to do so by the physician, because this can precipitate bleeding.

➤ Patients should avoid taking antacids with these medications or space the dosing of the two at least 2 hours apart. The concurrent use of digoxin and ticlopidine will result in decreased digitalis levels.

POINTS TO REMEMBER

Coagulation Modifiers

- Work by (1) preventing clot formation, (2) promoting clot formation, (3) lysing a preformed clot, or (4) reversing the action of anticoagulants.
- Anticoagulants, antiplatelet agents, antifibrinolytics, thrombolytics, and reversal agents are all examples.

Coagulation System

- Clot formation going on at same time as clot destruction.
- Clot destruction is governed by the fibrinolytic system.
- Clot formation is accomplished by the coagulation pathway, of which there is an extrinsic and an intrinsic pathway.
- The extrinsic pathway is initiated by blood vessels.
- The intrinsic pathway is initiated by blood cells.

warfarin (Coumadin)

- Prevents clot formation by inhibiting vitamin K-dependent clotting factors (II, VII, IX, and X).

- Used prophylactically to prevent clots from forming.
- Cannot lyse preformed clots.
- The degree of anticoagulation or "thinning of the blood" is monitored by the prothrombin time.

heparin

- Prevents clot formation by binding to antithrombin III and by doing so turns off certain activating factors.
- Overall effect is to turn off the coagulation pathway and prevent clots from forming.
- Cannot lyse or break down a clot.

Antiplatelet Agents

- Prevent clot formation by preventing platelet involvement in clot formation.
- Aspirin, dipyridamole, pentoxifylline, and ticlopidine all affect normal platelet function.

- Aspirin is the primary antiplatelet agent.
- At high doses works by inhibiting cyclooxygenase in platelets as well as blood vessels.

Antifibrinolytics

- Prevent lysis of fibrin, thus promoting clot formation.
- Have opposite effects of anticoagulants.
- Examples of agents include aminocaproic acid, tranexamic acid, aprotinin, and desmopressin.
- Work in opposition to anticoagulants, antiplatelets, and thrombolytics.
- Used to arrest oozing of blood from surgical sites such as chest tubes and to reduce total blood loss volume postoperatively.

Thrombolytics

- Anticoagulants that break down or lyse *preformed* clots in blood vessels that supply the heart with blood.
- Examples of agents include streptokinase (SK), urokinase, t–PA, and APSAC.

- SK derived from group A beta-hemolytic streptococci.
- Converts plasminogen to plasmin, which breaks down thrombi.
- Therapeutic effects include improved tissue perfusion, decreased chest pain, and prevention of further myocardial damage.
- Adverse effects include nausea, vomiting, and hypotension.

Nursing Considerations

- Therapeutic effects of most coagulation modifier agents include improved circulation, tissue perfusion, decreased pain, and prevention of further tissue damage.
- Before using any of these agents, it is important to perform a thorough physical assessment and record findings as well as monitor any pertinent laboratory values.
- Patients should be monitored for bleeding from all orifices as well as for easy bruising.

REVIEW QUESTIONS

1. Which of the following are the most frequent undesirable effects of thrombolytic treatment?
   a. Allergic reactions
   b. Nausea and vomiting
   c. Diaphoretic reactions
   d. Internal and even external bleeding
2. Which of the following is the antidote to an overdose of warfarin therapy?
   a. Vitamin C
   b. Vitamin K
   c. Protamine sulfate
   d. Potassium chloride
3. Which of the following reflect appropriate nursing interventions when administering heparin subcutaneously?
   a. Aspiration with injection
   b. Application of heat or cold to the site

   c. Use of a 5/8-inch needle that is 26-28 gauge
   d. Massaging of the site thoroughly after injection
4. Which of the following is the antidote to heparin?
   a. Vitamin C
   b. Vitamin K
   c. Protamine sulfate
   d. Potassium sulfate
5. Which of the following statements is correct about dipyridamole (Persantine)?
   a. It is used to reverse the effects of thrombolytic drugs.
   b. It has antiinflammatory effects that are useful with TIAs.
   c. It is often used as an adjunct to warfarin to prevent postoperative thromboembolic complications.
   d. It is usually indicated for reducing the risk of fatal strokes and decreasing any major complications.

For Answers see www.harcourthealth.com/MERLIN/Lilley/.

CRITICAL THINKING Activities

1. L.P. is a 69-year-old woman who has just had hip replacement surgery. Her orthopedic surgeon has prescribed 5000 U of subcutaneous heparin to be given twice a day for 7 days because she is at high risk for the development of a pulmonary embolism. The concentration of heparin for subcutaneous injections is 2500 U/ml, and it comes in a 10-ml vial. How many vials of subcutaneous heparin will be needed to complete L.P.'s 7-day course of therapy?

2. There are many side effects of the anticoagulant heparin. One of your patients has been on IV heparin for 72 hours. She is complaining of numbness and tingling of the extremities and fell when you got her out of bed, an activity she tolerated 6 hours before. What would your first action be and why? What would be some other data to collect on this patient at this time?
3. Explain the rationale for a patient to receive warfarin and heparin.

For Answers see www.harcourthealth.com/MERLIN/Lilley/.

bibliography

Albanese J, Nutz P: *Mosby's 2001 nursing drug reference and review cards,* St Louis, 2001, Mosby.

American Hospital Formulary Service: *AHFS drug information,* Bethesda, Md, 2000, American Society of Health-System Pharmacists.

Anderson PO, Knoben JE, Troutman WG: *Handbook of clinical drug data 1999-2000,* ed 9, New York, 1999, McGraw-Hill.

Johns Hopkins Hospital, Department of Pediatrics et al: *The Harriet Lane handbook,* ed 15, St Louis, 2000, Mosby.

Keen JH: *Critical care and emergency drug reference,* ed 3, St Louis, 1996, Mosby.

Medical Letter: Cilostazol for intermittent claudication 41(1052):44, May 7, 1999.

Medical Letter: Clopidogrel for reduction of atherosclerotic events 40(1028):59, June 5, 1998.

Mosby's GenRx: a comprehensive reference for generic and brand drugs, ed 10, St Louis, 2000, Mosby.

National Institute of Neurological Disorders and Stroke rt-PA Stroke Study Group: Tissue plasminogen activator for acute ischemic stroke, *N Engl J Med* 333(24):1581, 1995.

Skidmore-Roth L: *Mosby's 2001 nursing drug reference,* St Louis, 2001, Mosby.

Turkoski BB: *Drug information handbook for nursing 1999-2000: including assessment, administration, monitoring guidelines, and patient education,* ed 2, Cleveland, 1999, Lexi-Comp.

United States Pharmacopeial Convention: *USP DI: drug information for the health care professional,* vol. 1, ed 20, Englewood, Colo, 2000, Micromedex.

Remember to check the **Online Worksheet** for additional learning opportunities: **www.harcourthealth.com/MERLIN/Lilley/**

Chapter 27

Antilipemic Agents

When you reach the end of this chapter, you should be able to do the following:

1 Explain the nature of hyperlipidemia.

2 Discuss the different types of lipoproteins.

3 List the various antilipemic agents commonly used to treat hyperlipidemia.

4 Explain the rationale for antilipemic treatment and cite the dosages, side effects, cautions, contraindications, and drug interactions associated with the use of the various antilipemics.

5 Develop a nursing care plan that includes all phases of the nursing process for patients receiving antilipemics.

6 Cite the therapeutic responses produced by antilipemic agents.

www.harcourthealth.com/MERLIN/Lilley/

Look for this symbol for
topics covered in the
Online Worksheet

---

drug profiles

atorvastatin, p. 440	**fenofibrate**, p. 441
cholestyramine, p. 438	**gemfibrozil**, p. 441
colestipol	**niacin**, p. 442
hydrochloride, p. 438	**probucol**, p. 443

○── Key drug.

---

glossary

Antilipemic (an′ ti li pe′ mik) Drug that reduces lipid levels. (p. 433)

Apoproteins (ap′ o pro ten) A polypeptide chain not yet complexed to its specific prosthetic group. (p. 434)

Cholesterol (kə les′ tər ol) A fat-soluble crystalline steroid alcohol found in animal fats and oils and egg yolk and widely distributed in the body, especially in the bile, blood, brain tissue, liver, kidneys, adrenal glands, and myelin sheaths of nerve fibers. (p. 433)

Chylomicrons (ki′ lo mi′ kron) Minute droplets of lipoproteins. Chylomicrons consist of about 90% triglycerides and small amounts of cholesterol, phospholipids, and proteins. (p. 434)

Exogenous lipids (ek soj′ ə nəs / lip′ idz) Lipids originating outside the body or an organ or produced as the result of external causes, such as a disease caused by a bacterial or viral agent foreign to the body. (p. 434)

Foam cells The characteristic initial lesion of atherosclerosis, also known as the fatty streak. (p. 434)

HMG-CoA reductase inhibitors A class of cholesterol-lowering drugs that work by inhibiting the rate-limiting step in cholesterol synthesis. (p. 438)

Hypercholesterolemia (hi′ pər kə les tər ol e me ə) A condition in which greater-than-normal amounts of cholesterol are present in the blood. High levels of cholesterol and other lipids may lead to the development of atherosclerosis. (p. 434)

Lipoproteins (lip′ o pro tenz) Conjugated proteins in which lipids form an integral part of the molecule. They are synthesized primarily in the liver; contain varying amounts of triglycerides, cholesterol, phospholipids, and protein; and are classified according to their composition and density. (p. 433)

Statins A class of cholesterol-lowering drugs that are more formally known as *HMG-CoA reductase inhibitors.* (p. 438)

Triglycerides (tri glis′ ər id) A compound consisting of a fatty acid (oleic, palmitic, or stearic) and glycerol. Triglycerides make up most animal and vegetable fats and are the principal lipids in the blood, where they circulate bound to a protein, forming high- and low-density lipoproteins. (p. 433)

An understanding of **antilipemic** drugs begins with an understanding of how **cholesterol** and **triglycerides** are transported and used in the human body and how **lipoproteins,** apolipoproteins, receptors, and enzyme systems are involved in these processes. Also essential is an understanding of the basic mechanisms underlying lipid abnormalities and the link between hyperlipidemia and coronary heart disease (CHD). Armed with this knowledge, the clinician can develop and implement a rational approach to treatment using both nonpharmacologic and pharmacologic interventions.

LIPIDS AND LIPID ABNORMALITIES

PRIMARY FORMS OF LIPIDS

Triglycerides and cholesterol are the two primary forms of lipids in the blood. Triglycerides function as an energy source and are stored in adipose (fat) tissue. Cholesterol is primarily used to make steroid hormones, cell membranes, and bile acids. Triglycerides and cholesterol are both water-insoluble fats that must be bound to specialized lipid-carrying proteins called **apoproteins.** This combination of triglycerides and cholesterol with an apoprotein is referred to as a lipoprotein. Lipoproteins transport lipids via the blood. They are made up of a lipid core of triglycerides or cholesterol esters, or both, which is surrounded by a thin layer of phospholipids, apoproteins, and cholesterol. There are various types of lipoproteins, and they are classified according to their density and the type of apoproteins they contain. These various types of lipoproteins and their classification are listed in Table 27-1.

CHOLESTEROL HOMEOSTASIS

Fats are taken into the body through the diet and are broken down in the small intestine to form triglycerides. These triglycerides are in turn incorporated into chylomicrons, which are taken up into the lymphatic system. The primary purpose of **chylomicrons** is to transport lipids obtained from dietary sources **(exogenous lipids)** from the intestines to the liver to be used to make steroid hormones, peripheral cells, and bile acids.

The liver is the major organ where lipid metabolism occurs. The liver produces very-low-density lipoprotein (VLDL) from both endogenous and exogenous sources. The major role of VLDL is the transport of endogenous lipids to peripheral cells. Once VLDL is circulating, it is enzymatically cleaved by lipoprotein lipase and loses triglycerides. This creates intermediate-density lipoprotein (IDL), which is soon also cleaved by lipoprotein lipase, creating low-density lipoprotein (LDL). Cholesterol is almost all that is left in LDL after this process. Any tissues that require LDL, such as endocrine cells, possess LDL receptors. LDL and about half of IDL are returned to the liver by means of LDL receptors on the liver.

High-density lipoprotein (HDL) is produced in the liver and intestines and is also formed when chylomicrons are broken down. Lipids that are not used by peripheral cells are transferred as cholesterol esters to HDL. HDL then transfers the cholesterol esters to IDL to be returned to the liver. HDL is responsible for the "recycling" of cholesterol. HDL is sometimes referred to as the *good lipid* because it is believed to be cardioprotective.

If the liver has an excess amount of cholesterol, the number of LDL receptors on the liver decreases, resulting in an accumulation of LDL in the blood. One explanation for **hypercholesterolemia** (cholesterol in the blood) therefore is this down-regulation of hepatic LDL receptors. A major function of the liver is to manufacture cholesterol, a process that requires acetyl coenzyme A (CoA) reductase. Inhibition of this enzyme thus results in decreased cholesterol production by the liver. The entire process of cholesterol homeostasis is illustrated in Figure 27-1.

ATHEROSCLEROTIC PLAQUE FORMATION

Fundamental to the study of hyperlipidemia is an understanding of the processes by which lipids and lipoproteins participate in the formation of atherosclerotic plaque and subsequently the development of CHD. When the serum cholesterol levels are elevated, circulating monocytes adhere to the smooth endothelial surface of the coronary vasculature. These monocytes burrow into the next layer of the blood vessel (subendothelial tissue) and change into macrophage cells, which then take up cholesterol from circulating lipoproteins until they become filled with fat. Soon they become what are known as **foam cells,** the characteristic precursor lesion of atherosclerosis, also known as the *fatty streak.* Once this process is established, it is usually present throughout the coronary and systemic circulation.

LINK BETWEEN CHOLESTEROL AND CORONARY HEART DISEASE

Numerous epidemiologic trials have shown that as blood cholesterol levels increase in the members of a population, the incidence of death and disability related to CHD also increases. The risk of CHD in patients with cholesterol levels of 300 mg/dl is three to four times greater than that in patients with levels less than 200 mg/dl. The absolute incidence of CHD in premenopausal women and women on estrogen replacement therapy is approximately 25% less than that of men. This is thought to be secondary to the effects of estrogen, because the risk of CHD climbs considerably in postmenopausal women.

Table 27-1	Lipoprotein Classification	
Lipid Content	**Lipoprotein Classification**	**Protein Content**
Most ↑ Least	Chylomicron Very-low-density lipoprotein Low-density lipoprotein Intermediate-density lipoprotein High-density lipoprotein	Least ↓ **Most**

Statistics show that half of all Americans, both male and female, will die of a heart attack. Thus the thrust of treatment is two pronged: primary prevention of cardiac events in patients with risk factors, and secondary prevention of subsequent cardiac events in individuals who have previously suffered a cardiac event (e.g., myocardial infarction [MI]). The benefits of primary prevention as it refers to cholesterol reduction have been illustrated in a variety of recent trials. Some of the larger and more recent trials are the Lipid Research Clinics (LRC) Coronary Primary Prevention Trial, the Helsinki Heart Study, and the West of Scotland Coronary Prevention Study (WOS). The LRC trial used the drug cholestyramine, the Helsinki study used the drug gemfibrozil, and the WOS used the hydroxymethylglutaryl (HMG)–CoA reductase inhibitor pravastatin. These studies help reinforce the belief that in patients with known risk factors for CHD, drug therapy with an antilipemic agent can reduce the occurrence of CHD. First-time heart attack and death caused by heart disease can be reduced with drug therapy.

The benefits of secondary prevention as it refers to cholesterol reduction have been illustrated in a variety of recent trials as well. Some of the larger and more recent trials are the Cholesterol Lowering Atherosclerosis Study (CLAS), the Familial Atherosclerosis Treatment Study, and the Scandinavian Simvastatin Survival Study (4S trial). CLAS used the drugs colestipol and niacin, the Familial Atherosclerosis Treatment Study used the drugs niacin/colestipol and lovastatin/colestipol, and

the 4S trial used the drug simvastatin. These secondary prevention trials showed that in patients with documented CHD treatment with a cholesterol-lowering drug has many positive outcomes. Some of these are decreased coronary events, regression of coronary atherosclerotic lesions, and prolonged survival.

Measures taken early in a person's life to reduce and maintain cholesterol levels in a desirable range should have a dramatic effect in terms of preventing CHD and the death and disability it causes.

HYPERLIPIDEMIAS AND TREATMENT GUIDELINES

The decision to prescribe hyperlipemic drugs as an adjunct to diet therapy in patients with an elevated cholesterol level should be based on the patient's clinical profile. This includes the patient's age, sex, menopausal status (if the patient is a woman), family history, and response to dietary treatment, as well as the presence of risk factors (other than hyperlipidemia) for premature CHD and the cause, duration, and the phenotypic pattern of the patient's hyperlipidemia.

A major source of guidance for antilipemic treatment at the disposal of health care professionals in the United States has been the National Cholesterol Education Program (NCEP), which has been developed in close cooperation with other major professional organizations such as the American Heart Association. This program has two main thrusts, both aimed at reducing the total

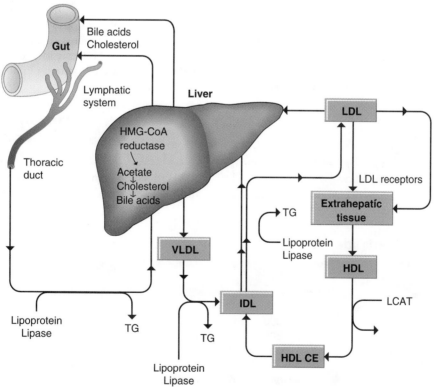

Fig. 27-1 Cholesterol homeostasis. *CE,* Cholesterol ester; *HDL,* high-density lipoprotein; *HMG–CoA,* hydroxymethylglutaryl-coenzyme A; *IDL,* intermediate-density lipoprotein; *LCAT,* lecithin cholesterol acetyltransferase; *LDL,* low-density lipoprotein; *TG,* triglyceride; *VLDL,* very-low-density lipoprotein.

risk of CHD in the population of the United States. One is focused on the entire population and consists of general guidelines for the prevention of CHD. It emphasizes the appropriate dietary intake of total cholesterol and saturated fat, weight control, physical activity, and the control of other lifestyle risk factors. The other aspect is focused on the management of individual patients who are at increased risk for CHD. The original guidelines for the detection, evaluation, and treatment of high serum cholesterol levels in adults were published in 1988, and revised guidelines were made available in June 1993. In these guidelines, the selection of diet and drug therapy options is determined by whether certain risk factors are present. These risk factors are listed in Box 27-1.

When the decision to institute drug therapy has been made, the choice of drug should then be determined by the specific lipid profile of the patient. There are four patterns of hyperlipidemia, and possibly a fifth, and these are determined by the nature of the plasma (serum) concentrations of total cholesterol and triglycerides. These various types of hyperlipidemias are listed in Table 27-2. The process of determining a patient's specific cholesterol profile is referred to as *phenotyping*.

One of the basic tenets of the NCEP guidelines is that all reasonable nonpharmaceutical means of controlling the blood cholesterol level (diet, exercise, and so on) should be tried and found to fail before drug therapy is considered. However, generally this means that diet modifications have been tried for at least 6 months and failed. Because the drug therapy for hyperlipidemias entails a long-term commitment to the therapy, factors that should be considered before the initiation of therapy should be the magnitude of hypercholesterolemia, the age and lifestyle of the patient, the relative contraindications to the first-choice drug, potential drug interactions, side effects, and the overall cost of therapy. The NCEP guidelines recommend that all patients with LDL cholesterol levels exceeding 190 mg/dl and those with LDL cholesterol levels between 160 and 190 mg/dl who have CHD or two or more risk factors be considered for drug therapy after an adequate trial of dietary and other nondrug therapies has proved ineffective. The treatment decisions that should be made based on the LDL cholesterol levels are listed in Table 27-3.

The major classes of drugs are the bile acid sequestrants (cholestyramine, colestipol), niacin, and the hepatic HMG-CoA reductase inhibitors (lovastatin, pravastatin, simvastatin, fluvastatin, atorvastatin, and cerivastatin). Other classes of drugs include fibric acid derivatives (gemfibrozil, clofibrate, and fenofibrate) and probucol.

Estrogen replacement therapy for postmenopausal women may also be considered. Ongoing studies are evaluating the use of estrogen in all patients at high risk for CHD regardless of sex or menopausal status.

BOX 27-1 High Blood Cholesterol: Risk Factors

POSITIVE RISK FACTORS

Age
   Male: ≥45 years
   Female: ≥55 years or women with premature menopause not on estrogen replacement therapy
Family history
   History of premature CHD (e.g., myocardial infarction or sudden death before 55 years of age in father or other male first-degree relative, or before 65 years of age in mother or other female first-degree relative.)
Current cigarette smoker
Hypertension: ≥140/90 mm Hg, or on antihypertensive medication
Low HDL cholesterol level: <35 mg/dl
Diabetes mellitus

NEGATIVE RISK FACTORS

High HDL cholesterol: ≥60 mg/dl—if the HDL cholesterol is ≥60 mg/dl, subtract one risk factor.

ANTILIPEMIC AGENTS

BILE ACID SEQUESTRANTS

Bile acid sequestrants, also called *bile acid–binding resins* and *ion-exchange resins*, are cholestyramine and colestipol.

TABLE 27-2 Types of Hyperlipidemias

| Phenotype | Lipoprotein Elevated | Lipid Composition | |
		Cholesterol (mg/dl)	Triglyceride
I	Chylomicrons	>300	>3000
IIa	LDL	>300	Normal ≅ 148
IIb	LDL, VLDL	>300	Normal ≅ 148
III	IDL	>400	>600 [1–3 × higher than cholesterol]
IV	VLDL	Normal or mildly elevated ≅ 250	>400
V	VLDL, chylomicrons	>300	>2000

LDL, Low-density lipoprotein; *VLDL*, very-low-density lipoprotein; *IDL*, intermediate-density lipoprotein.

Both these agents have been used widely for more than 20 years and have been evaluated extensively in well-controlled clinical trials. Generally these drugs lower the plasma concentrations of LDL cholesterol by 15% to 30%. They also increase the HDL cholesterol level by 3% to 8% and increase hepatic triglyceride and VLDL production, which may result in a 10% to 50% increase in the triglyceride level.

Mechanism of Action

Bile acid resins bind bile, preventing the resorption of the bile acids from the small intestine. Bile acids are necessary for the absorption and enterohepatic resorption of cholesterol. The hepatic synthesis of bile acids from cholesterol is stimulated by the depletion of the bile acid pool, resulting in a decreased pool of cholesterol in the liver. To compensate for this, both cholesterol biosynthesis and the number of high-affinity LDL receptors expressed on the liver's surface are increased, resulting in an increased rate of LDL catabolism (increased removal of LDL from the bloodstream). In this way, the bile acid sequestrants lower the plasma LDL levels by enhancing the efficiency of the receptor-mediated removal of LDL from plasma. The result of ion-exchange resin binding to bile acids is an insoluble resin–bile acid complex that is excreted by means of the feces.

Drug Effects

The fecal excretion of bile acids leads to a proportional breakdown of cholesterol into bile acids, which in turn lowers the serum cholesterol and LDL levels.

These drugs may also cause mild increases in the triglyceride levels and lower the absorption of fat-soluble vitamins.

Therapeutic Uses

Bile acid sequestrants are used as adjuncts in the management of type II hyperlipoproteinemia. In addition, cholestyramine is used to relieve the pruritus associated with partial biliary obstruction.

Side Effects and Adverse Effects

The adverse effects of colestipol and cholestyramine are similar; constipation is a frequent problem and may be accompanied by heartburn, nausea, belching, and bloating. These adverse effects tend to disappear over time, however. Many patients require extra education and support to help them deal with the gastrointestinal effects and comply with the medication regimen. It is important to initiate therapy with low doses and instruct patients to take the drugs with meals to reduce the side effects. Increasing the dietary fiber intake or taking a fiber supplement such as psyllium (Metamucil and others) as well as increasing fluid intake may relieve constipation and bloating. The most common side effects and adverse effects of the bile acid sequestrants are listed in Table 27-4.

Toxicity and Management of Overdose

Because the bile acid sequestrants are not absorbed, an overdose could cause obstruction of the gastrointestinal tract. Therefore treatment of an overdose involves restoring gut motility.

Interactions

The significant drug interactions associated with the use of bile acid sequestrants are limited to the absorption of concurrently administered drugs. All drugs should be taken at least 1 hour before or 4 to 6 hours after the administration of ion-exchange resins. In addition, high doses of a bile acid sequestrant will decrease the absorption of fat-soluble vitamins (A, D, E, and K).

Dosages

For dosage information on cholestyramine and colestipol hydrochloride, see the dosages table on p. 438.

Table 27-3	Treatment Decisions Based on LDL Cholesterol Level	
Patient Category	**Initiation Level**	**LDL Goal**
DIETARY THERAPY		
Without CHD and with fewer than two risk factors	≥160 mg/dl (4.1 mmol/L)	<160 mg/dl (4.1 mmol/L)
Without CHD and with two or more risk factors	≥130 mg/dl (3.4 mmol/L)	<130 mg/dl (3.4 mmol/L)
With CHD	≥100 mg/dl (2.6 mmol/L)	<100 mg/dl (2.6 mmol/L)
DRUG THERAPY		
Without CHD and with fewer than two risk factors	≥190 mg/dl (4.9 mmol/L)	<160 mg/dl (4.1 mmol/L)
Without CHD and with two or more risk factors	≥160 mg/dl (4.1 mmol/L)	<130 mg/dl (3.4 mmol/L)
With CHD	≥130 mg/dl (3.4 mmol/L)	<100 mg/dl (2.6 mmol/L)

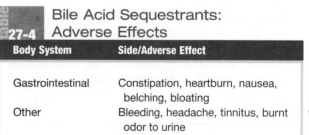

Table 27-4	Bile Acid Sequestrants: Adverse Effects
Body System	**Side/Adverse Effect**
Gastrointestinal	Constipation, heartburn, nausea, belching, bloating
Other	Bleeding, headache, tinnitus, burnt odor to urine

Activity

DOSAGES Selected Antilipemic Agents

agent	pharmacologic class	dosage range	purpose
atorvastatin (Lipitor)	HMG-CoA reductase inhibitors	*Adult* PO: 10-80 mg daily	Hyperlipidemia
cholestyramine (Questran)	Antilipemic ion-exchange resin	*Adult* PO: powder, 9 g 1-6 times/day	Hyperlipidemia
clofibrate (Atromid-S)	Fibric acid derivative	*Adult* PO: 2 g/day in four divided doses	Hyperlipidemia
colestipol hydrochloride (Colestid)	Antilipemic ion-exchange resin	*Adult* PO: granules, 5-30 g/day once or in divided doses; tablets 2-16 g/day	Hyperlipidemia
fenofibrate (Tricor)	Fibric acid derivative	*Adult* PO: 67 mg qd; max 201 mg daily	Hyperlipidemia
gemfibrozil (Lopid)	Fibric acid derivative	*Adult* PO: 600 mg bid 30 min ac in AM and PM	Hyperlipidemia
simvastatin (Zocor)	HMG-CoA reductase inhibitors	*Adult* PO: 10-80 mg daily	Hyperlipidemia

drug profiles

The bile acid sequestrants cholestyramine and colestipol are indicated for the treatment of type IIa and IIb hyperlipidemia. They lower the cholesterol level, in particular the LDL cholesterol level, by increasing the destruction of LDL. However, their use may result in increases in the VLDL cholesterol level. Because of the high incidence of gastrointestinal side effects in patients taking these agents, compliance with the prescribed dosage schedules is often poor. Therefore educating the patient to the purpose of therapy and expected side effects of the therapy and their treatment can foster improved compliance. Because of the pronounced drug interactions that can result from the concurrent administration of other drugs with bile acid sequestrants, patients must also be warned about this and the need to take these other drugs at other times of the day. The importance of patient education in the recipients of bile acid sequestrants cannot be overemphasized.

cholestyramine

Cholestyramine (Questran, Questran Light) is a prescription-only drug that is contraindicated in patients with a known hypersensitivity to it and in those suffering from complete biliary obstruction. It may interfere with the distribution of the proper amounts of fat-soluble vitamins to the fetus or nursing infant of pregnant or nursing women taking the agent. It is therefore classified as a pregnancy category C agent. The drug is only available orally as 4- and 9-g packets of powder to be taken as an oral suspension. The recommended dosages are given in the dosages table above.

colestipol hydrochloride

Colestipol hydrochloride (Colestid) is a prescription-only drug. It is contraindicated in patients who have shown a hypersensitivity reaction to it. It may interfere with the distribution of the proper amounts of fat-soluble vitamins to the fetus or nursing infant of pregnant or nursing women taking the agent. This drug is available in 5-g packets or bottles of 300 and 500. The recommended dosages of colestipol are given in the dosages table above. Pregnancy category B.

HMG–CoA REDUCTASE INHIBITORS

The specific competitive inhibitors of the rate-limiting enzyme in cholesterol synthesis, HMG–CoA reductase, are the most potent of the drugs available for reducing plasma concentrations of LDL cholesterol. Lovastatin was the first agent in this drug class to be approved for use, and this occurred in 1987. More recently, five other **HMG–CoA reductase inhibitors** have come available: pravastatin, simvastatin, atorvastatin, cerivastatin, and fluvastatin. The HMGs, or **statins** as they are sometimes called, are more effective than other types of antilipemic drugs in lowering the plasma concentrations of LDL and total cholesterol. The maximum extent to which these lipid levels are lowered does not occur until 6 to 8 weeks after the start of therapy. The findings from few direct comparisons of the HMGs have been published. However, the authors of the published account of one such study concluded that the following doses of agents would yield the same reduction in the LDL cholesterol level: simvastatin, 10 mg; pravastatin, 20 mg; and lovastatin, 20 mg. This particular study did not assess fluvastatin, atorvastatin, or cerivastatin. HMGs are primarily used in

Fluvastatin

It has been reported that maximal therapeutic effects associated with the use of fluvastatin (Lescol) usually occur in approximately 1 month. The adult dose is 20 mg taken in the evening. Because of drug interactions, especially with cimetidine (Tagamet), ranitidine (Zantac), and omeprazole (Prilosec), it is recommended that other medications be taken 2 hours after fluvastatin.

Table 27-5 HMG–CoA Reductase Inhibitors: Common Adverse Effects

Body System	Side/Adverse Effect
Central nervous system	Headache, dizziness, blurred vision, ophthalmoplegia, fatigue, nightmares, insomnia
Gastrointestinal	Constipation, cramps, diarrhea, nausea, changes in bowel function
Other	Myalgias, skin rashes

the treatment of type IIa and IIb hyperlipidemias and can be used in combination with gimfibrozil or niacin for type II hypercholesterolemia. However, the combination of HMGs with gemfibrozil or niacin increases the risk of myopathy.

Mechanism of Action

HMGs lower the blood cholesterol level by decreasing the rate of cholesterol production. The liver requires HMG–CoA reductase to produce cholesterol. It is the rate-limiting enzyme in the reactions needed to make cholesterol. The statins inhibit HMG–CoA reductase, thereby decreasing cholesterol production. When less cholesterol is produced, the liver increases the number of LDL receptors in order to augment the recycling of LDL from the circulation back into the liver, where it is needed for the synthesis of other needed substances such as steroids, bile acids, and cell membranes. Lovastatin and simvastatin are administered as inactive drugs or prodrugs that must be biotransformed into their active metabolites in the liver. In contrast, pravastatin is administered in its active form.

Therapeutic Uses

The HMG–CoA reductase inhibitors appear to be equally effective in their ability to reduce LDL cholesterol concentrations. However, simvastatin and atorvastatin are more potent on a milligram basis. Atorvastatin appears to be more effective in lowering triglycerides than other HMG–CoA reductase inhibitors. They are primarily indicated for the treatment of type IIa and IIb hyperlipidemias and have been shown to reduce the plasma concentrations of LDL cholesterol by 30% to 40%. Their cholesterol-lowering properties are dose dependent, in that the larger the dose, the greater the cholesterol-lowering effects. A 10% to 30% decrease in the concentrations of plasma triglycerides has been observed in patients receiving any of these drugs. Another very important therapeutic effect of the HMGs is an overall tendency for the HDL cholesterol level to increase by 2% to 15%.

Side Effects and Adverse Effects

The HMG–CoA reductase inhibitors available for clinical use have proved to be well tolerated, with significant side effects being fairly uncommon. Mild, transient gastrointestinal disturbances, rash, and headache have been the

most common problems. The common undesirable effects of the HMGs are listed in Table 27-5. Less common but still clinically important side effects include myopathy (muscle pain) and elevations in liver enzyme activity. The myopathy is uncommon (<0.1%) during monotherapy but appears to be dose dependent and is more common in patients receiving an HMG–CoA reductase inhibitor in combination with cyclosporin, niacin, genfibrozil, or erythromycin. The serum creatine phosphokinase concentrations may be increased by more than ten times the normal level in patients receiving these agents. Dose-dependent elevations in liver enzyme activity to values greater than three times the upper limit of normal have been noted in 0.4% to 1.9% of patients taking HMG–CoA reductase inhibitors. Most of these patients have remained asymptomatic, however.

Toxicity and Management of Overdose

Very limited data are available on the nature of toxicity and overdose in patients taking HMG–CoA reductase inhibitors. Treatment, if needed, is supportive.

Interactions

HMG–CoA reductase inhibitors should be used cautiously in patients taking oral anticoagulants. In addition, the coadministration of these drugs with erythromycin, gemfibrozil, or niacin has been observed to rarely lead to the development of rhabdomyolysis.

Laboratory interactions that can occur include increases in the SGOT levels and activated clotting time, thrombocytopenia, and transient eosinophilia.

Dosages

For dosage information on atorvastatin, see the following drug profile.

Activity

drug profiles

The HMG–CoA reductase inhibitors, or "statins," are all potent inhibitors of the enzyme that catalyzes the rate-limiting step in the synthesis of cholesterol. There are currently five statins: atorvastatin (Lipitor), fluvastatin (Lescol), lovastatin (Mevacor), pravastatin (Pravachol), and simvastatin (Zocor). There are some minor differences between agents in this class of antilipemics; the most dramatic difference is that of potency. All six agents are prescription-only drugs and are contraindicated in pregnant or lactating women and in those suffering from active liver dysfunction or with elevated serum transaminase levels of unknown cause. They are pregnancy category X agents. There is little evidence to recommend one agent over another.

atorvastatin

Atorvastatin (Lipitor) is one of the most frequently used agents in this class of cholesterol-lowering drugs. It is used primarily to lower total and LDL cholesterol as well as triglycerides. It is indicated for the treatment of type IIa and IIb hyperlipidemias. Atorvastatin has also been shown to raise good cholesterol, the HDL component. The recommended dosage for atorvastatin is 10 to 80 mg daily. It is a pregnancy category X agent.

PHARMACOKINETICS

HALF-LIFE	ONSET	PEAK	DURATION
14 hr	1-2 hr	2 wk*	Unknown

*Maximum therapeutic effect.

FIBRIC ACID DERIVATIVES

Until recently, clofibrate and gemfibrozil were the only two fibric acid antilipemics approved for clinical use in the United States. Fenofibrate has been added to this class of antilipemics. These agents primarily affect the triglyceride levels but may also lower the total cholesterol and LDL cholesterol levels and raise the HDL cholesterol level.

Mechanism of Action

Fibric acid agents are believed to work by activating lipoprotein lipase, an enzyme responsible for the breakdown of cholesterol. This enzyme usually cleaves off a triglyceride molecule from VLDL or LDL, leaving behind lipoproteins. Fibric acid derivatives can also suppress the release of free fatty acid from adipose tissue, inhibit the synthesis of triglycerides in the liver, and increase the secretion of cholesterol into bile.

Drug Effects

Fibric acid derivatives have been shown to reduce triglyceride levels. They have also been shown to reduce serum VLDL and LDL concentrations. Independent of their lipid-lowering actions, fibric acid derivatives can also induce changes in blood coagulation. This involves a tendency for them to decrease platelet adhesiveness. They can also increase plasma fibrinolysis, the process that causes fibrin and therefore clots to be broken down. Clofibrate has also been reported to increase the release of antidiuretic hormone from the posterior pituitary, to block

arginine-induced insulin and glucagon secretion by the pancreas, and to lower fasting blood glucose concentrations and serum insulin concentrations in patients with diabetes mellitus.

Therapeutic Uses

The fibric acid derivatives gemfibrozil, clofibrate, and fenofibrate all decrease the triglyceride levels and increase the HDL cholesterol level by as much as 25%. Both decrease the LDL concentrations in patients with type IIa and IIb hyperlipidemias but increase the LDL levels in patients with type IV and V hyperlipemias. They are indicated for the treatment of type III, IV, and V hyperlipidemias, and in some cases the type IIb form.

Side Effects and Adverse Effects

As a class, the most common adverse effects of the fibric acid derivatives are abdominal discomfort, diarrhea, nausea, headache, blurred vision, increased risk of gallstones, and prolonged prothrombin time. Liver function tests may also show increased function. The more common side effects and adverse effects are listed in Table 27-6.

Toxicity and Management of Overdose

Supportive therapy is called for in the management of an overdose of clofibrate. The pharmacokinetic data for clofibrate are very limited. The oral absorption of the drug is good, and its ability to bind to protein is high (>95%). It is excreted in the urine, primarily as metabolites.

The management of gemfibrozil overdose is also supportive. The drug is well absorbed, and the levels peak in 1 to 2 hours.

Interactions

Careful dosage adjustment of oral anticoagulants is necessary in patients also receiving clofibrate because clofibrate enhances their action. Furosemide can also displace clofibrate from inactive storage sites.

Gemfibrozil can also enhance the action of oral anticoagulants, thus also necessitating careful dose adjustments of these latter agents. When it is given in conjunction with an HMA–CoA reductase inhibitor, the risk of myositis, myalgias, and rhabdomyolysis is increased.

Laboratory test interactions that can occur in patients taking gemfibrozil include a decrease in the hemoglobin level, hematocrit value, and white blood cell count. In addition, the SGOT, activated clotting time (ACT), lactate dehydrogenase, and bilirubin levels can be increased. Clofibrate may increase SGOT (AST), SGPT (ALT), amylase, CPK, and LDH as well as decrease fibrinogen levels.

Dosages

For dosage information on gemfibrozil and fenofibrate, see the dosages table on p. 438.

Table 27-6 Fibric Acid Derivatives: Common Adverse Effects

Body System	Side/Adverse Effect
Gastrointestinal	Nausea, vomiting, diarrhea, gallstones, acute appendicitis
Genitourinary	Impotence, decreased urine output, hematuria, increased risk of urinary tract infections and viral infections
Other	Drowsiness, dizziness, rash, pruritus, alopecia, eczema, vertigo, headache

Table 27-7 Nicotinic Acid: Common Adverse Effects

Body System	Side/Adverse Effect
Gastrointestinal	Abdominal discomfort, gastrointestinal distress
Integumentary	Cutaneous flushing, pruritus, hyperpigmentation
Other	Blurred vision, glucose intolerance, hyperuricemia, rarely dry eyes, hepatotoxicity

drug profiles

The fibric acid derivatives gemfibrozil and fenofibrate are prescription-only drugs. They are both pregnancy category C agents and are contraindicated in the settings of hypersensitivity, preexisting gallbladder disease, significant hepatic or renal dysfunction, and primary biliary cirrhosis. Both agents decrease the triglyceride and increase the HDL levels by as much as 25%. They are good agents for the treatment of mixed hyperlipidemias.

fenofibrate

Fenofibrate (Tricor), a fibric acid derivative structurally similar to clofibrate (Atromid-S), has recently been approved by the FDA for treatment of hypertriglyceridemia. The standard tablet formulation has been available outside the United States for many years. The new micronized form is more rapidly and completely absorbed, especially when taken with food. It is more convenient to take than gemfibrozil and may have more favorable effects on LDL cholesterol; however, more direct comparisons are needed.

Fenofibrate is classified as a pregnancy category C agent and is contraindicated in patient with a known hypersensitivity to it. Fenofibrate is available as a 67-mg capsule. Recommended dosages are given in the dosages table on p. 438.

PHARMACOKINETICS

HALF-LIFE	ONSET	PEAK	DURATION
20 hr	Unknown	6-8 hr	Unknown

gemfibrozil

Gemfibrozil (Lopid) is a fibric acid derivative that decreases the synthesis of apolipoprotein B and lowers the VLDL level. It can also increase the HDL level. In addition, it is highly effective for lowering plasma triglyceride levels. In a very large trial, the Helsinki study, the triglyceride levels of the group receiving gemfibrozil were reduced by as much as 43% compared with the control group. The total cholesterol and LDL levels were reduced by 11% and 10%, respectively, and the high-density lipoprotein level was increased by 10%.

Gemfibrozil is indicated for the treatment of type IV and V hyperlipidemias and in some cases of the type IIb form. Gemfibrozil is only available orally as a 600-mg film-coated tablet. The specific dosing recommendations are given in the dosages table on p. 438. Pregnancy category C.

PHARMACOKINETICS

HALF-LIFE	ONSET	PEAK	DURATION
1.3-1.5 hr	Unknown	1-2 hr	Unknown

Activity

NIACIN

Niacin, or nicotinic acid, is not only a very unique lipid-lowering agent, it is also a vitamin. For its unique lipid-lowering properties to be realized, much larger doses of the agent are required than are commonly given when it is used as a vitamin. Niacin is a B vitamin, specifically vitamin B_3. It is an effective and inexpensive medication that exerts favorable effects on the plasma concentrations of all lipoproteins. Niacin is often given in combination with other antilipemic drugs to enhance the lipid-lowering effects.

Mechanism of Action

Although the exact mechanism of action of niacin is unknown, the beneficial effects are believed to be related to its ability to inhibit lipolysis in adipose tissue, decrease esterification of triglycerides in the liver, and increase the activity of lipoprotein lipase.

Drug Effects

The drug effects of are primarily limited to its ability to reduce the metabolism or catabolism of cholesterol and triglycerides. Niacin decreases the LDL levels moderately (10% to 20%), decreases the triglyceride levels (30% to 70%), and increases the HDL levels moderately (20% to 35%). Niacin is also a vitamin needed for many bodily processes. In large doses it may produce vasodilation that is limited to the cutaneous vessels. This effect seems to be induced by prostaglandins. Niacin also causes the release of histamine, resulting in an increase in gastric motility and acid secretion. Niacin may also stimulate the fibrinolytic system to break down fibrin clots.

Therapeutic Uses

Niacin has been shown to be effective in lowering lipid levels. This includes triglyceride, total serum cholesterol, and LDL cholesterol levels. It also brings about an increase in the HDL cholesterol levels. Niacin may also lower the lipoprotein (a) level, except in patients with severe hypertriglyceridemia. It has been shown to be effective in the treatment of types IIa, IIb, III, IV, and V hyperlipidemias.

Niacin's effects on triglyceride levels begin to be noticed after 1 to 4 days of therapy, with the decrease in the levels ranging from 20% to 80%. The decline in the LDL levels is less, with the maximum decrease ranging from 10% to 15%. The maximum effects of niacin are seen after 3 to 5 weeks of continuous therapy.

Side Effects and Adverse Effects

Niacin can cause flushing, pruritus, and gastrointestinal distress. Small doses of aspirin or nonsteroidal antiinflammatory drugs (NSAIDs) may be taken 30 minutes before niacin to minimize the cutaneous flushing. These undesirable effects can also be minimized by starting patients on a low initial dosage and increasing it gradually and having patients take the drug with meals. The most common side effects and adverse effects associated with niacin therapy are listed in Table 27-7.

Interactions

The major drug interactions associated with niacin are minimal. Niacin reportedly potentiates the hypotensive effects of ganglionic blockers (discussed in Chapter 23). In addition, when niacin is taken concomitantly with an HMG–CoA reductase inhibitor, the likelihood of myopathy developing is greatly increased.

Dosages

For dosage information on niacin, see the following drug profile for this agent.

drug profiles

niacin

Used alone or in combination with other lipid-lowering drugs, niacin (Nicobid, Slo-Niacin) is a very effective, inexpensive medication that, as previously mentioned, has beneficial effects on LDL cholesterol, triglyceride, and HDL cholesterol levels. Drug therapy with niacin is usually initiated at a small daily dose taken with or after meals to minimize the side effects previously discussed. Liver dysfunction has been observed in individu-

als taking sustained-release forms of niacin, not immediate-release forms.

Niacin is a pregnancy category C agent that is contraindicated in patients who have shown a hypersensitivity to it, in those with peptic ulcer, hepatic disease, hemorrhage, or severe hypotension, and in lactating women. Niacin is available over the counter (OTC) as well as by prescription. Niacin is only available orally as 25-, 50-, 100-, 250-, 500-, and 750-mg tablets and is commonly given in 2 to 4 divided doses of 1.5 to 6 g/day.

PHARMACOKINETICS

HALF-LIFE	ONSET	PEAK	DURATION
45 min	Unknown	30-70 min	Unknown

PROBUCOL

Three other drugs that can be considered in the treatment of selected patients with hypercholesterolemia are probucol, neomycin, and D-thyroxine. Of these three, only probucol is discussed here. Probucol (Lorelco) does not fit into any of the general categories of cholesterol-lowering agents. It is a synthetic lipophilic antioxidant that has been used as an antilipemic agent for almost 20 years. It is not frequently prescribed because it actually lowers the HDL level even more than it does the LDL level. The HDL level is lowered by as much as 30%, and the LDL level is often lowered by less than 10%; the total cholesterol level is lowered by 10% to 15%.

Mechanism of Action

The mechanism of action of probucol is uncertain, but it does not affect the production or degradation of LDL as many of the other antilipemic agents do. Instead it prevents unoxidized LDL from being oxidized and taken up by macrophages. By doing so, probucol prevents the formation of foam cells, which, as previously discussed, are the precursors of atheromas and atherosclerosis.

Drug Effects

The drug effects of probucol are limited to its ability to lower the cholesterol level, primarily the HDL and LDL levels. It has antioxidant properties as well. It may also affect the cardiac conduction system and cause prolongation of the QT interval, which is an occasional effect of membrane-stabilizing drugs such as the class I antidysrhythmics.

Therapeutic Uses

The therapeutic effects of probucol are cholesterol lowering. Probucol can decrease the LDL cholesterol level by approximately 8% to 15%, but unfortunately it also decreases the HDL cholesterol level by as much as 25%. The role of probucol in the management of hyperlipidemia remains controversial. It may be best considered a second-line drug in the treatment of primary types IIa and IIb hypercholesterolemias.

Side Effects and Adverse Effects

Probucol is generally well tolerated. The most common undesirable effects include abdominal pain, changes in bowel function, and nausea, but these occur in less than 8% of patients taking it. The drug should not be used in patients with an initially prolonged QT interval or in those with a history of ventricular dysrhythmias.

Interactions

Specific drug interaction information is unavailable. However, because antilipemic agents in general reduce or delay the absorption of other oral medications, probucol should be taken either 1 hour before or 4 to 6 hours after these agents.

Patients taking probucol have been found to have low hemoglobin and hematocrit values.

Dosages

For dosage information on probucol, see the following drug profile.

---

drug profiles

probucol

As of 1995, the antilipemic agent known as probucol (Lorelco) is no longer distributed in the United States. The product is still be available in other countries.

Probucol (Lorelco) is indicated for the treatment of type IIa and IIb hyperlipidemias and should probably be reserved for those patients who have failed to respond to other more effective antilipemic agents. Probucol has little if any effect on triglyceride levels. Probucol is a pregnancy category B agent that is contraindicated in patients with a known hypersensitivity to it. It should be used cautiously in patients with a history of dysrhythmias. It is available orally as 250- and 500-mg film-coated tablets. A common dosage is a 500-mg tablet given twice a day, once in the morning and once in the evening with meals.

PHARMACOKINETICS

HALF-LIFE	ONSET	PEAK	DURATION
2-3 mo*	5-11 days†	Unknown	25 days*

*Until serum cholesterol levels are back to baseline values.
†Until therapeutic effect.

---

nursing process

● Assessment

Before initiating antilipemic therapy in a patient, the nurse should obtain a thorough health and medication history, including the nature of any hypersensitivity reactions. The patient's dietary patterns; the exercise programs he or she is involved in; his or her weight, height, and vital signs; the nature of tobacco and alcohol use; and the patient's family history are important data to be used for developing a nursing care plan in patients receiving these medications.

Contraindications to the use of antilipemics include hypersensitivity to them, biliary obstruction, liver dysfunction, and active liver disease. Cautious use is indicated in children and in lactating or pregnant women. Some of the major drug interactions that can occur involve other antilipemics, insulin, oral antidiabetic agents, and oral anticoagulants.

● Nursing Diagnoses

Nursing diagnoses in the patient receiving an antilipemic agent include the following:
- Imbalanced nutrition, more than body requirements, related to poor dietary habits of high fat intake.
- Deficient knowledge related to an understanding of hyperlipidemia, the risks of CHD, and the need for lifestyle changes.
- Deficient knowledge related to an understanding of drug therapy and the therapeutic as opposed to the toxic effects.
- Ineffective therapeutic regimen management related to lack of experience with lifestyle changes and medication protocols.

● Planning

Goals for the patient receiving antilipemics include the following:
- Patient remains compliant with both nonpharmacologic and pharmacologic therapy.

---

research

Is the Rate of Procedures Linked to Outcomes?

According to a study conducted by Noraloo Roos and colleagues at the University of Manitoba, in some instances at least as many deaths could be prevented by decreasing an area's surgical rates to the US average as by improving the quality of technology and associated care with which procedures are performed. In a study of adverse outcomes associated with CABG surgery experienced by elderly residents of US cities in 1986, it was found that death rates were strongly associated with both the technical quality of the surgery and the surgical rate of the specific geographic area. The death rate per 1000 Medicare enrollees was 0.09 for the 30 cities (43.7 deaths or less per 1000 procedures) with the best technical quality as compared with a death rate of 0.23 per 1000 population in an area where the procedure was performed most frequently. The communities with the lowest surgical rates had about half the rates of adverse outcomes. ■

From Roos NP et al: A population-based approach to monitoring adverse outcomes of medical care, *Med Care* 33(2):127, 1995.

- Patient remains free of the complications associated with antilipemics because of appropriate use of the drug.
- Patient sees physician regularly and as indicated for the treatment of hyperlipidemia and to repeat laboratory studies.

Outcome Criteria

Outcome criteria related to the administration of antilipemics include the following:
- Patient will state importance of pharmacologic and nonpharmacologic therapy to his or her overall health and safety such as decreasing the risk of CHD.
- Patient will state the rationale of therapy as well as its side effects and expected therapeutic effects (i.e., decreasing lipid levels; gastrointestinal side effects; and therapeutic response of improved lipid profile).
- Patient will state those conditions that may arise of which the physician should be notified such as jaundice and abdominal pain.
- Patient will state importance of follow-up care with physician so as to monitor for changes in liver function studies as well as lipid levels.

● Implementation

Patients receiving any of these agents long term may require supplemental fat-soluble vitamins A, D, and K. Clofibrate often causes constipation, so patients need to increase fiber and fluid intake to offset this effect. Probucol, however, causes diarrhea. If either of these problems occurs and cannot be managed at home, the physician should be consulted. Niacin may result in pruritus and flushing, but these may be minimized by starting patients on decreased doses, with gradual increases in the dose as ordered by the physician. Nicotinic acid is better tolerated with meals.

Bile acid sequestrants such as cholestyramine and colestipol are in powder form and should be mixed thoroughly with food, fruit (e.g., crushed pineapple), or fluids (at least 2 ounces of fluid) before taking the mixture. The powder may not mix totally. Make sure that the patient is aware that it may not totally dissolve in the fluid and that more fluid may need to be added.

When mixing them with liquids, the powders need to be dissolved slowly, without stirring, for at least 1 minute because stirring causes the powder to clump. These medications must also be taken 1 hour before or 4 to 6 hours after other medications because of their ability to interact with other medications and food.

Many antilipemics take a while to reach effective levels and get at an effective dosage. For example, fenofibrate may be increased at 4- to 8-week intervals depending on the triglyceride levels but with a maximum dose of 201 mg. In addition, some of these agents should be taken with meals or at other times of the day. For example, it is recommended that fluvastatin, lovastatin, pravastatin, and simvastatin be taken once a day in the evening. These drugs are all HMG–CoA reductase inhibitors (also called *statins*). The bile acid sequestraints cholestyramine and colestipol should be taken before meals. The fibric acid derivatives, such as clofibrate and fenofibrate, and gemfibrozil are generally taken with meals or 30 minutes before throughout the morning and evening meals.

Patient teaching tips for these agents are below.

● Evaluation

Patients receiving an antilipemic agent need to be monitored for therapeutic and side effects during their therapy. The therapeutic effects of both nonpharmacologic and pharmacologic measures would be evidenced by a decrease to normal cholesterol and triglyceride levels. The nonpharmacologic measures include a low-fat, low-cholesterol diet; supervised, moderate exercise; weight loss; cessation of smoking or drinking; and relaxation therapy. If there is no response to pharmacologic therapy after about 3 months, then the medication is generally withdrawn. Tricor or fenofibrate may be increased at 4- to 8-week intervals depending on the triglyceride levels. Adverse effects for which to monitor include gastrointestinal upset, dyspepsia, increased liver enzyme levels, hepatomegaly, flatulence, weight gain, cholelithiasis, rash, fatigue, leukopenia, anemia, bleeding, dizziness, decreased libido, impotence, hematuria, myalgias, angina, and pulmonary emboli. Patients should also be closely monitored for the development of liver or renal dysfunction.

✒ patient teaching tips

Antilipemic Agents

➤ Patients should take these medications as ordered, and the dosing should not be changed without the physician's approval.

➤ Patients should not stop taking the medication without the physician's approval.

➤ Patients must be counseled concerning diet and nutrition. This is an important part of antilipemic therapy.

➤ Patients should be told they must take powder forms with a liquid. These should be mixed thoroughly but not stirred!

➤ Other medications should be taken 1 hour before or 4 to 6 hours after antilipemics because they can interfere with the absorption of antilipemics.

➤ The patient should notify the physician of the occurrence of any new or troublesome symptoms or of persistent gastrointestinal upset, constipation, gas, bloating, heartburn, nausea, vomiting, abnormal or unusual bleeding, and yellow discoloration of the skin. Other symptoms to report include decreased sex drive, impotence, and difficulty urinating.

➤ These medications, as with all medications, should be kept out of the reach of children.

➤ Patients should eat lots of raw vegetables, fruit, and bran and drink at least 2 quarts (2 liters) of fluids a day to prevent the constipation associated with anti-lipemic use.

➤ It has been observed that high-fiber foods also bring about a decrease in cholesterol levels, so this is an added benefit of the high-fiber foods consumed to prevent constipation.

➤ Women receiving these agents should check with their physician about the possible interaction with oral birth control pills, should they be taking them.

➤ Taking these medications with meals will help decrease any associated gastrointestinal upset.

➤ Patients should eat less animal fat and red meat while taking these medications if their cholesterol levels are high.

➤ Patients should engage in moderate daily exercise, but only with their physician's approval.

➤ If a once-a-day dosage scheme is chosen, the medications should be taken at night with the evening meal.

POINTS TO REMEMBER

Lipids

• Two primary forms of lipids are triglycerides and cholesterol.
• Triglycerides function as an energy source and are stored in adipose (fat) tissue.
• Cholesterol is primarily used to make steroid hormones, cell membranes, and bile acids.
• Lipoproteins transport lipids via the blood.

Link between Cholesterol and CHD

• Lipids and lipoproteins participate in the formation of atherosclerotic plaques, which leads to CHD.
• Lipids or plaque form in the blood vessels that supply the heart with needed oxygen and nutrients.
• They eventually decrease the lumen size of these blood vessels, reducing the amounts of these substances that can reach the heart

Antilipemics

• Drugs used to lower high levels of lipid (triglycerides and cholesterol).
• Major classes of antilipemics: (1) bile acid sequestrants, (2) fibric acid derivatives, and (3) HMG–CoA reductase inhibitors.
• The mechanism of action differs for each agent.

HMG–CoA Reductase Inhibitors

• Lower blood cholesterol level by decreasing the rate of cholesterol production.
• Inhibit the enzyme necessary for the liver to produce cholesterol.
• Have very few side effects.
• Six agents: lovastatin, pravastatin, simvastatin, fluvastatin, atorvastatin, and cerivastatin

Nursing Considerations

• Contraindications to the use of antilipemics include hypersensitivity, biliary obstruction, liver dysfunction, and active liver disease.
• While taking a nursing history it is important to find out whether the patient is taking drugs that interact with antilipemics, such as insulin, oral antidiabetic agents, or oral anticoagulants.
• Fat-soluble vitamins may need to be prescribed for patients taking these medications long term.
• Powder or granules must be mixed with noncarbonated liquid and *never* taken dry.
• Monitoring for side effects as well as liver and renal function is important.

REVIEW QUESTIONS

1. Cholestyramine is most likely to be effective in the treatment of which of the following?
   a. Mixed hyperlipidemias
   b. All types of hyperlipidemias
   c. Type IV and V hyperlipidemias
   d. Type IIa and Type IIb hyperlipidemias
2. Side effects of nicotinic acid may often be decreased if the patient:
   a. Takes it on an empty stomach.
   b. Makes sure to take it before breakfast each morning.
   c. Titrates the dose upward and takes only with water at night.

   d. Takes the medication with meals and with a low initial dose.
3. Which of the following are important to emphasize to a patient about his or her antilipemic medication?
   a. Take several hours before meals.
   b. Eating extra servings of fruit and vegetables may help prevent constipation.
   c. The drug should be used only as tolerated even if the dose is every other day.
   d. The drug should be taken with a double dose of Metamucil to prevent constipation.

4. Which of the following is associated with antilipemic medications?
   a. Diabetes insipidus
   b. Pulmonary fibrosis
   c. Liver malfunctioning
   d. Fatty deposits in the skin

5. Side effects of antilipemics include all of the following except:
   a. GI upset.
   b. Dizziness.
   c. Skin rashes.
   d. Constipation.

For Answers see www.harcourthealth.com/MERLIN/Lilley/.

CRITICAL THINKING Activities

1. Flushing of the face and neck may occur with the administration of nicotinic acid. What would you suggest to a patient to help decrease these reactions and their unpleasantness?
2. Is the following statement true or false? Explain your answer. *Antilipemics may be safely taken without con-* *cern of other medications, especially prescribed medications, and may be discontinued abruptly.*
3. Your patient has just informed you that he was told that it was okay to take his colestipol powder without fluids. Are you concerned about this? Explain your answer.

For Answers see www.harcourthealth.com/MERLIN/Lilley/.

bibliography

Albanese J, Nutz P: *Mosby's 2001 nursing drug reference and review cards,* St Louis, 2001, Mosby.

American Hospital Formulary Service: *AHFS drug information,* Bethesda, Md, 2000, American Society of Health-System Pharmacists.

Anderson PO, Knoben JE, Troutman WG: *Handbook of clinical drug data 1999-2000,* ed 9, New York, 1999, McGraw-Hill.

Atorvastin: a new lipid-lowering drug, *Med Lett Drugs Ther* 39(997): 29, 1997.

Choice of lipid-lowering drugs, *Med Lett Drugs Ther* 38(980):67, 1996.

Johns Hopkins Hospital, Department of Pediatrics et al: *The Harriet Lane handbook,* ed 15, St Louis, 2000, Mosby.

Keen JH: *Critical care and emergency drug reference,* ed 3, St Louis, 1996, Mosby.

Medical Letter: Cerivastatin for hypercholesterolemia 40(1018):13, January 16, 1998.

Medical Letter: Choice of lipid-lowering drugs 40(1042):117, December 18, 1998.

Medical Letter: Fenofibrate for hypertriglyceridemia 40(1030):68, July 3, 1998.

Mosby's GenRx: a comprehensive reference for generic and brand drugs, ed 10, St Louis, 2000, Mosby.

Skidmore-Roth L: *Mosby's 2001 nursing drug reference,* St Louis, 2001, Mosby.

Turkoski BB: *Drug information handbook for nursing 1999-2000: including assessment, administration, monitoring guidelines, and patient education,* ed 2, Cleveland, 1999, Lexi-Comp.

United States Pharmacopeial Convention: *USP DI: advice for the patient: drug information in lay language,* vol. 1I, ed 20, Englewood, Colo, 2000a, Micromedex.

United States Pharmacopeial Convention: *USP DI: drug information for the health care professional,* vol. 1, ed 20, Englewood, Colo, 2000b, Micromedex.

West of Scotland Coronary Prevention Study Group: Prevention of coronary heart disease with pravastatin in men with hypercholesterolemia, *N Engl J Med* 333:1301, 1995.

Activity

Remember to check the **Online Worksheet** for additional learning opportunities: **www.harcourthealth.com/MERLIN/Lilley/**

Part five

Drugs Affecting the Endocrine System: Study Skills Tips

- Questioning Strategy

QUESTIONING STRATEGY

One of the most important activities for learning is to become actively involved with the text. The best way to achieve this involvement is to develop the habit of asking questions. These questions can be generated using a number of different cues and structures that are part of the part and chapter structure. Some of what you anticipate as related material will not be correct. You will adjust your expectations as you read the material. For now focus on asking a lot of questions and making use of everything you know, which can help start the process of answering your questions.

Part Title

As you begin each new part, ask a question to focus your attention. What do all the chapters in this part have in common? In Part Five this question is: "What is the endocrine system?" This same question could be asked of Parts Two through Nine by simply replacing "endocrine" with the appropriate system for the specific part. Looking at the chapter titles in the part tells us that the endocrine system has to do with the pituitary agents, thyroid and antithyroid agents, antidiabetic and hypoglycemic agents, adrenal agents, women's health agents, and male reproductive agents. Although this answer is far too general to demonstrate any real understanding of the endocrine system, it is a beginning and helps keep you aware of what you need to learn from each chapter.

Chapter Titles

Chapter titles provide the first mechanism that can be used to generate questions. The first question to ask

about each chapter is a very basic one. What is this chapter about? That question is also answered immediately. "What is Chapter 28 about?" It is about pituitary agents.

The next question is equally obvious but also extremely important. The question to ask next is: "To what do pituitary (Chapter 28), thyroid and antithyroid (Chapter 29), antidiabetic and hypoglycemic (Chapter 30), adrenal (Chapter 31), women's health (Chapter 32), and men's health (Chapter 33) refer?" Take the chapter title and state it as a question. What do you know about these subjects?

Chapter Objectives

To enhance your study, turn each chapter objective into one or more questions. Here are some possible questions using the objectives from Chapter 30.

Objective 1
Discuss the normal actions and functions of the pancreas and the feedback system that regulates it.
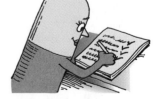
- What are the normal actions and functions of the pancreas?
- What is the feedback system for the pancreas?

Objective 2
Describe the differences between the hyposecretion and hypersecretion of insulin and the difference between Type 1 and Type 2 diabetes mellitus.
- What does *hypo-* mean?

- What does *hyper-* mean?
- What is hypersecretion of insulin?
- What is hyposecretion of insulin?
- What are the differences between hyposecretion and hypersecretion?

Since the objectives tell you what the authors expected you to know at the end of the chapter, starting out with questions based on the objectives will improve your learning and probably save you time.

Chapter Headings

The same principle can be applied to each of the topic headings set out in the chapter. Continuing to use Chapter 30 as a model, here are some samples of questions that might be useful as preparation for reading.

Type 1 Diabetes Mellitus

- What is Type 1 diabetes?
- What is mellitus?

As you start to process the chapter headings, you should also notice that they begin to answer some of the questions from the chapter objectives. This is a good time to begin setting up vocabulary cards.

Mechanism of Action

- What is the mechanism of action in Type 1 diabetes mellitus?
- Is there more than one mechanism?

Drug Effects

- What are the most important drug effects in Type 1 diabetes mellitus?
- Where do these effects take place?
- What is the evidence of these effects?

The idea is to focus on the major content of the chapter, and establish a guide for learning as you read.

Print Conventions Within the Body of the Chapter

Print conventions are useful in this study skills strategy. The use of *italics*, **bold**, <u>underlining</u>, and multiple colors of ink are examples of print conventions. They are designed to catch your attention. Use them as a basis for questions.

Chapter 30

In the first paragraph of this chapter the first obvious print convention is the word **glucose.** It is printed in bold. If you let your eyes float down the page and do not read anything, this word stands out. It must be important.

- What is glucose?
- What is the relationship between glucose and Type 1 diabetes mellitus?

There are more words on the first page of the chapter text that are in the same print style. Apply the same procedure to these terms. Also, notice that two of the terms, glycogen and glycogenolysis, must have some direct relationship, since the second term contains the first word. The basic question in each case is, "What does the term mean?" However, there should be more to your questions than just the basics. Glycogenolysis seems to mean that there is some operation or activity taking place. Ask yourself the following:

- What happens in glycogenolysis?
- Where does glycogenolysis occur?
- When does glycogenolysis occur?
- How does it relate to Type 1 diabetes mellitus?

Chapter Tables

Tables serve as a summary of information discussed in the chapter. You can learn a great deal from tables if you take the time.

Look at Table 30-1. The table summarizes characteristics of Type 1 and Type 2 diabetes. There are two obvious questions for each type.

- What is Type 1 (Type 2) diabetes?
- What are its characteristics?

Use these questions to study Table 30-1 and you will find that all the information you need to respond to these questions is found here. It may be useful to make a first pass throughout the chapter focusing only on the tables before you begin to read. You will learn a great deal about some of the topics, and you will have established background information that will help you ask better questions and read with better understanding.

The time you spend asking questions makes the reading and learning go more quickly. Another benefit is that some of the questions you ask appear on tests. These

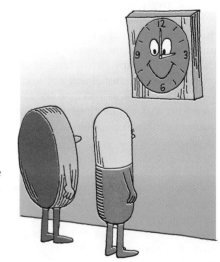

questions will be easy for you to answer. This promotes test-taking confidence, and better scores result in better grades. If you have not been using questioning strategy up to this point in your text, begin now. After you use the strategy for two or three chapters, you will find that the benefits far outweigh the time it takes.

Chapter 28

Pituitary Agents

www.harcourthealth.com/MERLIN/Lilley/

objectives

When you reach the end of this chapter, you should be able to do the following:

1 Describe the normal function of the anterior and posterior aspects of the pituitary gland.

2 Identify the various pituitary agents.

3 Discuss the mechanisms of action, indications, side effects, and contraindications related to pituitary agents.

4 Develop a nursing care plan that includes all phases of the nursing process for patients receiving pituitary agents.

Look for this symbol for topics covered in the **Online Worksheet**

---

drug profiles

corticotropin, p. 453
☞ **desmopressin,** p. 453
lypressin, p. 453
☞ **octreotide,** p. 453

somatropin and somatrem, p. 453
☞ **vasopressin,** p. 454

☞Key drug.

---

glossary

Negative feedback A way in which hormone secretion is regulated that involves a decrease in function in response to a stimulus. (p. 450)

Neuroendocrine system (nur o en′ də krən) The system that regulates the reactions of the organism to both internal and external stimuli and involves the integrated activities of the endocrine glands and nervous system. (p. 449)

Pituitary gland (pi too′ i tar′ e) An endocrine gland suspended beneath the brain that supplies numerous hormones that control many vital processes. (p. 449)

ENDOCRINE SYSTEM

The maintenance of physiologic stability is the main goal of the endocrine system, and it must accomplish this task despite constant changes in the internal and external environments. Every cell, and hence organ, in the body comes under its influence. The endocrine system communicates with the nearly fifty million target cells in the body using a chemical "language" called *hormones.* These are natural substances that are secreted into the bloodstream in response to the body's needs, which then conveys them to their site of action—the target cell.

For decades the pituitary gland was believed to be the master gland that regulated and controlled the other endocrine glands in this very diverse system. However, the discovery of strong evidence that the central nervous system (CNS), specifically the hypothalamus, controls the pituitary has caused this old belief to be discarded. The hypothalamus and pituitary are now viewed as functioning together as an integrated unit, with the primary direction coming from the hypothalamus. For this reason, the system is now frequently referred to as the **neuroendocrine system.** In fact, the endocrine system can be considered in much the same way as the CNS. Each is basically a system for signaling, and each operates in a stimulus-and-response manner. Together these two systems essentially govern all bodily functions.

The **pituitary gland** is made up of two distinct glands—the anterior (adenohypophysis) and posterior (neurohypophysis) pituitary. They are individually linked to and communicate with the hypothalamus, and each gland secretes its own set of hormones. These various hormones are listed in Box 28-1 and shown in Fig. 28-1.

Hormones are either water- or lipid soluble. The water-soluble hormones are protein-based substances such as the catecholamines norepinephrine and epinephrine. The receptors for these hormones are usually located on cell membranes. These hormones bind to their receptors on the cell surface, whereupon they either directly activate the cell to perform a function or cause a signal to be sent by means of a "second messenger" to generate an appropriate cellular response. The lipid-soluble hormones consist of the steroid and thyroid hormones. They are capable of crossing the plasma membrane through the process of simple diffusion and of binding with receptors within the cell nucleus, where they stimulate a specific cellular response.

The activity of the endocrine system is regulated by a system of surveillance and signaling usually dictated by the body's needs. Hormone secretion is commonly regulated by the process of **negative feedback.** This is best explained using a fictional example: When gland X releases hormone X, this stimulates target cells to release hormone Y. When there is an excess of hormone Y, gland X "senses" this and inhibits the release of hormone X.

BOX 28-1	Hormones of the Anterior and Posterior Pituitary

ANTERIOR PITUITARY (ADENOHYPOPHYSIS)
Adrenocorticotropic hormone (ACTH)
Follicle-stimulating hormone (FSH)
Growth hormone (GH)
Luteinizing hormone (LH)
Prolactin (PH)
Thyroid-stimulating hormone (TSH)

POSTERIOR PITUITARY (NEUROHYPOPHYSIS)
Antidiuretic hormone (ADH)
Oxytocin

PITUITARY AGENTS

There is a variety of drugs that affect the pituitary gland. They are generally used for the following purposes: as replacement therapy to make up for a hormone deficiency, as drug therapy to produce a particular hormone response, in a patient with a specific disorder, and as diagnostic aids to determine whether there is hypofunction or hyperfunction of hormones. The currently identified anterior and posterior pituitary hormones and the drugs that mimic or antagonize their actions are listed in Box 28-2. Many of these hormones have been synthesized, and some of them have already been discussed in other chapters.

The anterior pituitary drugs discussed in this chapter include corticotropin, somatotropin, somatrem, and octreotide; the posterior pituitary drugs discussed in this chapter consist of vasopressin, lypressin, and desmopressin. The many other drugs that have effects on the pituitary are covered in depth in other chapters.

Mechanism of Action

The mechanisms of action of the various pituitary agents differ depending on the agent, but overall they either augment or antagonize the natural effects of the pituitary

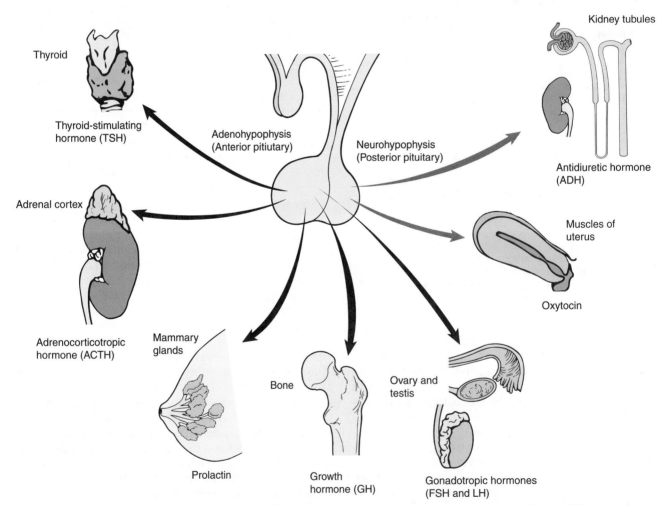

Fig. 28-1 Pituitary hormones. (From McKenry LM, Salerno E: *Mosby's pharmacology in nursing,* ed 21, St Louis, 2001, Mosby.)

hormones. Exogenously administered corticotropin elicits all the same pharmacologic responses as those elecited by the endogenous corticotropin, or ACTH. Regardless of whether it is exogenous or endogenous in origin, corticotropin travels to the adrenal cortex located just above the kidneys and stimulates the secretion of the mineralocorticoid cortisol (hydrocortisone), corticosterone, several weakly androgenic substances, and, to a very limited extent, aldosterone.

The drugs that mimic GH are somatropin and somatrem. These agents promote growth by stimulating the anabolic processes that cause growth. A drug that antagonizes the effects of the natural GH is octreotide, and it does so by inhibiting GH release. It is a synthetic polypeptide that is structurally and pharmacologically similar to GH release–inhibiting factor.

The drugs that affect the posterior pituitary such as vasopressin, lypressin, and desmopressin mimic the actions of the naturally occurring ADH. Exogenous vasopressin elicits all the same pharmacologic responses as those elicited by endogenous vasopressin (ADH). It increases water resorption in the distal tubules and collecting ducts of the nephrons, concentrates urine, and is a potent vasoconstrictor. It does all these by increasing the resorption of sodium and water in the distal tubules and collecting ducts of the kidneys.

Drug Effects

The drug effects of the various pituitary drugs also differ depending on the agent. Many of the effects are the same as those of the pituitary hormones. By stimulating the cortex of the adrenal gland to secrete cortisol, corticotropin causes sodium to be retained, resulting in edema and hypertension. Cortisol can also decrease inflammation by preventing the release of destructive substances from leukocytes. It also inhibits macrophage accumulation in inflamed areas, reduces leukocyte adhesion to capillary walls, and reduces capillary wall permeability and edema formation. Other effects of corticotropin are a decrease in the level of complement components, the antagonism of histamine activity, a reduction in fibroblast proliferation, the deposition of collagen, and the subsequent formation of scar tissue.

Somatropin and somatrem have pharmacologic effects equivalent to those of human GH. They both promote linear growth in children who lack normal amounts of the endogenous hormone. In addition, they cause increased cellular protein synthesis, nitrogen retention,

---

BOX 28-2 Anterior and Posterior Pituitary Hormones and Drugs

Hormone	Function/Mimicking Drug
ANTERIOR PITUITARY	
Adrenocorticotropic hormone	Targets adrenal gland; mediates adaptation to physical and emotional stress and starvation; redistributes body nutrients; promotes synthesis of adrenocortical hormone (glucocorticoids, mineralocorticoids, androgens); involved in skin pigmentation.
	Corticotropin: diagnosis of adrenocortical insufficiency.
Follicle-stimulating hormone	Stimulates oogenesis and follicular growth in females and spermatogenesis in males.
	Menotropins: same pharmacologic effects as FSH; many of the other gonadotropins also stimulate FSH (Chapter 32).
Growth hormone	Regulates anabolic processes related to growth and adaptation to stressors; promotes skeletal and muscle growth; increases protein synthesis; increases liver glycogenolysis; increases fat mobilization.
	Somatotropin: human GH for hypopituitary dwarfism.
	Octreotide: a synthetic polypeptide structurally and pharmacologically similar to growth hormone release–inhibiting factor; it inhibits GH.
Luteinizing hormone	Stimulates ovulation and estrogen release by ovaries in females; stimulates interstitial cells in males to promote spermatogenesis and testosterone secretion.
	Gonadotropins: many of the agents discussed in Chapter 32 stimulate LH.
Prolactin	Targets mammary glands; stimulates lactogenesis and breast growth.
	Bromocriptine: inhibits action of PH and therefore inhibits lactogenesis (Chapter 13).
Thyroid-stimulating hormone	Stimulates secretion of thyroid hormones (triiodothyronine [T3] and thyroxine [T4] by the thyroid.
	Thyrotropin: increases the production and secretion of thyroid hormones (Chapter 29).
POSTERIOR PITUITARY	
Antidiuretic hormone	Increases water resorption in distal tubules and collecting duct of nephron; concentrates urine; causes potent vasoconstriction.
	Vasopressin: ADH; performs all the physiologic functions of ADH.
	Lypressin: a synthetic vasopressin; has uses similar to those of vasopressin.
	Desmopressin: a synthetic vasopressin.
Oxytocin	Targets mammary glands; stimulates ejection of milk and contraction of uterine smooth muscle.
	Pitocin: has all the physiologic actions of oxytocin (Chapter 32).

Activity

liver glycogenolysis, impaired glucose tolerance, lipid mobilization, a reduction in body fat stores, and increased plasma levels of fatty acids. GH derivatives also cause the retention of sodium, potassium, and phosphorus.

Octreotide is a synthetic polypeptide that is structurally and pharmacologically related to somatostatin (GH release–inhibiting factor). It can eliminate or alleviate certain symptoms of carcinoid tumors (e.g., severe diarrhea, flushing). It is also effective in the management of the potentially life-threatening hypotension associated with a carcinoid crisis. Octreotide decreases the stool volume, electrolyte loss, and plasma concentrations of vasoactive intestinal polypeptide (VIP), a substance secreted by VIPomas that causes profuse watery diarrhea.

The synthetically made hormones that are structurally identical or similar to ADH are vasopressin, lypressin, and desmopressin. By increasing the resorption of sodium and water in the distal tubules and collecting duct of the nephron, they decrease the urinary flow rate, thereby causing as much as 90% of the water that might otherwise be excreted in the urine to be conserved. In large doses, vasopressin directly stimulates the contraction of smooth muscle, particularly of the capillaries and small arterioles, causing vasoconstriction. Desmopressin causes a dose-dependent increase in the plasma levels of factor VIII (antihemophilic factor, or von Willebrand's factor) and tissue plasminogen activator.

Therapeutic Uses

Corticotropin's primary therapeutic effect is the stimulation of the release of cortisol from the adrenal cortex, making it an excellent agent in the diagnosis of adrenocortical insufficiency. It is also used for the treatment of multiple sclerosis and corticotropin insufficiency caused by long-term corticosteroid use. Its antiinflammatory and immunosuppressant properties may be therapeutic in patients with normal adrenocortical function. Somatropin and somatrem are recombinantly made human GH. They are effective in stimulating skeletal growth in patients suffering from an inadequate secretion of normal endogenous GH, such as those with hypopituitary dwarfism. Octreotide is a synthetic polypeptide that is structurally and pharmacologically related to somatostatin (GH release–inhibiting factor). It is of benefit in alleviating or eliminating certain symptoms of carcinoid tumors stemming from the secretion of VIP. (These symptoms have been described in the previous section.) Vasopressin, lypressin, and desmopressin are used to prevent or control polydipsia, polyuria, and dehydration in patients with diabetes insipidus caused by a deficiency of endogenous ADH. Because of their vasoconstrictor properties, they are useful in the treatment of various types of bleeding, in particular gastrointestinal hemorrhage. Because of its unique ability to increase the plasma level of factor VIII (von Willebrand's factor) and tissue plasminogen activator, desmopressin is especially useful in the treatment of hemophilia A and type I von Willebrand's disease. They are occasionally used after cranial surgery that may involve the pituitary gland.

Side Effects and Adverse Effects

Many of the adverse effects of the pituitary drugs are specific to the individual agents. Those agents possessing similar hormonal effects generally have similar adverse effects. The most common adverse effects of the pituitary drugs described here are listed in Tables 28-1 to 28-3.

Interactions

An additive potassium-lowering effect can be seen when ACTH is given with diuretics or amphotericin B. Desmopressin when given with carbamazepine, chlorpropamide, and clofibrate may result in additive therapeutic effects

Table 28-1 Corticotropin: Common Adverse Effects

Body System	Side/Adverse Effect
Central nervous system	Convulsions, dizziness, euphoria, insomnia, headache, depression, psychosis
Gastrointestinal	Nausea, vomiting, peptic ulcer perforation, pancreatitis
Genitourinary	Water and sodium retention, hypokalemia
Other	Sweating, acne, hyperpigmentation, weakness, muscle atrophy, myalgia, arthralgia

Table 28-2 Desmopressin, Lypressin, and Vasopressin: Common Adverse Effects

Body System	Side/Adverse Effect
Cardiovascular	Increased blood pressure
Central nervous system	Drowsiness, headache, lethargy, flushing
Gastrointestinal	Nausea, heartburn, cramps
Genitourinary	Uterine cramping
Other	Nasal irritation and congestion, tremor, sweating, vertigo

Table 28-3 Drugs That Affect Growth Hormone: Common Adverse Effects

Body System	Side/Adverse Effect
Central nervous system	Headache
Endocrine	Hyperglycemia, ketosis, hypothyroidism
Genitourinary	Hypercalciuria
Other	Rash, urticaria, antibodies to GH, inflammation at injection site

Activity

of desmopressin. Lithium, alcohol, demeclocycline, and heparin when coadministered with desmopressin may result in decreased therapeutic effects of desmopressin.

Dosages

For the recommended dosages of pituitary agents, see the dosages table on p. 454.

drug profiles

corticotropin

Corticotropin (Acthar, H.P. Acthar Gel) is classified as a pregnancy category C agent. It is contraindicated in patients who have shown a hypersensitivity to it, in those with scleroderma, osteoporosis, congestive heart failure (CHF), peptic ulcer disease, hypertension, or primary adrenocortical insufficiency or hyperfunction, and in those who have undergone recent surgery. It is available in two parenteral forms, a regular form that may be given by IV, IM, or SC injection, and a repository form, which may be given intramuscularly or subcutaneously, that has more prolonged effects. The parenteral form is available in 25- and 40-U strengths and the repository form in 40- and 80-U/ml strengths. Common dosages are listed in the dosages table on p. 454.

PHARMACOKINETICS

HALF-LIFE	ONSET	PEAK	DURATION
Unknown	Rapid	1 hr	3 days*

*For repository form.

desmopressin

Desmopressin (DDAVP) is a synthetically made hormone that is structurally related to the endogenous hormone arginine vasopressin (ADH), but its effects differ slightly from those of the natural vasopressin (see the Drug Effects and Therapeutic Uses sections). It is classified as a pregnancy category B agent and is contraindicated in patients who have shown a hypersensitivity to it and in those with nephrogenic diabetes insipidus. It is available as a 10-μg/0.1 ml and a 100-μg/ml metered-dose nasal spray and a 4-μg/ml parenteral injection. For optimal control of the patient's disease, consistent timing of their intranasal dose is important. Common dosages are listed in the dosages table on p. 454.

PHARMACOKINETICS

HALF-LIFE	ONSET	PEAK	DURATION
IV: 1.5-2.5 hr	IV: 30 min	IV: 1.5-2 hr	IN: 12 hr

IN, Intranasal.

lypressin

Lypressin (Diapid) is lysine vasopressin, and it is identical to the vasopressin produced naturally in swine (pig) pituitaries. However, this synthetic vasopressin differs from that produced in humans in that it contains lysine instead of arginine in its structure, although the principal pharmacologic action of the two is similar. They both increase the resorption of sodium and water in the distal tubules and collecting duct of the nephron and in so doing block diuresis.

Lypressin is classified as a pregnancy B agent and is contraindicated in patients who have shown a hypersensitivity to it and in those with nephrogenic diabetes insipidus. It is available as a 185-μg/ml nasal spray. Common dosages are listed in the dosages table on p. 454.

PHARMACOKINETICS

HALF-LIFE	ONSET	PEAK	DURATION
15 min	Rapid	0.5-2 hr	3-8 hr

octreotide

Octreotide (Sandostatin) is contraindicated only in patients who have shown a hypersensitivity to it. It is only available parenterally as 50-, 100-, 200-, 500-, and 1000-μg/ml injections. Also available as a 10-, 20-, and 30-mg depot injection. Common dosages are listed in the dosages table on p. 454. Pregnancy category B.

PHARMACOKINETICS

HALF-LIFE	ONSET	PEAK	DURATION
1.7 hr	Unknown	15-30 min	12 hr

somatropin and somatrem

Somatropin (Genotropin, Humatrope, Nutropin, Nutropin AQ) and somatrem (Protropin) are both made by recombinant DNA techniques. They are contraindicated in anyone whose bones have stopped growing (i.e., those with closed epiphyses). They should also not be used in any patient showing evidence of an active tumor. All of the somatropin products and somatrem are given as subcutaneous injections. They differ in the types of formulations and the available dosages. Genotropin comes as a 1.5-mg (approximately 4 IU) two-chamber cartridge or a 5.8-mg (approximately 15 IU) two-chamber cartridge and a "Pen 5" injection device. Humatrope is available as a 5-mg (approximately 13-15 IU) lyophilized powder. Nutropin comes as a subcutaneous injection in 5-mg (approximately 15 IU) or 10 mg (approximately 30 IU) lyophilized sterile somatropinper vial or Nutropin AQ a 10-mg (approximately 30 IU) sterile liquid. Somatrem (Protropin) comes in 5 mg (approximately 15 IU) or 10 mg (approximately 30 IU) lyophilized sterile somatrem per vial. Common dosages are listed in the dosages table on p. 454. Both are pregnancy category C agents.

PHARMACOKINETICS

HALF-LIFE	ONSET	PEAK	DURATION
<30 min	SC: 3-6 hr	SC: 3-5 hr	Variable

○⇁vasopressin

Vasopressin (Pitressin) is a synthetic arginine vasopressin that structurally is identical to endogenous vasopressin (ADH) and produces all the same effects as the endogenous hormone. It is classified as

a pregnancy C agent and is contraindicated in patients who have shown a hypersensitivity to it and in those with chronic nephritis. It is available as a 20-U/ml parenteral injection. Common dosages are listed in the dosages table below.

PHARMACOKINETICS

HALF-LIFE	ONSET	PEAK	DURATION
10-35 min	Unknown	Unknown	2-8 hr

DOSAGES Selected Pituitary Drugs

agent	pharmacologic class	dosage range	purpose
corticotropin (Acthar)	Adrenal cortex stimulating hormone	*Pediatric* Suggested dose, 1.6 µg/kg/day or 50 µg/m²/day in 3-4 divided doses *Adult* IM/SC: 20 µg qid IM: 80-120 µg/day in divided doses for 2-3 wk IV: 10-25 µg in 500 ml of a suitable IV fluid (usually 5% dextrose) infused over 8 hr IV: up to 100 µg over 8 hr for 10 days	Replacement or therapeutic Antiinflammatory immunosuppressant Exacerbation of multiple sclerosis Diagnosis of adrenocortical insufficiency Myasthenia gravis
repository injection (H.P. Acthar Gel)		*Adult* IM: 40-80 µg q24-72h IM: 80-120 µg/day for 14-21 days	Antiinflammatory immunosuppressant Exacerbation of multiple sclerosis
desmopressin acetate (DDAVP)	Antidiuretic antihemophilic hormone	*Pediatric* ≥6 y/o: 0.2 ml (20 µg) of the nasal spray hs, with ½ dose administered to each nostril 3 mo-12 y/o: 0.05-0.3 ml (5-30 µg) of the nasal spray/day hs *Adult/Pediatric* ≥3 mo: IV: 0.3 µg/kg over 30 min *Adult* 0.1-0.4 ml (10-40 µg) of the spray hs or divided	Primary nocturnal enuresis Diabetes insipidus Hemophilia A, type 1 von Willebrand's disease Diabetes insipidus
lypressin (Diapid)	Synthetic antidiuretic hormone	*Adult/Pediatric* 1-2 sprays (7-14 µg) of the nasal spray administered 1-2 times in each nostril qid	Diabetes insipidus
○⇁octreotide (Sandostatin)	Growth hormone inhibitor	*Adult* IV/SC: 50 µg tid and adjust IV/SC: 100-600 µg/day in 2-4 divided doses IV/SC: 200-300 µg/day in 2-4 divided doses	Treatment of acromegaly Carcinoid tumors VIPoma
somatrem (Protropin)	Growth hormone	*Pediatric* IV/SC: Up to 0.1 mg/kg (0.26 µl/kg) 3 times/wk	Growth failure due to inadequate levels of natural GH
somatropin (Humatrope, Nutropin)	Growth hormone	*Pediatric* IV/SC: Up to 0.06 mg/kg (0.16 µl/kg) 2 times/wk	
○⇁vasopressin (Pitressin)	Antidiuretic hormone	*Pediatric* IM/SC: 5-10 U 3-4 times/day *Adult* IM/SC: 5 U to start and up to 10 U prn IM/SC: 10 U given 2 hr and ½ hr before procedure	Diabetes insipidus Postop abdominal distention Abdominal x-ray study

nursing process

● Assessment

Before administering any of the pituitary agents, the nurse should perform a thorough nursing assessment, obtain a complete medication history, and document the findings. There are many contraindications and cautions to the use of these agents and many drugs that interact with them, and all of this should be checked for before their administration. A hypersensitivity reaction to any of these medications is also a contraindication to their use. Further assessment data are provided in Box 28-3.

● Nursing Diagnoses

Nursing diagnoses related to the administration of pituitary agents include the following:
- Disturbed body image related to specific disease processes and their influence on physical characteristics.
- Excess fluid volume related to side effects of various pituitary agents.
- Fatigue related to use of various pituitary agents.
- Ineffective tissue perfusion related to drug-induced hypertension.

BOX 28-3

Pituitary Agents: Assessment Data

Assessment Parameters	Cautions and Drug Interactions	Contraindications
CORTICOTROPIN		
Baseline vital signs	*Cautions:*	Allergy
Electrolyte values	Pregnancy	Osteoporosis
Blood glucose levels	Lactation	CHF
Chest x-ray study	Liver disease	Ulcer disease
CBC, I&O, weight	Mental illness	Scleroderma
Cortisol levels	Myasthenia gravis	Fungal infections
Allergy to pork, because of cross-sensitivity	Gout	Recent surgery
	Hypothyroidism	Adrenocortical hypo/hyper function
	Latent tuberculosis	(primary)
	Drug interactions:	
	Alcohol	
	Aspirin	
	Steroids	
	Diuretics	
	Amphotericin B	
DESMOPRESSIN		
Vital signs with BP lying and standing q4h	*Cautions:*	Allergy to drug or to tricyclic antidepressants
	Depression or suicidal tendencies	
CBC: leukocytes	Narrow-angle glaucoma	Glaucoma
Cardiac enzymes	Increased intraocular pressure	MI (recovery phase)
Liver enzymes	Seizure disorder	BPH
Weight every week	Children under 12 years of age	Seizure disorder
ECG		Children under 12 years of age
SOMATROPIN AND SOMATREM		
Thyroid function studies	*Cautions:*	Drug allergy
GH antibodies	Diabetes mellitus	Intracerebral lesions
	Hypothyroidism	Closed epiphyseal plates
	Pregnancy	
	Drug interactions:	
	Glucocorticoids	
	Androgens	
	Thyroid hormones	
VASOPRESSIN AND LYPRESSIN		
Pulse-vital signs, especially with IM/IV dosage forms	*Cautions:*	Allergy
	Coronary artery disease	Chronic renal disease
I&O	Pregnancy	
Weight		
Edema		

CBC, Complete blood count; *I&O*, intake and output; *CHF*, congestive heart failure; *MI*, myocardial infarction; *BPH*, benign prostatic hypertrophy.

- Acute pain related to ulcerogenic side effects of various pituitary agents.
- Deficient knowledge related to new treatment with various pituitary agents.

Planning

Goals pertaining to patients receiving pituitary medications include the following:
- Patient maintains positive body image.
- Patient maintains normal fluid volume and electrolyte status while on various pituitary agents.
- Patient returns to normal or pretherapy levels of activity.
- Patient maintains adequate tissue perfusion.
- Patient experiences little to no pain related to medication-induced gastrointestinal upset or epigastric distress.
- Patient remains compliant with medication therapy.
- Patient is without self-injury related to adverse effects of medications.

Outcome Criteria

The outcome criteria for patients receiving pituitary agents include the following:
- Patient will openly verbalize fears, anxieties, and concerns with health care professionals regarding body image changes related to disease process and medication therapy.
- Patient's sodium level will be within normal limits while on medication therapy.
- Patient will state ways to decrease edema caused by medication such as dietary precautions.
- Patient will experience minimal gastrointestinal upset and gastric distress by taking medication with food or at mealtimes.
- Patient will state measures to employ to diminish the risk of falls related to the musculoskeletal and neurologic (seizures) side effects of medication.
- Patient will perform activities of daily living and other normal activity without difficulty.
- Patient will state importance of follow-up visits to the physician such as monitoring compliance, therapeutic effects, and adverse reactions.

Implementation

Corticotropin is available in IM, SC, and IV forms as well as in gel and repository forms. Gel forms should be at room temperature when administered, and IM injections should be administered using a 21-gauge needle. IV injections should be given over 2 minutes, or as designated in the packaging insert, and should be diluted with the recommended amounts of normal saline solution. The patient's protein intake should be increased because of the protein loss and the potential negative nitrogen balance that can occur. Patients are usually encouraged to decrease their sodium intake and increase their potassium intake to counteract the side effects of the medication. Instructions should be given about the various forms of lypressin and vasopressin (e.g., nasal spray). Vital signs should be monitored during administration of vasopressin. Injection sites for somatropin should be rotated. Desmopressin should be administered per physician's orders since it may vary per indication (i.e., diabetes insipidus versus other forms of pituitary dysfunction).

Teaching tips for patients receiving pituitary agents are presented in the box below.

Evaluation

Following are the therapeutic responses expected in patients receiving pituitary agents:
- Corticotropin should eliminate the pain associated with inflammation and produce increased comfort and muscle strength in patients with myasthenia gravis
- Somatropin should increase growth in children
- Desmopressin, lypressin, and vasopressin should eliminate severe thirst and decrease urinary output.

Side effects for which to monitor in patients receiving corticotropin include dependent edema, moon face, pulmonary edema, infection, and mental status changes that include increased aggressive behavior and irritability. Allergic reactions to corticotropin include rash, urticaria, fever, and dyspnea. If these occur, the drug should be discontinued and the physician notified. The side effects of somatropin include hypercalciuria. Desmopressin, lypressin, and vasopressin cause similar side effects, including hypertension, nausea, gastrointestinal upset, tremors, respiratory distress, and drowsiness.

---

patient teaching tips

Pituitary Agents

Corticotropin
- ➤ Patients receiving corticotropin and corticotropin-like drugs should be encouraged to maintain adequate hydration of up to 2000 ml per day, unless this is contraindicated.
- ➤ Patients receiving corticotropin should avoid vaccinations during drug therapy.
- ➤ Patients should not take any over-the-counter medications during therapy.
- ➤ Patients should avoid consuming alcohol.

- ➤ Patients should be told not to discontinue the medication abruptly.
- ➤ Patients should wear a MedicAlert tag at all times, naming the medication they are taking.
- ➤ Patients should be informed that the medication does not lead to a cure but does help alleviate the symptoms of the disease.
- ➤ Patients should notify their physician should they experience infection, fever, sore throat, joint pain, or muscular pain.

➤ Patients should tell all other health care professionals, such as dentists, that they are taking corticotropin.

Somatropin

➤ Patients should be given instructions regarding the dosage form and amount and the importance of compliance with therapy.

➤ Discolored or cloudy solutions should not be used.

➤ Show the parents of children receiving the agent how to keep a journal of the growth measurements.

Desmopressin

➤ The technique for nasal instillation should be demonstrated to the child and caregiver and reevaluated at later visits, with repeat demonstrations if necessary. Written instructions should also be provided.

➤ The patient should not take any over-the-counter medications for colds, cough, allergies, or hay fever because

of the epinephrine in these preparations that can interact with the desmopressin.

➤ Patients should avoid consuming alcohol.

➤ A MedicAlert bracelet or necklace should be worn at all times, naming the medication being taken.

Lypressin

➤ Patients should be encouraged to carry the medication with them at all times.

➤ The nasal spray should be used according to instructions and only after patients have cleared their nasal passages. The spray should not be INHALED!

Octreotide

➤ Inform patients with carcinoid tumors who are taking this drug that symptoms of flushing and severe diarrhea will improve or be eliminated.

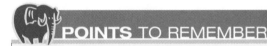

POINTS TO REMEMBER

Pituitary Gland

• Composed of two distinct glands: anterior and posterior.

• Each has its own set of hormones: anterior: TSH, GH, ACTH, PH, FSH, LH; posterior: ADH, oxytocin.

Pituitary Drugs

Mimic or antagonize action of endogenous pituitary hormones. Drugs that **mimic:**

• corticotropin

• somatropin: made by recombinant DNA synthesis

• somatrem: made by recombinant DNA synthesis

• vasopressin

• lypressin

• desmopressin:

– Synthetically-made hormone that is structurally related to endogenous arginine vasopressin, also known as antidiuretic hormone (ADH)

– Increases plasma levels of factor VIII (von Willebrand's factor) and tissue plasminogen activator

– Used in the treatment of hemophilia A and type I von Willebrand's disease

Drugs that **antagonize:**

• octreotide:

– Suppresses or inhibits certain symptoms of carcinoid tumors

– Decreases plasma concentration of vasoactive intestinal polypeptide (VIP)

Nursing Considerations

• Assessment in patients receiving corticotropin should include baseline vital signs, electrolyte values, blood glucose levels, chest x-ray studies, weight, cortisol levels, and allergy to pork because of cross-sensitivity.

• Assessment in patients receiving somatropin should include thyroid function and GH levels.

• Assessment in patients receiving desmopressin should include vital signs with lying and standing blood pressures, CBCs, cardiac and liver enzyme activity, ECG, and weight.

• Assessment in patients receiving vasopressin or lypressin should include vital signs, intake and output amounts, weight, and presence and status of edema.

REVIEW QUESTIONS

1. One of your patients at the clinic is complaining about the growth of a nodule on the back of his arm. He states that it has been getting larger over the last several weeks. His medications include somatropin. What should your next intervention be with consideration of these assessment findings?

   a. The growth should be incised and the somatropin increased.

   b. The medication should be abruptly discontinued and the growth will go away.

   c. The patient should assess the growth for the next 3 months and report to the physician if further increase in size occurs.

   d. Somatropin should not be used in patients with any type of "growths"; the patient should contact the physician immediately.

2. Which of the following should be included in the patient teaching of the nasal spray form of lypressin?
   a. Use the spray only when symptoms are present.
   b. Use the spray as directed and only after cleaning the nose but without inhaling the spray.
   c. Inhale the medication after two strong sprays, and then take a deep breath after inhalation of the dosage.
   d. The nostrils should be cleansed, but one side should be pinched during a very strong inhalation into the lungs.
3. Which of the following is a therapeutic response to vasopressin?
   a. Increased urinary output
   b. Increased albumin levels and anuria
   c. Decreased albumin levels and proteinuria
   d. Decreased urinary output and decreased thirst

4. A therapeutic response to lypressin therapy includes which of the following?
   a. Edema
   b. Oliguria
   c. Dysphagia
   d. Excitability
5. Tom is taking corticotropin but is now worried about the appearance of a new growth on the back of his hand. When you inquire about it, he tells you that it has been there for several weeks but has recently increased in size. What should your next action be?
   a. Immediately take Tom off of the corticotropin, and begin him on lypressin.
   b. Contact the physician about the new finding, but do not alter the drug unless ordered.
   c. Instruct Tom to increase the dose of corticotropin, which will help the inflammation.
   d. Lance the growth to see if it is infected, and begin weaning Tom off of the corticotropin.

For Answers see www.harcourthealth.com/MERLIN/Lilley/.

CRITICAL THINKING Activities

1. Vasopressin, lypressin, and desmopressin are structurally identical or similar to what endogenous hormone?
2. What are the two recombinantly made human GH products?

3. Your patient is excited that he is beginning therapy with pituitary agents and is positive about a cure. What would be your most appropriate response and why?

For Answers see www.harcourthealth.com/MERLIN/Lilley/.

bibliography

Albanese J, Nutz P: *Mosby's 2001 nursing drug reference and review cards,* St Louis, 2001, Mosby.

American Hospital Formulary Service: *AHFS drug information,* Bethesda, Md, 2000, American Society of Health-System Pharmacists.

Anderson PO, Knoben JE, Troutman WG: *Handbook of clinical drug data 1999-2000,* ed 9, New York, 1999, McGraw-Hill.

Johns Hopkins Hospital, Department of Pediatrics et al: *The Harriet Lane handbook,* ed 15, St Louis, 2000, Mosby.

Keen JH: *Critical care and emergency drug reference,* ed 3, St Louis, 1996, Mosby.

Mosby's GenRx: a comprehensive reference for generic and brand drugs, ed 10, St Louis, 2000, Mosby.

Skidmore-Roth L: *Mosby's 2001 nursing drug reference,* St Louis, 2001, Mosby.

Remember to check the **Online Worksheet** for additional learning opportunities: **www.harcourthealth.com/MERLIN/Lilley/**

Thyroid and Antithyroid Agents

www.harcourthealth.com/MERLIN/Lilley/

Look for this symbol for
topics covered in the
Online Worksheet
Activity

objectives

When you reach the end of this chapter, you should be able to do the following:

1 Discuss the normal actions and functions of the thyroid hormones.

2 Describe the differences in the diseases resulting from the hyposecretion and hypersecretion of the thyroid hormones.

3 Identify the various agents that are used to manage the hyposecretion and hypersecretion states.

4 Discuss the mechanisms of action, indications, contraindications and cautions, and side effects related to thyroid agents.

5 Develop a nursing care plan that includes all phases of the nursing process for patients receiving thyroid or antithyroid agents.

6 Identify the teaching guidelines for patients receiving thyroid or antithyroid agents.

drug profiles

○—**levothyroxine,** p. 462	○—**propylthiouracil,** p. 464
liothyronine, p. 462	**thyroglobulin,** p. 463
liotrix, p. 462	**thyroid,** p. 463
methimazole, p. 464	

○—Key drug.

glossary

Hyperthyroidism (hi′ pər thi′ roid iz əm) Condition characterized by excessive production of the thyroid hormones. (p. 460)

Hypothyroidism Condition characterized by decreased activity of the thyroid gland. (p. 460)

Thyroid-stimulating hormone Endogenous substance secreted by the pituitary gland that controls the release of thyroid hormone and is necessary for the growth and function of the thyroid gland. (p. 460)

Thyrotropin (thi ro′ tro pin) Thyroid preparation that increases the uptake of radioactive iodine in the thyroid and the secretion of thyroxine by the thyroid. (p. 460)

Thyroxine (thi rok′ sen) Thyroid hormone that influences the metabolic rate. (p. 459)

Triiodothyronine (tri i′ o do thi′ ro nen) Hormone that helps regulate growth, development, metabolism, and body temperature and inhibits the secretion of thyrotropin by the pituitary. (p. 459)

THYROID FUNCTION

The thyroid gland lies on either side of the neck and is responsible for the secretion of three hormones essential for the proper regulation of metabolism: **thyroxine** (T_4), **triiodothyronine** (T_3), and calcitonin. It is close to and communicates with the parathyroid gland, which lies just above and behind it. The parathyroid gland is a bean-shaped gland and consists of two pairs. These glands are made up of encapsulated cells, which are responsible for maintaining adequate levels of calcium in the extracellular fluid, primarily by mobilizing calcium from bone.

T_4 and T_3 are produced in the thyroid gland through the iodination and coupling of the amino acid tyrosine. The iodide needed for this process is acquired from our diet, and for normal function to be maintained, we need about 1 mg of iodide per week. This iodide is sequestered by the thyroid gland, where it is trapped and concentrated to twenty times its potency in blood. It is here that it is also converted to iodine, which is combined with the tyrosine to make diiodotyrosine. The combination of two molecules of diiodotyrosine causes the formation of thyronine, which therefore has four iodine molecules in its structure (T_4). Triiodothyronine is formed by the coupling of one molecule of diiodotyrosine with one molecule of monoiodotyrosine, thus it has three iodine molecules in its structure (T_3). The biologic potency of T_3 is about four times greater than that of T_4, but T_4 is present in much greater quantities. After the synthesis of these two thyroid hormones, they are stored in a complex with thyroglobulin (a protein that contains tyrosine and an amino acid) in the follicles in the thyroid gland called the colloid. When the thyroid gland is signaled to do so, the thyroglobulin—thyroid hormone complex is then enzymatically broken down to release either T_3 or T_4 into the circulation. This entire process is triggered by **thyroid-stimulating hormone** (TSH), also called **thyrotropin.** Its release from the anterior pituitary is stimulated when the blood levels of T_3 and T_4 are low.

The thyroid hormones are involved in a wide variety of bodily processes. They regulate lipid and carbohydrate metabolism, they are essential for normal growth and development, they control the heat-regulating system (thermoregulatory center), and they have multiple effects on the cardiovascular, endocrine, and neuromuscular systems. Therefore hyperfunction or hypofunction of the thyroid gland can lead to a wide range of serious consequences.

HYPOTHYROIDISM

A deficiency in thyroid hormones can be caused by a number of different diseases that affect the thyroid in different ways. There are three types of **hypothyroidism.** *Primary hypothyroidism* stems from an abnormality in the thyroid gland itself and occurs when the thyroid gland is not able to perform one of its many functions, such as releasing the thyroid hormones from their storage sites, coupling iodine with tyrosine, trapping iodide, or converting iodide to iodine, or any combination of these defects. It is the most common of the three. *Secondary hypothyroidism* results when the pituitary gland is dysfunctional and does not secrete the TSH needed to trigger the release of the T_3 and T_4 stored there. *Tertiary hypothyroidism* is similar to the secondary form in that the stimulus needed to trigger the secretion of the next hormone is absent. However, the source of the problem is that the level of the thyrotropin-releasing hormone (TRH) secreted from the hypothalamus is reduced, which in turn results in decreased TSH levels and hence decreased thyroid hormone levels. Knowledge of the underlying cause of the hypothyroidism allows one to treat the cause and by so doing eliminate the deficiency.

Hypothyroidism can also be classified by when it occurs in life. Hyposecretion of thyroid hormone during youth may lead to cretinism. Cretinism is a condition characterized by low metabolic rate, retarded growth and sexual development, and possibly mental retardation. Hyposecretion of thyroid hormone as an adult may lead to myxedema. Myxedema is a condition characterized by decreased metabolic rate but also involves loss of mental and physical stamina, gain in weight, loss of hair, firm edema, and yellow dullness of the skin.

Some forms of hypothyroidism may result in the formation of a goiter, which is an enlargement of the thyroid gland resulting from its overstimulation by elevated levels of TSH. The TSH level is elevated because of little or no thyroid hormone in the circulation. Common symptoms of hypothyroidism are thickened skin, hair loss, lethargy, constipation, anorexia, and many others.

HYPERTHYROIDISM

The excessive secretion of thyroid hormones, or **hyperthyroidism,** may be caused by several different diseases and drugs. Some of the more common diseases are Graves' disease, which is the most common cause; Plummer's disease, which is also known as *toxic nodular disease* and is the least common cause; multinodular disease; and thyroid storm, which is usually induced by stress or infection.

Hyperthyroidism can affect multiple body systems, resulting in an overall increase in metabolism. Frequently reported symptoms are diarrhea, flushing, increased appetite, muscle weakness, fatigue, palpitations, irritability, nervousness, sleep disorders, heat intolerance, and altered menstrual flow.

THYROID AGENTS

All three types of hypothyroidism are amenable to thyroid hormone replacement using various thyroid preparations. These agents can be either natural or synthetic in origin. The natural thyroid preparations are derived from the thyroids of animals such as cattle and hogs and include thyroid and thyroglobulin. All the natural prepara-

Reprinted with permission from Harrell GB, Murray PD: Diagnosis and management of congenital hypothyroidism, *J Perinat Neonat Nurs* 11:75, ©1998, Aspen Publishers.

---

research

Diagnosis of Hypothyroidism

Hypothyroidism is diagnosed by very careful assessment of the thyroid gland and through the use of several tests. These tests include serum T_4, free thyroxine (FT_4), free T_3, serum T_3, reverse T_3, serum TSH, thyroid-stimulating immunoglobulin, and thyroid uptake of radioiodine. With primary hypothyroidism, the diagnosis requires that a patient have lower-than-normal thyroid hormone levels and elevated TSH. Other tests to be done include direct TSH with T_3 or T_4, serum T_4, and T_3 uptake. Thyroidal uptake of iodine is decreased with hypothyroidism. Secondary and tertiary hypothyroidism may be differentiated from primary disease by taking TSH levels. With primary forms of the disease, the TSH is elevated because of the natural negative feedback system in an attempt to increase thyroid hormone levels. With the other forms of the disease, TSH levels are usually low or undetectable.

BOX 29-1	Thyroid Drugs: Clinically Equivalent Doses	
Thyroid Drug	**Approximate Equivalent Dose**
Natural thyroid preparations	
Thyroid	60-65 mg (1 grain)
Synthetic thyroid preparations	
Levothyroxine	100 μg or less
Liothyronine	25 μg
Liotrix	50 μg/12.5 μg

tions are standardized according to their iodine content. These agents are used infrequently. The synthetic thyroid preparations include levothyroxine, liothyronine, and liotrix, the latter agent containing a combination of T_4 and T_3 in a 4:1 ratio. The approximate clinically equivalent doses of the agents are given in Box 29-1, and this information is useful for guiding dosage adjustments when switching a patient from one thyroid hormone to another.

Mechanism of Action

The thyroid preparations are given to replace what the thyroid gland cannot itself produce in order to achieve normal thyroid levels (euthyroid). The thyroid drugs work in the same manner as the endogenous thyroid hormone. At the cellular level they work to induce changes in the metabolic rates, stimulate the cardiovascular system, and increase oxygen consumption, body temperature, blood volume, growth, and overall cellular growth.

Drug Effects

The drugs that are used to treat hypothyroid conditions affect many body systems, and they do this in the same way the endogenous thyroid hormones do. The principal pharmacologic effect of the drugs is an increase in the rate of protein, carbohydrate, and lipid metabolism. Thyroid hormones are also involved in the regulation of cell growth and differentiation and have a cardiostimulatory effect, which involves increasing the sensitivity of the heart to catecholamines or increasing the number of myocardial beta-adrenergic receptors, or both. In addition, thyroid hormones increase cardiac output, renal blood flow, and the glomerular filtration rate, which results in a diuretic effect.

Therapeutic Uses

The various thyroid preparations are used in the treatment of all three forms of hypothyroidism, although levothyroxine is generally the preferred agent because its hormonal content is standardized and its effect is therefore predictable. The thyroid drugs can also be used for the diagnosis of suspected hyperthyroidism and in the prevention or treatment of various types of goiters.

Side Effects and Adverse Effects

The adverse effects of thyroid medications are usually the result of overdose. The most significant adverse effect is cardiac dysrhythmia. Other more common undesirable effects are listed in Table 29-1.

Interactions

When thyroid preparations are taken in conjunction with oral anticoagulants, the activity of the oral anticoagulants may be increased, thus necessitating reduced anticoagulant doses. Thyroid preparations, when taken concomitantly with digitalis glycosides, may decrease serum digitalis levels. Cholestyramine binds to thyroid hormone in the gastrointestinal tract. This prevents the thyroid hormone from being absorbed into the bloodstream, which is necessary to produce its desired effect. Their concurrent use with cholestyramine results in reduced oral absorption of the antilipemic, and diabetic patients taking a thyroid agent may require increased doses of their hypoglycemic agents. In addition, their use with epinephrine in patients with coronary disease may induce coronary insufficiency.

Dosages

For the recommended dosages of the thyroid agents, see the dosages table on p. 462.

Activity

drug profiles

As previously mentioned, there is a variety of agents that may be used for the treatment of hypothyroidism. Natural agents are seldom used today, whereas the most commonly used are synthetic agents. There are many factors that must be considered before the initiation of drug therapy with a thyroid agent. These include the proportion of T_3 to T_4 desired, the cost, and the desired dura-

Thyroid Drugs: Common Adverse Effects

Table 29-1

Body System	Side/Adverse Effect
Cardiovascular	Tachycardia, palpitations, angina, dysrhythmias, hypertension, cardiac arrest
Central nervous system	Insomnia, tremors, headache, anxiety
Gastrointestinal	Nausea, diarrhea, increased or decreased appetite, cramps
Other	Menstrual irregularities, weight loss, sweating, heat intolerance, fever, thyroid storm

geriatric considerations

Thyroid Hormones

- The elderly patient is much more sensitive to thyroid hormone replacement therapy and also more liable to suffer more adverse reactions to thyroid hormones than patients in any other age group.
- Make sure that the medication regimen in an elderly patient is highly individualized. Often the dose in elderly patients must be 25% less than that given to patients of other age groups.
- Because the symptoms of hypothyroidism may be confused with the symptoms of other diseases, nonspecific symptoms such as stumbling, falling, depression, incontinence, cold intolerance, and weight gain should be thoroughly evaluated and documented before a diagnosis of hypothyroidism is rendered.

tion of effect. The thyroid drugs are classified as pregnancy category A agents. They are all contraindicated in patients who have had a hypersensitivity reaction to them in the past and in those suffering from adrenal insufficiency, myocardial infarction, or thyrotoxicosis.

Activity

levothyroxine

Levothyroxine (Levoxine, Levothroid, Synthyroid), or T_4, is the most commonly prescribed synthetic thyroid hormone. One advantage it has over the natural thyroid preparations is that it is chemically pure, being 100% T_4. Its half-life is also long enough that it only needs to be administered once a day. It is available orally as 12.5-, 25-, 50-, 75-, 88-, 100-, 112-, 125-, 150-, 175-, 200-, and 300-μg tablets and parenterally as a 200- and 500-μg injection. Common dosages are given in the dosages table below. Pregnancy category A.

PHARMACOKINETICS

HALF-LIFE	ONSET	PEAK*	DURATION*
9-10 days	2 days	3-4 wk	1-3 wk

*Therapeutic effects.

liothyronine

Liothyronine (Cytomel, Triostat) is also a chemically pure synthetic thyroid hormone preparation, but it is 100% T_3. Another way in which it differs from levothyroxine is that it has a rapid onset and a short duration of action. These pharmacokinetic differences are important because they make liothyronine the preferred agent when either a rapid effect or a rapidly reversible effect is desired, such as for diagnostic procedures requiring short-term thyrotropin suppression or for the treatment of myxedema coma. On the other hand, its more pronounced adverse cardiovascular effects along with its short duration of action make it less likely to be used for long-term use. It is only available orally as 5-, 25-, and 50-μg tablets and as a 10-μg/ml injection. Common dosages are given in the dosages table below. Pregnancy category A.

PHARMACOKINETICS

HALF-LIFE	ONSET	PEAK*	DURATION*
1-1.5 days	2 days	48-72 hr	72 hr

*Therapeutic effects.

liotrix

Liotrix (Thyrolar, Euthroid) is another synthetic thyroid hormone that is essentially a combination of the other two synthetic thyroid hormones, levothyroxine (T_4) and liothyronine (T_3). In the standard dose of liotrix, which is equivalent to 60 mg of thyroid, the respective amounts of T_3 and T_4 in the two commercial preparations differ slightly. Thyrolar contains 50 μg of T_4 and 12.5 μg of T_3. Euthroid contains 60 μg of T_4 and 15 μg of T_3. The clinical significance of this is questionable. Liotrix is only

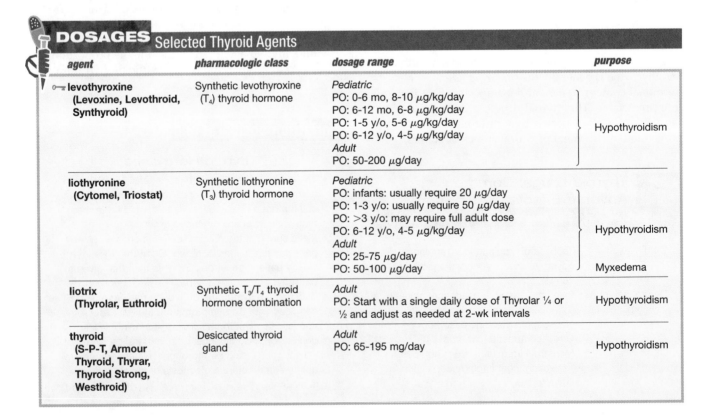

DOSAGES Selected Thyroid Agents

agent	pharmacologic class	dosage range	purpose
levothyroxine (Levoxine, Levothroid, Synthyroid)	Synthetic levothyroxine (T_4) thyroid hormone	*Pediatric* PO: 0-6 mo, 8-10 μg/kg/day PO: 6-12 mo, 6-8 μg/kg/day PO: 1-5 y/o, 5-6 μg/kg/day PO: 6-12 y/o, 4-5 μg/kg/day *Adult* PO: 50-200 μg/day	Hypothyroidism
liothyronine (Cytomel, Triostat)	Synthetic liothyronine (T_3) thyroid hormone	*Pediatric* PO: infants: usually require 20 μg/day PO: 1-3 y/o: usually require 50 μg/day PO: >3 y/o: may require full adult dose PO: 6-12 y/o, 4-5 μg/kg/day *Adult* PO: 25-75 μg/day PO: 50-100 μg/day	Hypothyroidism Myxedema
liotrix (Thyrolar, Euthroid)	Synthetic T_3/T_4 thyroid hormone combination	*Adult* PO: Start with a single daily dose of Thyrolar ¼ or ½ and adjust as needed at 2-wk intervals	Hypothyroidism
thyroid (S-P-T, Armour Thyroid, Thyrar, Thyroid Strong, Westhroid)	Desiccated thyroid gland	*Adult* PO: 65-195 mg/day	Hypothyroidism

available orally as tablets that contain T_4 and T_3 in the following amounts:

LEVOTHYROXINE (μG)	LIOTHYRONINE (μG)	TRADE NAME
12.5	3.1	Thyrolar ¼
25	6.25	Thyrolar ½
30	7.5	Euthyroid ½
50	12.5	Thyrolar-1
60	15	Euthyroid-1
100	25	Thyrolar-2
120	30	Euthyroid-2
150	37.5	Thyrolar-3
180	45	Euthyroid-3

Common dosages are given in the dosages table on p. 462. Pregnancy category A.

PHARMACOKINETICS

HALF-LIFE	ONSET	PEAK	DURATION
6-7 days	2-3 days	8-10 days	3-5 days

thyroglobulin

Thyroglobulin (Proloid) is a purified extract obtained from the thyroid of hogs. To ensure certain biologic activity, it has been standardized to contain a ratio of T_4 to T_3 of 2.5:1. It is only available as an oral preparation in the form of 32-, 65-, 100-, 130-, and 200-mg tablets.

PHARAMACOKINETICS

HALF-LIFE	ONSET	PEAK*	DURATION*
6-7 days	2 days	3-4 wk	1-3 wk

*Therapeutic effects.

thyroid

Thyroid (S-P-T, Armour Thyroid, Thyrar, Thyroid Strong, Westhroid) is the cleaned, dried, and powdered thyroid gland of domesticated animals, usually hogs, and it is a combination of both T_3 and T_4 in a normal physiologic ratio. Each 60 to 65 mg of thyroid is approximately equivalent to 100 mg or less of T_4 or 25 mg of T_3. There is also a Thyroid Strong preparation that is 50% more potent than regular thyroid. Thyroid is not considered the drug of choice for treating hypothyroidism because of lack of purity, uniformity, and stability in the formulation. It is the oldest and generally the least expensive of the available preparations. Thyroid is only available orally as 60-, 120-, 180-, and 300-mg capsules; 15-, 30-, 60-, 65-, 90-, 120-, 130-, 180-, 240-, and 300-mg tablets; 30-, 60-, and 120-mg bovine (cattle-derived) tablets; 15-, 30-, 60-, 120-, 200-, 250-, and 300-mg pork (hog-derived) tablets; 60- and 120-mg enteric-coated tablets; and 32.5-, 65-, 130-, and 200-mg Thyroid Strong tablets. Common dosages are given in the dosages table on p. 462. Pregnancy category A.

PHARMACOKINETICS

HALF-LIFE	ONSET	PEAK*	DURATION*
6-7 days	2 days	3-4 wk	1-3 wk

*Therapeutic effects.

ANTITHYROID AGENTS

The treatment of hyperthyroidism may be aimed at treating either the primary cause or the symptoms of the disease. Antithyroid drugs, iodides, ionic inhibitors, and radioactive isotopes of iodine are used to treat the underlying cause, and drugs such as beta-blockers are used to treat the symptoms. The focus of the discussion here is on the antithyroid drugs called the *thioamide derivatives*, which mainly consist of methimazole and propylthiouracil. Besides the thiamides, radioactive iodine may be used to treat hyperthyroidism. Radioactive iodine works by destroying the thyroid gland. It does this by emitting destructive beta rays once it is taken up into the follicles of the thyroid gland. Surgery is a nonpharmacologic means of treating hyperthyroidism and involves removal of part of the thyroid gland. It is usually a very effective way to treat hyperthyroidism.

Mechanism of Action

Methimazole and propylthiouracil act by inhibiting the incorporation of iodine molecules into the amino acid tyrosine, a process required to make both monoiodotyrosine and diiodotyrosine, the precursors of T_3 and T_4. By doing this, the formation of thyroid hormone is impeded. Propylthiouracil has the added ability to inhibit the conversion of T_4 to T_3 in the peripheral circulation. Neither drug can inactivate already existing thyroid hormone, however.

Drug Effects

The drug effects of methimazole and propylthiouracil are primarily limited to the thyroid gland, their overall effect being a decrease in the thyroid hormone level. The administration of these medications to patients suffering from hyperthyroidism lowers the high levels of thyroid hormone, thereby normalizing the overall metabolic rate.

Therapeutic Uses

Antithyroid agents are used to palliate hyperthyroidism and to prevent the surge in thyroid hormones that occurs after the surgical treatment of or during the radioactive iodine therapy for hyperthyroidism. In some types of hyperthyroidism such as that seen in the Graves' disease, the long-term administration of these agents (several years) may induce a spontaneous remission. However, most patients eventually require surgery or radioactive iodine therapy to ablate the condition.

Side Effects and Adverse Effects

The most damaging or serious adverse effects of the two antithyroid medications are liver and bone marrow toxicity. These and the more common adverse effects of methimazole and propylthiouracil are listed in Table 29-2.

Interactions

Drug interactions that occur with antithyroid agents include an additive agranulocytosis when they are taken in

Table 29-2 Antithyroid Drugs: Common Adverse Effects

Body System	Side/Adverse Effect
Central nervous system	Drowsiness, headache, vertigo, fever, paresthesia
Gastrointestinal	Nausea, vomiting, diarrhea, jaundice, hepatitis, loss of taste
Genitourinary	Smoky colored urine, decreased urine output
Hematologic	Agranulocytosis, leukopenia, thrombocytopenia, hypothrombinemia, lymphadenopathy, bleeding
Integumentary	Rash, pruritus, hyperpigmentation
Musculoskeletal	Myalgia, arthralgia, nocturnal muscle cramps
Renal	BUN and serum creatinine increased
Other	Enlarged thyroid, nephritis

conjunction with other bone marrow depressants and an increase in the activity of oral anticoagulants.

Dosages

See the dosages table on p. 465 for the recommended dosages of methimazole and propylthiouracil.

drug profiles

methimazole

Methimazole (Tapazole) is one of the two thioamide antithyroid agents and is rated as a pregnancy category D agent. It is contraindicated in patients who have shown a hypersensitivity to it and in pregnant women during the third trimester. It is only available orally as a 5- and 10-mg tablet. Common dosages are given in the dosages table on p. 465.

PHARMACOKINETICS

HALF-LIFE	ONSET	PEAK*	DURATION
5-13 hr	5 days	7 wk	2-4 hr

*Therapeutic effects.

propylthiouracil

Propylthiouracil (PTU) is the other thioamide antithyroid agents and is also rated as a pregnancy category D agent. The contraindications to its use are the same as those for methimazole. About 2 weeks of therapy with propylthiouracil may be necessary before symptoms improve. It is only available orally as a 50-mg tablet. Common dosages are given in the dosages table on p. 465.

PHARAMCOKINETICS

HALF-LIFE	ONSET	PEAK*	DURATION
1-2 hr	5 days	17 wk	2-4 hr

Activity *Therapeutic effects.

nursing process

● Assessment

Before administering any of the thyroid agents, the nurse should assess the patient for contraindications, which include adrenal insufficiency, myocardial infarction, and hyperthyroidism. Cautious use is recommended in patients with coronary heart disease, hypertension, angina, or cardiac disease, and in pregnant women.

The antithyroid hormones methimazole and propylthiouracil are contraindicated in patients who have shown a hypersensitivity to the medication and in pregnant women during the third trimester. Cautious use is recommended in patients with liver disease, infections, or bone marrow disease (because of the agranulocytosis and other blood dyscrasias they can cause) and during the first and second trimesters of pregnancy.

Baseline weights, vital signs, and intake and output should be obtained and recorded in patients receiving either a thyroid or antithyroid preparation.

● Nursing Diagnoses

Nursing diagnoses appropriate to patients receiving a thyroid or antithyroid preparation include the following:
- Risk for injury related to the side effects of the medications.
- Risk for infection related to the bone marrow depression caused by antithyroid medications.
- Acute pain related to the side effects of the medications.
- Decreased cardiac output related to side effects of the thyroid agents.
- Deficient knowledge related to lack of experience with self-administration of the medication.

● Planning

Goals pertaining to patients receiving a thyroid or antithyroid preparation include the following:
- Patient remains free from injury as the result of the side effects of the medications.
- Patient is monitored closely (e.g., for thyroid levels) while taking the medication.
- Patient remains free of infection while receiving antithyroid medication.
- Patient maintains normal energy levels while on thyroid agents.
- Patient experiences minimal side effects resulting from the medications.
- Patient demonstrates an understanding of the use of the thyroid agent and its side effects and need for compliance by stating such information.

Outcome Criteria

Outcome criteria that pertain to patients receiving a thyroid or antithyroid preparation include the following:
- Patient will state measures to implement to decrease the likelihood of self-injury related to the drug's side effects such as frequent laboratory checks and monitoring vital signs.

DOSAGES Selected Antithyroid Agents

agent	pharmacologic class	dosage range	purpose
methimazole (Tapazole)		*Pediatric* PO: 0.4 mg/kg/day in three divided doses q8h; usual maintenance dose is half initial dose; max 30 mg/day *Adult* PO: 15-60 mg in three divided doses q8h; maintenance dose is 5-10 mg/day; max 60 mg/day	Hyperthyroidism
propylthiouracil (PTU)	Antithyroid	*Pediatric* PO: 6-10 y/o: 50-150 mg/day in three divided doses q8h; maintenance dose depends on response >12 y/o; 150-300 mg in three divided doses q8h *Adult* PO: 300-900 mg/day in three divided doses q8h; usual maintenance dose is 100-150 mg/day in divided doses q8-12h	Hyperthyroidism

• Patient will state the importance of follow-up appointments with the physician for frequent blood studies and monitoring of therapeutic effects.

• Patient will state ways to decrease the risk of infection while receiving an antithyroid medication such as avoiding persons with infections and eating a proper diet and getting adequate rest.

• Patient will use relaxation techniques to deal with the nervousness and irritability caused by the agents or the diseases.

● Implementation

When administering thyroid agents, it is important to give the medication at the same time each day in order to maintain consistent blood levels of the agent. If possible, it is also best to administer thyroid agents given once a day in the morning to decrease the likelihood of insomnia that may result from evening dosing. If administering levothyroxine intravenously, the nurse should follow the manufacturer's guidelines regarding the dilutional substances and the rate of administration. If the patient is scheduled to undergo any radioactive isotope studies, the thyroid medication is usually discontinued about 4 weeks before the test, but only with a physician's order.

Antithyroid medications are better tolerated orally when taken with meals. These agents should also be given at the same time every day to maintain consistent blood levels of the agent. In addition, these medications should never be withdrawn abruptly.

Teaching tips for patients receiving thyroid or antithyroid agents are presented in the box at right.

● Evaluation

A therapeutic response to thyroid agents is reflected by the disappearance of the symptoms of hypothyroidism, including depression, constipation, loss of appetite, weight gain, cold intolerance, syncope, and dry and brittle hair. Increased nervousness, irritability, mood changes, angina, and palpitations are side effects that need to be reported to the physician immediately. Clues to the fact that a patient is receiving inadequate doses include a return of the symptoms of hypothyroidism (see previous discussion).

A therapeutic response to antithyroid medications would be characterized by weight gain, decreased pulse, a return to a normal blood pressure, and decreased serum levels of T_4. Symptoms of overdose include cold intolerance, depression, and edema. The patient should be encouraged to report the development of any swelling, sore throat, lesions, or other signs of inflammation. Clues to the fact that a patient is not receiving adequate doses include tachycardia, insomnia, irritability, fever, and diarrhea.

Activity

patient teaching tips

Thyroid and Antithyroid Agents

➤ Patients should never discontinue their medication without the physician's approval or order.

➤ It is important for patients taking thyroid agents to take the medication exactly as prescribed, at the same time everyday, and not to switch brands, unless approved by the physician.

➤ Too high of a dose of a thyroid agent will result in nervousness, irritability, and insomnia.

➤ Patients taking thyroid agents should report any unusual symptoms, chest pain, or heart palpitations.

➤ Patients taking either thyroid or antithyroid drugs should not take any over-the-counter medications without physician approval.

➤ Patients taking antithyroid medications may be advised to avoid eating foods high in iodine, such as soy, tofu, turnip, seafood, and some breads, as well as to avoid using iodized salt.

➤ Patients should understand that the therapeutic effects of thyroid agents may take several months to occur.

➤ Patients taking thyroid and antithyroid agents should keep a log or journal of their responses to the therapy and a graph of their pulse, weight, and mood status.

➤ Encourage patients to keep a journal of daily energy levels and appetite during the initiation of drug therapy. This information will assist in evaluating the effectiveness of the medication regimen.

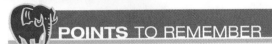

POINTS TO REMEMBER

Thyroid Hormone

- Thyroxine (T_4) and triiodothyronine (T_3) are the two hormones produced by the thyroid gland.
- Made by iodination and coupling with the amino acid tyrosine.
- T_4 is made by combining two molecules of diiodotyrosine (it has four iodine molecules).
- T_3 is formed by coupling one molecule of diiodotyrosine with one molecule of monoiodotyrosine (it has three iodine molecules).
- T_3 is about four times more biologically potent than thyroxine.

Hypothyroidism

- Primary hypothyroidism caused by an abnormality in the thyroid gland itself.
- Secondary hypothyroidism may result from a dysfunctional pituitary gland (lowered TSH level).
- Tertiary hypothyroidism similar to secondary in that the stimulus needed for secretion of thyroid hormone is absent.
- Tertiary hypothyroidism is due to hypothalamic rather than pituitary dysfunction (lowered TRH level).

Thyroid Replacement

- Natural and synthetic thyroid hormone.
- Natural preparations are derived from animal thyroid and include thyroid and thyroglobulin.
- Synthetic preparations include levothyroxine, liothyronine, and liotrix.

Hyperthyroidism

- Caused by excessive secretion of thyroid hormone from the thyroid gland.
- Due to different diseases or drugs.
- Diseases: Graves' disease, Plummer's disease, and multinodular disease.

Antithyroid Drugs

- Called *thioamide derivatives* and consist of mainly methimazole and propylthiouracil.
- Surgery is a nondrug therapy for hyperthyroidism.
- Drugs act by inhibiting the incorporation of iodine molecules into the amino acid tyrosine.
- By inhibiting the formation of the precursors of thyroid hormone they prevent its formation.

Nursing Considerations

- Children taking thyroid replacement hormones will show almost immediate behavior and personality changes reflecting their improved thyroid state.
- Patients on thyroid hormone replacement therapy should avoid iodine food containing iodized salt, soybeans, tofu, turnips, some types of seafood, and some breads. A nutritional consult is recommended as part of the therapy protocol.
- Patients should report the occurrence of excitability, irritability, or anxiety to their physician or health care provider, as these may indicate toxicity.
- Hair loss in children taking thyroid replacements is temporary.

REVIEW QUESTIONS

1. Dietary instructions for patients taking thyroid hormone replacement include which of the following?
   a. Use iodized salt at all times.
   b. Avoid all foods containing iodine.
   c. Fluid intake should equal up to 4500 ml per day.
   d. Increase sodium, potassium, and magnesium levels.
2. Which of the following agents may be used for short-term, rapid, and reversible thyrotropin suppressant therapy?
   a. Thyroid
   b. Liothyronine
   c. Thyroglobulin
   d. Mevothyroglobulin
3. Which of the following are expected side effects of thyroid hormone agents?
   a. Leukopenia, anemia, and dermatitis
   b. Anuria, tachycardia, and weight gain
   c. Bleeding, polyuria, and skin darkening
   d. Dysrhythmias, weight loss, and possibly fever

4. In an attempt to control the insomnia associated with thyroid hormone replacement therapy, the patient may be encouraged to do which of the following?
   a. Take the medication in the morning, if possible.
   b. Try lowering the dose every day by one-fourth until the insomnia is gone.
   c. Take one-half of the dose in the morning and the other half at dinner or bedtime.
   d. Try to switch the dosing to every other day, and if this is unsuccessful in relieving the insomnia, notify the physician of the problem.
5. The advantage of levothyroxine over natural forms is that:
   a. There are no side effects with levothyroxine.
   b. It only requires IM administration once monthly.
   c. Natural forms are not helpful and should not be considered at all.
   d. It requires administration only once daily orally because of long half-life.

CRITICAL THINKING Activities

1. Your patient has been taking thyroid agents for about 16 months and has recently noted palpitations and some heat intolerance. Should you be concerned about this? Explain your answer.

2. D.W. is a 63-year-old woman who has just had her thyroid gland removed and is being started on thyroid hormone replacement with levothyroxine (Synthroid) at a dose of 200 μg once a day.
    a. How much is 200 μg of levothyroxine in milligrams?
    b. How many grains of thyroid would this be equivalent to?

3. You are caring for a patient who has just been transferred to your floor from the intensive care unit. The patient underwent a thyroidectomy 2 days ago, and the transfer orders instruct that he should be started on his home medications. The written orders specify that 25 μg of levothyroxine should be given once daily. However, the pharmacy has sent 25 μg of liothyronine, another thyroid replacement product. Because the dose of each is the same, is it okay to administer the liothyronine?

For Answers see www.harcourthealth.com/MERLIN/Lilley/.

bibliography

Albanese J, Nutz P: *Mosby's 2001 nursing drug reference and review cards,* St Louis, 2001, Mosby.

American Hospital Formulary Service: *AHFS drug information,* Bethesda, Md, 2000, American Society of Health-System Pharmacists.

Anderson PO, Knoben JE, Troutman WG: *Handbook of clinical drug data 1999-2000,* ed 9, New York, 1999, McGraw-Hill.

Johns Hopkins Hospital, Department of Pediatrics et al: *The Harriet Lane handbook,* ed 15, St Louis, 2000, Mosby.

Keen JH: *Critical care and emergency drug reference,* ed 3, St Louis, 1996, Mosby.

Mosby's GenRx: a comprehensive reference for generic and brand drugs, ed 10, St Louis, 2000, Mosby.

Skidmore-Roth L: *Mosby's 2001 nursing drug reference,* St Louis, 2001, Mosby.

Turkoski BB: *Drug information handbook for nursing 1999-2000: including assessment, administration, monitoring guidelines, and patient education,* ed 2, Cleveland, 1999, Lexi-Comp.

MERLIN

Activity

Remember to check the **Online Worksheet** for additional learning opportunities: **www.harcourthealth.com/MERLIN/Lilley/**

Chapter 30

Antidiabetic and Hypoglycemic Agents

objectives

www.harcourthealth.com/MERLIN/Lilley/

Look for this symbol for topics covered in the **Online Worksheet**

When you reach the end of this chapter, you should be able to do the following:

1 Discuss the normal actions and functions of the pancreas and the feedback system that regulates it.

2 Describe the differences between the hyposecretion and hypersecretion of insulin and the difference between Type 1 and Type 2 diabetes mellitus.

3 Describe the various factors influencing the blood glucose levels in the presence or absence of diabetes mellitus.

4 Identify the various agents used to manage Type 1 and Type 2 diabetes mellitus.

5 Identify the signs and symptoms of hypoglycemia and hyperglycemia.

6 Discuss the mechanisms of action, indications, contraindications and cautions, and side effects relating to the insulin, oral antidiabetic, and hypoglycemic agents.

7 Develop a nursing care plan that includes all phases of the nursing process for patients receiving insulin, oral antidiabetic agents, or hypoglycemic agents.

8 Identify the teaching guidelines for patients receiving insulin, oral antidiabetic agents, or hypoglycemic agents.

---

drug profiles

acarbose, p. 479

chlorpropamide, p. 477

fixed-combination insulins, p. 473

o─ glipizide, p. 478

o─ glyburide, p. 478

intermediate-acting insulin, p. 472

long-acting insulin, p. 473

metformin, p. 479

rapid-acting insulin, p. 472

rosiglitazone, p. 479

sliding scale insulin, p. 473

o─ Key drug.

---

glossary

Diabetes mellitus (di ə be′ tēz me′ lə təs) Complex disorder of carbohydrate, fat, and protein metabolism primarily resulting from the lack of insulin secretion by the beta cells of the pancreas or from defects of the insulin receptors. (p. 469)

Diabetic ketoacidosis (ke′ to as i do′ sis) Diabetic coma. (p. 470)

Gestational diabetes A type of glucose intolerance that develops during pregnancy. (p. 470)

Glucagon (gloo′ kə gon) Hormone produced by the alpha cells in the islets of Langerhans that stimulates the conversion of glycogen to glucose in the liver. (p. 469)

Glucose (gloo′ kōs) One of the simple sugars found in fruits that serve as a major source of energy. (p. 469)

Glycogen (gli′ co jən) A polysaccharide that is the major carbohydrate stored in animal cells. (p. 469)

Glycogenolysis (gli′ co jə nol′ ə sis) Breakdown of glycogen to glucose. (p. 469)

Hyperglycemia (hi′ pər gli se′ me ə) Greater than 120 mg/dl of glucose in the blood. (p. 469)

Hypoglycemia Less than 40 mg/dl of glucose in the blood. (p. 470)

Insulin (in′ sə lin) Naturally occurring hormone secreted by the beta cells of the islands of Langerhans in response to increased levels of glucose in the blood. (p. 469)

Ketones (ke′ tōnz) Organic chemical compound produced through the oxidation of secondary alcohols. (p. 470)

Nephropathy (nə frop′ ə the) Disorder of the kidney that includes inflammatory, degenerative, and sclerotic conditions. (p. 470)

Neuropathy (nŏŏ rop′ ə the) Inflammation or degeneration of the peripheral nerves. (p. 470)

Polydipsia (pol i dip′ se ə) Chronic excessive intake of water. (p. 469)

Polyphagia (pol e fa′ jə) Excessive eating. (p. 469)

Polyuria (pol e u′ re ə) Increased frequency of urinary output, a characteristic of diabetes. (p. 469)

Retinopathy (ret i nop′ ə the) Noninflammatory eye disorder resulting from changes in the retinal blood vessels. (p. 469)

Type 1 diabetes mellitus An inability to metabolize carbohydrate caused by an overt insulin deficiency that occurs in children and adults. (p. 469)

Type 2 diabetes mellitus Type of diabetes in which patients are not insulin dependent but they may take insulin to correct the hyperglycemia. (p. 469)

PANCREAS

The pancreas is a large, elongated organ that is located behind the stomach. It is both an exocrine (secreting digestive enzymes) and endocrine organ, but it is its endocrine function that is relevant to the discussion here. There are two main hormones produced by the pancreas—insulin and glucagon. Both hormones play an important role in the regulation of the endocrine system, specifically the utilization, mobilization, and storage of **glucose,** which is one of the primary sources of energy for the cells of our body. There is a normal amount of glucose that circulates in the blood to meet quick energy requirements. However, not all the glucose we consume is needed. When the quantity of glucose in the blood is sufficient, the excess is stored as **glycogen** in the liver, where it remains until the body needs it.

When blood glucose is needed, the glycogen in the storage sites in the liver is converted back to glucose through a process called **glycogenolysis.** The hormone responsible for initiating this process is **glucagon.**

At the same time that the glucagon is released from the alpha cells of the islets of Langerhans in the pancreas, the beta cells of these same islets secrete insulin, a protein hormone composed of two chains (acidic A chain and basic B chain) joined by a disulfide linkage. The actions of **insulin** oppose those of glucagon. Essentially insulin takes the excess glucose from the blood and places it in the liver for storage. It also inhibits further glucagon release. These opposing actions of insulin and glucagon serve as a check and balance for each other, and both are needed to maintain normal glucose levels in the blood.

Two other substances that function as glucose regulators are cortisol and epinephrine. These work synergistically with glucagon to counter the effects of insulin and cause increases in the blood glucose level. Insulin actually serves many important functions in the body, all of them related to metabolism. It stimulates carbohydrate metabolism in skeletal and cardiac muscle and adipose tissue by facilitating the transport of glucose into these cells. In the liver, insulin facilitates the phosphorylation of glucose to glucose-6-phosphate, which is then converted to glycogen for storage. By causing glucose to be stored in the liver as glycogen, insulin keeps the kidney free of glucose. Without insulin the kidney could contain spillage substances such as glucose, ketones, and other substances that would otherwise draw water into the nephron, causing **polydipsia, polyuria,** and **polyphagia.**

Insulin also has a direct effect on fat metabolism. It stimulates lipogenesis and inhibits lipolysis and the release of fatty acids from adipose cells. In addition, insulin stimulates protein synthesis and promotes the intracellular shift of potassium and magnesium, thereby decreasing elevated blood concentrations of these electrolytes. The actions of insulin are antagonized by the following body substances: somatropin (growth hormone), epinephrine, adrenocortical hormones, thyroid hormones, and estrogens.

DIABETES MELLITUS

Hyperglycemia is the state in which there is too much glucose in the blood and results when the counterbalancing actions of glucagon and insulin go away. Hyperglycemia may also be defined numerically as a fasting plasma glucose (FPG) of greater than 126 mg/dl. One of the most common causes is a syndrome known as diabetes mellitus. **Diabetes mellitus** is primarily a disorder of carbohydrate metabolism that involves either a deficiency of insulin, a resistance to insulin, or both. Whatever the cause of the diabetes, the result is hyperglycemia.

Diabetes mellitus has been recognized since 1550 BC when Egyptians wrote of a malady they called *honeyed urine.* The first step toward discerning the cause of diabetes mellitus occurred in 1788 when Thomas Cawley, an English physician, voiced his suspicion that the source of the illness lay in the pancreas. However, it took over a century to prove this, and it took even longer to discover the substance, insulin, that is secreted from the pancreas, the lack of which is responsible for causing the disease. It was known that the substance, whatever it was, was needed by those afflicted with the illness, but the substance could not be isolated. It was not until the early 1920s that insulin was finally discovered. Its discovery is now considered one of the greatest triumphs of twentieth-century medicine, and its use in the therapy for diabetes mellitus has proved to be a life-saving remedy for millions.

Diabetes mellitus is not actually a single disease, however, but a group of diseases. This is why it is often regarded as a syndrome rather than a disease. The relative or absolute lack of insulin is believed to result from the destruction of beta cells in the pancreas such that insulin can neither be produced nor secreted. Hyperglycemia can also be caused by insulin receptor-defects. When the receptors that normally function in coordination with insulin in removing glucose from the blood are defective, they no longer recognize insulin and therefore the glucose remains in the blood. In addition, other cells throughout the body that are supposed to recognize insulin may become insulin resistant and refuse to use circulating insulin. These differences in the source of the hyperglycemia account for the two types of diabetes mellitus that have been recognized: **Type 1 diabetes mellitus** (insulin-dependent, or IDDM) and **Type 2 diabetes mellitus** (non–insulin-dependent, or NIDDM). There are also three categories of diabetes mellitus; these are secondary diabetes, gestational diabetes, and impaired glucose tolerance. The differences between Type 1 and Type 2 diabetes mellitus are listed in Table 30-1.

Type 1 Diabetes Mellitus

Type 1 diabetes mellitus (formerly known as insulin-dependent diabetes mellitus [IDDM]) is characterized by a lack of insulin production or by the production of a defective insulin, and affected patients require exogenous insulin to treat and prevent its many complications. Common complications of the disorder are the destruction of the retina of the eye **(retinopathy),** the destruction of

Table 30-1 Type 1 and 2 Diabetes: Characteristics		
Characteristic	**Type 1 (IDDM)**	**Type 2 (NIDDM)**
Onset	Juvenile-onset diabetes, <20 y/o	Maturity-onset diabetes, >40 y/o
Endogenous insulin	Little or none	Normal
Treatment	Insulin	Weight loss, diet and exercise, oral hypogly-cemics; only a third of patients need insulin
Incidence	10%	90%
Receptors	Normal	Decreased or defective
Body weight	Usually nonobese	Obese (80%)
Etiology	Autoimmune destruction of beta cells in the pancreas	Multifactorial genetic defects; strong association with obesity and insulin resistance resulting from a reduction in insulin receptors

nerves **(neuropathy),** and the destruction of the nephrons of the kidney **(nephropathy).** At times glucose is broken down into fatty acids that are converted to **ketones.** These in turn cause the development of **diabetic ketoacidosis** (DKA), a complex multisystem disorder and a common complication of uncontrolled Type 1 diabetes mellitus that results in coma. The person experiencing DKA is suffering from extreme hyperglycemia, positive serum ketone levels, acidosis, dehydration, and electrolyte imbalances. Approximately 25% to 30% of patients with Type 1 diabetes mellitus present with DKA, the most common precipitator of DKA being physical or emotional stress. The stress triggers it by causing the release of the counterregulatory hormones cortisol and epinephrine, which then mobilize glucagon and release glucose from the storage sites in the liver, further adding to the already elevated levels of glucose in the blood.

Type 2 Diabetes Mellitus

Type 2 diabetes mellitus, which was once thought to be a mild form of Type 1 diabetes mellitus, is an important but poorly treated disorder. Of all the forms of diabetes mellitus, it is by far the most common, accounting for about 85% of all the cases of diabetes mellitus and affecting as much as 10% of the population over 70 years of age. There are many common and dangerous misconceptions regarding Type 2 diabetes mellitus: that it is a mild diabetes, that it is easy to treat, and that tight metabolic control is unnecessary because these patients, being mostly old, will die before diabetic complications develop. None of these are true, however.

Type 2 diabetes mellitus is due to both insulin resistance and insulin deficiency. As prevously noted, one of insulin's normal roles is to take circulating glucose and transport it to tissues to be used as energy. In the setting of Type 2 diabetes mellitus, all the main target tissues of insulin (muscle, liver, and adipose tissue) are hyporesponsive (resistant) to the effects of the hormone. Not only is the absolute number of insulin receptors on these tissues reduced, but their sensitivity and responsiveness

to insulin are reduced as well. Therefore it is possible for a patient with Type 2 diabetes mellitus to have normal or even elevated levels of insulin yet have high blood glucose levels. The reason for this paradoxic situation is that the altered insulin-sensing mechanism causes the liver to overproduce glucose, adding to the already present hyperglycemic condition.

The reduction in insulin secretion that can occur in patients with Type 2 diabetes mellitus is the result of a loss of the response of the beta cells in the pancreas to the elevated blood glucose levels and other stimuli. If these beta cells do not recognize glucose, they do not secrete insulin, and glucose is not transported into cells or tissues nor is it stored in the liver. There also seems to be an alteration in the response to meals in patients with Type 2 diabetes mellitus. Either insulin resistance or insulin deficiency may lead to or induce the other.

Although Type 2 diabetes mellitus is a multifaceted disorder, lipid abnormalities, obesity, and hypertension are the primary findings in most persons afflicted with it. The dyslipidemias of Type 2 diabetes mellitus typically involve hypertriglyceridemia and the atherogenic combination of decreased high-density lipoprotein (HDL) and elevated low-density lipoprotein (LDL) cholesterol.

Gestational diabetes is a type of glucose intolerance that develops during pregnancy. It occurs in about 2% of pregnancies. The use of insulin is necessary to decrease risks of birth defects. In most cases it subsides after delivery. However, as many as 30% of these women are estimated to develop Type 2 diabetes within 10 to 15 years.

HYPOGLYCEMIA

Hypoglycemia is the condition in which the blood glucose level is abnormally low (generally below 40 mg/dl). When the cause is organic and the effects mild, treatment usually consists of dietary modifications, primarily a high intake of protein and low intake of carbohydrates. The condition can also be caused by the antidiabetic agents and occurs when the effect of these agents is greater than that expected. There are also other drugs that can cause it.

legal & ethical principles

Use of Abbreviations

Medication errors often occur as a result of misinterpretation of abbreviations. We are to always ensure safe medication administration to our patients to prevent undue injury or harm. Therefore the National Coordinating Council for Medication Error Reporting and Prevention recommends that the following abbreviations be written out IN FULL and the abbreviation avoided:

Abbreviation	Intended Meaning	Common Error
U	Units	Mistaken as a zero, a four (4), and cc
μg	Micrograms	Mistaken for mg (milligrams)
Q.D.	Latin abbreviation for every day	The period after the "Q" has been mistaken for an "I" and results in medications being given "QID" (four times daily) versus once daily
Q.O.D.	Latin abbreviation for every other day	Misinterpreted as "QD" (daily) or QID. If "O" is poorly written it may look like a period or "I".
D/C	Discharge or discontinue	Medications have been prematurely discontinued when D/C (intended to mean "discharge") was misinterpreted as "discontinue" because it was followed by a list of drugs.
HS	Half strength	Misinterpretation as the Latin abbreviation "HS" (hour of sleep).
cc	Cubic centimeters	Mistaken as "U" (units) when written poorly
AU, AS, AD	Both ears, left ear, right ear	Misinterpreted as the Latin abbreviation "OU" (both eyes), "OS" (left eye), "OD" (right eye)

Common symptoms of the disorder when it is more severe are confusion, sweating, hypothermia, tremor, headache, irritability, hallucinations, convulsions, and ultimately coma and death if it is not treated. Because the brain needs a constant amount of glucose to function, often some of the first symptoms of hypoglycemia are the central nervous system (CNS) manifestations of confusion, irritability, sweating, and so on.

Activity

ANTIDIABETIC AGENTS

The two largest classes of drugs used to treat diabetes mellitus are the insulins and the oral hypoglycemics. These drugs may broadly be referred to as *antidiabetic agents* because they are aimed at preventing the hyperglycemia induced by diabetes mellitus.

INSULINS

The primary treatment for Type 1 diabetes mellitus is insulin therapy. There are currently two main sources of insulin. It can be extracted from domesticated animals or synthesized in laboratories using recombinant DNA technology. The two insulins that come from animal sources are cattle (bovine) insulin, which differs from the human form by only two amino acids, and pig (porcine) insulin, which differs from human insulin by only one amino acid. Recombinantly made insulin is produced by feeding bacteria or yeast the genetic information necessary for them to reproduce an insulin that is exactly like human insulin. The pharmacokinetic properties of exogenous insulin (onset of action, peak effect, and duration of action) have been manipulated so that there are now five different insulin preparations. Several combination preparations are also available. This manipulation of insulin activity was required to help meet the various time-oriented metabolic demands for insulin in diabetic patients. Further modifications can be accomplished by mixing compatible insulin preparations before administration. Regular insulin can be mixed with any insulin preparation. Semilente is compatible with Lente and Ultralente insulin.

Mechanism of Action

Exogenous insulin elicits all the same physiologic responses as those usually elicited by the endogenous hormone and is administered to replace either what is not made or is made defectively.

Drug Effects

The drug effects of exogenously administered insulin are many and affect many body systems. They are the same as those of normal endogenous insulin. That is, exogenously administered insulin restores the diabetic's ability to metabolize carbohydrates, fats, and proteins; to store glucose in the liver; and to convert glycogen to fat.

Therapeutic Uses

As previously discussed, endogenous insulin has many positive effects on several body systems. Its primary therapeutic effect, however, is maintaining normal blood levels of glucose (60 to 120 mg/dl). By causing the appropriate utilization, mobilization, and storage of glucose, exogenous insulin can serve as a replacement for the defective or insufficient natural hormone. Insulin may also be used in patients with Type 2 diabetes. The most common scenarios of when this would be appropriate are when a patient with Type 2 diabetes becomes acutely ill and hospitalized, when he or she cannot take medications by mouth, or when his or her pancreas can no longer produce enough insulin.

30-2 Insulin: Common Adverse Effects

Body System	Side/Adverse Effect
Cardiovascular	Tachycardia, palpitations
Central nervous system	Headache, lethargy, tremors, weakness, fatigue, delirium, sweating
Metabolic	Hypoglycemia
Other	Blurred vision, dry mouth, hunger, nausea, flushing, rash, urticaria, anaphylaxis

Side Effects and Adverse Effects

Hypoglycemia resulting from an insulin overdose can result in shock and possibly death. This is the most immediate and serious adverse effect of insulin. Other more common adverse effects of insulin therapy are listed in Table 30-2.

Interactions

Drug interactions that can occur with the insulins are significant. Chlorthalidone, corticosteroids, diazoxide, epinephrine, ethacrynic acid, furosemide, phenytoin, thiazides, and thyroid hormones can all antagonize the hypoglycemic effects of insulin. Alcohol, anabolic steroids, guanethidine, monoamine oxidase (MAO) inhibitors, propranolol, and the salicylates can all increase insulin's hypoglycemic effects.

Dosages

See the dosages table on p. 473 for the recommended dosages of the various insulin agents.

drug profiles

The primary treatment for Type 1 diabetes mellitus is insulin therapy, and there are three basic types of insulin, as determined by their pharmacokinetic properties—rapid, intermediate, and long acting. They are classified as pregnancy category B agents and are contraindicated in patients who have shown hypersensitivity reactions to them.

rapid-acting insulin

Many rapid-acting insulin products are available, including Humulin, Novolin, Lispro, Iletin, and Velosulin. A Regular and a Semilente insulin come from each of the three main sources: beef, pork, and human. Both the Regular and Semilente forms are considered rapid acting because of their rapid onset of action. Regular insulin is also the only insulin that is clear. All other insulins are cloudy. Their effects are most like those of the endogenous insulin produced from the pancreas in response to a meal. After a meal, the glucose that is ingested stimulates the pancreas to secrete insulin. This insulin then takes

the excess glucose and stores it in the liver as glycogen. In people with diabetes mellitus, the insulin response to meals is deficient, so a rapid-acting insulin product such as Regular or Semilente is used.

All the currently available beef, pork, and human Regular and Semilente insulins are available in a strength of 100 U/ml. Iletin II, from purified pork, also is available in a 500-U/ml strength. The usually recommended doses are given in the dosages table on p. 473. Pregnancy category B.

PHARMACOKINETICS

	ONSET	PEAK	DURATION
Regular:	0.5-1 hr	2-3 hr	8 hr
Semilente:	0.5-1.5 hr	5-10 hr	12-16 hr

intermediate-acting insulin

There are two main types of intermediate-acting insulin products—Lente and Neutral Protamine Hagedorn (NPH insulin). There is an intermediate-acting agent from each of the three main sources: beef, pork, and human. As the experience with the Regular insulins grew, a search was mounted for a longer-acting insulin that would eliminate the need for relatively frequent dosing. It was found that the duration of the effects of insulin could be prolonged through the addition of a basic protein such as protamine or a substance such as zinc. This led to the development in the late 1930s and 1940s of protamine-zinc insulin (PZI) and NPH insulin.

In 1996 the United States Food and Drug Administration (FDA) approved the first new insulin in 14 years called Humalog. Humalog is insulin lispro (rDNA origin) indicated for treatment of diabetes mellitus. It is a new type of insulin that more closely mimics the body's natural rapid insulin output after eating a meal. Insulin lispro is a human insulin analog that is a rapid-acting, parenteral blood glucose-lowering agent. Chemically it is Lys(B28), Pro(B29) human insulin analog, created when the amino acids at positions 28 and 29 on the insulin B-chain are reversed. Insulin lispro is made from a special strain of *Escherichia coli* bacteria. This *E. coli* bacteria strain has been genetically altered to not cause infection, but to make insulin lispro.

Lente insulin is an intermediate-acting insulin that contains zinc, 70% of which is long-acting insulin zinc (Ultralente) and 30% of which is rapid-acting insulin zinc (Semilente). The result is a cloudy insulin solution with a usual onset of action of about 1 to 2.5 hours. NPH insulin, also known as isophane insulin, is a sterile suspension of zinc insulin crystals and protamine sulfate in buffered water for injection. The resulting suspension is a cloudy or milky suspension.

Because of their intermediate onset of action, the effects of these insulins are slower in onset and more

DOSAGES Insulins

agent	pharmacologic class	dosage range	purpose
combination insulins (NPH/regular) (Humulin 70/30*, Humulin 50/50, Mextard 70/30*, Novolin 70/30*)	Rapid/intermediate-acting insulin mixture	SC: Must be individualized to patient's needs	Diabetes
extended insulin zinc (Ultralente, Iletin)	Long-acting insulin zinc suspension	SC: Usual starting dose, 7-26 U 30-60 min before breakfast and adjusted	Diabetes
insulin injection (regular) (Humulin BR, Iletin, Velosulin)	Rapid-acting insulin (unmodified)	SC: Must be individualized to patient's needs	Diabetes and diabetic coma Hypertension
insulin zinc (Lente)	Intermediate-acting insulin zinc suspension	SC: Usual starting dose, 7-26 U 30-60 min before breakfast and adjusted	Diabetes
isophane insulin (NPH) (Humulin N, Iletin NPH, Novolin-N)	Intermediate-acting insulin zinc suspension	SC: Usual starting dose, 7-26 U 30-60 min before breakfast and adjusted	Diabetes
prompt insulin zinc (Semilente)	Rapid-acting insulin zinc suspension	SC: Usual starting dose, 10-20 U bid and adjusted	Diabetes

*In Canada, combination insulins are listed 30/70.

prolonged than those of endogenous insulin. Both of these intermediate-acting insulins area available in a strength of 100 U/ml. The usually recommended dosages are given in the dosages table above. Pregnancy category B.

PHARMACOKINETICS

ONSET	PEAK	DURATION
Lente: 1-2.5 hr	7-15 hr	18-24 hr
Isophane: 1-2 hr	4-12 hr	18-24 hr

long-acting insulin

There is only one type of long-acting insulin product—Ultralente insulin. It is available as both a human and beef insulin in a 100 U/ml strength. Its duration of action was prolonged through the addition of even more zinc, specifically zinc chloride, than that added to create the intermediate-acting insulins.

Ultralente insulin, or extended insulin zinc, is a sterile suspension of insulin in buffered water that is given by injection. The resulting suspension is cloudy or milky. The Ultralente insulins have an onset of action that exceeds 4 hours. Besides being slower in onset, their effects are also more prolonged than those of endogenous insulin. The usually recommended dosages are given in the dosages table above. Pregnancy category B.

PHARMACOKINETICS

ONSET	PEAK	DURATION
4 hr	10-30 hr	36 hr

fixed-combination insulins

Fixed-combination insulins (Humulin 50/50 and 70/30, Mextard 70/30, Novolin 70/30) were developed to more closely simulate the varying levels of endogenous insulin that occur normally in nondiabetic people. To maintain constant blood glucose levels both after and between meals, insulin must be present. In some insulin regimens, patients take a combination of a rapid-acting insulin to deal with the surges in glucose that occur after meals and an intermediate or long-acting insulin for in between meals when the glucose levels are less. However, this requires the mixing of insulins and the use of different types of insulins. Fixed-combination products were developed in an attempt to simplify matters. These agents can more closely simulate the body's own varying levels of insulin.

The fixed-combination insulin products from a human source are available in the following combinations: 50 U of isophane insulin (intermediate-acting) with 50 U of Regular (short-acting) insulin and 70 U of isophane insulin with 30 U of Regular insulin. The fixed-combination insulin product from a pork source contains 70 U of pork isophane insulin and 30 U of Regular pork insulin.

The available insulin products are classified by their source and pharmacokinetic characteristics in Table 30-3. Pregnancy category B.

sliding scale insulin

An important method for dosing insulin is referred to as the *sliding scale method*. With this method,

Available Insulin Products

Table 30-3

Type	Beef	Pork	Human
Rapid-acting			
Regular	Iletin 1*	Iletin II	Humulin R
	Iletin II	Regular Pork	Novolin R
Intermediate-acting			
Lente	Iletin I Lente*	Iletin II Lente	Humulin L
NPH	Lente Beef	Lente Pork	Novolin L
	Iletin I NPH*	Iletin II NPH	Humulin N
	NPH Beef	NPH Pork	Novolin N
		Insulated NPH	
Long-acting			
EZI	Iletin I Ultralente*	—	Humulin U
	Ultralente Beef		
PZI	Semilente	Iletin I Semilente*	—

*PZI, Protamine zinc insulin; EZI, extended zinc insulin.
*Iletin I is a combination of beef and pork regular insulin.

Insulin Mixing Compatibilities

Table 30-4

Insulin Type	Compatible With
Regular	All insulins
Semilente	Regular and Lente
Isophane	Regular only
Lente	Regular and Semilente
Ultralente	Regular and Semilente
Isophane 70% with Regular 30%	Premixed; do not mix with other insulins

subcutaneous Regular insulin doses are adjusted according to blood glucose test results. They are typically used in hospitalized diabetic patients whose insulin requirements may vary drastically because of stress (e.g., infections, surgery, acute illness), inactivity, or variable caloric intake. Sliding scale insulin scales may also be used in Type 1 patients on intensive insulin therapy. When an individual is on a sliding scale insulin regimen, blood glucose concentrations are determined several times a day (e.g., every four hours, every 6 hours, or at specified times: 7 AM, 11 AM, 4 PM, and midnight). This enables one to obtain fasting blood glucose values and values before meals. Subcutaneously administered Regular insulin is then ordered in an amount that increases with the increase in blood glucose. Two examples of sliding scale insulin orders are as follows:

Example One:
• No insulin for a blood glucose less than 200 mg/dl
• 4 U for a blood glucose of 200 to 249 mg/dl
• 6 U for a blood glucose of 250 to 299 mg/dl
• 8 U for a value of 300 mg/dl or greater.

Example Two:
Blood glucose minus 100 divided by 30 equals the number of units of insulin that should be given after every blood glucose determination (divide by 20 when an individual is unstable).

Any reasonable scale and/or dose can be used. The patient's sensitivity to insulin, the severity of the hyperglycemia, and several other factors should be taken into account. When the patient's insulin requirement has stabilized over 2 to 3 days, the number of units required during the last 24 hours is totaled. The patient can then be given any one of several different dosing regimens utilizing intermediate-acting insulins, short-acting insulins, or a combination of the two.

The mixing of insulins with different pharmacokinetic differences has many advantages. A rapid-acting insulin can be mixed in the same syringe with an intermediate-acting or long-acting insulin. Two advantages to this method of mixing insulins are that it reduces the total number of injections the patient must take and it prevents highs and lows in blood glucose levels. To ensure optimal results when mixing insulins, there are a few precautions that should be taken. These precautions are to first ensure compatibility (Table 30-4), withdraw Regular insulin first, and never mix various sources of insulin (e.g., beef, pork, biosynthetic).

The nurse must be aware that the onset of the action of Regular insulin is delayed when mixed with other insulins. This interaction of Regular and NPH insulin occurs within 15 minutes after mixing. This is also true for Regular and Lente mixtures. Regular and Lente mixtures require up to 24 hours for this interaction. Once mixed, these combinations will remain at this stability for 30 days at room temperature and 90 days if refrigerated. Patients stabilized on this premixed insulin combination will have a different response if they inject the two insulins separately.

Activity

Table
30-5

Sulfonylurea Agents

Agent	Potency	Onset of Action	Duration of Action	Active Metabolite
FIRST GENERATION				
chlorpropamide	Low	Slow	Very long	Yes
tolazamide	Low	Slow	Short	Yes
tolbutamide	Low	Fast	Short	Yes
SECOND GENERATION				
glimepiride	High	Fast	Long	No
glipizide	High	Very fast	Short	No
glyburide	High	Intermediate	Long	Yes

ORAL ANTIDIABETIC AGENTS

The treatment of Type 2 diabetes mellitus is a multi-pronged one. Because of the dyslipidemia of Type 2 diabetes mellitus, most (75%) of the patients with it are obese at the time of its initial diagnosis, and the obesity only worsens the insulin resistance. Therefore the initial treatment of Type 2 diabetes mellitus should consist of weight loss and lifestyle changes. The benefits of weight loss are that it lowers not only the blood glucose and lipid levels in these patients, but it also reduces the high blood pressure common in them. The lifestyle changes include stopping smoking, decreasing alcohol consumption, and exercising regularly. The reason why smoking should be stopped is that it doubles the risk of cardiovascular disease in these patients. In fact, stopping smoking would probably save far more lives than antihypertensive or antilipemic drug treatment together!

There is a strong correlation between diabetes mellitus and heart disease. Microvascular problems are now recognized at FPG levels of 126 mg/dl. It is recommended by the American Diabetic Association, the National Institute of Diabetes and Digestive and Kidney Disease, and the Centers for Disease Control and Prevention to test all adults 45 years of older for FPG levels every 3 years. Decreasing alcohol consumption is helpful because alcohol is broken down in the body to simple carbohydrates, which leads to increases in blood glucose. Regular exercise has tremendous benefit in that it increases insulin sensitivity, one of the primary problems in Type 2 diabetes mellitus.

If normal blood glucose levels are not achieved after 2 to 3 months of these dietary and lifestyle modifications, treatment with a sulfonylurea is indicated. However, these agents should never be used in lieu of dietary regulation, but only as a supplement.

The sulfonylureas are a group of oral antidiabetic agents that are able to stimulate insulin secretion from the beta cells of the pancreas. This increased insulin then helps transport the glucose out of the blood and into the tissues, cells, and organs where it is needed. Because of these actions, the sulfonylureas may also be broadly considered oral hypoglycemic agents. These agents have many other beneficial effects besides their ability to stimulate insulin release from the pancreas. They may also enhance the actions of insulin in muscle, liver, and adipose tissue, allowing these tissues to take up and store glucose more easily as a later source of energy. They may also increase the availability of insulin by preventing the liver from breaking it down as fast as it ordinarily would (reduced hepatic clearance). In summary, the overall effect of the sulfonylureas is that they improve both insulin secretion and the sensitivity to insulin in tissues. Repaglinide (Prandin) is structurally different from the sulfonylureas but shares a similar mechanism of action with the sulfonylureas. It also increases insulin secretion.

The sulfonylureas have been the backbone of the oral pharmacologic therapy for Type 2 diabetes mellitus for more than 30 years. Because their primary beneficial effect in patients with Type 2 diabetes mellitus is that they stimulate insulin secretion from beta cells in the pancreas, for them to work there must be functioning beta cells to stimulate. Thus these drugs work best during the early stages of the disease when there is preserved beta cell function. The commonly used sulfonylurea drugs are listed in Table 30-5.

Three new drug categories have recently emerged for the oral treatment of Type 2 diabetes mellitus. Late in 1994 metformin, a drug that had been used abroad since the 1950s, was approved for use in the United States. Metformin (Glucophage) belongs to a group of oral drugs used to treat Type 2 diabetes mellitus called *biguanides.* Metformin differs significantly from the sulfonylureas in that it does not increase insulin secretion from the pancreas and thus does not cause hypoglycemia. The biguanide metformin works by decreasing the production of glucose as well as increasing its uptake. The *alpha-glucosidase* inhibitors were next to become available. Acarbose (Precose) and miglitol (Glyset) are two oral agents that are alpha-glucosidase inhibitors. They are indicated for the management of hyperglycemia secondary to Type 2 diabetes mellitus. The third new drug category to emerge for the oral treatment of Type 2 diabetes mellitus is the *thiazolidinediones.* The first agent for use in the United States was troglitazone (Rezulin). It has recently been removed from the market over concerns of liver toxicity. The two newest thiazolidinediones are pioglitazone and rosiglitazone. They offer efficacy similar to that of troglitazone with less risk of toxicity. These agents work by decreasing insulin resistance. They may also be referred to as *insulin-sensitizing agents.* They are known to directly stimulate peripheral glucose uptake and storage as well as inhibit glucose and triglyceride production in the liver.

Activity

Mechanism of Action

As previously noted, sulfonylurea compounds exert their antidiabetic activity by stimulating the beta cells of the pancreas to secrete insulin. In patients with Type 2 diabetes mellitus this forces the extra glucose out of the blood (where it does all its harm) and into cells, tissues, and organs (where it can be used as energy or stored as fuel). The sulfonylurea compounds also increase the sensitivity of the cells of the muscles, liver, and fat to the effects of insulin. Repaglinide also increases insulin secretion from the pancreas, but it does this by binding to ATP-sensitive potassium channels on pancreatic beta cells.

The biguanide metformin is believed to exert its beneficial effects in Type 2 diabetes mellitus via three mechanisms: decreases glucose production by the liver; decreases intestinal absorption of glucose, and improves insulin sensitivity. It improves insulin sensitivity by increasing peripheral glucose uptake and utilization. Unlike sulfonylureas, glucophage does not produce hypoglycemia.

Alpha-glucosidase inhibitors work by reversibly inhibiting an enzyme called alpha-glucosidase. This enzyme is found in the brush border of the small intestine. Alpha-glucosidase is responsible for the hydrolysis of oligosaccharides and disaccharides to glucose and other monosaccharides. By blocking this enzyme, glucose absorption is delayed. The timing of administration of the alpha-glucosidase inhibitors is important. The beneficial effects of these agents are seen when they can blunt blood glucose elevations that are common after ingestion of food. By taking an alpha-glucosidase inhibitor with meals, this elevation can be blunted.

Thiazolidinediones, also known as *glitazones,* work by decreasing insulin resistance by making insulin receptors in such areas as the liver, skeletal muscle, and adipose tissue more sensitive to the effects of insulin. This results in enhanced glucose uptake and storage. Glitazones work at two of the primary sites in the body that are abnormal in patients with Type 2 diabetes mellitus: the liver and the skeletal muscle. In the presence of endogenous or exogenous insulin, glitazones decrease gluconeogenesis, glucose output, and triglyceride synthesis in the liver. They increase glucose uptake and utilization in skeletal muscle, and they increase glucose uptake and decrease fatty acid output in adipose tissue. It has no known effect on insulin secretion.

Drug Effects

The primary drug effects of sulfonylurea compounds are on the pancreas. Here, as previously mentioned, they stimulate the secretion of insulin from the beta cells. In addition, by enhancing the actions of insulin on muscle, liver, and adipose tissue, they cause these tissues to take up and store glucose more easily. This is of benefit in those cases of Type 2 diabetes mellitus in which there is plenty of insulin to transport the glucose out of the blood and into the tissues. However, the tissues are not sensitive to the effects of insulin and therefore do not accept the glucose. By preventing the liver from breaking insulin down, they also cause more insulin to be available.

The drug effects of metformin involve the liver, the intestine, skeletal muscle, and adipose tissue. Metformin decreases hepatic glucose production and the production of triglycerides and cholesterol from the liver. The liver, skeletal muscle, and adipose tissue become more sensitive to the effects of insulin in the presence of metformin. Metformin also affects the intestines by decreasing the absorption of glucose.

The alpha-glucosidase inhibitors acarbose and miglitol primarily affect the small intestine and the pancreas. These agents inhibit the enzyme alpha-amylase found in the pancreas. They also inhibit another enzyme found in the lumen of the small intestine. This enzyme is known as *alpha-glucoside hydrolase.*

The drug effects of the glitazones involve the liver, skeletal muscle, and adipose tissue. In the liver, the glitazones decrease gluconeogenesis, glucose output, and triglyceride synthesis. At the level of the skeletal muscle, the glitazones increase the rate of glucose uptake and utilization. The glitazones also effect adipose tissue by increasing glucose uptake and decreasing fatty acid output.

Therapeutic Uses

Sulfonylurea drugs are used to lower the blood glucose levels in patients when diet and lifestyle changes have failed to do so, although beta cell function must be preserved for this to happen.

The biguanide metformin and the alpha-glucosidase inhibitors are indicated as monotherapy in patients with Type 2 diabetes mellitus. They are indicated as an adjunct to a diet to lower blood glucose when hyperglycemia cannot be satisfactorily managed on diet alone. Metformin may be used concomitantly with a sulfonylurea when diet and glucophage or a sulfonylurea alone does not result in adequate glycemic control. This is true for alpha-glucosidase inhibitors as well. The glitazones are most commonly used alone or with a sulfonylurea, metformin, or insulin in patients with Type 2 diabetes mellitus.

Side Effects and Adverse Effects

The most serious adverse effects of sulfonylureas involve the hematologic system and include agranulocytosis, hemolytic anemia, thrombocytopenia, and cholestatic jaundice. Effects on the gastrointestinal system include nausea, epigastric fullness, and heartburn. Erythrema, photosensitivity, hypoglycemia, and morbilliform and maculopapular eruptions are other undesirable effects.

The biguanide metformin primarily affects the gastrointestinal tract. The most common side effects of therapy with metformin are abdominal bloating, nausea, cramping, a feeling of fullness, and diarrhea. These all are usually self-limiting, transient, and can be lessened by starting with low doses, titrating up slowly, and taking the medication with food. Less common side effects with metformin are metallic taste and reduction in vitamin B_{12} levels. Lactic acidosis is extremely rare with metformin and is lethal in 50% of the cases. Unlike sulfonylureas, metformin does not cause hypoglycemia.

The alpha-glucosidase inhibitors acarbose and miglitol also have side effects that primarily involve the gastrointestinal tract. They can cause flatulence, diarrhea, and abdominal pain. At high doses they may also elevate hepatic enzymes (transaminases). Unlike sulfonylureas they do not cause hypoglycemia, hyperinsulinemia, or weight gain.

Rosiglitazone and pioglitazone both may cause moderate weight gain, edema, and mild anemia, possibly as a result of fluid retention. The safe use of the glitazones during pregnancy, in children, and in patients with CHF has not been established. There is concern that hepatic toxicity may be a class effect of glitazones. For this reason the glitazones' package insert advises measuring ALT before beginning treatment, every 2 months for 1 year, and periodically thereafter.

Interactions

The potential drug interactions that can occur with sulfonylureas are significant. Their hypoglycemic effect is increased when taken concurrently with alcohol, anabolic steroids, beta-blockers, chloramphenicol, guanethidine, MAO inhibitors, oral anticogulants, phenylbutazone, and sulfonamides.

Drugs that are capable of reducing the hypoglycemic effect of sulfonylureas include adrenergics, corticosteroids, thiazides, and thyroid preparations. Metformin concentrations can be increased when it is concomitantly given with furosemide and nifedipine. When it is given with cationic drugs such as cimetidine or digoxin, competition for renal tubular secretion occurs, resulting in increased metformin concentrations. Alpha-glucosidase inhibitors potentially interact with intestinal adsorbents (e.g., charcoal) and digestive enzyme preparations containing carbohydrase-splitting enzymes (e.g., amylase, pancreatin). When these drugs are concomitantly administered with an alpha-glucosidase inhibitor they may reduce the effect of them. Clinically important interactions between rosiglitazone and other drugs have not been reported. LDL and HDL cholesterol increased between 12% and 19% in individuals taking rosiglitazone, and triglyceride levels may actually decrease. Pioglitazone, on the other hand, is partly metabolized by CYP3A4. Serum concentrations of pioglitazone may be increased if taken concurrently with a 3A4 inhibitor such as ketoconazole. However, pioglitazone raises LDL cholesterol only slightly and lowers serum triglyceride concentrations.

Dosages

For the recommended dosages of oral antidiabetic agents, see the dosages table on p. 478.

drug profiles

Over the past 5 years several new oral agents have been approved for the treatment of Type 2 diabetes mellitus. Sulfonylurea drugs are the oldest class of these agents.

There are two classes, or generations, of sulfonylurea drugs. The first-generation sulfonylureas are the older, low-potency drugs acetohexamide, tolbutamide, chlorpropamide, and tolazamide. The second-generation sulfonylureas are the newer, high-potency drugs glyburide and glipizide.

The agents glyburide, glipizide, and chlorpropamide are by far the most prescribed of the sulfonylurea compounds. The newest sulfonylurea compound, approved in 1995, is glimepiride (Amaryl). There are also several new drug categories of oral agents used to patients with Type 2 diabetes mellitus. The biguanides, alpha-glucosidase inhibitors, and thiazolidinediones are three of these new drug categories. Currently the only biguanide used in the United States is metformin (Glucophage). There are two currently available alpha-glucosidase inhibitors, acarbose (Precose) and miglitol (Glyset). The newest drug class to treat patients with Type 2 diabetes mellitus are the thiazolidinediones. Ciglitazone, englitazone, pioglitazone, and troglitazone all belong to this class of agents. Currently rosiglitazone and pioglitazone are the only glitazones available.

chlorpropamide

Chlorpropamide (Diabinese) is a first-generation sulfonylurea agent that is structurally similar to the other first-generation agents acetohexamide, tolazamide, and tolbutamide and is the most commonly used of the first-generation agents. It differs from the other first-generation agents in that it has a very long duration of action. The chlorpropamide-induced decrease in the blood glucose level may be prolonged in patients with decreased renal function because the drug is dependent on the kidneys for elimination. Like the other first-generation agents, it has active metabolites that can accumulate if they are not eliminated by the kidneys, resulting in a prolongation of their effects and possible toxicity. This would be manifested by hypoglycemia.

Chlorpropamide is classified as a pregnancy category D drug and is contraindicated in patients with a known hypersensitivity to sulfonylureas, patients with juvenile or brittle diabetes, or patients experiencing renal failure. Profound flushing of the skin and in particular the face occurs if it is taken with alcohol. Although this can occur with any of the sulfonylurea compounds, it is most prominent with chlorpropamide use and is called the *chlorpropamide-alcohol flush*. Facial temperature can also increase. Chlorpropamide is available orally as a 100- and

DOSAGES Selected Oral Antidiabetic Agents

agent	pharmacologic class	dosage range	purpose
acarbose (Precose)	Alpha-glucosidase inhibitor	*Adult* PO: 25-100 mg three times a day with first bite of meal	Type 2 diabetes mellitus
chlorpropamide (Diabinese)	1st-generation sulfonylurea (oral hypoglycemic)	*Adult* PO: 100-500 mg/day as a single dose	Type 2 diabetes mellitus
glipizide (Glucotrol, Glucotrol XL)	2nd-generation sulfonylurea (oral hypoglycemic)	*Adult* PO: 2.5-5.0 mg/day up to 40 mg/day max	Type 2 diabetes mellitus
glyburide (DiaBeta, Micronase, Glynase Prestab)	2nd-generation sulfonylurea (oral hypoglycemic)	*Adult* PO: 1.25-20 mg/day as a single dose	Type 2 diabetes mellitus
metformin (Glucophage)	Biguanide	*Adult* PO: 500-2500 mg as a single or twice daily dose	Type 2 diabetes mellitus
rosiglitazone (Avandia)	Glitazones	*Adult* PO: 4 to 8 mg once or 2 to 4 mg bid	Type 2 diabetes mellitus

250-mg tablet. Common dosages are listed in the dosages table above.

PHARMACOKINETICS

HALF-LIFE	ONSET	PEAK	DURATION
24-48 hr	1 hr	3-6 hr	60 hr

glipizide

Glipizide (Glucotrol, Glucotrol XL) is a second-generation sulfonylurea agent with a potency much greater than that of the first-generation agents. This explains why the common doses of glipizide are 5 and 10 mg compared with the 100- to 500-mg doses of the first-generation agents. In contrast to the other second-generation agent glyburide, glipizide has a very rapid onset and short duration of action with no active metabolites. This confers many benefits. The rapid onset of action allows it to function much like the body's normal response to meals when greater levels of insulin are rapidly required to deal with the increased glucose in the blood. When a patient with Type 2 diabetes mellitus takes glipizide, it rapidly stimulates the pancreas to release insulin and transport the extra glucose in the blood to the muscles, liver, and adipose tissues.

Its short duration of action compared with that of glyburide prevents the long-term stimulation of the beta cells in the pancreas, which may otherwise cause the beta cells to become resistant to the effects of the sulfonylurea agents. It may also cause them to make too much insulin, thereby inducing hyperinsulinemia, which can cause the muscle, liver, and fat tissues to become resistant to the effects of insulin. Glipizide also does not have any active metabolites.

Glipizide is a pregnancy category C drug that has the same contraindications as chlorpropamide, except that it is not contraindicated in patients with renal failure. It works best if given 30 minutes before meals. This allows the timing of the insulin secretion induced by the glipizide to correspond to the elevation in the blood glucose level induced by the meal in much the same way as the endogenous levels are raised in a person without diabetes. It is only available orally as 5- and 10-mg regular-release and extended-release (XL) tablets. Common dosages are listed in the dosages table above.

PHARMACOKINETICS

HALF-LIFE	ONSET	PEAK	DURATION
2-4 hr	1-1.5 hr	1-3 hr	10-24 hr

glyburide

Glyburide (DiaBeta, Micronase, Glynase Prestab) is the other second-generation sulfonylurea drug. It differs from the first-generation oral hypoglycemic agents in its greater potency and from glipizide in its slower onset and longer duration of action and the fact that it has active metabolites. These differences can have significant consequences. Because of its relatively slow onset of action, glyburide is less desirable for the treatment of the short-term elevations in the blood glucose levels that occur after meals. However, its longer duration of action make it better for the long-term, constant stimulation of the pancreas, causing it to release a constant amount of insulin. This may be beneficial in controlling blood glucose levels during the night and/or throughout the day. Because of the varying glucose levels, it is possible and therefore rational to use glipizide and glyburide together, with glyburide dosed either in the morning or in the morning and the evening to control the blood glucose levels throughout the day or evening, and with glipizide dosed 30 minutes before meals to deal with the elevations in the blood glucose levels after meals.

Glyburide is a pregnancy category B drug with the same contraindications as those for glipizide. It is only available orally as 1.25-, 2.5-, and 5-mg tablets. Also available as 1.5-, 3-, 4.5-, and 6-mg micronized tablets (Glynase Pres-Tab). Common dosages are listed in the dosages table on p. 478.

PHARMACOKINETICS

HALF-LIFE*	ONSET	PEAK	DURATION
2-4 hr	1-1.5 hr	4 hr	20-24 hr

*When assays have been performed to measure the metabolite levels, the terminal elimination half-life has been found to average 10 hours.

metformin

Metformin (Glucophage) is a biguanide, oral antidiabetic agent. It works primarily by inhibiting hepatic glucose production and increasing sensitivity of peripheral tissue to insulin. Because of its different mechanism of action from sulfonylurea agents, it may be given concomitantly with sulfonylurea agents.

Metformin is a pregnancy category B drug and is contraindicated in patients with a hypersensitivity to biguanides, hepatic or renal disease, alcoholism, and cardiopulmonary disease. It is only available orally as 500-, 850-, and 1000-mg tablets. Common dosages are listed in the dosages table on p. 478.

PHARMACOKINETICS

HALF-LIFE	ONSET	PEAK	DURATION
1.5-5 hr	<1 hr	1-3 hr	24 hr

acarbose

Acarbose (Precose) is one of the two currently available alpha-glucosidase inhibitors. The other agent in this drug category is miglitol (Glyset). These agents work by blunting elevated blood sugar levels after a meal. To optimally work, it is taken with the first bite of each meal. It too may be taken concomitantly with sulfonylurea agents or with metformin.

Acarbose is a pregnancy category B drug and contraindicated in patients with a hypersensitivity to alpha-glucosidase inhibitors, diabetic ketoacidosis, cirrhosis, inflammatory bowel disease, colonic ulceration, partial intestinal obstruction, or chronic intestinal disease. It is only available orally as 50- and 100-mg tablets. Common dosages are listed in dosages table on p. 478.

PHARMACOKINETICS

HALF-LIFE	ONSET	PEAK	DURATION
2-3 hr	1-1.5 hr	14-24 hr	9-15 hr

rosiglitazone

Rosiglitazone (Avandia) is classified as a "glitazone" or thiazolidinedione derivative. It is marketed for the treatment of patients with Type 2 diabetes. Rosiglitazone and pioglitazone are used alone or with a sulfonylurea, metformin, or insulin. Glitazone antidiabetic agents work by decreasing insulin resistance.

The safe use of glitazones during pregnancy, in children, and in patients with CHF has not been established. Thre is concern that hepatic toxicity may be a class effect of glitazones. For this reason the glitazones' package insert advises measuring ALT before beginning treatment, every 2 months for 1 year and periodically thereafter. Rosiglitazone is available as a 2-, 4-, and 8-mg unscored tablet. It is classified as a pregnancy category C agent. Recommended dosages are given in the dosage table on p. 478.

PHARMACOKINETICS

HALF-LIFE	ONSET	PEAK	DURATION
3-4 hr	Unknown	1 hr	Unknown

Activity

GLUCOSE-ELEVATING DRUGS

Two drugs are used for the treatment of hypoglycemia. Glucagon, a natural hormone secreted by the pancreas, has also been synthesized in the laboratory and is now available as a tablet to be given when a quick response to hypoglycemia is needed. Diazoxide is another agent that may be given to correct abnormally low blood glucose levels. It works by inhibiting the release of insulin from the pancreas and is most commonly given to patients with long-term illnesses that are causing hypoglycemia. An example of such an illness is pancreatic cancers that cause the pancreas to oversecrete insulin, resulting in too much insulin in the blood, or hyperinsulinemia. The oral form of diazoxide is used for the treatment of hypoglycemia. The IV form is used for the treatment of hypertensive emergencies (very high blood pressures).

nursing process

● Assessment

Before administering any type of insulin, it is important to question patients about allergies they may have to insulin, beef, or pork and whether they are taking drugs that interact with insulin. Those that produce a greater hypoglycemic effect include alcohol, steroids, oral hypoglycemic agents, and MAO inhibitors. The use of insulin with thyroid hormones, oral contraceptives, and steroids results in a decreased hypoglycemic effect. Lispro is contraindicated in patients with episodes of hypoglycemia or allergies to the product.

Oral antidiabetic agents are contraindicated in patients with allergies to the medication proper or to the sulfonylureas in general. The oral agents are also contraindicated in the treatment of juvenile-onset diabetes because these patients have no functioning beta cells in the pancreas, which is where the oral agents work. The oral agents should be administered with caution to elderly patients or to anyone with cardiac, renal, hepatic, or thyroid disease. Drugs that interact with them include warfarin sodium, aspirin, digoxin, insulin, diuretics, beta-blockers, calcium channel blockers, corticosteroids, phenobarbital, and phenytoin, to name just a few. Because of the many drugs with which oral antidiabetic agents interact, it is crucial for the nurse to check what other medications a patient who is to receive an oral antidiabetic is also taking.

With acarbose, miglitol, and other related oral hypoglycemics, overdosage of the agent may not necessarily cause hypoglycemia. However, it may lead to GI symptoms requiring medical treatment, so be cautious with those individuals who have a history of GI disorders. Drug interactions of acarbose and miglitol include the drugs that are generally listed as interacting with oral hypoglycemics (such as corticosteroids and thiazide diuretics) and intestinal adsorbents. With glitazones, such as rosiglitazone, safe use during pregnancy, in children, and in patients with CHF has not been established. There is concern that hepatic toxicity may be a class effect of glitazones. Therefore their package insert advises measuring ALT before beginning treatment, every 2 months for 1 year, and periodically thereafter.

With metformin, there are several drug interactions for which to assess before administering the agent. Cimetidine may increase metformin levels and anticoagulant levels may be decreased if oral anticoagulants are given concurrently with metformin. If patients taking metformin need a procedure performed with contrast media (such as with an angiogram) there may be increased risk for renal dysfunction, therefore the metformin should be discontinued just before the procedure and restarted as ordered only after renal function has been reevaluated.

Questions about the patient's medical history are important in determining whether the patient's diabetes is well controlled or whether there are problems with polyuria, polydipsia, polyphagia, weight loss, visual changes, and fatigue. The nurse should ask about problems with hypoglycemia such as the acute onset of nervousness, sweating, lethargy, weakness, cold and clammy skin, and a change in sensorium. Symptoms of hyperglycemia include tachycardia, blood glucose levels that exceed 150 mg/dl, and a change in respiration (Kussmaul's).

Before administering any glucose elevating drug, a thorough history should be obtained and documented. Baseline vital signs and blood glucose levels as well as the patient's sensorium should also be documented.

Nursing Diagnoses

Nursing diagnoses in patients receiving antidiabetic agents include the following:
- Risk for injury related to changes in sensorium and the pathophysiologic impact of diabetes.
- Risk for infection related to diabetes.
- Imbalanced nutrition, more than body requirements, related to the disease process.
- Deficient knowledge related to diabetes mellitus, its management, and the prevention of its complications.
- Ineffective management of therapeutic regimen related to lack of experience with diabetic treatment regimen.

Planning

Goals in patients receiving antidiabetic agents include the following:
- Patient remains free of self-injury and complications of diabetes.
- Patient remains free from infection.
- Patient maintains adequate weight control and dietary habits in the overall management of diabetes.
- Patient states the effects of diabetes on body function.
- Patient remains compliant with the medical regimen.
- Patient states the importance of compliance to medication regimens, lifestyle changes, dietary restrictions, and high-risk behaviors.
- Patient states the action and side effects of insulin or the oral hypoglycemic agents.

Outcome Criteria

Outcome criteria in patients receiving antidiabetic agents include the following:
- Patient will perform self-assessment and foot care as directed and as needed to maintain healthy skin.
- Patient will immediately report elevated temperature, difficult-to-heal lesions or sores, and any unusual redness of an area to their health care provider.

- Patient will observe the diet recommended by the American Diabetic Association or other dietary consultant per the physician's orders or nutritional consult.
- Patient will eat a healthy diet, get sufficient rest and relaxation, and notify the physician should any unusual problems occur with changes in usual activity (problems such as nausea and vomiting).
- Patient will keep all scheduled appointments with health care providers to monitor therapeutic effectiveness or for complications of therapy.
- Patient will take medication as scheduled, monitor blood glucose levels, and watch for any signs and symptoms of hyperglycemia or hypoglycemia.

● Implementation

In any patient who is to receive insulin or the oral antidiabetic agents, it is critical to always check the blood glucose levels before administering the agent so that there is an accurate baseline reading. Always check the order at least three times before administering the medication and always have another registered nurse check the injection you prepare to make sure it is in accordance with the physician's order. Roll the vial, do not shake it, before withdrawing the medication. Insulin may be stored at room temperature if it is to be used within 1 month, otherwise it needs to be refrigerated. Never use insulin that is discolored or past its expiration date. Administer the insulin subcutaneously and at a 90-degree angle, unless the patient is emaciated. Only Regular insulin can be administered intravenously. A 25- to 28-gauge needle should be used, and always use an insulin syringe, which is calibrated in units. If mixing insulins, always withdraw the Regular or rapid-acting (unmodified) insulin first and then the intermediate-acting or NPH (modified) insulin.

When administering SQ insulin lispro it is important to remember that it is absorbed more rapidly than Regular insulin with a peak effect of 30 to 90 minutes. It is also important to remember that lispro must be given 15 minutes before meals versus 30 to 60 minutes before meals with Regular insulin. This is a very important point to remember in the administration of lispro. Lispro mixtures with Humulin N or Humulin U should be given 15 minutes before meals and immediately after mixing of the agents. A good rule of thumb to remember about lispro is that 1 Unit of lispro has the same glucose lowering effect as 1 Unit of Regular insulin; however, the effect with lispro is a more rapid onset and shorter duration of action. The physician may also order an increase in carbohydrates and a decrease in high fat intake to avoid postprandial hypoglycemia.

Insulin is usually given about 15 to 30 minutes before meals, so be sure that the meal trays are either on their way to the unit or are already there. Oral antidiabetic agents should be administered at least 30 minutes before meals.

Metformin should be taken with meals to minimize nausea or diarrhea. With metformin, it is important (as with any antidiabetic agent or insulin) to know what to do if symptoms of hypoglycemia occur, such as using glucagon; eating glucose tablets or gel, corn syrup, or honey; drinking fruit juice or nondiet soft drink; or eating a small snack such as crackers or half of a sandwich. Rosiglitazone and pioglitazone may both cause moderate weight gain, edema, and mild anemia. Therefore during therapy the patient needs to monitor and record his or her weight and have regular follow-up appointments with the physician or health care provider. All of the oral agents are to be taken exactly as prescribed. For rosiglitazone, the dosage is 4 to 8 mg once daily, or 2 to 4 mg bid for the Type 2 diabetic. For more information to share with your patients, you can just type in the drug name in a search engine on the Internet. Searching under the drug manufacturer's name may also be helpful. In addition, a helpful Internet site to share with patients is www.usp.org, where many conditions, diseases, and treatment modalities are discussed.

With oral antidiabetic agents, when a patient is NPO (nothing by mouth) and hospitalized, the physician should be contacted for any further orders. The physician should also be contacted when a patient becomes ill at home and unable to take the usual dosage of oral agent. Patients on oral agents or insulin should also be encouraged to have a MedicAlert bracelet or ID band.

Patients taking insulin injections should be instructed to rotate sites within the same location for about 1 week (so that all injections would be rotated in one area, such as the right arm, before rotating to a new location, such as the abdomen) but at least ½ to 1 inch away from the previous site. Some practitioners may recommend only using the abdomen because of more complete absorption.

Patient education is crucial to ensure the safe and effective use of the antidiabetic agents. Patient teaching tips for these agents are listed in the box on p. 482.

● Evaluation

A therapeutic response to any of the antidiabetic agents includes a decrease in the blood glucose levels to the level prescribed by the physician, one at which the patient is free of the symptoms of hyperglycemia and hypoglycemia. Patients with diabetes need to be monitored to make sure they are complying with therapy, and the nurse also needs to watch for the manifestations of hypoglycemia or hyperglycemia. An insulin allergy is manifested by local swelling, itching, and redness at the injection site.

With insulin lispro, since the onset is more rapid than with Regular insulin and there is a shorter duration of action, it is crucial to monitor and have the patient monitor the blood glucose level more closely until the dosage is regulated and blood glucose is at the level the physician desires. Should patients be switched from Regular insulin to lispro, once again, it is important to monitor glucose levels closely.

With metformin, side effects for which to monitor include a metallic taste, epigastric discomfort, weight loss, nausea, vomiting, or diarrhea. Evaluate the patient for lactic acidosis. Therapeutic effects would include better control of blood glucose levels.

A therapeutic response to glucose-elevating drugs includes elevation of blood glucose levels to within normal limits (fasting blood sugar >60, <120, or a level designated by the physician).

Activity

patient teaching tips

Insulin and Antidiabetic Agents

➤ Patients need to have a thorough understanding of their type of diabetes and its specific management, including special diets and exercise, as ordered by the physician. Provide the patient with any available literature, pamphlets, and videos on diabetes. The American Diabetic Association can also provide the patient with information on diabetes and other resources available.

➤ Patients should always carry an identification card and wear a MedicAlert bracelet or necklace that identifies them as diabetics, and also carry a supply of readily available sugar.

➤ Patients should know the signs and symptoms of hyperglycemia, such as an increased pulse rate, abnormal breathing, and a fruity, acetone odor to their breath.

➤ Patients should know the signs and symptoms of hypoglycemia, such as weakness, nervousness, cold and clammy skin, sweating, paleness of the skin, and shallow, rapid breathing. The physician or health care provider should be notified if any of these symptoms occur!

➤ Patients taking oral antidiabetic agents should know how to measure their blood glucose level with a glucometer and perform this as ordered by their physician.

➤ Patients should notify their physician should they note yellow discoloration of the skin, dark urine, fever, sore throat, weakness or any unusual bleeding, or easy bruising.

➤ Patients taking insulin should always carry an extra supply of medication, syringes, needles, and alcohol or antiseptic swabs when traveling.

➤ Diabetics are very sensitive to changes in blood glucose levels when they are ill, have an infection, are vomiting or not able to eat, or under stress. If any of these conditions occur, patients may require a change in their diabetic treatment. They should therefore notify their physician should any of these illnesses or stressors occur.

➤ Diabetic patients should avoid consuming alcohol because it will make their blood glucose level drop, causing them to become very ill.

➤ There are many drug interactions that patients should be educated about when taking insulin or an antidiabetic agent.

➤ Always educate patients regarding the drug interactions for oral hypoglycemics and insulin.

POINTS TO REMEMBER

Antidiabetic Agents

- Drugs that affect the pancreas (insulin and oral hypoglycemics).
- Insulin takes glucose from the blood and puts it in the liver to be stored.
- Oral hypoglycemics stimulate insulin secretion from the beta cells of the pancreas as well as enhance insulin's effectiveness.

Glucagon

- The second hormone secreted by the pancreas.
- Responsible for initiating glycogenolysis.
- Glycogenolysis opposes the action of insulin; it increases the blood glucose level.

Glycogen

- The storage form of glucose.
- Most is stored in the liver.
- Broken down by the synergistic actions of glucagon, cortisol, and epinephrine.

Types of Diabetes

- Type 1 diabetes mellitus:
  - Also known as insulin-dependent diabetes (IDDM) or juvenile-onset diabetes.
  - Little or no endogenous insulin produced.

  - Much less common—about 10% of all diabetics.
  - Patients are usually nonobese.
- Type 2 diabetes mellitus:
  - Also known as non–insulin-dependent diabetes (NIDDM) or adult-onset diabetes.
  - Insulin secretion is usually normal.
  - Much more common—about 90% of all diabetics.
  - 80% of patients are obese.

Complications Associated with Diabetes

- Retinopathy, neuropathy, nephropathy.
- Severe complication of uncontrolled diabetes is diabetic ketoacidosis (DKA).
- DKA is due to the body utilizing other sources of energy besides glucose, such as fatty acids.
- Fatty acids are broken down into ketones, which leads to acidosis.

Nursing Considerations

- Always check for allergies to specific medications and to beef and pork insulins before initiating therapy.
- Correct diet is an important component of the entire medical treatment regimen for a diabetic.
- Patients need to learn about their disease and the type of insulin they are taking—its onset of action, peak effect, and duration of action, as well as the im-

portance of always having a rapidly active form of sugar available.
- Patients also need to learn the signs and symptoms of hypoglycemia and hyperglycemia and the methods of treating it at home, as well as when to contact their physician.

- Foot care and the prevention of infection should be part of the patient education given to diabetics.
- Drug interactions for Rezulin include birth control pills and may reduce their efficacy as much as 30%.

REVIEW QUESTIONS

1. Which of the following statements is true about Humulin NPH?
   a. It is a rapid-acting insulin.
   b. It is an interemediate-acting insulin.
   c. There are no reactions associated with this synthetic insulin.
   d. There are no problems with hypoglycemia with these forms of insulin.
2. Which of the following is important to include in the patient teaching for patients taking insulin or any oral hypoglycemic agents?
   a. Oral agents may be used with Type 1 diabetes.
   b. Insulin is only indicated for adult-onset diabetes.
   c. Alcohol consumed with the oral agents may cause an antabuse reaction.
   d. If mixing insulins, one should draw up the intermediate before the rapid.
3. A therapeutic response to glucose-elevating drugs would result in what type of results?
   a. Glucose readings of about 30 mg/dl
   b. Glucose readings of about 50 mg/dl

   c. Elevation of glucose to over 350 or 400 mg/dl
   d. Elevation of glucose to between 60 and 200 mg/dl
4. One of the preoperative same-day surgery patients is a Type 2 diabetic. She is NPO and has not eaten since approximately 9:00 PM the previous night. What would be your most appropriate intervention regarding the administration of her oral hypoglycemic medication that she takes twice daily?
   a. Hold all medications until after surgery.
   b. Administer a small dose of insulin instead.
   c. Contact her physician regarding any further orders.
   d. Administer the medication with 30 ml of fluids.
5. When is the best time for an elderly patient to take an oral hypoglycemic agent?
   a. At bedtime
   b. Before lunch
   c. In the morning before breakfast
   d. With the oral agents, the time of day is not of concern

For Answers see www.harcourthealth.com/MERLIN/Lilley/.

CRITICAL THINKING Activities

1. Type 1 diabetes mellitus has recently been diagnosed in a 240-pound, 45-year-old woman. When she is admitted to your unit for additional testing and control of her diabetes, she is placed on a 1500-calorie diabetic diet and on 30 U of NPH insulin to be given every day at 7:30 AM. At 4 PM on the first day of therapy she becomes diaphoretic, weak, and pale. How would you explain these symptoms to this patient?

2. Which of the following substances would eliminate the polydipsia, polyuria, and a low specific gravity of urine in a diabetic: insulin, glucagon, ADH, or aldosterone? Explain your answer.
3. What actions would be necessary in the nursing care of the Type 1 diabetes mellitus patient who is NPO for surgery but with orders for the usual AM (before breakfast) Regular and NPH insulin? Explain your answer.

For Answers see www.harcourthealth.com/MERLIN/Lilley/.

bibliography

Albanese J, Nutz P: *Mosby's 2001 nursing drug reference and review cards*, St Louis, 2001, Mosby.
American Hospital Formulary Service: *AHFS drug information*, Bethesda, Md, 2000, American Society of Health-System Pharmacists.
Anderson PO, Knoben JE, Troutman WG: *Handbook of clinical drug data 1999-2000*, ed 9, New York, 1999, McGraw-Hill.
Bliss M: The history of insulin, *Diabetes Care* 16[suppl 3]:4, 1993.

Johns Hopkins Hospital, Department of Pediatrics et al: *The Harriet Lane handbook*, ed 15, St Louis, 2000, Mosby.
Keen JH: *Critical care and emergency drug reference*, ed 3, St Louis, 1996, Mosby.
Lilley LL, Guanci R: Mederrors: know your antidiabetic agents, *Am J Nurs* 97(1):19, 1997.
McKenry LM, Salerno E: *Mosby's pharmacology in nursing*, ed 21, St Louis, 2001, Mosby.

Medical Letter: Miglitol for type 2 diabetes mellitus 41(1053):49, May 21, 1999.

Medical Letter: Pioglitazone (Actos) 41(1066):112, November 19, 1999.

Medical Letter: Repaglinide for type 2 diabetes mellitus 40(1027):55, May 22, 1998.

Medical Letter: Rosiglitazone for type 2 diabetes mellitus 41(1059):71, August 13, 1999.

Medical Letter: Troglitazone for non-insulin-dependent diabetes mellitus 39(1001):49, 1997.

Mosby's GenRx: a comprehensive reference for generic and brand drugs, ed 10, St Louis, 2000, Mosby.

Saleil AR, Olefsky JM: Thiazolidinediones in the treatment of insulin resistance and Type II diabetes, *Diabetes* 45:1661, 1996.

Skidmore-Roth L: *Mosby's 2001 nursing drug reference,* St Louis, 2001, Mosby.

Tsai SC, Burnakis TG: Aldose reductase inhibitors: an update, *Ann Pharmacother* 27:751, 1993.

United States Pharmacopeial Convention: *USP DI: advice for the patient: drug information in lay language, vol. 1I,* ed 20, Englewood, Colo, 2000, Micromedex.

United States Pharmacopeial Convention: *USP DI: drug information for the health care professional, vol. 1,* ed 20, Englewood, Colo, 2000, Micromedex.

Activity

Remember to check the **Online Worksheet** for additional learning opportunities: **www.harcourthealth.com/MERLIN/Lilley/**

Chapter 31

Adrenal Agents

objectives

When you reach the end of this chapter, you should be able to do the following:

1 Discuss the normal actions and functions of the adrenal system and its feedback mechanism.

2 Describe the differences between the hyposecretion and hypersecretion of the adrenal hormones.

3 Describe the various diseases that are attributed to the hyposecretion and hypersecretion of adrenal hormones.

4 Identify the various agents used to manage the hyposecretion and hypersecretion of adrenal hormones as well as other indications for the use of adrenal agents.

5 Discuss the mechanisms of action of, indications for, contraindications and cautions to, and side effects of adrenal medications.

6 Develop a nursing care plan that includes all phases of the nursing process for patients receiving adrenal medications.

7 Identify the teaching guidelines for patients receiving adrenal medications.

www.harcourthealth.com/MERLIN/Lilley/

Look for this symbol for topics covered in the **Online Worksheet** Activity

drug profiles

aminoglutethimide, p. 490

dexamethasone, p. 489

fludrocortisone, p. 489

○—**hydrocortisone,** p. 489

○—**prednisone,** p. 489

○— Key drug.

glossary

Addison's disease Life-threatening condition caused by failure of adrenocortical function. (p. 486)

Adrenal cortex (ə dre′ nəl kor′ teks) Outer portion of the adrenal gland. (p. 485)

Adrenal medulla (ə dre′ nəl mə dul′ə) Inner portion of the adrenal gland. (p. 485)

Aldosterone (al dos′ tər ōn) Mineralocorticoid hormone produced by the adrenal cortex that acts on the renal tubule to regulate sodium and potassium balance in the blood. (p. 486)

Cortex Outer layer of a body organ or other structure. (p. 486)

Corticosteroid (kor ti ko ster′ oid) Any one of the natural or synthetic adrenocortical hormones (p. 486)

Cushing's syndrome Metabolic disorder characterized by abnormally increased secretion of the adrenocortical steroids caused by any one of several sources: ACTH-dependent adrenocotical hyperplasia or tumor, ectopic ACTH-secreting tumor, or excessive administration of steroids. (p. 486)

Epinephrine (ep′ ĭ nef′ rin) Endogenous adrenal hormone and synthetic adrenergic vasoconstrictor. (p. 485)

Norepinephrine (nor′ ep ĭ nef′ rin) Adrenergic hormone that increases blood pressure by causing vasoconstriction but does not affect cardiac output. (p. 485)

ADRENAL SYSTEM

The adrenal gland is an endocrine organ that sits on top of the kidneys like a cap. It is composed of two distinct parts called the **adrenal cortex** and the **adrenal medulla** that both structurally and functionally are very different. The adrenal cortex is made up of regular endocrine tissue, and the adrenal medulla is made up of neurosecretory tissue. Therefore the adrenal gland actually functions as two different endocrine glands, with each secreting different hormones.

The adrenal medulla secretes two important hormones, both of which are catecholamines. These are **epinephrine,** or adrenaline, which accounts for about 80% of the secretion, and **norepinephrine,** or noradrenaline, which accounts for the other 20%. (Both of these hormones are discussed in Chapter 16 and will not be discussed further here in any detail.) The differences between the adrenal cortex and the adrenal medulla and the various hormones secreted by each are listed in Table 31-1.

The hormones secreted from the adrenal cortex, which are the focus of this chapter, are broadly referred to as

Table 31-1　Adrenal Gland: Characteristics

Type of Tissue	Type of Hormone	Specific Drugs/Hormones
ADRENAL CORTEX		
Endocrine	Glucocorticoids	betamethasone, corticotropin (ACTH), cortisone, dexamethasone, hydrocortisone, methylprednisolone, paramethasone, prednisolone, triamcinolone
	Mineralocorticoids	aldosterone, fludrocortisone, desoxycorticosterone
ADRENAL MEDULLA		
Neuroendocrine	Catecholamines	epinephrine, norepinephrine

Box 31-1　Adrenal Cortex Hormones: Biologic Functions

GLUCOCORTICOIDS
Antiinflammatory actions
Maintenance of normal blood pressure
Carbohydrate and protein metabolism
Fat metabolism
Stress effects

MINERALOCORTICOIDS
Sodium and water resorption
Blood pressure control
Potassium levels and pH of blood

corticosteroids because they arise from the **cortex** and they are made from the crystalline *steroid* alcohol cholesterol. There are two types of corticosteroids—glucocorticoids and mineralocorticoids. These are secreted by two different layers, or zones, of the cortex. The zona glomerulosa, which is the outer layer, secretes the mineralocorticoids, and the zona fasciculata, which lies under the zona glomerulosa, secretes the glucocorticoids. A third, inner layer, the zona reticularis, secretes small amounts of sex hormones. All the hormones secreted by the adrenal cortex are steroid hormones.

The mineralocorticoids get their name from the fact that they play an important role in regulating mineral salts (electrolytes) in the body. In humans the only physiologically important mineralocorticoid is **aldosterone.** Its primary role is to maintain normal levels of sodium in the blood (sodium homeostasis) by causing sodium to be resorbed from the urine back into the blood in exchange for potassium and hydrogen ions. In this way aldosterone not only regulates the blood sodium levels but also influences the potassium levels of the blood and its pH.

Overall, the corticosteroids are necessary for many vital bodily functions, and some of the important ones are listed in Box 31-1. Without these hormones, life-threatening consequences may arise.

Adrenal corticosteroids are synthesized as needed; the body does not store them as it does other hormones. The body levels of these hormones are regulated by the hypothalamus-pituitary-adrenal (HPA) axis in much the same way as the levels of hormones secreted by the previously discussed endocrine glands (pancreas, thyroid, and pituitary) are regulated. As the name implies, this axis consists of a very organized system of communication between the adrenal gland, the pituitary, and the hypothalamus and, as is the case for the other endocrine glands, uses hormones as the messengers and a negative feedback mechanism as the controller and maintainer of the process. This feedback process operates as follows: When the level of a particular corticosteroid is low, corticotropin-releasing hormone is released from the hypothalamus into the bloodstream and travels to the anterior pituitary, where it triggers the release of corticotropin (ACTH). The corticotropin is then transported in the blood to the adrenal cortex, where it stimulates the production of the corticosteroid. The corticosteroid is then released into the bloodstream, and when it reaches a peak level, this sends a signal (negative feedback) to the hypothalamus, and the HPA axis is inhibited until the level of the corticosteriod is depleted, whereupon the axis is stimulated once again.

The oversecretion (hypersecretion) of adrenocortical hormones can lead to a collection of signs and symptoms called **Cushing's syndrome.** The hypersecretion of glucocorticoids results in the redistribution of body fat from the arms and legs to the face, shoulders, trunk, and abdomen, resulting in the "moon face" characteristic. The hypersecretion of aldosterone, or primary aldosteronism, leads to increased water retention and muscle weakness resulting from the potassium loss.

The undersecretion (hyposecretion) of adrenocortical hormones causes a condition referred to as **Addison's disease.** It is associated with increased blood sodium levels, decreased blood glucose and potassium levels, dehydration, and weight loss. The combination of a mineralocorticoid (fludrocortisone) and a glucocorticoid (prednisone or some other suitable agent) are used for treatment.

ADRENAL AGENTS

All the naturally occurring corticosteroids are available as exogenous agents, and there are also higher-potency synthetic analogues. The adrenal glucocorticoids are an extremely large group of steroids, and they are classified in various ways. They can be classified by whether they are a natural or synthetic corticosteroid; by the method of administration (e.g., systemic, topical); by their salt and water retention potential (mineralocorticoid activity); by

Table 31-2   Available Synthetic Corticosteroids

Hormone Type	Method of Administration	Individual Drugs
Adrenal steroid inhibitor	Systemic	aminoglutethimide, trilostane, mitotane, ketoconazole, metyrapone
Glucocorticoid	Topical	alclometasone dipropionate, amcinonide, betamethasone benzoate, betamethasone dipropionate, betamethasone valerate, clobestasol propionate, clocortolone pivalate desonide, desoximethasone, dexamethasone sodium phosphate, diflorasone diacetate, fluocinolone acetonide, fluocinonide, flurandrenolide, fluticasone propionate, halobitasol propionate, halcinonide, hydrocortisone acetate, hydrocortisone valerate, methylprednisolone acetate, mometasone furoate, triamcinolone
	Systemic	betamethasone, cortisone, dexamethasone, hydrocortisone, methylprednisolone, prednisolone, prednisone, triamcinolone
	Inhaled	beclomethasone, dexamethasone, flunisolide, triamcinolone acetonide, fluticasone
	Nasal	beclomethasone dipropionate, dexamethasone sodium phosphate, flunisolide, triamcinolone acetonide
Mineralocorticoid	Systemic	fludrocortisone acetate

their duration of action (i.e., short, intermediate, or long acting), or by some combination of these schemes. The only corticoisteroid with exclusive mineralocorticoid activity is fludrocortisone. The currently available synthetic adrenal hormones and adrenal steroid inhibitors are listed in Table 31-2.

Mechanism of Action

The action of the corticosteroids is related to their involvement in the synthesis of specific proteins. There are several steps to this process. Initially the steroid hormones bind to a receptor on the surface of a target cell to form a steroid-receptor complex, which is then transported to the nucleus of that target cell. Once inside the nucleus of the target cell, the complex stimulates the cell's DNA to produce messenger-RNA, which is then used as a template for the synthesis of a specific protein. It is these proteins that exert specific drug effects.

Drug Effects

Most of the corticosteroids exert their effects by modifying enzyme activity, so their role is more intermediary than direct.

As previously mentioned, the naturally occurring mineralocorticoid aldosterone affects electrolyte and fluid balance by working on the distal renal tubule to promote sodium resorption from the nephron into the blood, which pulls water and fluid along with it. In doing so it causes fluid and water retention, which leads to edema and hypertension. It may also promote potassium and hydrogen excretion.

The naturally occurring glucocorticoids hydrocortisone (cortisol) and cortisone have some mineralocorticoid activity and therefore have some of the same effects as aldosterone (i.e., fluid and water retention). Their other main effect is the inhibition of inflammatory and immune responses. Glucocorticoids primarily inhibit or help control the inflammatory response by stabilizing the cell membranes of inflammatory cells called *lysosomes*, decreasing the permeability of capillaries to the inflammatory cells, and decreasing the migration of white blood cells (WBCs) into already inflamed areas. They may also lower fever by reducing the release of interleukin-1 from WBCs. They do this by stimulating the cells that eventually become red blood cells called erythroid cells. The stimulation of these cells in the bone marrow prolongs the survival of erythrocytes (RBCs and platelets). The glucocorticoids also promote the breakdown (catabolism) of protein, the production of glycogen (gluconeogenesis), and the redistribution of fat from peripheral to central areas of the body.

Therapeutic Uses

All the systemically administered glucocorticoids have a similar clinical efficacy but differ in their potency and duration of action and in the extent to which they cause salt and fluid retention (Table 31-3). They are indicated in the treatment of the following conditions:

- Adrenocortical deficiency
- Adrenogenital syndrome
- Bacterial meningitis (particularly in infants)
- Cerebral edema
- Collagen diseases (e.g., systemic lupus erythematosus)
- Dermatologic diseases (e.g., exfoliative dermatitis, pemphigus)
- Endocrine disorders (thyroiditis)
- Gastrointestinal diseases (ulcerative colitis, regional enteritis)
- Hematologic disorders (reduce bleeding tendencies)
- Ophthalmic disorders (nonpyogenic inflammations)
- Organ transplant recipients (decrease immune response)
- Palliative management of leukemias and lymphomas

Systemic Glucocorticoids: A Comparison

31-3

Drug	Origin	Duration of Action	Equivalent Dose (mg)	Salt and Water Retention Potential
betamethasone	Synthetic	Long	0.75	Very low
cortisone	Natural	Short	25.0	High
dexamethasone	Synthetic	Long	0.75	Very low
hydrocortisone	Natural	Short	20.0	High
methylprednisolone	Synthetic	Intermediate	4.0	Low
prednisone	Synthetic	Intermediate	5.0	Low
prednisolone	Synthetic	Intermediate	5.0	Low
triamcinolone	Synthetic	Intermediate	4.0	Very low

Corticosteroids: Common Adverse Effects

31-4

Body System	Side/Adverse Effects
Cardiovascular	Congestive heart failure, cardiac edema, hypertension—all due to electrolyte imbalances
Central nervous system	Convulsions, headache, vertigo, mood swings, psychic impairment, nervousness, insomnia,
Endocrine	Growth suppression, Cushing's syndrome, menstrual irregularities, carbohydrate intolerance, hyperglycemia, HPA axis suppression
Gastrointestinal	Peptic ulcers with possible perforation, pancreatitis, ulcerative esophagitis, abdominal distention
Integumentary	Fragile skin, petechiae, ecchymosies, facial erythema, poor wound healing, hirsutism, urticaria
Musculoskeletal	Muscle weakness, loss of muscle mass, osteoporosis
Ocular	Increased intraocular pressure, glaucoma, exophthalmos, cataracts
Other	Weight gain

- Remission of proteinurea in nephrotic syndrome
- Spinal cord injury

Glucocorticoids are administered by inhalation for the control of steroid-responsive bronchospastic states. Nasally administered glucocorticoids are used in the management of rhinitis and to prevent the recurrence of polyps after surgical removal. The topical steroids are the largest group and are used in the management of inflammations in the eye, ear, and skin.

Side Effects and Adverse Effects

The potent metabolic, physiologic, and pharmacologic effects of the corticosteroids can influence every body system, with the result that they can produce a wide variety of significant undesirable effects. The more common of these are summarized in Table 31-4.

Interactions

The systematically administered corticosteroids can interact with many agents:

- Their use with non–potassium-sparing diuretics (e.g., thiazides, loop diuretics) can lead to severe hypocalcemia and hypokalemia.
- Their use with aspirin, other nonsteroidal antiinflammatory drugs (NSAIDs), and other ulcerogenic drugs produces additive gastrointestinal effects.
- Their use with anticholinesterase drugs produces weakness in patients with myasthenia gravis.
- Their use with immunizing biologicals inhibits the immune response to the biological.
- Their use with antidiabetic agents may reduce the hypoglycemic affect.
- Oral hypoglycemics or insulin may need increased dose adjustments.

Dosages

For information on the recommended dosages of adrenal agents, see the dosages table on p. 490.

drug profiles

CORTICOSTEROIDS

The systemic corticosteroids consist of 13 chemically different but pharmacologically similar hormones. They all exert varying degrees of glucocorticoid and mineralocorticoid effects. Their differences arise out of slight changes in their chemical structures.

Corticosteroids can cross the placenta and produce fetal abnormalities. For this reason, they are classified as pregnancy category C agents. They may also be secreted in breast milk and cause abnormalities in the nursing infant. They are contraindicated in patients who have exhibited hypersensitivity reactions to them in the past as well as in patients with fungal or bacterial infections. Short- or long-term use can lead to a condition known as *steroid psychosis*. In addition, the cessation of long-term treatment with these agents requires a tapering of the daily dose because the administration of the exogenous hormones causes the endogenous production of the hormones to stop. Tapering daily doses allows the HPA axis the time it needs to recover and start to stimulate the normal production of the endogenous hormones.

dexamethasone

Dexamethasone (Decadron, Hexadrol, Dexone, Solurex, Dexaject-LA) is one of the three long-acting glucocorticoids, the other two being betamethasone and paramethasone. These agents have half-lives that range from 3 to 5 hours and durations of action of 36 to 54 hours. Usually dexamethasone and the other long-acting corticosteroids are used for antiinflammatory or immunosuppressant purposes. They have only minimal mineralocorticoid properties and therefore alone are inadequate for the management of adrenocortical insufficiency. Dexamethasone may be administered by inhalation for the treatment of bronchial asthma. A dexamethasone suppression test may be performed to establish the diagnosis of Cushing's syndrome or an adrenal adenoma. Dexamethasone inhibits the release of corticotropin (ACTH) from the pituitary gland and decreases the output of endogenous corticosteroids. Dexamethasone has also been shown to be very effective in preventing the nausea and vomiting associated with emetogenic cancer chemotherapy.

Dexamethasone is available orally as a 0.5-mg/5 ml oral elixir; as a 0.5-mg/5 ml solution; and as 0.25-, 0.5-, 0.75-, 1-, 1.5-, 2-, 4-, and 6-mg tablets. Dexamethasone as an acetate salt is given intramuscularly and is available as a 8- and 16-mg injection. Dexamethasone sodium phosphate is given either intramuscularly, intraarticularly, or intravenously as a 4-, 10-, 20-, or 24- mg/ml injection. Recommended dosages are given in the dosages table on p. 490. Pregnancy category C.

PHARMACOKINETICS

HALF-LIFE	ONSET	PEAK	DURATION
36-54 hr	Unknown	1-2 hr	66 hr

fludrocortisone

Fludrocortisone (Florinef) is a synthetic mineralocorticoid with very weak glucocorticoid but very potent mineralocorticoid activity. It is used for oral replacement therapy in patients suffering from an adrenocortical insufficiency such as Addison's disease. It has also been used to increase systolic and diastolic blood pressure in patients suffering from chronic severe postural hypotension. It is only available as a 0.1-mg oral tablet. Recommended dosages are given in the dosages table on p. 490.

PHARMACOKINETICS

HALF-LIFE	ONSET	PEAK	DURATION
18-36 hr	10-20 min	PO: 1.7 hr	Unknown

hydrocortisone

Hydrocortisone (Cortef, Hydrocortone, Solu-Cortef) is a short-acting adrenocortical steroid. Both it and cortisone are the only two short-acting agents. Compared with other glucocorticoids they have the strongest mineralocorticoid actions (potassium excretion and sodium and water retention) and weakest glucocorticoid actions (antiinflammatory, immunosuppressant, and metabolic-type effects). They have relatively short half-lives (0.5 to 2 hours) and therefore short durations of action. Because they have both glucocorticoid and mineralocorticoid properties, either hydrocortisone or cortisone is usually the corticosteroid of choice for replacement therapy in patients with adrenocortical insufficiency.

Hydrocortisone is available in oral, injectable, and topical preparations. It is available orally as 5-, 10-, and 20-mg tablets and as a 10-mg/5 mg oral suspension; parenterally as a 25-, 50-, 100-, 250-, 500-, and 1000-mg injection; and topically as a cream, lotion, ointment, and spray preparation. Recommended dosages are given in the dosages table on p. 490. Pregnancy category C.

PHARMACOKINETICS

HALF-LIFE	ONSET	PEAK	DURATION
0.5-2 hr	Unknown	1 hr	30-36 hr

prednisone

Prednisone (Orasone, Meticorten, Deltasone, Cortan, Sterapred) is one of the four intermediate-acting glucocorticoids, the others being methylprednisolone, prednisolone, and triamcinolone. These agents have half-lives that are more than double those of the short-acting corticosteroids (2 to 5 hours), and therefore they have much longer durations of action. Prednisone is the preferred oral glucocorticoid for antiinflammatory or immunosuppressant purposes. This agent has only minimal mineralocorticoid properties and therefore alone is inadequate for the management of adrenocortical insufficiency (Addison's disease).

Prednisone is available orally as a 5-mg/5 ml oral solution; as a 5-mg/5 ml syrup; as 1-, 2.5-, 5-, 10-, 20-, 25-, and 50-mg tablets; and as a 5-mg film-coated tablet. Recommended dosages are given in the dosages table on p. 490. Pregnancy category C.

PHARMACOKINETICS

HALF-LIFE	ONSET	PEAK	DURATION
18-36 hr	Unknown	1-2 hr	36 hr

ANTIADRENALS

Aminoglutethimide, metyrapone, and trilostane are antiadrenals, or adrenal steroid inhibitors. They inhibit the normal actions or function of the adrenal cortex by inhibiting the conversion of cholesterol into adrenal corticosteroids. They are indicated for the treatment of Cushing's syndrome, which results from an overproduction of corticosteroids by the adrenal gland. They are contraindicated in patients who have shown a previous hypersensitivity reaction to them, and many are classified as pregnancy category X agents. Their most common adverse effects are nausea, anorexia, dizziness, and skin rash.

aminoglutethimide

Aminoglutethimide (Cytadren) is the most commonly used of the three antiadrenal drugs in the treatment of Cushing's syndrome, metastatic breast cancer, and adrenal cancer. It is only available orally as a 250-mg tablet. Recommended dosages are given in the dosages table below. Pregnancy category D.

PHARMACOKINETICS

HALF-LIFE	ONSET	PEAK	DURATION
9 hr	Unknown	Unknown	Unknown

DOSAGES Selected Corticosteroid and Antiadrenal Agents

agent	pharmacologic class	dosage range	purpose
aminoglutethimide (Cytadren)	Adrenal corticosteroid inhibitor	*Adult* PO: Start with 250 mg qid and adjust according to response; max 2 g/day	Selected cases of Cushing's syndrome
dexamethasone (Decadron, Hexadrol, Dexone, Solurex, Dexeject-LA)	Synthetic long-acting glucocorticoid	*Pediatric* PO: 0.025-0.35 mg/day in divided dose q6-12h *Adult* PO: 0.75-9 mg/day in divided dose q6-12h	Allergic, autoimmune, collagen, inflammatory conditions; cerebral edema; immunosuppression; palliation of selected neoplasms
dexamethasone acetate (Decadron-LA, Dexeject-LA, Solurex LA)	Synthetic long-acting repository glucocorticoid	*Adult* IM: 8-16 mg every 1-3 wk prn for systemic effects Intraarticular: 4-16 mg every 1-3 wk prn Intralesional: 0.8-1.6 mg/injection site	Same as dexamethasone Antiinflammatory Antiinflammatory
fludrocortisone (Florinef)	Synthetic glucocorticoid mineralocorticoid	*Adult* PO: 0.1 mg 3 times/wk to 0.2 mg/day PO: 0.1-0.2 mg/day	Addison's disease Salt-dosing adrenogenital syndrome
hydrocortisone (Cortef, Hydrocortone)	Natural short-acting glucocorticoid	*Pediatric* PO: 0.56-8 mg/day in 3-4 divided doses *Adult* PO: 10-320 mg/day in 3-4 divided doses	Adrenocortical insufficiency
hydrocortisone sodium succinate (Solu-Cortef)	Natural water-soluble, short-acting glucocorticoid	*Pediatric* IM/IV: 0.16-1 mg/kg administered 1-2 times/day *Adult* IM/IV: 100 mg-8 g/day	Adrenocortical insufficiency
prednisone (Orasone, Meticorten, Deltasone, Cortan, Sterapred)	Synthetic intermediate-acting glucocorticoid	*Pediatric* PO: 0.05-2 mg/kg/day divided 1-2 times/day *Adult* PO: 5-60 mg/day daily *or* divided 1-2 times/day	Allergic, autoimmune, collagen, inflammatory conditions; cerebral edema; immunosuppression; palliation of selected neoplasms

nursing process

● Assessment

Before administering any of the adrenal agents, the nurse should perform a thorough physical assessment to determine the patient's baseline weight, intake and output status, vital signs (especially blood pressure), hydration status, skin condition, and immune status. Important baseline laboratory values include the serum Na, K, BUN, and Hgb levels and Hct. All this is crucial for ensuring the safe and most effective use of these adrenal agents and for identifying any specific cautions or contraindications in advance of treatment, as well as for monitoring the patient's response to the treatment. Any edema or electrolyte imbalances need to be documented and brought to the attention of the physician. Because glucocorticoids can elevate a patient's blood glucose level, a baseline level must be determined. Because corticosteroids often aggravate peptic ulcer disease, the nurse should find out whether the patient has a history of ulcer disease, gastritis, or heartburn.

There are many drugs that interact with corticosteroids (see previous discussion), so the nurse should always find out what prescription and over-the-counter (OTC) medications the patient is currently taking to prevent these interactions from occurring.

Antiadrenal agents are contraindicated in patients with a known hypersensitivity to them.

● Nursing Diagnoses

Nursing diagnoses appropriate to the patient receiving adrenal agents include the following:
- Imbalanced nutrition, more than body requirements, related to changes in appetite resulting from corticosteroid therapy or antiadrenal agents.
- Disturbed body image related to the physiologic influence of diseases of the adrenal gland on the body.
- Excess fluid volume related to increased cardiac output from increased volume and/or fluid retention associated with mineralocorticoids.
- Risk for infection related to side effects of glucocorticoid therapy.
- Impaired skin integrity related to side effects of glucocorticoids.
- Risk for injury stemming from changes in sensorium and possible confusion related to side effects of corticosteroid therapy or from adverse reactions of antiadrenal agents.

● Planning

The goals in patients receiving corticosteroids or antiadrenals include:
- Patient describes the healthy diet to observe during treatment.
- Patient experiences minimal body image disturbances.
- Patient exhibits minimal complications resulting from the fluid retention caused by mineralocorticoid therapy.

- Patient is free of infection during corticosteroid therapy.
- Patient's skin and mucous membranes remains intact during treatment.
- Patient maintains normal electrolyte levels.
- Patient remains free of changes in sensorium and possible confusion or dizziness from adrenal or antiadrenal therapy.
- Patient states symptoms to report immediately to the physician should they occur.

Outcome Criteria

Outcome criteria for patients receiving adrenal agents include the following:
- Patient will eat adequate foods according to the food guide pyramid and maintain weight within normal range with adequate menu planning.
- Patient will openly verbalize fears about body image disturbances to health care providers.
- Patient will experience minimal problems with fluid volume excess and not gain more than 2 lb/week.
- Patient will notify the physician if fever ($>100.0°$ F or $38°$ C) occurs.
- Patient will perform frequent mouth and skin care to prevent infections and maintain intactness.
- Patient will implement measures to minimize major electrolyte imbalances during corticosteroid or mineralocorticoid therapy such as forcing fluids and possible salt restrictions or additives as ordered.
- Patient will change positions slowly and walk carefully to prevent injuries from dizziness or syncope.
- Patient will identify symptoms to report to the physician such as a weight gain of more than 2 lb/week, shortness of breath, edema, dizziness, or syncope.
- Patient must be weaned off corticosteroids to prevent Addison's disease.

● Implementation

Some of the systemic forms of adrenal agents, such as hydrocortisone and prednisone, may be given by the oral, IM, IV, or rectal route. Parenteral forms of these agents should be diluted according to the manufacturer's guidelines and administered over the recommended time span; for example, hydrocortisone should be given at a rate of 25 mg or less per minute. All liquid and parenteral forms should be mixed thoroughly before administration. IM forms should always be administered in a large-muscle (e.g., gluteal) site as opposed to the deltoid muscle, and the sites rotated to prevent tissue trauma and damage. Oral forms should be given with food or milk so as to minimize gastrointestinal upset. Injections should not be given subcutaneously because this may lead to tissue damage.

Topical agents should be applied as ordered and only according to the instructions in the package insert, which, for example, may specify the use of an occlusive dressing. The skin should be clean and dry before application, and the nurse should wear gloves and apply the medication with either a sterile tongue depressor or cotton-tipped applicator, if the skin is intact. A sterile technique should be used if the skin is not intact!

Beclomethasone is a nasally administered synthetic corticosteroid that should be used as ordered. Any written instructions that come with the product should be read and followed carefully. Before administering a nasal corticosteroid, the patient should clear the nasal passages, and this may require a decongestant, which the physician may need to prescribe. See Chapter 8 for more instructions on nasal sprays.

Steroid inhalers should be used as ordered and the patient adequately taught the technique for administration (also covered in Chapter 8). It is important to emphasize to patients receiving them that, once the inhaler has been used, they should clean out the oral cavity with mouthwash to prevent possible oral fungal infections from developing.

Patients receiving fludrocortisone should take it with food or milk to minimize gastrointestinal upset. Weight gain of more than 5 pounds (2.25 kg) a week during mineralocorticoid therapy should be reported to the physician. Abrupt withdrawal is not recommended because this may precipitate an adrenal crisis.

Aminoglutethimide should be taken with an antacid (before the steroid) to minimize gastrointestinal up-

set. Because this drug is often used in patients with malignant tumors, it is also important to enhance the patient's nutritional and general well-being during therapy, such as by giving him or her nutritional supplements or vitamins.

See the box below for more teaching tips for patients receiving adrenal agents.

● Evaluation

A therapeutic response to corticosteroids includes a resolution of the underlying manifestations of the disease, such as a decrease in inflammation. Adverse effects for which to monitor include weight gain; increased blood pressure; pulse irregularities; mental status changes such as aggression, depression, or psychosis; electrolyte disturbances; elevated glucose levels; decreased healing; gastrointestinal upset; and ulcer-related symptoms. The systemic agents may cause potassium depletion, and this is manifested by fatigue, nausea, vomiting, muscle weakness, and dysrhythmias.

A therapeutic response to aminoglutethimide includes a decrease in the size of the tumor or a decrease in the Cushing's syndrome. Side effects to watch for include jaundice, skin lesions, hypotension, headache, lethargy, weakness, gastrointestinal upset, and hepatotoxicity.

---

patient teaching tips

Adrenal Agents

➤ Because of their suppressed immune system, patients taking corticosteroids should avoid people with infections and report any fever, increased weakness and lethargy, or sore throat.

➤ Encourage patients to tell the nurse and other members of the health care team about unpleasant side effects and changes in appearance.

➤ Encourage patients to get adequate rest, exercise, and nutrition.

➤ Patients should understand the importance of monitoring of their nutritional status, weight, fluid volume, electrolyte status, skin turgor, and glucose levels during therapy.

➤ Encourage patients to keep a daily log of their general feelings of well-being and any response to the medication, along with any questions for the physician.

➤ Emphasize the importance of not discontinuing any of the corticosteroids and of keeping all medications out of the reach of children.

➤ Patients should take all adrenal medications exactly as prescribed and at the same time every day. Oral agents are to be taken with meals or food.

➤ Topical corticosteroids should be applied as recommended by the manufacturer as well as according to the physician's orders.

➤ Hydrocortisone and prednisone should be taken exactly as ordered, and one daily AM dose is recom-

mended, if ordered by the physician, to minimize adrenal suppression. Sudden discontinuation of these agents can precipitate an adrenal crisis caused by a sudden drop in the serum levels of cortisone. Cushingoid symptoms include moon face, weight gain, muscle wasting, and increased deposition of fat in the trunk area, leading to truncal obesity. Patients should notify the physician of any weakness, joint pain, dyspnea, fever, dysrhythmias, depression, edema, or any other unusual symptom.

➤ Topical agents should be applied as ordered, and often the site should be covered with an occlusive dressing; the method for doing this should be demonstrated to the patient. The skin should be clean and dry before topical administrations.

➤ Nasal sprays should be administered per the manufacturer's guidelines and the physician's orders. (See Chapter 8 for more information on the administration of nasal agents.)

➤ Aminoglutethimide should be administered as ordered and careful attention paid to the overall nutritional status and well-being of the patient. In addition, the patient should report the development of jaundice, rash, fever, or skin lesions. If masculinization occurs, this will disappear once the therapy is stopped.

➤ Patients should wear MedicAlert tags at all times.

POINTS TO REMEMBER

Adrenal Gland

- An endocrine organ that sits on top of the kidneys.
- Composed of two distinct tissues: the adrenal cortex and the adrenal medulla.
- Adrenal medulla secretes two important hormones: epinephrine (80%) and norepinephrine (20%).
- Adrenal cortex secretes hormones known as *corticosteroids:* glucocorticoids and mineralocorticoids.

Corticosteroids

- Glucocorticoid biologic functions: antiinflammatory actions, maintenance of normal blood pressure, carbohydrate and protein metabolism, fat metabolism, and stress effects.
- Mineralocorticoid biologic functions: sodium and water resorption, blood pressure control, and potassium levels in and pH of blood.

Nursing Considerations

- Adrenal agents may be administered orally, intramuscularly, or intravenously; some are also administered by means of a rectal enema.

- Parenteral forms should be diluted and administered according to the manufacturer's guidelines.
- Intramuscular forms of adrenal agents should be administered deep into a large muscle such as in the gluteal area.
- Steroid inhalers should be used as ordered and only after adequate patient education.
- Adverse effects to monitor for include weight gain (if more than 5 pounds [2.25 kg] in a week), increase in blood pressure, pulse irregularities, mental status changes such as aggression or depression, electrolyte disturbances, elevated glucose levels, decreased healing, gastrointestinal tract upset, and ulcer-related symptoms.
- Patients should be monitored frequently for weight gain, changes in nutritional status, electrolyte imbalances, and fluid volume excess.
- Patients should not be taken off these agents abruptly.
- Once-a-day dosing corticosteroids should be administered between 6 and 9 AM to minimize adrenal suppression, and this needs to be explained to the patient.
- Patients taking antiadrenal agents should be monitored carefully for development of jaundice, rash, fever, or skin lesions.

REVIEW QUESTIONS

1. Which of the following statements is correct about corticosteroids?
   a. Have few side effects
   b. Often used for their antiinflammatory effects
   c. May be administered only by inhalant dosage forms
   d. May be used long term without major complications
2. Which of the following drugs interact adversely with corticosteroids?
   a. NSAIDs
   b. Antibiotics
   c. Acetaminophen
   d. Opioid derivatives
3. Which of the following is considered one of the classical features or characteristics of increased levels of corticosteroids or Cushing's syndrome?
   a. Weight loss
   b. "Moon face"
   c. Muscle thickening
   d. Increased thoracic subcutaneous tissue

4. Your patient is taking fludrocortisone (Florinef Acetate) for treatment of autonomic dysfunction with symptoms of posturally related syncope. Which of the following statements is **true** about fludrocortisone?
   a. Food and milk may help minimize GI upset.
   b. It may worsen hypotension if taken long term.
   c. Weight gain of about 10 to 15 pounds is expected.
   d. It may be initiated and withdrawn without regard to any time frame.
5. Steroid inhalers have some specific instructions, such as which of the following?:
   a. Will always result in systemic effects and Cushing's syndrome.
   b. Should be taken only when symptomatic for preventive treatment for asthma.
   c. Patients should rinse their mouths with mouthwash after each use to prevent oral thrush.
   d. May be used up to 8 times a day with only two puffs at a time for maintenance dosing.

For Answers see www.harcourthealth.com/MERLIN/Lilley/.

CRITICAL THINKING Activities

1. A 19-year-old man is admitted through the emergency room after a motorcycle accident. He is conscious upon admission, has stable vital signs, and minimal cuts and abrasions on the left side of his body. You perform a thorough neurologic examination and find absence of sensation to light touch and pinprick and lower extremity paralysis. Reflexes are absent below the groin area. The physician orders a high dose IV

methylprednisolone. What is the purpose of this medication and what should you, as the nurse, watch for while the patient is receiving this medication?

2. You are caring for a patient who is taking 100 mg of hydrocortisone orally. The physician decides that he is more familiar with prednisone and wants to change the patient over to the equivalent oral dose of prednisone. What should you recommend?

3. Discuss the influence of hyperaldosteronism on the body and the indicated treatment.

For Answers see www.harcourthealth.com/MERLIN/Lilley/.

bibliography

Albanese J, Nutz P: *Mosby's 2001 nursing drug reference and review cards,* St Louis, 2001, Mosby.

American Hospital Formulary Service: *AHFS drug information,* Bethesda, Md, 2000, American Society of Health-System Pharmacists.

Anderson PO, Knoben JE, Troutman WG: *Handbook of clinical drug data 1999-2000,* ed 9, New York, 1999, McGraw-Hill.

Brenner ZR, Cannito M: Administering steroids, *Nursing 98* 28(3):34, 1998.

Brody TM, Larner J, Minneman KP: *Human pharmacology: molecular to clinical,* ed 3, St Louis, 1997, Mosby.

Johns Hopkins Hospital, Department of Pediatrics et al: *The Harriet Lane handbook,* ed 15, St Louis, 2000, Mosby.

Keen JH: *Critical care and emergency drug reference,* ed 3, St Louis, 1996, Mosby.

Mosby's GenRx: a comprehensive reference for generic and brand drugs, ed 10, St Louis, 2000, Mosby.

Skidmore-Roth L: *Mosby's 2001 nursing drug reference,* St Louis, 2001, Mosby.

Thibodeau GA, Patton KT: *Anatomy and physiology,* ed 4, St Louis, 1999, Mosby.

United States Pharmacopeial Convention: *USP DI: advice for the patient: drug information in lay language, vol 1I,* ed 20, Englewood, Colo, 2000, Micromedex.

Remember to check the **Online Worksheet** for additional learning opportunities: **www.harcourthealth.com/MERLIN/Lilley/**

Activity

Chapter 32

Women's Health Agents

www.harcourthealth.com/MERLIN/Lilley/

Look for this symbol for topics covered in the **Online Worksheet** Activity

objectives

When you reach the end of this chapter, you should be able to do the following:

1 Discuss the variety of disorders that are treated with estrogens and progestins.

2 Discuss the normal hormonally mediated feedback system and how it regulates the female reproductive system.

3 Describe the rationale for the various treatments and cite dosages, side effects, cautions, contraindications, and drug interactions associated with estrogen and progestin therapy, selective estrogen receptor modulators, and drugs used in labor and delivery.

4 Develop a nursing care plan that includes all phases of the nursing process for the patient receiving estrogens, progestins, oral contraceptives, and drugs used in labor and delivery.

5 Discuss combined oral contraceptives and selective estrogen receptor modulators.

6 List the expected therapeutic responses to the various women's health agents.

7 Describe the therapeutic responses to uterine stimulants and relaxants, as well as their mechanism of actions, side effects, contraindications, and drug interactions.

drug profiles

alendronate, p. 503

chorionic gonadotropin, p. 511

o— clomiphene, p. 511

dinoprostone, p. 507

ergonovine and methylergonovine, p. 508

estrogen, p. 498

medroxyprogesterone, p. 501

o— megestrol, p. 501

menotropins, p. 511

oxytocin, p. 508

raloxifene, p. 504

ritodrine, p. 509

terbutaline, p. 509

o— Key drug.

glossary

Corpus luteum (kor′ pəs loo′ te əm) Structure that forms on the surface of the ovary after every ovulation and acts as a short-lived endocrine organ that secretes progesterone. (p. 510)

Endocrine gland (en′ do krin) Part of a system of glands that secrete hormones into the blood. (p. 496)

Endometrium (en′ do me′ tre əm) Mucous membrane lining the uterus. (p. 496)

Fallopian tube (fə lo′ pe ən) Passage through which an ovum is carried to the uterus. (p. 496)

Gonadotropin (gon′ə do tro′ pin) Hormone that stimulates the testes and ovaries. (p. 496)

Implantation The attachment, penetration, and embedding of the blastocyst in the lining of the uterine wall. (p. 496)

Menarche (mə nahr′ ke) The first menstruation and the beginning of cyclic menstrual function. (p. 497)

Menopause (men′ o pawz) The cessation of menses. (p. 497)

Menses (men′ sēz) The normal flow of blood that occurs during menstruation. (p. 497)

Menstrual cycle (men′ stroo əl) The recurring cycle of changes in the endometrium when the decidual layer is shed, regrows, proliferates, is maintained for several days, and is shed again at menstruation. (p. 497)

Nucleic acid (noo kle′ ik) Compound involved in energy storage and release and in the determination and transmission of genetic characteristics. (p. 497)

Osteoporosis (os′ tē ō pə rō′ sis) A condition characterized by the progressive loss of bone density and thinning of bone tissue. (p. 502)

Ova (o′ və) Female reproductive or germ cells. (p. 496)

Ovaries (o′ və rez) Pair of female gonads located on each side of the lower abdomen beside the uterus. (p. 496)

Puberty (pu′ bər te) Period of life when the ability to reproduce begins. (p. 497)

Uterus (u′ tər əs) Hollow, pear-shaped female organ in which the fertilized ovum is implanted and the fetus develops. (p. 496)

Vagina (və ji′ nə) Part of the female genitalia that forms a canal from the orifice through the vestibule to the uterine cervix. (p. 496)

FEMALE REPRODUCTIVE SYSTEM

The female reproductive system consists of the ovaries, fallopian tubes, uterus, vagina, and an external structure (vulva). The development of these primary sex characteristics, their subsequent reproductive functions (starting at puberty), and their maintenance are controlled by pituitary **gonadotropins** and the female steroid sex hormones, estrogens. Estrogens are also responsible for stimulating the development of secondary female sex characteristics.

The **ovaries** (female gonads) are paired glands located on each side of the uterus and function both as an **endocrine gland** and as a reproductive gland. As a reproductive gland they produce mature **ova** from ovarian follicles, which are then ovulated and transported down the **fallopian tube** to the uterus. As an endocrine gland the ovaries are responsible for producing estrogens and progesterone.

The **uterus** consists primarily of smooth muscle and an inner layer called the **endometrium.** It is a mucous membrane and the site of the following:

- **Implantation** of a fertilized ovum and the subsequent development of the fetus
- Initiation of labor and birthing of the infant
- Menstruation

The **vagina** serves as a common passageway for birthing and menstrual flow. In addition, it is a receptacle for the penis during sexual intercourse and the sperm after male ejaculation.

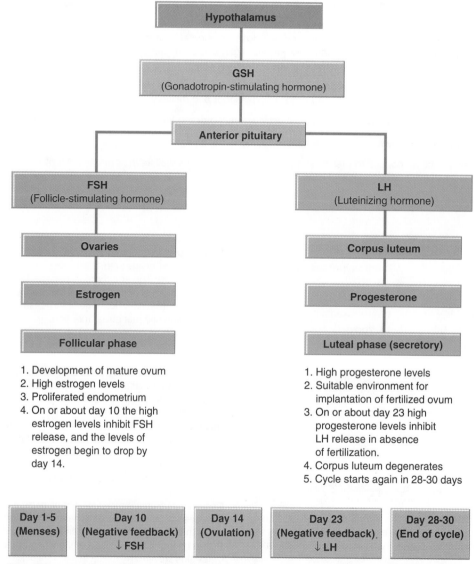

Fig. 32-1 Hormonal activity during ovulation. Gonadotropin-stimulating hormone (GSH) from the hypothalamus stimulates the pituitary gland, causing a surge in the production of follicle-stimulating hormone (FSH). When the level of estrogen reaches an appropriately high level, it stimulates the hypothalamus and pituitary gland to secrete luteinizing hormone (LH). The LH brings the follicle to full maturation, causing it to release an ovum. In the absence of a fertilized ovum, estrogen and progesterone are then secreted by the ovary, which inhibits the production of LH and ends the cycle.

The **menstrual cycle** usually takes 1 month to complete. It commences during puberty with the first menses **(menarche)** and ceases with **menopause,** which in most women occurs between 45 and 55 years of age. The hormonally controlled menstrual cycle consists of three distinct but interrelated phases:

- **Phase 1.** The menstrual phase, which initiates the cycle and lasts from 5 to 7 days.
- **Phase 2.** The follicular phase, during which a mature ovum develops from an ovarian follicle. This phase is also called the proliferative or preovulatory phase. It terminates on or about day 14 of the cycle.
- **Phase 3.** The final phase of the cycle is called the luteal or postovulatory phase. It is when the corpus luteum forms from the ruptured graafian follicle and progesterone is produced. The endometrium is developed to receive the fertilized ovum, and it is here that it is implanted. If fertilization does not occur, the corpus luteum degenerates and the cycle begins again on or about day 28.

Figure 32-1 illustrates the sequence of hormone secretions and related events that take place during the menstrual cycle.

FEMALE SEX HORMONES

ESTROGENS

There are three major endogenous estrogens: estradiol, estrone, and estriol. All are synthesized from cholesterol in the ovarian follicles and have the basic structure of a steroid. For this reason they are sometimes referred to as *steroid hormones.* Estradiol is the principal and most active of the three and represents the end-product of estrogen synthesis.

The exogenous estrogenic agents, those used for therapeutic reasons, were developed because most of the endogenous estrogens are inactive orally. These synthetic agents fall into two categories: steroidal and nonsteroidal, and the agents in the two categories are as follows:

Steroidal
- conjugated estrogens (Premarin)
- esterified estrogens (Estratab, Menest)
- estradiol transdermal (Estraderm, Estrace)
- estradiol cypionate (Depoestradiol, Depogen)
- estradiol valerate (Delestrogen, Duragen)
- ethinyl estradiol (Estinyl, Feminone)
- estrone (Gynogen, Theelin aqueous)
- estropipate (Ogen)
- quinestrol (Estrovis)

Nonsteroidal
- chlorotrianisene (TACE)
- dienestrol (DV)
- diethylstilbestrol
- diethylstilbestrol diphosphate (Stilphostrol)

The natural (steroidal) estrogenic agent obtained from the urine of pregnant mares is Premarin (*pregnant mare urine*). There is another source now for this conjugated estrogen product. A product called Cenestin is actually conjugated estrogens obtained from soy and yam plants. Ethinyl estradiol is one of the most potent of these estrogens. Nonsteroidal agents do not have the basic steroid structure but can still act on estrogenic tissues throughout the body.

Mechanism of Action

The binding of estrogen to estrogen receptors stimulates the synthesis of **nucleic acid** (DNA and RNA) and proteins, which are the building blocks for all living tissue. Estrogens are also required at **puberty** for the development and maintenance of the female reproductive system and the development of secondary sex characteristics (feminization). A new class of agents, called *selective estrogen receptor modulators* (SERMs), has emerged. SERMs have a variety of actions throughout the body. Their therapeutic effects are derived from their agonist effects on the estrogen receptors on bones. Simultaneously they have antagonist effects on both breast and uterus estrogen receptors. This is believed to be beneficial in that these tissues would not be stimulated, potentially leading to cancer of the breast and uterus.

Drug Effects

Estrogens produce their effects in estrogen-responsive tissues, which have a high content of estrogen receptors. These tissues comprise the female genital organs, the breasts, the pituitary gland, and the hypothalamus.

At the time of puberty the production of estrogen increases greatly. This causes **menses** to be initiated, the breasts to develop, body fat to be redistributed, soft skin to form, and other feminizing changes to occur. Estrogens play a role in the shaping of body contours and the skeleton. For instance, long bones are usually inhibited from growing, with the result that females are usually shorter than males.

Therapeutic Uses

Estrogens are utilized in the treatment or prevention of an assortment of disorders that primarily result from estrogen deficiency. These conditions are listed in Box 32-1.

BOX 32-1   Indications for Estrogen Therapy

- Atrophic vaginitis (shrinkage of the vagina and/or urethra)
- Hypogonadism
- Oral contraception (in combination with a progestin)
- Ovarian failure or castration
- Uterine bleeding
- Breast/prostate cancer (palliative treatment of advanced inoperable cases)
- Kraurosis vulvae (atrophy and shrinkage of the skin of the vagina and vulva)
- Osteoporosis and prophylaxis
- Postpartum lactation (prevention of)
- Dysmenorrhea (painful or difficult menstruation)

Side Effects and Adverse Effects

The most serious side and adverse effects of the estrogens are thromboembolic events. Rarely they can cause erythema multiforme, a rare skin disorder in which acute eruptions of macules, papules, or subdermal vesicles that exhibit a multiforme appearance appear on the hands and forearms. It can be recurrent or may run a severe course and fatally terminate in Stevens-Johnson syndrome. The most common undesirable effect of estrogens is nausea. Other undesirable effects are listed in Table 32-1.

Interactions

Estrogens can decrease the activity of the oral anticoagulants, and their concurrent use with rifampin can decrease the estrogenic effect. Their use with tricyclic antidepressants (TCAs) may result in a toxic response. Smoking during estrogen therapy should be avoided because this too can diminish the estrogenic effect and add to the risk of a thrombosis.

Dosages

See the dosages table on p. 499 for the recommended dosages of estrogens.

PROGESTINS

Progestational agents consist of both natural and synthetic agents. *Progesterone* is the principal natural proges-

---

drug profiles

estrogen

Estrogen replacement is indicated for the treatment of many clinical conditions, but primarily those resulting from estrogen deficiency (see Box 32-1). Therefore it follows that many of these conditions occur around menopause when the endogenous estradiol level is declining. Any estrogen capable of binding to the estrogen receptors in target organs can alleviate these menopausal symptoms. As a general rule, however, the smallest dose of estrogen that alleviates the symptoms or prevents the condition is used for the shortest possible time.

BOX 32-2 Diethylstibestrol (DES)

Between 1940 and 1971, an estimated 6 million mothers and their fetuses were exposed to diethylstilbestrol (DES). It was used to prevent reproductive problems such as miscarriage, premature delivery, intrauterine fetal death, and toxemia. This use resulted in significant complications of the reproductive system in both female and male offspring. Two large groups have been established to monitor these complications: the Registry for Research on Hormonal Transplacental Carcinogenesis and the Diethylstilbestrol Adenosis (DESAD) Project.

Estrogenic agents are contraindicated in the following clinical settings: hypersensitivity, active or history of estrogen-associated thromboembolic disorders (except for cancer palliation), abnormal genital bleeding, estrogen-dependent neoplasms, and breast cancer. These agents are also classified as pregnancy category X agents by the FDA.

The principal pharmacologic effects of all the estrogens are similar because there are only slight differences in their chemical structure. These differences make for different potencies, which in turn make them useful for a variety of indications. They also allow the agents to be given by different routes of administration.

Many fixed estrogen/progestin combination products have emerged over the years. These are commonly referred to as *continuous-combined hormone replacement therapy* (CCHRT). The rationale for the development of these agents is that the use of unopposed estrogen therapy has been associated with an increased risk of endometrial hyperplasia, a possible precursor of endometrial adenocarcinoma. The addition of continuous administration of progestin to an estrogen regimen reduces the incidence of endometrial hyperplasia associated with the use of unopposed estrogen therapy. Examples of these fixed combinations are conjugated estrogens with medroxyprogesterone (Prempro and Premphase), norethindrone acetate with ethinyl estradiol (Femhrt), and estradiol with norethindrone (CombiPatch).

Activity

---

tational hormone. It is produced by the corpus luteum and during pregnancy by the placenta. Because orally administered progesterone is relatively inactive and parenterally administered progesterone causes local reactions and pain, chemical derivatives were developed that are effective orally and also more potent. Their actions are also more specific and of longer duration. These are the progestins, and the commonly used ones are as follows:

- hydroxyprogesterone (Duralutin, Gesterol LA)
- medroxyprogesterone (Amen, Cycrin, Provera, Depo-Provera)

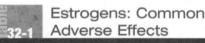

Table 32-1 Estrogens: Common Adverse Effects

Body System	Side/Adverse Effects
Cardiovascular	Hypertension, thrombophlebitis, edema
Gastrointestinal	Nausea, vomiting, diarrhea, constipation, abdominal pain
Genitourinary	Amenorrhea, breakthrough uterine bleeding, enlarged uterine fibromyomas
Other	Tender breasts, fluid retention, decreased carbohydrate tolerance, headaches

DOSAGES Selected Estrogenic Agents

agent	pharmacologic class	dosage range	purpose
STEROIDAL			
conjugated estrogens (Cenestin, Premarin) and esterified estrogens (Estratab, Menest)	Estrogenic hormone mixture	*Adult* PO: 0.3-1.25 mg/day cyclically Intravaginal: 2-4 g/day cyclically	Atropic vaginitis, kraurosis vulvae, vasomotor symptoms of menopause
		PO: 10 mg tid for at least 3 mo PO: 1.25 mg/day cyclically or continuously PO: 2.5-7.5 mg/day divided for 20 days, followed by a 10-day rest period PO: 3.75 mg q4h for 5 doses or 1.25 mg q4h for 5 days PO: 1.25-2.5 mg tid IM/IV: 25 mg repeat in 6-12 hr prn	Breast cancer Castration, ovarian failure Female hypogonadism Postpartum breast engorgement Prostate cancer Abnormal uterine bleeding
estradiol (Estrace)	Estrogenic hormone	*Adult* PO: 1-2 mg/day cyclically Intravaginal: 2-4 g/day for 12 wk with 1 g 1-3 times/wk PO: 10 mg tid for at least 3 mo PO: 1-2 mg/day tid PO: 0.5 mg/day cyclically for 3 wk, then off 1 wk Topical (patch): 2-4 g once daily	Atropic vaginitis, kraurosis vulvae, vasomotor symptoms of menopause Breast cancer Prostate cancer Osteoporosis prophylaxis Atropic vaginitis or kraurosis vulvae
estradiol cypionate (Dep Gynogen, Depogen)	Estrogenic hormone	*Adult* IM: 1-5 mg every 3-4 wk IM: 1.5-2 mg every mo for 3 wk, then off 1 wk	Symptoms of menopause Female hypogonadism
estradiol transdermal (Estraderm, FemPatch, Vivelle, Climara)	Estrogenic hormone	*Adult* Topical: Apply 0.05 mg system to abdominal skin twice weekly, either cyclically (intact uterus) or continuously (nonintact uterus). Dosage must be adjusted.	Symptoms of menopause
estradiol valerate (Delestrogen, Duragen, Valergen)	Estrogenic hormone	*Adult* IM: 10-20 mg every 4 wk IM: 10-25 mg administered at first stage of labor IM: 30 mg or more every 1-2 wk	Symptoms of menopause Postpartum breast engorgement Prostate cancer
estropipate (Ogen)	Estrogenic hormone (solubilized estrone)	*Adult* PO: 0.625-5 mg/day cyclically Intravaginal: 2-4 g/day cyclically PO: 1-25-7.5 mg/day for 21 days, then off 7 days PO: 0.625 mg/day for 25 days of a 31-day cycle	Atrophic vaginitis, kraurosis vulvae, symptoms of menopause Female castration, hypogonadism, primary ovarian failure Osteoporosis prophylaxis
ethinyl estradiol (Estinyl)	Estrogenic hormone	*Adult* PO: 0.02-1.5 mg/day cyclically PO: 0.05 mg 1-3 times/day for 2 wk, followed by progesterone for 2 wk. Continue this regimen for 3-6 mo. PO: 1 mg tid PO: 0.15-2 mg/day Vaginal (extended-release insert): once every 3 mo	Symptoms of menopause Female hypogonadism Breast cancer Prostate cancer Urogenital atrophy
quinestrol (Estrovis)	Synthetic estrogenic hormone	*Adult* PO: 100 μg/day for 7 days, then 100 μg weekly as maintenance	Atrophic vaginitis, kraurosis, vulvae, female castration/hypogonadism, primary ovarian failure, symptoms of menopause

Continued

DOSAGES Selected Estrogenic Agents—cont'd

agent	pharmacologic class	dosage range	purpose
NONSTEROIDAL chlorotrianisene (TACE)	Synthetic nonsteroidal estrogenic agent	*Adult* PO: 12-25 mg/day in 28 day cycles (1-21, off 22-28) PO: 12 mg qid for 7 days or 50 mg q6h for 6 doses PO: 12-25 mg/day	Atrophic vaginitis, kraurosis vulvae, symptoms of menopause Postpartum breast engorgement Prostate cancer
dienestrol (DV)	Synthetic nonsteroidal estrogenic agent	*Adult* Intravaginal: apply 1-2 applicators full/day for 1-2 wk. Reduce dosage as indicated. Usual maintenance dose is 1 applicator full 1-3 times/day for 3-6 mo	Atrophic vaginitis, kraurosis vulvae
diethylstilbestrol (DES, Honvol, Stilboestrol)	Synthetic nonsteroidal estrogenic agent	*Adult* PO: 15 mg/day PO: 1-3 mg/day	Breast cancer Prostate cancer
diethylstilbestrol diphosphate (Stilphostrol)	Synthetic nonsteroidal estrogenic agent	*Adult* PO: 50 mg tid and adjusted; do not exceed 1 g/day IV: 0.5 g/day and increase to 1 g on next ≥5 days, followed by 0.25-0.5 g maintenance dose 1-2 times/wk	Prostate cancer

- norethindrone (Norlutin, Micronor)
- norethindrone acetate (Aygestin, Norlutate)
- norgestrel (Ovrette, Ovral)
- megestrol (Megace)
- progesterone (Gesterol 50, Prometrium)

Progestins produce all the same responses as those produced by progesterone. These include inducing secretory changes in the endometrium, increasing the basal body temperature, producing changes in the vaginal epithelium, relaxing uterine smooth muscle, stimulating mammary alveolar tissue growth, inhibiting the pituitary, and producing withdrawal bleeding in the presence of estrogen.

Mechanism of Action

When exogenous progestins are given, the body senses that it does not need to produce and release more progestins. These progestins in the blood signal the pituitary gland to inhibit gonadotropin. This mechanism is called *feedback inhibition.*

Drug Effects

Progestins affect the pituitary gland, uterus (especially during the menstrual cycle) vaginal mucosa, and mammary glands. Because gonadotropin normally stimulates the ovaries, its suppressed release as the result of feedback inhibition causes the function of the ovaries to be suppressed. The subsequent effects on the uterus include an increase in the secretory (luteal) phase of endometrial development during the menstrual cycle and relaxation of uterine smooth muscle during pregnancy. In addition, the vaginal mucosa increases in thickness and mammary tissue growth is stimulated during therapy with progestins. Progestins are known to decrease endometrial tissue proliferation.

Therapeutic Uses

Progestins are useful in the treatment of functional uterine bleeding caused by a hormonal imbalance, fibroids, or uterine cancer; the treatment of primary and secondary amenorrhea; the adjunctive and palliative treatment of some cancers and endometriosis; and alone or in combination with estrogens for the prevention of conception. They may also be useful to prevent a threatened miscarriage and alleviate the symptoms of premenstrual syndrome (PMS). Specifically, medroxyprogesterone, hydroxyprogesterone, norethindrone, and progesterone have all been used to treat hormone imbalance, primary or secondary amenorrhea, and functional bleeding of the uterus, although medroxyprogesterone is the one most commonly used for this. Norethindrone and norgestrel may be used to treat female hormone imbalance and endometriosis but are more commonly used alone or in combination with estrogens as contraceptives to prevent pregnancy. Megestrol is commonly used to treat breast and endometrial cancers. When estrogen replacement therapy is used after menopause, progestins may be used to decrease endometrial proliferation that can be caused by unopposed estrogen.

Side Effects and Adverse Effects

The most serious undesirable effects of progestins include liver dysfunction, commonly manifested as cholestatic jaundice; thrombophlebitis; and thromboembolic disorders such as pulmonary embolism. The more common of these effects are listed in Table 32-2.

Interactions

Reports of possible decreases in glucose tolerance when progestins are taken with antidiabetic agents may require

research

Emergency Postcoital Contraception

Emergency contraception (EC) is one way that female rape victims may be treated without the impact of unwanted pregnancies. However, its use in the United States is not well known. It has been used in specific settings, such as college health centers and family planning clinics for patients with unwanted pregnancies who have had no or poor prenatal care and for rape victims in emergency rooms. The use of EC has many ethical and religious implications, making its use controversial in many professional arenas. However, all women should have all options, including EC, presented to them when they are confronted with the aforementioned situations.

EC is available in several forms. EC pills are high-dose hormones and are not considered to be "abortifacient." The mechanism of action of this drug may be through its inhibition of ovulation and a disruption of the corpus luteum. In addition, it decreases the luteal phase and inhibits the secretion of pituitary hormones while making the cervical mucus impossible to penetrate. EC pills also decrease the function of endometrial hormones and have an effect on the endometrium that makes implantation of the egg impossible. Contraindications include a history of thromboembolic disorders, cerebrovascular accident, and tumors of the liver and breast. Females who have a history of migraines, liver disease, and high blood pressure are at a higher risk for complications with use of EC pills. Side effects include nausea and vomiting. If taken more than 72 hours after the rape or unprotected intercourse, the rate of effectiveness declines to 85% or lower. For more information about EC, the Emergency Contraceptive Hotline can be contacted toll-free at 888-NOT-2-LATE.

Data from Schnare SM: Emergency postcoital contraception, *Am J Nurse Pract* 4(2): 15, 2000.

that the dose of the antidiabetic agent be adjusted. The concurrent use of medroxyprogesterone or norethindrone with aminoglutethimide or rifampin induces increased metabolism of the progestin.

Dosages

For recommended dosages of the progestins, see the dosages table on p. 502.

drug profiles

medroxyprogesterone

Medroxyprogesterone (Amen, Cycrin, Provera, Depo-Provera) inhibits the secretion of pituitary gonadotropins, which prevents follicular maturation and ovulation; stimulates the growth of mammary tissue; and has an antineoplastic action against endometrial cancer. It is used to treat uterine bleeding, secondary amenorrhea, endometrial cancer, and re-

Table 32-2 Progestins: Common Adverse Effects

Body System	Side/Adverse Effects
Gastrointestinal	Nausea, vomiting
Genitourinary	Amenorrhea, breakthrough uterine bleeding, spotting, changes in menstrual flow, changes in cervical erosion and secretions
Other	Edema, weight gain or loss, allergic rash, pyrexia, somnolence or insomnia, mental depression

nal cancer, and is also used as a contraceptive. Its most common use is to prevent endometrial cancer caused by estrogen replacement. It is classified as a pregnancy category X agent and is contraindicated in patients with a history of thrombophlebitis, thromboembolic disorders, cerebral apoplexy, liver disease, undiagnosed vaginal bleeding, suspected breast cancer, or drug hypersensitivity.

Medroxyprogesterone is available in both oral and parenteral preparations. Orally it is available as 2.5-, 5-, and 10-mg tablets. Parenterally it is available as a 100-, 150-, and 400-mg/ml sterile suspension for IM injection. Recommended dosages are given in the dosages table on p. 502.

PHARMACOKINETICS

HALF-LIFE	ONSET	PEAK	DURATION
14.5 hr	Unknown	IM: 2-7 hr	IM: 3 mo

megestrol

Megestrol (Megace) is a synthetic progestin that differs structurally from progesterone only in the addition of a methyl group on the steroid nucleus and a double bond. Although megestrol shares the actions of the progestins, it is primarily used in the palliative management of recurrent, inoperable, or metastatic endometrial or breast cancer. It has also been used in the management of anorexia, cachexia, or an unexplained, substantial weight loss in patients with acquired immunodeficiency syndrome (AIDS). In addition, it may be used to stimulate appetite and promote weight gain in patients with cancer. It is also classified as a pregnancy category X agent, and the contraindications to its use are the same as those of the other progestins. It is only available orally as a 200-mg/5 ml oral suspension and as 20- and 40-mg tablets. Recommended dosages are given in the dosages table on p. 502.

PHARMACOKINETICS

HALF-LIFE	ONSET	PEAK	DURATION
34 hr	6-8 wk	Unknown	4-10 mo

Activity

DOSAGES Selected Progestational Agents and Selective Estrogen Receptor Modulators (SERMs)

agent	pharmacologic class	dosage range	purpose
hydroxyprogesterone caproate (Hy-Gestrone, Hylutin, Hyprogest, Prodox)	Progestin	*Adult* IM: 375 mg	Amenorrhea, uterine bleeding
medroxyprogesterone acetate (Amen, Cycrin, Provera, Depo-Provera)	Progestin	*Adult* PO: 5-10 mg/day for 5-10 day; withdrawal bleeding usually starts 3-7 days after ending therapy PO: 5-10 mg each day for 5-10 days beginning on calculated day 16 or 21 of cycle IM: 400-1000 mg/wk	Amenorrhea Uterine bleeding Metastatic endometrial or renal cancer
megestrol acetate (Megace)	Progestin	*Adult* PO: 400-800 mg/day PO: 40 mg qid PO: 40-320 mg/day in divided doses	Weight loss in AIDS patients Breast cancer Endometrial cancer
norethindrone (Norlutin)	Progestin	*Adult* PO: 5-20 mg starting on day 5 and ending on day 25 of the cycle PO: 10 mg/day for 2 wk and increase by 5 mg every 2 wk until 30 mg/day is reached, then continue for 6-9 mo; if breakthrough bleeding occurs, therapy should be stopped temporarily	Amenorrhea, uterine bleeding Endometriosis
norethindrone acetate (Aygestin, Norlutate)	Progestin	*Adult* PO: 2.5-10 mg daily for 5-10 days PO: 5 mg/day for 2 wk and increase by 2.5 mg every 2 wk until 15 mg/day is reached, then continue for 6-9 mo; if breakthrough bleeding occurs, therapy should be stopped temporarily	Amenorrhea, uterine bleeding Endometriosis
progesterone (Progestasert, Gesterol 50)	Progestin	*Adult* IM: 5-10 mg/day for 6-8 days IM: 5-10 mg/day for 6 days	Amenorrhea Uterine bleeding
raloxifene (Evista)	SERM	*Adult* PO: 60 mg daily	Osteoporosis prevention

SELECTIVE ESTROGEN RECEPTOR MODULATORS AND RELATED AGENTS

A new class of agents that work primarily on estrogen receptors have emerged for the prevention of postmenopausal **osteoporosis.** Selective estrogen receptor modulators (SERMs) act as estrogen receptor agonists at the estrogen receptors on bones while simulatneously blocking or antagonizing estrogen receptors on breast and uterine tissue.

Currently raloxifene (Evista) and tamoxifen (Novadex) are the available SERMs. Tamoxifen has been available for many years. It has primarily been used alone as an adjunct to surgery and radiation therapy for the treatment of breast cancer in women with negative axillary lymph nodes and in postmenopausal women with positive axillary lymph nodes. Adjuvant tamoxifen therapy reduces the occurrence of contralateral breast cancer in premenopausal or postmenopausal women with breast cancer. It has also been shown to be beneficial in women at high risk of developing breast cancer for primary prevention.

Raloxifene, the newest SERM, has primarily been studied for prevention of osteoporosis, although many studies suggest that it may be beneficial in the treatment of osteoporosis as well. Other agents that have also shown beneficial results in the prevention and/or treatment of osteoporosis are estrogens such as estradiol (Climara), bisphosphonates such as alendronate (Fosamax) or tiludronate (Skelid), calcium supplementation, and calcitonin.

Approximately 23 million women in the United States currently are affected by osteoporosis or have low bone mass. Nearly 40% of women over 50 years of age will develop an osteoporotic fracture, and the annual costs to society equal nearly $11 billion. Supplemental calcium should be added to the diet if daily intake is inadequate. Risk factors for postmenopausal osteoporosis include Caucasian or Asian descent, slender body build, early estrogen deficiency, smoking, alcohol consumption, low calcium diet, sedentary lifestyle, and family history of osteoporosis.

Mechanism of Action

Tamoxifen stimulates estrogen receptors on bone and blocks estrogen receptors on the breast. It is primarily used as an adjuvant agent in the prevention and treatment of breast cancer. Raloxifene also stimulates estrogen receptors on bone and blocks estrogen receptors on breast tissue. The difference is that raloxifene also blocks the estrogen receptors of the uterus.

Drug Effects

SERMs have different degrees of estrogen agonist or antagonist effects in different tissues. The three-dimensional configuration of a drug determines which of these effects the drug will have. Tamoxifen acts as an estrogen receptor agonist on bone and an estrogen antagonist on the breast. Antagonism of breast tissue in estrogen-receptor-positive patients helps reduce the incidence and reoccurrence of breast cancer. Tamoxifen acts as a partial estrogen agonist on the uterus. The influence of this stimulation is still unknown. Raloxifene has an estrogen agonist effect on bone and an antagonist effect on both the breast and the uterus. SERMs have positive effects on lipid metabolism. They decrease total and LDL cholesterol. Stimulation of estrogen receptors on bone, seen with both tamoxifen and raloxifene, helps prevent bone loss by increasing bone mineral density.

Therapeutic Uses

Raloxifene is primarily used for the prevention of postmenopausal osteoporosis. Its use for the treatment of osteoporosis or the prevention of breast cancer is unknown at this point. Tamoxifen on the other hand is used for the treatment and prevention of breast cancer.

Side Effects and Adverse Effects

The primary side effects of SERMs are hot flashes and leg cramps. Like estrogens they can increase the risk of venous thromboembolism and they are teratogenic. Postmenopausal women taking raloxifene were no more likely to develop breast, uterine, or ovarian cancer than women taking a placebo.

Interactions

Cholestyramine and ampicillin decrease the absorption of raloxifene, and raloxifene can decrease the effects of warfarin.

Dosages

For the recommended dosage of raloxifene, see the dosages table on p. 502.

---

case study **Osteoporosis**

T.L. is a relatively healthy 73-year-old female with newly diagnosed postmenopausal osteoporosis. She has been prescribed treatment with alendronate (Fosamax) 10 mg orally every day. Approximately 5 days after initiating treatment, T.L. experiences dysphagia and odynophagia. She is scheduled for an endoscopy in the morning to rule out ulcerative esophagitis.

- *What is Fosamax and what are its indications?*
- *How could the adverse reaction to this medication administration have been prevented?*
- *What drug interactions are significant with Fosamax?*

For Answers see www.harcourthealth.com/MERLIN/Lilley/.

---

drug profiles

alendronate

Alendronate (Fosamax) is an oral bisphosphonate that is indicated for the prevention and treatment of osteoporosis in men and postmenopausal women. It is also indicated for the treatment of glucocorticoidinduced osteoporosis in men and women and for treatment of Paget's disease. It works by inhibiting osteoclast-mediated bone resorption. Osteoclasts break down bone, reabsorbing calcium back into the circulation, and eventually leading to osteoporosis if not controlled. Alendronate was the first nonestrogen, nonhormonal option for preventing bone loss. Recently a second oral bisphosphonate, tiludronate (Skelid), was approved. Tiludronate is currently indicated only for the treatment of Paget's disease.

Data show that alendronate may reduce the risk of hip fracture by 51%, spinal fracture by 47%, and wrist fracture by 48%. It is contraindicated in women known to be hypersensitive to alendronate. Precaution should be taken in patients with dysphagia, esophagitis, esophageal ulcer, or gastric ulcer because it can be very irritating. Case reports of esophageal erosions have been published. It is recommended that alendronate be given first thing in the morning upon rising with an 8-ounce glass of water and that the patient not lie down for at least 30 minutes after taking. When patients stabilized on alendronate are hospitalized and cannot comply with these recommendations, the medication is often withheld. Alendronate has an extremely long terminal half-life, and going several days without taking a dose will do little if anything to the therapeutic efficacy of the drug.

Alendronate is available in 5-, 10-, and 40-mg tablets. It is dosed 5-40 mg daily. The normal dose for treatment and prevention of osteoporosis is 10 mg daily, and the normal dose for treatment of Paget's disease is 40 mg daily. It recently became available in a 35- and 70-mg tablet for once weekly dosing.

PHARMACOKINETICS

HALF-LIFE	ONSET	PEAK	DURATION
10 yr	3 wk*	Unknown	Unknown

*Therapeutic effect.

raloxifene

Raloxifene (Evista) is an SERM. It is used primarily for the prevention of postmenopausal osteoporosis. Raloxifene has positive effects on cholesterol, decreasing total and LDL cholesterol without effecting HDL or triglycerides. Raloxifene helps prevent osteoporosis by stimulating estrogen receptors on bone and increasing bone density. Raloxifene is contraindicated in women who are or may become pregnant and in women with active or past history of venous thromboembolic events, including deep vein thrombosis, pulmonary embolism, and retinal vein thrombosis. It is also contraindicated in women known to be hypersensitive to raloxifene or other constituents of the tablets. It is available in 60-mg film-coated tablets. Recommended dosages are listed in the dosages table on p. 502.

PHARMACOKINETICS

HALF-LIFE	ONSET	PEAK	DURATION
27 hr	Unknown	Unknown	Unknown

ORAL CONTRACEPTIVES

Oral contraceptives are the most effective form of birth control currently available. Estrogen-progestin combinations, sometimes referred to as "the pill," are oral contraceptives that contain both estrogenic and progestinic steroids. The estrogenic component is either ethinyl estradiol or mestranol. Ethinyl estradiol is a semisynthetic steroidal estrogen, and as previously noted, it is the most orally active estrogenic drug currently available. It is about twenty times more potent than diethylstilbestrol. Mestranol is slightly less active. The progestinic component is desogestrel, ethynodiol diacetate, levonorgestrel, norethindrone, norethindrone acetate, norethynodrel, or norgestrel.

The currently available oral contraceptives may be biphasic or triphasic in terms of the doses taken at different times in the menstrual cycle. The biphasic agents contain a fixed estrogen dose but a low progestin dose for the first 10 days and a higher dose for the rest of the cycle in 21- or 28-day dosage packages. The triphasic oral contraceptives contain three different estrogen-progestin dose ratios that are administered sequentially during the cycle in 21- or 28-day dosage packs. The triphasic products closely duplicate the normal hormonal levels of the female cycle. These contraceptives also come in a monophasic form, in which the estrogen and progestin doses are the same throughout the cycle. There are also oral contraceptives that are progestin-only agents.

Oral Contraceptives: Common Adverse Effects

Table 32-3

Body System	Side/Adverse Effects
Cardiovascular	Hypotension, thrombophlebitis, edema, thromboembolism, pulmonary embolism, myocardial infarction
Central nervous system	Dizziness, headache, migraines, depression, stroke
Gastrointestinal	Nausea, vomiting, diarrhea, anorexia, pancreatitis, cramps, constipation, increased appetite, increased weight, cholestatic jaundice
Genitourinary	Amenorrhea, cervical erosion, breakthrough bleeding, dysmenorrhea, breast changes

Mechanism of Action

Oral contraceptives prevent ovulation by inhibiting the release of gonadotropins and by increasing uterine mucous viscosity resulting in (1) decreased sperm movement and fertilization of the ovum, and (2) possible inhibition of implantation of fertilized egg (zygote).

Drug Effects

Oral contraceptives have many of the same effects as those normally produced by the endogenous estrogens and progesterone. The contraceptive effect mainly results from the suppression of the hypothalamic-pituitary system they induce, which in turn prevents ovulation. Other incidental benefits to their use are that they improve menstrual cycle regularity and decrease blood loss during menstruation. A decreased incidence of functional ovarian cysts and ectopic pregnancies has also been associated with their use. Drawbacks to their use include hypertension, thromboembolism, alterations in carbohydrate and lipid metabolism, increases in serum hormone concentrations, and alterations in serum metal and plasma protein levels. It is the estrogen component that appears to be the source of most of these metabolic effects.

Therapeutic Uses

Oral contraceptives are primarily used to prevent pregnancy. In addition, they are used to treat endometriosis and hypermenorrhea and to produce cyclic withdrawal bleeding. Occasionally combination oral contraceptives (COCs) are used to provide postcoital emergency contraception. Emergency contraception pills (ECPs) are not effective if the woman is pregnant and should be taken within 72 hours of unprotected intercourse with a follow-up dose 12 hours after the first dose. They are intended to prevent pregnancy after known or suspected contraceptive failure or unprotected intercourse. Preven and Alesse are two ethinyl estradiol/levonorgestrel combination agents that are commonly used for this indication.

DOSAGES Selected Oral Contraceptive Agents

agent	pharmacologic class	dosage range	purpose
Biphasic (Nelova LO/11 Ortho-Novum 10/11 21, Orth-Novum 10/11-28)	Fixed estrogen-variable progestin 21- or 28-day products		
Monophasic (Brevicon, Demulen, Genora, Levlen, Lo/Orval Norinyl, Ortho Novum, Orval)	Fixed estrogen-progestin 21- or 28-day products; 28-day products contain 7 inert tablets	Take exactly as directed by physician/patient product insert (21/28 day programs) and at intervals not exceeding 24 hr.	Contraception
Triphasic (Ortho-Novum 7/7/7 21; Ortho-Novum 7/7/7 28; Tri-Levlen 21, 28; Triphasil-21, -28; Tri-Norinyl 21, 28 day)	Three fixed estrogen-progestin combination		

Side Effects and Adverse Effects

Common side effects and adverse effects associated with the use of oral contraceptives are listed in Table 32-3.

Interactions

There are many drugs that decrease the effectiveness of oral contraceptives. The drugs that have clinically relevant interactions with oral contraceptives are few and include the following:

- Antibiotics
- Barbiturates
- griseofulvin
- isoniazid
- rifampin

Drugs that may have reduced effectiveness when taken with oral contraceptives include the following:

- Anticonvulsants
- Beta-blockers
- guanethidine
- Hypnotics
- Hypoglycemic agents
- Oral anticoagulants
- theophylline
- TCAs
- Vitamins

Dosages

For the recommended dosages of oral contraceptives, see the dosages table above.

drug profiles

Oral contraceptives are contraindicated in the following settings: known or suspected breast cancer, estrogen neoplasia, pregnancy, present or past thrombophlebotic disorders, undiagnosed abnormal genital bleeding, cerebrovascular and coronary disease, and benign or malignant liver tumors associated with estrogen use. Oral contraceptives are classified as pregnancy category X agents.

LABOR AND DELIVERY DRUGS

Many drugs can be used during labor and delivery. There are agents that stimulate uterine contraction, those that relax the uterus, those that stimulate ovulation, those that inhibit lactation, and those that suppress the immune response. Many of these drugs have other uses and may be discussed in greater detail in other chapters, but all are discussed briefly here.

UTERINE STIMULANTS

There are three types of drugs that are used to stimulate uterine contractions: ergot derivatives, prostaglandins, oxytocin. All work on the uterus, a highly muscular organ that has a complex network of smooth muscle fibers and a large blood supply. The uterus undergoes several changes during normal gestation and childbirth that at different times make it either resistant or susceptible to various hormones and drugs. These agents are sometimes referred to as oxytocic agents, named after the naturally occurring hormone oxytocin whose action they mimic. It is one of the two hormones secreted by the posterior pituitary. The other is vasopressin, or antidiuretic hormone. The uterus of a woman who is not pregnant is relatively insensitive to oxytocin, but during pregnancy the uterus becomes more sensitive to oxytocin, being most sensitive at term (the end of gestation).

During childbirth, oxytocin stimulates uterine contraction, and during lactation it promotes the movement of milk from the mammary glands to the nipples. Oxytocin is available in a synthetic form called *Pitocin*. This agent is used to induce labor at or near full-term gestation and to stimulate labor when uterine contractions are weak and ineffective. Oxytocic agents are also used to prevent or control uterine bleeding after delivery, to complete an incomplete abortion, and to promote milk ejection during lactation.

Another class of oxytocic agents are the prostaglandins, natural hormones involved in regulating the muscles of the uterus, referred to as the *myometrium*. These hormones cause very potent contractions of the myometrium and may be responsible for the natural induction of labor.

When the prostaglandin concentrations increase during the final few weeks of pregnancy, this stimulates mild myometrial contractions, commonly known as *Braxton Hicks contractions*. The prostaglandins may be used therapeutically to induce labor and enhance uterine muscle tone. They may also be used to stimulate the myometrium to induce abortion during the second trimester when the uterus is resistant to oxytocin.

The third class of oxytocic agents are the ergot alkaloids, which are also potent simulators of uterine muscle. These agents increase the force and frequency of uterine contractions and are used after delivery of the infant and placenta to prevent postpartum uterine atony and hemorrhage.

Mechanism of Action

The mechanisms of action of the various oxytocic agents vary depending on the agent. One common characteristic of all three classes of agents is that they stimulate uterine smooth muscle contraction. As previously noted, Pitocin is the synthetic form of oxytocin and has all the pharmacologic properties of the endogenously produced hormone. It indirectly stimulates contraction of uterine smooth muscle by increasing the sodium permeability of uterine myobrils. In the term uterus, oxytocin increases the amplitude and frequency of uterine contractions; decreases cervical activity, producing dilation; and impedes uterine blood flow. During lactation, oxytocin causes the cells surrounding the alveoli of the breast to contract, forcing milk from the alveoli into the larger ducts and thus facilitating milk ejection. Prostaglandins such as dinoprostone directly stimulate uterine and gastrointestinal smooth muscle. Like Pitocin, dinoprostone increases the frequency and amplitude of uterine contractions but the uterus is more responsive to it than to Pitocin in early pregnancy. This is why it may be used to induce abortion. Dinoprostone-induced uterine contractions are usually sufficient to cause evacuation of both the fetus and the placenta. It also produces cervical dilation and softening.

legal & ethical principles

Administration of Oxytocin

A patient is admitted to labor and delivery for the delivery of her third child and is given oxytocin for induction of labor. The patient eventually ended up with a hysterectomy because of a uterine tear, which resulted in uncontrolled heavy uterine bleeding that did not stop with repair of the tear. During the hysterectomy, the patient received several blood transfusions and subsequently developed hepatitis. The hospital, nurses, and physicians were sued for negligence and malpractice, and a verdict was made on behalf of the patient. The health care professionals and the hospital were cited as failing to properly monitor and adhere to the standards of care for administration of oxytocin. What nursing actions could have easily been implemented to ensure patient and fetal safety and prevent harm or injury during drug administration? Would documentation of monitoring also be necessary?

Ergot alkaloids such as ergonovine and methylergonovine are pharmacologically similar; both directly stimulate contractions of uterine and vascular smooth muscle. In large doses they elicit sustained, forceful contractions of the uterus. Like the other two classes of oxytocic drugs, ergot alkaloids also increase the amplitude and frequency of uterine contractions and uterine tone, which together impedes uterine blood flow. Ergonovine and methylergonovine also increase contractions of the cervix.

Drug Effects

The drug effects of the oxytocic agents are primarily limited to the uterine smooth muscle. The drug effects other than those on the uterus vary depending on the agent. Pitocin stimulates the smooth muscle of the uterus, causing uterine contraction and decreased uterine blood flow. It also facilitates milk ejection and may also produce vasodilation of vascular smooth muscle, thereby increasing renal, coronary, and cerebral blood flow. However, an initial decrease in blood pressure that it may produce is usually followed by a small but sustained increase in blood pressure. Prostaglandins such as dinoprostone directly stimulate uterine and gastrointestinal smooth muscle. Its effects on the uterus are similar to those of oxytocin, but it has the unique feature of being able to stimulate the uterine smooth muscle before full gestation. This makes it useful in abortions. Dinoprostone may also stimulate the circular smooth muscle of the gastrointestinal tract and increase gastrointestinal motility. When inhaled, dinoprostone causes bronchodilation. It may also cause increases in body temperature. Ergot alkaloids such as ergonovine and methylergonovine directly stimulate contractions of uterine and vascular smooth muscle and produce vasoconstriction. This vasoconstriction causes increases in the central venous pressure, blood pressure, and rarely peripheral ischemia, resulting in gangrene.

Therapeutic Uses

The therapeutic uses of the oxytocic agents vary depending on the particular agent. Pitocin is commonly used to induce labor in near-term or term pregnancies, to augment labor and promote contractions if labor is prolonged, to promote expulsion of the placenta and control uterine bleeding postpartum, to facilitate the completion

Table 32-4 Oxytocic Agents: Most Common Adverse Effects

Body System	Side/Adverse Effects
Cardiovascular	Hypotension or hypertension, chest pain
Central nervous system	Headache, dizziness, fainting
Gastrointestinal	Nausea, vomiting, diarrhea,
Genitourinary	Vaginitis, vaginal pain, cramping
Other	Leg cramps, joint swelling, chills, fever, weakness, blurred vision

of incomplete abortions after prostaglandin induction of the abortion, to promote milk ejection when the milk supply is inadequate, and to reduce postpartum breast engorgement. Prostaglandins such as dinoprostone are administered intravaginally to induce abortion during the second trimester (beyond the twelfth week of gestation). Dinoprostone cervical gel may also be used to improve cervical inducibility (cervical "ripening") near or at term in women with a medical or obstetric need for labor induction. This agent prepares the cervix for the induction of labor and makes the process easier. Intranasally administered dinoprostone may also be used to dilate the bronchi in patients with bronchial asthma, but its effects in this setting have been inconsistent, thus limiting its use for this purpose. Ergot alkaloids such as ergonovine and methylergonovine are primarily used for the prevention and treatment of postpartum and postabortion hemorrhage caused by uterine atony or subinvolution.

Side Effects and Adverse Effects

The most common undesirable effects of dinoprostone, ergonovine, methylergonovine, and oxytocin are listed in Table 32-4.

Interactions

There are few clinically significant drug interactions that occur with the oxytocic agents. The most common and important of these involve sympathomimetic drugs. The combination of drugs that produce vasoconstriction, such as sympathomimetics, with the oxytocic agents can result in severe hypertension.

Dosages

For the recommended dosages of selected oxytocic agents, see the dosages table below.

---

drug profiles

dinoprostone

Dinoprostone (Prostin E_2, Cervidil, Prepidil) is a synthetic derivative of the naturally occurring hormone prostaglandin E_2. It is used for the termination of pregnancy from the twelfth through the twentieth gestational weeks, for evacuation of the uterine contents in the management of missed abortion or intrauterine fetal death up to 28 weeks of gestational age, for the management of nonmetastatic gestational trophoblastic disease, and for ripening of an unfavorable cervix in pregnant women at or near term with a medical or obstetrical need for labor induction. The use of dinoprostone is contraindicated in the following settings: hypersensitivity, uterine fibrosis, cervical stenosis, pelvic inflammatory disease, and respiratory disease. It is also contraindicated in patients who have undergone pelvic operations. It is available as a 20-mg vaginal suppository (Prostin E_2), a 0.3-mg/hr vaginal insert (Cervidil), and a 0.5-mg/3 g vaginal gel. It is considered a pregnancy catgory C agent. Commonly recommended dosages are given in the dosages table below.

PHARMACOKINETICS

HALF-LIFE	ONSET	PEAK	DURATION
Gel			
N/A	Rapid	30-45 min	Unavailable
Suppository (vaginal)			
N/A	10 min	Unavailable	2-3 hr

DOSAGES Selected Uterine Stimulants

agent	pharmacologic class	dosage range	purpose
dinoprostone (Prostin E₂, Cervidil, Prepidil)	Prostaglandin E_2 abortifacient oxytoxic	*Adult* Vaginal: Insert one suppository (20 mg) q3-5h until abortion occurs; max 240 mg or 2 days	Abortion induction
		Cervical gel: 0.5 mg q6h until cervical/uterine response; max daily dose 1.5 mg	Labor induction
methylergonovine (Methergine)	Oxytoxic ergot alkaloid	*Adult* PO: 0.2-0.4 mg q6-12h for 2-7 days IM: 0.2 mg after delivery of placenta and repeated q2-4h prn for a total of 5 doses IV: Reserved for excessive bleeding; dosage the same as for IM route	Postpartum uterine atony and hemorrhage
oxytocin (Pitocin, Syntocinon)	Oxytoxic hypothalamic hormone	*Adult* IV: Infusion rate 1-2 mU/min; can be increased slowly until contractions reach desired rate/intensity	Labor induction
		IV: 10-40 U in 1000 ml infused at a rate sufficient to control uterine atony IM: 3-10 U after delivery of placenta	Postpartum uterine atony and hemorrhage
		Intranasal spray: 1 spray in one/both nostrils 2-3 min before nursing/pumping breast	Assist postpartum milk ejection

ergonovine and methylergonovine

The ergot alkaloids ergonovine (Ergotrate) and methylergonovine (Methergine) are pharmacologically similar. Their use is contraindicated in patients with a known hypersensitivity to ergot medications and in those with pelvic inflammatory disease. They also should not be used to augment labor, before delivery of the placenta, or during a spontaneous abortion.

Methylergonovine is available orally as 0.2-mg tablets and is a pregnancy category C agent. It is also available parenterally as a 0.2-mg/ml injection. Ergonovine is no longer being produced by the manufacturer and is a pregnancy category X agent. Commonly recommended dosages are given in the dosages table on p. 507.

PHARMACOKINETICS

HALF-LIFE	ONSET	PEAK	DURATION
<2 hr	PO: 5-15 min IM: <5 min	30 min	3 hr

oxytocin

Oxytocin (Pitocin and Syntocinon) is the synthetic form of the endogenous hormone oxytocin and has all of its pharmacologic properties. Oxytocin is contraindicated in patients with a history of hypersensitivity to the drug. Use of the nasal spray is contraindicated during pregnancy. Commonly recommended dosages are given in the dosages table on p. 507.

PHARMACOKINETICS

HALF-LIFE	ONSET	PEAK	DURATION
3-5 min	IV: Immediate IM: <5 min	IV: Immediate IM: Immediate	IV: 2-3 hr IM: 2-3 hr

UTERINE RELAXANTS

When contractions of the uterus begin before term, it may be desirable to stop labor, because premature birth, or labor before term, can have many detrimental effects, death of the neonate being the most serious consequence. Postponing delivery by relaxing the uterine smooth muscles and helping prevent contractions and the induction of labor increases the likelihood of the infant's survival. However, this measure is generally only employed after the twentieth week of gestation because spontaneous labor occurring before the twentieth week is frequently associated with a defective fetus and thus is usually not interrupted. Only uterine contractions occurring between about 20 and 37 weeks of gestation are considered premature labor.

The nonpharmacologic treatment of premature labor includes bed rest, sedation, and hydration. Drugs given to inhibit labor and maintain the pregnancy are called *tocolytics*. The three most commonly used tocolytics are ritodrine, terbutaline, and magnesium sulfate. Terbutaline and ritodrine are classified as beta-adrenergic agents (see Chapter 16) and work by directly relaxing uterine smooth muscle. Magnesium sulfate is most commonly used as an anticonvulsant in the treatment of pregnancy-induced hypertension (preeclampsia), but it is also an effective tocolytic agent.

Mechanism of Action

One common characteristic of all three tocolytics is that they relax uterine smooth muscle and stop the uterus from contracting. As previously mentioned, terbutaline and ritodrine work by directly relaxing uterine smooth muscle. They do so by stimulating beta-adrenergic receptors located on the bronchial tree, peripheral vasculature, and uterine smooth muscles. These are believed to be primarily beta$_2$-adrenergic receptors. (The beta$_1$-adrenergic receptors are located on the heart and are not stimulated by terbutaline or ritodrine except at high doses.)

Drug Effects

The drug effects of terbutaline and ritodrine are related to their beta-adrenergic effects. When the bronchial beta-adrenergic receptors are stimulated by these beta agonists, the bronchi dilate and airway resistance decreases. When the beta-adrenergic receptors of the peripheral vasculature are stimulated by these beta agonists, these blood vessels dilate and blood pressure decreases. Finally, when the beta-adrenergic receptors located on the uterine smooth muscle are stimulated by the beta agonists terbutaline and ritodrine, the uterine smooth muscle relaxes, thus stopping premature contractions.

Therapeutic Uses

Both terbutaline and ritodrine are used to inhibit uterine contractions in preterm labor. However, this is generally done only after the twentieth week of gestation, because

---

cultural implications

Use of Oral Contraceptives

A study done in 1997 found that African-American women are twice as likely as Caucasian women to *not* use a contraceptive method. With some 40 million females being at risk for unintended conception, more than half of unintended pregnancies occur in those females not using contraception. Previous research also shows that there is a great misunderstanding about the pill and how to take it for effectiveness.

Data from Libbus K, Arps CA: Beliefs related to the use of oral contraceptives by African-American women, Ages 18-35, *J Natl Black Nurses Assoc* 9(1):29, 1997

as previously noted, spontaneous labor before the twentieth week is frequently associated with a defective fetus and therefore is usually not interrupted. Terbutaline may also be used as a bronchodilator in the symptomatic treatment of bronchial asthma and reversible bronchospasm.

Side Effects and Adverse Effects

The most common adverse effects of terbutaline and ritodrine are listed in Table 32-5.

Toxicity and Management of Overdose

The toxicity stemming from an overdose of oxolytics and its management are similar to those of the other adrenergic agents and are discussed in Chapter 16.

Interactions

Few drug interactions occur with uterine relaxants. The most notable are sympathomimetic agents and beta-blockers. Sympathomimetic agents when given with uterine relaxants may have additive cardiovascular effects, and beta-blockers when given with uterine relaxants may have antagonistic effects.

Dosages

For the recommended dosages of ritodrine and terbutaline, see the dosages table below.

📋 drug profiles

Ritodrine and terbutaline are contraindicated in the following settings: hypersensitivity, eclampsia, hypertension, dysrhythmias, thyrotoxicosis, before the twentieth week of pregnancy, antepartum hemorrhage, intrauterine fetal death, maternal cardiac disease, pulmonary hypertension, and uncontrolled diabetes.

ritodrine

Ritodrine (Yutopar) is indicated for the prevention of preterm labor. Parenterally it is available as a 10- and 15-mg/ml injection for IV infusion, and orally it is available as a 10-mg tablet. Commonly recommended dosages are given in the dosages table below. Pregnancy category B.

PHARMACOKINETICS

HALF-LIFE	ONSET	PEAK	DURATION
IM/IV: 2-3 hr	IM: <15 min	IM: 20-40 min	IM: Unknown
PO: 2 hr	PO: <1 hr	PO: 30-60 min	PO: Unknown

terbutaline

Terbutaline (Brethine, Bricanyl) is indicated for the prevention of preterm labor and may also be used as a bronchodilator in the symptomatic treatment of bronchial asthma and occasionally in the treatment of hyperkalemia. It is available parenterally as a 1-mg/ml injection for SC administration and orally as a 2.5- and 5-mg tablet. It is also available as a 200-mg/metered spray for oral inhalation. Commonly recommended dosages are given in the dosages table below. Pregnancy category B.

PHARMACOKINETICS

HALF-LIFE	ONSET	PEAK	DURATION
PO: 20 hr	PO: 30-45 min	PO: 1-2 hr	PO: 6-8 hr
IV: 20 hr	IV: 5 min	IV: 30-60 min	IV: 1.5-4 hr
INH: Unknown	INH: 5-30 min	INH: 1-2 hr	INH: 3-4 hr

Activity

Tocolytic Agents: Most Common Adverse Effects

Table 32-5

Body System	Side/Adverse Effects
Cardiovascular	Palpitations, tachycardia, hypertension, dysrhythmias, altered maternal and fetal heart rate and blood pressure, chest pain
Central nervous system	Tremors, anxiety, insomnia, headache, dizziness, nervousness
Gastrointestinal	Nausea, vomiting, anorexia, bloating, constipation, diarrhea
Metabolic	Hyperglycemia, hypokalemia
Other	Rash, dyspnea, hyperventilation, glycosuria, lactic acidosis

DOSAGES Selected Uterine Relaxants

agent	pharmacologic class	dosage range	purpose
terbutaline sulfate (Brethine, Bricanyl)	Beta adrenergic	*Adult* 10 μg/min to a max of 80 μg/min IV if needed; 2.5 mg PO q4-6h for maintenance	Unlabeled management of preterm labor
ritodrine (Yutopar)	Beta adrenergic	*Adult* Starting IV infusion dose, 50-100 μg/min; usual effective dose, 150-350 μg/min	Management of preterm labor

FERTILITY AGENTS

Loss of fertility in women occurs for various reasons, and some of these disorders are amenable to treatment with fertility agents. These agents are bromocriptine, clomiphene, gonadorelin, chorionic gonadotropin, menotropins, and urofollitrophin.

In cases of infertility in which the hypophysis (pituitary gland) and the ovaries are normal but the stimulus that activates follicular development is absent, clomiphene can stimulate the hypothalamus and thus the ovaries to develop ovarian follicles. In women who are infertile because they cannot supply sufficient gonadotropins to properly stimulate the ovary, the hypophysis or pituitary gland is usually dysfunctional. Menotropins, gonadorelin, chorionic gonadotropin, and urofollitrophin may be useful in treating this form of infertility because they stimulate the release of follicule-stimulating hormone (FSH) and luteinizing hormone (LH). Chorionic gonadotropin and gonadorelin are used when primarily LH release must be stimulated.

Mechanism of Action

The mechanisms of action of the various fertility agents vary depending on the agent. Chorionic gonadotropin and gonadorelin have the principal pharmacologic effects of human chorionic gonadotropin (hCG). In fact, gonadorelin has the same amino acid sequence as hCG. The pharmacologic effects and mechanisms of action of the two agents are identical to those of LH. They may also have a minimal effect on FSH. During the normal menstrual cycle, LH and FSH are responsible for stimulating the development and maturation of the normal ovarian follicle. The abrupt midcycle increase in the LH concentration triggers ovulation. Because gonadotropin and gonadorelin can substitute for LH in this function, they can cause ovulation as well.

Menotropins and urofollitrophins have pharmacologic effects similar to those of FSH, which stimulates the development and maturation of the ovarian follicle. They also have properties similar to those of LH, which causes ovulation and stimulates the development of the **corpus**

Table 32-6 Fertility Agents: Most Common Adverse Effects

Body System	Side/Adverse Effects
Cardiovascular	Tachycardia, phlebitis, deep vein thrombosis, hypovolemia
Central nervous system	Dizziness, headache, flushing, depression, restlessness, anxiety, nervousness, fatigue, fever
Gastrointestinal	Nausea, bloating, constipation, abdominal pain, vomiting, anorexia
Other	Urticaria, ovarian hyperstimulation, multiple pregnancies, blurred vision, diplopia, photophobia, breast pain

luteum. The administration of menotropins for 9 to 12 consecutive days stimulates ovarian follicular growth and maturation in women whose infertility is not due to primary ovarian failure. To induce ovulation, a single, large dose of gonadotropin, which has LH activity, is then given when the clinical assessment shows that sufficient follicular maturation has occurred.

Clomiphene appears to stimulate the release of FSH and LH, which results in the development and maturation of the ovarian follicle, induces ovulation, and causes the subsequent development and function of the corpus luteum. Gonadotropin release may result either from direct stimulation of the hypothalamic-pituitary axis or from a decreased inhibitory influence of estrogens on the hypothalamic-pituitary axis, the latter occurring because of the competing influence of the endogenous estrogens from the uterus, pituitary, or hypothalamus. Clomiphene may also directly affect the biosynthesis of ovarian hormones.

Drug Effects

The drug effects of the ovulation stimulants, or fertility agents, are primarily the same as the effects of FSH and LH. By manipulating these drugs in various ways, they can be made to mimic these hormones' natural effects. They may also stimulate spermatogenesis in men.

Therapeutic Uses

The ovulation stimulants are primarily used in the treatment of female infertility. Clomiphene is used chiefly to induce ovulation in women who do not ovulate but want to get pregnant. It is also used in the treatment of other disorders, ranging from menstrual abnormalities to gynecomastia to fibrocystic disease of the breast. Gonadotropin and gonadorelin are customarily used in conjunction with menotropins in the treatment of infertility. Their action is almost identical to that of pituitary LH, and they may also have slight FSH activity. In addition, they may be used in men for the treatment of various conditions such asprepubertal cryptorchidism and hypogonadotropic hypogonadism. Menotropin is used to induce ovulation in women who do not ovulate. It also stimulates spermatogenesis in men. Urofollitrophin is pharmacologically similar to menotropins and therefore has similar therapeutic effects.

Side Effects and Adverse Effects

The most common adverse effects of the ovulation stimulants are listed in Table 32-6. Some of the agents may cause more and some fewer undesirable effects.

Interactions

Few drug interactions occur with fertility agents. The most notable are tricyclic antidepressants, butyrophenones, methyldopa, phenothiazines, and reserpine. When any of these agents are used with the fertility agents, increased prolactin concentrations can be seen. Additive hypotensive effects are seen when antihypertensives are given with bromocriptine.

Dosages

For recommended dosages of the fertility agents, see the dosages table below.

drug profiles

clomiphene

Clomiphene (Clomid, Serophene) is primarily used to stimulate the production of pituitary gonadotropins, which in turn induces the maturation of the ovarian follicle and eventually ovulation. It is contraindicated in women with a known hypersensitivity to it and in those with hepatic disease or undiagnosed vaginal bleeding. It is classified as a pregnancy category X agent and is available as a 50-mg oral tablet. Commonly recommended dosages are given in the dosages table below.

PHARMACOKINETICS

HALF-LIFE	ONSET	PEAK	DURATION
5 days	4-12 days	Unknown	1 mo

chorionic gonadotropin

Chorionic gonadotropin (A.P.L., Chorex-5, Follutein, Gonic, Pregnyl, Profasi HP) is a hormone that is normally secreted by the placenta, and its principal pharmacologic effects are the same as hCG's. It is classified as a pregnancy category B agent and is contraindicated in patients with a

known hypersensitivity to it, in patients with ovarian cysts or hormonally dependent tumors, and in those with anovulation stemming from causes other than those of hypothalamic origin. It is only available parenterally as 5000-, 10,000-, and 20,000-unit injections. Commonly recommended dosages are given in the dosages table below.

PHARMACOKINETICS

HALF-LIFE	ONSET	PEAK	DURATION
5.6 hr	2 hr	6 hr	36 hr

menotropins

Menotropins (Pergonal) is a purified preparation of gonadotropins extracted from the urine of postmenopausal women. It is classified as a pregnancy category C agent and is contraindicated in the settings of primary ovarian failure, abnormal bleeding, thyroid or adrenal dysfunction, an organic intracranial lesion, ovarian cysts, and primary testicular failure. It is only available as a parenteral injection in the following potencies: 75 IU of FSH activity with 75 IU of LH activity, or 150 IU of FSH activity with 150 IU of LH activity. Commonly recommended dosages are given in the dosages table below.

PHARMACOKINETICS

HALF-LIFE	ONSET	PEAK	DURATION
Unknown	Unknown	Unknown	Unknown

DOSAGES Selected Fertility Agents

agent	pharmacologic class	dosage range	purpose
chorionic gonadotropin (A.P.L., Follutein, Chorex-5, Gonic, Pregnyl, Profasi HP)	Gonotropin (placental) ovulation stimulant	*Adult* IM: 4000 units 3 times/wk for 3 wk IM: 500-1000 units 3 times/wk for 3 wk followed by same dose 2/wk for 3 wk IM: 5000-10,000 units given 1 day after the last dose of menotropins	Prepubertal cryptorchidism Hypogonadotropic hypogonadism Female infertility
clomiphene (Clomid, Serophene)	Ovulation stimulant	*Women* PO: 50 mg/day for 5 days. If ovulation does not occur, a second course of 100 mg/day for 5 days and a third and final course of 100 mg/day for 5 days can be administered	Female infertility in selected patients
menotropins (Pergonal, Humegon)	Gonadotropins (FSH/LH) ovulation stimulant	*Adult* IM: 1 ampule (75 IU of FSH/LH) for 9-12 days followed by 5000-10,000 U of hCG 1 day after the last dose of menotropins. Repeat course if required with 1 ampule of 150 IU of FSH/LH for 9-12 days followed by 10,000 U of hCG. A third and final course may be required. *Adult* IM: after pretreatment with hCG, administer 1 ampule (75 IU of FSH/LH) 3 times/wk with 2000 U of hCG 2 times/wk for a least 6 mo	Female infertility Male infertility

nursing process

• Assessment

Before administering estrogen or progesterone agents, the nurse should determine whether the patient has any contraindications to its use. These include a history of breast cancer, thromboembolic disorders, malignancies of the reproductive tract, or abnormal vaginal bleeding. They also should not be used in breast-feeding or pregnant women. Cautious use of the estrogens and progestins is called for in patients with hypertension, asthma, blood dyscrasias, diabetes, headaches, congestive heart failure, depressive disorders, seizure disorders, liver disease, renal disease, or a family history of breast or reproductive tract cancer.

Combination oral contraceptives (COCs) are used in emergency situations of postcoital conception. They have the same cautions and contraindications but are generally only a one-time-use agent.

The patient's baseline blood pressure, weight, blood glucose levels, liver function, and urinary output should also be determined and documented. It is important to assess the patient's smoking history and status, including the number of packs per day and number of years. Drug allergies and any prescription and nonprescription drugs being used should also be recorded. Drugs that interact with estrogens include anticoagulants, oral antidiabetic agents, TCAs, anticonvulsants, barbiturates, and steroids. Drugs that interact with progestins include anticoagulants, oral antidiabetic agents, TCAs, anticonvulsants, barbiturates, and steroids.

Dinoprostone, a new synthetic prostaglandin E_2 hormone, is indicated in specific situations requiring termination of pregnancy. Its use has many specific guidelines (e.g., to use between 12 and 20 weeks). It is contraindicated with fibroids, PID, pelvic stenosis, respiratory disease, and pelvic operation. It is also contraindicated in females with a history of pelvic operations.

Before administering uterine stimulants such as oxytocin and prostaglandins, the nurse should determine and document the patient's blood pressure, pulse, and respiration. The fetal heart rate and contraction fetal heart rate should also be determined and recorded. The same considerations apply to ergot alkaloids, with assessment of the patient being particularly critical because these agents are most often used for the prevention and control of postpartum and postabortion hemorrhage. The most notable drug interaction that occurs is that resulting from their concurrent use with sympathomimetic drugs, which can precipitate severe hypertension.

As previously mentioned, uterine relaxants such as ritodrine, terbutaline, and magnesium sulfate should only be used in women presenting in premature labor who are in their twentieth to thirty-seventh week of gestation. Cautious administration is recommended in any patient receiving them, but especially in women who have other complications of pregnancy or any condition such as seizures, hypertension, diabetes, a cardiac dysrhythmia, angina, or hypokalemia. Contraindications to their use include allergies, eclampsia, hypertension, thyrotoxicosis, antepartum hemorrhage, intrauterine fetal death, and other conditions listed earlier in this chapter. Testing of reflexes and a head-to-toe neurologic assessment are also necessary before magnesium sulfate therapy is initiated.

Before any of the fertility agents are administered, it is important to determine whether there are any contraindications to their use and to identify any cautions. Contraindications include allergies, pregnancy, liver disease, and undiagnosed vaginal bleeding. Cautious use is recommended in patients with hypertension, seizure disorders, or diabetes mellitus.

SERMs, including raloxifene (blocks breast and uterine estrogen receptors, but used only for postmenopausal osteoporosis because it increases bone density) and tamoxifen (used only to treat and prevent breast cancers of an estrogen-receptor–stimulating type) are used cautiously in patients with leukopenia, thrombocytopenia, or cataracts and those who are lactating. Contraindications include thrombophlebitis (active or history of), hypersensitivity, and pregnancy. CBCs and platelets should be drawn and the physician contacted if WBC count is less than 3500 or platelet count is less than 100,000. Also assess for bleeding, such as hematuria, blood in the stool, petechiae, etc. Drug interactions for which to assess include ampicillin, oral anticoagulants, and cholestyramine.

• Nursing Diagnoses

Nursing diagnoses in patients receiving estrogens, progestins COCs, or SERMs include the following:
- Risk for infection related to possible drop in WBCs due to effects of the SERM.
- Disturbed body image related to physiologic or pathologic effects stemming from changes in the female hormone levels, osteoporosis, or effects of breast cancer and its treatment.
- Deficient knowledge related to first-time therapy.

Nursing diagnoses in patients receiving drugs to promote labor and delivery include the following:
- Acute pain related to delivery and associated abnormalities.
- Disturbed body image related to abnormal pregnancy or associated complications.
- Anxiety related to possible fetal death or the complications of labor and pregnancy.
- Deficient knowledge related to unknown events and outcome of pregnancy.

Nursing diagnoses related to the use of fertility drugs include the following:
- Disturbed body image related to inability to conceive.
- Anxiety related to unknown effects of treatment.
- Deficient knowledge related to the new treatment.

• Planning

Goals in patients receiving drugs for the treatment of various disorders and conditions of the female reproductive tract include the following:
- Patient is free of body image disturbances.
- Patient states the rationale for hormonal replacement, COCs, SERMs, uterine relaxants, or fertility drugs.

- Patient states the side effects of specific medications.
- Patient states the importance of compliance with hormonal therapy and other recommended pharmacologic and nonpharmacologic measures for the treatment of premature labor, preeclampsia, or fertility disorders.

Outcome Criteria

Outcome criteria in patients receiving agents used to treat various disorders and conditions of the female reproductive tract include the following:

- Patient will openly verbalize her concerns, fears, and anxieties with staff about body image changes and the need for medication.
- Patient will be compliant with pharmacologic and nonpharmacologic therapy with successful management of osteoporosis, breast cancer, infertility, preeclampsia, or premature labor, or he or she will experience effective birth control.
- Patient will be free of complications and disturbing side effects associated with each group of drugs, such as chest pain, leg pain, blurred vision, thrombophlebitis, and leukopenia.
- Patient will return for regular follow-up visits with physician to monitor therapeutic and adverse effects of treatment.

● Implementation

Both estrogens and progestins should be administered in the lowest doses possible and then the doses titrated as needed. IM doses should be given deep in large muscle masses and the injection sites rotated. Oral forms should be taken with food or milk to minimize gastrointestinal upset. Dinoprostone, the synthetic prostaglandin E_2, is available in gel, suppository, and vaginal insert forms. Patient teaching tips are given in the box on p. 514.

Ritodrine should be administered using an IV infusion pump or orally, as ordered. Only clear parenteral solutions should be used and administered only after accurate dilutions have been mixed in such solutions as 5% dextrose in water or normal saline. Generally they should only be infused at a rate of 0.3 mg/min, with a dilution of 150 mg/500 ml given at a rate of 0.1 mg/min, or as ordered. The patient should be positioned in the left lateral recumbent position to minimize hypotension and increase renal blood flow.

Oxytocin should only be administered using an IV infusion pump and after dilution in 5% dextrose in water or 0.9% normal saline at a rate of 20 to 40 mU/min, or as ordered for completing an incomplete abortion; at no greater than 20 mU/min for stimulating labor; and at 20 to 40 mU/min for controlling postpartum bleeding. A crash cart should be kept on the unit, and magnesium sulfate should be kept at the patient's bedside.

Fertility agents such as clomiphene are often self-administered. Specific instructions regarding their administration at home and the way to monitor drug effectiveness are very important to enhancing the success of treatment.

Teaching tips for patients receiving COCs, SERMs, uterine stimulants, uterine relaxants, and fertility agents are presented in the box on p. 514.

● Evaluation

Therapeutic responses to estrogens include the disappearance of menopausal symptoms, absence of breast engorgement, and a decrease in the size of prostatic tumors. The side effects of estrogens include thromboembolism, edema, jaundice, abnormal vaginal bleeding, hyperglycemia, nausea, vomiting, increased appetite, and weight gain.

Therapeutic responses to progestins include a decrease in abnormal uterine bleeding and disappearance of menstrual disorders such as amenorrhea. The side effects of progestins include edema, hypertension, cardiac symptoms, depression, changes in mood and affect, and jaundice.

Therapeutic effects of SERMs include increased bone density (with raloxifene) and improvement in or prevention of breast cancers (estrogen-receptor positive). Side effects include leukopenia, decreased platelets, risk for thrombophlebitis, hot flashes, and leg cramps.

Therapeutic effects of oxytocin and other uterine stimulants include stimulation of labor and control of postpartum bleeding. Adverse reactions include changes in vital signs with bradycardia, dysrhythmias and premature ventricular contractions, severe abdominal pain and shocklike symptoms with a decrease in blood pressure, and increased pulse. All of these indicate possible uterine rupture and fetal distress. The patient should also be closely monitored for the occurrence of acceleration or deceleration as well as for the signs and symptoms of water intoxication. In addition, the physician should be notified if contractions last longer than 1 minute or do not occur.

The primary therapeutic effect of the uterine relaxants is the absence of preterm labor. Adverse maternal effects for which to monitor include palpitations, nausea, vomiting, headache, jitteriness, tremors, chest pain, cardiac dysrhythmias, and anxiety. Adverse neonatal effects include hypoglycemia, ileus, hypotension, and hypocalcemia. Both maternal and fetal heart rates as well as the maternal blood pressure should be closely monitored either as set out in the institutional policy and procedure manual, as ordered by the physician, or as the needs of the patient dictate. Nursing actions in the latter instance should be documented in the nurses' notes on the patient. The IV fluid rate and volume must also be closely monitored so that fluid volume overload is not allowed to occur.

The therapeutic effect of fertility agents would be the successful fertilization of an ovum and resultant pregnancy. Adverse reactions for which to monitor in patients receiving these agents include hot flashes, abdominal discomfort, blurred vision, gastrointestinal upset, nervousness, depression, weight gain, and hair loss. Multiple births and birth defects are other possible consequences of therapy. Therapeutic effects of dinoprostone include effective and therapeutic (physically and emotionally) termination of pregnancy in the previously mentioned section of this chapter.

patient teaching tips

Women's Health Agents

Estrogens and Progestins

➤ Patients should take oral forms of hormones with food or milk to minimize GI upset.

➤ Patients should perform regular breast examinations and report any unusual lumps or bumps.

➤ Patients should report chest pain, leg pain, blurred vision, headache, neck stiffness and pain, edema, yellow discoloration of the skin or sclera, clay-colored stools, and vaginal bleeding.

➤ Breast-feeding is not recommended in patients on estrogen therapy.

➤ Patients should report any weight gain of more than 5 pounds (2.25 kg) in a week.

➤ While on estrogen therapy, patients should avoid sunlight or wear sunscreen because these agents make the skin more susceptible to sunburn. Patients should be informed of the increased sensitivity to sunlight and ultraviolet light.

➤ These agents should be discontinued by the physician if pregnancy is suspected.

➤ If a dose is missed, it is important to NOT double-up on medication. Take the pills when the omission is remembered, and utilize another form of birth control for that cycle of pills.

➤ Follow-up Pap smears and gynecological check-ups are important.

Uterine Relaxants

➤ Patients should understand the rationale for treatment with a uterine relaxant.

➤ Patients should understand the need for complying with other aspects of treatment such as bed rest while experiencing premature onset of labor (POL).

➤ Tell the patient that the oral preparation of ritodrine is often used as a form of maintenance treatment, if needed.

➤ It is important for patients on maintenance ritodrine therapy to understand the importance of regular monitoring of the blood glucose and electrolyte levels.

➤ Patients should report any increase in the intensity, duration, or frequency of their contractions as well as palpitations, anxiety, shortness of breath, vomiting, dizziness, or tachycardia to the nurse or physician.

➤ Any loss of fetal movement should be immediately reported to the physician or nurse.

Uterine Stimulants

➤ Specific instructions for the use of oxytocin should be reviewed for patients administering it intranasally. They should be told to blow their nose, sit upright, hold the container upright, insert it into the nostril, and squeeze it during inspiration.

➤ The physician should be notified immediately by the patient if she begins to experience excessively strong contractions, edema or other symptoms of water intoxication, palpitations, chest pain, or changes in fetal movement.

➤ Patients should receive explicit instructions regarding the self-administration of these drugs.

Fertility Agents

➤ Patients should keep a journal of all medications, body changes and any other changes, their emotional and physical status, and any related signs and symptoms.

➤ It is important to emphasize the importance of regular follow-up visits to the physician in patients undergoing treatment for infertility.

➤ Make sure patients understand all instructions regarding the treatment regimen and the medication (use, dose, route, timing, side effects, drug interactions, and so on), because this is critical to ensuring compliance and safe self-administration.

➤ Teach patients how to monitor for the therapeutic effects and side effects.

COCs

➤ These agents are used for postcoital emergency contraception.

➤ They are *not* effective if the female is pregnant.

➤ COCs should be taken within 72 hours of unprotected intercourse with a follow-up dose 12 hours later.

SERMs

➤ Postmenopausal women are at no greater risk for gynecological cancers.

➤ Patients should have periodic CBC with a differential and platelet counts performed.

➤ Warnings about the risk of thrombophlebitis should be emphasized.

➤ Antacids, before the oral forms, may help with the GI upset, nausea, and vomiting.

POINTS TO REMEMBER

Menstrual Cycle

• First menses or menstrual cycle is called *menarche,* which then occurs once a month until it ceases with menopause.

• Consists of three phases: menstrual phase (1st), follicular phase (2nd), and luteal phase (3rd).

• Follicular phase associated with high levels of estrogen.

• Luteal phase associated with high levels of progesterone.

Estrogens

• Three major estrogens are synthesized in the ovaries: estradiol (principal estrogen), estrone, and estriol.

- Exogenous estrogens can be broken down into two main groups: steroidal estrogens (e.g., conjugated estrogens, esterified estrogens, estradiol) and non-steroidal estrogens (e.g., chlorotrianisene, dienestrol, diethylstilbestrol).
- Work by binding to and interacting with the estrogen receptors, increasing the synthesis of DNA and RNA.
- Ethinyl estradiol is a semisynthetic steroidal estrogen and the most orally active estrogenic drug.

Progestins

- Progesterone is a hormone secreted by the corpus luteum.
- Progesterone is the principal natural progestational hormone.
- Chemical derivatives of progesterone are called *progestins.*
- Have a variety of uses: uterine bleeding, amenorrhea, adjunctive and palliative treatment of some cancers, and others.

Oral Contraceptives

- Most effective form of birth control currently available.
- Combinations of both estrogenic and progestinic steroids.

Labor and Delivery Drugs

- Uterine stimulants: ergot derivatives, prostaglandins, and oxytocin.
- Uterine stimulants are sometimes called *oxytocic agents.*
- Uterine relaxants: used to stop preterm labor and maintain pregnancy by stopping uterine contractions.
- Uterine relaxants are sometimes called *tocolytics.*

Nursing Considerations

- A thorough nursing assessment is necessary to ensure the safe and effective use of female reproductive agents, including information on the patient's past medical problems, history of menses and problems with menstrual cycle, medications taken (prescribed and over-the-counter), the number of pregnancies and miscarriages, the last menstrual period, and any related surgical or medical treatments.
- Patient education should focus on the medication therapy and its importance to the management of the specific disease or disorder and also on means to ensure a positive self-image and open communication.

REVIEW QUESTIONS

1. Oral estrogen therapy must include adequate patient teaching for it to be a successful hormonal replacement. Which of the following statements is important to include in such teaching?
   a. Sunbathing and use of tanning beds is not a concern.
   b. A milky or blood-tinged discharge from the breast is to be expected.
   c. Taking the medication with food will have no effect on decreasing GI upset.
   d. The patient should report a weight gain of 5 pounds per week to his or her health care provider.
2. Oral estrogens are contraindicated in which of the following patients? Those with:
   a. Acne.
   b. Postpartum "blues."
   c. History of skin cancer.
   d. History of deep vein thrombosis (DVT).
3. Oxytocin (Pitocin) is used to _____ and should be administered _____.

   a. induce delivery; by IV bolus only
   b. induce labor; via IV infusion pump
   c. induce miosis; to those who are to have a cesarean section
   d. induce emesis; to those who have overdosed on estrogen
4. What are some of the side effects of the fertility agents?
   a. Anuria
   b. Polyuria
   c. Diabetes
   d. Dizziness
5. Which of the following would be a contraindication for the use of estrogen hormonal replacement for a 48-year-old female with symptoms of menopause?
   a. Diabetes
   b. "Hot flashes"
   c. Uterine bleeding
   d. Thrombophlebitis

For Answers see www.harcourthealth.com/MERLIN/Lilley/.

CRITICAL THINKING Activities

1. K.T. has spent 14 hours in labor with her first pregnancy and has made little progress. She is becoming exhausted, and the uterine contractions have decreased in strength. Oxytocin is ordered to be given at a rate of 1 mU/min. The normal concentration of oxytocin is 10 mU/ml. What rate (in milliliters per hour) should the infusion be run at to deliver 1 mU/min?

2. Why are oxytocics such as Pitocin and Ergotrate used to treat postpartum and postabortion bleeding caused by uterine relaxation and enlargement?
3. What is the primary mechanism by which oral contraceptives prevent pregnancy?

For Answers see www.harcourthealth.com/MERLIN/Lilley/.

bibliography

Albanese J, Nutz P: *Mosby's 2001 nursing drug reference and review cards,* St Louis, 2001, Mosby.

American Hospital Formulary Service: *AHFS drug information,* Bethesday, Md, 2000, American Society of Health-System Pharmacists.

Anderson PO, Knoben JE, Troutman WG: *Handbook of clinical drug data 1999-2000,* ed 9, New York, 1999, McGraw-Hill.

Briggs GG, Freeman RK, Yaffe SJ: *Drugs in pregnancy and lactation: a reference guide to fetal and neonatal risk,* ed 5, Philadelphia, 1998, Lippincott Williams & Wilkins.

Johns Hopkins Hospital, Department of Pediatrics et al: *The Harriet Lane handbook,* ed 15, St Louis, 2000, Mosby.

Keen JH: *Critical care and emergency drug reference,* ed 3, St Louis, 1996, Mosby.

McKenry LM, Salerno E: *Mosby's pharmacology in nursing,* ed 21, St Louis, 2001, Mosby.

Medical Letter: Raloxifene for postmenopausal osteoporosis 40(1022):29, March 13, 1998.

Mosby's GenRx: a comprehensive reference for generic and brand drugs, ed 10, St Louis, 2000, Mosby.

Skidmore-Roth L: *Mosby's 2001 nursing drug reference,* St Louis, 2001, Mosby.

Smith A, Hughes P: The estrogen dilema, *AJN* 98(4):17, 1998.

United States Pharmacopeial Convention: *USP DI drug information for the health care professional, vol. 1,* ed 20, Englewood, Colo, 2000, Micromedex.

United States Pharmacopeial Convention: *USP DI: Advice for the patient, vol. II,* ed 20, Englewood, Colo, 2000, Micromedex.

Remember to check the **Online Worksheet** for additional learning opportunities: **www.harcourthealth.com/MERLIN/Lilley/**

Activity

Chapter 33

Men's Health Agents

www.harcourthealth.com/MERLIN/Lilley/

objectives

When you reach the end of this chapter, you should be able to do the following:

1 Discuss the normal anatomy and physiology of the male reproductive system.

2 Identify the various male reproductive agents and their indications with rationale for use.

3 Discuss the mechanisms of action, dosages, side effects, cautions, contraindications, and drug interactions for the various agents that affect the male reproductive system.

4 Develop a nursing care plan that includes all phases of the nursing process for the patient receiving agents that affect the male reproductive system.

Look for this symbol for topics covered in the **Online Worksheet Activity**

drug profiles

○━ **danazol**, p. 520
finasteride, p. 520
fluoxymesterone, p. 520

methyltestosterone, p. 520
sildenafil, p. 520
testosterone, p. 520

○━ Key drug.

glossary

Anabolic activity (ə nab′ ə lik) The activity produced by testosterone that causes the development of bone and muscle tissue. (p. 517)

Androgenic activity (an dro jen′ ik) The activity produced by testosterone that causes the development and maintenance of the male reproductive system. (p. 517)

Androgens Male sex hormones responsible for mediating the development and maintenance of male sex characteristics. (p. 517)

Benign prostatic hypertrophy Enlargement of the prostate gland. (p. 518)

Erythropoietic effect (ə rith′ ro poi et′ ik) Effect that stimulates the production of red blood cells. (p. 517)

Prostate cancer A malignant tumor growth within the prostate gland. (p. 518)

Testosterone (təs tos′ tə rōn) The main androgenic hormone. (p. 517)

MALE REPRODUCTIVE SYSTEM

The male reproductive system consists of several structures, the testes and seminiferous tubules being the most important to this discussion. The testes are the male gonads, and they are a pair of oval glands located in the scrotal sac. They are the site of both reproductive (andro-genic) and endocrine activity. The seminiferous tubules, which are channels in the testes, are the site of spermatogenesis, which is the process by which mature sperm cells are produced.

The normal development and maintenance of the primary male sex characteristics (normal male anatomy) as well as the secondary ones (growth and maturation of the prostate, seminal vesicles, penis, and scrotum; male hair distribution, such as facial, pubic, chest, and axillary hair; laryngeal enlargement and thickening of the vocal cords; and defining of body musculature and fat distribution) are mediated by the male sex hormones called **androgens.** Androgens must be secreted in adequate amounts for these characteristics to appear. One of the primary androgens is **testosterone.** It is produced from clusters of interstitial cells located between the seminiferous tubules. Besides its **androgenic activity,** testosterone is also involved in the development of bone and muscle tissue; inhibition of protein catabolism (its breakdown); and retention of nitrogen, phosphorus, potassium, and sodium. These contribute to its **anabolic activity.** The hormone initiates the synthesis of specific proteins needed for androgenic and anabolic activity by binding to chromatin in the nucleus of interstitial cells. In addition, testosterone appears to have an **erythropoietic effect** in that it stimulates the production of red blood cells.

MALE REPRODUCTIVE AGENTS

There are several synthetic derivatives of testosterone, and these were developed with the intention of improving on the pharmacokinetic and pharmacodynamic characteristics of the naturally occurring hormone. One way this was accomplished was by combining various esters with testosterone, resulting in a prolonged duration of action of the hormone. For example, testosterone propionate is formulated in an oily solution and its hormonal effects last for 2 to 3 days; the effects of testosterone cypionate and testosterone enanthate in oil last even longer. They can be administered once every 2 to 4 weeks. Orally administered testosterone has very poor pharmacokinetic and pharmacodynamic characteristics because most its dose is metabolized and destroyed by the liver before it can reach the circulation. To circumvent this problem, researchers developed methyltestosterone. Both the serum levels and effectiveness of buccally administered methyltestosterone are increased. Fluoxymesterone, another testosterone derivative, is effective when administered orally.

There are other chemical derivatives of the naturally occurring testosterone known as *anabolic steroids.* These are synthetic agents that closely resemble the natural hormone, but they possess high anabolic activity. Anabolic steroids have a great potential for being misused by athletes, especially body builders and weight lifters, because of their muscle-building properties. Improper use of these substances can have many serious consequences. For this reason, anabolic steroids are currently classified as controlled (schedule III) substances by the U.S. Drug Enforcement Administration. (This classification implies that misuse of the agent can lead to psychologic or physical dependence, or both.)

Androgen inhibitors are agents that block the effects of naturally occurring (endogenous) androgens. The specific enzyme they inhibit is 5-alpha-reductase. For this reason, they are called *5-alpha-reductase inhibitors.* As previously mentioned, androgens maintain secondary sex characteristics, one of which is the growth and maintenance of the prostate. When androgens are secreted in excessive amounts, the prostate enlarges, a condition known as **benign prostatic hypertrophy** (BPH). BPH is amenable to treatment with a 5-alpha-reductase inhibitor. Currently, however, the only such agent available is finasteride.

There are also two other classes of androgen inhibitors. The first is the antiandrogen flutamide. Flutamide works by physically blocking the binding of androgens to the androgen receptors. The second is the gonadotropin-releasing hormone (GnRH) analogs leuprolide and goserelin. These agents work by inhibiting the secretion of pituitary gonadotropin, which eventually leads to a decrease in testosterone production. Another class of agents that may be used to help alleviate the symptoms of obstruction due to BPH are the alpha$_1$-adrenergic blockers. These agents are discussed in greater detail in Chapter 17. The alpha$_1$-adrenergic blockers that are most commonly used for symptomatic relief of obstruction secondary to BPH are terazosin (Hytrin), doxazosin (Cardura), and tamsulosin (Flomax). Tamsulosin appears to have a greater specificity for the alpha$_1$ receptors on the prostate and thus may cause less hypotension. All four of these drug classes (5-alpha-reductase inhibitors, antiandrogens, GnRH analogs, and alpha$_1$-adrenergic blockers) can be used to treat BPH. GnRH analogs are more frequently used to treat **prostate cancer.**

The currently available natural and synthetic androgens, synthetic anabolic steroids, antiandrogens, 5-alpha-reductase inhibitors, and GnRH analogs are listed in Box 33-1.

Sildenafil (Viagra) is the first oral drug approved for the treatment of erectile dysfunction (ED). Another agent, alprostadil, is also indicated for ED; however, this agent must be given by injection or pushed into the urethra. Sildenafil is considered a phosphodiesterase inhibitor and is listed with other commonly used male health agents in Box 33-1. Apomorphine (Uprima), a dopamine agonist, is one of the newest medications indicated for ED.

Mechanism of Action

Androgens such as testosterone stimulate the synthesis of RNA. This reduces the substance that stimulates the prostate to grow. Over time the prostate will decrease in size. The increased synthesis of protein aids in the formation and maintenance of muscular and skeletal proteins. Another potent anabolic, or building, effect of androgens is the retention of nitrogen, a substance essential for the manufacture of protein. Nitrogen also promotes the storage of inorganic phosphorus, sulfate, sodium, and potassium.

Finasteride works by inhibiting the enzymatic process responsible for converting testosterone to 5-alpha-dihydrotestosterone (DHT), which is the principal an-

BOX 33-1 Currently Available Men's Health Agents

ALPHA$_1$-ADRENERGIC BLOCKERS
terazosin
doxazosin
tamsulosin

ANABOLIC STEROIDS
nandrolone
oxymetholone
stanozolol

ANDROGENS
danazol
fluoxymesterone
methyltestosterone
testosterone

ANTIANDROGEN
flutamide

DOPAMINE AGONIST
apomorphine

5-ALPHA-REDUCTASE INHIBITOR
finasteride

GnRH ANALOGS
leuprolide
goserelin

PERIPHERAL VASODILATOR
minoxidil

drogen responsible for stimulating prostatic growth. Finasteride can dramatically lower the prostatic DHT concentrations. Apomorphine (Uprima) works by stimulating dopamine receptors in the CNS. The stimulation of D_1 and D_2 receptors initiates and enhances erection. It also improves blood flow to the penis.

Drug Effects

The natural and synthetic androgens and the synthetic anabolic steroids have effects similar to those of the endogenous androgens. These are stimulation of the normal growth and development of the male sex organs (primary sex characteristics) and maintenance of the secondary sex characteristics. They also cause retention of the substances needed for the building of proteins (nitrogen, potassium, and phosphorus) and retard the breakdown of amino acids. This may result in weight gain and an increase in musculature and strength. The administration of exogenous androgens causes the release of endogenous testosterone to be inhibited as the result of the feedback inhibition of pituitary luteinizing hormone (LH). Large doses of exogenous androgens may also suppress sperm production as the result of the feedback inhibition of pituitary follicle-stimulating hormone (FSH). Androgens also stimulate the production of erythrocytes by promoting the production of erythropoietic stimulating factor.

The drug effects of finasteride are limited primarily to the prostate, but this agent may also affect 5-alpha-reductase processes elsewhere in the body, such as hair follicles, skin, and liver. Inhibition of this enzyme system leads to a dramatic reduction of prostate size in men with BPH. It has also been noted that men taking finasteride experience increased hair growth as well.

Finasteride is also indicated for the treatment of both male- and female-pattern baldness. Results are encouraging. The inhibition of 5-alpha-reductase prevents the thinning of hair caused by increased levels of DHT.

Therapeutic Uses

The primary use for androgens is replacement therapy. However, there is a variety of other uses for these agents listed in Box 33-2.

Side Effects and Adverse Effects

Although rare, some of the most devastating effects of steroids occur in the liver, where they cause the formation of blood-filled cavities, a condition known as *peliosis of the liver.* This is a potential consequence of the long-term administration of androgenic anabolic steroids and can be life-threatening. Other serious hepatic effects are hepatic neoplasms, cholestatic hepatitis, jaundice, and abnormal liver function. Fluid retention is another undesirable effect of androgens and may account for some of the weight gain seen in persons taking them. The serious adverse effects that can be caused by the androgens far outweigh the advantages to be gained from their use in those seeking improved athletic ability.

Other less serious adverse effects of androgens are listed in Table 33-1. These effects can be seen with all androgens with 17-alpha-alkyl substitutions to their structure (fluoxymesterone, methandrostenolone, methyltestosterone, oxandrolone, oxymetholone, and stanozolol).

Sildenafil has a relatively safe side effect profile. In patients with preexisting cardiovascular disease, especially those on nitrates, sildenafil lowers blood pressure substantially and can lead to serious adverse events. Headache, flushing, and dyspepsia have been the most common adverse effects reported.

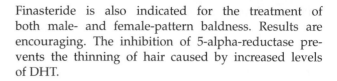

Box 33-2 Men's Health Agents: Therapeutic Uses

Androgen or Androgen Inhibitor	Therapeutic Use
apomorphine	Erectile dysfunction
danazol	Endometriosis
	Fibrocystic breast disease
danazol and stanozolol	Hereditary angioedema
finasteride	Benign prostatic hypertrophy
	Male androgenetic alopecia
fluoxymesterone and methyltestosterone	Inoperable breast cancer
	Male hypogonadism
	Postpartum breast engorgement
methyltestosterone	Postpubertal cryptorchidism
minoxidil	Hypertension
	Male androgenetic alopecia
nandrolone	Metastatic breast cancer
oxymetholone	Various anemias
sildenafil	Erectile dysfunction
testosterone	Primary or secondary hypogonadism

Table 33-1 Androgens: Common Adverse Effects

Body System	Side/Adverse Effects
Central nervous system	Headache, anxiety, mental depression, generalized paresthesias
Endocrine	Acne, gynecomastia, amenorrhea, menstrual irregularities, and virilization (deepening of voice, hirsutism, and clitoral enlargement)
Hematologic	Polycythemia; suppression of clotting factors II, V, VII, X; increased serum cholesterol level
Other	Priapism or excessive sexual stimulation in males; male-pattern baldness; water retention, along with retention of sodium, chloride, potassium, and inorganic phosphates; stomatitis; hypercalcemia from osteolysis

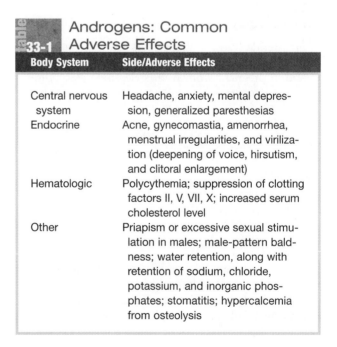

Activity

Finasteride has been reported to cause loss of libido, loss of erection, ejaculatory dysfunction, hypersensitivity reactions, gynecomastia, and severe myopathy. The drug has also caused a 50% decrease in prostatic specific antigen (PSA) concentrations. Pregnant women should not handle crushed or broken tablets on a regular basis because of the possibility of topic absorption, which can lead to teratogenic effects.

Minoxidil causes tachycardia, angina pectoris, and marked fluid retention when taken orally. The topical formulation may cause some of these adverse effects. The most common are dizziness and tachycardia. Local irritation, itching, dryness, and erythema are more common, especially with the stronger 5% topical formulation. Allergic contact dermatitis has also been reported.

MERLIN
Activity

Interactions

All androgens, when used with oral anticoagulants, can significantly increase anticoagulant activity.

Dosages

For recommended dosages of the male reproductive agents, see the dosages table on p. 521.

drug profiles

⊶danazol

Danazol (Danocrine) is a synthetic derivative of ethisterone that possesses weak androgenic activity. It is classified as a pregnancy category C agent, and its use is contraindicated in patients with significant cardiac, hepatic, or renal dysfunction and those with porphyria; in women with undiagnosed abnormal vaginal bleeding; and in pregnant or lactating women. Refer to the dosages table on p. 521 for dosage information.

finasteride

Finasteride (Proscar, Propecia) is contraindicated in patients who have shown a hypersensitivity to it and in pregnant women. It is classified as a pregnancy category X agent. Refer to the dosages table on p. 521 for dosage information.

PHARMACOKINETICS

HALF-LIFE	ONSET	PEAK	DURATION
4-15 hr*	Unknown 3-12 mo†	8 hr‡	Unknown

*Varies with age.
†To lower DHT concentrations.
‡To reduce prostate size.

fluoxymesterone

Fluoxymesterone (Halotestin) is a synthetic androgen hormone that is contraindicated in patients with significant cardiac, hepatic, or renal dysfunction; pregnant or breast-feeding women (pregnancy

category X); and men with breast carcinoma or known or suspected prostate cancer. For recommended dosages, see the dosages table on p. 521.

PHARMACOKINETICS

HALF-LIFE	ONSET	PEAK	DURATION
9.2 hr	Unknown	Unknown	Unknown

methyltestosterone

Methyltestosterone (Android, Oreton-M) is contraindicated in patients with significant cardiac, hepatic, or renal dysfunction; pregnant or breast-feeding women; and men with breast carcinoma or known or suspected prostate cancer. It is a pregnancy category X agent. Refer to the dosages table on p. 521 for the recommended dosages.

PHARMACOKINETICS

HALF-LIFE	ONSET	PEAK	DURATION
10-100 min	Unknown	1-2 hr (serum)	Unknown

sildenafil

Sildenafil (Viagra) is the first oral drug approved by the FDA for treatment of ED. Other currently available agents for the treatment of ED include alprostadil (Caverject and Muse) and apomorphine (Uprima). Sildenafil potentiates the physiologic response, causing penile erection after sexual arousal by relaxing smooth muscle and increasing blood flow.

Sildenafil is contraindicated in patients with a known hypersensitivity to it and is considered a pregnancy category B agent. Sildenafil can potentiate the hypotensive effects of nitrates, and its administration to patients who are using organic nitrates, either regularly and/or intermittently, in any form is therefore contraindicated. It is available as 25-, 50-, and 100-mg tablets. Common dosages are listed in the dosages table on p. 521.

PHARMACOKINETICS

HALF-LIFE	ONSET	PEAK	DURATION
4 hr	0.5-1 hr	1 hr	4 hr

testosterone

Testosterone (Androderm, Delatestryl, Depo-Testosterone, Testoderm, Virilon) is a naturally occurring anabolic steroid. It is used for primary and secondary hypogonadism but may also be used to treat oligospermia and breast cancer. When used as replacement therapy, a transdermal product is desirable. There are presently two transdermal patches. They attempt to mimic the normal circadian variation in testosterone concentration seen in young healthy men where the maximum testosterone levels occur in the early morning hours and minimum concentrations in the evening. Of the two available transdermal delivery systems, Testoderm is always applied to

DOSAGES Selected Male Health Agents

agent	pharmacologic class	dosage range	purpose
danazol (Danocrine)	Synthetic androgenic hormone	*Adult* PO: 200-800 mg/day in 2 divided doses and reduced to a dose that maintains amenorrhea. Therapy requires 3-9 mo. 100-400 mg/day in 2 divided doses for 4-6 mo 200 mg 2-3 times/day and reduced by 50% after a favorable response at 1- to 3-mo intervals	Endometriosis Fibrocystic breast disease Hereditary angioedema
finasteride (Proscar, Propecia)	5-alpha-reductase inhibitor	*Adult* PO: 1 mg daily for alopecia and 5 mg daily for BPH	Benign prostatic hypertrophy Male androgenetic alopecia
fluoxymesterone (Halotestin)	Synthetic androgenic hormone	*Adult* PO: 10-40 mg/day divided doses for 1-3 mo 2.5 mg after delivery followed by 5-10 mg/day divided for 4-5 days 5-20 mg/day divided	Breast cancer Postpartum breast pain/ engorgement Male hypogonadism
methyltestosterone (Android, Oreton-M)	Synthetic androgenic hormone	*Adult* PO: 10-50 mg/day or 5-25 mg/day—buccal tablets 50-200 mg/day or 25-50 mg/day—buccal tablets 80 mg/day for 3-5 days after delivery	Male hypogonadism Breast cancer Postpartum breast pain/ engorgement
minoxidil (Rogaine)	Vasodilator	*Adult* Topical: 2%-5% solution applied to scalp twice daily	Male androgenetic alopecia
sildenafil (Viagra)	Phosphodiesterase inhibitor	*Adult* PO: 25-100 mg 1 hr before intercourse	Erectile dysfunction
testosterone cypionate (Dep-Android, Depo-Testosterone, Virilon, Delatestryl)	Natural androgenic hormone	*Adult* IM: 50-500 mg every 2-4 wk 200-400 mg every 2-4 wk	Male hypogonadism Breast cancer
testosterne transdermal (Testoderm, Androderm)	Natural androgenic hormone	*Adult* Skin: 2.5-, 4-, or 6-mg system applied Testoderm: apply only to scrotum Androderm: never apply to scrotum	Male hypogonadism

the scrotal skin, whereas Androderm is always applied to the body skin and never to the scrotal skin.

Testosterone is pregnancy category X drug and contraindicated for use in patients with severe renal, cardiac, or hepatic disease; hypersensitivity; pregnancy; lactation, and genital bleeding. Testosterone is considered a schedule III controlled substance under the Anabolic Steroids Control Act. It is available as a 100- and 200- mg/ml IM injection and as 2.5-, 4-, and 6-mg/day transdermal patches. Common dosages are listed in the dosages table above.

PHARMACOKINETICS*

HALF-LIFE	ONSET	PEAK	DURATION
10-100 min	1-2 hr	2-4 hr	2 hr

*Serum concentrations when testosterone is delivered via the transdermal route.

nursing process

● Assessment

Androgenic agents are used for the treatment of a variety of disorders and diseases, including malignancies of the male reproductive system. Before administering any male reproductive agent to a patient, the purpose for its use, the patient's urinary patterns, and any difficulty in urination should be assessed and documented. Contraindications to the use of testosterone and related products include an allergy to the medication; renal, cardiac, or liver disease; and pregnancy. Cautious use is recommended in patients with diabetes and those with a history of cardiovascular disease or myocardial infarction (MI). Because androgenic anabolic steroids such as testosterone and nandrolone increase weight and raise the potassium, chloride, nitrogen and phosphorus levels, it is important to determine and record the patient's baseline weight, height, vital signs, and serum electrolyte levels. It is also important to look at the results of laboratory tests that assess renal, cardiac and liver functions, such as the blood urea nitrogen (BUN), creatinine, SGOT, lactate dehydrogenase, creatine phosphokinase, and bilirubin levels. Prostatic specific antigen (PSA) levels are often ordered before treatment with agents such as finasteride.

Specifically, danazol is contraindicated in patients with significant cardiac, hepatic, or renal dysfunction; in pregnant or lactating women; and in women with abnormal vaginal bleeding. Finasteride is contraindicated in patients with known allergies to the medication. Finasteride also carries the caution for it not to be used in pregnant women because of teratogenic effects, so pregnant females should not even handle this agent. Nandrolone is contraindicated in patients with severe cardiac, liver, or renal disease; pregnant women and those with abnormal vaginal bleeding; and men with breast or prostate cancer. Sildenafil should be used cautiously in patients with cardiovascular disease, especially if they are also taking nitrates due to enhanced postural hypotensive effects and potential syncope. Androgenic agents interact with oral anticoagulants, steroids, insulin, and oral antidiabetic agents.

● Nursing Diagnoses

Nursing diagnoses relevant to patients receiving androgenic agents include the following:
- Disturbed body image related to sexual dysfunction, ED, or malignancies.
- Fatigue related to side effects of androgenic agents.
- Excess fluid volume related to sodium retention caused by large dosages of androgenic agent.
- Disturbed body image related to sexual dysfunction associated with side effects (decreased libido, impotence) of agents affecting the male reproductive system.
- Situational low self-esteem related to sexual dysfunction secondary to drugs used to treat disorders of the male reproductive system.
- Deficient knowledge related to self-administration of agents altering the male reproductive system.

● Planning

Goals for patients receiving androgenic agents include the following:
- Patient maintains positive body image.
- Patient maintains normal activity levels during androgenic therapy.
- Patient maintains normal sodium and fluid volume levels.
- Patient experiences minimal alterations in sexual integrity and function during androgenic therapy.
- Patient remains compliant with androgenic therapy.
- Patient verbalizes feelings and concerns about actual or perceived changes in sexual patterns.

Outcome Criteria

Outcome criteria related to the administration of androgenic agents include the following:
- Patient will verbalize feelings, fears, and anxieties concerning potential for alteration in body image related to disease process or the side effects of androgenic therapy.

- Patient will maintain healthy activity level during androgenic therapy and suffer minimal fatigue with increased activities of daily living.
- Patient will state measures to be taken to minimize edema related to sodium retention stemming from use of large dosages of androgens such as dietary cautions.
- Patient will verbalize feelings, anxieties, and fears of alteration in their sexual integrity or function during androgenic therapy and seek counseling if needed.
- Patient will take medications as prescribed.

● Implementation

When administered intramuscularly, testosterone and related products should be injected deep into the upper outer quadrant of the gluteus muscle injection site. Generally the lowest dose possible is prescribed to prevent as many side effects as possible. Other dosage forms, such as sublingual or oral ones, need to be given exactly as instructed. The manufacturer's guidelines for the administration of some of the sublingual or buccal forms of androgenic agents recommend that the patient not swallow, chew, eat, or drink the buccal tablet but must let it be completely absorbed.

Finasteride should be given orally without regard to meals. The medication should be protected from light and heat. In addition, finasteride should not be handled by a pregnant woman because of teratogenic effects. Fluoxymesterone should be given with milk or food to decrease gastrointestinal upset. Patients taking sildenafil should be warned about potential side effects, such as flushing and headache. Minoxidil, in topical forms, may also lead to local reactions, and excessive rash or redness should be reported.

geriatric considerations

Viagra and the Elderly

Over 10 million men suffer from erectile dysfunction (ED). ED occurs with an increasing incidence as men age, with about 2% of patients being in their forties and 23% 65 years of age. Sildenafil (Viagra) is a prescription medication that is being commonly ordered for ED but not without concerns and cautions for the patient. This is especially true for elderly patients who generally have other medical conditions (e.g., renal disorders, hypertension, diabetes) and are taking usually more than one other prescribed medication. Older individuals also have a declining liver function, so drugs may not be as effectively metabolized as when they were younger. In addition, Viagra is highly protein-bound, causing it to stay around in the body longer and creating more drug interactions. A decreased dosage of Viagra, initially at 25 mg per day, is generally indicated for patients over 65 years of age and for those with liver or renal impairment. Side effects to be concerned about in all patients, particularly with older patients, include headache, flushing, urinary tract infection, diarrhea, rash, and dizziness. Cautious use includes patients who have cardiac disease and angina. These patients are at greater risk of complications and even more so if they are also on nitrates for their cardiovascular disease. This is especially problematic for the patient over 65 years of age who is self-medicating.

From Catania PN: Viagra for home care patients, *Home Care Provider* 3(4):197, 1998.

Danazole should be taken with food or milk to minimize the gastric upset often associated with its use. Finasteride is an antiprostatitis agent that is used in the management of BPH. It is administered orally for 6 to 12 months and then the condition is reevaluated. For finasteride, it may take up to 6 months for effectiveness in treating BPH.

Nandrolone, an anabolic steroid, should be taken exactly as ordered and at the lowest possible dose. If edema occurs, a low sodium diet may be recommended. See also the Herbal Interactions box for Saw Palmetto, an herbal supplement taken to relieve symptoms of enlarged prostate.

Teaching tips for patients receiving androgenic medications are presented in the box at right.

• Evaluation

The therapeutic effect of androgenic agents is essentially the amelioration of whatever condition they are being used to treat. Some of the therapeutic effects may not be seen for 3 or 4 months, such as in the case of osteoporosis. It may also take up to 4 weeks for some of these medications, such as testosterone, to take effect. It is important to observe and monitor the patient for side effects of these medications, such as hypercalcemia, hypoglycemia, hypertension, edema, changes in sexual functioning, and mood changes. Therapeutic effects of sildenafil include improved sexual functioning, with side effects of dizziness, flushing of the face, and headache. Minoxidil has therapeutic effects of increased hair growth and side effects of topical irritation and even some systemic effects, if absorbed, such as edema.

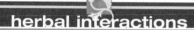

herbal interactions

Saw Palmetto

BENEFIT OF HERB
Relieves symptoms of enlarged prostate

POTENTIAL INTERACTIONS
None known

CAUTIONS AND NOTES
Does not reduce size of prostate; can cause stomach disturbances and headache; high doses can cause diarrhea

patient teaching tips

Androgenic Treatment

➤ Patients taking an androgenic or any type of hormone-related agent should be told *never* to abruptly stop taking the medication. Discontinuing the medication should only be done with a physician's order, and the patient monitored over the several weeks during which the dose is tapered.

➤ Female patients taking danazol should report any abnormal vaginal discharge or bleeding and should perform routine breast examinations.

➤ Patients taking finasteride should understand the rationale for therapy and know its side effects.

➤ Patients taking any of the androgenic medications should always be careful about taking other prescription or over-the-counter medications or eating foods that interact with these agents.

➤ A woman taking nandrolone should notify her physician of any menstrual irregularities or of any decrease in the therapeutic effects.

➤ Patients being given testosterone intramuscularly should be aware of the indicated route of administration and the proper technique of administration.

POINTS TO REMEMBER

Androgens

- Male sex hormones.
- Responsible for normal development and maintenance of male sex characteristics.
- Primary androgen is testosterone.
- Danazol, fluoxymesterone, methyltestosterone, and testosterone are exogenous agents.

Testosterone

- Responsible for development and maintenance of male reproductive system and secondary sex characteristics.
- Oral testosterone has very poor pharmacokinetic and pharmacodynamic characteristics.
- Administered by parenteral route and by topical patch.
- Methyltestosterone was developed to circumvent the problems associated with oral administration.

Anabolic Steroids

- Nandrolone, oxymetholone, and stanozolol.
- Chemical derivatives of testosterone.
- Responsible for bone and muscle development and decreased protein breakdown.

- Classified as controlled substances by the U.S. Drug Enforcement Administration (Schedule III).

Androgen Inhibitors

- Used to block the effects of naturally occurring androgens.
- Also called *5-alpha-reductase inhibitors* because of the enzyme they block, the enzyme needed to form testosterone.
- Currently the only agent is finasteride (Proscar and Propecia).
- Used to stop growth of the prostate in men with BPH and with male androgenic alopecia.
- Finasteride should not be handled by pregnant females.

Nursing Considerations

- Testosterone and related products, if administered intramuscularly, should be given deep in the upper outer quadrant of the gluteus muscle injection site.
- Therapeutic effects of androgenic agents often take 3 to 4 months to appear.
- These agents should never be withdrawn abruptly.

REVIEW QUESTIONS

1. In monitoring the patient at home who is on Viagra, which of the following are crucial to assess for patient safety while using this medication?
   a. Daily weights, I&O, and weekly creatines should be assessed.
   b. The one major side effect is polyuria, so I&O would be needed.
   c. Blood pressure and drug interactions must be monitored.
   d. There is no reason to monitor any vital signs because this is a benign medication.

2. Which of the following would NOT be a contraindication for Viagra use?
   a. Angina
   b. Hypotension
   c. Being 65 years of age
   d. Cardiovascular diseases

3. Excessive amounts of androgen in the male patient would probably be characterized by which of the following?
   a. Weight loss
   b. Bradycardia
   c. Fluid retention
   d. Decreased facial hair growth

4. One of your clinic patients has BPH and is receiving finasteride as treatment. What are the expected side effects of this medication?
   a. Alopecia
   b. Hair growth
   c. Urinary retention
   d. Urinary tract infection

5. Which of the following would NOT be appropriate nursing interventions when administering testosterone cypionate IM 75 mg for the treatment of male hypogonadism?
   a. Treatments with the parenteral forms usually occur at 2-week intervals.
   b. Inform the patient that it may take up to 4 months for the therapeutic effects.
   c. Injections should be given deep IM in the upper-outer quadrant of the gluteus muscle group.
   d. Since IM injections may be painful, you may ask the physician to change the order to 150 mg of oral testosterone.

For Answers see www.harcourthealth.com/MERLIN/Lilley/.

CRITICAL THINKING Activities

1. How do finasteride and methyltestosterone differ in their mechanisms of action?
2. Why might an androgen be prescribed in a patient suffering from anemia?
3. Develop a teaching plan about the risks of anabolic steroids for an 18-year-old male football player and weight-lifter.

For Answers see www.harcourthealth.com/MERLIN/Lilley/.

bibliography

Albanese J, Nutz P: *Mosby's 2001 nursing drug reference and review cards,* St Louis, 2001, Mosby.

American Hospital Formulary Service: *AHFS drug information,* Bethesda, Md, 2000, American Society of Health-System Pharmacists.

Anderson PO, Knoben JE, Troutman WG: *Handbook of clinical drug data 1999-2000,* ed 9, New York, 1999, McGraw-Hill.

Arky R: *Physician's desk reference,* Montvale, NJ, 1998, Medical Economics.

Catania, PN: Viagra for home care patients, *Home Care Provider* 3(4):197, 1998.

Johns Hopkins Hospital, Department of Pediatrics et al: *The Harriet Lane handbook,* ed 15, St Louis, 2000, Mosby.

Keen JH: *Critical care and emergency drug reference,* ed 3, St Louis, 1996, Mosby.

The Medical Letter: Propecia and Rogaine extra strength for alopecia 40(1021):25, 1998.

The Medical Letter: Sildenafil: an oral drug for impotence 40(1026):51, 1998.

The Medical Letter: Tamsulosin for benign prostatic hyperplasia 39(1011):96, 1997.

Mosby's GenRx: a comprehensive reference for generic and brand drugs, ed 10, St Louis, 2000, Mosby.

The Record: FDA issues repeat Viagra warning, p. A8, June 10, 1998.

Skidmore-Roth L: *Mosby's 2001 nursing drug reference,* St Louis, 2001, Mosby.

Turkoski BB: *Drug information handbook for nursing 1999-2000: including assessment, administration, monitoring guidelines, and patient education,* ed 2, Cleveland, 1999, Lexi-Comp.

Activity

Remember to check the **Online Worksheet** for additional learning opportunities: **www.harcourthealth.com/MERLIN/Lilley/**

Part Six

Drugs Affecting the Respiratory System: Study Skills Tips

- Study on the Run, PURR

STUDY ON THE RUN, PURR

The basic approach in applying Study on the Run (SOTR) is to make use of small blocks of time that are otherwise nonproductive. Plan, Rehearse, and Review do not require that the entire chapter be covered in one study session. These steps produce their benefits by promoting repetition of learning.

Where Is the Time?

SOTR time is everywhere. In the course of a single day you might have an hour or more that can be used for SOTR actions. It is just a matter of becoming aware of little bits and pieces of your day that can ordinarily slip away without being productive. Small blocks of time are everywhere in your day; it just takes a little creativity on your part to become aware of them. Finishing an exam early, standing in the checkout line, waiting for the teakettle to boil, or even waiting for the washing machine to finish the last spin before you change loads can be time used for SOTR. Get creative and be flexible. Remember, every minute of time you use this way is a minute of time you will not have to find later.

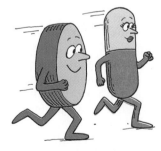

SOTR and Plan

I have repeatedly stressed the importance of questioning as an essential component in Plan. Look at the chapter objectives for Chapter 35. There are seven objectives presented for this chapter. Work on the questions for as many of these objectives as can be accomplished in the time you have. If you complete questions for only two objectives, do not look upon it as failure to complete something. Instead learn to view what you have done as that much less to do later. The time you spend now frees up that much more time during your large blocks of study time for intense study reading.

Will you forget the questions you generated in this session before you have the opportunity to read the chapter? If you make it a habit to ask questions as a continuing part of all study, you will find that you remember the focus questions very well. If you have trouble remembering your own questions, use a pencil. Write questions in the margins of the text. Gradually you will find questioning becomes such an automatic procedure that you will be able to dispense with writing questions. You will remember them.

SOTR and Vocabulary

One of the most challenging aspects of a course like this is the almost overwhelming vocabulary load. If the new vocabulary load is not enough, there is also the need to keep reviewing previous parts and chapters because some term that was introduced three chapters ago has reappeared and you do not remember it clearly. Creating your own vocabulary cards is a perfect SOTR activity.

The basic card model is simple. The word, common form, prefix, or suffix appears on the card front. The back of the card may have just a little information, the minimum being a definition of what is on the front, or the back of the card may contain considerable information. I recommend that you include part, chapter, and page number on the back so that you can locate the term quickly if the need arises. In addition, you may want to add a specific example from the text or of your own creation to help clarify the term. Put as much information on the back as you find useful.

Creating Vocabulary Cards with SOTR

Use the time between classes to create several personal vocabulary cards. Grab your text and your blank note cards. Open to the next chapter you will be studying. Flip over to the glossary pages. Write the first word from the glossary on the front of a blank note card. Flip the card over. Write the part and chapter numbers and the page number for the glossary on the card. Pick a standard location for this. Put these numbers in a top corner or a bottom corner, but make sure you put them in the same corner every time. Eventually this becomes a habit and makes the preparation process faster. It also helps when you are making use of the cards because you will know exactly what information you put on the card and where you put it. Put this card aside and repeat the process with the next term in the glossary. In those few minutes before you go to class you can have completed the basic preparation for a full set of cards covering the 21 terms in the Chapter 35 glossary.

Notice that all I proposed was that you copy the term and the location information. I did not tell you to copy the definition in the glossary at this time. The term, used in the context of a sentence and a paragraph, may be much easier to understand. If, as you read the chapter, you feel that the glossary definition is also useful to have on this card, you can always flip back using the location information you put on the card.

SOTR and Vocabulary Review

Your vocabulary cards are ideal for SOTR action. Carry a deck of cards with you at all times. Whenever you have even a minute or two, you can pull out a stack of cards—cards from previous chapters or the current chapter. Use the oral ask-and-answer method discussed in the *Study Guide*. For instance, the first term in the glossary for Chapter 35 is *allergen*. Ask yourself aloud, "What is an allergen?" Then try to 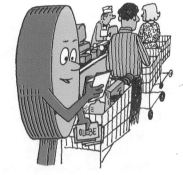 answer the question aloud. Answer: "An allergen is a substance that produces an allergic reaction." It is not necessary to recall the exact answer presented in the glossary and/or chapter. What is important is that you re-spond with a clear and meaningful answer. The answer given above is not exactly the same as that stated in the glossary, but the general concept is the same. Once you have stated your answer, turn the card over and check to make sure that you were correct. Each time you do this with a term, you are strengthening your long-term memory and will find that it takes less and less time to recall the terms you need.

SOTR and Chapter Review

It can be overwhelming if you think that review means rereading the material and therefore you need large blocks of uninterrupted time. There is a much more efficient way to review, and it works well in short time blocks, which makes it a perfect technique for SOTR.

Look at the first page of Chapter 34. You should instantly see a number of visible structures that make it easy to review key terms and concepts without rereading the entire block of material. First, there is the chapter title: *Antihistamines, Decongestants, Antitussives, and Expectorants.* What are antihistamines? This is a question you would have generated when you were engaged in the Plan step of PURR. Now that you have read the chapter, repeat the question and answer it aloud. Answer aloud because you will hear what you say, and will either know the material or need to mark it to come back and reread. Now ask a more complex question: "What is the role of antihistamines? What do they do?" Now try to answer these questions. If you can, then you do not need to reread to find out what antihistamines are. Next, looking at p. 528 you will notice some things in **bold print.** Apply the same process. Using the bold face words and phrases as stimulus, ask questions and try to answer them to your own satisfaction. If you cannot develop a satisfactory answer, then you know that some rereading is needed. But it is very focused. You are not trying to reread everything on the page, only the material right there associated with the term.

Looking further down the page you will see a list. Look at the previous sentence: "This explains why, when excessive amounts of histamine are released, this can lead to anaphylaxis and severe allergic symptoms and result in any or all of the following physiologic changes." Ask questions. If you can answer, no reading is necessary. If you cannot answer, you know that the answers are found immediately after this sentence in the indented list. Use the structures in the chapter to accomplish focused review. Comprehension is improved, long-term memory is strengthened, and your test grades will reflect this.

The benefits of SOTR are enormous. There is no drawback. You are using time that otherwise would be "wasted." This time now becomes productive study time. The more active you become in looking for SOTR opportunities, the more you will find. The more SOTR time you spend the better student you will become.

34

Antihistamines, Decongestants, Antitussives, and Expectorants

objectives

www.harcourthealth.com/MERLIN/Lilley/

When you reach the end of this chapter, you should be able to do the following:

Look for this symbol for topics covered in the **Online Worksheet**

1 Identify the various agents representative of antihistamines, decongestatnts, antitussives, and expectorants.

2 Discuss the mechanisms of actions and indications for the use of antihistamines, decongestants, antitussives, and expectorants.

3 Discuss the contraindications, adverse effects, and various dosage forms for antihistamines, decongestants, antitussives, and expectorants.

4 Develop a nursing care plan that includes all phases of the nursing process for patients taking antihistamines, decongestants, antitussives, and expectorants.

drug profiles

benzonatate, p. 536	**fexofenadine**, p. 531
codeine, p. 537	⚬━ **guaifenesin**, p. 538
⚬━ **dextromethorphan**, p. 537	⚬━ **loratadine**, p. 531
diphenhydramine, p. 532	**naphazoline**, p. 535

⚬━ Key drug.

glossary

Adrenergics (sympathomimetics) (a drə nər' jiks) Of or pertaining to sympathetic nerve fibers of the autonomic nervous system that use epinephrine or epinephrine-like substances as neurotransmitters. (p. 534)

Antagonist (an tag' ə nist) Any agent that exerts an action opposite to that of another or competes for the same receptor sites. (p. 528)

Anticholinergics (parasympatholytics) (an tĭ co lin'ər jiks) Of or pertaining to the blockade of acetylcholine receptors that results in the inhibition of the transmission of parasympathetic nerve impulses. (p. 534)

Antihistamines (an' tĭ his' tə min) Any substance capable of reducing the physiologic and pharmacologic effects of histamine, including a wide variety of drugs that block histamine receptors. (p. 528)

Benzonatate (ben zo' nə tāt) A nonopiate antitussive. (p. 536)

Corticosteroids Any one of the natural or synthetic hormones produced by the adrenal cortex. They influence or control key processes of the body, such as carbohydrate and protein metabolism; the maintenance of serum glucose levels; electrolyte and water balance; and the functions of the cardiovascular system, skeletal muscle, the kidneys, and other organs. (p. 534)

Dextromethorphan (deks' tro məth or' fan) An antitussive derived from morphine but lacking opioid effects. (p. 536)

Empiric therapy (em pir' ik) A method of treating disease based on observations and experience without an understanding of the cause of or mechanism responsible for the disorder or the way in which the therapeutic agent or procedure effects improvement or cure. (p. 533)

Expectorant (ek spek' tə rənt) An agent that increases the flow of fluid in the respiratory tract, reducing the viscosity of bronchial and tracheal secretions and facilitating their removal by the cough reflex and ciliary action. (p. 537)

Guaifenesin (gwi' fen' əsin) Glyceryl guaiacolate, a white to slightly gray powder with a bitter taste and faint odor. It is widely used as an expectorant. (p. 537)

Histamine antagonist (his' tə mēn) Drug that competes with histamine for histamine receptors. (p. 528)

Influenza Highly contagious infection of the respiratory tract caused by a myxovirus and transmitted by airborne droplets. (p. 533)

Iodinated glycerol (i o' dĭ nā ted / glis' ər ol) One of the substances that makes up iodine. (p. 537)

Nonsedating antihistamines Substances that work peripherally to block the actions of histamine and therefore do not have the central nervous system effects that many of the older antihistamines have. (p. 530)

Peripherally acting antihistamines Another name for nonsedating antihistamines. (p. 530)

Potassium iodide One of the products that makes up iodine. (p. 537)

Reflex stimulation An irritation of the respiratory tract occurring in response to an irritation of the gastrointestinal tract. (p. 537)

Rhinovirus (ri' no vi' rəs) Any of about 100 serologically distinct, small RNA viruses that cause about 40% of acute respiratory illnesses. (p. 533)

Sympathomimetic A pharmacologic agent that causes effects that mimick those resulting from stimulation of organs and structures by the sympathetic nervous system. They do this by occupying adrenergic receptor sites and acting as an agonist or by increasing the release of norepinephrine at postganglionic nerve endings. (p. 534)

Terpin hydrate (tər' pin / hī' drāt) Diminishes secretions and promotes healing of the mucous membrane. (p. 537)

Upper respiratory tract infection Any infectious disease of the upper respiratory tract, including the common cold, laryngitis, pharyngitis, rhinitis, sinusitis, and tonsillitis. (p. 533)

HISTAMINE AND ANTIHISTAMINES

Histamine is a bodily substance that performs many functions. It is involved in central nervous system (CNS) transmission, dilation of capillaries, contraction of smooth muscles, stimulation of gastric secretion, and acceleration of the heart rate. There are two types of cellular receptors for histamine. Histamine$_1$ (H$_1$) receptors mediate smooth muscle contraction and dilation of capillaries, and histamine$_2$ (H$_2$) receptors mediate the acceleration of the heart rate and gastric acid secretion. This explains why, when excessive amounts of histamine are released, this can lead to anaphylaxis and severe allergic symptoms and result in any or all of the following physiologic changes:

- Constriction of smooth muscle, especially in the stomach and lungs
- Increase in body secretions
- Vasodilation and increased capillary permeability resulting in fluid movement out of the blood vessels and into the tissues, causing a drop in blood pressure and edema
- Dramatic decrease in blood pressure

Antihistamines are drugs that directly compete with histamine for specific receptor sites. For this reason they are also called **antagonists.** Antihistamines that compete with histamine for the H$_2$ receptors are called **histamine$_2$ antagonists** (also called *H$_2$ blockers*) and include such agents as cimetidine, ranitidine, famotidine, and nizatidine. Because they act on the gastrointestinal system, they are discussed in detail in Part Nine, which focuses on the agents that affect this system. The focus of this chapter is on the **histamine$_1$ antagonists** (also called *H$_1$ blockers*); these are the agents more commonly known as *antihistamines.* They are very useful agents because approximately 10% to 20% of the general population is sensitive to various environmental allergies. Histamine mediates many disorders, such as allergic rhinitis (e.g., hay fever, mold and dust allergies), anaphylaxis, angioneurotic edema, drug fevers, insect bite reactions, and urticaria (itching).

H$_1$ antagonists include such drugs as diphenhydramine, chlorpheniramine, and fexofenadine. They are of greatest value in the treatment of nasal allergies, particularly seasonal hay fever. They are also given to relieve the symptoms of the common cold, such as sneezing and running nose. In this regard they are palliative, not curative; that is, they can help alleviate the symptoms of a cold but can do nothing to destroy the virus causing it.

The clinical efficacy of the more than a dozen different antihistamines is extremely similar, although they all have varying degrees of antihistaminic, anticholinergic, and sedating properties. The particular actions of, and hence indications for, a particular antihistamine are determined by its specific chemical make-up. All antihistamines compete with histamine for the H$_1$ receptors in areas such as the smooth muscle surrounding blood vessels and bronchioles. They also affect the secretions of the lacrimal, salivary, and respiratory mucosal glands. These are primarily anticholinergic actions of antihistamines.

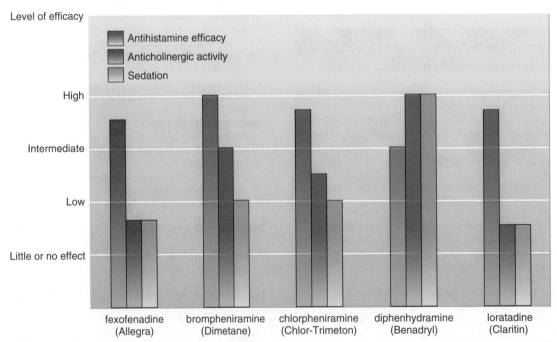

Fig. 34-1 Comparison of efficacy and side effects of selected antihistamines. (Modified from McKenry LM, Salerno E: *Mosby's pharmacology in nursing,* ed 19, St Louis, 1995, Mosby.

Because of their antihistamic properties, they are indicated for the treatment of allergies. These agents also differ from each other in their potency and their adverse effects, especially in the degree of drowsiness they produce. The antihistaminic, anticholinergic, and sedative properties of some of the commonly used antihistamines are summarized in Fig. 34-1. Some of the commonly used antihistamines are listed in Table 34-1 along with their various anticholinergic and sedative effects. These effects make them useful for the treatment of such problems as vertigo, motion sickness, insomnia, and cough.

Mechanism of Action

H_1 blockers (antihistamines) work by blocking or inhibiting the action of histamine throughout the body. They do not push off histamine that is already bound to its receptor but compete with the substance for unoccupied receptors. Therefore these agents are most beneficial when given early in a reaction before all the histamine binds to receptors. This binding of H_1 blockers to these receptors prevents the adverse consequences of histamine stimulation—vasodilation, increased gastrointestinal and respiratory secretions, and increased capillary permeability.

Drug Effects

During allergic reactions, histamine and other substances are released from mast cells, basophils, and other cells in response to antigens (foreign substances) circulating in the blood. It then binds to and activates specific receptors in the nose, eyes, respiratory tract, and skin, producing the characteristic allergic signs and symptoms. Antihistamines can prevent or alleviate these reactions. The various drug effects of antihistamines are listed in Table 34-2. By blocking the H_1 receptors and thereby preventing histamine from acting on the cell, antihistamines have the opposite effects of histamine. Histamine causes extravascular smooth muscle (e.g., in the bronchial tree) to contract, whereas antihistamines cause it to relax. They also prevent or reduce salivary, gastric, lacrimal, and bronchial secretions. Histamine causes pruritus by stimulating nerve endings. Antihistamines can prevent or alleviate the itching. Histamine causes microvascular dilation (involves both H_1 and H_2 receptors) and increased vascular permeability (involves only H_1 receptors). Antihistamines have the opposite effect.

Therapeutic Uses

Antihistamines are more effective in preventing the actions of histamine than in reversing them once they have taken place. Because of their anticholinergic actions, they have a drying effect and reduce nasal, salivary, and lacrimal gland hypersecretion (runny nose and tearing and itching eyes). In the skin they block capillary permeability, wheal-and-flare formation, and itching. Antihistamines are most beneficial in the management of nasal

Table 34-1 Effects of Various Antihistamines

Chemical Class	Anticholinergic Effects	Sedative Effects	Comments
Alkylamines			
brompheniramine	Moderate	Low	Cause less drowsiness and more CNS stimulation; suitable for daytime use.
chlorpheniramine	Moderate	Low	
dexchlorpheniramine	Moderate	Low	
Ethanolamines			
clemastine	High	Moderate	Substantial anticholinergic effects; commonly cause sedation; with usual doses drowsiness occurs in about 50% of patients; diphenhydramine and dimenhydrinate also used as antiemetics.
diphenhydramine	High	High	
dimenhydrinate	High	High	
Ethylenediamines			
pyrilamine	Low to none	Low	Weak sedative effects, but adverse gastrointestinal effects are common.
tripelennamine	Low to none	Moderatae	
Phenothiazines			
promethazine	High	High	Principally used as antipsychotics; some are useful as antihistamines, antipruritics, and antiemetics.
trimeprazine	High	Moderate	
Piperadines			
azatadine	Moderate	Moderate	Commonly used in the treatment of motion sickness; hydroxyzine is used as a tranquilizer, sedative, antipruritic, and antiemetic.
cyproheptadine	Moderate	Low	
hydroxyzine	Moderate	Moderate	
phenindamine	Moderate	Low to none	
Miscellaneous			
fexofenadine	Low to none	Low to none	Very few adverse effects from anticholinergic or sedative effects; almost exclusively antihistaminic effects, can take during day because no sedative effects. In general they are longer acting and have fewer side effects.
loratadine	Low to none	Low to none	

Table 34-2 Antihistamines: Drug Effects

Body System	Histamine Effects	Antihistamine Effects
Cardiovascular system (small blood vessels)	Dilation of blood vessels, increased blood vessel permeability (allows substances to leak into tissues).	Prevents dilation of blood vessels and increased permeability.
Immune system (release of various substances commonly associated with allergic reactions)	Mast cells release histamine and several other substances, resulting in allergic reactions.	Do not stabilize mast cells nor do they prevent the release of the substances such as histamine, but they bind to histamine receptors and prevent the actions of histamine.
Smooth muscle (on exocrine glands)	Stimulates salivary, gastric, lacrimal, and bronchial secretions.	Prevents salivary, gastric, lacrimal, and bronchial secretions.

Table 34-3 Antihistamines: Common Adverse Effects

Body System	Side/Adverse Effects
Cardiovascular	Local anesthetic (quinidine-like) effect on the cardiac conduction system resulting in dysrhythmias, arrest, hypotension, palpitations, syncope, dizziness, death (see Interactions section)
Central nervous system	Sedation (mild drowsiness to deep sleep), dizziness, muscular weakness, paradoxical excitement, restlessness, insomnia, nervousness, seizures
Gastrointestinal	Anorexia, nausea, vomiting, diarrhea or constipation, hepatitis, jaundice
Other	Dryness of mouth, nose, and throat; urinary retention; impotence; vertigo; visual disturbances; blurred vision; tinnitus; headache; rarely agranulocytosis, hemolytic anemia, leukopenia, thrombocytopenia, pancytopenia

allergies, seasonal or perennial allergic rhinitis (e.g., hay fever), and some of the typical symptoms of the common cold. They are also very useful in the treatment of allergic reactions, motion sickness, Parkinson's disease, and vertigo. In addition, they have been used as sleep aids.

Side Effects and Adverse Effects

Drowsiness is usually the chief complaint of people who take antihistamines, but these sedative effects vary from class to class (see Table 34-1). The anticholinergic (drying) effects of antihistamines can cause such side effects as dry mouth, changes in vision, difficulty urinating, and constipation. The most frequent side effects and adverse effects of the antihistamines are listed in Table 34-3.

Ketoconazole and erythromycin may increase concentrations of loratadine. Alcohol, monoamine oxidase (MAO) inhibitors, and CNS depressants may increase CNS depressant effects of diphenhydramine and cetirizine.

Interactions

Fexofenadine, when given with erythromycin or ketoconazole, can increase fexofenadine concentrations. The major difference between fexofenadine and terfenadine is that these increased levels of fexofenadine do not result in severe cardiac rhythm disturbances.

Dosages

For the recommended dosages for selected antihistamines, see the dosages table on p. 531.

drug profiles

Although some antihistamines are prescription drugs, most are available over the counter (OTC). Antihistamines are available in many dosage forms to be administered orally, intramuscularly, intravenously, or topically.

NONSEDATING ANTIHISTAMINES

A major advance in antihistamine therapy occurred with the development of the **nonsedating antihistamines** fexofenadine and loratadine. These agents were developed in part to eliminate many of the unwanted side effects of the older antihistamines (mainly sedation). These agents work peripherally to block the actions of histamine and therefore do not have the CNS effects that many older antihistamines have. For this reason these agents are also called **peripherally acting antihistamines.** Another advantage these agents have over the older antihistamines is that they have longer durations of action, which allows some of them to be taken only once a day. This further increases compliance. Unlike many older antihistamines, nonsedating antihistamines are only available by prescription, in part because of some of the life-threatening drug interactions associated with these agents.

DOSAGES　Selected Antihistamines

agent	pharmacologic class	dosage range	purpose
NONSEDATING ANTIHISTAMINES			
fexofenadine (Allegra)	H₁ antihistamine	*Adult* PO: 60 mg twice daily	Allergic rhinitis
loratadine (Claritin)	H₁ antihistamine	*Pediatric <80 kg* PO: 5 mg once/day *Adult/Pediatric ≥12 y/o* PO: 10 mg ac once/day	Allergic rhinitis
TRADITIONAL ANTIHISTAMINE			
diphenhydramine (Benadryl)	H₁ antihistamine	*Pediatric >20 lb (9 kg)* PO/IM/IV: 6.25-25 mg 3-4 times/day (1 mg/kg/dose 3-4 times day); max 300 mg/day	Allergic disorders, nighttime sleep aid, motion sickness
		PO: 2-12 y/o: 1 mg/kg hs *Adult*	Nighttime sleep aid
		PO: 25-50 mg 3-4 times/day max 400 mg/day	Allergic disorders, motion sickness
		IM/IV: 10-50 mg q4h; max 400 mg/day PO: 50 mg hs	Nighttime sleep aid

The dosage range column subscripts use H_1 antihistamine.

fexofenadine

Fexofenadine (Allegra) is the active metabolite of terfenadine (Seldane). Terfenadine has numerous interactions with other drugs that are metabolized via the cytochrome P-450 3A4 enzyme system. These other drugs, such as erythromycin (an antibiotic) and ketoconazole (an antifungal drug), can lead to terfenadine build-up in the blood. There is a resulting potential for serious, sometimes fatal, cardiac dysrhythmias. The FDA determined that terfenadine was no longer considered safe and has therefore removed it from the market. The FDA has determined that drugs containing terfenadine are no longer shown to be safe because fexofenadine is now available. Terfenadine is a prodrug. Fexofenadine is the active metabolite of terfenadine produced in the body, and it provides nearly all of terfenadine's therapeutic effect. It does not, however, block cardiac potassium channels or cause QT prolongation or ventricular arrhythmias (notably torsades de pointes type ventricular tachycardia) as terfenadine can at greater than usual blood levels. Terfenadine has been voluntarily withdrawn from the market by its manufacturer and replaced by fexofenadine.

Fexofenadine is indicated for the relief of symptoms associated with seasonal allergic rhinitis in adults and children 12 years of age and older. It is contraindicated in patients with known hypersensitivity to fexofenadine or any of its ingredients. Fexofenadine is classified as a pregnancy category C agent. Fexofenadine is only available as an oral 60-mg capsule. See the dosages table above for dosage information.

PHARMACOKINETICS

HALF-LIFE	ONSET	PEAK	DURATION
14-16 hr	1-2 hr	2-3 hr	10-12 hr

loratadine

Loratadine (Claritin) is another nonsedating antihistamine. It also only needs to be taken once a day. Structurally it is similar to cyproheptadine and azatadine, but unlike these other agents, it cannot distribute into the CNS. Loratadine is used to relieve the symptoms of seasonal allergic rhinitis (e.g., hay fever).

Loratadine is classified as a pregnancy category B agent and is contraindicated in patients who have shown a hypersensitivity to it, those suffering from an acute asthma attack, and those with lower respiratory tract diseases. Loratadine is available orally as a 10-mg tablet, as syrup and as rapidly disintegrating tablets. See the dosages table above for dosage information.

PHARMACOKINETICS

HALF-LIFE	ONSET	PEAK	DURATION
8.4-24 hr	1-3 hr	8-12 hr	24 hr

TRADITIONAL ANTIHISTAMINES

The traditional antihistamines are the older agents that work both peripherally and centrally. They also have anticholinergic effects, which in some cases make them more effective than nonsedating antihistamines. Some of these commonly used older agents are diphenhydramine, brompheniramine, chlorpheniramine, dimenhydrinate, doxylamine, meclinzine, and promethazine. These agents are used either alone or in combination with other drugs in the symptomatic relief of many disorders ranging from insomnia to motion sickness. Many patients respond to and tolerate the older agents quite well, and because many are generically available, they are much less expensive. These agents are available both OTC and by prescription.

diphenhydramine

Diphenhydramine (Benadryl) is an older, traditional antihistamine that works both peripherally and centrally. It also has potent anticholinergic effects. It is one of the most commonly used antihistamines, in part because of its excellent safety profile and efficacy. It has the greatest range of therapeutic indications of any antihistamines available. It is used for the relief or prevention of histamine-mediated allergies and motion sickness, the treatment of Parkinson's disease, and as a sleep-aid. It is also used in conjunction with epinephrine in the management of anaphylaxis and in the treatment of acute dystonic reactions.

Diphenhydramine is classified as a pregnancy category B agent and is contraindicated in patients with a known hypersensitivity to it, nursing mothers, neonates, and patients with lower respiratory tract symptoms. It is available in oral, parenteral, and topical preparations. Orally, diphenhydramine is available as a 25- and 50-mg capsules and regular and film-coated tablets; as a 12.5-mg/5 ml elixir; and in several combination products that contain other cough and cold medications. Parenterally, diphenhydramine is available as a 10- and 50-mg/ml injection. Topically, diphenhydramine is available as a 1% and 2% cream. It also is available in combination with several other drugs that are commonly given topically, such as calamine, camphor, and zinc oxide. These combination preparations are available as aerosols, creams, gels, and lotions. The recommended dosages are given in the dosages table on p. 531.

PHARMACOKINETICS

HALF-LIFE	ONSET	PEAK	DURATION
2-7 hr	15-30 min	1-2 hr	4 hr

OTHER ANTIHISTAMINES

Brompheniramine and chlorpheniramine are other antihistamines commonly used alone or in combination with other drugs as OTC cough and cold preparations. Dimenhydrinate is commonly used in the treatment of motion sickness. It is available as a chewable tablet that can be quickly absorbed, making its onset of action rapid. This is of use in patients suffering from vertigo or motion sickness of sudden onset. Because of its potent sedating effects, doxylamine is very frequently used in combination with cough and cold medications such as acetamin-

ophen (Tylenol) to induce sleep in cold sufferers. Meclizine, which is used for the treatment of vertigo, is available both OTC and by prescription in higher doses. One of the most commonly used antiemetic agents is an antihistamine. This agent, promethazine, is commonly given for the treatment of various types of nausea and vomiting. It is available in oral and rectal preparations and as an injection. Following is a listing of all the antihistamines, including the commonly recommended dosages and other pertinent information:

- **azatadine** (Optimine) Available by prescription as 1-mg tablets. The recommended dosage is 1 to 2 mg twice daily, given with a full glass of water. It is rated as a pregnancy category B agent.
- **azelastine** (Astelin) Currently the only antihistamine formulated as a metered spray solution for intranasal administration. Each azelastine hydrochloride nasal spray, 137 μg, bottle contains 17 mg (1 mg/ml) of azelastine hydrochloride to be used with the supplied metered-dose spray pump unit. Each bottle can deliver 100 metered sprays. Each spray delivers a mean of 0.137 ml solution containing 137 μg of azelastine hydrochloride. The recommended dose of Astelin nasal spray in adults and children 12 years and older is two sprays per nostril twice daily. Before initial use, special instructions for priming the pump unit and delivery system must be followed. Azelastine is a pregnancy category C agent.
- **brompheniramine** (Dimetane) Available as a 2-mg/5 ml elixir and as 4-, 8-, and 12-mg tablets. These dosage forms may be either obtained by prescription or OTC, depending on the dose and dosage instructions. The recommended oral dosage is 4 to 8 mg three to four times daily, taken with a full glass of water. It is rated as a pregnancy category C agent.
- **buclizine** (Bucladin-S, Softabs) Available by prescription as 50-mg tablets. The usual adult dosage is 50 mg taken one half hour before travel and repeated after 4 to 6 hours, if needed. It has no pregnancy category designation.
- **cetirizine** (Zyrtec) Active metabolite of hydroxyzine. It is indicated for the treatment of perennial allergic rhinitis (year-round allergies), seasonal allergic rhinitis, and chronic urticaria (itching and hives). Cetirizine is available in 5- and 10-mg tablets and is given as a single daily dose with or without food. Cetirizine is a pregnancy category B agent.
- **chlorpheniramine** (Chlor-Trimeton) Available as 4-, 8-, and 12-mg tablets. These dosage forms are available either by prescription or OTC, depending on the dose and dosage instructions. The recommended oral dosage is 4 mg every 4 to 6 hours, given with a full glass of water. It is rated as a pregnancy category B agent.

- **clemastine** (Tavist) Available by prescription or OTC as a 0.67-mg/5 ml syrup and in 1.34- and 2.68-mg tablets. The recommended oral adult dosage is 1.34 to 2.68 mg one to three times daily, given with a full glass of water. It is rated as a pregnancy category B agent.
- **cyclizine** (Marezine) Available OTC as 50-mg tablets. The recommended adult dosage is 50 mg taken one half hour before travel and repeated after 4 to 6 hours, if needed. The total daily dose should not exceed 200 mg. The recommended dosage in 6- to 12-year-old children is 25 mg, given up to three times per day. It is rated as pregnancy category B agent.
- **cyproheptadine** (Periactin) Available as a 2-mg/5 ml syrup and as 4-mg tablets. The usual adult dosage is 4 mg three to four times per day, given with a full glass of water. It is rated as a pregnancy category B agent.
- **dexchlorpheniramine** (Polaramine) A prescription drug available as a 2-mg/5 ml syrup and as 2-, 4-, and 6-mg tablets. The recommended adult dosage is 2 mg four to six times per day, given with a full glass of water. It is rated as a pregnancy category B drug.
- **dimenhydrinate** (Dramamine) A prescription drug available as 50-mg tablets. The recommended oral adult dosage is 50 to 100 mg every 4 to 6 hours, taken one half hour before travel. The recommended dosage for 6- to 12-year-old children is 25 to 50 mg every 6 to 8 hours, taken one half hour before travel. It is rated as a pregnancy category B drug.
- **doxylamine** (Unisom) An OTC drug available as 25-mg tablets. The recommended adult dosage is 25 mg at bedtime, taken with a full glass of water. It is rated as a pregnancy category B drug.
- **hydroxyzine** (Atarax, Vistaril) The hydrochloride salt of hydroxyzine is known as Atarax, and the pamoate salt is known as Vistaril. Hydroxyzine is considered a weak anxiolytic. It has sedative and mild antianxiety activity similar to that of diphenhydramine. It is a prescription-only drug and is available as 10-, 25-, 50-, and 100-mg tablets; 25-, 50-, and 100-mg capsules; a 10-mg/5 ml syrup; a 25-mg/5 ml suspension; and a 25- and 50-mg/ml injection. It is rated as a pregnancy category C drug.
- **meclizine** (Antivert, Bonine) Available as 12.5-, 25-, and 50-mg tablets and as 25-mg chewable tablets, either by prescription or OTC, depending on the dose and dosage instructions. The recommended adult oral dosage is 25 to 50 mg, repeated once daily and given with a full glass of water. It is rated as a pregnancy category B drug.
- **methdilazine** (Tacaryl) Available by prescription as a 4-mg/5 ml syrup and as 4- and 8-mg tablets.

The recommended adult dosage is 8 mg, taken with a full glass of water two to four times per day. It is rated as a pregnancy category B drug.

- **promethazine** (Phenergan) A prescription drug available as a 25- and 50-mg/ml injection, as a 6.25- and 25-mg/5 ml syrup, and as 12.5-, 25-, and 50-mg tablets. The recommended adult dosage is 12.5 to 25 mg three times daily, taken with a full glass of water. It is rated as a pregnancy category C drug.
- **trimeprazine** (Temaril) A prescription drug available as 5-mg capsules, 2.5-mg tablets, and a 2.5-mg/5 ml syrup. The recommended adult dosage is 2.5 mg four times a day, given with a full glass of water. It has no pregnancy category designation.
- **tripelennamine** (PBZ) A prescription drug available as 25-, 50-, and 100-mg tablets. The recommended adult dosage is 25 to 50 mg every 4 to 6 hours, given with a full glass of water. It has no pregnancy category designation.
- **triprolidine** (Actidil) An OTC drug available as a 1.25-mg/5 ml syrup and 2.5-mg tablet. The recommended adult dosage is 2.5 mg every 4 to 6 hours, taken with a full glass of water. It is rated as a pregnancy category C drug.

COLD MEDICATIONS

The agents used to treat the symptoms of the common cold are decongestants, antitussives (cough suppressants), and expectorants. Most common colds are due to a viral infection, most often a **rhinovirus** or an **influenza** virus such as myxovirus. These viruses normally invade the tissues (mucosa) of the upper respiratory tract (nose, pharynx, and larynx) to cause an **upper respiratory tract infection** (URI). The inflammatory response elicited by these invading viruses stimulates excessive mucus production. This fluid drips down the pharynx and into the esophagus and lower respiratory tract, which leads to symptoms typical of cold—sore throat, coughing, and upset stomach. The irritation of the nasal mucosa often triggers the sneeze reflex and also causes the release of several inflammatory and vasoactive substances, which results in the dilation of the small blood vessels in the nasal sinuses and leads to nasal congestion. The treatment of the common symptoms of URIs involves the combined use of antihistamines, nasal decongestants, antitussives, and expectorants. However, they can only relieve the symptoms of URIs. They can do nothing to eliminate the causative pathogen. Antivirals and antibiotics are currently the only agents that can do this, but treatment with these is often hampered by the fact that the viral or bacterial cause cannot be readily identified. Because of this, the treatment rendered can only be determined on the basis of what is believed to be the most likely cause. This is called **empiric therapy.**

DECONGESTANTS

Nasal congestion is due to excessive nasal secretions and inflamed and swollen nasal mucosa. The primary causes of nasal congestion are allergies and URIs, especially the common cold. There are three separate groups of nasal decongestants: **adrenergics (sympathomimetics),** which are the largest group; **anticholinergics (parasympatholytics),** which are rarely used; and selected topical **corticosteroids** (intranasal steroids).

Nasal decongestants can be taken orally to produce a systemic effect, inhaled, or administered topically to the nose. Each method of administration has its advantages and disadvantages.

Decongestants administered by the oral route include the following:
- phenylephrine (Neo-Synephrine)
- pseudoephedrine* (Sudafed)

Agents administered by the oral route produce prolonged decongestant effects, but the onset of activity is more delayed and the effect less potent than those of decongestants applied topically. However, the clinical problem of rebound congestion associated with topically administered agents is almost nonexistent with oral doses.

Decongestants suitable for being inhaled must be aromatic and include the following:
- deoxyephedrine (Vicks inhaler)
- propylhexedrine (Benzedrex inhaler)

The topical administration of adrenergics and intranasal steroids produces a potent decongestant effect with a prompt onset of action. However, sustained use of these agents for several days causes a rebound congestion, which only exacerbates the condition. Decongestants suitable for being inhaled include the following:

Adrenergics
- ephedrine (Vicks, Vatronol)
- naphazoline (Privine)
- oxymetazoline (Afrin, Sinex Long-Acting)
- phenylephrine (Neo-Synephrine)
- tetrahydrozoline (Tyzine, Tyzine Pediatric)

Intranasal steroids
- beclomethasone dipropionate (Beconase, Vancenase)
- dexamethasone sodium phosphate (Decadron Phosphate Turbinase)
- flunisolide (Nasalide)

Mechanism of Action

Nasal decongestants are most commonly used for their ability to shrink engorged nasal mucous membranes and relieve nasal stuffiness. Adrenergic agents (e.g., ephedrine, oxymetazoline) accomplish this by constricting the small blood vessels that supply the structures of the upper respiratory tract, the primary ones being the blood vessels surrounding the nasal sinuses. When these blood vessels are stimulated by alpha-adrenergic drugs, they

*Pseudoephedrine is an alpha-beta agent, but the alpha activity is the greater of the two.

constrict. Because sympathetic nervous system (SNS) stimulation produces the same effect, these agents are sometimes referred to as **sympathomimetics.** Once these blood vessels shrink, the nasal secretions in the swollen mucous membranes are better able to drain.

Nasal steroids are aimed at the inflammatory response elicited by the invading organisms (viruses and bacteria), which the body responds to by producing inflammation, walling off the area, and attracting various cells of the immune system. Steroids exert their antiinflammatory effect by causing these cells to be turned off or rendered unresponsive.

Drug Effects

The drug effects of topical alpha-adrenergic agents are predominantly limited to the mucosal surface on which they are administered. They constrict the arterioles in the mucous membranes, resulting in local vasoconstriction of the dilated blood vessels and a subsequent reduction in blood flow and nasal congestion. The drug effects of intranasal steroids are discussed in Chapter 35.

Therapeutic Uses

Nasal decongestants relieve the nasal congestion associated with acute or chronic rhinitis, the common cold, sinusitis, and hay fever or other allergies. They may also be used to reduce swelling of the nasal passage and to facilitate visualization of the nasal and pharyngeal membranes before surgery or diagnostic procedures.

Side Effects and Adverse Effects

Adrenergic agents are usually well tolerated. Rare adverse effects of these agents include nervousness, insomnia, palpitations, and tremor.

Occasionally a topically applied adrenergic nasal decongestant is somewhat absorbed into the bloodstream, producing drug effects elsewhere in the body. These include cardiovascular effects such as hypertension and palpitations and CNS effects such as headache, nervous-

DOSAGES Selected Decongestant, Expectorant, and Antitussive Agents

agent	pharmacologic class	dosage range	purpose
benzonatate (Tessalon Perles)	Nonopioid antitussive	Adult/Pediatric >10 y/o PO: 100 mg tid; do not exceed 600 mg/day	Cough suppression
codeine (Dimetane-DC, Tussar SF, Novahistine DH, Robitussin A-C, others)	Opioid antitussive	Pediatric PO: 2-6 y/o: 2.5-5 mg q4-6h; do not exceed 30 mg/day PO: 6-12 y/o: 5-10 mg q4-6h; do not exceed 60 mg/day Adult PO: 10-20 mg q4-6h; do not exceed 120 mg/day	Cough suppression
dextromethorphan (Vicks Formula 44, Robitussin-DM, others)	Nonopioid antitussive	Pediatric PO: 2-6 y/o; 2.5-7.5 mg q4-8h; do not exceed 30 mg/day PO: 6-12 y/o: 5-10 mg q4h or 15 mg q6-8h; do not exceed 60 mg/day Adult/Pediatric >12 y/o PO: 10-30 mg q4-8 h; do not exceed 120 mg/day	Cough suppression
guaifenesin (glyceryl guaiacolate) (Guiatuss, Humibid, Robitussin, others)	Expectorant	Pediatric PO: 2-6 y/o: 50-100 mg q4h; do not exceed 600 mg/day PO: 6-12 y/o: 100-200 mg q4h; do not exceed 1200 mg/day Adult/Pediatric ≥12 y/o PO: 100-400 mg q4h; do not exceed 2400 mg/day	Respiratory congestion
naphazoline (Privine)	Alpha-adrenergic vasoconstrictor	Adult/Pediatric ≥12 y/o 0.05% solution 1-2 drops or sprays in each nostril q6h prn; max 3-5 days	Nasal decongestant

ness, and dizziness. These systemic effects are the result of alpha-adrenergic stimulation of the heart, blood vessels, and CNS. The most common side effects of intranasal steroids include local mucosal irritation and dryness.

Interactions

There are few significant drug interactions with the nasal decongestants. Sympathomimetics and nasal decongestants can increase toxicity when given together. MAO inhibitors may result in additive pressor effects when given with nasal decongestants.

Dosages

For the recommended dosages of naphazoline, the only nasal decongestant profiled, see the dosages table above.

drug profiles

Many of the decongestants are OTC agents, but the more potent agents that can cause serious side effects are available only by prescription. Adrenergic agents are usually contraindicated in patients with diabetes, hypertension, cardiac disease, thyroid dysfunction, prostatitis, or a known hypersensitivity to them. Although nasal steroids are relatively safe, they too are contraindicated in some circumstances, specifically nasal mucosal infections and drug hypersensitivity.

Many adrenergic agents (phenylephrine, prophylhexedrine, and pseudoephedrine) and some steroids (beclomethasone, dexamethasone, and flunisolide) are discussed in greater detail in other chapters. The adrenergic agents such as naphazoline are discussed here. These are usually the first-line agents used in the treatment of nasal congestion because they are available OTC.

naphazoline

Naphazoline (Privine) is chemically and pharmacologically very similar to the other sympathomimetic agents oxymetazoline, tetrahydrozoline, and xylometazoline. When these agents are administered intranasally, they cause dilated arterioles to constrict, thereby reducing nasal blood flow and congestion. During a cold the blood vessels that surround the nasal sinus are usually dilated or swollen and engorged with white blood cells, histamines, and many other cells that are involved in fighting infections of the respiratory tract. This swelling, or dilation, blocks the nasal passage, resulting in the nasal congestion. When agents such as naphazoline are applied to this area, they relieve this swelling and congestion by constricting these blood vessels.

Naphazoline and its chemically related cousins are classified as pregnancy category C agents and have the same contraindications as the other nasal decongestants. Nasally administered naphazoline is available as a 0.05% nasal solution and is meant to be instilled into each nostril. Common dosages for this agent are given in the dosages table on p. 535.

PHARMACOKINETICS

HALF-LIFE	ONSET	PEAK	DURATION
Unknown	5-10 min	Unknown	2-6 hr

ANTITUSSIVES

Coughing is a normal physiologic function and serves the purpose of removing potentially harmful foreign substances and excessive secretions from the respiratory tract. The cough reflex is stimulated when receptors in the bronchi, alveoli, and pleura (lining of the lungs) are stretched. This causes a signal to be sent to the cough center in the medulla of the brain, which in turn stimulates the cough. Although most of the time coughing is a beneficial response, there are times when it is not useful and may even be harmful (e.g., after a surgery such as hernia repair). In these situations, this otherwise normal response must be stopped or inhibited through the use of an antitussive agent. There are two main categories of these agents—opioid and nonopioid antitussives.

Although all opioid agents have antitussive effects, only codeine and its semisynthetic derivative hydrocodone are used as antitussives. Both agents are effective in suppressing the cough reflex and, if used in the prescribed manner, their use should not lead to dependency. The two drugs are usually incorporated into various dosage formulations and are rarely used as sole agents.

Nonopioid antitussive drugs are less effective than opioid ones and are available either alone or in combination with other agents in an array of OTC cold and cough preparations. Dextromethorphan is the most widely used of these antitussive agents and is a derivative of the synthetic opioid levorphanol. Benzonatate is another nonopioid agent.

Mechanism of Action

The opioid antitussives codeine and hydrocodone suppress the cough reflex through a direct action on the cough center. The nonopioid cough suppressant **dextromethorphan** works in the same way. However, because it is not an opioid, it does not have analgesic properties nor does it cause addiction or CNS depression. Another nonopioid antitussive is **benzonatate.** Its mechanism of action is entirely different from that of the other agents. Benzonatate suppresses the cough reflex by anesthetizing (numbing) the stretch receptors and thus keeping the cough reflex from being stimulated in the medulla.

Drug Effects

Codeine, hydrocodone, and dextromethorphan directly suppress the cough reflex, whereas benzonatate anesthetizes, or numbs, the stretch receptors. Opioid antitussives also provide analgesia and have a drying effect on the mucosa of the respiratory tract. They also tend to increase the viscosity of the bronchial secretions.

Therapeutic Uses

Although they have other properties, such as the analgesic effect of opioid agents, antitussives are used primarily to stop the cough reflex when the cough is nonproductive and/or harmful.

Side Effects and Adverse Effects

Following are the side effects and adverse effects of selected antitussive agents:
- benzonatate: dizziness, headache, sedation, nausea, constipation, pruritus, and nasal congestion
- codeine: sedation, nausea, vomiting, lightheadedness, and constipation
- dextromethorpan: dizziness, drowsiness, and nausea
- diphenhydramine: sedation, dry mouth, and other anticholinergic effects
- hydrocodone: sedation, nausea, vomiting, lightheadedness, and constipation

Interactions

There are very few drug interactions that occur with benzonatate, although there are some associated with the use of opioid antitussives and dextromethorphan. Opioid antitussives (codeine and hydrocodone) may potentiate the effects of other opioids, general anesthetics, tranquilizers, sedatives and hypnotics, tricyclic antidepressants (TCAs), monoamine oxidase (MAO) inhibitors, alcohol, and other CNS depressants. Dextromethorphan should not be given in conjunction with MAO inhibitors.

Dosages

For the recommended dosages of selected antitussive agents, see the dosages table on p. 535.

drug profiles

Antitussives come in many oral dosage forms and are available both with and without a prescription. Most of the narcotic antitussives are available only by prescription because of the associated abuse potential. Dextromethorphan is the most popular nonnarcotic antitussive available OTC.

benzonatate

Benzonatate (Tessalon) is a nonopioid antitussive agent that is thought to work by anesthetizing or numbing the cough receptors. It is only available with a prescription and only as a 100-mg capsule, to be taken orally. It is classified as a pregnancy category C agent and is contraindicated in patients with a known hypersensitivity to it. Common dosages are listed in the dosages table on p. 535.

PHARMACOKINETICS

HALF-LIFE	ONSET	PEAK	DURATION
Unknown	15-20 min	Unknown	3-8 hr

codeine

Codeine (Dimetane-DC, Tussar SF, Novahistine DH, Robitussin A-C, and many others) is a very popular opioid antitussive agent. It is used in combination with many other common cough and cold medications in the treatment of coughs. Because it is an opioid, it is potentially addictive and can depress respirations and the CNS. For this reason, codeine-containing cough suppressants are more tightly controlled substances. These cough suppressants are available in many oral dosage forms—solutions, tablets, capsules, and suspensions. They are classified as pregnancy category C agents and are contraindicated in patients with a known hypersensitivity to opiates, and those suffering from respiratory depression, increased intracranial pressure, seizure disorders, or severe respiratory disorders. Common dosages are listed in the dosages table on p. 535.

PHARMACOKINETICS

HALF-LIFE	ONSET	PEAK	DURATION
2.9 hr (plasma)	30-60 min	1-2 hr	4-6 hr

dextromethorphan

Dextromethorphan (Vicks Formula 44, Robitussin-DM, and many others) is a nonopioid antitussive that is available alone or in combination with many other cough and cold preparations. It is widely used because it is safe and nonaddicting and does not cause respiratory and CNS depression. It is classified as a pregnancy category C agent and is contraindicated in the following: hypersensitivity, asthma and emphysema, and persistent headache. Dextromethrophan is available as lozenges, a solution, liquid-filled capsules, granules, tablets (oral, chewable, extended-release, and film-coated), and an extended-release suspension. Common dosages are listed in the dosages table on p. 535.

PHARMACOKINETICS

HALF-LIFE	ONSET	PEAK	DURATION
Unknown	15-30 min	Unknown	3-6 hr

Activity

EXPECTORANTS

Expectorants aid in the expectoration (removal) of excessive mucus that has accumulated in the respiratory tract by disintegrating and thinning out the secretion. They are administered orally either as single agents or in combination with other drugs to facilitate the flow of respiratory secretions by reducing the viscosity of tenacious secretions. The actual clinical effectiveness of expectorants is highly questionable, however. Placebo-controlled clinical evaluations have failed to show that expectorants reduce the viscosity of sputum. Despite this, expectorants are popular drugs and are contained in most OTC cold and cough preparations. The most common expectorant in OTC products is guaifenesin (formerly known as glyceryl guaiacolate). The various expectorants include the following:

- ammonium chloride
- guaifenesin (Robitussin)
- iodinated glycerol (Organidin)
- potassium iodide (Pima syrup)
- terpin hydrate elixir

Mechanism of Action

Expectorants work by means of one of two different mechanisms of action, depending on the agent. The first is **reflex stimulation,** in which loosening and thinning of the respiratory tract secretions occurs in response to an irritation of the gastrointestinal tract produced by the agent. **Guaifenesin** is one of the most commonly used of these agents. The secretory glands can also be stimulated directly to increase their production of respiratory tract fluids. **Terpin hydrate** works in this way. Iodine-containing products (**iodinated glycerol** and **potassium iodide**) have been conjectured to work by both directly and indirectly stimulating the production of respiratory tract fluids.

Drug Effects

Expectorants primarily affect the gastrointestinal and respiratory tracts, either directly by stimulating the respiratory tract or indirectly by irritating the gastrointestinal tract.

Therapeutic Uses

Expectorants are used for the relief of the nonproductive coughs commonly associated with the common cold, bronchitis, laryngitis, pharyngitis, pertussis, influenza, and measles. They may also be used for the suppression of coughs caused by chronic paranasal sinusitis. By loosening and thinning sputum and the bronchial secretions, they may indirectly diminish the tendency to cough.

Side Effects and Adverse Effects

The side effects and adverse effects of expectorants are minimal. The most common side effects of the individual expectorants are listed in Table 34-4.

Interactions

The drug interactions most commonly seen in conjunction with expectorant use occur with the iodinated products. They may produce an additive or synergistic hypothyroid effect when used concurrently with lithium. Their use with antithyroid agents may result in an additive hypothyroid effect, and their use with potassium iodide, potassium-containing drugs, or potassium-sparing

Table 34-4 Expectorants: Common Adverse Effects

Expectorant	Side/Adverse Effects
ammonium chloride	Nausea, vomiting, metabolic acidosis, acidification of urine
guaifenesin	Nausea, vomiting, gastric irritation
iodinated glycerol	Gastrointestinal irritation, rash, enlarged thyroid gland
potassium iodide	Iodism, nausea, vomiting, taste perversion
terpin hydrate	Gastric upset; elixir also has a high alcohol content

case study   Asthma

A 13-year-old female, K.L., has had well controlled asthma since 6 years of age. Her daily regimen consists of cromolyn Na (Intal) by nebulizer and Aerobid inhaler. Loratidine (Claritin) has now been added to her treatment regimen. Since early spring, she has been suffering from seasonal rhinitis. Her dose of Claritin is 10 mg once a day.

- *What type of patient education tips should you share with K.L. about Claritin?*
- *Why is it recommended that Claritin be given on a empty stomach?*
- *What directions should you give K.L. about taking Claritin in relation to meal times?*

For Answers see www.harcourthealth.com/MERLIN/Lilley/.

diuretics may lead to the development of hyperkalemia, which can result in cardiac dysrhythmias or cardiac arrest.

Dosages

The recommended dosages of guaifenesin, the only expectorant profiled, are given in the dosages table on p. 535.

drug profiles

guaifenesin

Guaifenesin (Guiatuss, Humibid, Robitussin, and many others) is a very commonly used expectorant that is available in several different oral dosage forms—capsules, tablets, solutions, and granules. It is used in the symptomatic management of coughs of varying origin. It is beneficial in the treatment of productive coughs because it thins difficult-to-cough-up mucus in the respiratory tract. Pharmacokinetics for guaifenesin are not available. See the dosages table on p. 535 for the common dosages. Pregnancy category C.

nursing process

• Assessment

Assessment should begin with gathering data about the condition or allergic reaction for which the agent is indicated. For example, an allergic reaction to a drug, food, or substance may include signs and symptoms such as hives, wheezing or bonchospasm, tachycardia, or hypotension.

Before administering antihistamines, the nurse must ensure that the patient has no allergies to this group of medications, even though these agents are actually used mostly for the treatment of drug allergies and other allergic symptoms. They are also contraindicated in patients suffering from an acute asthma attack and those with lower respiratory tract disease. Cautious use or very close monitoring is

called for in patients with a history of increased intraocular pressure; those with cardiac or renal disease, hypertension, bronchial asthma, chronic obstructive pulmonary disease, peptic ulcer disease, convulsive disorders, or benign prostatic hypertrophy; and pregnant women.

The one contraindication to the use of nonsedating antihistamines is hypersensitivity. They should not be given concurrently with erythromycin, ketoconazole, or itraconazole because of the serious cardiovascular disorders this can precipitate. Cautious use is called for in patients with impaired liver function.

Before administering an antitussive agent, the patient should be assessed for hypersensitivity to the agent, and a respiratory and cough assessment should be performed and documented. Decongestants may result in hypertension, palpitations, and CNS stimulation, and their use may be contraindicated in patients with disorders of these systems. Expectorants should be used with caution in the elderly or debilitated patient or in those individuals with asthma or respiratory insufficiency.

• Nursing Diagnoses

Nursing diagnoses appropriate to patients receiving any of the respiratory agents include the following:

- Impaired gas exchange related to the disorders affecting the respiratory system with increased congestion.
- Deficient knowledge related to the effective use of cold and other related products due to lack of information and patient teaching.
- Risk for injury related to the sedating side effects of many of these respiratory agents (antihistamines, antitussives).

• Planning

Goals for patients receiving any of these respiratory-related agents include the following:

- Patient states rationale for the use of antihistamines, expectorants, antitussives, or decongestants.
- Patient states the side effects of medication.
- Patient states the importance of compliance with therapy.

- Patient identifies symptoms to report to the physician.
- Patient states the importance of follow-up appointments with the physician.
- Patient states relief of symptoms with treatment.

Outcome Criteria

Outcome criteria pertaining to patients receiving any of these respiratory-related agents include the following:

- Patient will remain compliant with antihistamine therapy until symptoms are resolved or by physician's order.
- Patient will take medications exactly as prescribed, no more and no less, to avoid complications of therapy and to experience maximal effectiveness.
- Patient will report any of the following symptoms to the physician immediately: increase in cough, congestion, shortness of breath, chest pain fever (>100.0° F), or any change in sputum production or color (i.e., if not clear).
- Patient will report resolution of symptoms and an improved health status.

● Implementation

Patients on antihistamines should take the medications as prescribed, and most of these medications are best tolerated when taken with meals. Even though this slightly minimizes absorption of the agent, it has the benefit of also minimizing the gastrointestinal upset it can cause. If patients complain of dry mouth, they can suck on candy or chew gum, preferably sugarless, and perform frequent mouth care to ease the discomfort. OTC medications and other prescribed medications should not be taken with an antihistamine unless approved by the physician because of the serious drug interactions that can occur. Patients re-

ceiving any of the newer agents such as nonsedating agents should follow directions carefully on self-administration.

Patients taking expectorants should receive more fluids, unless contraindicated, to help loosen and liquify secretions and to help with expectoration. Any cough or symptoms of fever (>100.0° F) should be reported to the physician.

Patients taking chewable or lozenge antitussive agents should avoid fluid for 30 to 35 minutes after their use to prevent "washing away" their effect. Drowsiness or dizziness may occur with the use of antitussives, so patients should be cautioned against driving a car or operating heavy machinery until they feel back to normal.

Patient teaching tips for these agents are presented in the box below.

● Evaluation

A therapeutic response to respiratory agents would include a decrease in the symptoms of the condition for which they were prescribed. These include cough; congestion; nasal, salivary, and lacrimal gland hypersecretion; motion sickness; allergic rhinitis; Parkinson's disease; and vertigo. Some of the antihistamines, such as diphenhydramine, are also helpful as sleep aids, and a therapeutic response would of course be successful induction of sleep. Adverse effects for which to monitor in patients using an antitussive, antihistamine, expectorant, or decongestant include excessive dry mouth, drowsiness, oversedation, dizziness (lightheadedness), paradoxical excitement, nervousness, dysrhythmias, palpitations, gastrointestinal upset, urinary retention, fever, dyspnea, chest pain, palpitations, headache, or insomnia depending on the agent prescribed. (See Table 34-3 for other common side effects.)

---

patient teaching tips

Antihistamine Agents

➤ Patients should be encouraged to contact the physician or other health care provider should excessive sedation, confusion, or hypotension occur.

➤ Patients taking any of the cold products or antihistamines should be told to avoid driving or operating heavy machinery.

➤ Patients taking antihistamines should not consume alcohol or take other CNS depressants.

➤ Patients should be thoroughly educated regarding the purpose of the medication, the expected side effects, and the drugs with which they interact.

➤ Patients taking nonsedating antihistamines should always inform their physician or health care provider, including dentists, that they are taking this medication because some of these agents interact adversely with erythromycin, ketoconazole, and itraconazole.

➤ Patients should always check the package inserts that come with OTC cold preparations to find out the drugs they may interact with.

Decongestants and Expectorants

➤ Patients should report a fever (>100.0° F), cough, or other symptoms lasting longer than a week to their physician.

➤ Patients taking expectorants should force fluids, unless contraindicated, to increase expectoration of sputum.

➤ Some decongestants cause cardiac and CNS stimulating effects that may result in palpitations, insomnia, restlessness, and nervousness.

➤ Patients should avoid caffeine and caffeine-containing products.

Antitussive Agents

➤ Because nonopioid antitussives may cause sedation, drowsiness, or dizziness, patients taking them should be told to avoid driving or operating heavy machinery.

➤ Patients should report any of the following symptoms to their physician: a cough that lasts longer than a week, a persistent headache, fever, and/or a rash.

➤ Patients taking antitussive lozenges or chewable tablets should not drink liquids for 30 to 35 minutes afterwards.

POINTS TO REMEMBER

Antihistamines

- Two types of histamine blockers: histamine$_1$ (H$_1$) blockers and histamine$_2$ (H$_2$) blockers.
- H$_2$ blockers are used in the treatment of gastric acid disorders such as ulcers.
- H$_1$ blockers are the agents most people are referring to when they use the term *antihistamine*.
- H$_1$ blockers prevent the harmful effects of histamine.
- Used for treatment of seasonal allergic rhinitis, anaphylaxis, insect reactions, etc.

Nonsedating Antihistamines

- Drugs such as loratadine (Claritin) and fexofenadine (Allegra).
- Devoid of the sedating effect that most antihistamines have.
- Nonsedating because they avoid the central nervous system and work peripherally.

Decongestants

- Consist of adrenergics and corticosteroids.
- Most are adrenergic drugs such as pseudoephedrine and phenylephrine.
- The adrenergics work by stimulating engorged and swollen blood vessels in the sinuses to constrict, which decreases pressure and allows mucous membranes to drain.

Antitussives

- Antitussives are used to stop or reduce coughing.
- Are either opioid or nonopioid.
- Opioid agents: codeine and hydrocodone.

- Nonopioid antitussives: benzonatate and dextromethorphan.

Expectorants

- Drugs that aid in expectoration or removal of mucus.
- Work by reducing the viscosity of secretion by thinning them down.
- Guaifenesin and terpin hydrate are two common expectorants.
- Their mechanism of action is related to their ability to irritate the gastrointestinal tract and to cause reflex stimulation or irritation of the respiratory tract.

Nursing Considerations

- Contraindications to the use of antihistamines include hypersensitivity, acute asthma attack, and lower respiratory tract disease.
- Cautious use of antihistamines or use with very close monitoring of the patient is called for in patients with a history of increased intraocular pressure or those with cardiac or renal disease, hypertension, bronchial asthma, COPD, peptic ulcer disease, convulsive disorders, or BPH, as well as in pregnant women.
- Nonsedating antihistamines have important contraindications to their use, such as their concurrent use with erythromycin, ketoconazole, or itraconazole.
- If patients are taking any of the cold products or antihistamines, they should avoid driving and operating heavy machinery.
- Patients should avoid consuming alcohol and taking other CNS depressants while they are taking antihistamine agents.

REVIEW QUESTIONS

1. Which of the following side effects is most commonly associated with loratadine (Claritin)?
   a. Dysphagia
   b. Drowsiness
   c. Reflex tachycardia
   d. Increased sexual desire
2. Decongestants that have beta-stimulating effects may also result in which of these adverse effects?
   a. Fever
   b. Bradycardia
   c. Hypertension
   d. CNS depression
3. Antihistamines have all of the following therapeutic effects except:
   a. Prevention of the dilation of blood vessels.
   b. Prevention of increased vascular permeability.

   c. Stimulation of salivary, gastric, lacrimal, and bronchial secretions.
   d. Ability to bind to receptors and prevent histamine from being released from mast cells.
4. Antitussives are drugs that are used to:
   a. Stop or reduce coughing.
   b. Constrict the blood vessels and relieve congestion.
   c. Block the effects of histamine on the blood vessels.
   d. Aid in the removal of mucus by reducing the viscosity of secretions.
5. The binding of H$_1$ blockers (antihistamines) to the unoccupied receptors prevents which of the following consequences of histamine stimulation?
   a. Vasodilation
   b. Leukopenic infiltration
   c. Decreased capillary permeability
   d. Diminished gastrointestinal secretions

CRITICAL THINKING Activities

1. Why should antihistamines be used with caution in asthmatic patients?

2. Discuss the problem of rebound congestion when overusing nasal spray decongestants. Does this phe-nomenon also occur with oral decongestants? Explain your answer.

3. What additional nursing interventions would be helpful for an older patient, without major medical problems, who is taking guaifenesin?

For Answers see www.harcourthealth.com/MERLIN/Lilley/.

bibliography

Albanese J, Nutz P: *Mosby's 2001 nursing drug reference and review cards*, St Louis, 2001, Mosby.

American Hospital Formulary Service: *AHFS drug information*, Bethesda, Md, 2000, American Society of Health-System Pharmacists.

Anderson PO, Knoben JE, Troutman WG: *Handbook of clinical drug data 1999-2000*, ed 9, New York, 1999, McGraw-Hill.

Johns Hopkins Hospital, Department of Pediatrics et al: *The Harriet Lane handbook*, ed 15, St Louis, 2000, Mosby.

Keen JH: *Critical care and emergency drug reference*, ed 3, St Louis, 1996, Mosby.

Mosby's GenRx: a comprehensive reference for generic and brand drugs, ed 10, St Louis, 2000, Mosby.

Skidmore-Roth L: *Mosby's 2001 nursing drug reference*, St Louis, 2001, Mosby.

Turkoski BB: *Drug information handbook for nursing 1999-2000: including assessment, administration, monitoring guidelines, and patient education*, ed 2, Cleveland, 1999, Lexi-Comp.

Activity

Remember to check the **Online Worksheet** for additional learning opportunities: **www.harcourthealth.com/MERLIN/Lilley/**

Chapter 35

Bronchodilators and Other Respiratory Agents

objectives

www.harcourthealth.com/MERLIN/Lilley/

Look for this symbol for topics covered in the **Online Worksheet** Activity

When you reach the end of this chapter, you should be able to do the following:

1 Describe the anatomy and physiology of the respiratory system.

2 Describe how lower respiratory tract diseases affect the respiratory system.

3 Discuss the manifestations of lower respiratory tract diseases.

4 Identify the factors that precipitate lower respiratory tract diseases.

5 Identify the various respiratory agents, both the classes and specific agents, used in the treatment of lower respiratory tract disease.

6 Discuss the mechanisms of action, indications, contraindications, dosages, side effects and toxic effects, and therapeutic effects associated with the agents used to treat lower respiratory tract diseases.

7 Explain the nursing process as it relates to patients with lower respiratory tract diseases.

---

drug profiles

○━ **albuterol,** p. 549

beclomethasone dipropionate, p. 554

○━ **cromolyn,** p. 556

○━ **epinephrine, ephedrine, ethylnorepinephrine,** p. 549

metaproterenol, p. 550

montelukast, p. 552

nedocromil, p. 556

theophylline, p. 546

zafirlukast, p. 552

zileuton, p. 552

○━ Key drug.

---

glossary

Allergen (al′ ər jen) Any substance that evokes an allergic response. (p. 544)

Allergic asthma (as′ mə) Asthma caused by hypersensitivity to an allergen or allergens. (p. 544)

Alveoli (al′ ve o li) Microscopic sacs where oxygen is exchanged for carbon dioxide. (p. 543)

Antibody (an′ ti bod′ e) An immunoglobulin produced by lymphocytes in response to bacteria, viruses, or other antigenic substances. (p. 544)

Antigen (an′ ti jən) Substance, usually a protein, that causes the formation of an antibody and reacts specifically with that antibody. (p. 544)

Asthma attack Onset of wheezing together with difficulty breathing (p. 543)

Bronchial asthma (brong′ ke əl) Recurrent and reversible shortness of breath resulting from narrowing of the bronchi and bronchioles. (p. 543)

Chronic bronchitis (brong ki′ tis) Chronic inflammation of the bronchi. (p. 543)

Emphysema (em′ fə se′ mə) Condition of the lungs resulting from enlargement of the air spaces distal to the bronchioles. (p. 543)

Idiopathic asthma (id′ e ə pa′ thik) Asthmatic condition for which no specific cause has been truly identified; also called *intrinsic asthma.* (p. 544)

Immunoglobulin (im′ u no glob′ u lin) Any of five structurally and antigenically distinct antibodies present in the serum and external secretions of the body. (p. 544)

Intrinsic asthma (in trin′ sik) Asthmatic condition for which no specific cause has been truly identified; also called *idiopathic asthma.* (p. 544)

Ipratropium bromide (ip′ rə tro′ pe əm / bro′ mid) The only anticholinergic drug used in the treatment of asthma. (p. 550)

Lower respiratory tract Division of the respiratory system composed of organs located almost entirely within the chest. (p. 543)

Mast cell stabilizers Drugs such as cromolyn and nedocromil that stabilize the membranes of cells that normally release very harmful bronchoconstricting substances. (p. 554)

Nonseasonal allergic asthma Asthmatic condition caused by the continuous presence of an allergen such as animal dander, mold, or dust. (p. 544)

Seasonal asthma Asthmatic condition caused by the periodic appearance of a particular allergen. (p. 544)

Status asthmaticus (sta′ təs / az mat′ ik əs) A prolonged asthma attack. (p. 543)

Sympathomimetic bronchodilators Group of drugs commonly used during the acute phase of an asthmatic attack to quickly reduce airway constriction and restore normal airflow; also called *beta-agonists.* (p. 547)

Upper respiratory tract Division of the respiratory system composed of organs located outside the chest cavity (thorax). (p. 543)

Xanthine bronchodilators (zan' thēn / brong' ko di la' torz) Xanthine derivatives that produce bronchodilation by competitively inhibiting the enzyme phosphodiesterase and increasing the cyclic adenosine monophosphate level. (p. 544)

RESPIRATORY SYSTEM

The main function of the respiratory system is to deliver oxygen to the cells that make up the body and then to remove carbon dioxide from these cells. To perform this deceptively simple task requires a very intricate system of tissues, muscles, and organs called the *respiratory system*. It consists of two divisions, or tracts—the upper and lower respiratory tracts. The **upper respiratory tract** (URT) is composed of the structures that are located outside the chest cavity (thorax). These are the nose, nasopharynx, oropharynx, laryngopharynx, and larynx. The **lower respiratory tract** (LRT) is located almost entirely within the chest, and it is composed of the trachea, all segments of the bronchial tree, and the lungs. The URT and LRT have four main accessory structures that aid in their overall function. These are the oral cavity (mouth), the rib cage, the muscle of the rib cage (intercostal muscles), and the diaphragm. The URT and LRT together with the accessory structures make up the respiratory system, and they are in constant communication with each other as they perform the vital function of respiration and the exchange of oxygen for carbon dioxide.

The air we breathe is a mixture of many gases. The lungs are able to extract the oxygen needed for sustaining life by filtering, warming, and humidifying the air. The oxygen is actually delivered to the cells by the blood vessels that make up the circulatory system, and the transfer of oxygen from the respiratory system to the circulatory system takes place in the microscopic sacs at the end of the bronchial tree called **alveoli**. It is here that the respiratory system "hands off" the oxygen it has extracted from inhaled air to the hemoglobin in red blood cells (RBCs). It is also here that carbon dioxide that has been deposited in the blood by the cells and transported back to the lungs by the circulatory system is diffused back into the respiratory system and then exhaled into the air.

The respiratory system performs a vital function by exchanging oxygen and carbon dioxide. Other important functions of the respiratory system are speech, smell, and regulation of pH (acid-base balance).

DISEASES OF THE RESPIRATORY SYSTEM

Several diseases and disorders impair the function of the respiratory system. Those that affect the URT include colds, rhinitis, and hay fever, and they and the agents used to treat them are discussed in Chapter 34. The diseases that impair the function of the LRT include asthma, **emphysema,** and **chronic bronchitis.** The one feature these diseases have in common is that they all involve the obstruction of airflow through the airways. *Chronic obstructive pulmonary disease* (COPD) is the name applied collectively to emphysema and chronic bronchitis because the obstruction is relatively constant. Asthma that is persistent and present most of the time despite treatment is also considered a COPD. Cystic fibrosis and infant respiratory distress syndrome are other disorders that affect the LRT, but because the treatment for them places more emphasis on nonpharmacologic than on pharmacologic measures, they are not a focus of the discussion in this chapter.

ASTHMA

Bronchial asthma is defined as a recurrent and reversible shortness of breath and occurs when the airways of the lung (bronchi and bronchioles) become narrow as a result of bronchospasm, inflammation and edema of the bronchial mucosa, and the production of viscid mucus. The alveolar ducts and alveoli distal to the bronchioles remain open, but the obstruction to the airflow in the airways prevents carbon dioxide from getting out of the air spaces and oxygen from getting into them. Wheezing and difficulty breathing are the symptoms, and because of the sudden and dramatic onset of these episodes, they are commonly referred to as **asthma attacks.** Most of the attacks are short, and normal breathing is subsequently recovered. However, an asthma attack may be prolonged for days to weeks, a condition known as **status asthmaticus.** The onset of asthma occurs before 10 years of age in 50% of patients and before 40 years of age in about 30%.

There are three categories of asthma: allergic, idiopathic, and mixed allergic/idiopathic asthma, and approximately

pediatric considerations

Respiratory Agents

- Bronchodilators are often used in children but should be used with *extreme caution* in these young patients. Monitor for adverse effects such as tremors, restlessness, gastrointestinal tract upset, hallucinations, dizziness, palpitations, and tachycardia.
- Xanthine derivatives should be used very cautiously in children 6 months of age and older, with close monitoring of the blood levels and response to the medication. CNS-stimulating effects may be enhanced in children, and these effects should be watched for.
- Cromolyn sodium is generally used in children older than 6 years of age and should be used only if the child and parent or caregiver can accurately demonstrate the correct use of the nebulizer and how to care for the equipment. They should also show themselves capable of monitoring for the adverse effects.
- A daily journal or graph should be kept in which the date, time, drug used, signs and symptoms, and peak flowmeter results are documented. This will help chart the patient's compliance with the regimen and whether therapeutic effects are present or absent.

Steps Involved in an Attack of Allergic Asthma

- The offending allergen provokes the production of hypersensitive antibodies (most commonly IgE) that are specific to the allergen. This immunologic response initiates patient sensitivity.
- The IgE antibodies are homocytotrophic and collect on the surface of mast cells, thus sensitizing the patient to the allergen.
- Subsequent allergen contact provokes the antigen-antibody reaction on the surface of mast cells.
- Mast cell integrity is then violated, and these cells release chemical mediators. They also synthesize and then release other chemical mediators. These mediators include bradykinin, eosinophil chemotactic factor of anaphylaxis (ECF-A), histamine, prostaglandins, and slow-reacting substance of anaphylaxis (SRS-A).
- The released chemical mediators, especially histamine and SRS-A, trigger the bronchial constriction and the asthma attack.

Types of Asthma

Type of Asthma	Most Likely Cause
Allergic	Allergens (antigens) such as animal dander, dust, and molds.
Idiopathic	Poorly defined etiologic factors; may be induced by stress, respiratory infections, or strenuous exercise.
Mixed	Combination of allergens and some of the idiopathic factors.

Classifications of Agents Used to Treat Asthma

Long-Term Control	Quick-Relief
antileukotriene agents	short-acting inhaled beta$_2$-agonists
cromolyn	systemic corticosteroids
inhaled steroids	
ipratropium	
long-acting beta$_2$-agonists	
nedocromil	
theophylline	

2% of the general population is affected by one of the three types. Allergic asthma accounts for approximately 30% to 35% of the cases of asthma and idiopathic asthma for about 35% to 50%, with the mixed form accounting for the remaining cases.

Allergic asthma is caused by a hypersensitivity to an allergen or allergens in the environment. An **allergen** is any substance that elicits on allergic reaction. In patients with **seasonal asthma** the allergen is a substance such as pollen, which is present only periodically (seasonally). The offending allergens in patients with **nonseasonal asthma** are substances such as dust, mold, and animal danders, which are present in the environment throughout the year. Exposure to the offending allergen in a patient with either type of allergic asthma causes an immediate allergic reaction (asthma attack). This is mediated by hypersensitive antibodies already present in the patient's body that sense the allergen to be a foreign substance, or **antigen.** The **antibody** in asthma sufferers is usually **immunoglobulin** E (IgE), which is one of the five types of antibodies in the body (the others are IgG, IgA, IgM, and IgD). Upon exposure to the allergen, the patient's body responds by mounting an immediate and potent antigen-antibody reaction. This reaction occurs on the surface of cells such as mast cells that are rich in histamines and other mediators and stimulates the release of histamine, which, as shown in the previous chapter, triggers the allergic reaction (in this case the asthma attack). The sequence of events that occurs in a patient with allergic asthma is listed in Box 35-1.

The specific cause of **idiopathic,** or **intrinsic, asthma** is unknown. It is not mediated by IgE, and there is no family history of allergies in affected patients. There are, however, certain factors that have been noted to precipitate asthma attacks in these patients, including respiratory infections, stress, cold weather, and strenuous work or exercise.

As the name implies, mixed allergic/idiopathic asthma results from a combination of allergic and idiopathic factors.

The three types of asthma and their most likely causes are summarized in Box 35-2.

The National Asthma Education and Prevention Program established guidelines for the diagnosis and management of asthma. The current set of guidelines is the second published on the management of asthma and was published in early 1997. With respect to pharmacologic therapy, drugs are no longer classified as either antiinflammatory or bronchodilators but as long-term control and quick-relief medications. The specific agents in each classifications are listed in Box 35-3.

The guidelines advocate the use of a stepwise approach to the treatment of asthma. The particular steps and recommended drug classifications for each step are listed in Table 35-1.

CHRONIC BRONCHITIS

Chronic bronchitis is a continuous inflammation of the bronchi, although it is the inflammation of the bronchioles that occurs in the disorder that is responsible for the obstruction to airflow. The disease can arise as the result of repeated attacks of acute bronchitis or in the context of chronic generalized diseases. It is usually precipitated by prolonged exposure to bronchial irritants. One of the most common is cigarette smoke. Some patients acquire the disease by other predisposing factors such as viral or bacterial pulmonary infections during childhood. Others may have mild impairment of the ability to inactivate proteolytic enzymes. Unknown genetic characteristics may be responsible as well. Patho-

Table 35-1 Stepwise Therapy for the Management of Asthma

Step	Drug Classification
Step 1: Mild intermittent	Short-acting inhaled beta$_2$ agonists as needed
Step 2: Mild persistent	Cromolyn or nedocromil (particularly in children) and low-dose inhaled corticosteroids (preferred) plus short-acting inhaled beta$_2$-agonists as needed
	Theophylline and antileukotriene agents considered second line
Step 3: Moderate persistent	Medium-dose inhaled corticosteroids
	Long-acting bronchodilator (salmeterol preferred)
	Short-acting inhaled beta$_2$-agonists as needed
Step 4: Severe persistent	High-dose inhaled corticosteroids
	Long-acting bronchodilators
	Systemic corticosteroids
	Short-acting inhaled beta$_2$-agonists as needed

Box 35-4 Mechanisms of Antiasthmatic Drugs

Antiasthmatic	Mechanism in Asthma Relief
Anticholinergics	Block cholinergic receptors, thus preventing the binding of cholinergic substances that cause constriction.
Antileukotriene agents	Modify or inhibit the activity of leukotrienes, which decreases arachidonic acid-induced inflammation and allergen-induced bronchoconstriction.
Beta-agonists and xanthine derivatives	Raise intracellular levels of cAMP, which in turn produces smooth muscle relaxation and dilates the constricted bronchi and bronchioles.
Corticosteroids	Prevent the inflammation commonly provoked by the substances released from mast cells.
Mast cell stabilizers (cromolyn and nedocromil)	Stabilize the cell membranes that the antigen-antibody reactions take place on (the mast cell), thereby preventing the release of substances such as histamine that cause constriction.

logically it involves the excessive secretion of mucus and certain structural changes in the bronchi.

EMPHYSEMA

Emphysema is the condition that results when the air spaces enlarge as a result of the destruction of the alveolar walls. This appears to stem from the effect of proteolytic enzymes released from leukocytes in the setting of alveolar inflammation. Because the alveolar walls are then partially destroyed, the area where oxygen and carbon dioxide exchange takes place is reduced, thus impairing effective respiration. As with chronic bronchitis, smoking appears to be the primary irritant responsible for precipitating the underlying inflammation that leads to the development of emphysema.

TREATMENT OF DISEASES OF THE LOWER RESPIRATORY TRACT

In the past, the treatment of asthma and other COPDs involved drugs that cause airways to dilate. Now there is a greater understanding of the pathophysiology of asthma. The emphasis of research has shifted from the bronchoconstriction component of the disease to the inflammatory one. The role played by inflammatory cells and their mediators has become just as important as the bronchoconstriction component of the disease. *Leukotrienes* (LTs) are believed to be the key mediators in the inflammatory response that occurs in asthma.

These various classes of bronchodilating agents include beta-agonists, selected anticholinergics, xanthine derivatives, corticosteroids, and indirect-acting antiasthmatic drugs such as cromolyn sodium and nedocromil sodium. The antileukotriene agents include the 5-lipoxygenase inhibitor zileuton (Zyflo), a 5-lipoxygenase-activating protein inhibitor montelukast (Singulair), and three leukotriene receptor antagonists (LRAs), zafirlukast (Acculate), pranlukast, and verlukast. A synopsis of how these agents work is provided in Box 35-4.

BRONCHODILATORS

Bronchodilator drugs are an important part of the pharmacotherapy for the COPDs such as asthma, chronic bronchitis, and emphysema. As their name implies, they are able to dilate the bronchi and bronchioles that are narrowed as a result of the disease process. There are two classes of such agents: **xanthine derivatives** and beta-agonists.

XANTHINE DERIVATIVES

The natural xanthines consist of the plant alkaloids caffeine, theobromine, and theophylline, but only theophylline and its chemical derivatives are used as bronchodilators. Caffeine is primarily utilized as a central nervous system (CNS) stimulant (analeptic) and theobromine as a diuretic. Besides theophylline, the other xanthine bronchodilators used clinically for the treatment of bronchoconstriction are aminophylline, dyphylline, and oxtriphylline.

Because of their relatively slow onset of action, xanthines are used more for the prevention of asthmatic symptoms than for the relief of acute asthma attacks. They are also used as bronchodilators in the symptomatic treatment of the asthma and reversible bronchospasm that may occur in patients with chronic bronchitis or emphysema. Aminophylline is used in patients with status asthmaticus who have not responded to fast-acting beta-agonists such as epinephrine.

Mechanism of Action

The mechanisms of action of theophylline and its chemical derivatives are similar. They all cause bronchodilation by increasing the levels of the energy-producing substance cyclic adenosine monophosphate (cAMP). They do this by competitively inhibiting phosphodiesterase (PDE), the enzyme responsible for breaking down cAMP. cAMP plays an integral role in the maintenance of an open airway in patients with COPD because its intracellular concentration determines smooth muscle relaxation and the inhibition of the IgE-induced release of the chemical mediators (histamine, SRS-A, and others) that are responsible for causing an allergic reaction. An accumulation of cAMP therefore causes the constricted airways of the lung to dilate.

Drug Effects

Xanthines have many beneficial drug effects other than those beneficial to the respiratory system. In the respiratory system they mostly cause the airways of the lungs to dilate by relaxing the smooth muscle of the respiratory tract, thereby relieving bronchospasm and allowing greater airflow into and out of the lungs. Xanthines also stimulate all levels of the CNS, but to a lesser degree than caffeine, another xanthine. This stimulation of the CNS has the beneficial effect of directly stimulating the medullary respiratory center. In large doses, theophylline and its derivatives may stimulate the cardiovascular system, resulting in both an increased force of contraction (positive inotrope) and an increased heart rate (positive chronotrope). The increased force of contraction increases cardiac output and hence blood flow to the kidneys. This in combination with the xanthines' ability to dilate blood vessels in and around the kidney, thus increasing the glomerular filtration rate, results in a diuretic effect.

Therapeutic Uses

Theophylline and the other xanthine derivatives are used to dilate the airways in patients with asthma, chronic bronchitis, or emphysema. They may be used in mild to moderate cases of acute asthma and as an adjunct agent in the management of a COPD. The combination of their ability to increase the force of contraction in a failing heart and to dilate the airways also makes them useful as adjunctive therapy for the relief of the pulmonary edema and paroxysmal nocturnal dyspnea in patients with left-sided heart failure. Aminophylline may be used to increase urine out-

put. Their ability to increase cardiac output and thus the blood flow to the kidneys causes diuresis.

Side Effects and Adverse Effects

The common side effects of the xanthine derivatives include nausea, vomiting, and anorexia. In addition, gastroesophageal reflux has been observed to occur during sleep in patients taking them. Cardiac side effects include sinus tachycardia, extrasystole, palpitations, and ventricular dysrhythmias. Transient increased urination and hyperglycemia are other side effects.

Interactions

The use of xanthine derivatives with any of the following agents causes the serum level of the xanthine derivative to be increased: allopurinol, cimetidine, erythromycin, flu vaccine, and oral contraceptives. Their use with sympathomimetics can produce additive cardiac and CNS stimulation.

Dosages

For the recommended dosages of theophylline, the only xanthine derivative profiled, see the dosages table on p. 547.

---

geriatric considerations

Xanthine Derivatives

- Xanthine derivatives should be given cautiously with careful monitoring in elderly patients because of the increased sensitivity to these drugs (due to decreased drug metabolism).
- Assess elderly patients for signs of toxicity: restlessness, insomnia, irritability, tremors, nausea, and vomiting. Be careful to assess restlessness and its cause since it could also be due to hypoxia.
- Inform elderly patients to not chew or crush sustained released forms and to be careful of drug interactions.
- Encourage elderly patients never to omit doses or double-up on doses. They should contact their physician or health care provider should one of these occur.
- Lower doses in the elderly should be used initially with close monitoring for adverse effects.

---

drug profiles

theophylline

Theophylline (Bronkodyl, Elixophyllin, Slo-bid, Theo-Dur, Theo-24, Quibron-T, Uniphyl) is one of the most commonly used of all the xanthine derivatives as well as of all the bronchodilators. It is used most frequently in the treatment of chronic respiratory disorders but may also be used for the relief of mild to moderate acute asthmatic attacks. Theophylline is

drug	pharmacologic class	dosage range	purpose
theophylline (Bronkodyl, Elixophyllin, Slo-bid, Theo-Dur, Theo-24, Quibron-T, Uniphyl)	Xanthine derivative	*Pediatric* PO: usual dose is 2.5 mg/kg q6h *Adult* PO: usual dose is ≥160 mg q6h*	Asthma

*Adjust dosage to achieve optimal patient response.

available in oral, rectal, parenteral, and topical dosage forms, but only with a prescription. These various preparations are listed in Box 35-5.

Theophylline is classified as a pregnancy category C agent and is contraindicated in patients with a known hypersensitivity to xanthines and in patients with tachyarrhythmias. Its beneficial effects can be maximized by maintaining levels in the blood within a certain target range. If these levels become too high, then many unwanted adverse effects can occur. If the levels become too low, then the patient receives little therapeutic benefit. Although the optimal level may vary from patient to patient, the common therapeutic range for theophylline in the blood is 10 to 20 μg/ml. The commonly recommended dosages are given in the dosages table above.

PHARMACOKINETICS

HALF-LIFE	ONSET	PEAK	DURATION
7-9 hr	Unknown	1-2 hr	Varies with dosage form

BETA-AGONISTS

Beta-agonists are a large group of drugs that are commonly used during the acute phase of an asthmatic attack to quickly reduce airway constriction and restore airflow to normal. They are agonists or stimulators of the sympathetic nervous system (SNS) receptors (beta- and alpha-adrenergic receptors discussed in depth in Part III). These drugs imitate the effects of norepinephrine on these receptors. For this reason, they are also called **sympathomimetic bronchodilators.** For a beta-agonist to dilate the airways of the lungs, it must stimulate the beta$_2$-adrenergic receptors located throughout the lungs. When these receptors are stimulated, the constricted airways dilate; conversely, a nonspecific beta-blocker would cause the airways to constrict.

Beta-agonists, or sympathomimetic bronchodilators, are categorized according to the specific receptors they stimulate, and there are as a result three types of these bronchodilators:

1. Nonselective adrenergic drugs, which stimulate the alpha, beta$_1$ (cardiac), and beta$_2$ (respiratory) receptors. Example: epinephrine.

Available Theophylline Preparations
box 35-5

Dosage Form	Strengths
ORAL	
Capsules	100 and 200 mg
Extended-release capsules	50, 60, 65, 75, 100, 125, 130, 200, 250, 260, and 300 mg
Solution	27 and 50 mg/5 ml
Tablets	100, 125, 200, 250, and 300 mg
Extended-release tablets	100, 200, 250, 300, 400, 450, and 500 mg
PARENTERAL	
Injection	25, 2500, and 5000 mg/ml
Injection for infusion	0.4, 0.8, 1.6, 2, 3.2, and 4 mg/ml
RECTAL	
Suppository	250 and 500 mg

2. Nonselective beta-adrenergic drugs, which stimulate both beta$_1$ and beta$_2$ receptors. Example: isoproterenol (Isuprel).
3. Selective beta$_2$ drugs, which only stimulate the beta$_2$ receptors. Example: albuterol.

These drugs can also be categorized according to the route of administration as oral, parenteral, or inhalational agents. The various beta-agonist bronchodilators are listed in Table 35-2.

Mechanism of Action

The mechanism of action of beta-agonist bronchodilators begins at the specific receptor stimulated and ends with the dilation of the airways, but many reactions must take place at the cellular level for this bronchodilation to occur. When a beta$_2$-adrenergic receptor is stimulated by a beta-agonist, adenylate cyclase, an enzyme needed to make cAMP, is activated. The bronchioles, which are the small airways that precede the alveoli, are surrounded by smooth muscle. If this smooth muscle contracts, the airways are narrowed and the amount of oxygen and carbon dioxide exchanged is reduced. The increased levels of cAMP made available by adenylate cyclase cause these smooth muscles to relax, which results in bronchial dilation and increased airflow into and out of the lungs.

Drugs such as epinephrine stimulate alpha-adrenergic receptors causing vasoconstriction. This vasoconstriction reduces the amount of edema or swelling in the mucous

Table 35-2 Beta-Agonist Bronchodilators

Drug	Type	Brand Names	Route of Administration
albuterol	Beta$_2$	Proventil, Ventolin	PO, inhalation
bitolterol	Beta$_2$	Tornalate	Inhalation
ephedrine	Alpha-beta	None	PO, IM, IV, SC
epinephrine	Alpha-beta	Adrenalin, Primatene, Bronkaid, Bronitin, Medihaler-Epi	SC, IM, inhalation
ethylnorepinephrine	Alpha-beta	Bronkephrine	IM, SC
isoetharine	Beta$_1$-beta$_2$	Arm-a-Med Isoetharine	Inhalation
isoproterenol	Beta$_1$-beta$_2$	Isuprel, Medihaler-Iso	IV, sublingual, inhalation
levalbuterol	Beta$_2$	Xopenex	Inhalation
metaproterenol	Beta$_1$-beta$_2$	Alupent, Metaprel	PO, inhalation
pirbuterol	Beta$_2$	Maxair	Inhalation
salmeterol	Beta$_2$	Serevent, Serevent Diskus	Inhalation
terbutaline	Beta$_2$	Brethine, Bricanyl	PO, SC, inhalation

membranes and limits the quantity of secretions normally secreted from these membranes. However, beta$_1$-receptor stimulation also results in unwanted cardiac side effects such as an increased heart rate and force of contraction.

Drug Effects

Drugs such as albuterol that predominantly stimulate the beta$_2$-receptors have more specific drug effects. By predominantly stimulating the beta$_2$-adrenergic receptors of the bronchial, uterine, and vascular smooth muscles, they cause bronchodilation as one of the desirable effects. They may also have a dilating effect on the peripheral vasculature, resulting in a decrease in diastolic blood pressure. By stimulating intracellular shifts of potassium from the blood, the beta$_2$ stimulants are thought to stimulate Na$^+$/K$^+$-ATPase, resulting in a temporary decrease in potassium levels. This makes them useful in treating patients with hyperkalemia.

Some beta-agonist bronchodilators partially stimulate beta$_1$ receptors, causing CNS and cardiovascular system stimulation. This may result in nervousness, tremors, a fast heart rate, and elevated blood pressure.

Other beta-agonist bronchodilators may stimulate both alpha and beta receptors. This stimulation of the alpha-adrenergic receptors mostly results in constriction, specifically of the arterioles in the skin, mucous membranes, and organs. However, it also results in the dilation of the arterioles in skeletal muscles. Some of this vasoconstriction can be beneficial in the management of certain respiratory disorders. For instance, a beta-agonist such as ephedrine that also stimulates alpha receptors may also cause dilated blood vessels in the nasal mucosa to constrict, thereby producing nasal decongestion.

Therapeutic Uses

The therapeutic effects of the beta-agonists are mostly confined to the treatment of various pulmonary disorders. However, because they have effects outside the respiratory system, they may also be used for the management of other disorders. The primary respiratory system-related therapeutic effects are the relief of bronchospasm, bronchial asthma, bronchitis, and other pulmonary diseases.

Because some of these agents have the ability to stimulate both beta$_1$- and alpha-adrenergic receptors, they may be used to treat hypotension and shock. The agents that stimulate alpha receptors cause the blood vessels surrounding the nasal passages to constrict. This results in the relief of nasal congestion and stuffiness.

Because terbutaline has the added ability to stimulate the beta$_1$-receptors on the uterus that control uterine contractions, it is used to produce uterine relaxation and prevent premature labor in pregnant women.

By stimulating a shift of potassium out of the blood and into cells, beta$_2$-agonists can be used to treat the hyperkalemia that often afflicts patients with renal failure.

Side Effects and Adverse Effects

Alpha-beta agonists produce the greatest array of undesirable effects. These include insomnia, restlessness, anorexia, cardiac stimulation, tremor, and vascular headache. The side effects of the nonselective beta-agonists are limited to beta-adrenergic effects, including cardiac stimulation, tremor, anginal pain, and vascular headache. Beta$_2$ agents can cause hypotension, vascular headaches, and tremor.

Interactions

The use of beta-agonist bronchodilators with a nonselective beta-adrenergic blocker antagonizes the bronchodilation. Their use with a monoamine oxidase (MAO) inhibitor and other sympathomimetics is best avoided. Diabetics may require an adjustment in the dose of their hypoglycemic agent, especially patients taking epinephrine, because of the increased blood glucose levels that can occur.

Dosages

For recommended dosages of selected beta-agonists, see the dosages table on p. 549.

DOSAGES Selected Beta-Agonists

agent	pharmacologic class	dosage range	purpose
albuterol (Proventil, Proventil Repetabs, Ventolin, Volmax)	Beta$_2$-agonist	*Pediatric* PO: 2-6 y/o: 0.1 mg/kg tid PO: 6-12 y/o: 2 mg 3-4 time/day *Adult/Pediatric* ≥12 y/o PO: 2-4 mg 3-4 times/day Solution: 2.5 mg/inhalation 3-4 times/day *Adult/Pediatric* ≥4 y/o Aerosol: 2 inhalations q4-6h Powder: 200 μg/inhalation q4-6h	Asthma
epinephrine (Adrenalin, Primatene, Bronkaid, Bronitin, Medihaler-Epi)	Alpha-beta agonist	*Pediatric* SC: 10 μg/kg/dose *Adult* SC/IM: 100 μg-1 mg IV: 25-400 μg Aerosol: 0.2 mg per inhalation prn	Asthma
metaproterenol (Alupent, Metaprel)	Beta$_1$-beta$_2$-agonist	*Pediatric* PO: 6-9 y/o: 10 mg 3-4 times/day PO: >9 y/o: 20 mg 3-4 times/day *Adult* PO: 20 mg 3-4 times/day *Adult/Pediatric* Aerosol: 2-3 inhalations (0.65 mg/dose) q3-4h	Asthma

Activity

drug profiles

Although beta-agonists are commonly used in the treatment of an acute asthmatic attack, they are also used to treat hypotension and shock, as decongestants, to relax uterine muscles and prevent premature labor, and to lower serum potassium levels in patients with hyperkalemia.

albuterol

Albuterol (Proventil, Proventil Repetabs, Ventolin, Volmax) is one of six beta$_2$-specific bronchodilating beta-agonists. The others are bitolterol, levalbuterol, pirbuterol, salmeterol, and terbutaline. Salmeterol (Serevent and Serevent Diskus) is being used more often. This is because its unique 12-hour duration of action makes it an attractive alternative. Albuterol is most commonly used in the treatment of acute attacks of bronchial asthma but may also be used in the prevention of such attacks. If used too frequently, dose-related adverse effects may be seen as a result of albuterol losing its beta$_2$-specific actions at larger doses. The consequence of this is that the beta$_1$ receptors are stimulated, causing nausea, increased anxiety, palpitations, tremors, and an increased heart rate.

Albuterol is classified as a pregnancy category C agent and is contraindicated in patients with a hypersensitivity to sympathomimetics, tachyarrhythmias, and severe cardiac disease. It is only available with a prescription as an oral solution and tablet as well as an inhalational agent. Orally, albuterol

is available as a 2-mg/5 ml syrup, 2- and 4-mg tablets, 4- and 8-mg extended-release tablets, and 4-mg extended-release film-coated tablets. As an inhalational agent it is available in a metered-dose inhaler that releases 90-μg per spray, a 200-μg powder contained in a capsule, and a 0.083% solution and a 0.5% concentrated solution for nebulization. Commonly recommended dosages are given in the dosages table above.

PHARMACOKINETICS

HALF-LIFE	ONSET	PEAK	DURATION
2.7-5 hr	PO: 5-15 min	2-3 hr	4-8 hr

epinephrine, ephedrine, ethylnorepinephrine

Epinephrine (Primatene, Bronkaid, Adrenalin, Medihaler-Epi, Bronitin), ephedrine, and ethylnorepinephrine are all beta-agonist bronchodilators that work by stimulating both beta and alpha receptors. Their beta$_2$-stimulating properties result in the bronchodilation, but by also stimulating alpha receptors, they have effects elsewhere in the body. One of these is arteriolar constriction in the mucous membranes, making them useful as nasal decongestants.

Epinephrine is available with or without a prescription. Ephedrine and ethylnorepinephrine are available only with a prescription. All three agents are available in several dosage forms and are used to treat a variety of respiratory and nonrespiratory

Update on Metered Dose Inhalers

The global treaties curbing ozone-depleting chlorofluoro-carbons (CFCs) have spurred the U.S. Food and Drug Administration (FDA) to propose a strategy for phasing out asthma inhalers that use CFCs as propellants. The FDA published an *Advance Notice of Proposed Rulemaking* (ANPR) on March 5, 1997. The purpose of the ANPR is to allow interested persons or groups to comment on a proposed phase-out strategy before the development of a proposed rule. The ANPR is only the first stage of a multistage process that would result in CFC-containing inhalers to be phased out. Pharmaceutical companies have proactively responded by developing new alternative propellants like hydrofluoroalkane (HFA) and dry powder inhalers, which are activated by inspiration and thus do not require a propellant. Examples of both are listed below:

HFAs or
hydrofluorocarbons (HFCs)
- Proventil HFA

Dry powder
- Pulmicort Turbuhaler
- Flovent Rotodisk
- Serevent Diskus

disorders. However, those preparations used for the treatment of respiratory disorders are generally given by the inhalational or oral route. Epinephrine given for this purpose comes in a metered-dose inhaler that releases 160, 200, 220, and 250 μg per spray for oral inhalation and as a 1%, 1.83%, and 2.25% solution for nebulization. Commonly recommended dosages of epinephrine are given in the dosages table on p. 549.

PHARMACOKINETICS

HALF-LIFE	ONSET	DURATION	PEAK
Unknown	Inhalation: 1-5 hr	1-3 hr	Rapid

metaproterenol

Metaproterenol (Alupent, Metaprel) is a synthetic sympathomimetic bronchodilator that stimulates both beta$_1$ and beta$_2$ receptors. Other similar bronchodilating beta-agonists are isoetharine and isoproterenol. These agents produce dilation of the airways, but they also have beta$_1$-stimulating properties that are more pronounced at higher doses. CNS and cardiovascular system stimulation is the result.

Metaproterenol is only available with a prescription and is classified as a pregnancy category C agent. The contraindications to its use are the same as those for the beta$_2$-agonists such as albuterol, but it is also contraindicated in patients with narrow-

angle glaucoma. Metaproterenol is available in both oral and inhalational preparations. Orally it is available as a 10-mg/5 ml solution and as 10- and 25-mg tablets. As an inhalational agent it is available in a metered-dose inhaler that releases 0.65 mg per spray. It also is available in a 0.4%, 0.6%, and 5% solution for nebulization. Common dosage recommendations are given in the dosages table on p. 549.

PHARMACOKINETICS

HALF-LIFE	ONSET	PEAK	DURATION
Unknown	PO: 15-30 min	1 hr	4 hr

OTHER RESPIRATORY AGENTS

Bronchodilators are just one type of agent used to treat asthma, chronic bronchitis, and emphysema. There are also other agents that are effective in suppressing various underlying causes of some of these respiratory illnesses. These drugs include antileukotriene agents (zileuton, montelukast, and zafirlukast), anticholinergics (ipratropium and azelastine), corticosteroids (beclomethasone, budesonide, dexamethasone, flunisolide, fluticasone, and triamcinolone), and mast cell stabilizers (cromolyn and nedocromil).

ANTICHOLINERGICS

Currently the only anticholinergic agent that is used in the treatment of asthma is **ipratropium bromide** (Atrovent). Many patients benefit from both a beta$_2$-agonist and an anticholinergic agent. Now there is a combination product containing both albuterol and ipratropium called Combivent. Chemically it is very similar to atropine and produces local bronchodilation after inhalation. On the surface of the bronchial tree are receptors for acetylcholine (ACh), the neurotransmitter for the parasympathetic nervous system (PSNS). When the PSNS releases ACh from its nerve endings, the neurotransmitter binds to the ACh receptors on the surface of the bronchial tree, resulting in bronchial constriction and narrowing of the airways. An anticholinergic drug such as ipratropium bromide prevents this bronchoconstriction, thereby causing the airways to dilate. Because its actions are slow and prolonged, ipratropium is used for prevention of the bronchospasm associated with the COPDs (chronic bronchitis or emphysema), not for the management of acute exacerbations.

The most commonly reported adverse effects of ipratropium therapy are dry mouth or throat, gastrointestinal distress, headache, coughing, and anxiety. It is classified as a pregnancy category B agent and is contraindicated in patients with a known hypersensitivity to it, atropine, or any of its derivatives. There are currently no drugs that are known to interact with ipratropium. The usual adolescent or adult dose is one or two inhalations three to four times daily.

PHARMACOKINETICS

HALF-LIFE	ONSET	PEAK	DURATION
1.6 hr	5-15 min	1-2 hr	4-5 hr

ANTILEUKOTRIENE AGENTS

A new class of asthma medications called *leukotriene receptor antagonists* (LTRAs), or antileukotriene agents, are available. Antileukotriene agents are the first new class of asthma medications to be introduced in the United States in more than 20 years. They offer asthma sufferers a new treatment option to help control their disease.

Before the use of antileukotriene agents, most asthma treatments focused on relaxing the squeeze of bronchial muscles with bronchodilators. In the last decade, researchers have begun to understand how asthma symptoms are caused by the immune system at the cellular level. A chain reaction starts when a trigger, such as cat hair or dust, starts a series of chemical reactions in the body. This produces several substances, including a family of molecules known as *leukotrienes*. In people with asthma, these leukotrienes cause inflammation, bronchoconstriction, and mucus production. This in turn leads to coughing, wheezing, and shortness of breath. Antileukotriene agents prevent leukotrienes from attaching to receptors located on circulating cells as well as cells within the lungs. This blocks inflammation in the lungs, which leads to asthma symptoms. The research responsible for the discovery of these agents is the direct result of a Nobel Prize-winning discovery made by scientist Ben Samuelsson in 1979.

Currently there are three subcategories of antileukotriene agents. Each subcategory attempts to modify or inhibit the activity of LTs and thus relieve the inflammatory process underlying asthma. These subcategories are classified by the mechanisms by which these agents block the inflammatory process in asthma. The first class of antileukotriene agents is inhibitors of the enzyme 5-lipoxygenase (zileuton and ICI-D2138). Zileuton (Zyflo) is the only one currently available. The second subcategory of antileukotriene agents is inhibitors of 5-lipoxygenase-activating protein (MK-886, MK-591, and BAY-X-1005). Presently none of these agents are available. The third subcategory of antileukotriene agents is the LTD4-receptor blockers (montelukast, pobilukast, pranlukast, tomelukast, verlukast, and zafirlukast). Montelukast (Singulair) and zafirlukast (Accolate) are the only members of this category currently available.

Mechanism of Action

The currently available antileukotriene agents are montelukast, zafirlukast, and zileuton. They all work by blocking the action of LTs. Zileuton differs from zafirlukast and montelukast in that it actually inhibits the enzyme 5-lipoxygenase. This enzyme is responsible for the metabolism of arachidonic acid. By blocking it, all production of leukotrienes is halted. For this reason, zileuton may be

referred to as an *antiinflammatory drug*. Montelukast and zafirkast, on the other hand, allow 5-lipoxygenase to break down arachidonic acid to various LTs. The antiinflammatory action of montelukast and zafirlukast come from their ability to block specific LTs called *crystinyl leukotrienes*. These LTs are thought to be important mediators of asthma. Montelukast and zafirlukast block receptors on cells and lung tissue for these special LTs. This in turn prevents inflammation in the lung.

Drug Effects

The drug effects of antileukotriene agents are primarily limited to the lungs. Through their blocking action on LTs, they prevent smooth muscle contraction of the bronchial airways. Blocking LTs decreases mucus secretion and prevents vascular permeability as well. Other LTs that these agents block prevent the mobilization and migration of such cells as neutrophils and leukocytes into the lungs. Decreased neutrophil and leukocyte infiltration to the lungs prevents inflammation in the lungs.

Therapeutic Uses

The antileukotriene agents montelukast, zarfirlukast, and zileuton are used for the prophylaxis and chronic treatment of asthma in adults and children 12 years of age and older. These agents are not meant for management of acute asthmatic attacks. Improvement with their use is typically seen in about 1 week.

Side Effects and Adverse Effects

The side effects of antileukotriene agents differ depending upon the specific agent. Zileuton and zafirlukast both can cause headaches. The most frequently reported adverse effects with zileuton after headaches are dyspepsia, nausea, dizziness, and insomnia. With zafirlukast after headaches, nausea and diarrhea are the most common side effects. Zafirlukast as well as zileuton may also lead to liver dysfunction.

Toxicity and Management of Overdose

Limited information regarding human experience of acute overdose with zileuton or zafirlukast exists. It is recommended in an event of toxicity or overdose of these agents that symptomatic and supportive measures be taken.

Interactions

Montelukast has fewer drug interactions than zafirlukast or zileuton. It does not interact with theophylline, warfarin, digoxin, prednisone, or either the estrogen or progestin components of combination oral contraceptives. Phenobarbital decreases montelukast concentrations. For information on the drugs that interact with zafirlukast and zileuton, see Table 35-3.

Dosages

For recommended dosages of montelukast, zafirlukast, and zileuton, see the dosages table on p. 553.

35-3 Drug Interactions: Antileukotriene Agents

Drug	Mechanism	Result
ZAFIRLUKAST (ACCOLATE)		
aspirin	Decreased clearance	Increased zafirlukast levels
erythromycin	Decreased bioavailability	Decreased zafirlukast levels
tolbutamide, phenytoin, and carbamazepine	Inhibited metabolism	Increased tolbutamide, phenytoin, and carbamazepine levels
warfarin	Decreased clearance	Increased warfarin levels
ZILEUTON (ZYFLO)		
propranolol	Decreased clearance	Increased propranolol levels
theophylline	Decreased clearance	Increased theophylline levels
warfarin	Decreased clearance	Increased warfarin levels

drug profiles

Antileukotriene agents are a new class of asthma medications. Currently there are three antileukotriene agents available—zileuton, zafirlukast, and montelukast. They are primarily used for oral prophylaxis and chronic treatment of asthma. These agents are not recommended for treatment of acute asthma attacks.

montelukast

Montelukast (Singulair) is the third agent to become available in the antileukotriene class. It belongs to the same subcategory of antileukotriene agents as zafirlukast. Montelukast and zafirlukast work by blocking LTD4-receptors to augment the inflammatory response. Montelukast offers the advantage of being FDA approved for use in children 2 years of age and older. It also has fewer side effects and drug interactions than zafirlukast.

Montelukast is contraindicated in patients with a known hypersensitivity to it and is considered a pregnancy category B agent. It is available in 4- and 5-mg chewable tablet and a 10-mg film-coated tablet. Common dosages are listed in the dosages table on p. 553.

PHARMACOKINETICS

HALF-LIFE	ONSET	PEAK	DURATION
2.7-5.5 hr	30 min	3-4 hr 2.5 hr*	24 hr

*2.5 hours for the chewable tablet.

zafirlukast

Zafirlukast (Accolate) is an LTD4-receptor blocker. It is currently the only member of the LTD4-receptor blockers available. It is currently indicated for the prophylaxis and chronic treatment of asthma in adults and children 12 years of age and older. Zafirlukast is classified as a pregnancy category B agent and is contraindicated in pa-tients with a hypersensitivity to zafirlukast. It is available as a 20-mg oral tablet. Common dosages are listed in the dosages table on p. 553.

PHARMACOKINETICS

HALF-LIFE	ONSET	PEAK	DURATION
10 hr	30 min	3-4 hr	12 hr

zileuton

Zileuton (Zyflo) is a 5-lipoxygenase inhibitor. It prevents inflammation in the lungs caused by the production of LTs. It is currently indicated for the prophylaxis and chronic treatment of asthma in adults and children 12 years of age and older. Zileuton is classified as a pregnancy category C agent and is contraindicated in patients with active liver disease or transaminase elevations greater than or equal to three times the upper limit of normal and in patients with a hypersensitivity to zileuton. It is available as a 600-mg oral filmtab. Common dosages are listed in the dosages table on p. 553.

PHARMACOKINETICS

HALF-LIFE	ONSET	PEAK	DURATION
2.5 hr	30 min	2-4 hr	5-8 hr

CORTICOSTEROIDS

Corticosteroids are used in the treatment of chronic asthma for their antiinflammatory effects, which lead to decreased airway obstruction. As with ipratroprium bromide, corticosteroids also do not relieve the symptoms of acute asthmatic attacks but are used prophylactically to prevent an attack. Corticosteroids do this by preventing the release of substances that produce inflammation in the lungs. They can be given by inhalation or by the oral route in severe cases of asthma when the agent cannot get to the airways because of the obstruction. Corticosteroids administered by inhalation have an advantage over orally administered corticosteroids in that their action is

DOSAGES Selected Antileukotriene Agents

agent	pharmacologic class	dosage range	purpose
montelukast (Singulair)	Antileukotriene agent	*Adult* 10 mg daily *Pediatric (6-14 y/o)* 5 mg daily	Asthma
zarfirlukast (Accolate)	Antileukotriene agent	*Adult/Pediatric >12 y/o* 20 mg twice daily	Asthma
zileuton (Zyflo)	Antileukotriene agent	*Adult/Pediatric >12 y/o* 600 mg four times a day *Pediatric 2-5 y/o* 4 mg daily	Asthma

Table 35-4 White Blood Cells (Leukocytes)

Specific WBC*	Role in Inflammation	Corticosteroid Effect
GRANULOCYTES		
Neutrophils (65%)	Contain powerful lysosomes, which are digestive-like enzymes; release chemicals that destroy invading organisms and also attack other WBCs.	Stabilize their cell membranes so that inflammation-causing substances not released.
Eosinophils (2%-5%)	Main function is in allergic reactions and in protecting against parasitic infections; ingest inflammatory chemicals and antigen-antibody complexes.	Little if any effect.
Basophils (0.5%-1%)	Contain histamine, an inflammation-causing substance, and heparin, an anticoagulant.	Stabilize their cell membranes so that histamine not released.
AGRANULOCYTES		
Lymphocytes (25%)	Two types: T-lymphocytes and B-lymphocytes; T-cells attack infecting or cancerous cells; B-cells produce antibodies against specific antigens.	Decrease activity of the lymphocytes.
Monocytes (3%-5%)	Produce macrophages, which can migrate out of the bloodstream to such places as mucous membranes, where they are capable of engulfing large bacteria or virus-infected cells.	Inhibited macrophage accumulation in already inflamed areas, thus preventing more inflammation.

*Percentage in parentheses is the proportion of the total number of leukocytes they constitute.

limited to the topical site of action—the lungs. This prevents systemic effects. The chemical structures of the corticosteroids given by inhalation have also been slightly altered so as to limit their systemic absorption from the respiratory tract. The corticosteroids administered by inhalation include the following:

- beclomethasone dipropionate (Beclovent, Vanceril)
- budesonide (Pulmicort Turbuhaler, Rhinocort)
- dexamethasone sodium phosphate (Decadron Phosphate Respihaler)
- flunisolide (AeroBid, AeroBid-M)
- fluticasone (Flonase, Cutivate, Flovent, Flovent Rotadisk)
- triamcinolone acetonide (Azmacort)

Mechanism of Action

Although the exact mechanism of action of the corticosteroids has not been determined, it is conjectured that they have the dual effect of both reducing inflammation and enhancing the activity of beta-agonists.

The corticosteroids previously mentioned produce their antiinflammatory effects through a complex sequence of actions. They essentially work by stabilizing the membranes of cells that normally release very harmful bronchoconstricting substances (e.g., histamine, SRS-A). These cells are called *leukocytes*, which is another name for white blood cells (WBCs), and there are five different types of these cells, each with their own specific characteristics. The five types of WBCs, their role in the inflammatory process, and the way in which corticosteroids inhibit their normal action, combat inflammation, and produce bronchodilation are summarized in Table 35-4.

Corticosteroids have also been shown to restore or increase the responsiveness of bronchial smooth muscle to beta-adrenergic receptor stimulation, which results in more pronounced stimulation of the beta$_2$ receptors by beta agonist drugs such as albuterol. It may take several weeks of continuous therapy before the full effects of the corticosteroids are realized.

Drug Effects

Most of the drug effects of inhaled corticosteroids are limited to their topical site of action in the lungs. Because of the chemical structure of corticosteroids, there is very little systemic absorption of the agents when they are administered by inhalation. When there is significant systemic absorption (absorption into the bloodstream), corticosteroids can affect any of the organ systems in the body. Some of these systemic-drug effects include adrenocortical insufficiency, increased susceptibility to infection, fluid and electrolyte disturbances, endocrine effects, dermatologic effects, and nervous system effects.

Therapeutic Uses

Inhaled corticosteroids are used for the treatment of bronchospastic disorders that are not adequately controlled by the conventional bronchodilators (beta-agonists and xanthine derivatives). They are not considered first-line agents for the management of acute asthmatic attacks or status asthmaticus.

Side Effects and Adverse Effects

The main undesirable local effects of corticosteroids on the respiratory system include pharyngeal irritation, coughing, dry mouth, and oral fungal infections. Systemic effects are rare (see Chapter 31) because of the low doses used for inhalation therapy.

Interactions

Inhaled corticosteroids are capable of causing few or no drug interactions. This is due in part to the fact that they are administered by inhalation and so are delivered directly to the site of action in the respiratory tract. Because they are not administered systemically, they neither have systemic effects nor can they interact with other systemically administered drugs.

Dosages

For recommended dosages of selected corticosteroids, see the dosages table on p. 554.

---

drug profiles

Inhaled corticosteroids are contraindicated in patients who are hypersensitive to glucocorticoids, patients whose sputum is positive for *Candida* organisms, and patients with systemic fungal infection. All four of the inhaled corticosteroids are classified as pregnancy category C agents and are only available with a prescription.

beclomethasone dipropionate

Beclomethasone dipropionate (Beclovent, Vanceril) is administered by oral inhalation for the treatment of bronchial asthma in patients who require corticosteroids on a long-term basis for the control of symptoms. It may also be used in patients who have not responded to an adequate trial of conventional therapy, usually xanthines and beta-agonists, as well as in the management of patients with a COPD (such as chronic bronchitis) whose disease has been stabilized with oral corticosteroid therapy. Beclomethasone in an oral solution or rectal suspension has also been used in the management of inflammatory diseases of the gastrointestinal tract.

When beclomethasone is administered by oral inhalation, the primary sites of action are the bronchi and the bronchioles. Very little drug reaches the bloodstream through the respiratory tract because it is metabolically inactivated. Compared with dexamethasone, another inhaled corticosteroid, beclomethasone appears to have greater topical anti-inflammatory activity and to cause fewer adverse systemic effects. The use of an inhaled corticosteroid frequently allows for a reduction in the daily dose of the systemic corticosteroids often taken by patients with chronic bronchial asthma. Beclomethasone is available as an aerosolized mist in a metered-dose inhaler that releases 42 mg per spray and is given by oral inhalation. The available inhaled corticosteroids, their various dosage strengths, and their pharmacokinetic properties are summarized below. Commonly recommended dosages are listed in the dosages table on p. 554. Pregnancy category C.

PHARMACOKINETICS

beclomethasone dipropionate (42 μg/metered spray)

HALF-LIFE	ONSET	PEAK	DURATION
3-15 hr	10 min	15-30 min	4-6 hr

dexamethasone sodium phosphate (100 μg/metered spray)

HALF-LIFE	ONSET	PEAK	DURATION
36-54 hr*	10-15 min	15-30 min	4-6 hr

flunisolide (250 μg/metered spray)

HALF-LIFE	ONSET	PEAK	DURATION
1-2 hr	Unknown	Unknown	1 hr

triamcinolone (100 μg/metered spray)

HALF-LIFE	ONSET	PEAK	DURATION
Unknown	Unknown	Unknown	Unknown

*Biologic half-life.

MAST CELL STABILIZERS

The **mast cell stabilizers** cromolyn and nedocromil are additional agents that can be used in the treatment of COPDs such as asthma, chronic bronchitis, and emphysema. Cromolyn and nedocromil are considered indirect acting because they prevent the release of the various chemical substances that cause bronchospasm. They have

agent	pharmacologic class	dosage range	purpose
beclomethasone (Beclovent, Vanceril)	Synthetic glucocorticoid	*Adult/Pediatric 6-12 y/o* 1-2 inhalations 3-4 times/day. Each inhalation delivers 42 μg; do not exceed 840 μg/day	Asthma
dexamethasone sodium phosphate (Decadron Phosphate Respihaler)	Synthetic glucocorticoid	*Pediatric* 2 inhalations 3-4 times/day. Each inhalation delivers 100 μg; do not exceed 800 μg/day (8 inhalations/day) *Adult* 3 inhalations 3-4 times/day; do not exceed 1200 μg (1.2 mg)/day (12 inhalations/day)	Asthma
flunisolide (AeroBid, AeroBid-M)	Synthetic glucocorticoid	*Pediatric 6-12 y/o* 1-2 inhalations 3-4 times/day. Each inhalation delivers 250 μg; do not exceed 1200 μm (1.2 mg)/day. *Adult* 2 inhalations bid in AM and PM; do not exceed 2000 μg (2 mg)/day	Asthma
triamcinolone acetonide (Azmacort)	Synthetic glucocorticoid	*Pediatric 6-12 y/o* 1-2 inhalations 3-4 times/day. Each inhalation delivers 100 μg; do not exceed 1200 μg (1.2 mg)/day (12 inhalations/day) *Adult* 2 inhalations 3-4 times/day; do not exceed 1600 μg (1.6 mg)/day (16 inhalations/day)	Asthma

no direct bronchodilator activity and are used only prophylactically. They are most effective in preventing the asthma caused by extrinsic factors such as allergens and that caused by exercise.

Mechanism of Action

Both cromolyn and nedocromil are called mast cell stabilizers. The cells that these two indirect-acting antiasthmatic agents affect are those listed and described in Table 35-4. As previously mentioned, these cells release the vasoconstrictive substances (e.g., histamine, SRS-A) responsible for causing the bronchoconstrictive disorders such as asthma. Cromolyn and nedocromil exert their actions by stabilizing the membranes of the cells that normally release these harmful substances in response to an antigen-antibody reaction, thereby suppressing the release of the substances.

Nedocromil and cromolyn share many of the pharmacologic effects previously mentioned, but nedocromil is more potent on a weight basis in inhibiting mediator release and the bronchoconstriction induced by various stimuli. Nedocromil also appears to affect a broader range of inflammatory cells (eosinophils, neutrophils, macrophages, mast cells, monocytes, and platelets). Nedocromil can inhibit both an acute bronchoconstrictor response and a delayed inflammatory response to inhaled antigens and irritants. It may also suppress cough by inhibiting the neuronal reflexes in airways.

Drug Effects

The drug effects of cromolyn and nedocromil are primarily limited to the lungs, and when administered into the lungs, very little if any of the agents gets into the blood-stream to cause systemic effects. The primary drug effect of these agents is on the surface of cell membranes. Because these drugs can be administered by several different routes (orally, inhaled, and in the eye), they can get to all areas of the body where there are inflammatory cells (e.g., mast cells, monocytes, macrophages, neutrophils) and stabilize their cell membranes, thereby preventing the release of the harmful cellular contents that cause inflammation. Cromolyn and nedocromil may also inhibit the movement of some cells into and out of the tissues and blood vessels.

Therapeutic Uses

Cromolyn and nedocromil are used as adjuncts to the overall management of patients with COPDs and are used solely for prophylaxis. These agents are of no value in the treatment of acute asthma attacks, and the types of asthma they are used in the prevention of are exercise-induced bronchospasm and the bronchospasm induced by exposure to other known precipitating factors such as cold dry air, environmental pollutants, and allergens. They may also be used for the symptomatic prevention and treatment of seasonal or perennial allergic rhinitis. Cromolyn may be used to relieve allergic eye disorders that result in itching, tearing, redness, and discharge. It has also been administered orally for the prophylactic management of food allergies and for the treatment of chronic inflammatory bowel disease (Crohn's disease and ulcerative colitis).

Side Effects and Adverse Effects

Most of the side effects of cromolyn and nedocromil affect the respiratory system and include coughing, sore throat,

Cromolyn Sodium

- Children over 6 years of age who are being treated with cromolyn sodium administered by nasal spray should be given only ONE spray in each nostril tid or qid BUT only as ordered by the physician and NOT to exceed six doses in 24 hours. This type of spray is usually indicated for the treatment of allergic rhinitis.
- Children over 5 years of age being treated for bronchospasms with inhaled forms are usually given 20 mg administered over less than 1 hour qid and nebulizer forms at a dose of 20 mg qid.
- Children over 5 years of age being treated for bronchial asthma are generally prescribed inhaler and nebulizer forms at a dose of 20 mg qid. Children are usually very willing and eager to learn about ways to prevent respiratory difficulty, so it is important to show them AND family members or caregivers the proper inhalation technique, which is as follows: Have the child exhale, then put the inhaler in place. Have the child inhale deeply with the head tipped back so as to maximize the opening of the air passages. The cromolyn sodium should be administered during this deep inhalation. After inhaling, instruct the child to remove the inhaler while holding the breath, than exhale when needed and repeat as instructed.

- Children should be told that capsules ARE NOT TO BE chewed.
- Be sure that the child, parents, or caregivers know that cromolyn sodium is preventive, not curative, treatment, that it must be used year-round, and that it may take up to 4 weeks before therapeutic effects are noticed.
- Nebulizer forms of cromolyn sodium should be administered as instructed and according to the physician's orders. All equipment, including the filter and tubing, should be kept clean. Filters need to be purchased or ordered well ahead of time, and manufacturer's guidelines suggest changing them when they begin to appear gray. The tubing and mouthpieces should be cleaned according to the manufacturer's guidelines using water and white vinegar. Specific instructions should be followed regarding the use of the machine and proper breathing during use of the machine. Once the nebulizer session is over, the mouthpiece should be rinsed. The child should also rinse out his or her mouth with water.
- Use of a spacer device may be indicated

rhinitis, and bronchospasm. Other effects include taste changes, dizziness, and headache.

Dosages

For the recommended dosages of cromolyn and nedocromil, see the dosages table on p. 557.

⊙⊷ cromolyn

Cromolyn (Nasalcrom, Opticrom, Gastrocrom, Intal) is a mast cell stabilizer that is indicated for the prevention of bronchospasms and bronchial asthmatic attacks. It differs from nedocromil in that it seems to stabilize fewer cell types and is less potent. It was the first of the two agents in this drug class to be discovered and used in clinical practice.

Cromolyn is classified as a pregnancy category B drug and is contraindicated in patients who are hypersensitive to the drug or to its lactose filler. Patients who have lactose intolerance may exhibit symptoms of this disorder after the inhalation of cromolyn. Cromolyn is also contraindicated in patients who have status asthmaticus. It is available for both oral and ophthalmic administration as well as for nasal and oral inhalation, and because of its many dosage formulations, it may be used for the treatment of many disorders. The nasal solution delivers 5.2 mg per metered spray; the ophthalmic

solution is a 4% solution; the oral capsules contain 100 mg of the agent; the aerosolized oral inhalation agent delivers 800 μg per metered spray; the powder for oral inhalation is available as a 20-mg capsule; and the solution for nebulization has a concentration of 20 mg/2 ml. Recommended dosages are given in the dosages table on p. 557.

PHARMACOKINETICS

HALF-LIFE	ONSET	PEAK	DURATION
1.5 hr	Unknown	15 min	4-6 hr

nedocromil

Nedocromil (Tilade) is indicated for the prevention of bronchospasms and bronchial asthma attacks. The contraindications to its use are the same as those for cromolyn, and it is also a pregnancy category B agent. Its particular mechanism of action has already been described. Nedocromil is only available as an aerosolized inhaler, and it is only used as an adjunct agent in the overall management of patients with mild to moderate bronchial asthma. It too is only available with a prescription. It comes in a metered-dose inhaler that delivers 1.75 mg per spray for oral inhalation. Recommended dosages are given in the dosages table on p. 557.

PHARMACOKINETICS

HALF-LIFE	ONSET	PEAK	DURATION
1.5 hr	Unknown	15 min	4-6 hr

DOSAGES Cromolyn and Nedocromil

agent	pharmacologic class	dosage range	purpose
cromolyn (Nasalcrom, Intal)	Mast cell stabilizer	*Adult/Pediatric* ≥5 y/o Inhalation: 5-20 mg 4 times/day Nasal solution: 1 spray 3-4 times/day	Asthma Rhinitis
nedocromil (Tilade)	Mast cell stabilizer	*Adult/Pediatric* ≥12 y/o Up to 14 mg/day; spray delivers 1.75 mg per dose administered 3-4 times/day	Asthma

nursing process

● Assessment

The net drug effect of all the bronchodilators (beta-agonists, anticholinergics, xanthine derivatives, indirect-acting antiasthmatics, and corticosteroids) is relaxation of the bronchial smooth muscle. There are many indications for their use, but there are also many cautions and contraindications to their use, and these can be identified by means of thorough patient assessments. Beta-agonists are contraindicated in patients with a history of cardiac disease, dysrhythymias, angina, coronary artery disease, hypertension, diabetes, or convulsive disorders. Anticholinergic agents used as bronchodilators are contraindicated in patients with a history of benign prostatic hypertrophy or glaucoma. Xanthine derivatives such as aminophylline are contraindicated in patients with a history of peptic ulcer disease or gastrointestinal disorders, and cautious use (with close monitoring) is recommended in patients with a history of a cardiac disorder. Corticosteroids are contraindicated in patients with an allergy to the drug, a psychosis, fungal infections, AIDS, tuberculosis, or idiopathic thrombocytopenia, as well as in children under 2 years of age. Cautious use is recommended in patients with diabetes mellitus, glaucoma, osteoporosis, ulcer disease, renal disease, congestive heart failure, edema, myasthenia gravis, seizure disorders, or esophagitis. A baseline assessment of blood pressure and pulse with respirations (rate and depth) and auscultation of lung sounds is needed before and during treatment with any respiratory agents.

With antileukotrienes (e.g., zileuton, montelukast, and zafirlukast), it is important to assess that the drug has been indicated for chronic treatment because these agents are for chronic, not acute, asthma. Zileuton is contraindicated in patients who are allergic to the agent, who have hepatic dysfunction, or whose transaminase is elevated to equal or greater than three times the normal level. Zafirlukast is contraindicated in patients who are allergic to the medication. There are also significant drug interactions. Levels of zileuton are increased if given with theophylline, warfarin, or propranolol. With zafirlukast, warfarin, tolbutamide, phenytoin, and carbamazepine will all have increased levels. Also, levels of zafirlukast will decrease if given with erythromycin, and

levels will decrease if given with aspirin. Phenobarbital decreases the effects of montelukast.

Cromolyn sodium is used in the management of asthma but only as preventive treatment, not for the control of acute exacerbations of asthma, so acute exacerbations represent a contraindication to its use. Use of the inhaled form of this medication in children younger than 5 years of age and in pregnant or lactating women is not recommended.

In a thorough assessment of patients receiving any of the respiratory agents, the patient's skin color, temperature, and respirations (rate [<12 or >24 breaths/min] and rhythm) must be checked. The nurse should also find out whether the patient is having problems with cough, dyspnea, orthopnea, or respiratory distress; whether he or she has or is suffering from sternal retraction, cyanosis, restlessness, activity intolerance, or cardiac symptoms such as palpitations, hypertension, and tachycardia; and whether he or she is using accessory muscles to breathe. In addition, the nurse should ask patients whether they have a history of allergies and, if so, what they are, whether there is sputum production, and what other medications and nondrug therapies they are using. Patients should also be asked to give a thorough history of their respiratory disease. The type of asthma attack also needs to be assessed and documented because of different indications for specific drugs.

Activity

● Nursing Diagnoses

Nursing diagnoses related to the administration of respiratory agents include the following:
- Impaired gas exchange related to pathophysiologic changes caused by respiratory disease.
- Fatigue related to disease process.
- Risk for injury related to side effects of medication.
- Anxiety related to disease process and medication therapy.
- Disturbed thought processes related to the CNS stimulation caused by bronchodilators.
- Deficient knowledge related to unfamiliar treatment regimen.
- Deficient knowledge related to the disease process and its precipitating factors.
- Deficient knowledge related to the medication therapy.
- Noncompliance related to side effects of medication therapy.

NURSING CARE PLAN Asthma

Jennifer, a 13-year-old girl recently diagnosed with asthma, is to begin nebulizer treatments with cromolyn sodium (Intal) twice daily. She has been compliant with her steroid inhaler and with other treatments for her asthma, so the physician believes that the cromolyn sodium will help prevent some of her asthmatic attacks. Since you are the nurse on the "well" side of the pediatrician's office today, you are to tell her about the medication and its use.

assessment	***Nursing Diagnosis***	Deficient knowledge related to new diagnoses of asthma treatment and minimal patient teaching
	Subjective Data	"I'm not sure that this stuff will work"
	Objective Data	• 13-year-old newly diagnosed asthmatic
		• Success with other therapies
		• Listens and comprehends well
		• Anxious to get asthma under control
		• RR20
		• Lungs clear
		• BP 100/60
		• P66
planning and outcome criteria	***Goals***	Patient will remain compliant to new asthma treatment within 1 mo
	Outcome Criteria	Patient will state the following about cromolyn sodium therapy:
		• Use
		• Side effects
		• Cautions
		• Side effects to report to the physician
implementation		Patient teaching should include the following:
		• Remember that this medication is to be given by nebulizer for the time being and should be taken directly as ordered (bid).
		• Make sure that after you do the treatment that you rinse your mouth out and gargle to prevent irritation to the mouth and throat.
		• You may not see its full effects for about 4 wk because it takes that long to get to its therapeutic effects of preventing some of your episodes of asthma.
		• Keep machinery clean as recommended by the manufacturer.
		• Once we have discussed the medication, you will be all set to go because you already know how to use the machine.
		• Side effects associated with cromolyn sodium include the following: throat irritation, cough, nasal stuffiness, burning of the eyes, headache, nausea, dry mouth, bitter taste.
		• Call the physician if you should experience severe headaches, dizziness, rash, or joint pain or swelling.
evaluation		Patient will display a therapeutic response to cromolyn sodium as evidenced by:
		• Decrease in asthmatic symptoms
		• Decreased chest tightness and wheezing
		• Decrease in cough
		• Fewer asthma attacks
		• Regular respiratory rate and rhythm
		• No dyspnea
		Patient will experience minimal side effects and report those indicated.

● Planning

Goals for the patient receiving respiratory agents include the following:
- Patient experiences minimal exacerbations of the disease while compliant with medication regimen.
- Patient states the importance of rest to recovery.
- Patient will be free of self-injury related to either the disease or the side effects of the medication.
- Patient remains compliant with the medication regimen as well as with nonpharmacologic therapies.
- Patient follows up with health care providers as instructed by the physician.

Use of Inhalers

PATIENTS RECEIVING ALBUTEROL

- Instructions to patients regarding the proper use of inhaled forms of medications are crucial to ensuring their safe and effective use. Make sure to have patients demonstrate the technique for using an inhaler or nebulizer.
- Instructions regarding the care of the inhaler or nebulizer and associated equipment are also important. This involves washing the inhaler in warm water every day and drying it before reuse or washing the tubing, and other apparatus used with the nebulizer. White vinegar can be used to rinse out the tubing of nebulizers. Always encourage patients to follow the manufacturer's recommendations regarding the use, storage, and cleaning of any equipment used.
- Patients must be warned not to let the inhaler spray get in their eyes.
- A therapeutic response to albuterol inhaler use includes absence of wheezing and dyspnea.
- Patients must be instructed and reminded during home health care visits to use these medications EXACTLY as prescribed and that an overdose may precipitate palpitations, angina, hypertension, or dysrhythmias.

HOW TO CHECK VOLUME OF MEDICATION LEFT IN A CANISTER (E.G., FOR INHALERS)

Metered-dose inhalers (MDIs) may be checked for residual amounts of medication so that the patient can always be aware of when the medication may be "running out" in the inhaler. First, obtain a container that is wider and longer than the inhaler and fill up to ¾ full with water. Drop the inhaler into the container with the water, but be sure that the mouthpiece is not on the inhaler. If the canister drops to the bottom and lies on its side, then it is full. If it drops to the bottom and lands with the bottom of the inhaler pointing upward then it is about ¾ full. If it lands in the water with about ¼ of the bottom of the inhaler exposed, then it is approxi-

mately ½ full. If the canister "leans" to its side and is submerged except for about ¼ of the bottom of the inhaler, then it is most likely about ¼ full. Once the canister "floats" on *top* of the water line, then it is most likely near empty. Remember to educate patients about this little "check" on their inhalers, but also remind them that it is merely an estimate!*

GENERAL NURSING CONSIDERATIONS FOR PATIENTS USING A METERED-DOSE INHALER

The nurse must inform all patients who are using MDIs about their function and how they help people with asthma in delivering medication directly to the lungs. Also explain that the pressurized canister contains measured doses of the medication. Instructions should include the following:

- Shake the container thoroughly and then breathe out fully through your mouth.
- Place the inhaler mouthpiece in front of your mouth with your lips around it or follow directions for using a spacer device, if provided.
- Activate the inhaler by pressing down on it at the *same* time that you are breathing in *slowly* and very deeply.
- Counting to 5 seconds while breathing in may help, and then hold for an additional *10 seconds before* breathing out or exhaling.
- If a second dose is recommended, repeat the directions above *but* wait 1 to 2 minutes between doses.

To avoid any type of mouth infection from the use of an inhaled corticosteroid, the nurse must inform patients to gargle with water and cleanse out the mouth after the treatment. Often the directions may vary on the inhaler's instructions, so the nurse must demonstrate the technique to patients and clarify any other type of instructions with their health care provider. Children 6 years of age and older are usually able to be trained to use these MDIs properly, but adult supervision is recommended.

*From Blonshine S: Patient education: the key to asthma management, *Home Care Provider* 3(3):157, 1998.
Recommended Internet sites: www.mayohealth.org and www.drkoop.com.

- Patient does not increase or decrease dose or stop taking the medication without approval of physician.
- Patient's respiratory status will improve because of compliance with medication therapy.

Outcome Criteria

Outcome criteria for patients receiving respiratory agents include the following:

- Patient will briefly describe the disease process, its signs and symptoms, and the precipitating factors.
- Patient will state measures to take to prevent self-injury resulting from the disease or the side effects of the medication such as taking medications as prescribed.
- Patient will be well rested, with plans to rest during periods of exacerbation.
- Patient will state the expected side effects of the drug such as palpitations, nervousness, mood changes, and insomnia.

- Patient will contact the physician with increased dyspnea, shortness of breath, increased cough, or fever.
- Patient will state the importance of taking the medication as prescribed, the reasons for not increasing or decreasing the dose of the agent, and the importance of not stopping the drug therapy to prevent complications and exacerbations related to disease or side effects of medications.

● Implementation

Nursing interventions that apply to patients with a COPD in general include patient education and an emphasis on prevention, in addition to implementing the drug therapy prescribed. Measures to take to prevent, relieve, or decrease the manifestations of the disease should be emphasized to the patient at all times during treatment. Bronchodilators should be given exactly as prescribed and by the prescribed route (such as parenterally or orally or by intermittent positive pressure breathing). The proper method for administering the inhaled forms of these agents should be demonstrated to the patient, and the patient asked to demonstrate the method back. Patients should also be strongly discouraged from taking more than the prescribed dose of the beta-agonists because of the excessive cardiac demands (hypertension and tachycardia) this can cause. The nurse should always find out what other medications patients are taking to make sure that they are not taking one that can interact with any of the bronchodilators or antiasthmatic agents. Home health and community care implications applicable to patients receiving albuterol are given in the box on p. 559.

Xanthine derivatives should be given exactly as prescribed. If they are to be given parenterally, the nurse should always determine the correct diluent to be used, the amount of the agent, and the time to infuse medication. Timed-release preparations should not be crushed or chewed because of the irritating effects they can have on the gastric mucosa. Suppository forms of the drug should be refrigerated, and patients should be told to notify their physician if rectal burning, itching, or irritation occurs in association with their use.

Corticosteroid inhalers should be used as prescribed, with cautions against overuse. All equipment, inhalers or nebulizers, should be kept clean and filters cleaned and changed (nebulizers) and in good working condition. Rinsing of the mouth after using the inhaler or nebulizer is recommended. Pediatric patients may need a physician's order to have these medications "on hand" at school and during athletic events or physical education. Peak flow meter use is also encouraged to help patients better regulate their disease.

Cromolyn sodium, although not a bronchodilator, does have a role to play in the *preventive* treatment of asthma. It is available as a powder contained in a capsule that is administered by a specific type of inhaler, but in both adults and children, it is most popularly administered by a nebulizer. During a treatment session using either delivery system, the patient may experience bronchospasms. If they continue, the patient's condition should be stabilized, the session discontinued, and the physician notified. The proper technique for inhalant administration is presented in the Pediatric Considerations box pertaining to cromolyn sodium therapy (see p. 556). Other interventions such as forcing fluids and avoiding precipitating factors are also recommended.

The antileukotrienes zileuton, montelukast, and zafirlukast are given orally. Of most concern are the montelukast chewable tablets, which contain aspartame and approximately 0.842 mg of phenylamine per 5 mg tablet. Patient education for the leukotriene receptor antagonists should include how they are indicated for chronic, and *not* acute, asthma. These agents should be taken every night on a continuous schedule, even if symptoms improve.

Patient teaching tips for bronchodilators and other respiratory agents are presented on p. 561.

Miscellaneous pediatric considerations relevant to treatment with the various respiratory agents are discussed in the box on p. 543. See the Case Study below to test your understanding of the nursing process in a hospitalized patient with a COPD.

● Evaluation

The therapeutic effects of any of the agents used to treat or prevent respiratory diseases include decreased dyspnea; decreased wheezing, restlessness, and anxiety; improved respiratory patterns with return to normal rate and quality; improved activity tolerance and arterial blood gas levels; increased quality of life; and decreased severity and incidence of respiratory symptoms. The therapeutic effects of bronchodilating agents such as xanthine derivatives or beta-agonists, include decreased symptoms and increased ease of breathing. Peak flow meters are easy to use and help monitor *early on* the decrease in peak flow due to bronchospasms. The respiratory rate, rhythm, depth, and lung fields should also return to normal. Other antiasthmatic or bronchodilating agents should produce the same therapeutic effects.

Adverse effects for which to monitor in patients receiving beta-agonists include tachyarrhythmias, chest pain, restlessness, agitation, nervousness, and insomnia. Adverse effects of anticholinergic agents consist of dry mouth, constipation, headache, nervousness, nausea, and blurred vision. The xanthine derivatives may cause palpitations, tachydysrhythmias, chest pain, gas-

---

case study **Chronic Obstructive Pulmonary Disease**

Ms. Brown is a 73-year-old woman who worked in the local traffic tunnel for about 25 years and has had a COPD for 10 years caused by her exposure to environmental pollutants while on the job and her cigarette smoking. She is now retired and is frequently admitted to the hospital for treatment of her condition. She quit smoking about 8 years ago. She is now in the hospital for treatment of an acute exacerbation of her COPD and an upper respiratory tract infection. The physician has ordered the following: Aminophylline IV per respiratory therapy protocol, IV continuous infusion at a rate of 0.8 mg/kg/hr; chest physiotherapy bid and as needed; cephalothin antibiotic therapy, 1 g IV in 30 ml NS q8h; I&O; daily weights; VS with breath sounds q2h and as needed until stable; and albuterol inhaler, two puffs q4h per respiratory therapy protocol.

- *What nursing interventions would be most appropriate for helping this patient conserve energy while enhancing O_2 and CO_2 gas exchange?*
- *What is the rationale for using the continuous IV infusion of aminophylline?*
- *What are the reasons for prescribing the albuterol inhaler and the antibiotic? Be specific about the reasons for each.*
- *What would be the most important patient education guidelines to impart to Ms. Brown concerning the use of oral aminophylline and the albuterol inhaler at home?*

For Answers see www.harcourthealth.com/MERLIN/Lilley/.

trointestinal upset, agitation, headache, insomnia, and restlessness. Besides watching for the side effects of xanthine derivatives, the therapeutic blood levels should also be checked. That for theophylline is 10-20 $\mu g/ml$. Any level above this is considered toxic and may cause fatal reactions. The adverse effects of cromolyn sodium include hypotension, bitter taste, dizziness, nausea, vomiting, dysrhythmias, and restlessness.

Adverse effects for which to monitor in patients taking antileukotrienes include headache, dyspepsia, nausea, dizziness, and insomnia. Therapeutic effects include an improvement in the control of chronic asthma.

---

patient teaching tips

Bronchodilators and Other Respiratory Agents

➤ Patients should be encouraged to take measures that promote a generally good state of health and that can prevent, relieve, or decrease symptoms of COPD. Such measures include avoiding exposure to conditions (e.g., allergens, stress, smoking, air pollutants) that can precipitate bronchoconstriction or that can worsen the symptoms; adequate fluid intake (at least 3000 ml/day, unless contraindicated, to thin the mucus); compliance with medical treatment, including frequent follow-up visits; and proper diet. They should also be told to avoid excessive fatigue, heat, and extremes in temperature and to avoid consuming caffeine-containing beverages, because these may increase bronchoconstriction.

➤ Patients should use the medications as ordered to prevent bronchoconstriction if they anticipate respiratory difficulty, such as using their inhaler before aerobic exercise.

➤ Patients should be encouraged to get prompt treatment for flu or other illnesses, especially respiratory illnesses, and to get vaccinated against pneumonia or flu, unless this is contraindicated.

➤ Encourage patients to always check with their physician before taking any other medication, even OTC medications.

➤ Corticosteroid treatment in patients with a COPD requires much patience on the part of the nurse as well as much patient education. Patients should first be made aware that abruptly *discontinuing* these medications can lead to serious consequences and that the agent should be weaned gradually over 1 to 2 weeks, and only under a physician's care and recommendation. They should wear an ID bracelet or necklace and carry a card at all times that identifies them as a steroid user. Patients should be told about the cushingoid symptoms that can be caused by steroids. These include moon face, acne, an increase in fat pads, and edema. Should they occur, the physician should be notified immediately. It is important to explain to the patient that these symptoms are the result of excess steroid levels. The signs and symptoms of Addison's disease, or adrenal insufficiency, resulting from inadequate steroid levels include nausea, dyspnea, joint pain, weakness, and fatigue and should also be reported to the physician. Drugs that can interact with corticosteroids, and that therefore should be avoided, include aspirin, alcohol, barbiturates, phenytoin, theophylline, anticoagulants, anticonvulsants, antidiabetic agents, antituberculin agents, antifungal agents, digitalis, diuretics, NSAIDs, oral contraceptives, estrogens, and macrolide antibiotics. *Patients should re-*

port any weight gain of more than 5 pounds (2.25 kg) a week or the occurrence of chest pain to their physician.

➤ Patients taking a beta-agonist should be told to take the medication exactly as prescribed by the physician with no omissions or double dosing. Patients should notify the physician should they experience insomnia, jitteriness, restlessness, palpitations, chest pain, or any change in symptoms.

➤ Patients should be told to take xanthine derivatives exactly as ordered and to notify their physician should they experience palpitations, nausea, vomiting, weakness, dizziness, chest pain, or convulsions. The concurrent use of xanthine derivatives with other medications, such as cimetidine, allopurinol, oral contraceptives, and flu vaccine, or with large amounts of caffeine, which is also a xanthine, can have deleterious effects. Patients should never double up on doses if they have missed a dose; however, they may take it if only 1 hour has passed, but not if more than an hour has passed. They should never crush or chew sustained-released tablets, pills, or capsules.

➤ Patients should be told that cromolyn sodium needs to be administered consistently for the therapeutic effects to occur and that it may take up to 4 weeks before any of these effects are seen. Patients should be taught how to administer the medication and told to gargle and rinse the mouth with water afterward to minimize irritation to the throat and oral mucosa. Side effects include throat irritation, cough, headache, a bitter or bad taste in the mouth, and dry mouth.

➤ Inhaled forms of respiratory medications should be administered after patients have exhaled and then as they inhale deeply with the head tipped backward to produce maximal opening of the airway. Patients should then remove the inhaler and hold their breath for as much as 10 seconds, then exhale. Patients should be taught how to use a nebulizer and how to care for the equipment, such as changing the filters when they become discolored (grayish) and cleaning the tubing and mouthpieces frequently with soap, water, and white vinegar. Disposable tubing and mouthpieces are available.

➤ If a canister (MDI) is being used for the first time or if it has not been used in a while and has been stored in an upright position, teach the patient to activate the canister at least once into the air before administering the dose as ordered. This will help make sure that the first dose from an MDI will contain the adequate amount of medication.

POINTS TO REMEMBER

Beta-Agonists

- Work by stimulating adenylate cyclase, which produces more cAMP and in turn causes relaxation of the smooth muscle that surrounds the airways.
- Beta-agonists may stimulate alpha and beta receptors, $beta_1$ and $beta_2$ receptors, or just $beta_1$ receptors.
- $Beta_2$ stimulants are the most specific for the lungs and have the fewest side effects.

Xanthines

- Caffeine, theobromine, and theophylline are examples of xanthines.
- Work by inhibiting phosphodiesterase.
- Phosphodiesterase breaks down cAMP, which is needed to relax smooth muscles.
- Theophylline is the most common; aminophylline is the parenteral form of theophylline.

Anticholinergics

- Ipratropium bromide (Atrovent) is only agent used for treatment of COPD.
- Used for maintenance and not for relief of acute bronchospasms.
- Work by blocking the bronchoconstrictive effects of acetylcholine.

Corticosteroids

- Beclomethasone, dexamethasone, flunisolide, and triamcinolone are examples.

- Work by stabilizing the membranes of cells that release harmful bronchoconstricting substances.

Indirect-Acting Agents

- Cromolyn (Nasalcrom) and nedocromil (Tilade).
- Only used prophylactically; used for management of chronic pulmonary disease.
- Work by stabilizing the mast cell wall, thereby preventing potentially harmful vasoconstrictive substances from being released.

Nursing Considerations

- Contraindications to beta-agonist use include history of cardiac disease, dysrhythmias, angina, coronary artery disease, hypertension, and seizure disorders.
- Anticholinergics are contraindicated in patients with BPH or glaucoma.
- Xanthine derivatives are contraindicated in patients with a history of gastrointestinal tract disorders or peptic ulcer disease.
- Cromolyn sodium is used to prevent asthma, and treatment with this medication must be adhered to year-round.
- All respiratory agents should be given exactly as ordered and the diluent checked in terms of the proper amount and type of solution.
- Antileukotriene agents zileuton and zafirlukast are given orally.
- Side effects of antileukotriene include headache, dizziness, insomnia, and dyspepsia.

REVIEW QUESTIONS

1. The physician prescribes cromolyn sodium (Intal) to be given by nebulizer at home for an 11-year-old girl with a 9-year history of asthma. The rationale for the use of this medication is that it:
   a. Inhibits histamine release.
   b. Inhibits mast cell degeneration.
   c. Stimulates the release of bronchospastic agents.
   d. Stimulates the substances that release acetylcholine.
2. Albuterol is a _____ type of beta-agonist that works by increasing the level of _____, which causes _____ of smooth muscle in the respiratory tract.
   1. nonselective adrenergic
   2. nonselective beta-adrenergic
   3. selective $beta_2$
   4. vasoconstriction
   5. cAMP
   6. relaxation
   7. stimulation
   8. potassium

   a. 1, 4, and 7
   b. 2, 8, and 6
   c. 3, 5, and 6
   d. 3, 8, and 6
3. Side effects associated with xanthine derivatives include which of the following?
   a. CNS depression
   b. Sinus tachycardia
   c. Increased appetite
   d. Temporary urinary retention
4. Indirect-acting agents (cromolyn and nedocromil), corticosteroids (e.g., triamcilone), and anticholinergics (e.g., ipratroprium bromide) are all used _____ for patients with airway diseases such as asthma, chronic bronchitis, and emphysema.
   a. Acutely
   b. As needed
   c. Emergently
   d. Prophylactically

5. Your patient is changed from a xanthine to an antileu-kotriene (zileuton) for treatment of her asthma. Which of the following would be a contraindication to its use?

a. Polyuria
b. Liver dysfunction
c. Diabetes insipidus
d. Transient urinary frequency

For Answers see www.harcourthealth.com/MERLIN/Lilley/.

CRITICAL THINKING Activities

1. Your patient is taking a xanthine derivative and should not ingest xanthine-containing beverages. What are examples of these beverages, and why is it important to avoid consuming them while taking a xanthine derivative?

2. Discuss the necessary patient education for the use of leukotreine modifiers, especially the rationale for the important emphasis of taking the medication daily as ordered.

3. State the general guidelines for the use of a MDI, especially when it is new.

For Answers see www.harcourthealth.com/MERLIN/Lilley/.

bibliography

Albanese J, Nutz P: *Mosby's 2001 nursing drug reference and review cards,* St Louis, 2001, Mosby.

American Hospital Formulary Service: *AHFS drug information,* Bethesda, Md, 2000, American Society of Health-System Pharmacists.

Anderson PO, Knoben JE, Troutman WG: *Handbook of clinical drug data 1999-2000,* ed 9, New York, 1999, McGraw-Hill.

Holgate ST et al: Leukotriene antagonists and synthesis inhibitors: new directions in asthma therapy, *Allergy Clin Immunol* 98(1):1, 1996.

Johns Hopkins Hospital, Department of Pediatrics et al: *The Harriet Lane handbook,* ed 15, St Louis, 2000, Mosby.

Keen JH: *Critical care and emergency drug reference,* ed 3, St Louis, 1996, Mosby.

Larsen JS, Jackson SK: Antileukotriene therapy for asthma, *Am J Health Syst Pharmacol* 53(1):2821, 1996.

Medical Letter: Budesonide turbuhaler for asthma 40(1018):15, January 16, 1998.

Medical Letter: Montelukast for persistent asthma 40(1031):71, July 17, 1998.

Mosby's GenRx: a comprehensive reference for generic and brand drugs, ed 10, St Louis, 2000, Mosby.

Skidmore-Roth L: *Mosby's 2001 drug reference,* St Louis, 2001, Mosby.

Spector SL: Leukotriene inhibitors and antagonists in asthma, *Ann Allergy Asthma Immunol* 75(6 Part I):463, 1996.

Turkoski BB: *Drug information handbook for nursing 1999-2000: including assessment, administration, monitoring guidelines, and patient education,* ed 2, Cleveland, 1999, Lexi-Comp.

United States Pharmacopeial Convention: *USP DI: drug information for the health care professional, vol. 1,* ed 20, Englewood, Colo, 2000, Micromedex.

Remember to check the **Online Worksheet** for additional learning opportunities: **www.harcourthealth.com/MERLIN/Lilley/**

Activity

Part 7

Antiinfective and Antiinflammatory Agents: Study Skills Tips

- Nursing Process
- Assessment
- Nursing Diagnoses
- Evaluation

This study model focuses on the Nursing Process section in Chapter 36. Since there is a Nursing Process section at the end of each chapter, the discussion of the example in Chapter 36 is applicable to all chapters.

NURSING PROCESS

Look at the opening paragraph of this section, which introduces the focus for the section and serves as your preliminary focus for learning.

"The discussion of the nursing process will <u>focus</u> on each <u>major classification of antibiotics</u> so that there is an <u>awareness of general and specific information</u> about the various antibiotics."

The underlining in this paragraph is intended to point out the important information found in this paragraph. The Nursing Process section focuses on major classifications. Another critical piece of this paragraph is the need to see both *general* and *specific* information about the classifications. Although the paragraph is only one sentence in length, it clearly defines what you, as the student, need to keep in mind as you study this section.

ASSESSMENT

What is the purpose of this section? Each time you begin to read the Nursing Process section of a chapter, you need to ask this question. What are you supposed to learn? What are you supposed to know? What are you supposed to be able to do? All these questions relate to your role as a nurse. Consider the following sentence from this section in Chapter 36.

"<u>Before the administration</u> of any antibiotic, it is <u>crucial to ensuring</u> the effectiveness and <u>appropriateness of</u> <u>treatment for the nurse to collect</u> data on the <u>patient regarding his or her age; hypersensitivity to drugs; hepatic (SGOT, SGPT), renal, and cardiac function (i.e., pertinent laboratory test results); culture and sensitivity results; and CBC, Hgb, and Hct values.</u>"

Assessment clearly has to do with patient care. You are assessing the patient as he or she relates to the pharmacologic interventions that this chapter discusses. I have done some underlining in this section to bring into sharper focus some of the things that you must be very aware of as you study.

First, notice the use of the word *crucial* in the first line. Something is so important at this point that it cannot be ignored. Immediately the questioning process should be activated. What is crucial? The answer follows immediately in the sentence. You must have data collected on the patient. The sentence goes on to identify the kind of data that should be available, and the sentence makes it clear that it has to be done "before administration." Each of the data factors is important, and each relates to other parts and chapters in this text.

The patient's age should be known. Chapter 3 deals with pediatric and geriatric concerns. Children and elderly patients respond to drugs differently than adults. This would directly affect dosage and possibly even the choice of antibiotics to be administered. This also ties directly to "effectiveness of treatment" referred to in this sentence.

The next data item is hypersensitivities. Some individuals are "allergic" to certain antibiotics. It would be dangerous and possibly fatal to administer an antibiotic to a patient if he or she is hypersensitive. This connects with the "appropriateness of treatment," which is the other crucial element specified in this sentence. As you consider each of the underlined elements in this sentence, you must keep in mind its relationship to effectiveness and appropriateness.

Another data item specifies hepatic-renal-cardiac functioning. As you read this you should instantly think to what hepatic, renal, and cardiac refer. Then you should try to recall information from this chapter that related the specific antibiotics to these functions. Learning is cumulative. The Nursing Process section assumes you have read and understood what was presented earlier in the chapter.

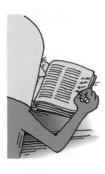

One more aspect of this sentence is the use of standard medical abbreviations. In earlier Study Skills Tips it has beeen suggested that you prepare vocabulary cards for these abbreviations to help you in a situation such as this. You need to know what CBC, Hgb, and Hct mean, what they measure, and how they relate to appropriate and effective administration of antibiotics. If these letters are not meaningful to you, then you will not be able to link what you know about the antibiotics with what you must know about administering them as a nurse. Many test questions on nursing examinations use the standard abbreviations, and you must know them instantly and be able to relate them to the situation covered. As you look at antibiotic administration and CBC, Hgb, and Hct, think what a test question might ask about these data elements in a real application in patient care? This is what the nursing process is all about.

• NURSING DIAGNOSES

The same first question applies here as in every other section. What am I supposed to learn? Since the focus is on administration of antibiotics, the expectation you should bring to this is an awareness of your role in diagnosis. What should you look for in working with patients that affects the administration of antibiotics?

This same procedure should be applied to the sections on Planning, Outcome Criteria, and Implementation. Consider what each of these headings suggests about the nursing process, and read and evaluate the information, relating it to what you have already learned. Also consider the implications of the information as possible test questions that may ask you to do more than recall specific facts. As an example, consider the following case:

Patient A, age 23, has a fever of 100.8° F. She was admitted yesterday and delivered a healthy infant 8 hours ago. She is breast feeding the newborn. What antibiotics might be administered for the fever? What specific antibiotics should be used with caution or eliminated from consideration?

This case demonstrates the need to read and think critically. You need to remember not only the specific facts from the chapter, but also be able to take a case study example and apply those facts to that specific situation.

• EVALUATION

This is the final section under Nursing Process. What are you supposed to evaluate?

"The therapeutic effects of antibiotics in general include a decrease in the signs and symptoms of the infection; a return to normal vital signs, including temperature and negative results of culture and sensitivity tests; a decrease to a normal CBC; and improved appetite, energy level, and sense of well-being." This sentence makes it clear that you are evaluating the patient and his or her response to the antibiotics being administered. In evaluating the patient, what should you look for? Given the focus in nursing process on contraindications, cautions, hypersensitivity, and reactions related to the administration of antibiotics, you should be evaluating two aspects of the patient.

First you should look for the positive responses set forth in the above text sample that indicate the patient is responding favorably to the treatment. But when you read the next sentence in this section, you see: "Common adverse reactions for which to monitor . . . " This says your role in evaluation is to monitor the patient for negative responses and be prepared to educate the patient as to the effects he or she is experiencing and possible steps to help alleviate the symptoms.

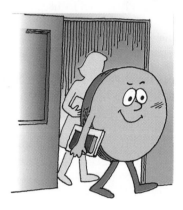

The Nursing Process section in each chapter should be read carefully and thoughtfully because it is in this section where you begin to see how the complex pharmacologic material presented earlier in the chapter fits into your role as a nurse. This material should be read with the same concern and care that you have given to the highly complex materials earlier in the chapter, as this is the section in which you must think about **application** of all you have learned. Apply the PURR model and be an active questioner and reader, and you will be successful in working with Nursing Process in each chapter.

www.harcourthealth.com/MERLIN/Lilley/

objectives

When you reach the end of this chapter, you should be able to do the following:

1 Discuss the general principles of antibiotic therapy.

2 Explain how antibiotics work to rid the body of infection.

3 Discuss the pros and cons of antibiotic usage.

4 Describe the various concerns with overuse of antibiotics.

5 Discuss the indications, cautions, contraindications, mechanisms of action, side effects, and toxicity associated with the various antibiotic groups.

6 Classify the various antibiotics with examples of specific drugs in each classification grouping.

7 Develop a nursing cae plan that includes all phases of the nursing process for the patient receiving antibiotics.

Look for this symbol for topics covered in the **Online Worksheet** Activity

drug profiles

amikacin, p. 583

ampicillin, p. 574

amoxicillin, p. 574

azithromycin and clarithromycin, p. 588

aztreonam, p. 589

cefazolin sodium, p. 576

cefepime, p. 579

cefixime, p. 578

cefoxitin, p. 577

ceftazidime, p. 578

ceftriaxone, p. 578

cefuroxime, p. 578

cephalexin, p. 576

ciprofloxacin, p. 585

clindamycin, p. 589

demeclocycline, p. 580

doxycycline, p. 581

erythromycin, p. 587

gentamicin, p. 583

imipenem-cilastatin, p. 590

linezolid, p. 590

methicillin, p. 573

penicillin G and penicillin V potassium, p. 573

quinupristin/ dalfopristin, p. 590

sulfamethoxazole, p. 570

sulfisoxazole, p. 571

vancomycin, p. 591

°—= Key drug.

glossary

Antibiotic Of or pertaining to the ability to destroy or interfere with the development of a living organism. (p. 568)

Bactericidal antibiotics Antibiotics that kill bacteria. (p. 581)

Bacteriostatic antibiotics Antibiotics that do not actually kill but rather inhibit the growth of bacteria. (p. 569)

Beta-lactams (lak′ təmz) The chemical structure of penicillins. (p. 571)

Empiric therapy When pertaining to antibiotic therapy, involves the treatment of an infection before specific culture information has been reported or obtained. (p. 568)

Glucose-6-phosphate dehydrogenase deficiency An inherited disorder in which the red blood cells are partially or completely deficient in glucose-6-phosphate dehydrogenase, a critical enzyme in the aerobic glycolysis process. A sex-linked disorder, the defect is fully expressed in affected males despite a heterozygous pattern of inheritance. (p. 569)

Host factors Particular factors pertinent to patient with infection. (p. 569)

Prophylactic Antibiotics taken before exposure to an infectious organism in efforts to prevent the development of infection. (p. 568)

Slow acetylator (ə set′ ə la′ tor) A common genetic host factor. A peripheral neuropathy may develop in affected persons given isoniazid. (p. 569)

Subtherapeutic Referring to treatment that is considered ineffective because of an inadequate amount of drug at the site of infection. (p. 568)

Superinfection An infection occurring during antimicrobial treatment for another infection, resulting in overgrowth of nonsusceptible organism. (p. 568)

Teratogens (ter′ ə to jənz) Any substance, agent, or process that interferes with normal prenatal development and causes one or more developmental abnormalities in the fetus. (p. 569)

Therapeutic Of or relating to treatment that is considered beneficial. (p. 568)

INFECTION

A person is able to remain healthy and resistant to the microorganisms that cause infection because of the existence of certain host defenses. These defenses take various forms. They can be actual physical barriers such as intact skin or the ciliated respiratory mucosa. They can be physiologic defenses such as the gastric acid in the stomach and immune factors such as antibodies. They can also be the phagocytic cells (macrophages and polymorphonuclear neutrophils) that are part of the reticuloendothelial system.

Microorganisms are everywhere in both the external environment as well as the internal environment of our bodies. They can be intrinsically harmful to humans, or they can be innocuous and even beneficial under normal circumstances but become harmful when these conditions are altered in some way. An example of an intrinsically harmful microorganism is *Rickettsia rickettsii*, which causes Rocky Mountain spotted fever. Certain species of *Streptococcus* are normally present on the body. They normally do not cause harm, but under certain circumstances they can cause endocarditis in patients whose heart valves have been damaged as a result of rheumatic fever.

When a person's normal host defenses are breached or somehow compromised, that person becomes susceptible to infection. The microorganisms invade and multiply in the body tissues, and if the infective process overwhelms the body's own defense system, the infection becomes clinically apparent. The patient then manifests the characteristic signs and symptoms of infection—fever, chills, sweats, redness, pain and swelling, fatigue, weight loss, increased white blood cell (WBC) count, and the formation of pus. Not all patients will exhibit signs of infection. This is especially true in elderly and immunocompromised patients.

To help the body and its normal host defenses combat an infection, antibiotic therapy is often required. Antibiotics are most effective when their actions are combined with the body's multiple defense mechanisms. However, before considering the specific agents and the therapy proper, there are certain general principles pertaining to antibiotic therapy that should be explained and understood first.

GENERAL PRINCIPLES OF ANTIBIOTIC THERAPY

Therapy should begin with an initial assessment of the patient to determine whether he or she has the common signs and symptoms of infection previously mentioned. The patient should also be assessed during and after antibiotic therapy to make certain the therapy is working, the infection is not recurring, and there are no untoward problems with the therapy.

Often the signs and symptoms of an infection appear long before an organism can be identified. When this happens and the risk of life-threatening or severe complications is high, an **antibiotic** is given to the patient immediately. The antibiotic selected is one that can best kill the microorganisms known to be the most common causes of infection. This is defined as **empiric therapy.** Before the start of empiric antibiotic therapy, suspected areas of infection should be cultured in an attempt to identify a causative organism. If an organism is identified, it is then tested for various antibiotic susceptibilities. The results of these tests can confirm whether the empiric therapy chosen is appropriate for eradicating the organism identified. If not, therapy can be adjusted or streamlined to optimize efficacy.

Antibiotics are also given for **prophylactic** reasons. This is done when patients are scheduled to have a procedure in which the likelihood of microorganisms being present is high. Prophylactic antibiotic therapy is used to prevent an infection. However, the risk of infection varies depending on the procedure being performed. For example, the risk of infection in a patient undergoing coronary artery bypass surgery is relatively low compared with that in a person undergoing intraabdominal surgery for the treatment of injuries suffered in a motor vehicle accident. In the latter case, it is highly likely that the bacteria that normally live in the gastrointestinal tract will be present in the area of surgery. This would constitute a contaminated or dirty surgical field, and therefore the likelihood of infection would be high.

To optimize antibiotic therapy, the patient should be continuously monitored both to determine the effectiveness of therapy and whether the therapy is having any adverse effects. A **therapeutic** response to antibiotics is one in which there is a decrease in the specific signs and symptoms of infection compared with the baseline findings (e.g., fever, elevated WBC count, redness, inflammation, drainage, pain). Antibiotic therapy is said to be **subtherapeutic** when it is ineffective. This can result from using an incorrect route of administration, inadequate drainage of abscess, poor antibiotic penetration to the infected area, subtherapeutic serum levels of the agent, or bacterial resistance to the antibiotic. Antibiotic therapy is considered *toxic* when the serum levels of the antibiotic are too high, when the patient has an allergic reaction to the antibiotic, or when the patient experiences an adverse reaction to the drug. These include rash, itching, hives, fever, chills, joint pain, difficulty breathing, or wheezing.

Superinfections and antibiotic interactions with food and other drugs are other problems to be watched for in patients taking antibiotics. Superinfections occur when antibiotics reduce or completely eliminate the normal bacterial flora. This consists of certain bacteria and fungi that are needed to maintain normal function in various organs. When these bacteria or fungi are killed by antibiotics, this permits other bacteria or fungi to take over and cause infection. An example of a superinfection caused by antibiotics is the development of vaginal yeast infections when the normal vaginal flora is reduced and yeast growth is no longer suppressed. The chemical makeup of antibiotics can also cause the body to react in many ways. Food-drug and drug-drug interactions are frequent problems in patients taking antibiotics. One of the more common food-drug interactions is that between milk or cheese and tetracycline, resulting in decreased levels of tetracycline. An example of an antibiotic-drug interaction is that between quinolone antibiotics and antacids, resulting in decreased absorption of quinolone antibiotics.

Other important factors that are essential to the appropriate use of antibiotics are host-specific factors, or **host factors.** These are the particular factors that pertain to the infected patient and that can have an important bearing on the success or failure of antibiotic therapy. Some of these host factors are age, allergy history, organ function (kidneys and liver), pregnancy status, genetic characteristics, site of infection, and host defenses.

Age-related host factors are those that apply to patients at either end of the age spectrum. For instance, infants and children may not be able to take certain antibiotics such as tetracyclines because of their effects on developing teeth or bones; quinolones, which may also affect bone development in children; and sulfonamides, which may displace bilirubin from albumin and precipitate kernicterus in young patients. The aging process affects the function of various organ systems. As we age, there is a gradual decline in the function of such organs as the kidneys and liver, the organs responsible for eliminating and breaking down various antibiotics. Thus giving older patients antibiotics in doses appropriate only for younger patients could result in antibiotic toxicities.

If a patient has a history of an allergic reaction to an antibiotic, this plays an important role in the selection of the most appropriate antibiotic for that patient. Penicillins and sulfonamides are two broad categories of antibiotics to which many people have allergic or anaphylactic reactions.

Pregnancy-related host factors are also important when it comes to selecting appropriate antibiotics since several antibiotics can pass through the placenta to the fetus and cause harm to the developing fetus. Such drugs are called **teratogens.** Their use in pregnant women can result in birth defects.

Many drugs, including certain antibiotics, depend on specific enzyme systems to break them down so that they can be eliminated. However, some patients have certain genetic abnormalities that may result in deficiencies of the enzymes needed by these systems, with the result that the antibiotic has abnormal effects. Two common examples of such genetic host factors are **glucose-6-phosphate dehydrogenase** (G6PD) **deficiency** and **slow acetylator** status. The administration of such antibiotics as sulfonamides, nitrofurantoin, pyrimethamine, and chloramphenicol to a person with G6PD deficiency will result in the hemolysis, or destruction, of red blood cells (RBCs). A peripheral neuropathy may develop in a slow acetylator given isoniazid.

The anatomic site of the infection is another important host factor to consider when determining not only which antibiotic to use but also the dose, route of administration, and duration of therapy.

Consideration of these host factors helps ensure that the most appropriate antibiotic is selected for a particular patient. Appropriate assessment and routine monitoring of antibiotic therapy increase the likelihood that the antibiotic therapy is safe and effective.

ANTIBIOTICS

Antibiotics can be broken down into many broad categories based on their chemical structures. Some of the more common of these categories are sulfonamides, penicillins, cephalosporins, macrolides, and quinolones. There are, however, many more such categories, (aminoglycosides, tetracyclines, and other miscellaneous agents) that do not easily fit into one of the broad categories. The characteristics that distinguish one class of agents from the next are the antibacterial spectrum, mechanism of action, potency, toxicity, and pharmacokinetic properties shared by the agents in that class.

SULFONAMIDES

Sulfonamides are a chemically related group of antibiotics that are all synthetic derivatives of sulfanilamide. They were one of the first group of drugs used as antibiotics, and some of the more commonly prescribed agents are sulfadiazine, sulfamethizole, sulfamethoxazole, and sulfisoxazole. Sulfasalazine, another sulfonamide, is used for other indications besides infections. Their antibiotic activity is the result of their ability to antagonize or inhibit an enzyme that is essential for the growth and proliferation of certain bacteria, and there are a wide range of organisms that sulfonamide antibiotics are effective in combating. These antibiotics achieve very high concentrations in the kidneys, through which they are eliminated. Therefore they are primarily used in the treatment of urinary tract infections (UTIs). Sulfonamides are also used in the treatment of mild to moderate ulcerative colitis, active Crohn's disease, and rheumatoid arthritis. In addition, they may be combined with other antibiotics to increase their antibiotic potency.

Mechanism of Action

Sulfonamides do not actually destroy bacteria but inhibit their growth. For this reason they are considered **bacteriostatic antibiotics.** They inhibit the growth of susceptible bacteria by preventing the synthesis of a folic acid, a B-complex vitamin that is required for the proper synthesis of purines and nucleic acid. It is composed of a molecule of para-aminobenzoic acid (PABA), pteridine, and glutamic acid. Specifically, sulfonamides compete (competitive inhibition) with the PABA for the enzyme that incorporates the PABA into the folic acid molecule during biosynthesis. Because sulfonamides are capable of blocking a specific step in a biosynthetic pathway, they are also considered antimetabolites. However, those microorganisms that can utilize preformed folic acid are not affected by the sulfonamides.

As previously mentioned, greater effectiveness of the sulfonamides' antibiotic potency is achieved by combining the sulfonamide agent sulfamethoxazole with trimethoprim (a nonsulfonamide). The resulting combination is called *co-trimoxazole.* Together the two antibiotics are capable of blocking two successive steps in the bacterial folic acid pathway. Unfortunately, however, many organisms once susceptible to the sulfonamides are now resistant to them.

Drug Effects

Only microorganisms that synthesize their own folic acid are inhibited by sulfonamides. Those animals and bacteria that are capable of utilizing folic acid precursors or preformed folic acid are not affected by them. Human cells can utilize preformed folic acid and are therefore not affected by sulfonamides.

Therapeutic Uses

The sulfonamides are used for the treatment of UTIs caused by susceptible strains of *Enterobacter* spp., *Escherichia coli, Klebsiella* spp., *Proteus mirabilis, Proteus vulgaris,* and *Staphylococcus aureus.*

In addition, sulfonamides are the drugs of choice for the treatment of nocardiosis, *Pneumocystis carinii,* and infections secondary to the bacteria *Stenotrophomonas maltophilia.* They are also excellent drugs for the treatment of upper respiratory tract infections. Sulfonamides are used as adjuncts in the treatment of malaria and toxoplasmosis and as alternative agents for the management of chlamydial infections and dermatitis herpetiformis. Following are the specific indications for the various sulfonamides: sulfapyridine is used for the treatment of dermatitis herpetiformis; sulfadiazine, sulfisoxazole, sulfamethoxazole, and triple sulfa are all used for the treatment of nocardiosis; and sulfasalazine is used to treat ulcerative colitis. Systemic antibacterial agents include sulfacytine, sulfadiazine, sulfamethiazole, sulfamethoxazole, sulfisoxazole, and triple sulfa.

Side Effects and Adverse Effects

Sulfonamide drugs are a common cause of allergic reactions. These agents are included in several drug classes, including antimicrobials, diuretics, oral hypoglycemics, and carbonic anhydrase inhibitors. Although immediate reactions can occur, sulfonamides typically cause delayed cutaneous reactions. These reactions often begin with fever followed by a rash (morbilliform eruptions, erythema multiforme, or toxic epidermal necrolysis). Other reactions to sulfonamides include mucocutaneous, gastrointestinal, hepatic, renal, or hematologic complications, which may be fatal. It is believed that sulfonamide reactions are immune mediated and involve the production of reactive metabolites. It is important to differentiate between sulfites and sulfonamides. Sulfites are commonly used as preservatives in everything from wine to food to injectable drugs. The most common side effects are listed in Table 36-1.

Activity

Interactions

Sulfonamides produce a fairly wide array of interactions when taken in conjunction with oral anticoagulants, PABA preparations, and urinary acidifiers.

Table 36-1	Sulfonamides: Common Adverse Effects	
Body System	**Side/Adverse Effects**
Blood	Agranulocytosis, aplastic anemia, hemolytic anemia, thrombocytopenia
Gastrointestinal	Nausea, vomiting, diarrhea, pancreatitis
Integumentary	Epidermal necrolysis, exfoliative dermatitis, Stevens-Johnson syndrome, photosensitivity
Other	Convulsions, crystalluria, toxic nephrosis, headache, peripheral neuritis, urticaria

Laboratory Test Interactions

Sulfonamides can increase the serum levels of aspartate aminotransferase, acetyltransferase, and alkaline phosphatase.

Dosages

For recommended dosages of selected sulfonamides, see the dosages table on p. 571.

---

drug profiles

Sulfonamides are classified as pregnancy category C agents and are contraindicated in patients with a known hypersensitivity to sulfonamides, in pregnant women at term, and in infants under 2 months of age.

sulfamethoxazole

Sulfamethoxazole (Gantanol, Azo-Gantanol, Bactrim) is a sulfonamide antibiotic. Because it is eliminated by means of the kidneys and reaches very high concentrations there, it is commonly used to treat UTIs caused by susceptible organisms. It is combined with phenazopyridine in a preparation known as Azo-Gantanol. The phenazopyridine is an analgesic-anesthetic that affects the mucosa of the urinary tract. Together the two agents not only inhibit susceptible bacteria in UTIs but also relieve any pain associated with the infection. Sulfamethoxazole by itself is available as a 500-mg/5 ml oral suspension and a 500-mg tablet. In combination with phenazopyridine it is available as a film-coated tablet containing 500 mg of sulfamethoxazole and 100 mg of phenazopyridine.

Sulfamethoxazole is also combined with the antimetabolite trimethoprim in a fixed combination containing a 5:1 ratio of sulfamethoxazole to trimethoprim. As explained earlier, this combination of agents sequentially inhibits two steps in the folic acid pathway, giving it antibacterial synergism. It is

DOSAGES Selected Sulfonamides

agent	pharmacologic class	dosage range	purpose
sulfamethoxazole (Gantanol, Azo-Gantanol, Bactrim)	Sulfonamide	*Pediatric >2 mo* PO: 50-60 mg/kg loading dose, followed by 25-30 mg/kg q12h; do not exceed 75 mg/kg/day. *Adult* PO: 2 g loading dose, followed by 1-2 g 2-3 times/day. The dose for Azo-Gantanol is the same. Do not exceed 2 days of treatment	Nocardiosis, UTIs, adjunct for toxoplasmosis
sulfisoxazole (Gantrisin, Azo-Gantrisin, Pediazole)	Sulfonamide	*Pediatric >2 mo* PO: 75 mg/kg loading dose, followed by 150 mg/kg/day in 4-6 doses *Adult* PO: 2-4 g loading dose, followed by 4-8 g/day in 4-6 doses	Nocardosis, UTIs, adjunct for toxoplasmosis

commonly used in the treatment of UTIs caused by susceptible bacteria, *Pneumocystis carinii* pneumonia, ear infections (otitis media), bronchitis, gonorrhea, and many other infectious conditions. It is also used for prophylaxis in HIV-infected patients. This fixed combination of sulfamethoxazole and trimethoprim is available as a 40-mg/5 ml oral suspension and in two strengths of oral tablets containing 80 and 400 mg and 160 and 800 mg of trimethoprim and sulfamethoxazole, respectively. It is also available in a fixed-combination agent containing 16 mg/ml of trimethoprim and 80 mg/ml of sulfamethoxazole to be given as an IV injection. Recommended dosages of the sulfamethoxazole products are listed in the dosages table above. Pregnancy category C.

PHARMACOKINETICS

HALF-LIFE	ONSET	PEAK	DURATION
7-12 hr	Variable	2-4 hr (plasma)	Up to 12 hr

sulfisoxazole

Sulfisoxazole (Gantrisin, Azo-Gantrisin, Pediazole) is a short-acting sulfonamide antibiotic that is primarily used for its ability to effectively inhibit organisms in the urinary tract. It also is available as a fixed-combination product containing either phenazopyridine (Azo-Gantrisin) or erythromycin (Pediazole). It has good activity against those organisms that commonly cause ear infections (otitis media) in small children, so it is also available in an oral suspension for this purpose.

Unlike sulfamethoxazole, it is not available as a parenteral agent. It is available as a 500-mg tablet (Gantrisin); as a fixed-combination product containing 500 mg of sulfisoxazole and 50 mg of phenazopyridine (Azo-Gantrisin); as a 500-mg/5 ml oral solution and oral suspension; and as a fixed-combination product containing 600 mg of

sulfisoxazole and 200 mg of erythromycin per 5 ml of the inert substance (Pediazole, E.S.P., or Eryzole). Recommeded dosages are given in the dosages table above. Pregnancy category C.

PHARMACOKINETICS

HALF-LIFE	ONSET	PEAK	DURATION
4.6-7.8 hr	Variable	1-4 hr (plasma)	4-6 hr

PENICILLINS

The penicillins are a very large group of chemically related antibiotics that are derived from a fungus, or mold, often seen on bread or fruit. Penicillins may also be called **beta-lactams,** a term that refers to their chemical structure. The penicillins can be divided into four groups based on their structure and the bacteria they kill. These four groups are natural penicillins, penicillinase-resistant penicillins, aminopenicillins, and extended-spectrum penicillins. Examples of antibiotics in each group and a brief description of their characteristics are given in Box 36-1.

Penicillins were first introduced onto the market in the early 1940s, and to this day they have remained very effective and safe antibiotics. They are bactericidal and can kill a wide variety of gram-positive and some gram-negative bacteria. Penicillins work by inhibiting bacterial cell wall synthesis, which they accomplish by interfering with the biosynthesis of structural substances needed in the cell walls of bacteria. However, bacteria have acquired the capacity to produce enzymes capable of destroying penicillins. These enzymes are called *beta-lactamases,* and they can destroy the structural component of the penicillin called the *beta-lactam ring.* This was a problem until chemicals were synthesized that inhibit these enzymes. Three of these beta-lactamase inhibitors are clavulanic acid, tazobactam, and sulbactam. By binding with the beta-lactamase they prevent the enzyme from breaking down the penicillin. Examples

Box 36-1 Penicillins: Classification

Class	Antibiotics	Description
Aminopenicillins	amoxicillin, ampicillin, bacampicillin	Have an amino group attached to their penicillin nucleus that enhances their activity against gram-negative bacteria compared with natural penicillins.
Extended-spectrum agents	piperacillin, ticarcillin, carbenicillin, mezlocillin	Have wider spectra of activity than that of all the above types of penicillins.
Penicillinase-resistant agents	cloxacillin, dicloxacillin, methicillin, nafcillin, oxacillin	Stable against hydrolysis by most staphylococcal penicillinases (enzymes that normally break down the natural penicillins).
Penicillins	penicillin G, penicillin V	Various natural penicillins have been produced by changing different side chains; penicillin exists as F, G, N, O, V, and X; only penicillin G and V are currently used clinically.

Table 36-2 Penicillins: Common Adverse Effects

Body System	Side/Adverse Effects
Central nervous system	Lethargy, hallucinations, anxiety, depression, twitching, coma, convulsions
Gastrointestinal	Nausea, vomiting, diarrhea, increased AST and ALT (liver function tests), abdominal pain, colitis
Hematologic	Anemia, increased bleeding time, bone marrow depression, granulocytopenia
Metabolic	Hyperkalemia, hypokalemia, alkalosis
Other	Taste alterations, sore mouth, dark, discolored, or sore tongue, hives, rash

of currently available penicillin–beta-lactamase inhibitor combinations are as follows:
- ampicillin + sulbactam = Unasyn
- amoxicillin + clavulanic acid = Augmentin
- ticarcillin + clavulanic acid = Timentin
- piperacillin + tazobactam = Zosyn

Mechanism of Action

The mechanism of action of penicillins involves several steps that together result in the inhibition of bacterial cell wall synthesis. In the first step, penicillins slide through the bacteria's cell walls to get to their site of action. However, some penicillins are too large to pass through these openings in the cell walls, and because they cannot get to their site of action, they cannot kill the bacteria. On the other hand, some bacteria can make the openings in their cell walls smaller so that the penicillin cannot get through to kill them. The penicillin that does gain entry into the bacteria must then find the appropriate binding site, in this case an area called the *penicillin-binding protein*. By binding to this protein the penicillin interferes with the normal cell wall synthesis, causing the formation of defective cell walls that are unstable and easily broken down. Bacteria death usually results from lysis.

Drug Effects

Penicillins only inhibit the cell wall synthesis of bacteria, not that of other cells in the body. Therefore the drug effects of penicillins are limited to the killing of bacteria. In humans this has the therapeutic effect of destroying invading bacteria that are responsible for infections.

Therapeutic Uses

Penicillins are indicated for the prevention and treatment of infections caused by susceptible bacteria. The microorganisms most commonly destroyed by penicillins are gram-positive bacteria, including the *Streptococcus, Enterococcus,* and *Staphylococcus* species. Most penicillins have little if any ability to kill gram-negative bacteria, although some of the extended-spectrum penicillins can.

Side Effects and Adverse Effects

Allergic reactions to penicillin occur in 0.7% to 8% of treatment courses. The most common reactions to penicillin include urticaria, pruritus, and angioedema. About 10% of allergic reactions are life-threatening, and 10% of these are fatal. A wide variety of idiopathic reactions occur, such as maculopapular eruptions, eosinophilia, Stevens-Johnson syndrome, and exfoliative dermatitis. Maculopapular rash occurs in about 2% of treatment courses with penicillin and 5.2% to 9.5% with ampicillin. Patients who are allergic to penicillins may also be sensitive to other beta-lactams. The exact incidence of cross-reactivity between cephalosporins and penicillins is not known; however, it is believed to be low.

Penicillins are generally well tolerated and associated with very few adverse effects. As with many drugs, the most common ones are gastrointestinal in nature. Their most common side effects and adverse effects are listed in Table 36-2.

Penicillins: Drug Interactions

36-3

Drug	Mechanism	Result
Aminoglycosides and clavulanic acid	Additive	More effective killing of bacteria
NSAIDs	Compete for protein binding	More free and active penicillin
Oral contraceptives	Decrease effectiveness	May decrease efficacy of the contraceptive
probenecid	Competes for elimination	Prolongs the effects of penicillins
rifampin	Inhibition	May inhibit the killing activity of penicillins
warfarin	Increases metabolism	Penicillins may increase metabolism of warfarin, decreasing its effect

Interactions

There are many drugs that interact with penicillins; some have positive effects, and others have harmful effects. The most common and clinically significant drug interactions associated with penicillin use are listed in Table 36-3.

Dosages

For dosage information on selected penicillins, see the dosages table on p. 575.

drug profiles

Penicillins are classified as pregnancy category B agents. They are very safe antibiotics and are only contraindicated in patients with a hypersensitivity to them. Because of their relatively safe side effect profile, there are otherwise very few contraindications to their use.

NATURAL PENICILLINS

penicillin G and penicillin V potassium

Penicillin G has four salt forms: benzathine; potassium, procaine, and sodium. All of these forms are given parenterally, either intravenously or intramuscularly. Penicillin G and its various salt forms are rarely given any more. Other forms of penicillin are more frequently used.

Penicillin V potassium (Pen-Vee K, Beepen-VK, V-Cillin K, Ledercillin VK, Veetids) is only available in oral preparations. It too is not used as often as other forms of penicillin. It is contraindicated in patients who are hypertensive to it and in newborns, and it is also a pregnancy category C agent. It is available as a 125- and 250-mg/5 ml oral solution; 250- and 500-mg tablets; and 125-, 250-, and 500-mg film-coated tablets. Commonly recommended dosages are given in the dosages table on p. 575.

PHARMACOKINETICS

HALF-LIFE	ONSET	PEAK	DURATION
30 min	Variable	30-60 min (plasma)	4-6 hr

PENICILLINASE-RESISTANT PENICILLINS

methicillin

Methicillin (Staphcillin) is one of the five currently available penicillinase-resistant penicillins, the other four being cloxacillin, dicloxacillin, nafcillin, and oxacillin. The penicillinase-resistant penicillins are able to resist the breakdown of the penicillin-destroying enzyme (penicillinase) commonly produced by bacteria such as staphylococci. For this reason, they may also be referred to as *antistaphylococcal penicillins.* They accomplish this by attaching a large, bulky side chain around the beta-lactam ring that hinders the penicillinase and prevents it from attacking the beta-lactam ring, thus destroying the antibiotic. There are, however, certain strains of staphylococci, specifically *Staphylococcus aureus,* that are methicillin resistant. This bacteria can resist the actions of methicillin and therefore survive. Methicillin has the same contraindications and pregnancy rating as the natural penicillins. It is only available parenterally as a 1-, 4-, 6-, and 10-g injection. Commonly recommended dosages are given in the dosages table on p. 575.

PHARMACOKINETICS

HALF-LIFE	ONSET	PEAK	DURATION
20-30 min	Variable	30-60 min	6 hr

AMINOPENICILLINS

There are three aminopenicillins—amoxicillin, ampicillin, and bacampicillin. Because of the presence of a free amino group on the penicillin nucleus, aminopenicillins have enhanced activity against gram-negative bacteria, against which the natural and penicillinase-resistant penicillins are relatively ineffective. Amoxicillin is an analogue of ampicillin, and bacampicillin is a prodrug of ampicillin. Bacampicillin has no antibacterial activity until hydrolyzed to ampicillin in the body. Aminopenicillins have the same contraindications and pregnancy ratings (B) as the other penicillins.

amoxicillin

Amoxicillin (Amoxil, Polymox, Trimox, Wymox) is a very commonly prescribed aminopenicillin. Amoxicillin is used to treat infections caused by susceptible organisms in the ears, nose, throat, genitourinary tract, skin, and skin structures. It is available as 125-, 200-, 250-, and 400-mg chewable tablets; 500- and 875-mg tablets; 250- and 500-mg capsules; and 50-, 125-, 200-, 250-, and 400-mg/5 ml powder for oral suspension. Commonly recommended dosages are given in the dosages table on p. 575.

PHARMACOKINETICS

HALF-LIFE	ONSET	PEAK	DURATION
1-1.3 hr	0.5-1 hr	1-2 hr	6-8 hr

ampicillin

Ampicillin is the prototypical aminopenicillin, and it differs from penicillin G only in that it has the amino group on the penicillin nucleus. It is available in three different salt forms—anhydrous, trihydrate, and sodium. Like penicillin G, each salt form allows it to be administered by a different route. Ampicillin anhydrous and trihydrate are both administered orally, and ampicillin sodium is given parenterally. Anhydrous ampicillin (Omnipen) is available as 250- and 500-mg capsules and as a 250-mg/5 ml suspension. Trihydrate ampicillin (Polycillin, Principen, and Totacillin) is available as 250- and 500-mg capsules and 125-, 250-, and 500-mg/5 ml suspensions. Sodium ampicillin (Ampicillin sodium, Omnipen-N, and Totacillin-N) is available as 125-, 250-, 500-, 1000-, 2000-, and 10,000-mg vials for injection. Commonly recommended dosages are given in the dosages table on p. 575.

PHARMACOKINETICS

HALF-LIFE	ONSET	PEAK	DURATION
PO: 0.7-1.4 hr	Variable	1-2 hr (serum)	4-6 hr

EXTENDED-SPECTRUM PENICILLINS

By making a few changes in the basic penicillin structure, agents were produced with a wider spectrum of activity than that possessed by either of the other two classes of semisynthetic penicillins (penicillinase-resistant penicillins and aminopenicillins) or by the natural penicillins. There are four of these extended-spectrum penicillins currently available—carbenicillin, piperacillin, ticarcillin, and mezlocillin. These can be broken down into two main classes, as determined by their structure. These are as follows:

- Carboxypenicillins = carbenicillin and ticarcillin
- Acylaminopenicillins = piperacillin and mezlocillin

Carboxypenicillins have a carboxylic acid group attached to the basic penicillin nucleus, which has endowed it with new activity against some bacteria that the other classes of penicillins cannot kill, such as the *Pseudomonas* spp., as well as with stability against the beta-lactams produced by *Proteus* organisms. Acylaminopenicillins have a basic group on one of the side chains off the main penicillin nucleus, giving them even greater activity against *Pseudomonas* spp. and Enterobacteriaceae than the carboxypenicillins. Carbenicillin differs structurally from ampicillin only in the substitution of a carboxy group for an amino group on the penicillin nucleus. Ticarcillin is an analogue of carbenicillin with a B-thienyl group, and mezlocillin is an ampicillin derivative that contains a ureido group on the penicillin nucleus. Piperacillin is a piperazine derivative of ampicillin. The result is that small changes in the natural penicillin structure have translated into big changes in activity against new bacteria.

All the extended-spectrum penicillins are given parenterally (IV) except for carbenicillin, which is only given orally. The contraindications to their use are the same as those of the other penicillins, and they are also all pregnancy category C agents. Both ticarcillin and piperacillin are available in fixed-combination products that include beta-lactamase inhibitors. The ticarcillin fixed-combination product (Timentin) includes clavulanate potassium. Piperacillin is combined with tazobactam in a product called Zosyn. Common dosage recommendations for ticarcillin (Ticar) are listed in the dosages table on p. 575.

PHARMACOKINETICS

carbenicillin indanyl sodium (Geocillin): 382-mg film-coated tablets

HALF-LIFE	ONSET	PEAK	DURATION
0.8-1 hr	Variable	0.5-2 hr*	6 hr

mezlocillin sodium (Mezlin): 1-, 2-, 3-, 4-, and 20-g vials for injection

HALF-LIFE	ONSET	PEAK	DURATION
0.7-1.3 hr	Variable	IV: 5 min*	Variable

piperacillin sodium (Pipracil): 2-, 3-, 4-, and 40-g vials for injection

HALF-LIFE	ONSET	PEAK	DURATION
0.6-1.3 hr	Variable	IV: 5 min*	Variable

ticarcillin disodium (Ticar): 1-, 3-, 6-, and 20-g vials for injection

HALF-LIFE	ONSET	PEAK	DURATION
0.9-1.3 hr	Variable	IV: 5 min*	Variable

*Serum.

DOSAGES Selected Penicillins

agent	pharmacologic class	dosage range	purpose
amoxicillin (Amoxil, Polymox, Trimox, Wymox)	Aminopenicillin	*Child >20 kg* PO: 40 mg/kg/day in divided doses q8h *Adult/child >20 kg* PO: 250-500 mg q8h	Antiinfective
ampicillin (anhydrous, trihydrate, and sodium salt form)	Aminopenicillin	*Pediatric <20 kg* PO: 50-100 mg/kg divided q6-8h *Pediatric >20 kg* PO: 250-500 mg qid IM/IV: 25-50 mg/kg divided *Adult* PO: 250-500 mg qid IM/IV: 25-50 mg qid	Antiinfective
methicillin (Staphcillin)	Penicillinase-resistant penicillin	*Pediatric* IM: 25 mg/kg q6h *Adult* IM: 1 g q4 or 6h IV: 1 g q6h	Penicillinase-producing staph infections
penicillin V potassium (Pen-Vee K, Beepen-VK, V-Cillin, Ledercillin VK, and Veetids)	Acid-stable penicillin	*Pediatric <12 y/o* PO: 15-50 mg/kg/day in 3-6 doses *Adult* PO: 250-500 mg 3-4 times/day	Antiinfective; tachyarrhythmias
ticarcillin disodium (Ticar)	Extended-spectrum penicillin	*Neonatal <2000 g* IM/IV: 75 mg/kg/12 hr for first 4 days; after 7 days of age, 75 mg/kg/8 hr *Neonatal >2000 g* IM/IV: 75 mg/kg/8 h for first 7 days; after 7 days of age, 100 mg/kg/8 hr *Pediatric* <40 kg IM/IV: 50-100 mg/kg/day divided *Adult/Pediatric >40 kg* IM/IV: 150-300 mg/kg/day divided	Antiinfective

CEPHALOSPORINS

Cephalosporins are semisynthetic antibiotic derivatives of cephalosporin C, a substance produced by a fungus but synthetically altered to produce an antibiotic. These chemically altered derivatives of this fungus are broadly referred to as cephalosporins, and they are structurally and pharmacologically related to penicillins. Like penicillins, cephalosporins are also bactericidal and work by interfering with bacterial cell wall synthesis. They also bind to similar PBPs inside bacteria.

Cephalosporins have a broad spectrum of bacteria they can destroy, and this is directly related to the chemical changes that have been made to their basic cephalosporin structure. Broadly they are active against many gram-positive bacteria, some gram-negative bacteria, and some anaerobic bacteria. They are not active against fungi and viruses. The cephalosporins have thus far been divided into three generations of agents according to the differences in their antimicrobial activity. Each generation has certain chemical similarities and thus similar spectrums of bacteria that they kill. In general, first-generation cephalosporins have the best gram-positive coverage but

poor gram-negative coverage. On the other hand, third-generation cephalosporins have the best gram-negative coverage but poor gram-positive coverage. Over the past several years, cephalosporins with a broader spectrum of antibacterial activity than third-generation cephalosporins have emerged. This has prompted classification of these agents into a new group called *fourth-generation cephalosporins*. These agents typically have more activity against gram-positive bacteria that third-generation cephalosporins. They still maintain good gram-negative coverage as well. Cefepime, cefpirome, and cefdinir are three fourth-generation cephalosporins. The currently available parenteral and oral cephalosporin antibiotics are listed in Box 36-2.

The safety profiles, contraindications, and pregnancy ratings of the cephalosporins are very similar to those of the penicillins. The most frequently reported side effects include mild diarrhea, abdominal cramps or distress, rash, pruritus, redness, and edema. Because cephalosporins are chemically very similar to penicillins, a person who has had an allergic reaction to penicillin may also have an allergic reaction to a cephalosporin. This is

Cephalosporins: Parenteral and Oral Preparations

BOX 36-2

First Generation		Second Generation		Third Generation		Fourth Generation	
IV	PO	IV	PO	IV	PO	IV	PO
cefazolin	cefadroxil	cefamandole	cefaclor	cefoperazone	cefixime	cefepime	cefdinir
cephalothin	cephalexin	cefoxitin	cefuroxime	cefotaxime	cefpodoxime proxetil	cefpirome	
cephradine	cephradine	cefuroxime	cefprozil	ceftizoxime	ceftibuten		
cephapirin		cefonicid		ceftriaxone			
		ceforanide		ceftazidime			
		cefmetazole		moxalactam			
		cefotetan					

referred to as *cross-sensitivity.* Various investigators have observed that the incidence of cross-sensitivity between penicillins and cephalosporins is between 1% and 18%. However, only those patients who have had a serious anaphylactic reaction to penicillin should not be given cephalosporins. As a class the cephalosporins are very safe and effective antibiotics, and they should not be unnecessarily avoided out of overly cautious concern about possible cross-sensitivity.

Penicillins and cephalosporins are practically identical in their mechanism of action, drug effects, therapeutic effects, side effects and adverse effects, and drug interactions. For that reason this information is not repeated for the cephalosporins and the reader is referred to the pertinent discussion in the section on the penicillin agents. Cephalosporins of all generations are very safe agents that are categorized as pregnancy category B drugs. They are contraindicated in patients who have shown a hypersensitivity to them and in infants younger than 1 month of age. The prototypical first-, second-, third-, and fourth-generation cephalosporins are described in the following drug profiles section.

Dosages

For the recommended dosages of selected cephalosporin agents, see the dosages table on p. 577.

---

drug profiles

FIRST-GENERATION CEPHALOSPORINS

First-generation cephalosporins are usually active against gram-positive bacteria and have limited activity against gram-negative bacteria. They are available both in parenteral and oral forms. One of the most frequently used parenteral first-generation cephalosporins is cefazolin; cephalexin is a very frequently used oral first-generation cephalosporin.

cefazolin sodium

Cefazolin (Ancef, Kefzol) is a prototypical first-generation cephalosporin. As with all first-generation

cephalosporins, it has excellent coverage against gram-positive bacteria but limited coverage against gram-negative bacteria. It is only available in a parenteral formulation that 500- and 1000-mg vials for IM or IV injection. Commonly recommended dosages are given in the dosages table on p. 577.

PHARMACOKINETICS

HALF-LIFE	ONSET	PEAK	DURATION
1.2-2.2 hr	Variable	1-2 hr	Variable

cephalexin

Cephalexin (Keflex, Keftab) is a prototypical oral first-generation cephalosporin. It also has excellent coverage against gram-positive bacteria but limited coverage against gram-negative bacteria. It is only available in oral formulations—250- and 500-mg capsules (Keflex pulvules); a 125- and 250-mg/5 ml oral suspension; 250-mg film-coated tablets (Keflex); and 250- and 500-mg tablets (Keftab). Commonly recommended dosages can be found in the dosages table on p. 577.

PHARMACOKINETICS

HALF-LIFE	ONSET	PEAK	DURATION
0.5-1.2 hr	Variable	1 hr	6-12 hr

SECOND-GENERATION CEPHALOSPORINS

Second-generation cephalosporins have similar coverage against gram-positive organisms as the first-generation cephalosporins but enhanced gram-negative coverage. They include both parenteral and oral formulations. Like first-generation agents, second-generation cephalosporins are also excellent prophylactic antibiotics because of their favorable safety profile, broad range of organisms they can kill, and relatively low cost. Currently there are seven parenteral second-generation cephalosporins (cefamandole, cefoxitin, cefuroxime, cefonicid, ceforanide, cefmetazole, and cefotetan) and three oral agents (cefaclor, cefuroxime axetil, and cefprozil).

DOSAGES Selected Cephalosporin Agents

agent	pharmacologic class	dosage range	purpose
cefazolin sodium (Ancef, Kefzol)	1st-generation cephalosporin	*Pediatric* IM/IV: 25-50 mg/kg/day in 3-4 doses; doses up to 100 mg/kg/day may be required. *Adult* IM/IV: 25- mg-1 g q8-12h; dose up to 1.5 g q6h may be required.	Antiinfective
cefepime (Maxipime)	4th-generation cephalosporin	*Adult* IV: 0.5-2 g q12h	Antiinfective
cefixime (Suprax)	3rd-generation cephalosporin	*Pediatric* PO: 8 mg/kg/day as a single dose or 4 mg/kg q12h *Adult* PO: 400 mg/day as a single dose or 200 mg q12h	Antiinfective
cefoxitin (Mefoxin)	2nd-generation cephalosporin	*Pediatric* IM/IV: 80-160 mg/kg/day in 4-6 equal doses *Adult* IM/IV: 1-3 g q4-8h	Antiinfective
ceftazidime (Ceptaz, Fortaz, Tazidime, Tazicef)	3rd-generation cephalosporin	*Neonatal* IV: 30 mg/kg q12h *Infant/Child* IV: 30-50 mg/kg q8h	Antiinfective
ceftriaxone (Rocephin)	3rd-generation cephalosporin	*Pediatric* IM/IV: 50-75 mg/kg/day divided q12h *Adult* IM/IV: 1-4 g/day as a single dose or divided	Antiinfective
cefuroxime (Ceftin, Kefurox, Zinacef)	2nd-generation cephalosporin	*Pediatric >3 mo* IM/IV: 50-100 mg/kg/day in 3-4 doses *Adult* IM/IV: 0.75-1.5 g q6-8h	Antiinfective
cephalexin (Keflex, Keftab)	1st-generation cephalosporin	*Pediatric* PO: 25-50 mg/kg/day divided; doses up to 100 mg/kg/day may be required *Adult* PO: 1-4 g/day divided	Antiinfective

These agents differ slightly with regard to their antibacterial coverage. Cefoxitin and cefotetan may have better coverage against various anaerobic bacteria such as *Bacteroides fragilis, Peptostreptococcus* spp., and *Clostridium* spp. than the other agents in this class. Three second-generation agents (cefoxitin, cefmetazole, and cefotetan) are structurally different from the other agents in the class by having a methoxy group rather than a hydrogen group on the beta-lactam ring of the cephalosporin nucleus. They are called *cephamycins.* Their unique structure enables them to kill certain bacteria that the other second-generation agents cannot.

cefoxitin

Cefoxitin (Mefoxin) is a parenteral second-generation cephalosporin that, because of its unique structure, is a cephamycin. Being a second-generation cephalosporin, it has excellent gram-positive coverage and better gram-negative coverage than the first-

generation agents. Because it is a cephamycin, it can kill anaerobic bacteria. Cefoxitin has been used extensively as a prophylactic antibiotic in patients undergoing such surgerical procedures as abdominal or colorectal operations because it can kill the bacteria that usually reside in these areas (gram-positive and gram-negative bacteria and anaerobes). Like the other cephalosporins, it is very safe and is rated as a pregnancy category B agent. Its contraindications are the same as those of the other cephalosporins. Cefoxitin is only available in parenteral preparations: 1-, 2-, and 10-g vials for injection and a 20- and 40-mg/ml frozen powder for injection. Commonly recommended dosages can be found in the dosages table above.

PHARMACOKINETICS

HALF-LIFE	ONSET	PEAK	DURATION
30-60 min	Variable	20-30 min	Variable

cefuroxime

Cefuroxime sodium (Kefurox, Zinacef) is the parenteral form of this second-generation cephalosporin. The oral form is a different salt of cefuroxime, cefuroxime axetil (Ceftin). Cefuroxime is a very versatile second-generation cephalosporin. It is also highly used as a prophylactic antibiotic for various surgical procedures. It has more activity against gram-negative bacteria than first-generation cephalosporins but a narrower spectrum of activity against gram-negative bacteria than third-generation cephalosporins. It differs from the cephamycins such as cefoxitin in that it does not kill anaerobic bacteria. Cefuroxime axetil is a prodrug. It has little antibacterial activity until it is hydrolyzed in the liver to its active form. It is available as 125-, 250-, and 500-mg film-coated tablets. Cefuroxime sodium is available as 750-mg, 1.5-g, and 7.5-g vials for injection. Commonly recommended dosages can be found in the dosages table on p. 577.

PHARMACOKINETICS

HALF-LIFE	ONSET	PEAK	DURATION
1.2 hr	Variable	2.2-3 hr	6-8 hr

THIRD-GENERATION CEPHALOSPORINS

Third-generation cephalosporins (cefoperazone, cefotaxime, ceftizoxime, ceftriaxone, ceftazidime, and cefixime) are the most potent of the three generations of cephalosporins in fighting gram-negative bacteria, but they generally have less activity than first- and second-generation agents when it comes to destroying gram-positive bacteria. Slight changes in the chemical structure have endowed specific agents with certain advantages over the others.

Because of specific changes in their basic cephalosporin structure, cefoperazone and ceftazidime have significant activity against *Pseudomonas* spp. In fact, these two third-generation agents have the best activity of all the cephalosporins against this difficult-to-treat gram-negative bacteria. Cefoperazone differs from ceftazidime in that it is principally excreted in the bile rather than the kidneys, as ceftazidime is. Ceftriaxone is an extremely long-acting third-generation agent that can be given only once a day in the treatment of most infections. It also has the unique characteristic of being able to pass easily through the blood-brain barrier. For this reason, it is one of the few cephalosporins that is indicated for the treatment of meningitis, an infection of the meninges of the brain. Cefixime, cefpodoxime proxetil, and ceftibuten are currently the only oral third-generation cephalosporins. All the other third-generation agents are only available in parenteral forms.

cefixime

Structurally, cefixime (Suprax) is similar to cefotaxime, ceftizoxime, and ceftriaxone, but it differs from these three agents in that one aspect of its structure allows for better gastrointestinal absorption. It has better activity against gram-negative bacteria than other oral cephalosporins such as cefaclor, cefuroxime axetil, or cefprozil, but its gram-negative activity is less than that of many of the other parenterally administered third-generation cephalosporins, especially against Enterobacteriaceae such as *Enterobacter* and *Pseudomonas* spp. Cefixime is a prescription-only drug that has the same pregnancy rating and contraindications as the other cephalosporins. Cefixime is available as a 100-mg/5 ml oral suspension and as 200- and 400-mg film-coated tablets. Commonly recommended dosages can be found in the dosages table on p. 577.

PHARMACOKINETICS

HALF-LIFE	ONSET	PEAK	DURATION
2.4-4 hr	Variable	3-4.4 hr	12-24 hr

ceftriaxone

Ceftriaxone (Rocephin) is a parenterally administered third-generation cephalosporin that differs from the other agents in that it has a very long half-life that allows it to be given once a day. Structurally it resembles other third-generation agents such as cefotaxime and ceftizoxime, but it has an acidic enol group that distinguishes it from these other agents. This is believed to be responsible for the long serum half-life of the drug. Ceftriaxone's spectrum of activity is similar to that of the other third-generation agents cefotaxime and ceftizoxime. It can be given both intravenously and intramuscularly. In some cases of infections, one IM injection can eradicate the infection. Ceftriaxone is 93% to 96% bound to plasma protein, an amount higher than that of many of the other cephalosporins. It can also easily pass through the meninges and diffuse into the cerebrospinal fluid (CSF), making it an excellent agent for the treatment of CNS infections. Ceftriaxone is available as an injection that can be given either intramuscularly or intravenously. It is available as 250-mg, 500-mg, 1-g, 2-g, and 10-g vials. Commonly recommended dosages can be found in the dosages table on p. 577.

PHARMACOKINETICS

HALF-LIFE	ONSET	PEAK	DURATION
4.3-8.7 hr	Variable	IM: 2-4 hr	24 hr

ceftazidime

Ceftazidime (Ceptaz, Fortaz, Tazidime, Tazicef) is a parenterally administered third-generation cephalosporin with excellent coverage against difficult-to-treat gram-negative bacteria such as *Pseudomonas* spp. It differs from its closest third-generation relative cefoperazone in that it is eliminated renally as opposed to by the biliary route. It is the third-generation cephalosporin of choice for many indications because of its excellent spectrum of activity and safety profile. It can be given either intramuscularly or intravenously and to children as well as adults. It is available as 500-mg, 1-g, 2-g, 6-g, and 10-g vials for injection. Ceptaz was created so that the amount of gas produced when it is reconstituted is decreased. The gas produced can be so great that it expels the needle directly out of the vial. Commonly recommended dosages are given in the dosages table on p. 577.

PHARMACOKINETICS

HALF-LIFE	ONSET	PEAK	DURATION
2 hr	Variable	IM: 1 hr	8-12 hr

FOURTH-GENERATION CEPHALOSPORINS

Fourth-generation cephalosporins (cefepime, cefpirome, and cefdinir) have a broader spectrum of antibacterial activity (specifically against against gram-positive bacteria) and than third-generation cephalosporins. They may also be more resistant to beta-lactamases, enzymes capable of destroying beta-lactam antibiotics like cephalosporins. Of the three fourth-generation cephalosporins, only cefepime is presently available in the United States. Cefepime and cefpirome are both parenteral antibiotics, whereas cefdinir is an oral agent. Cefdinir is presently the largest selling cephalosporin in Japan.

cefepime

Cefepime (Maxipime) is the prototypical fourth-generation cephalosporin. Cefepime is a broad-spectrum cephalosporin that most closely resembles ceftazidime in its spectrum of activity. It differs from ceftazidime in that it has increased activity against many enterobacter species and gram-positive organisms. This characteristic defines it as a fourth-generation cephalosporin. Cefepime is indicated for the treatment of uncomplicated and complicated UTIs, uncomplicated skin and skin-structure infections, and pneumonia. Cefepime is a prescription-only drug that is contraindicated in patients with a history of hypersensitivity to it or other cephalosporins. It is classified as a pregnancy category B agent. Cefepime is only available in parenteral preparations: 500-mg, 1-g, and 2-g vials for injection. Commonly recommended dosages can be found in the dosages table on p. 577.

PHARMACOKINETICS

HALF-LIFE	ONSET	PEAK	DURATION
2 hr	0.5 hr	0.5-1.5 hr	8-12 hr

TETRACYCLINES

The tetracyclines are a small chemically related group of five antibiotics, three of which are naturally occurring and two of which are semisynthetic. They are derivatives of *Streptomyces* organisms. Although the tetracyclines are bacteriostatic, the body's own host defense mechanisms are helping to kill bacteria as well. The three naturally occurring tetracyclines are demeclocycline, oxytetracycline, and tetracycline. The two semisynthetic tetracyclines are doxycycline and minocycline. The available tetracycline antibiotics and a brief description of them is given in Box 36-3.

Tetracyclines are chemically and pharmacologically similar to one another. The most significant chemical characteristic of these agents is their ability to bind (chelate) to divalent (Ca^{2+}, Mg^{2+}) and trivalent metallic (Al^{3+}) ions to form insoluble complexes. Therefore their coadministration with milk, antacids, or iron salts causes a considerable reduction in the oral absorption of the tetracycline. In addition, their strong affinity for calcium usually precludes their use in pediatric patients younger than 8 years of age, pregnant women, and nursing mothers (tetracyclines are present in breast milk).

Tetracyclines primarily differ from one another in the following ways:

- Oral absorption rates: all are adequately absorbed, but doxycycline and minocycline are absorbed the most.
- Body tissue penetration: doxycycline and minocycline possess the best penetration potential (brain and CSF).
- Half-life and resulting dosage schedule: see the dosages table on p. 581 and pharmacokinetics information in the drug profiles section.

Mechanism of Action

Tetracyclines work by inhibiting protein synthesis in susceptible bacteria. For this synthesis to occur, transfer RNA must bind to the messenger RNA ribosome. The tetracyclines obstruct this synthesis by binding to that portion of the ribosome called the *30S subunit*. This in turn shuts down many of the bacteria's essential functions, such as growth and repair, so that eventually the bacteria stops growing and dies.

BOX 36-3

Available Tetracycline Antibiotics

Tetracycline Product	Description
NATURAL TETRACYCLINES	
demeclocycline	All chemically derived from *Streptomyces* spp. by a fermentation process.
oxytetracycline	
tetracycline	
SEMISYNTHETIC TETRACYCLINES	
doxycycline	Chemical derivative of oxytetracycline.
minocycline	Chemical derivative of tetracycline.

Drug Effects

Tetracyclines are used primarily for their antibiotic effects. They inhibit the growth of and kill a very wide range of *Rickettsia, Chlamydia,* and *Mycoplasma* organisms, as well as a variety of gram-negative and gram-positive bacteria. They are also useful in the treatment of spirochetal infections such as syphilis and Lyme disease. Demeclocycline possesses a unique drug effect in that it inhibits the action of antidiuretic hormone, making it useful in the treatment of the syndrome of inappropriate antidiuretic hormone (SIADH). Another drug effect of tetracyclines is their ability to cause inflammation that results in fibrosis in the lungs. This is a useful property in patients with pleural or pericardial effusions caused by metastatic tumors, thoracentesis, or thoracastomy tubes, because when instilled into the pleural space of the lungs, they cause scar tissue to form, thereby reducing the fluid accumulation.

Therapeutic Uses

Tetracyclines have a wide range of activity and as a class have essentially the same antimicrobial spectrum. They inhibit the growth of many gram-negative and gram-positive organisms and even some protozoa. They are considered the drugs of choice for the treatment of the following infections caused by susceptible organisms:

- *Chlamydia:* lymphogranuloma venereum, psittacosis, and nonspecific endocervical, rectal, and urethral infections.
- *Mycoplasma:* Mycoplasma pneumonia.
- *Rickettsia:* Q fever, rickettsial pox, Rocky Mountain spotted fever, scrub typhus, typhus.
- *Other bacteria:* acne control, brucellosis, chancroid, cholera, granuloma inguinale, shigellosis, and spirochetal relapsing fever. In addition, it is used for the treatment of Lyme disease and as part of the treatment regimen for *Helicobacter pylori* infections associated with peptic ulcer disease. It is also used as an alternative agent in penicillin-allergic patients for treatment of gonorrhea and syphilis.
- *Protozoa:* balantidiasis.

Besides these antibiotic-related indications, as previously noted, demeclocycline is also used to treat SIADH as well as pleural and pericardial effusions.

Side Effects and Adverse Effects

Tetracyclines cause similar side effects and adverse effects. They can cause discoloration of the permanent teeth and tooth enamel hypoplasia in both fetuses and children and possibly retard fetal skeletal development if taken during pregnancy. Other clinically significant undesirable effects include photosensitivity, with the highest incidence of this seen in patients taking demeclocycline, and alteration of the intestinal flora, resulting in the following:

- Overgrowth of nonsusceptible organisms (superinfection), especially *Candida* and pediatric staphylococcal enteritis
- Diarrhea
- Pseudomembranous colitis

They can also alter the vaginal flora, resulting in moniliasis; cause reversible bulging fontanelles in neonates; precipitate thrombocytopenia, possible coagulation irregularities, and hemolytic anemia; and exacerbate systemic lupus erythematosus. Other effects include gastric upset, enterocolitis, and maculopapular rash.

Interactions

There are several significant drug interactions associated with the use of tetracyclines. When taken with antacids, antidiarrheal agents, dairy products, or iron preparations, the oral absorption of the tetracycline is reduced. Nephrotoxicity may occur when they are taken with methoxyflurane. Their use with oral anticoagulants requires caution, and they can also antagonize the effects of bactericidal antibiotics.

In addition, depending on the dose, they can cause the blood urea nitrogen (BUN) levels to be increased.

Dosages

For dosage information for selected tetracyclines, see the dosages table on p. 581.

drug profiles

Tetracyclines were one of the first class of antibiotics capable of a wide range of antibiotic coverage. They are also unique in that they are useful in the treatment of conditions other than bacterial infections. In this regard they are used for the treatment of SIADH and as sclerosing agents in the treatment of pleural effusions. They are prescription-only drugs that are potentially harmful to children younger than 8 years of age and that should not be given to pregnant women because by binding to calcium they can prevent normal bone growth and cause tooth enamel hypoplasia in the child or the fetus. They are also contraindicated in patients who have had hypersensitivity reactions to them in the past and in lactating women. Resistance to one tetracycline implies resistance to all tetracyclines. They are classified as pregnancy category D agents.

demeclocycline

Demeclocycline (Declomycin) is a naturally occurring tetracycline antibiotic that is derived from strains of *Streptomyces.* It is used both for its antibacterial action and for its ability to inhibit SIADH. Demeclocycline has all the characteristics of this class of tetracyclines. It is only available orally as 150- and 300-mg film-coated tablets. Commonly recommended dosages can be found in the dosages table on p. 581. Pregnancy category D.

PHARMACOKINETICS

HALF-LIFE	ONSET	PEAK	DURATION
10-17 hr	Variable	3-4 hr	6-12 hr

DOSAGES Selected Tetracycline Agents

agent	pharmacologic class	dosage range	purpose
demeclocycline (Declomycin)	Tetracycline	*Pediatric >8 y/o* PO: 6-12 mg/kg divided in 2-4 doses *Adult* PO: 150 mg q6h	Antiinfective
doxycycline (Doryx, Doxy-Caps, Doxy-Tabs Vibramycin, Vibra-Tabs)	Tetracycline	*Pediatric >8 y/o* PO/IV: 4.4 mg/kg/day in divided doses on day 1, then 2.2-4.4 mg/kg/day *Adult* PO: 200 mg day 1, followed by 100-200 mg/day	Antiinfective

doxycycline

Doxycycline (Doryx, Doxy-Caps, Doxy-Tabs, Vibramycin, Vibra-Tabs) is a semisynthetic tetracycline antibiotic that was made by altering the naturally occurring tetracycline oxytetracycline. Doxycycline is available in the following three salt forms: calcium, hyclate, and monohydrate. It is useful in the treatment of rickettsial infections such as Rocky Mountain spotted fever, chlamydial and mycoplasmal infections, gonorrhea, spirochetal infections, and many gram-negative infections. Doxycycline may also be used as a sclerosing agent in the treatment of pleural effusions.

It is available orally as a 25- and 50-mg/5 ml oral suspension; 50- and 100-mg capsules; 100-mg delayed-release capsules; and 100-mg film-coated tablets. It is also available as a parenteral agent in the form of 100- and 200-mg injections. Commonly recommended dosages can be found in the dosages table above. Pregnancy category D.

PHARMACOKINETICS

HALF-LIFE	ONSET	PEAK	DURATION
14-24 hr	Variable	1.5-4 hr	Up to 12 hr

AMINOGLYCOSIDES

The aminoglycosides are a group of natural and semisynthetic antibiotics that destroy bacteria rather than inhibit their growth, so they are **bactericidal antibiotics.** They are similar to the tetracyclines in that they are derived from *Streptomyces* organisms. The aminoglycoside antibiotics available for clinical use are listed in Box 36-4. These agents can be given by several different routes, but they are not given orally because of their poor oral absorption. An exception to this is the use of neomycin. When neomycin is administered orally, it is used to decontaminate the gastrointestinal tract.

Aminoglycosides are very potent antibiotics and are capable of potentially serious toxicities. As a result they are generally reserved for the treatment of more serious or life-threatening infections. They can kill both gram-positive and gram-negative bacteria but are customarily used to kill gram-negative bacteria such as *Pseudomonas* spp., *E. coli*, *Proteus* spp., *Klebsiella* spp., *Serratia* spp., and others because there are other less toxic antibiotics that are effective against the gram-positive bacteria they can kill. Often they are used in combination with other antibiotics such as cephalosporins, penicillins, or vancomycin in the treatment of various infections because the combined effect of the two antibiotics is greater than that of either agent alone. This is a phenomenon known as a *synergistic effect.*

Aminoglycosides work in a way that is similar to that of the tetracyclines in that they also bind to ribosomes and thereby prevent protein synthesis in bacteria. The three aminoglycosides most commonly used for the treatment of systemic infections are gentamicin, tobramycin, and amikacin. The serious toxicities of the aminoglycosides are renal failure and hearing loss (ototoxicity). Certain optimal drug blood levels are strived for to prevent these toxicities from occurring and to optimize the antibiotic killing power. Following are the levels for a few of these agents:

	Peak	Trough
Gentamicin and tobramycin	5-12 $\mu g/ml$	<2 $\mu g/ml$
Amikacin	20-35 $\mu g/ml$	<10 $\mu g/ml$

The ototoxicity associated with aminoglycoside use involves both auditory impairment and vestibular damage and is thought to be due in part to damage to the eighth cranial nerve inflicted by the agents proper. Symptoms include dizziness, tinnitus, and hearing loss. The nephrotoxicity, or renal failure, is manifested by urinary casts, proteinuria, and increased BUN and serum creatinine levels. In light of these potentially serious toxicities, patients receiving aminoglycosides should be monitored for the signs and symptoms of renal failure (rising BUN and creatinine levels) and hearing loss (fullness in ears, ringing in ears, and dizziness). The risk of these toxicities is greatest in patients with preexisting renal impairment, patients already receiving other renally toxic drugs, and patients on high doses of or prolonged aminoglycoside therapy.

Aminoglycosides should be administered with caution in premature and full-term neonates because of the renal

Box 36-4 Available Aminoglycoside Antibiotics

Origin	Aminoglycoside Product	Description
Natural	gentamicin kanamycin neomycin paromomycin streptomycin tobramycin	All chemically derived from *Streptomyces* spp. by a fermentation process.
Semisynthetic	amikacin netilmicin	Chemical derivative of kanamycin. Structurally related to gentamicin.

Box 36-5 Aminoglycosides: Specific Antibacterial Spectrums

Aminoglycoside	Spectrum
amikacin sulfate	*Acinetobacter* spp., *Enterobacter aerogenes*, *Escherichia coli*, *Klebsiella pneumoniae*, *Proteus* spp., *Providencia* spp., *Pseudomonas* spp., *Serratia* spp., *Staphylococcus* infections.
gentamicin sulfate	*E. aerogenes*, *E. coli*, *Klebsiella pneumoniae*, *Proteus* spp., *Pseudomonas* spp., *Salmonella* spp., *Serratia* spp. (nonpigmented), *Shigella* spp.
kanamycin sulfate	*Acinetobacter* spp., *E. coli*, *Klebsiella pneumoniae*, *Proteus* spp., *Serratia marcescens*. It is administered orally for the treatment of cirrhotic patients in hepatic coma caused by nitrogen-producing bacteria and for intestinal antisepsis.
neomycin sulfate	Toxicity limits use to gastrointestinal tract (hepatic coma, *E. coli* diarrhea, and antisepsis) and as a topical antibacterial.
netilmicin sulfate	*Citrobacter* spp., *Enterobacter* spp., *E. coli*, *Klebsiella pneumoniae*, *Proteus* spp., *Pseudomonas aeruginosa*, *Serratia* spp.
paromomycin sulfate	Amebic dysentery.
streptomycin sulfate	Granuloma inguinale, plague, tularemia, tuberculosis, nonhemolytic *Streptococcus* endocarditis.
tobramycin sulfate	*Citrobacter* spp., *Enterobacter* spp., *E. coli*, *Klebsiella* spp., *Proteus* spp., *Providencia* spp., *Pseudomonas aeruginosa*, *Serratia* spp.

immaturity of these patients, which can result in prolonged actions of the aminoglycosides and a greater risk of toxicities. Aminoglycosides have been shown to cross the placenta and cause fetal harm when administered to pregnant women. There have been several reports of total, irreversible bilateral congenital deafness in the children of women taking aminoglycosides during pregnancy. Therefore aminoglycosides should be used in pregnant women only in the event of life-threatening situations or severe infections when safer drugs either cannot be used or are ineffective. The pregnancy categories of the various aminoglycosides are as follows: gentamicin, C; tobramycin, D; amikacin, D; kanamycin, D; neomycin, C; netilmicin, D; and streptomycin, B. These antibiotics are also distributed in breast milk, so their use should be avoided in lactating women. Aminoglycosides are contraindicated in patients with a known hypersensitivity or a history of a serious toxic reaction to them.

Activity

Mechanism of Action

As previously mentioned, aminoglycosides kill bacteria by binding to and disrupting protein synthesis in bacteria. Specifically they do this by binding to both the 30S and 50S ribosomal subunits, structures that need to be functioning for protein synthesis to occur. When this process is disrupted, the bacterial cell eventually dies.

Drug Effects

The drug effects of the aminoglycosides are primarily limited to their ability to kill bacteria. They are active against many aerobic gram-negative bacteria and some aerobic gram-positive bacteria, but they are relatively inactive against fungi, viruses, and most anaerobic bacteria. Some aminoglycosides (e.g., streptomycin) are active against *Mycobacterium* spp. Other agents such as paromomycin are active against protozoal infections.

Therapeutic Uses

The toxicity associated with aminoglycosides restricts their use to the treatment of serious gram-negative infections and specific conditions involving gram-positive cocci, in which case gentamicin is usually given in combination with a penicillin. Paromomycin is used to treat amebic dysentery, a protozoal intestinal disease.

The selection of an aminoglycoside is based on the susceptibility of the causative organism. Serious *Pseudomonas* infections are treated with a suitable aminoglycoside and

DOSAGES Selected Aminoglycosides

agent	pharmacologic class	dosage range	purpose
amikacin (Amikin)	Aminoglycoside antibiotic	*Neonatal* IM/IV: 10-mg/kg loading dose, followed by 7.5 mg/kg q12h *Adult/Child* IM/IV: 15 mg/kg/day in 2-3 equal doses	Antiinfective
gentamicin (Garamycin, Gentamicin)	Aminoglycoside	*Neonatal <1 wk* IM/IV: 5 mg/kg/day *Neonatal/Infant* IM/IV: 7.5 mg/kg/day *Child* IM/IV: 6-7 mg/kg/day *Adult* IM/IV: 3-5 mg/kg/day	Antiinfective

an extended-spectrum penicillin. Refer to Box 36-5 for the antibacterial spectrums of specific aminoglycosides.

Side Effects and Adverse Effects

The most significant adverse effects of the aminoglycosides are ototoxicity and nephrotoxicity. Other undesirable effects include headache, paresthesia, neuromuscular blockade, dizziness, vertigo, skin rash, fever, and overgrowth of nonsusceptible organisms.

Interactions

There are several significant drug interactions associated with aminoglycoside use. Their use with neurotoxic or nephrotoxic drugs such as colistimethate, ethacrynic acid, furosemide, and polymyxin B should be avoided. The concurrent administration of dimenhydrinate can mask aminoglycoside toxicity, and the coadministration of a neuromuscular blocking agent can increase their activity. Calcium salts can be administered to reverse the blockade. In addition, their use with oral anticoagulants can increase the anticoagulant activity because they decrease intestinal vitamin K synthesis.

Dosages

For recommended dosages of selected aminoglycosides, see the dosages table above.

drug profiles

There are seven aminoglycoside antibiotics, but only three are commonly administered systemically—gentamicin, tobramycin, and amikacin. These agents should be used with extreme caution if at all in pregnant women and nursing mothers. Infants can tolerate aminoglycosides, but they should be given in smaller doses, the drug levels should be tightly monitored, and the infants should be closely watched for the occurrence of side effects. Aminoglycosides are frequently given in combination with other antibiotics such as penicillins, cephalosporins, and vancomycin.

amikacin

Amikacin (Amikin) is a semisynthetic aminoglycoside antibiotic derived by chemically altering kanamycin, a naturally occurring aminoglycoside. As previously noted, it differs from gentamicin and tobramycin in that its therapeutic drug levels are much higher than those of the other two agents. The peak levels should be between 20 and 35 μg/ml, and the trough level should be less than 10 μg/ml. Aiming for blood drug levels in this range accomplishes two essential goals. It (1) ensures that there will be sufficient antibiotic present to destroy the maximum amount of bacteria, and (2) prevents the unwanted nephrotoxicity and ototoxicity sometimes associated with aminoglycoside therapy.

Amikacin has the same contraindications as those mentioned for the aminoglycosides in general and is considered a pregnancy category D agent. It is available as a 50- and 250-mg/ml injection for IV administration. Commonly recommended dosages can be found in the dosages table above.

PHARMACOKINETICS

HALF-LIFE	ONSET	PEAK	DURATION
2-3 hr	Variable	1 hr	8-12 hr

gentamicin

Gentamicin (Garamycin, Gentamicin) is a naturally occurring aminoglycoside that is obtained from cultures of *Micromonospora purpurea*. It is one of the aminoglycosides most commonly used in clinical practice today. It has the same contraindications as the other aminoglycosides and is classified as a pregnancy C agent. It can be given either intravenously or intramuscularly, with the dosage the same for both routes. It is indicated for the treatment of several susceptible gram-positive and gram-negative bacteria. As previously discussed, the common therapeutic drug levels for gentamicin and tobramycin are lower than those for amikacin. Gentamicin is available in several dosage forms. It is available as a 10- and 40 mg/ml injection for IM or IV use; a 2-mg/ml injection for intrathecal use; and a 10-, 60-, 80-, and 100-mg/ml injection for IV infusion. It is also available as a 3% solution or ointment for ophthalmic use, and in this form is used for the treatment of eye infections. Gentamicin also is available as a 0.1% ointment for topical application on superficial skin infections, burns, and skin ulcers. Commonly recommended dosages can be found in the dosages table on p. 583.

PHARMACOKINETICS

HALF-LIFE	ONSET	PEAK	DURATION
2 hr	Variable	0.5-2 hr	8-12 hr

QUINOLONES

Quinolone antibiotics are very potent broad-spectrum antibiotics. They kill bacteria rather than inhibit their growth and are therefore bactericidal. The first of these agents to come available were cinoxacin and nalidixic acid. These two agents have narrower spectrums of activity (kill fewer kinds of bacteria) than the newer, more potent, and less toxic quinolones, and are therefore seldom used anymore. The newer quinolone antibiotics include, in order of their release onto the market, norfloxacin, ciprofloxacin, enoxacin, ofloxacin, lomefloxacin, perfloxacin, levofloxacin, and sparfloxacin. A fluorine atom was added onto the basic quinolone structure to create these newer agents, and this increased their antibacterial potency and made them able to kill a broader range of bacteria. Because of this chemical change, these agents are sometimes called *fluoroquinolones.*

Fluoroquinolones are active against a wide variety of gram-negative and selected gram-positive bacteria. Ciprofloxacin, norfloxacin, and ofloxacin are effective against an extensive spectrum of gram-negative bacteria. Enoxacin and lomefloxacin are effective against slightly fewer gram-negative bacteria, and of the gram-positive bacteria, they are only effective against *Staphylococcus* spp. Sparfloxacin and levofloxacin are the newest fluoroquinolone antimicrobials. Sparfloxacin and levofloxacin are somewhat more active than older fluoroquinolones against gram-positive organisms such as *S. pneumoniae,* including strains highly resistant to penicillin. *Enterococcus* and *Staphylococcus aureus* are also susceptible to sparfloxacin and levofloxacin. The characteristics of fluoroquinolone antibiotics and their therapeutic effects are summarized in Box 36-6.

Gatifloxacin and moxifloxacin have similar in vitro activity. Gatifloxacin is two to four times and moxifloxacin is four to eight times more active than levofloxacin against *S. pneumoniae,* including strains highly resistant to penicillin. It is uncertain whether these in vitro differences will mean anything clinically. Both gatifloxacin and moxifloxacin are active against some strains of *Staphy-loccus aureus* and enterococci, but methicillin-resistant staphylococci and vancomycin-resistant enterococci are generally also resistant to gatifloxacin and moxifloxacin. The activity of gatifloxacin and moxifloxacin against many enteric gram-negative bacteria and *Pseudomonas aeruginosa* is similar to that of levofloxacin and less than that of ciprofloxacin. Gatifloxacin and moxifloxacin have some in vitro activity anaerobes, although less than that of trovafloxacin (Trovan).

With the exception of norfloxacin, these antibiotics have excellent oral absorption. In many cases their oral absorption is as good as the rapidity with which the IV formulation is available. However, the concurrent use of antacids with fluoroquinolones causes their oral absorption to be greatly reduced. Fluoroquinolones are primarily excreted by the kidneys, which contain a high percentage of unchanged drug. Together with the fact that they have extensive gram-negative coverage, this makes them suitable for treating UTIs. Their use in children is not currently recommended because they have been shown to affect cartilage development in laboratory animals. The risks versus benefits must always be weighed when deciding whether to use a drug in this setting.

Mechanism of Action

Quinolone antibiotics destroy bacteria by altering their DNA. They accomplish this by interfering with DNA gyrase, the enzyme necessary for the synthesis of bacterial DNA. If bacteria cannot produce DNA, they die. Quinolones do not seem to affect the mammalian enzyme and therefore do not inhibit the production of human DNA.

Drug Effects

The drug effects of quinolone antibiotics are mostly limited to their effects on bacteria. They kill susceptible strains of mostly gram-negative organisms, and they are also capable of killing some gram-positive organisms. Some quinolones are also believed to diffuse into and concentrate themselves in human neutrophils, where some bacteria such as *Staphylococcus aureus, Serratia marcescens,* and *Mycobacterium fortuitum* reside. If they can do so to a sufficient extent, they can kill these bacteria.

Therapeutic Uses

Quinolone antibiotics are used in the treatment of various bacterial infections. The particular bacteria and the body site infected determine which quinolone is selected. Box 36-6 lists the available fluoroquinolone antibiotics, the broad range of bacteria they kill, and the indications for their use according to body site.

Side Effects and Adverse Effects

Fluoroquinolones are capable of causing some both serious and bothersome adverse effects, the most common of which are listed in Table 36-4. Bacterial overgrowth is another possible complication of quinolone therapy, but this is more commonly associated with long-term use.

Box 36-6   Fluoroquinolone Antibiotic Characteristics

Fluoroquinolone	Bacteria Killed	Indications
ciprofloxacin (Cipro)	Extensive gram-negative and selected gram-positive bacterial coverage	Lower respiratory tract infections, bone and joint infections, infectious diarrhea, urinary tract infections, skin infections
enoxacin (Penetrex)	Reduced gram-negative and gram-positive bacterial (*Staphylococcus*) coverage	Urinary tract infections, sexually transmitted diseases
lomefloxacin (Maxaquin)		Lower respiratory tract and urinary tract infections
norfloxacin (Noroxin)	Gram-negative and some gram-positive bacterial coverage	Urinary tract infections, sexually transmitted diseases
ofloxacin (Floxin)	Extensive gram-negative and selected gram-positive bacterial coverage	Urinary tract and lower respiratory tract infections, sexually transmitted diseases

Interactions

There are several drugs that interact with fluoroquinolones, with significant consequences. Their use with antacids, iron or zinc preparations, or sucralfate causes the oral absorption of the fluoroquinolone to be greatly reduced. Probenecid can reduce the renal excretion of the fluoroquinolone, and the use of some fluoroquinolones with theophylline may increase the toxicity of the bronchodilator. Nitrofurantoin can antagonize the antibacterial activity of the fluoroquinolones, and oral anticoagulants should be used with caution in patients receiving fluoroquinolones because of the antibiotic-induced alteration of the intestinal flora, which affects vitamin K synthesis.

drug profiles

Quinolones are broad-spectrum synthetic antibiotics with bactericidal activity. They are very effective in both their oral and parenteral forms and are used to treat a variety of infections, including urinary tract, lower respiratory tract, bone and joint, and skin and skin structure infections, as well as sexually transmitted diseases (STDs). Because of their excellent oral bioavailability, the oral forms of many of these quinolones are just as effective as their parenteral counterparts when given to patients with a functioning gastrointestinal tract. Quinolones are prescription-only agents that are classified as pregnancy category C agents. They are contraindicated in patients with a known hypersensitivity to them.

ciprofloxacin

Ciprofloxacin (Cipro) was one of the first of the newer broad-coverage, potent fluoroquinolones to come available. It was first marketed in an oral form and as such has the advantage and convenience of an oral medication. Also, because of its excellent bioavailability, it can work as well as many IV antibiotics. It is also capable of killing a wide range of gram-negative bacteria and is even effective against traditionally difficult to kill gram-negative bacteria such as *Pseudomonas*. Some anaerobic bacteria as

Table 36-4   Fluoroquinolones: Common Adverse Effects

Body System	Side/Adverse Effects
Central nervous system	Headache, dizziness, fatigue, insomnia, depression, restlessness, convulsions
Gastrointestinal	Nausea, constipation, increased AST (SGOT) and ALT (SGPT) (liver function tests), flatulence, heartburn, vomiting, diarrhea, oral candidiasis, dysphagia, pseudomembranous colitis
Integumentary	Rash, pruritus, urticaria, photosensitivity (with lomefloxacin), flushing
Other	Fever, chills, blurred vision, tinnitus

well as atypical organisms such as *Chlamydia, Mycoplasma,* and *Mycobacterium* can also be killed by ciprofloxacin. It is available in both oral and parenteral forms. Orally it is available as 250-, 500-, and 750-mg oral film-coated tablets. Parenterally it is available in doses of 200 and 400 mg contained in premixed bags for IV infusion or in a 10-mg/ml concentrate for IV injection. The common adult dosage of ciprofloxacin is 250 to 750 mg q12h. Also available as a 3.5-mg/ml ophthalmic solution and a 0.03% ophthalmic ointment.

PHARMACOKINETICS

HALF-LIFE	ONSET	PEAK	DURATION
3-4.8 hr	Variable	1-2.3 hr	Up to 12 hr

MACROLIDES

The macrolides are a large group of antibiotics that first became available in the early 1950s with the introduction of erythromycin. Macrolides are considered bacteriostatic; however, in high enough concentrations, they may be bactericidal in some susceptible bacteria. As with many of the other classes of antibiotics, macrolides inhibit the growth of bacteria by inhibiting protein synthesis, specifically by binding to the 50S ribosomal subunit.

There are five main macrolide antibiotics: azithromycin, clarithromycin, dirithromycin, erythromycin, and troleandomycin. Azithromycin and clarithromycin are two of the newer agents in the class. Although their spectrum of antibacterial activity is similar to that of erythromycin, they have longer durations of action than erythromycin, which allows them to be given less often; they produce fewer and less severe gastrointestinal tract side effects than erythromycin, and they need to be given for shorter lengths of time than many of the erythromycin products. They also exhibit better efficacy in eradicating various bacteria and are capable of better tissue penetration. Because erythromycin has a bitter taste and is quickly degraded by the acidity of the stomach, several salt forms and many dosage formulations were developed to circumvent these problems. These various salt forms and dosage formulations and the benefits of each are briefly summarized in Box 36-7.

Mechanism of Action

The mechanism of action of macrolide antibiotics is similar to that of other antibiotics. As previously mentioned, they bind to the 50S ribosomal subunit inside the cells of bacteria and by doing so prevent the production of the bacterial protein needed for the bacteria to grow, with the result that the bacteria eventually die. This action can immediately kill some susceptible strains of bacteria if the concentration of the macrolide is high enough.

Drug Effects

The drug effects of macrolide antibiotics are limited to their actions within bacteria. Macrolides are effective in the treatment of a wide range of infections. These include various infections of the upper and lower respiratory tract, skin, and soft tissue caused by some strains of *Streptococcus* and *Haemophilus*; spirochetal infections such as syphilis and Lyme disease; gonorrhea; *Chlamydia* and *Mycoplasma* infections; and *Listeria monocytogenes* and *Corynebacterium* infections. Because of its gastrointestinal tract–irritating properties, erythromycin affects the motility of the gastrointestinal tract. This property has been studied experimentally and may prove to be of benefit in increasing gastrointestinal motility in conditions such as delayed gastric emptying in diabetics.

Therapeutic Uses

The therapeutic effects of macrolide antibiotics are mostly limited to their antibacterial actions. Infections caused by *Streptococcus pyogenes* (group A beta-hemolytic streptococci) are inhibited by macrolides, as are mild to moderate upper and lower respiratory tract infections caused by *Haemophilus influenzae*. Spirochetal infections that are treated with erythromycins and other macrolides are syphilis and Lyme disease. Various forms of gonorrhea and *Chlamydia* and *Mycoplasma* infections are also susceptible to the effects of macrolides.

As previously noted, a therapeutic effect of erythromycin outside its antibiotic actions is its ability to irritate the gastrointestinal tract, which stimulates smooth muscle and gastrointestinal motility. This may be of benefit to patients who have decreased gastrointestinal motility. It has also been shown to be of some benefit for facilitating the passage of feeding tubes from the stomach into the small bowel. Azithromycin and clarithromycin have both been recently approved for the treatment of *Mycobacterium avium* complex (MAC) infections. Clarithromycin also has another new indication. It has been approved for use in combination with omeprazole for the treatment of patients with active ulcer associated with *Helicobacter pylori*.

Side Effects and Adverse Effects

Many of the older macrolide products, primarily erythromycin derivatives, have many side effects. Most affect the gastrointestinal tract, although the two newest macrolides, azithromycin and clarithromycin, seem to be as-

---

Box 36-7 Erythromycin Formulations

SALT FORMS

	BENEFIT
Stearate salt	Developed to overcome bitter
Estolate	taste of erythromycin
Ethylsuccinate ester	

DOSAGE FORMULATIONS

Film coated	Developed to overcome bitter
Enteric coated (pellets and particles)	taste and to protect the erythromycin from acid degradation in the stomach.

STRUCTURAL CHANGES

Semisynthetic macrolides:	Developed to improve
Azide group (azithromycin)	resistance to acid degradation in the stomach and increase
Methylation of hydroxy group (clarithromycin)	tissue penetration in order to improve antibiotic efficacy.

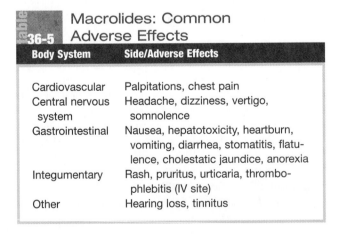

Table 36-5 Macrolides: Common Adverse Effects

Body System	Side/Adverse Effects
Cardiovascular	Palpitations, chest pain
Central nervous system	Headache, dizziness, vertigo, somnolence
Gastrointestinal	Nausea, hepatotoxicity, heartburn, vomiting, diarrhea, stomatitis, flatulence, cholestatic jaundice, anorexia
Integumentary	Rash, pruritus, urticaria, thrombophlebitis (IV site)
Other	Hearing loss, tinnitus

sociated with a lower incidence of these gastrointestinal tract complications. The most common of these adverse effects are listed in Table 36-5.

Interactions

The drugs that compete for hepatic metabolism with the macrolides are carbamazepine, cyclosporine, and warfarin. When these drugs are given with macrolides it results in enhanced effects. Sometimes this is done intentionally so that smaller doses of the drugs can be given, possibly decreasing the incidence of other less desirable side effects. Other times it is unintentional and can result in toxic effects. When theophylline and macrolides are given concurrently, there is a decreased clearance of theophylline, which can lead to increased theophylline effects. Two properties of macrolides that are the source of many of these interactions are that they are highly protein bound and they are metabolized in the liver. Drugs that are bound to protein are usually bound to albumin in the blood, making them inactive. When they are displaced from these binding sites on albumin and are then free and unbound, they become active. Therefore when a patient is given two or more drugs that compete for the same binding sites on albumin in the blood, one will not successfully bind, with the result that it is free in the blood and active. That drug will then have a greater action or effect in the body. A similar situation arises when two drugs are competing for metabolism in the liver. The result is a delay in the drugs' metabolism and thus a prolonged drug effect.

Dosages

For dosage information on selected macrolide antibiotics, see the dosages table below.

drug profiles

Macrolide antibiotics are used to treat a variety of infections ranging from Lyme disease to Legionnaire's disease. Of the four macrolide agents currently available, erythromycin has been around the longest and has been the mainstay of the treatment for various infections for more than four decades. Azithromycin and clarithromycin have fewer side effect profiles and a better pharmacokinetics profile than older agents.

All macrolides are prescription-only drugs and are rated as a pregnancy category C agents. They are contraindicated in patients with a known hypersensitivity to macrolides or with preexisting liver disease. As previously noted, because these agents are highly protein bound and metabolized in the liver, they may interfere with other drugs that are also highly protein bound or hepatically metabolized.

⊶erythromycin

Erythromycin, which goes by many product names, is the most frequently prescribed macrolide antibiotic. It is available in several different salt and dosage forms that were developed to circumvent some of the drawbacks it has chemically. (See Box 36-7 on erythromycin formulations that summarizes these benefits).

The absorption of oral erythromycin is enhanced if it is taken on an empty stomach, but because of the high incidence of stomach irritation associated with its use, many of the agents are taken after a meal or snack. The various salt forms and dosage formulations, their strengths, and product names are listed in Box 36-8.

DOSAGES   Selected Macrolide Antibiotic Agents

agent	pharmacologic class	dosage range	purpose
azithromycin (Zithromax)	Semisynthetic macrolide antibiotic	*Adult/Child >16 y/o* PO: 500 mg as a single dose on day 1 followed by 250 mg once/day 1 hr ac or 2 hr pc PO for MAC infections: Prophylaxis = 1200 mg once weekly treatment = 500 mg once daily IV: 500 mg qd for at least 2 days followed by PO at 500 mg qd for a 7-10 day course of therapy* *Child <16 y/o* PO: 10 mg/kg on day 1 followed by 5 mg/kg on days 2-5†	Antiinfective
clarithromycin (Biaxin)	Semisynthetic macrolide antibiotic	*Adult/Child >12 y/o* PO: 250-500 mg q12h PO for *H. pylori* infections: 500 mg q8h with omeprazole 40 mg daily for 14 days	Antiinfective
⊶erythromycin (many trade names)	Microbial antibiotic	*Child* PO: 30-100 mg/kg/day divided *Adult* PO: 250-500 mg qid	Antiinfective

MAC, Mycobacterium avium complex.
*Dosing of azithromycin for community-acquired pneumonia.
†Dosing of azithromycin for otitis media.

azithromycin and clarithromycin

Azithromycin (Zithromax) and clarithromycin (Biaxin) are semisynthetic macrolide antibiotics that differ structurally from erythromycin and as a result have advantages over erythromycin. These include better side effect profiles and pharmacokinetic properties. They also cause less gastrointestinal tract irritation. Both have very similar spectrums of activity that differ only slightly from that of erythromycin, and the two agents are used for the treatment of both upper and lower respiratory tract and skin and skin structure infections.

Azithromycin is capable of excellent tissue penetration, allowing it to reach high concentrations in infected tissues. It also has a long duration of action, allowing it to be dosed once daily. Azithromycin is available orally as 250- and 600-mg tablets; as 100-mg/5 ml, 200-mg/5 ml, and 1-g single dose pack oral suspension; and as a 500-mg vial for parenteral administration. Azithromycin is recommended for use in adults and children. Food decreases both the rate and extent of gastrointestinal absorption. Commonly recommended dosages can be found in the dosages table above.

Clarithromycin can be given only twice daily and is recommended for use in adults and children 12 years of age or older. Its safety and efficacy in younger patients has not been established. It is also available orally as 250- and 500-mg film-coated tablets and as 125-mg/5 ml and 250-mg/5 ml oral suspension. Common dosages are found in the dosages table on p. 587.

PHARMACOKINETICS

Azithromycin*

HALF-LIFE	ONSET	PEAK	DURATION
6-8 hr	Variable	2.5 hr	Up to 24 hr

Clarithromycin

HALF-LIFE	ONSET	PEAK	DURATION
3-7 hr	Variable	2 hr	Up to 12 hr

*For oral formulation.

MISCELLANEOUS ANTIBIOTICS

There are many categories of antibiotics, with aminoglycosides, cephalosporins, macrolides, penicillins, tetracyclines, quinolones, and sulfonamides representing the bulk of the antibiotics used in clin-

---

BOX 36-8   Erythromycin Dosage Forms and Product Names

Form	Strength	Product Name
ERYTHROMYCIN BASE (PO)		
Capsules		
Delayed release (enteric-coated pellets)	250 mg	ERYC, ERYC Sprinkle
Tablets		
Delayed release (enteric-coated particles)	333 and 500 mg	PCE Dispertab
Delayed release (enteric coated)	250, 333, and 500 mg	E-mycin, Ery-Tab, and E-base
Film-coated	250 and 500 mg	Erythromycin Base Filmtab
ERYTHROMYCIN ESTOLATE (PO)		
Capsules	250 mg	Ilosone Pulvules
Tablets	500 mg	Ilosone
Suspension	125 and 250 mg/5 ml	Ilosone Liquid
ERYTHROMYCIN ETHYLSUCCINATE (PO)		
Tablets		
Chewable	200 mg	Eryped
Film-coated	400 mg	E.E.S. 400 Filmtab
Suspension		
Drops	100 mg/2.5 ml	Eryped Drops
Oral suspension	200 and 400 mg/5 ml	Eryped 200 and 400
Oral liquid	200 and 400 mg/5 ml	E.E.S. 200 and 400
ERYTHROMYCIN GLUCEPTATE (IV)		
Parenteral	1 g	Ilotycin Gluceptate Intra Venous
ERYTHROMYCIN LACTOBIONATE (IV)		
Parenteral	500 mg and 1 g	Erythrocin Lactobionate IV, Erythrocin Piggyback
ERYTHROMYCIN STEARATE (PO)		
Tablets		
Film-coated	250 and 500 mg	Erythrocin Stearate Filmtab

ical practice. There are, however, some other important antibiotics that deserve quick mention. These are aztreonam, clindamycin, dapsone, imipenem, polypeptide antibiotics, and vancomycin. For common dosages, see the dosages table below.

aztreonam

Aztreonam (Azactam) is a synthetic monobactam antibiotic that is primarily active against aerobic gram-negative bacteria. Aztreonam is a bactericidal antibiotic, and it destroys bacteria by inhibiting bacterial cell wall synthesis, resulting in lysis. Aztreonam is indicated for the treatment of moderately severe systemic and urinary tract infections.

Aztreonam is a prescription-only drug that can be given either intramuscularly or intravenously. It is classified as a pregnancy category B agent and is contraindicated in patients with a known hypersensitivity to it, penicillin, or the cephalosporins. Only 6% to 16% of the agent is metabolized by the liver, with most of it excreted unchanged by the kidneys. Aztreonam is associated with no significant drug interactions worth mentioning. It is only available

in a parenteral form in 500-mg, 1-g, and 2-g vials for injection. Common dosages are found in the dosages table below.

PHARMACOKINETICS

HALF-LIFE	ONSET	PEAK	DURATION
1.5-2 hr	Variable	IM: 1 hr	6-12 hr

clindamycin

Clindamycin (Cleocin, Cleocin Pediatric, Cleocin Phosphate) is a semisynthetic derivative of lincomycin, an older antibiotic. Like many semisynthetic derivatives, it was improved over its predecessor agents through the addition of certain chemical groups to the basic structure, with the result that it is more effective and causes fewer adverse effects than its parent compound.

Clindamycin can be either bactericidal or bacteriostatic, depending on the concentration of the drug at the site of infection and on the infecting bacteria. It inhibits protein synthesis in bacteria by binding to the 50S ribosomal subunit, the same site as erythromycin. It is indicated for the treatment of chronic bone

DOSAGES Selected Miscellaneous Agents

agent	pharmacologic class	dosage range	purpose
aztreonam (Azactam)	Monobactam antibiotic	*Adult* IM/IV: 500 mg-2 g q8-12h	Antiinfective
clindamycin (Cleocin, Pediatric, Cleocin Phosphate)	Lincosamide antibiotic	*Neonatal* IM/IV: 15-20 mg/kg/day in 3-4 equal doses *Pediatric >1 mo* IM/IV: 20-40 mg/kg/day in 3-4 equal doses *Pediatric <10 kg* PO: 37.5 mg tid *Pediatric* PO: 8-25 mg/kg/day in 3-4 equal doses *Adult* PO: 15-450 mg q6h IV: 600-2700 mg/day in 2-4 equal doses	Antiinfective
imipenem-cilastatin (Primaxin)	Antibiotic combination	*Adult* IV: 250 mg-1 g q6-8h	Antiinfective
linezolid (Zyvox)	Oxazolidinone	*Adult* IV: 600 mg q12h	Antiinfective
quinupristin/ dalfopristin (Synercid)	Streptogramin antibiotic	*Adult* IV: 7.5 mg/kg/q8h	Antiinfective
vancomycin (Lyphocin, Vancocin, Vancoled)	Glycopeptide antibiotic	*Neonatal* IV: 15 mg/kg, followed by 10 mg/kg q12h for first week and q8h thereafter up to 1 mo of age *Pediatric* IV: 40 mg/kg/day divided PO: 40 mg/kg/day in 3-4 divided doses for 7-10 days IV: 15 mg/kg q12h *Adult* IV: 1 g q12h PO: 250-500 mg q6h	Antiinfective

infections, genitourinary tract infections, intraabdominal infections, anaerobic pneumonia, septicemia caused by streptococci and staphylococci, and serious skin and soft tissue infections caused by susceptible bacteria. Most aerobic gram-positive bacteria, including staphylococci, streptococci, and pneumococci, are susceptible to clindamycin's actions. It is also active against several anaerobic organisms.

Clindamycin is classified as a pregnancy category B agent and is contraindicated in patients with a known hypersensitivity to it, those with ulcerative colitis or enteritis, and infants younger than 1 month old. Gastrointestinal tract side effects are the most common and include nausea, vomiting, abdominal pain, diarrhea, pseudomembranous colitis, and anorexia. Clindamycin is available in both an oral and parenteral form. Orally it is available as 75-, 150-, and 300-mg capsules and as a 75-mg/5 ml oral suspension. Parenterally it is available in 300-, 600-, and 900-mg vials for injection. It is also available as a 2% vaginal cream, a lotion, and a topical solution. Common dosages are found in the dosages table on p. 589.

PHARMACOKINETICS

HALF-LIFE	ONSET	PEAK	DURATION
2.4 hr	Variable	45 min	6 hr

imipenem-cilastatin

Imipenem-cilastatin (Primaxin) is a fixed combination of imipenem, which is a semisynthetic carbapenem antibiotic similar to beta-lactam antibiotics, and cilastatin, an inhibitor of an enzyme that breaks down imipenem. Imipenem has a wide spectrum of activity against gram-positive and gram-negative aerobic and anaerobic bacteria. Cilastatin is a unique drug in that it inhibits an enzyme in the kidneys called *dihydropeptidase*, which if not inhibited quickly, would break down the imipenem. Cilastatin also blocks the renal tubular secretion of imipenem, which also prevents imipenem from being metabolized by the kidneys, the primary route of excretion of the agent. Meropenem (Merrem) is the second agent in this class of antibiotics called *carbapenems*. Meropenem appears to be somewhat less active against gram-positive organisms, more active against Enterobacteriaceae, and equally active against *Pseudomonas aeruginosa* than imipenem.

Imipenem exerts its antibacterial effect by binding to penicillin-binding proteins inside bacteria, which in turn inhibits bacterial cell wall synthesis. Imipenem kills bacteria and is therefore bactericidal. Unlike many of the penicillins and cephalosporins, imipenem is very resistant to the antibiotic-inhibiting actions of beta-lactamases. There are no significant drug interactions associated with imipenem use. The most serious adverse effect of imipenem therapy are seizures, which have been reported to occur in 1.5% of the patients receiving <500 mg q6h. However, in patients receiving high doses of the agent (>500 mg q6h), there is about a 10% incidence of seizures. Seizures are more likely in the elderly and the renally impaired.

Imipenem is indicated for the treatment of bone, joint, skin, and soft tissue infections; bacterial endocarditis caused by *S. aureus,* intraabdominal bacterial infections; pneumonia; urinary tract and pelvic infections; and bacterial septicemia caused by susceptible bacterial organisms. Imipenem is classified as a pregnancy C agent and is contraindicated in patients with a known hypersensitivity to it or to local anesthetics of the amide type. Imipenem is only available parenterally as 250- and 500-mg vials for IV injection and as 500- and 750-mg vials for IM injection. Common dosages are given in the dosages table on p. 589.

PHARMACOKINETICS

HALF-LIFE	ONSET	PEAK	DURATION
2-3 hr	Variable	2 hr	6-8 hr

linezolid

Linezolid (Zyvox) is the first antibacterial drug in a new class of antibiotics known as *oxazolidinones*. Linezolid is used to treat infections associated with vancomycin-resistant *Enterococcus faecium* (VREF), more commonly referred to as *VRE.* Linezolid has also received approval for treatment of hospital-acquired pneumonia and complicated skin and skin structure infections, including cases caused by methicillin-resistant *Staphylococcus aureus* (MRSA). In addition, aprpoval was granted for treatment of community-acquired pneumonia and uncomplicated skin and skin structure infections. The most frequently reported side effects attributed to linezolid are headache, nausea, diarrhea, and vomiting. It has also been shown to decrease platelet count. It is contraindicated in patients with a known hypersensitivity to it. It is considered a pregnancy category C agent. It is available as 200-mg/100 ml, 400-mg/200 ml, and 600-mg/300 ml plastic infusion bags; 400- and 600-mg tablets; and a 100-mg/5 ml-240 ml suspension. Common dosages are listed in the dosages table on p. 589.

PHARMACOKINETICS

HALF-LIFE	ONSET	PEAK	DURATION
5 hr	1–2 hr	1–2 hr	12 hr

quinupristin/dalfopristin

Quinupristin and dalfopristin (Synercid) are two streptogramin antibacterials marketed in a 30:70 combination. They are approved for IV treatment of bacteremia and life-threatening infection caused by VRE and for treatment of complicated skin and skin structure infections caused by *Staphylococcus aureus* and *Streptococcus pyogenes*. These two strep-togramin antibacterials work synergistically on the bacterial ribosome to disrupt protein synthesis.

Common side effects are arthralgias and myalgias, which may become severe. Adverse effects related to the infusion site, including pain, inflammation, edema, and thrombophlebitis, have developed in about 75% of patients treated through a peripheral IV. It is contraindicated in patients with a known hyper-sensitivity to it, pristinamycin, or virginiamycin. It is considered a pregnancy category B agent. It is avail-able a 500-mg powder for injection containing 350 mg of dalfopristin and 150 mg of quinupristin. Common dosages are listed in the dosages table on p. 589.

PHARMACOKINETICS

HALF-LIFE	ONSET	PEAK	DURATION
1-3 hr	1-2 hr	3-4 hr	8-12 hr

⊶vancomycin

Vancomycin (Lyphocin, Vancocin, Vancoled) is a natural bactericidal antibiotic structurally unrelated to any other commercially available antibiotics. It destroys bacteria by binding to the bacterial cell wall, producing immediate inhibition of cell wall synthesis and death. This mechanism differs from that of the penicillins and cephalosporins.

It is the antibiotic of choice for the treatment of methicillin-resistant *S. aureus* (MRSA) infection and infections caused by many other gram-positive bacteria. It is not active against gram-negative bac-teria, fungi, or yeast. Oral vancomycin is indicated for the treatment of antibiotic-induced pseudo-membranous colitis *(Clostridium difficile)* and for the treatment of staphylococcal enterocolitis. Because the oral formulation is poorly absorbed from the gastrointestinal tract, it is used for its local effects on the surface of the gastrointestinal tract. The par-enteral form is indicated for the treatment of bone and joint infections and bacterial bloodstream in-fections caused by *Staphylococcus* spp. Resistance to vancomycin has been noted with increasing fre-quency in patients with infections caused by *Ente-rococcus* organisms. These strains have been isolated most often from gastrointestinal tract infections but have also been isolated from skin, soft tissue, and bloodstream infections.

Vancomycin is classified as a pregnancy category B agent and is contraindicated in patients with a known hypersensitivity to it. It should be used with caution in those with preexisting renal dysfunction or hearing loss, as well as in elderly patients and neonates. Vancomycin is similar to the aminoglyco-sides in that there are very specific drug levels in the blood that are safe. If the levels are too low (<5 µg/ml), there is a risk of their being subthera-peutic, with the result that their antibacterial ef-ficacy is decreased. If the blood levels are too

high (>26 µg/ml), this may cause toxicities, the two most severe of which are ototoxicity (hearing loss) and nephrotoxicity (kidney damage). Optimal blood levels of vancomycin should be a peak level of 18 to 26 µg/ml and a trough level of 5 to 10 µg/ml. If these levels are obtained, then the antibacte-rial effect of the vancomycin will be optimal and the side effects minimal. Vancomycin is available in both oral and parenteral forms. Orally it is avail-able as 125- and 250-mg capsules and a 1- and 10-g solution. Parenterally it is available in 500-mg and 1-g vials for IV infusions. Common dosages are given in the dosages table on p. 589.

PHARMACOKINETICS

HALF-LIFE	ONSET	PEAK	DURATION
4-6 hr	Variable	1 hr	Up to 12 hr

nursing process

The discussion of the nursing process will focus on each major classification of antibiotics so that there is an awareness of general and specific information about the various antibiotics.

● Assessment

Before the administration of any antibiotic, it is crucial to ensuring the effectiveness and appropriateness of treat-ment for the nurse to collect data on the patient regarding his or her age; hypersensitivity to drugs; hepatic (AST [SGOT], ALT [SGPT]), renal, and cardiac function (i.e., pertinent laboratory test results); culture and sensitivity results; and CBC, Hgb, and Hct values. It may also be

case study Antibiotic Therapy

Mr. Garrison is a resident of an assisted care facility post LCVA for the last 5 years. His cardiovascular and cere-brovascular statuses are stable. However, he has had a productive cough for 2 days and a low-grade fever. Upon physical assessment and chest x-ray examination, the physician diagnoses him with LLL pneumonia. The physi-cian orders PO Cipro 200 mg q12h and PO Theo-Dur 300 mg q12h. Maalox has been ordered prn for gastrointesti-nal upset.

● *What concerns should the nurse caring for this patient have about the use of Cipro and any of the other medications ordered for Mr. Garrison? Are there other interactions with this medication?*

necessary to monitor bowel status and patterns. Assessing for bleeding, such as for ecchymosis (bleeding gums) may also be necessary. With any antibiotic therapy, it is important to assess for overgrowth of infection as evidenced by fever, lethargy, perineal itching, etc. The status of the patient's immune system and his or her overall condition is also important, because if the immune system is deficient in some way, the patient's ability to physically resist infection will be diminished. It is also important to obtain and document a list of all prescribed and over-the-counter (OTC) medications the patient is taking so that drug interactions can be averted. A culture and sensitivity should be obtained before beginning therapy.

Penicillins

Contraindications to the use of penicillins include a known hypersensitivity to them. Cautious use is generally recommended in neonates and in pregnant or lactating women. The patient must also be assessed for a history of asthma, a sensitivity to multiple allergens, or a sensitivity to cephalosporins, because a patient with any of these conditions may also be allergic to penicillin agents. In addition, a patient who is to be given a procaine penicillin should be assessed for any procaine hypersensitivity. The drugs that interact with these agents are listed in Table 36-3.

Cephalosporins

Before receiving any of the cephalosporins, the patient should be assessed thoroughly for the existence of any hypersensitivity, including a hypersensitivity to penicillins. Cautious use is recommended in patients who have a history of any type of drug allergy or who have impaired renal or liver function. In addition, cautious use, with careful and frequent monitoring of the patient's vital signs and any complaints of dyspnea, hives, and so on, is recommended for patients who are also taking furosemide, ethacrynic acid, colistin, or aminoglycosides. (See Table 36-3, which gives information on the drug interactions associated with the penicillins, but which are the same for the cephalosporins.)

Sulfonamides

Any patient who is to receive a sulfonamide agent should first be assessed for any drug allergies. Other contraindications include pregnancy, lactation, severe hepatitis, glomerular nephritis, and uremia. Cautious use is recommended in patients with impaired liver or renal function, severe allergies, or bronchial asthma, and in patients also taking anticoagulants or oral antidiabetic agents of the sulfonylurea group. There are many drug-drug interactions that need to be assessed for with this particular class of antibiotics, and they vary from drug to drug.

Tetracyclines

Contraindications to the use of tetracyclines include pregnancy and hypersensitivity. They should also not be given to children under 8 years of age. Cautious use is recommended in lactating women and in patients with renal or hepatic disease. Drugs and substances that interact with tetracyclines include antacids, dairy products, penicillins, and oral anticoagulants. Doxycyclines also have many drug-drug interactions that need to be assessed for before use, such as antacids, iron, phenytoin, anticoagulants, barbiturates, and oral contraceptives.

Aminoglycosides

Aminoglycosides should be used with caution in patients with impaired renal function. There are also many medications that interact with aminoglycosides and that should *not* be given in conjunction with this antibiotic group. These agents include oral anticoagulants, diuretics, cephalothins, skeletal muscle relaxants, and general anesthetic agents. The aminoglycosides are also ototoxic and nephrotoxic, so baseline hearing tests and renal function studies (BUN and serum and urine creatinine levels) should be performed and the results documented. Nephrotoxic effects are manifested by decreased urine creatinine clearance and increased serum creatinine levels.

Clindamycin

Hypersensitivity to either clindamycin or to its parent agent lincomycin is a contraindication to its use. It is also contraindicated in patients with ulcerative colitis or enteritis and in infants younger than 1 month of age. Cautious use of clindamycin is recommended in patients with renal disease, liver disease, or gastrointestinal disorders; in elderly patients; and in pregnant or lactating women. Drugs that interact with it include muscle relaxants, chloramphenicol, and erythromycin.

Quinolones

Quinolones (or fluoroquinolones) are used most commonly to treat urinary, gastrointestinal, and upper respiratory infections. They should not be used in patients who are allergic to any of the agents. Cautious use is recommended in patients who have seizure disorders or renal disease, in the elderly, and in children. They should also be used cautiously in pregnant or lactating women. There are many drug-drug interactions for which to assess before use; a few include antacids, anticoagulants, antineoplastics, and theophylline.

Macrolides

Macrolides are contraindicated in patients with a known allergy to drugs. They should be used cautiously in patients with impaired liver function. There are also many drug-drug interactions; a few examples include clindamycin, theophylline, antihistamines, penicillins, and oral anticoagulants.

Vancomycin

Vancomycin, a tricyclic glycopeptide, is contraindicated in patients with hearing loss and those who are allergic to the medication. Cautious use is recommended for the elderly, neonates, pregnant or lactating women, and patients with compromised renal function. Drugs that interact or are incompatible with vancomycin include the aminoglycosides, cephalosporins, polymyxin, cisplatin, and amphotericin B. The combined use of these agents with vancomycin may precipitate nephrotoxicity or ototoxicity.

Nursing Diagnoses

Nursing diagnoses appropriate to patients receiving any of the antibiotics include the following:

- Risk for infection related to the patient's compromised immune system status before treatment.
- Risk for injury (compromised organ function) related to side effects of medications (e.g., ototoxicity and nephrotoxicity) and from a weakened physical state.
- Acute pain related to infection and adverse reaction to medications.
- Deficient knowledge related to lack of information and experience with the medication regimen.
- Ineffective therapeutic regimen management related to lack of information about the proper use of antibiotics and the need for patient education.

Planning

Goals of nursing care in patients receiving antibiotics include the following:

- Patient is free of the signs and symptoms of infection once therapy is completed.
- Patient experiences minimal side effects of antibiotic therapy.
- Patient remains compliant with therapy.
- Patient returns for follow-up visits as recommended.
- Patient completes medical regimen of entire course of antibiotics as ordered.

Outcome Criteria

Goals related to the administration of all antibiotics are as follows:

- Patient will experience increased sense of well-being related to resolving infection.
- Patient will state the signs and symptoms of an infection (e.g., fever, pain, malaise) and report them if they occur while on antibiotics.
- Patient will be able to identify the side effects of antibiotic therapy such as gastrointestinal upset, nausea, and diarrhea (specific to each class).
- Patient will experience increased periods of comfort and improved energy levels related to a resolving infectious process and minimal side effects of therapy.
- Patient will state the reasons for compliance with therapy (i.e., to adequately irradicate bacteria).
- Patient will state the measures to take to minimize the gastrointestinal distress associated with antibiotic therapy, such as taking with yogurt or other foods, *as appropriate.*
- Patient will keep follow-up appointments with the physician or other health care provider to be evaluated for therapeutic effects or complications of therapy.

Implementation

There are some common nursing interventions that apply to the antibiotics as a whole as well as some very different interventions that apply to specific classes or agents.

Any patient taking a penicillin should be carefully monitored for at least 30 minutes after its administration so that an allergic reaction will not go undetected. Penicillin G binds to food and is poorly absorbed in an acidic medium, so it should be given 1 hour before or 2 hours after meals. In addition, the effectiveness of oral penicillins is decreased when they are taken concurrently with caffeine, citrus fruit, cola beverages, fruit juices, or tomato juice. The IM administration of a penicillin such as penicillin G benzathine may cause irritation to localized tissue, so it should be administered into a large muscle mass. IM medications should be diluted well in the diluent recommended by the manufacturer and the sites rotated. When administering IV ampicillin, it should be diluted according to the manufacturer's guidelines and infused over the recommended time. The IV sites should be assessed frequently and changed every 48 hours, or as dictated by institutional policy. IV administration is to be *avoided,* except for agents such as ampicillin, nafcillin, and methicillin. The nurse should always double-check to make sure that, if the medication has been ordered to be given intravenously, it indeed can be given by this route. IM administered imipenem-cilastin (Primaxin) is often reconstituted with lidocaine without epinephrine and is given in a deep, large muscle mass. IV imipenem-cilastin (Primaxin) must be mixed with appropriate diluents (0.9% NaCl, D5, .45 NaCl) and administered over 20 to 30 minutes (250-500 mg dose).

Should the patient experience an anaphylactic reaction to a penicillin, management often includes the IV or SC administration of epinephrine, maintenance of the patient's airway, and other supportive treatment such as the administration of steroids, vasopressors, or oxygen or implementation of cardiopulmonary resuscitation.

Orally administered cephalosporins should be given with food to decrease gastrointestinal upset, even though this will delay absorption. IM injections may be very irritating and so should be given deep in a large muscle mass. If accidental SC injection occurs, sterile abscesses may form. When cephradine is being given by infusion, it should not be mixed with lactated Ringer's solution. IV sites of administration should be assessed frequently for redness, swelling, and heat and changed every 48 hours, or as dictated by institutional policy. Alcohol, when used with some of the cephalosporins, may

---

case study **Viral vs. Bacterial Infections**

A pediatric patient's mother is continually demanding, in calls to the office or at visits where infections (e.g., viral versus bacterial infection) are not suspected, an order for an antibiotic for her 3-year-old son who has repeated viral throats. You think it may be helpful to discuss the issue of "drug resistance" with her in a tactful way.

- *What type of information would be helpful to share with her and why?*

For Answers see www.harcourthealth.com/MERLIN/Lilley/.

result in antabuse-like reactions, so always check for this contraindication before giving the medication. With the newer cephalosporins, it is necessary for patient safety to check names carefully since there are many agents that sound alike or are spelled alike.

Sulfonamides should always be given with plenty of fluids (at least 2000 to 2400 ml per day) to prevent the crystalluria that can occur with the oral forms. Oral forms will cause less gastrointestinal upset if taken with milk or food.

Tetracyclines should not be given with dairy products, antacids, sodium bicarbonate, kaolin-pectin, or iron because these chelate or bind with the tetracycline, resulting in a decreased antibiotic effect. These foods and drugs can be given 2 hours before or 3 hours after the tetracycline. Oral forms should be given with at least 8 ounces of fluid. IV tetracycline should be given per physician's orders and manufacturer's guidelines regarding diluents. IV administered doxycycline is very irritating to the veins, so the IV site should be checked daily and changed per policy every 72 hours. Diluents include 0.9% NaCl, Ringer's, LR, and D5/LR.

Quinolones should be taken exactly as prescribed and for the full course of treatment. The patient should limit his or her intake of alkaline foods and drugs such as antacids, dairy products, peanuts, vegetables, and sodium bicarbonate. Any of the quinoline agents should be administered only after culture and sensitivity testing has been done on a fresh urine sample from the patient. Fluid intake of up to 3 liters per day should be encouraged, unless contraindicated.

Oral fluoroquinolones are tolerated more easily with food. These agents are often phototoxic as well.

If an IV infusion of lincomycin is ordered, 1 g of the medication should be diluted in 100 ml or more of D5W or NS, but not to the extent that a rate of infusion of 100 ml/hr would be exceeded. IM injections should be given deep in the muscle and the sites rotated. Oral forms should be given with at least 8 ounces (240 ml) of fluid and on an empty stomach.

Vancomycin should be reconstituted for IV administration according to the manufacturer's guidelines and should be infused over at least 60 minutes. Extravasation may cause local skin irritation and damage, so frequent monitoring of the IV tube and site is needed. Sterile water for reconstitution is recommended, and if further IV dilution is needed, D5W or NS may be used. If Redman's syndrome occurs (decreased BP, flushing of neck and face), an antihistamine may need to be ordered. Adequate hydration (at least 2 L of fluids/24 hr unless contraindicated) is also important with vancomycin to prevent nephrotoxicity.

Clindamycin should be administered as ordered and if given intravenously should be given by infusion, not by an IV push. No more than 1200 mg should be infused in a single 1-hour infusion, and the usually recommended dilution and dosage is 300 mg per 50 ml of compatible fluids delivered over more than 10 minutes. IM injections of the agent should be given deep in a large muscle mass and the sites rotated. Oral forms should be given with at least 8 ounces (240 ml) of fluids.

Teaching guidelines for patients receiving antibiotics are listed in the box below.

● Evaluation

The therapeutic effects of antibiotics in general include a decrease in the signs and symptoms of the infection; a return to normal vital signs, including temperature and negative results of culture and sensitivity tests; a decrease to a normal CBC; and improved appetite, energy level, and sense of well-being.

Common adverse reactions for which to monitor in patients taking penicillins include rash, dermatitis, fever, joint pain, or itching. Patients taking cephalosporins should be watched for the occurrence of diarrhea, abdominal pain, colitis symptoms, headache, fever, chills, nausea, vomiting, rash, or dyspnea. Adverse reactions to the sulfonamides for which to monitor include leukopenia, nausea, vomiting, abdominal pain, hepatitis syndrome, renal failure, nephrosis, and Stevens-Johnson syndrome. Tetracyclines may cause diarrhea, hepatotoxicity, nausea, stomatitis, pericarditis, rash, fever, headache, and oral candidiasis or other superinfections. Quinolones may cause lethargy, dizziness, or confusion. Vancomycin may cause hearing loss and ringing or roaring in ears, and its use should be discontinued if these symptoms appear. The physician should be notified if any unusual side effects occur or if fever, sore throat, restlessness, wheezing, or tightness in the chest arises. Treatment with clindamycin, although an agent in a different class of antibiotics, requires similar nursing interventions, and the patient education guidelines are also similar.

✎ patient teaching tips

Antibiotics

➤ Patients should take any antibiotic exactly as prescribed and for the time specified.

➤ All oral antibiotics are absorbed better if taken with at least 6 to 8 ounces of water.

➤ MedicAlert tags, bracelets, or necklaces should be worn at all times by patients with drug allergies!

➤ Oral forms of penicillins are better absorbed if taken with 6 to 8 ounces of water and on an empty stomach. Patients should know to report any sore throat, fever, muscle weakness, or joint pain to the physician immediately.

➤ Cephalosporins should be taken with meals, when taken orally, to minimize gastrointestinal irritation and not taken concurrently with alcohol or alcohol-containing products (some cough syrups and mouth washes) because of the Antabuse-type reactions that can occur. Drugs that interact with cephalosporins include tetracyclines, erythromycin, aminoglycosides, probenecid, furosemide, and vancomycin. Yogurt or buttermilk products may be taken to help decrease the diarrhea that occurs secondary to the destruction of the normal intestinal flora. The medication should be taken exactly as prescribed and for the specified time. Should sore throat, bruising, bleeding, or joint pain develop, the patient should notify the physician of this immediately because this may indicate the occurrence of a blood dyscrasia.

➤ Sulfonamides should be taken with at least 2400 ml of fluid per day, unless contraindicated. Patients should avoid sunlight and using tanning beds because of the photosensitivity they cause. OTC medications should be avoided, especially vitamin C and aspirin, because these drugs interact with the sulfonamides. Patients taking oral contraceptives should use another form of contraception because sulfonamides decrease the contraceptive effect. Patients should know to take the full course of medication and in accordance with the physician's directions. The patient should notify the physician if fever, sore throat, mouth sores, easy bruising, or skin rash occurs.

➤ Tetracyclines cause photosensitivity, so patients taking them should avoid sun exposure and using tanning beds. Milk products, iron preparations, antacids, and other dairy products should be avoided because of the chelation that occurs, which decreases the effectiveness of the medication. All medications should be taken with at least 6 to 8 ounces of fluids, preferably water.

➤ Quinolones such as norfloxacin should be taken with at least 3 liters of fluids per day, unless otherwise specified by the physician. This helps to prevent crystallization of the drug in the kidneys. Should dizziness occur, the patient may need assistance in ambulating and performing other activities of daily living. The patient should notify the physician if rash, fever, sore throat, headache, agitation, or confusion occurs. Some of the agents are phototoxic.

➤ Oral forms of lincomycin should be taken with plenty of fluids and with food to minimize gastrointestinal distress. Patients should be informed of the importance of complying with therapy and of taking the full course of therapy. Sore throat, fever, or excessive fatigue should be reported to the physician. This drug is usually ordered to be taken around the clock to maintain therapeutic blood levels.

➤ Vancomycin should be taken exactly as prescribed and for the number of days specified to ensure that the infecting organism is destroyed. The medication should be administered around the clock to maintain steady blood levels. The patient should report any fever, sore throat, or rash to the physician.

POINTS TO REMEMBER

Antibiotic Classes

• Seven main classes of antibiotic agents: sulfonamides, penicillins, cephalosporins, macrolides, quinolones, aminoglycosides, and tetracyclines.
• Classes of antibiotics differ in the way in which they destroy bacteria.

Antibiotic Characteristics

• Antibiotics are either bacteriostatic or bactericidal.
• *Bacteriostatic* means that the antibiotic inhibits the growth of the bacteria but does not directly kill it.
• *Bactericidal* means that the antibiotic directly kills the bacteria.
• Most antibiotics work by inhibiting bacterial cell wall synthesis in some way.

Bacteria Characteristics

• Bacteria have survived for years because they can adapt to their surroundings.

• If a bacteria's surroundings include an antibiotic, over time it can mutate in such a way that it can survive an attack by an antibiotic.
• The production of beta-lactamases is one way in which bacteria can fend off the effects of antibiotics.

Nursing Considerations

• The most common side effects of antibiotics are nausea, vomiting, and diarrhea.
• Antibiotics should always be taken for the length of time prescribed.
• A therapeutic response to antibiotic treatment includes disappearance of fever, lethargy, drainage, and redness.
• Each class of antibiotics has specific side effects and drugs that the agents interact with and must be carefully assessed and monitored.
• Signs and symptoms of suprainfections include fever, perineal itching, cough, lethargy, or any unusual discharge.

REVIEW QUESTIONS

1. Your patient is scheduled for colorectal surgery tomorrow. He is not septic, his WBC count is normal, he has no fever, and he is otherwise in good health. The gastrointestinal surgeon asks you to recommend a cephalosporin for prophylaxis. What generation of cephalosporin would you recommend and why?
   a. A third-generation cephalosporin because it is the most potent
   b. A second-generation cephalosporin because it is the least toxic
   c. A first-generation cephalosporin because it kills the bacteria that are most common in this surgical field
   d. A second-generation cephalosporin because it kills the bacteria that are most common in this surgical field

2. You are caring for a 34-year-old man who has been admitted for the treatment of Rocky Mountain spotted fever (RMSF). He is placed on doxycycline, a tetracycline antibiotic, but is now complaining of gastrointestinal upset. The physician orders Maalox to be taken after each dose of the doxycycline. You call the physician and inform him that the gastrointestinal tract upset is caused by _____ and that the Maalox will result in _____ if continued.

a. the RMSF; toxic shock syndrome
b. the doxycycline; aluminum toxicity
c. the doxycycline; increased doxycycline efficacy
d. the doxycycline; decreased doxycycline efficacy

3. The quinolone antibiotics, such as Cipro and Floxin, are unique in their mechanism of action in that they _____.
   a. interfere with DNA gyrase
   b. prevent the synthesis of folic acid
   c. bind to penicillin-binding proteins
   d. bind to 30S and 50S ribosomal subunits

4. The two newest macrolide antibiotics, azithromycin and clarithromycin, differ from the prototype macrolide, erythromycin, in that they have _____.
   a. better efficacy
   b. better tissue penetration
   c. a longer duration of action
   d. all of the above

5. Which of the following are expected side effects of the aminoglycosides?
   a. Glaucoma
   b. Palpitations
   c. Nephrotoxicity
   d. Diabetes mellitus

For Answers see www.harcourthealth.com/MERLIN/Lilley/.

CRITICAL THINKING Activities

1. Explain the rationale for not taking dairy products, iron, or calcium with tetracycline. What would be recommended if these products are not taken out of the diet?
2. Ms. Smith is taking an aminoglycoside for the treatment of a recurrent UTI. What conditions should be assessed for or laboratory studies performed before the initiation of therapy?
3. What symptoms would alert you to the fact that a patient is suffering from a superinfection or overgrowth of normal flora stemming from the use of tetracycline?

For Answers see www.harcourthealth.com/MERLIN/Lilley/.

bibliography

Albanese J, Nutz P: *Mosby's 2001 nursing drug reference and review cards,* St Louis, 2001, Mosby.

American Hospital Formulary Service: *AHFS drug information,* Bethesda, Md, 2000, American Society of Health-System Pharmacists.

Anderson PO, Knoben JE, Troutman WG: *Handbook of clinical drug data 1999-2000,* ed 9, New York, 1999, McGraw-Hill.

Degan R: Pharmacology in practice: antibiotics, *RN* 60(10):49, 1997.

Fitzgerald M: Macrolide antibiotics, *Clin Excellence Nurse Prac* 1(1):71, 1997.

Johns Hopkins Hospital, Department of Pediatrics et al: *The Harriet Lane handbook,* ed 15, St Louis, 2000, Mosby.

Keen JH: *Critical care and emergency drug reference,* ed 3, St Louis, 1996, Mosby.

Medical Letter: Gatifloxacin and moxifloxacin: two new fluoroquinolones 42(1072):15, February 21, 2000.

Medical Letter: Quinupristin/dalfopristin 41(1066):109, November 19, 1999.

Medical Letter: Sparfloxacin and levofloxacin, 39(999):41, 1997.

Mosby's GenRx: a comprehensive reference for generic and brand drugs, ed 10, St Louis, 2000, Mosby.

Skidmore-Roth L: *Mosby's 2001 nursing drug reference,* St Louis, 2001, Mosby.

Activity

Remember to check the **Online Worksheet** for additional learning opportunities: **www.harcourthealth.com/MERLIN/Lilley/**

Chapter 37

Antiviral Agents

objectives

When you reach the end of this chapter, you should be able to do the following:

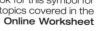

Look for this symbol for topics covered in the **Online Worksheet**

1 Discuss the effects of viruses on the human body.

2 Describe the process of immunosuppression in patients afflicted with viral infections, specifically those with human immunodeficiency virus.

3 Discuss the indications, contraindications, cautions, routes, mechanisms of action, side effects, toxicity, and therapeutic effects realeted to antiviral agents.

4 Identify the various antiviral agents and their specific indications.

5 Develop a nursing care plan that includes all phases of the nursing process for patients receiving antiviral agents.

drug profiles

○━**acyclovir,** p. 600
○━**amantadine,** p. 601
ganciclovir, p. 602
indinavir, p. 602
nevirapine, p. 603

oseltamivir and zanamivir, p. 606
ribavirin, p. 605
trifluridine, p. 605
○━**zidovudine,** p. 605

○━Key drug.

glossary

Antiviral agent Drug that destroys viruses. (p. 598)
Deoxyribonucleic acid (de ok' se ri' bo noo kle' ik) Nucleic acid composed of a sugar, a phosphate group, and a purine or pyridine nucleoside that carries genetic information and is found principally in the chromosomes of the nucleus of a cell. (p. 599)
Ribonucleic acid Nucleic acid composed of a sugar, a phosphate group, and a purine or a pyridine nucleoside that transmits genetic information and is found in both the nucleus and the cytoplasm of cells. (p. 599)
Synthetic purine nucleoside analogue (pu ren noo' kle o sid an' ə log) Substance that is both chemically made and a purine nucleoside and that resembles another in terms of its structure or constituents but has different effects. (p. 599)

ANTIVIRAL THERAPY

Antiviral agents kill viruses by inhibiting their ability to replicate, making it easier for the body's immune system to destroy the virus. There are currently only a few of the known viruses that can be destroyed by antiviral agents. Some of these viruses are as follows:

- Cytomegalovirus (CMV)
- Herpes simplex virus (HSV)
- Human immunodeficiency virus (HIV)
- Influenza A ("the flu")
- Respiratory syncytial virus (RSV)

One reason why only a few viruses can be killed with the agents currently available is that often by the time the signs and symptoms of a viral illness appear, the virus has finished replicating. Because it is only during viral replication that antiviral agents can work, it is then too late for them to be effective. So, even if there were effective agents to kill these viruses, unless this silent process can be detected and therapy instituted in time, they would otherwise be of no use. Another reason why there are so few agents is that because viruses live inside the body's cells and use them to replicate, any drug that kills a virus could also kill healthy cells. Thus for an antiviral agent to be effective *and* safe, it must kill only the virus and not unduly harm the body's cells. There are few agents that have met these criteria.

As previously mentioned, antiviral agents work by inhibiting viral replication. For a virus to replicate, it must first attach to and enter the healthy cell, where it makes use of the cell's energy to generate both DNA- and RNA-synthesizing pathways as well as its own protein-synthesizing pathways to make more viruses (Fig. 37-1). Antiviral agents inhibit this process in various ways. Some antiviral drugs are able to enter the same cells that the viruses enter. Once inside, the antiviral drugs interfere with viral nucleic acid synthesis, its

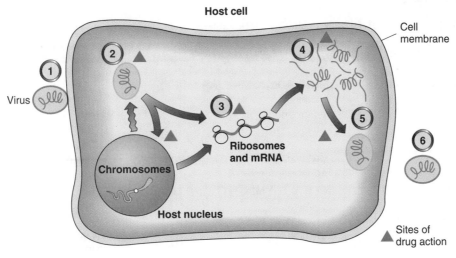

1. Attachment to host cell
2. Uncoating of virus
3. Control of DNA, RNA, and/or protein production
4. Production of viral subunits
5. Assembly of virions
6. Release of virions

Fig. 37-1 Virus replication. Some viruses integrate into host chromosome with development of latency. (Modified from Brody TM, Larner J, Minneman KP: *Human pharmacology: molecular to clinical,* ed 3, St Louis, 1998, Mosby.)

BOX 37-1 DNA and RNA Characteristics

Characteristic	DNA	RNA
Type of sugar	Deoxyribose	Ribose
Nucleoside pairing	cytosine with guanine	cytosine with guanine
	adenine with thymine	adenine with uracil

Purines: adenine and guanine; pyridines: cytosine, thymine, and uracil.

regulation, or both. Other antiviral drugs work by keeping a virus from binding to the cells. If a virus cannot then get into the cells, it cannot replicate, and it dies. Other antiviral agents stimulate the body's immune system to kill the virus.

The best antiviral response is seen in patients with a competent, well-functioning immune system. Such an immune system can work with the agent to eliminate or effectively destroy viruses. Those patients who become a host for a virus or viruses are frequently immunocompromised. Cancer patients with leukemia or lymphoma, organ transplant recipients, and AIDS patients are all examples of patients who are immunocompromised. These patients are prone to frequent and often severe viral infections, which may recur when antiviral drug therapy is stopped.

Most of the antivirals agents are **synthetic purine nucleoside analogues,** which means that they are chemically made (synthetic) purine nucleosides (adenine or guanine) that are chemically similar (analogues). There are two types of nucleic acid—**deoxyribonucleic acid** (DNA), which consists of a sugar (deoxyribose), a phosphate group, and a purine (adenine or guanine) or a pyrimidine (cytosine or thymine) nucleoside, and **ribonucleic acid** (RNA), which is made up of a sugar (ribose), a phosphate group, and a purine (adenine or gua-

nine) or a pyrimidine (cytosine or uracil) nucleoside. The differences between DNA and RNA are listed in Box 37-1, and the currently available antiviral agents their nucleoside type (purine verses pyridine), and their antiviral activity are summarized in Table 37-1.

Mechanism of Action

The different antiviral agents vary in the way in which they kill viruses. To replicate, the virus first attaches to and diffuses into the cell. Once in the cell it has its genetic makeup copied, after which the nucleus of the infected cell utilizes its DNA and RNA to make new viruses. An antiviral agent can work at any of these steps: attachment, reading of the virus' genetic makeup, and making of new virus. The overall effect of these agents, however, is the inhibition of viral replication. Many antivirals accomplish this by interfering with viral DNA polymerase; others inhibit reverse transcriptase.

Drug Effects

Antiviral agents are used to treat a variety of virus-related disorders ranging from HSV to HIV, but the agents exert varying degrees of activity against viruses. These drug effects, or antiviral activity, are summarized for the different agents in Box 37-2.

Characteristics of Nucleoside Analogues

table 37-1

Antiviral Agent	Nucleoside Analogue of	Antiviral Activity
PURINE NUCLEOSIDES (GUANINE [G] AND ADENOSINE [A])		
acyclovir	guanine	HSV 1 and 2, VZV
didanosine (ddI)	adenosine	HIV
ganciclovir (DHPG)	guanine	CMV retinitis and systemic CMV infection
ribavirin (RTCD)	guanine	Influenza type A and B, RSV, LV, HV
vidarabine (Ara-A)	adenosine	HSV, herpes zoster
PYRIMIDINE NUCLEOSIDES (CYTOSINE [C], THYMINE [T], AND URACIL [U])		
idoxuridine (IDU)	thymine	HSV
lamivudine (3TC)	cytosine	HIV
stavudine (d4T)	thymine	HIV
trifluridine	thymine	HSV
zalcitabine (ddC)	cytosine	HIV
zidovudine (AZT)	thymine	HIV

CMV, Cytomegalovirus; *HIV,* human immunodeficiency virus; *HSV,* herpes simplex virus (types 1 and 2); *HV,* hantavirus; *LV,* lassa virus; *RSV,* respiratory syncytial virus; *VZV,* varicella zoster virus.

Therapeutic Uses

The therapeutic effects of the antiviral agents vary greatly depending on the particular agent and its spectrum of activity. The increasing public awareness of one of the most devastating viruses known to humankind, HIV, has stimulated much research into antiviral agents. This has led to the development of many new and improved agents, though many of these agents also produce significant toxicities. The therapeutic effects of the various agents are also summarized in Box 37-2.

Side Effects and Adverse Effects

The side effects and adverse effects of the antiviral agents are as different as the agents themselves. Each has its own specific side effect profile. Because viruses reproduce in human cells and therefore have many of the same features as these cells, it makes it much harder to target a unique enzyme or feature of the virus. Selective killing is difficult, and as a result, more good human cells are killed in the process, resulting in more serious toxicities. These serious adverse effects are listed by agent in Table 37-2.

Interactions

The significant drug interactions that occur with the antiviral agents involve those agents administered systemically. Many of the antivirals are applied topically to the eye or body, and the incidence of drug interactions associated with these agents is low. The antiviral agents, the drugs they interact with, and the result of the interaction are listed in Box 37-3.

Dosages

See the dosages table on p. 604 for recommended dosages for selected antiviral agents.

drug profiles

There have been many new agents recently added to the antiviral drug class. This has in part been prompted by the growing concern over the devastating effects HIV infection (AIDS) has had on our population. Many new and improved antiviral agents have been developed, some of which have improved actions but greater toxicities. Others with similar actions but improved side effect profiles. Some of the prototypical antiviral agents are discussed here.

⊶ acyclovir

Acyclovir (Zovirax) is a synthetic nucleoside analogue of guanine that is mainly used to suppress the replication of HSV 1 and 2 as well as the varicella-zoster virus (VZV), commonly known as *chickenpox* and *shingles.* Acyclovir is considered the drug of choice for the treatment of both initial and recurrent episodes of both these viral infections. Another antiviral agent with properties similar to those of acyclovir is vidarabine. It was one of the first effective antiviral drugs available in an injectable formulation but differs from acyclovir in that it is an analogue of adenine.

Acyclovir is available in oral, topical, and parenteral formulations. It is available orally as 200-mg capsules, a 200-mg/5 ml suspension, and 400- and 800-mg tablets. Parenterally it is available as a 500-mg and 1-g injection for IV infusion. Topically it is available as a 5% ointment. Acyclovir is classified as a pregnancy category C drug and is contraindicated in patients hypersensitive to it. It is a prescription-only drug. Commonly recommended dosages can be found in the dosages table on p. 604.

BOX 37-2   Antiviral Therapeutic Effects

Antiviral	Viral Activity	Therapeutic Effect
acyclovir, famciclovir, valacyclovir, and vidarabine	HSV 1 and 2, VZV	Vidarabine was used primarily in treatment of herpes simplex encephalitis, disseminated or CNS herpes infections in the newborn, herpes keratitis (topically), and herpes zoster, but has been generally replaced by acyclovir, famciclovir, and valacyclovir. Acyclovir is used topically, orally, and intravenously for treatment of herpes simplex, encephalitis, and most other significant herpes infections. It is more efficacious and less toxic than vidarabine. Administration as soon as possible produces the best results. These agents reduce viral shedding, decrease local symptoms, and decrease severity and duration of illness
amantadine and rimantadine	Influenza A	Used for the treatment and prophylaxis of influenza A but ineffective against influenza B; most effective if given before exposure or within 48 hours of development of symptoms; reduces fever and palliates symptoms of influenza.
cidofovir, ganciclovir, and foscarnet	CMV	Ganciclovir is the older and more studied of these three agents. It now is available in a variety of formulations (oral, parenteral, and an ocular implant). It has been shown to be effective for not only CMV retinitis but also other CMV infections such as gastrointestinal infection and pneumonitis and for prevention of CMV in recipients of solid organ transplants and in patients with HIV infection. The primary dose-limiting toxicity of ganciclovir is bone marrow toxicity. Foscarnet and cidofovir are less toxic to the bone marrow but can cause renal failure. This can be minimized with the administration of probenecid tablets and hydration on the day of infusion.
delavirdine and nevirapine	HIV	In combination with nucleoside analogues, these two non-nucleoside reverse transcriptase inhibitors (NNRTI) are used to treat HIV-infected patients, including newly infected asymptomatic patients.
didanosine, lamivudine, stavudine, zalcitabine, and zidovudine	HIV	Approved for the treatment of HIV infections in the setting of AIDS and AIDS-related complex; they produce a significant reduction in mortality and incidence of opportunistic infections, improve physical performance, and significantly improve T-cell counts.
idoxuridine and trifluridine	HSV	Used to treat herpes simplex keratitis; are only used topically because of significant liver and bone marrow toxicity.
indinavir, ritonavir, saquinavir, and nelfinavir	HIV	Newer class of drugs for the treatment of HIV infection when antiretoviral therapy is warranted. Used in combination with nucleoside analogues. Ritonavir and indinavir may used as monotherapy. They are all potent inhibitors of the HIV protease enzyme, which is critical to replication of the virus that causes AIDS.
ribavirin and RSV immune globulin	Influenza A and B, RSV, Lassa virus, Hantavirus	Severe RSV bronchopneumonia can be treated using an aerosol (Ribavirin) or an IV infusion (RSV immune globulin). These products have been shown to improve oxygenation, decrease viral shedding, and alleviate pneumonia symptoms. Inhalation treatment with Ribavirin has also been shown to be effective in influenza A and B infections. Oral and parenteral treatment are effective for Lassa fever virus as well as Hantavirus.

CMV, Cytomegalovirus; *HSV,* herpes simplex virus; *RSV,* respiratory syncytial virus; *VZV,* varicella zoster virus.

PHARMACOKINETICS			
HALF-LIFE	ONSET	PEAK	DURATION
2.1-5 hr	Unknown	PO: 1.5-2 hr	4-5 hr

⊶amantadine

Amantadine (Symmetrel) has a narrow antiviral spectrum in that it is only active against influenza A viruses. It is used both prophylactically and thera-

peutically. It has been shown to be very effective, if not lifesaving, when used prophylactically in, for instance, elderly, chronically ill, or immunocompromised patients in whom an influenza A infection can be particularly devastating.

Rimantadine is a structural analogue of amantadine that has the same spectrum of activity, mechanism of action, and clinical indications. However,

Activity

Table 37-2 Selected Antivirals: Adverse Effects

Antiviral Agent	Side/Adverse Effects
acyclovir	Most common nausea, vomiting, diarrhea, headache, transient burning when topically applied
amantadine and rimantadine	CNS: insomnia, nervousness, lightheadedness; gastrointestinal; anorexia, nausea; anticholinergic effects
didanosine	Gastrointestinal: pancreatitis; CNS: peripheral neuropathies, seizures
foscarnet	CNS: headache, seizures; MET: hypocalcemia, hypophosphatemia, hyperphosphatemia, hypokalemia; GU: acute renal failure; HEM: bone marrow suppression; gastrointestinal: nausea, vomiting, diarrhea
ganciclovir	HEM: bone marrow toxicity; gastrointestinal: nausea, anorexia, vomiting, CNS: headache, seizures
idoxuridine	Nothing significant
indinavir	Nausea, abdominal pain, headache, diarrhea, vomiting, weakness or fatigue, insomnia, flank pain, taste changes, acid regurgitation, back pain, indirect hyperbilirubinemia, nephrotithiasis
nevirapine	Rash, fever, nausea, headache, increases in liver function tests
ribavirin	Rash, conjunctivitis, anemia, mild broncospashm
trifluridine	Burning, swelling, stinging, photophobia, pain
vidarabine	Ophthalmic effects: burning, lacrimation, keratitis, foreign body sensation, pain, protophobia, uveitis, stromal edema
zalcitabine	Peripheral neuropathy, rash, ulcers
zidovudine	Bone marrow suppression, nausea, headache

CNS, Central nervous system; *GU*, genitourinary system; *HEM*, hematologic; *MET*, metabolic.

it differs from amantadine in that it has a longer half-life and causes less CNS toxicity. Rimantadine has gastrointestinal side effects similar to those of amantadine.

Amantadine is classified as a pregnancy category C agent and is contraindicated in patients with a known hypersensitivity to it, lactating women, children under 12 months of age, and patients with an eczematic rash. Amantadine is only available orally as a 50-mg/5 ml solution and 100-mg liquid-filled capsules. Commonly recommended dosages can be found in the dosages table on p. 604.

PHARMACOKINETICS

HALF-LIFE	ONSET	PEAK	DURATION
24 hr	Unknown	1-4 hr	12-24 hr

ganciclovir

Like acyclovir, ganciclovir (Cytovene) is also a synthetic analogue of guanine, but it has a much different spectrum of antiviral activity. Ganciclovir, foscarnet, and cidofovir are the three antiviral agents that are used in the treatment of CMV infections. They also have activity against HSV 1 and 2, Epstein-Barr virus, and VZV but are not used for the treatment of infection caused by these viruses because there are other less toxic antiviral agents that are just as effective in inhibiting them.

Of the three antivirals, ganciclovir is the one more frequently used in the treatment of CMV infections. The most common site of CMV infections in the immunocompromised patient is the eye, and the result is CMV retinitis, a devastating viral infection that can lead to blindness. Disseminated CMV infections such as gastrointestinal tract infections and pneumonitis are other non–FDA-approved indications for ganciclovir treatment.

A dose-limiting toxicity of ganciclovir treatment is bone marrow suppression; that of foscarnet and cidofovir is renal toxicity. These toxicities should be kept in mind when deciding on which agent is more appropriate in a particular patient. For example, a heart transplant recipient who contracts CMV retinitis is immunocompromised because of immunosuppressant drug therapy and is most likely taking cyclosporine, which is nephrotoxic. Therefore using foscarnet in this patient is more dangerous than using ganciclovir. On the other hand, a patient who contracts a CMV infection and is immunocompromised because of a bone marrow transplant would be better treated using foscarnet.

Ganciclovir is available orally as a 250 mg capsule, as an ocular implant, and parenterally as a 500-mg injection for IV infusion. It is classified as a pregnancy category C agent and is contraindicated in patients with a hypersensitivity to either it or acyclovir. Commonly recommended dosages can be found in the dosages table on p. 604.

PHARMACOKINETICS

HALF-LIFE	ONSET	PEAK	DURATION
2.5-3.6 hr	Unknown	Variable	Variable

indinavir

Indinavir (Crixivan) belongs to a newer class of drugs for the treatment of advanced HIV. This class of antivirals is known as the protease inhibitors. Indinavir, ritonavir (Norvir), saquinavir (Invirase), nelfinavir (Viracept), and amprenavir (Agenerase) are potent inhibitors of the HIV protease enzyme.

BOX 37-3   Interactions of Antiviral Drugs

ACYCLOVIR WITH THE FOLLOWING:
- *zidovudine:* increased risk of neurotoxicity
- *probenecid:* increased acyclovir levels by decreasing renal clearance
- *interferon:* additive antiviral effects

AMANTADINE WITH THE FOLLOWING:
- *Anticholinergic drugs:* increased adverse anticholinergic effects
- *CNS stimulants:* additive CNS stimulant effects

DIDANOSINE WITH THE FOLLOWING:
- *Antacids:* increased absorption of didanosine, which is a positive effect
- *dapsone:* may interfere with gastrointestinal absorbtion of dapsone
- *itraconazole and ketoconazole:* didanosine decreases their absorption, give 2 hours before
- *Quinolones:* didanosine decreases absorption of some quinolone antibiotics
- *Tetracyclines:* decreased absorption of tetracyclines; give 2 hours before tetracyclines
- *zalcitabine:* additive toxicity (peripheral neuropathies); avoid giving together
- *zidovudine:* additive and synergistic effect against HIV

GANCICLOVIR WITH THE FOLLOWING:
- *zidovudine:* increased risk of hematologic toxicity, (i.e., bone marrow suppression)
- *foscarnet:* additive or synergistic effect against CMV and HSV-2
- *imipenem:* increased risk of seizures

INDINAVIR WITH THE FOLLOWING:
- *Drugs metabolized by the CYP3A4 hepatic microsomal enzyme system (astemizole, cisapride, triazolam, and midazolam):* competition for metabolism resulting in elevated blood levels and potential toxicity

- *rifabutin and ketoconazole:* increased plasma concentrations of rifabutin and ketoconazole
- *rifampin:* increased metabolism of indinavir
- *didanosine:* alters the optimal pH of the stomach for indinavir to be maximally absorbed
- *ketoconazole:* increased plasma concentrations of ganciclovir

NEVIRAPINE WITH THE FOLLOWING:
- *Drugs metabolized by the CYP3A4 hepatic microsomal enzyme system:* increased metabolism of these drugs
- *Protease inhibitors:* decreased plasma concentrations of protease inhibitors
- *Oral contraceptives:* decreased plasma concentrations of oral contraceptives
- *rifampin and rifabutin:* decreased nevirapine serum concentration

ZALCITABINE WITH THE FOLLOWING:
- *Antacids:* reduced zalcitabine absorption
- *cimefidine:* decreased zalcitabine renal elimination
- *Drugs associated with pancreatic, peripheral neuropathy, and renal toxicities:* should be avoided because of additive toxicities
- *zidovudine:* additive or synergistic effect against HIV

ZIDOVUDINE WITH THE FOLLOWING:
- *acyclovir:* increased neurotoxicity
- *didanosine and zalcitabine:* additive or synergistic effect against HIV
- *ganciclovir and ribavirin:* antagonize the antiviral action of zidovudine
- *Cytotoxic agents:* increased risk for hematologic toxicity
- *beta-interferon:* increased serum levels of zidovudine

Activity

This enzyme is critical to the replication of the virus that causes AIDS. Indinavir can be taken in combination with other anti-HIV therapies or alone. Indinavir produces increases in CD4 cell counts, an important measure of immune system function. It also produces significant reductions in viral load, or levels of HIV in the bloodstream. Indinavir, ritonavir, saquinavir, and nelfinavir are most commonly given in combination with two reverse-transcriptase inhibitors to maximize efficacy and decrease the incidence of resistance.

Indinavir is well tolerated in patients. Nephrolithiasis (defined as flank pain, blood in the urine, or kidney stones) can occur in approximately 4% of patients. People who take indinavir are encouraged to drink at least 48 ounces of liquids every day to maintain hydration and help avoid nephrolithiasis. Indinavir is classified as a pregnancy cate-

gory C drug and is contraindicated in patients with clinically significant hypersensitivity to any of its components. Indinavir is only available orally as 200- and 400-mg capsules. Commonly recommended dosage can be found in the dosages table on p. 604.

PHARMACOKINETICS

HALF-LIFE	ONSET*	PEAK	DURATION*
1.5-2.5 hr	2 wk	0.5-1 hr	6 mo

*Therapeutic effects.

nevirapine

Nevirapine (Viramune) is a non-nucleoside reverse transcriptase inhibitor [NNRTI]. This is a new class of antiviral agents indicated for the treatment of HIV-1 infection, the virus that causes AIDS. The currently available NNRTIs are nevirapine, delavirdine

DOSAGES Selected Antiviral Agents

agent	pharmacologic class	dosage range	purpose
acyclovir (Zovirax)	Purine nucleoside analogue antiviral	Topical: apply ointment q3h 6 times/day	HSV cutaneous infection
		Pediatric	Chickenpox
		PO: 20 mg/kg qid for 5 days	HSV-1, HSV-2 infection
		IV: 250 mg/m² for 1 hr q8h for 7 days	shingles
		500 mg/m² q8h for 10 days	HSV encephalitis and shingles
		Adult (acute treatment)	
		PO: 200 mg q4h 5 times/day for 10 days or 400 mg tid for 7-10 days	HSV-2 (genital herpes)
		800 mg q4h 5 times/day for 7-10 days	Shingles
amantadine (Symmetrel)	Antiviral	*Pediatric*	
		PO: 1-9 y/o: 2-4 mg/kg/day (max 150 mg/day) once daily or divided into 2 daily doses	
		9-12 y/o: 100 mg bid	Prophylaxis and treatment of influenza A
		Adult	
		PO: 100 mg bid or 200 mg once/day	
ganciclovir (Cytovene)	Purine nucleoside analogue antiviral	*Adult*	
		IV: 5 mg/kg q12h for 14-21 days; maintenance dose, 5 mg/kg over 1 hr/day or 6 mg/kg/day for 5 days every wk	CMV retinitis in immunocompromised
indinavir (Crixivan)	Protease inhibitor	*Adult*	HIV Infections
		PO: 800 mg q8h	
nevirapine (Viramune)	Non-nucleoside reverse transcriptase inhibitor	*Adult*	HIV Infections
		PO: 200 mg qd for 14 days; then 200 mg q12h	
ribavirin (Virazole)	Purine nucleoside analogue antiviral	*Infant/Pediatric*	Selected infant and pediatric patients with RSV infections
		Aerosol: treatment with SPAG-2 for 12-18 hr/day with drug concentration of 20 mg/ml in drug reservoir of unit; average aerosol concentration for 12 hr pd, 190 µg/L of air. Treatment should last at least 3 days and not more than 7 days	
trifluridine (Viroptic)	Pyrimidine nucleoside analogue antiviral	Ophthalmic solution: 1 gtt q2h while awake to affected eye to maximum of 9 gtt per day until re-epithealization, then 1 gtt q4h for another 7 days	HSV 1 and 2 keratoconjunctivitis, recurrent epithelial keratitis
zidovudine (Retrovir)	Pyrimidine nucleoside analogue antiviral	*Pediatric 3 mo-12 y/o*	
		PO: 180 mg/m² q6h (720 mg/m²/day); do not exceed 200 mg q6h	
		Adult	HIV infections
		PO: asymptomatic cases, 500 mg/day divided q4h; symptomatic cases, 600 mg/day divided q4h	
		IV: 1-2 mg/kg infused over 1 hr q4h	
		Maternal/Fetal	
		Mother: PO: 100 mg 5 times/day after 14 weeks of pregnancy; during labor switch to 2 mg/kg IV over 1 hr, followed by continuous infusion of 1 mg/kg/hr until cord is clamped	Fetal HIV prophylaxis
		Infant: PO: 2 mg/kg q6h starting within 12 hr after delivery and continued for 6 wk or	
		IV: 1.5 mg/kg over 30 min q6h	

SPAG, small particle aerosol generator.

(Rescriptor), and efavirenz (Sustiva). Another agent that works and looks similar to NNRTIs is abacavir (Ziagen). It is a carbocyclic nucleoside that is a potent and selective inhibitor of reverse transcriptase and is considered a nucleoside reverse transcriptase inhibitor (NRTI). These agents are used in combination with nucleoside analogues like zidovudine. They directly inactivate reverse transcriptase enzyme, whereas the nucleoside analogues prevent the growth of the DNA chain.

Nevirapine is well tolerated when compared with other therapies for HIV. The most frequent adverse events associated with nevirapine therapy are rash, fever, nausea, headache, and abnormal liver function tests. Nevirapine is classified as a pregnancy category C drug and is contraindicated in patients with clinically significant hypersensitivity to any of its components. Nevirapine is only available orally as a 200-mg tablet. Commonly recommended dosage can be found in the dosage table on p. 604. The recommended dosage in the dosages table is generally preceded by a lead-in period of one 200-mg tablet daily for the first 14 days. This is done to lessen the frequency of rash.

PHARMACOKINETICS

HALF-LIFE	ONSET*	PEAK	DURATION*
25-30 hr	2 hr	2-4 hr	24 hr

*Therapeutic effects.

ribavirin

Ribavirin (Virazole) is a unique antiviral agent in that it is only given by oral or nasal inhalation. It is a synthetic nucleoside analogue of guanosine, as are many of the other antiviral agents, but it has a spectrum of antiviral activity that is broader than that of other currently available antiviral agents. It interferes with both RNA and DNA synthesis and as a result inhibits both protein synthesis and viral replication.

Ribavirin is used for the treatment of severe lower respiratory tract infections caused by RSV. It is also useful in the treatment of both influenza A and B infections as well as Lassa fever and Hantavirus infections.

Because ribavirin may cause fetal toxicity when administered to pregnant women, it is a pregnancy category X agent. It is therefore contraindicated in pregnant women with RSV infections because the risk of teratogenic or embryocidal effects far outweighs any benefits to be gained in the treatment of these generally self-limiting infections. Ribavirin is only available in an inhalational form that is given either nasally or orally. Commonly recommended dosages can be found in the dosages table on p. 604.

PHARMACOKINETICS

HALF-LIFE	ONSET	PEAK	DURATION
1.4-2.5 hr*	Unknown	End of inhalation period	Variable

*In respiratory secretions.

trifluridine

Trifluridine (Viroptic) is an analogue of thymidine. Both are used to treat herpes simplex keratitis, but trifluridine is also indicated for the treatment of herpes simplex keratoconjunctivitis. They are applied only topically to the eye because of the significant liver and bone marrow toxicities they can cause when given orally.

Trifluridine is classified as a pregnancy category C agent and is contraindicated in patients with a known hypersensitivity to it. It is only available as a 1% ophthalmic solution. Commonly recommended dosages can be found in the dosages table on p. 604.

PHARMACOKINETICS

HALF-LIFE	ONSET	PEAK	DURATION
12 min	Unknown	Immediate	2 hr

zidovudine

Zidovudine (AZT, ZDV, Retrovir) is a synthetic nucleoside analogue of thymidine that has had an enormous impact on the treatment and quality of life of patients infected with HIV who have AIDS. HIV requires reverse transciptase for viral replication. This process is inhibited by zidovudine as well as the other reverse transcriptase inhibitors lamivudine (Epivir), zalcitabine (Hivid), didanosine (Videx), and stavudine (Zerit). Although there have been many new therapies approved recently, none currently available can eradicate the infection. They are effective in that they decrease the viral load and delay immunologic decline. However, HIV over time can become resistant to the effects of reverse transcriptase inhibitors. For this reason it is common practice to now use multiple agents in the treatment of HIV infection.

Besides its antiviral activity, zidovudine also has bactericidal activity against some gram-negative bacteria, particularly many Enterobacteriaceae. These five antiviral agents are all approved for the treatment of HIV infections in patients with AIDS or AIDS-related complex (ARC). Treatment leads to a significant reduction in mortality and the incidence of opportunistic infections, improves patient's physical performance, and significantly improves T-cell counts.

Zidovudine's major dose-limiting adverse effect is bone marrow suppression, and this is often the reason why a patient with an HIV infection has to be switched to another anti-HIV agent such as zalcitabine or didanosine. Some patients may be taking a combination of two of these agents to maximize their actions but also to cut back on the dose of both agents, thus decreasing the likelihood of toxicity. The combination of various nucleoside analogues is so common that pharmaceutical companies have begun to make combination products. An example is Combivir, which is a single tablet that combines 150 mg of lamivudine and 300 mg of zidovudine.

Zidovudine is classified as a pregnancy category C agent and is contraindicated in patients with a known hypersensitivity to it. It is available in both oral and parenteral formulations. Parenterally it is available as a 10-mg/ml injection for IV infusion. Orally it is available as 100- and 300-mg capsules and a 50-mg/5 ml solution. Commonly recommended dosages can be found in the dosages table on p. 604.

PHARMACOKINETICS

HALF-LIFE	ONSET	PEAK	DURATION
0.78-1.93 hr	Unknown	0.4-1.5 hr	3-5 hr

NEURAMINIDASE INHIBITORS
oseltamivir and zanamivir

Oseltamivir (Tamiflu) and zanamivir (Relenza) are two agents that belong to the newest class of antiviral agents known as *neuraminidase inhibitors*. These agents are active against influenza types A and B. They are indicated for the treatment of uncomplicated acute illness caused by influenza infection in adults. They have been shown to reduce the duration of influenza infection by several days. The neuraminidase enzyme enables budding virus to escape from infected cells and spread throughout the body. Neuraminidase inhibitors are designed to stop the spread of influenza.

The most frequently reported adverse events with oseltamivir are nausea or vomiting, and those with zanamivir are diarrhea, nausea, and sinusitis. Oseltamivir is available as a 75-mg capsule to be taken twice a day for 5 days. Zanamivir is available as a dry powder for inhalation. The typical dose is two inhalations twice a day for 5 days. Treatment with oseltamivir and zanamivir should begin within 2 days of influenza symptom onset. Oseltamivir and zanamivir are contraindicated in patients with known hypersensitivity to them.

nursing process

● Assessment

Before administering an antiviral agent the nurse should perform a thorough assessment to find out what underlying diseases the patient may have and his or her medical history. This is important to ensure safe medication use. The nurse should also find out whether the patient has any known allergies to the medication or whether he or she has suffered any side effects of the medication in the past. It is important to assess the patient's nutritional status and baseline vital signs as well because of the profound effects viral illnesses can have on them, especially if the patient is also immunosuppressed. Contraindications to the use of most of the antiviral agents include herpes zoster infection in immunosuppressed patients. Cautious use, with careful monitoring, is recommended in patients who have renal or hepatic disease, who are dehydrated or in electrolyte imbalance, who are pregnant or lactating, or who have seizure disorders. Specifically, nevirapine should be given cautiously with close monitoring in patients with liver dysfunction because it may cause abnormal liver function laboratory results.

Amantadine is contraindicated in children under 1 year of age and should be used cautiously in patients suffering from congestive heart failure (because of the cardiovascular side effects it causes) or orthostatic hypotension. Laboratory results that should also be obtained before the start of therapy include WBC, RBC, BUN, CPK, LDH, and creatinine clearance. Culture and sensitivity testing should also be done. Zidovudine has been used in patients with HIV infections, but it is associated with many side effects and is capable of significant drug interactions that may increase the risk of toxicity. The agents with which it interacts in this way are vincristine, adriamycin, amphotericin B, and interferon. Some of the NSAIDs, such as probenecid and indomethacin, as well as acetaminophen and aspirin may interact with it as well, also enhancing the potential for toxicity. Indinavir and nevirapine are contraindicated in

research

Recommendations for Occupational HIV Exposure Chemoprophylaxis

Type of Exposure	Source	Prophylaxis	Therapy
Percutaneous	Blood	Recommended	zidovudine + lamivudine + indinavir
			zidovudine + lamivudine +/− indinavir
	Fluid containing visible blood or other potentially infectious fluid or tissue	Offer	zidovudine + lamivudine
Mucus membrane	Blood	Offer	zidovudine + lamivudine +/− indinavir
	Fluid containing visible blood or other potentially infectious fluid or tissue	Offer	zidovudine +/− lamivudine
Skin (i.e., prolonged contact, extensive area, area without skin integrity)	Blood	Offer	zidovudine + lamivudine +/− indinavir

patients who are allergic to their chemical properties. Renal studies should be assessed before use of indinavir and hepatic function studies before use of nevirapine.

Nursing Diagnoses

Nursing diagnoses appropriate to patients receiving antiviral agents include the following:
- Acute pain related to the signs and symptoms of a viral infection.
- Risk for injury related to side effects of medication.
- Deficient knowledge related to the viral infection, its transmission, and treatment.
- Activity intolerance related to weakened state and influence of drug treatment.
- Risk for infection related to compromised physical status.

Planning

Goals pertaining to patients receiving antiviral agents include the following:
- Patient is free of symptoms of viral infection once therapy is completed.
- Patient remains compliant with therapy.
- Patient experiences improved energy and appetite and improved ability to engage in activities of daily living.
- Patient states the rationale for therapy for any sexual partners if diagnosed with genital herpes.
- Patient experiences minimal side effects of antiviral agent.

Outcome Criteria

Outcome criteria for patients receiving antiviral agents include the following:
- Patient will experience increased periods of comfort as a result of successful treatment of viral infection.
- Patient will state the effect of a viral infection on his or her state of health (e.g., compromised immune system) and need for appropriate treatment.
- Patient will state the rationale for self-treatment and any sexual partners if diagnosed with genital herpes,

as well as the importance of compliance with the treatment to prevent worsening of symptoms and decrease severity of episodes.
- Patient will identify possible side effects of antiviral agent such as diarrhea, headache, nausea, and insomnia.

Implementation

Nursing interventions pertinent to patients receiving antiviral agents include use of the appropriate technique of application or administration of ointment, aerosol powders, or IV or oral forms of medication. Handwashing before and after administration of the medication is necessary to prevent contamination of the site and spread of infection to others. In addition, strict adherence to standard precautions is important to the safety of both the patient and the nurse.

Topical antiviral agents such as acyclovir should be applied in accordance with the manufacturer's guidelines or physician's orders, and gloves must be used to prevent the spread of infection to others. Intravenously administered acyclovir should be diluted in recommended solutions such as sterile water for injection or in the solutions recommended by the manufacturer. IV administration is usually done over 1 hour, but all sources of drug information should be consulted first to make sure that this and not some other timing is called for.

Most antivirals should be administered with caution in those patients who have renal or hepatic dysfunction. Because zidovudine suppresses bone marrow functioning, it should not be used in conjunction with other agents that do the same because of the resulting additive adverse effects. Other drugs that interact with zidovudine

---

case study | Antiviral Therapy

One of your patients, Z.K., a 33-year-old biology professor, has just begun therapy with zidovudine for an ARC infection. She is to be dosed with 200 mg orally every 4 hours, and will be taking the medication at home. She is inquiring about the new medication regimen, drug interactions, side effects, and any other important medication and how it differs from other antivirals.
- *Develop a patient teaching guide for Z.K. emphasizing any specific cautions and symptoms to report to the health care provider.*
- *Compare and contrast the various antiviral agents.*
- *At what level with platelets and WBCs would there probably be a change or discontinuation of zidovudine?*

For Answers see www.harcourthealth.com/MERLIN/Lilley/.

---

home health/community points

Alternative Approaches to Treatment

Many alternative approaches to the traditional methods of treating various disease processes exist, including AIDS and HIV. Even though alternative approaches to traditional medicine may not be acknowledged by health care providers, the health care provider must provide patients with adequate resources so they can make the best informed decision. Several resources for patients that can be accessed on the Internet:

    www.nursingcenter.com
    www.projinf.org/cgi-bin/print_hit_bold.pl/hh/
      alternative.html
    www.healthy.net/hwlibraryarticles/ayurvedic/intro.htm
    www.rnweb.com

Other sources include journals and books, such as the following:

    AIDS Patient Care (journal)
    Alternative Therapy in Health and Medicine (journal)
    Spencer JW, Jacobs JJ: *Complementary/alternative medicine: an evidence-based approach,* St Louis, 1998, Mosby.

include aspirin, acetaminophen, benzodiazepines, cimetidine, morphine, and sulfonamides.

Acyclovir and many of the other antiviral agents also interact with several drugs, and these have been enumerated earlier in the section on drug interactions. Fluid intake of at least 2400 ml per day should be encouraged in patients receiving acyclovir, unless contraindicated. This is to prevent crystalluria and is also applicable to patients receiving it intravenously. IV infusions should be administered slowly over at least 1 hour and the IV sites watched closely for the development of redness, swelling, or heat. Acyclovir capsules may be given with food. Acyclovir sodium should not be administered subcutaneously, imtramuscularly, orally, or ophthalmically. There are many IV agents and solutions that are incompatible with IV acyclovir, and the nurse should check and recheck this before proceeding with the co-administration of other agents or solutions. Zanamivir is to be used, if indicated, within 2 days of the onset of flu symptoms. It comes in a powder for inhalant use.

Idinavir and nevirapine are administered orally. With indinavir, patients should drink at least 48 ounces of fluids every day to maintain adequate hydration and help prevent nephrolithiasis.

Orally administered didanosine should be given every 12 hours, or as ordered, and on an empty stomach 1 hour before meals or 2 hours after meals. Antifungals are incompatible with didanosine. Buffered powder solutions for oral administration should be mixed in at least 4 ounces of water, not fruit juice or acid-containing juices, and the solution should be drunk immediately after mixing.

Activity

Patient teaching tips for the antivial agents are presented in the box at right.

● Evaluation

The therapeutic effects of antiviral agents depend mainly on the type of viral infection and the immune and general status of the patient. This could range from delayed pro-

gression of AIDS and ARC to a decrease in flulike symptoms and the frequency of herpetic flare-ups and opportunistic infections. Herpetic lesions should crust over, and the frequency of recurrence should decrease. Adverse reactions to specific antiviral agents should be monitored for, and these specific reactions are listed in Table 37-2.

---

patient teaching tips

Antiviral Therapy

➤ Tell patients the importance of taking these medications exactly as prescribed and for the full course of therapy.

➤ Some antivirals may cause dizziness, so the patient should be cautioned about driving or participating in activities requiring alertness.

➤ Patients should consult the physician before taking any other prescribed or OTC medications.

➤ Patients in immunosuppressed states should avoid crowds and persons with infections.

➤ Standard precautions and safe sex should be advocated in patients who are HIV positive.

➤ Patients using acyclovir ointment for treatment of herpes simplex infection should not use any other additional creams or ointments on the site. The patient should wear a glove or finger cot when applying topical solutions to affected areas, which should be kept clean and dry.

➤ Patients with any type of viral infection should practice good hygiene.

➤ Inform patients that antiviral agents are not cures but do help to manage the related symptoms.

➤ With zidovudine, caution patients to take on an empty stomach and to use exactly as prescribed.

➤ Hair loss *may* occur with zidovudine, and patients should be aware of this rare adverse reaction so they can purchase a wig, hairpiece, or be prepared for this hair loss in their own way.

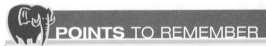

POINTS TO REMEMBER

Viruses

• Current viruses killed by antivirals: CMV, HSV, HIV, influenza A, RSV.
• Difficult to kill because they live inside human cells.
• Drugs work by inhibiting viral replication.

Antiviral Drugs

• Are synthetic purine and pyrimidine nucleoside analogues.
• They trick virus into thinking that they are either a purine (adenine or guanine) or a pyrimidine (cytosine or thymine) and then are taken up by the virus, which tries to use them to replicate itself and in doing so ends up dying.

• Must be able to enter cells infected with virus, interfere with ability of virus to bind to cells, and stimulate body's immune system.

Purine Analogue Antivirals

• Are synthetic analogues of purine nucleosides such as adenine and guanine.
• Most common examples are acyclovir, didanosine, and ganciclovir.

Pyrimidine Analogue Antivirals

• Are synthetic analogues of pyrimidine nucleoside such as cytosine and thymine.

- Most common examples are zalcitabine, zidovudine, and trifluridine.

Nursing Considerations

- Antiviral agents should be administered only after all physician orders are read and understood and after a thorough nursing assessment that includes an examination of the patient's nutritional status and baseline vital signs.

- Contraindications to the use of antiviral agents include herpes zoster in immunosuppressed patients.
- Cautious use is recommended in patients with renal, hepatic, or seizure disorders; pregnant or lactating women; and patients who are dehydrated or in electrolyte imbalance.
- There are many drugs that interact with the antiviral agents, so the nurse should always check to make sure the patient is taking none of these agents before administering the antiviral agent.

REVIEW QUESTIONS

1. Treatment with antiviral agents is often more difficult than it seems because of which of the following?
   a. Viral replication is not well understood.
   b. Often the symptoms appear only after the viral replication is finished.
   c. The virus develops a resistance to medication and a more porous permeable membrane.
   d. The virus develops a double-protein-layer wall, and this prevents penetration of the drug.

2. You are caring for a patient who has AIDS. He has been on AZT (zidovudine) for a year and a half, and his CD4 count has just recently started to drop below 125. The physician adds didanosine (ddl) to the patient's antiviral drug regimen. Which of the following statements regarding the patient's drug therapy is most accurate?
   a. The combination is appropriate because it consists of an antifungal and an antiviral drug.
   b. The combination of AZT and ddl in unnecessary because it consists of two drugs from the same class.
   c. The combination is appropriate because it consists of two antivirals with synergistic actions yet different side effect profiles.
   d. The combination of AZT and ddl is potentially harmful because both drugs have similar side effect profiles, which increases the chance of toxicity.

3. A month into therapy with the combination-drug regimen of AZT and ddl, a CBC reveals a low number of platelets, neutrophils, and other cells produced by the bone marrow. You recognize this as:
   a. Pancreatitis induced by AZT.
   b. A peripheral neuropathy induced by ddl.
   c. Bone marrow suppression induced by ddl.
   d. Bone marrow suppression induced by AZT.

4. The change of events that occurs in Question 3 prompts some adjustments in the patient's drug regimen. On the following day when you arrive to care for this patient, you notice that the physician on call over the weekend has stopped the AZT treatment and started ddC (zalcitabine) treatment. You call the physician to notify her that:
   a. ddl is an antifungal and ddC is an antiviral, and the combination is okay.
   b. ddl and ddC can both cause bone marrow suppression, and the combination is potentially dangerous.
   c. ddl and ddC are antagonistic to each other, and each will reduce the effectiveness of the other agent.
   d. ddl and ddC can both cause peripheral neuropathies, and the combination is potentially dangerous.

5. Which of the following are cautions or contraindications to the use of amantadine treatment?
   a. Polycythemia
   b. Diagnosis of influenza
   c. Congestive heart failure
   d. Severe CNS dysfunction

For Answers see www.harcourthealth.com/MERLIN/Lilley/.

CRITICAL THINKING Activities

1. What condition or problem would cause drug treatment in a patient with HIV to be switched to another drug that is also an anti-HIV agent? Explain your answer.

2. What antiviral agent would be best for a patient who has had a bone marrow transplant but has also contracted CMV? Why?

3. What is the benefit of rimantadine over amantadine?

For Answers see www.harcourthealth.com/MERLIN/Lilley/.

bibliography

Albanese J, Nutz P: *Mosby's 2001 nursing drug reference and review cards,* St Louis, 2001, Mosby.

American Hospital Formulary Service: *AHFS drug information,* Bethesda, Md, 2000, American Society of Health-System Pharmacists.

Anderson PO, Knoben JE, Troutman WG: *Handbook of clinical drug data 1999-2000,* ed 9, New York, 1999, McGraw-Hill.

Johns Hopkins Hospital, Department of Pediatrics et al: *The Harriet Lane handbook,* ed 15, St Louis, 2000, Mosby.

Keen JH: *Critical care and emergency drug reference,* ed 3, St Louis, 1996, Mosby.

Klaus BB, Grodesky MJ: HIV and HAART in 1997: highly effective antiretroviral therapy, *Nurse Pract* 22(8):139, 1997.

Lisanti P, Zwolski K: Understanding the devastation of AIDS, *Am J Nurs* 97(7):26, 1997.

Mosby's GenRx: a comprehensive reference for generic and brand drugs, ed 10, St Louis, 2000, Mosby.

Skidmore-Roth L: *Mosby's 2001 nursing drug reference,* St Louis, 2001, Mosby.

Remember to check the **Online Worksheet** for additional learning opportunities: **www.harcourthealth.com/MERLIN/Lilley/**

Activity

38

Antitubercular Agents

objectives

When you reach the end of this chapter, you should be able to do the following:

1 Identify the various first-line and second-line agents used for the treatment of tuberculosis.

2 Discuss the mechanisms of action, dosages, and side effects, indications for treatment, cautions, contraindications, and drug interactions associated with the various antitubercular agents.

3 Develop a nursing care plan that includes all phases of the nursing process for patients receiving antitubercular drugs.

4 Develop a teaching guide for patients receiving any of the antitubercular agents.

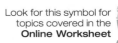

www.harcourthealth.com/MERLIN/Lilley/

Look for this symbol for topics covered in the **Online Worksheet**

---

drug profiles

ethambutol, p. 613 | rifampin, p. 615
o—= isoniazid, p. 614 | rifapentine, p. 616
pyrazinamide, p. 615 | streptomycin, p. 616

o—= Key drug.

---

glossary

Aerobic (a′ ro′ bik) Requiring oxygen for the maintenance of life. (p. 611)

Antitubercular agents (an′ ti too bər′ ku ler) Drugs used to treat infections caused by *Mycobacterium* spp. (p. 611)

Bacillus (bə sil′ us) Rod-shaped bacteria. (p. 611)

Isoniazid (i′ so ni′ ə zid) Primary and most frequently prescribed tuberculostatic agent. (p. 611)

Multi-drug–resistant TB Tuberculosis that demonstrates resistance to two or more drugs. (p. 612)

Primary (first-line) agents Class of drugs currently employed for the treatment of pulmonary tuberculosis; first choice drugs (p. 611)

Primary TB infection A patient's first tuberculosis infection. (p. 612)

Reinfection The most chronic form of tuberculosis. (p. 612)

Secondary (second-line) agents Class of drugs currently employed for the treatment of pulmonary tuberculosis; second choice drugs (p. 611)

Slow acetylators Someone with a genetic defect that causes a deficiency in the enzyme needed to break down isoniazid. (p. 615)

Tubercle bacilli (too′ bər ka′l) Rod-shaped tuberculosis bacteria. (p. 611)

TUBERCULOSIS

Mycobacterium tuberculosis is the bacteria that causes tuberculosis (TB). It is an **aerobic** bacillus, which means that it is a rod-shaped microorganism *(bacillus)* that requires a lot of oxygen for it to grow and flourish *(aerobic)*. This bacteria's need for a highly oxygenated body site explains why *Mycobacterium* infections most commonly affect the lungs, the growing ends of bones, and the brain (cerebral cortex), with the kidney, liver, and genitourinary tract other less common sites.

These **tubercle** (tuberculous) **bacilli** are transmitted from one of three sources: humans, cows (bovine), or birds (avian), although bovine and avian transmission are much less common than human transmission. Tubercle bacilli are conveyed in droplets expelled by infected people or animals during coughing or sneezing and then inhaled by the new host. After these infectious droplets are inhaled, the infection spreads to the susceptible organ sites by means of the blood and lymphatic system. However, tuberculosis does not develop in all people who inhale these infectious droplets. Instead, the bacteria become dormant or walled off by calcified or fibrous tissues. TB is a very slow-growing organism as well. All these characteristics can make TB an organism that is very difficult to treat. Many of the antibiotics used to treat TB work by inhibiting growth rather than directly killing the organism. Therefore the slower growing the organism the more difficult the organism can be to treat. At the other end of the spectrum are the infected people whose host defenses have been broken down as the result of immunosuppressive drug therapy, chemotherapy for cancer, or an immunosuppressive disease such as acquired immunodeficiency syndrome (AIDS). In these people the disease can inflict devastating and irreversible damage. The first infectious episode is considered the **primary TB infection; reinfection** represents the more chronic form of the disease.

Over the past decade there has been growing concern about the increasing number of cases of TB. This is evidenced by the 18% increase in the incidence of TB that took place between 1985 and 1991. It is now estimated that between 10 and 15 million people worldwide have some form of tuberculous infection.

Several factors are responsible for fomenting this health care crisis, but one very important source of the problem is the increasing number of people who are particularly susceptible to the infection—homeless and undernourished or malnourished people; AIDS victims; people taking immunosuppressant drugs; drug abusers; and people suffering from cancer. Those people at high risk of contracting the disease also tend to be members of minority groups (64% of all cases) and those who live in crowded and poorly sanitated facilities.

As great of a concern as the increasing number of TB cases has been the appearance of drug-resistant tuberculosis. For instance, the Centers for Disease Control and Prevention (CDC), which track and monitor the epidemiologic course of many diseases (TB being one of major importance), observed that in 1991 in New York City 33% of patients with TB were resistant to at least one antitubercular drug. Disease resistant to two or more drugs is called **multi-drug—resistant TB** (MDR-TB). There have already been outbreaks of such cases in nine institutional facilities, and the CDC has found that these occurred to a great extent (20% to 100%) in human immunodeficiency virus (HIV)-infected persons. They also found the mortality in these people with MDR-TB to range between 72% and 89%.

Activity

ANTITUBERCULAR AGENTS

The agents used to treat infections caused by all forms of *Mycobacterium* are called **antitubercular agents,** and these agents fall into two categories: **primary (first-line)** and **secondary (second-line) agents.** The antimycobacterial activity, efficacy, and potential adverse and toxic effects of the various agents determine the class to which they belong. **Isoniazid** (INH), a primary antitubercular drug, is the most frequently used antitubercular agent. It can be used either as the sole agent in the prophylaxis of TB or in combination with other antitubercular agents. The various first- and second-line antibiotics agents are listed in Box 38-1.

An important consideration during drug selection is the relative likelihood of drug-resistant organisms and drug toxicity. Following are other key elements important to the planning and implementation of the affective therapy:

1. Drug-susceptibility tests should be performed on the first-isolated *Mycobacterium* sp. (to prevent the development of MDR-TB).
2. Before the results of the susceptibility tests are known, the patient should be started on a four-drug regimen, consisting of isoniazid, rifampin, pyrazinamide, and ethambutol or streptomycin, which to-

---

BOX 38-1

First- and Second-Line Antitubercular Agents

PRIMARY
ethambutol
isoniazid
pyrazinamide (PZA)
rifampin
streptomycin

SECONDARY*
capreomycin
cycloserine
ethionamide
kanamycin
para-aminosalicyclic acid (PAS)

OTHER
rifabutin

*Multidrug regimens that include drugs such as streptomycin, kanamycin, and capreomycin, which have similar toxic effects, should include only one of these drugs.

---

gether are 95% effective in combating the infection. The use of multiple medications reduces the possibility of the organism becoming drug resistant.
3. Once drug susceptibility results are available, the regimen should be adjusted accordingly.
4. Patient compliance and the adverse effects of the prescribed regimen should be monitored closely because the incidence of both is high.

Despite all the agents available to combat TB and the efforts mounted to detect and treat victims of the disease, treatment has been made difficult by two problems previously mentioned: patient noncompliance with therapy and the growing incidence of drug-resistant organisms.

Mechanism of Action

The mechanisms of action of the various antitubercular drugs vary depending on the agent. These drugs act on *M. tuberculosis* in one of three ways: they inhibit either protein or cell wall synthesis or work by some other means. The antitubercular agents are listed in Box 38-2 by their mechanism of action.

Drug Effects

The drug effects of the antitubercular agents are primarily limited to their ability to kill *M. tuberculosis*, but other strains of *Mycobacterium* may also be susceptible to the killing actions of these drugs. They are used as the initial treatment for patients with uncomplicated pulmonary TB and for most children and adults with extrapulmonary TB. Antitubercular drug effects have not been fully tested in pregnant women, but the combination of isoniazid and ethambutol has been used to treat pregnant women with clinically apparent TB without teratogenic complications.

Besides being used for the initial treatment of TB, antitubercular agents have also proved effective in the management of treatment failures and relapses. Infection with species of *Mycobacterium* other than *M. tuberculosis* (also

Box 38-2   Antitubercular Agents: Mechanisms of Action

Drugs	Description
INHIBIT PROTEIN SYNTHESIS	
capreomycin	Streptomycin and kanamycin work by interfering with normal protein synthesis and production of
kanamycin	faulty proteins. Rifampin and capreomycin act at different points in the protein synthesis pathway
rifabutin	from streptomycin and kanamycin. Rifampin inhibits RNA synthesis and may also inhibit DNA
rifampin	synthesis. Human cells are not as sensitive as the mycobacterial cells and are not affected by
streptomycin	rifampin except at high drug concentrations. Capreomycin inhibits protein synthesis by preventing translocation on ribosomes.
INHIBIT CELL WALL SYNTHESIS	
cycloserine	Cycloserine acts by inhibiting the amino acid (D-Alanine) involved in the synthesis of cell walls.
ethionamide	Isoniazid and ethionamide also act at least partly to inhibit the synthesis of wall components,
isoniazid	but the mechanisms of these two agents are still not clearly understood.
OTHER MECHANISMS	
ethambutol	Other proposed MOAs for isoniazid exist. Isoniazid is taken up by mycobacteria cells and under-
ethionamide	goes hydrolysis to isonicotinic acid, which reacts with cofactor NAD to form a defective NAD that
isoniazid	is no longer active as a coenzyme for certain life-sustaining reactions in the *M. tuberculosis* or-
para-aminosalicylic acid	ganism. Ethionamide directly inhibits mycolic acid synthesis, which eventually has the same dele-
pyrazinamide	terious effects on the TB organism as isoniazid. Ethambutol affects lipid synthesis, resulting in the inhibition of mycolic acid incorporation into the cell wall, thus inhibiting protein synthesis. Para-aminosalicylic acid acts as a competitive inhibitor of para-aminobenzoic acid in the synthesis of folate. The MOA of pyrazinamide in the inhibition of TB is unknown. It can be either bacteriostatic or bactericidal, depending on the susceptibility of the particular *Mycobacterium* organism and the concentration of the drug attained at the site of infection.

MOA, Mechanism of action; *NAD,* nicotinamide adenine dinucleotide.

called *MOTT*) as well as atypical mycobacterial infections have also been successfully treated with these agents. Nontuberculous mycobacteria (NTM) may also be susceptible to antitubercular drugs. However, in general, antitubercular agents are not as effective against other species of *Mycobacterium* as they are against *M. tuberculosis*. Some of these other species that may be of particular concern in immunocompromised patients such as AIDS patients are *M. avium-intracellulare, M. flavescens, M. marinum,* and *M. kansasii*. Additional *Mycobacterium* infections that may respond to antitubercular agents are those caused by *M. fortuitum, M. chelonae, M. smegmatis, M. xenopi,* and *M. scrofulaceum*.

Therapeutic Uses

Antitubercular drugs are primarily used for the prophylaxis or treatment of TB. The effectiveness of these agents depends on the type of infection, adequate dosing, sufficient duration of treatment, drug compliance, and the selection of an effective drug combination. The therapeutic effects of the different antitubercular drugs are listed in Box 38-3.

Side Effects and Adverse Effects

Antitubercular agents are fairly well tolerated. Isoniazid, one of the mainstays of treatment, is noted for causing pyridoxine deficiency and liver toxicity. The most problematic drugs and their associated adverse effects are listed in Table 38-1.

Interactions

The drugs that can interact with antitubercular agents can cause significant effects. See Table 38-2 for a summary of these interactions. Besides these drug interactions, isoniazid can cause a false-positive Clinitest reading and an increase in the serum levels of the alanine aminotransferase (ALT) and aspartate aminotransferase (AST).

Dosages

For the recommended dosages of selected antitubercular agents, see the dosages table on p. 616.

drug profiles

Antitubercular drugs can only be obtained by prescription and are indicated for the treatment of many different *Mycobacterium* infections, including *M. tuberculosis*. the organism that causes TB. They are available in many different dosage forms, including orally, intravenously, and intramuscularly administered agents. Some of the primary and secondary agents that are commonly used in the treatment of TB are discussed here.

ethambutol

Ethambutol (Myambutol) is a primary bacteriostatic agent used in the treatment of TB that is

Antitubercular Agents: Therapeutic Uses

BOX 38-3

Drug	Therapeutic Use
capreomycin	• Used with other antitubercular agents for treatment of pulmonary TB caused by *M. tuberculosis* after primary agents fail, drug resistance appears, or drug toxicity occurs.
cycloserine	• Used with other antitubercular agents for treatment of active pulmonary and extrapulmonary TB after failure of primary agents.
ethambutol	• Indicated as a primary agent for the treatment of TB.
ethionamide	• Used with other antitubercular agents in the treatment of clinical TB after failure of primary agents and other mycobacterial diseases.
isoniazid	• Used alone or in combination with other antitubercular agents in the treatment and prevention of clinical TB.
kanamycin	• Used in combination with other antitubercular agents in treatment of clinical TB. It is not intended for long-term use.
para-aminosalicylate sodium	• Used in combination with other antitubercular agents for the treatment of pulmonary and extrapulmonary *M. tuberculosis* infection after failure of primary agents.
pyrazinamide	• Used with other antitubercular agents in the treatment of clinical TB.
rifabutin	• Used to prevent or delay the development of *M. avium-intracellulare* bacteremia and disseminated infections in patients with advanced HIV infections.
rifampin	• Used with other antitubercular agents in the treatment of clinical TB.
	• Used in treatment of diseases caused by mycobacteria other than *M. tuberculosis.*
	• Used for preventive therapy in patients exposed to isoniazid-resistant *M. tuberculosis.*
	• Used to eliminate meningococci from the nasopharynx of asymptomatic *Neisseria meningitidis* carriers when the risk of meningococcal meningitis is high.
	• Used for chemoprophylaxis in contacts of patients with *Haemophilus influenzae* type B (Hib) infection.
	• Used with at least one other antiinfective agent in the treatment of leprosy.
	• Used in the treatment of endocarditis caused by methicillin-resistant staphylococci, chronic staphylococcal prostatitis, and multiple-antiinfective–resistant pneumococci.
streptomycin	• Used in combination with other antitubercular agents in treatment of clinical TB and other mycobacterial diseases.

Antitubercular Agents: Common Adverse Effects

TABLE 38-1

Drug	Side/Adverse Effects
capreomycin	Ototoxicity, nephrotoxicity
cycloserine	Psychotic behavior, seizures
ethambutol	Retrobulbar neuritis, blindness
ethionamide	Gastrointestinal tract disturbances, hepatotoxicity
isoniazid	Peripheral neuritis, hepatotoxicity
kanamycin	Ototoxicity, nephrotoxicity
para-aminosalicylic acid	Gastrointestinal tract disturbances, hepatotoxicity
pyrazinamide	Hepatotoxicity, hyperuricemia
rifabutin	Gastrointestinal tract disturbances, rash, neutropenia, discolored urine
rifampin	Hepatitis, hematologic disorders, discoloration of urine, stools, saliva, tears, sweat, and sputum
streptomycin	Ototoxicity, nephrotoxicity, blood dyscrasias

believed to work by diffusing into the mycobacteria and suppressing RNA synthesis, thereby inhibiting protein synthesis. Ethambutol is included with isoniazid, streptomycin, and rifampin in many TB combination-drug therapies. It may also be used to treat other mycobacterial diseases. It is classified as a pregnancy category B agent and is contraindicated in patients with a hypersensitivity to it, those with optic neuritis, and children younger than 13 years of age. It is available only in oral forms as a 100-mg tablet and a 400-mg film-coated tablet. The usual recommended dosages are given in the dosages table on p. 616.

PHARMACOKINETICS

HALF-LIFE	ONSET	PEAK	DURATION
3.3 hr	Variable	2-4 hr	Up to 24 hr

isoniazid

Isoniazid (Laniazid, INH, Nydrazid) is not only the mainstay in the treatment of TB but also is the most widely used antitubercular agent. It may be given

Activity

38-2 Antitubercular Agents: Drug Interactions

Drug	Mechanism	Results
AMINOSALICYLATE		
probenecid	Reduces excretion	Increased aminosalicylate levels
Salicylates	Additive effects	Aminosalicylate toxicity
ISONIAZID		
Antacids	Reduces absorption	Decreased isoniazid levels
cycloserine, ethionamide, and rifampin	Additive effects	Increased CNS and hepatic toxicity
phenytoin + carbamazepine	Decreases metabolism	Increased phenytoin and carbamazepine effects
STREPTOMYCIN		
Nephrotoxic and neurotoxic drugs	Additive	Increased toxicity
Oral anticoagulants	Alter intestinal flora	Increased bleeding tendencies
RIFAMPIN		
Beta-blockers		
Benzodiazepines		
cyclosporine		
Oral anticogulants		
Oral antidiabetics	Increased metabolism	Decreased therapeutic effects of these drugs
Oral contraceptives		
phenytoin		
quinidine		
theophylline		

either as a single agent for prophylaxis or in combination with other antitubercular drugs for the treatment of active TB. It is a bactericidal agent that kills the mycobacteria by disrupting cell wall synthesis as well as essential cellular functions.

Isoniazid is metabolized in the liver through a process called *acetylation*, which requires a certain enzymatic pathway to break down the drug. However, some people have a genetic deficiency of the enzymes needed for this to occur. Such people are called **slow acetylators.** When isoniazid is taken by slow acetylators, the isoniazid accumulates because there is not enough of the enzymes to break down the isoniazid. Therefore the dosages of isoniazid may need to be adjusted downward in these patients.

Isoniazid is available in both oral and parenteral formulations. Orally it is available as a 50-mg/5 ml solution and as 50-, 100-, and 300-mg tablets. Parenterally it is available in a strength of 100 mg/ml for IM injection. There is also an oral formulation of isoniazid called *Rifamate* that includes rifampin. It is available as a fixed-dose capsule, and the respective amounts of isoniazid and rifampin are 150 mg and 300 mg.

Isoniazid is classified as a pregnancy category C agent. It is contraindicated in patients with a hypersensitivity to it, in those with optic neuritis, and in those with previous isoniazid-associated hepatic injury or acute liver disease. The usually recommended dosages of isoniazid are given in the dosages table on p. 616.

PHARMACOKINETICS

HALF-LIFE	ONSET	PEAK	DURATION
1-4 hr	Variable	1-2 hr	Up to 24 hr

pyrazinamide

Pyrazinamide is an antitubercular drug that can be either bacteriostatic or bactericidal, depending on its concentration at the site of infection and the particular susceptibility of the mycobacteria. It is frequently used in combination with other antitubercular drugs for the treatment of TB. Its mechanism of action is unknown, but it is believed to work by inhibiting lipid and nucleic acid synthesis in the mycobacteria. Pyrazinamide is only available as an oral formulation in a 500-mg tablet. It is classified as a pregnancy category C agent and is contraindicated in patients who have had a hypersensitivity reaction to it. The usually recommended dosages are given in the dosages table on p. 616.

PHARMACOKINETICS

HALF-LIFE	ONSET	PEAK	DURATION
9-10 hr	Variable	2 hr	Up to 24 hr

rifampin

Rifampin (Rifadin, Rimactane) is a synthetic antibiotic with activity against many forms of *Mycobacterium* as well as against meningococcus, *Haemophilus influenzae* type B, and leprosy. It is a

DOSAGES Selected Antitubercular Agents

agent	pharmacologic class	dosage range	purpose
ethambutol (Myambutol)	Synthetic primary antimycobacterial	*Adult* PO: 25 mg/kg/day for 2 months and then 15 mg/kg/day qd	
isoniazid (INH, Laniazid, Nydrazid)	Synthetic primary antimycobacterial	*Adult* PO: 300 mg once/day for prophylaxis and 5-10 mg/kg/day for active TB (max 300 mg/day)	
pyrazinamide (none)	Synthetic primary antimycobacterial	*Adult* PO: 15-30 mg/kg/day	For active TB
rifampin (Rifadin, Rimactane)	Semisynthetic primary antimycobacterial antibiotic	*Adult* PO: 600 mg/day	
streptomycin (many product names)	Antimycobacterial aminoglycoside antibiotic	*Adult* IM: 1 g/day initially for 60-90 days then 1 g 2-3 times/week	

broad-spectrum bactericidal agent that kills the offending organism by inhibiting protein synthesis. Rifampin is used either alone in the prevention of TB or in combination with other antitubercular agents in its treatment. A notable side effect of rifampin is that it can turn urine, feces, saliva, skin, sputum, sweat, or tears a red-orange to red-brown color.

Rifampin is available in both oral and parenteral formulations and, as previously mentioned, in combination with isoniazid (Rifamate). As an oral agent it is available as a 150- and 300-mg oral capsule. In its parenteral formulation it is available in a vial for injection that contains 600 mg of the agent. Rifampin is classified as a pregnancy category C agent and is contraindicated in patients with a known hypersensitivity to it. The usual recommended dosages are given in the dosages table above.

PHARMACOKINETICS

HALF-LIFE	ONSET	PEAK	DURATION
3 hr	Variable	2-4 hr	Up to 24 hr

rifapentine

Rifapentine (Prifitin) is a cyclopental derivative of rifampin. It offers advantages over rifampin in that it has a much longer duration of action and possibly better efficacy. It has been shown to have greater antimycobacterial efficacy and neutrophil penetration. It is indicated for pulmonary tuberculosis and comes as a 150-mg tablet. Rifapentine is dosed 600 mg twice weekly. It is classified as a pregnancy category C agent and is contraindicated in patients with a hypersensitivity to rifapentine.

PHARMACOKINETICS

HALF-LIFE	ONSET	PEAK	DURATION
14-17 hr	Unknown	5-6 hr	Unknown

streptomycin

Streptomycin is an aminoglycoside antibiotic that goes by many trade names. Introduced in 1944, it was the very first antitubercular drug to come available that could effectively treat TB. Mostly because of its toxicities it is today most frequently used only in combination-drug regimens for the treatment of MDR-TB infections.

Streptomycin is only available in a parenteral formulation: a 1- and 5-g injection as well as a 400-mg/ml injection. Streptomycin is classified as a pregnancy category D agent and is contraindicated in patients hypersensitive to it. The usually recommended dosages are given in the dosages table above.

PHARMACOKINETICS

HALF-LIFE	ONSET	PEAK	DURATION
2-3 hr	Variable	1-2 hr	Up to 24 hr

nursing process

● Assessment

Before administering any of the primary or secondary antitubercular agents, to ensure the safe and effective use of these medications, the nurse should obtain a thorough medical history on the patient and perform a complete assessment. Liver function studies should be performed in patients who used to receive isoniazid or rifampin because of the hepatic impairment these agents can cause. This is especially important in elderly patients and patients who consume alcohol daily because of the greater likelihood of liver disorders in such patients.

A thorough neurologic assessment is also called for because of the increased incidence of peripheral neuropathies of the feet and hands in patients taking isoniazid. It is also important to check the patient's CBC, Hgb level, and Hct value before administering isoniazid because of the hematologic disorders they can cause. Renal studies, such as the creatinine and BUN levels as well as urinalysis, should also be performed both at the start of isoniazid or rifampin therapy and during therapy. Contraindications to the use of rifampin include hypersensitivity. Contraindications to the use of isoniazid include allergy to the drug, liver or renal disease, pregnancy, lactation, and optic neuritis. The drugs that interact with these agents are listed in Table 38-2. Sputum cultures are routinely done as part of the workup in patients, so the nurse should always check these results before administering the specific antitubercular drugs to confirm that the appropriate agent is being given.

Pyrazinamide, ethambutol, and streptomycin are the other primary agents used in the treatment of TB. Baseline liver function tests should be performed in patients who are to be given pyrazinamide because of the hepatotoxicity it can cause. It can also cause hyperuricemia, so gout or flare-ups of gout may occur in susceptible patients. The Hgb levels and Hct values should also be checked. Contraindications to the use of any of these three agents include hypersensitivity.

Ethambutol may cause a decrease in visual acuity resulting from optic neuritis, so a thorough eye examination may be called for before the institution of therapy. In addition, the patient's baseline liver function status, Hgb levels, and Hct values should be determined before the initiation of therapy. Contraindications to the use of ethambutol include hypersensitivity and optic neuritis. Cautious use is called for in patients with liver or renal disease, hematologic disorders, or diabetes.

Streptomycin is contraindicated in patients with renal disease or those with a hypersensitivity to the agent. The patient's BUN and creatinine levels should be measured and urinalysis performed before the start of therapy. It should be used very carefully in the elderly and in patients with hearing disorders because of the ototoxicity it can cause.

The assessment aspect of the nursing care in patients being given any of the other secondary agents (see Box 38-3) is very similar.

Nursing Diagnoses

Nursing diagnoses pertaining to patients receiving antitubercular agents include the following:
- Risk for injury related to noncompliance to drug therapy and to an overall status of poor health.
- Ineffective therapeutic regimen management of TB related to poor compliance to therapy.
- Ineffective family therapeutic regimen management related to poor compliance and poor housing and living conditions.
- Deficient knowledge related to the disease process and treatment protocol.

Planning

Goals for patients receiving antitubercular agents are focused on patient safety and compliance with therapy, and these include the following:
- Patient experiences minimal side effects of the treatment for TB.
- Patient takes medication regularly and for the length of time prescribed.
- Patient remains free of injury related to drug interactions with the antitubercular drugs.
- Patient remains free of toxic effects or reports them to the physician immediately.
- Patient remains compliant with the drug therapy.

Outcome Criteria

The outcome criteria for patients receiving antitubercular agents are also focused on patient study and compliance. These include the following:
- Patient will state the therapeutic effects (improved signs and symptoms and killing of mycobacterium) as

For a project that received new funding, you and five of your community health nursing colleagues have been asked to give some minipresentations to various large work settings in the community. One place is in your health department with the nurses who work in the adult clinic.

- *What are some of the key components that you should include, as per OSHA's tuberculosis infection control guidelines, in your presentation to this staff.*
- *What information could then be used or what information could then be shared with patients in the adult clinic?*

For Answers see www.harcourthealth.com/MERLIN/Lilley/.

well as possible side effects (neuropathies, gastrointestinal upset) of the treatment.

- Patient will state the importance of taking the medication regularly and for the length of time prescribed to prevent complications, relapses, or recurrences.
- Patient will state the drugs that interact with antitubercular agent such as salicylates, antacids, and anticoagulants.
- Patient will report toxic effects such as renal or liver dysfunction, hearing loss, and blindness to the physician, should they occur.
- Patient will show improvement of disease state with a decreased cough, fever, and normal laboratory values.

Implementation

Because drug therapy is the mainstay of the treatment of TB and often lasts for up to a 24 months, patient education is critical, with a special emphasis on compliance. Simple, clear, and concise instructions should be given to the patient. This should include the fact that multiple drugs are generally used and that 90% cure rates can be achieved with combination therapy consisting of isoniazid and rifampin (if the patient is strictly compliant with therapy). All antitubercular agents should be given exactly as ordered and at the same time every day. Consistent use and dosing is critical in maintaining steady blood levels and in minimizing the chances of resistance to the drug therapy.

Generally speaking, oral preparations should be given with meals to diminish gastrointestinal tract upset, even though it is often recommended that they be given either 1 hour before or 2 hours after meals. An antiemetic may be necessary in some patients. Intramuscularly administered agents such as streptomycin, capreomycin sulfate, and kanamycin should be given deep in a large muscle mass and the sites rotated. Pyridoxine in doses of 200 to 300 mg per day may be ordered in patients taking cycloserine or isoniazid to prevent the associated neurotoxicity.

Patient teaching tips for antitubercular agents are presented in the box below.

Evaluation

The nurse should always document patients' responses, or lack of them, to therapy. The therapeutic response to antitubercular therapy is reflected by a decrease in the symptoms of TB, such as cough and fever, and by weight gain. The results of laboratory studies (culture and sensitivity tests) and the chest x-ray findings should confirm the clinical findings. Patients with drug-resistant disease do not show a clinical response to the therapy, and laboratory findings will confirm this.

Patients also need to be monitored for the occurrence of adverse reactions to antitubercular agents. These include fatigue, nausea, vomiting, numbness and tingling of the extremities, fever, loss of appetite, depression, and jaundice. The physician should be notified if they occur, and the incident should be documented accordingly.

---

patient teaching tips

Antitubercular Agents

➤ Patients should be told to take all medications directly as ordered by the physician.

➤ Patients should know that compliance with therapy means taking the medication as ordered and for the ordered length of time and that compliance is essential for achieving a cure. This includes keeping follow-up appointments with the physician.

➤ Patients should not consume alcohol while they are receiving these medications and should always check with their physician before taking any other type of medication.

➤ Diabetic patients taking isoniazid should monitor their blood glucose levels using a glucometer because of the hyperglycemia this medication can cause.

➤ Patients should take pyridoxine as prescribed by the physician to prevent some of the neurologic side effects of isoniazid such as numbness and tingling of extremities.

➤ Patients taking isoniazid or rifampin should report the following side effects to the physician immediately: fever, nausea, vomiting, loss of appetite, yellow tint to skin or eyes, unusual bleeding, or numbness and tingling of extremities.

➤ Women taking oral contraceptives who are prescribed rifampin must be switched to another form of birth control, because oral contraceptives become ineffective when given with rifampin.

➤ Patients who are taking rifampin should be told that their urine, stool, saliva, sputum, sweat, or tears may become reddish orange, and even contact lenses may be stained.

➤ Patients should see their health care provider at least monthly during treatment.

➤ Patients must be reminded that they are contagious during the initial period of the illness and its diagnosis, so they should make every effort to wash their hands and cover their mouths when coughing or sneezing.

They should also be careful about where they throw away dirty tissues.

➤ Patients being treated for TB need to always take care of themselves. This includes adequate nutrition, rest, and relaxation.

➤ Patients should keep all medications away from children.

➤ Patients should always wear a MedicAlert tag or bracelet naming the antitubercular medications they are taking.

POINTS TO REMEMBER

Antitubercular agents

- Primary (first-line) antitubercular agents include ethambutol, isoniazid, pyrazinamide (PZA), rifampin, streptomycin; secondary (second-line) agents include para-aminosalicylic acid (PAS), capreomycin, cycloserine, ethionamide, and kanamycin.
- Multidrug regimens include drugs such as streptomycin, kanamycin, and capreomycin, which have similar toxic effects. Only one of these agents should be used.
- Therapeutic effects include treatment of pulmonary and extrapulmonary *M. tuberculosis* infections. Depending on the agent used, these may also be used for disseminated infections in patients with advanced HIV infections and endocarditis.

Side effects

- PAS: gastrointestinal tract disturbances and hepatotoxicity
- capreomycin: ototoxicity and nephrotoxicity
- ethambutol: retrobulbar neuritis and blindness

- isoniazid: peripheral neuritis and hepatotoxicity
- rifabutin: gastrointestinal tract disturbances, rash, and neutropenia
- rifampin: hepatitis
- streptomycin: hepatotoxicity, ototoxicity, nephrotoxicity, and blood dyscrasias

Nursing considerations

- Patient education should include the importance of strict compliance to regimen for improvement of condition or cure.
- Patients should not consume alcohol while taking any of these medications.
- Vitamin B_6 is needed to combat peripheral neuritis associated with isoniazid.
- Women on oral contraceptive therapy and taking rifampin should be counseled on other forms of birth control because of the ineffectiveness of oral contraception while on rifampin.

REVIEW QUESTIONS

1. Which of the following side effects is expected with use of either isoniazid or rifampin?
   a. Headache and neck pain
   b. Glaucoma and gynecomastia
   c. Reddish-brown urine and emesis
   d. Numbness or tingling of extremities
2. Why would a patient need pyridoxine when taking INH?
   a. To improve energy
   b. To reduce GI side effects
   c. To combat cardiac abnormalities
   d. To prevent neurologic side effects
3. Women taking oral contraceptives with rifampin should:
   a. have an annual Pap smear.
   b. expect reddish-brown vaginal discharge.
   c. switch to an alternate form of birth control.
   d. experience increased energy level and breast discharge.

4. Patients are considered contagious:
   a. during any phase of the illness.
   b. any time up to 18 months after therapy.
   c. during the postictal phase of tuberculosis.
   d. during the initial period of the illness and its diagnosis.
5. Which of the following would be a therapeutic response to antitubercular drugs?
   a. The patient states that he or she is feeling much better.
   b. There is no fever, the WBC count is 21,000, and cough has subsided.
   c. The patient reports a decrease in cough and night sweats and few side effects.
   d. There is a decrease in symptoms supported by improved chest x-ray results, sputum culture, and sensitivity tests.

CRITICAL THINKING Activities

1. What is considered a therapeutic response to antituberculin drugs?

2. Is there any concern for the female taking oral contraception while taking rifampin? Explain your answer.

3. What parameters should be assessed while a patient is taking antituberculin drugs and why?

For Answers see www.harcourthealth.com/MERLIN/Lilley/.

bibliography

Albanese J, Nutz P: *Mosby's 2001 nursing drug reference and review cards,* St Louis, 2001, Mosby.

American Hospital Formulary Service: *AHFS drug information,* Bethesda, Md, 2000, American Society of Health-System Pharmacists.

Anderson PO, Knoben JE, Troutman WG: *Handbook of clinical drug data 1999-2000,* ed 9, New York, 1999, McGraw-Hill.

Block AB et al: Nationwide survey of drug-resistant tuberculosis in the United States, *JAMA* 271(9):665, 1994.

Center for Disease Control and Prevention: Outbreak of multi-drug resistant tuberculosis at a hospital-New York City, *MMWR Morb Mortal Wkly Rep* 42(22), 1993.

Cohen FL: Adherence to therapy in tuberculosis, *Ann Rev Nurs Res* 15:153, 1997.

Greenblatt D et al: Interaction of triazolam and ketoconazole, *Lancet* 345:191, 1995.

Johns Hopkins Hospital, Department of Pediatrics et al: *The Harriet Lane handbook,* ed 15, St Louis, 2000, Mosby.

Keen JH: *Critical care and emergency drug reference,* ed 3, St Louis, 1996, Mosby.

Mosby's GenRx: a comprehensive reference for generic and brand drugs, ed 10, St Louis, 2000, Mosby.

Skelskey C, Leshem OA: Tuberculosis surveillance in long-term care, *Am J Nurs* 97(10):16, 1997.

Skidmore-Roth L: *Mosby's 2001 nursing drug reference,* St Louis, 2001, Mosby.

Remember to check the **Online Worksheet** for additional learning opportunities: **www.harcourthealth.com/MERLIN/Lilley/**

Chapter 39

Antifungal Agents

www.harcourthealth.com/MERLIN/Lilley/

Look for this symbol for topics covered in the **Online Worksheet**

objectives

When you reach the end of this chapter, you should be able to do the following:

1 Identify the various antifungal medications.

2 Describe the mechanisms of action, indications, contraindications, routes of administration, side and toxic effects, and the drug interactions associated with the use of antifungal agents.

3 Develop a nursing care plan that includes all phases of the nursing process for patients taking antifungal medications.

4 Develop educational guidelines for patients receiving antifungal medications.

drug profiles

○━ **amphotericin B,** p. 624
○━ **fluconazole,** p. 624
nystatin, p. 626

○━ Key drug.

glossary

Antimetabolite (an′ ti mə tab′ o lit) Drug or other substance that is an antagonist or that resembles a normal human metabolite and interferes with its function in the body, usually by competing for the metabolite's receptors or enzymes. (p. 623)

Cytochrome P-450 system A group of enzymes in the liver that are responsible for the metabolism of a large number of medications. (p. 624)

Ergosterol (er gos′ tə rol′) Unsaturated hydrocarbon of the vitamin D group isolated from yeast, mushrooms, ergot, and other fungi; the main sterol in fungal membranes. (p. 623)

Flucytosine (floo si′ to sen) An antimetabolite that constitutes one of the four major groups of antifungal agents. It works by being taken up into the needed cellular metabolic pathway, thereby causing a malfunction in the normal pathway, which in turn shuts down the pathway. (p. 623)

Fungi (fun′ ji) A very large, diverse group of eukaryotic, thallus-forming microorganisms that require an external carbon source. Fungi consist of yeast and molds. (p. 621)

Griseofulvin (gris′ e o ful′ vin) One of the four major groups of antifungal agents. It acts by preventing susceptible fungi from reproducing. (p. 623)

Imidazoles (im′ id a zolz) One of the four major groups of antifungal agents. They include ketoconazole, miconazole, clotrimazole, econazole, and fluconazole and work by inhibiting a needed enzyme in susceptible fungi. (p. 623)

Molds Multicellular fungi characterized by long, branching filaments called *hyphae,* which entwine to form a mycelium. (p. 621)

Mycosis (mi ko′ sis) Infection caused by fungi. (p. 621)

Oral candidiasis (kan′ di di′ e sis) Overgrowth of *Candida albicans* occurring in the tissues of the mouth (also called *thrush*). (p. 622)

Pathologic fungi Fungi that cause mycoses. (p. 621)

Polyenes (pol e′ enz) One of the four major groups of antifungal agents. It includes amphotericin B and nystatin. Polyenes work by binding to sterols in fungal membranes, allowing potassium and magnesium ions to leak out of the cell and altering fungal cellular metabolism, which leads to death of the organism. (p. 623)

Sterol (ster′ ol) Substance in the cell membranes of fungi to which polyenes bind. (p. 623)

Yeast Single-celled fungi that reproduce by budding. (p. 622)

Yeast infection An infection caused by *Candida* (single-celled fungi). Most commonly infecting the mouth (thrush), esophagus, and genitourinary tract. (p. 622)

FUNGAL INFECTIONS

Fungi are a very large and diverse group of microorganisms that comprise both yeast and molds. Yeasts are single-celled fungi that reproduce by budding and are actually very useful organisms. They are used in baking and alcoholic beverages. **Molds** are multicellular and are characterized by long, branching filaments called *hyphae,* which entwine to form a "mat" called a *mycelium.* Some fungi are part of the normal flora of the skin, mouth, intestines, and vagina.

The infection caused by a fungus can also be called a **mycosis,** but there are very few fungi that cause such infections. Those that do are termed **pathologic fungi,** and the infections they cause range in severity from being mild and superficial to severe and life-threatening. These infections can be contracted by several different routes. They can be ingested orally, they can become implanted under the skin after injury, or if the fungal spores are airborne, they can be inhaled. There are four general types of mycotic infections: systemic, cutaneous, subcutaneous, and superficial. Many fungal infections are superficial and the symptoms primarily annoying; others are systemic and can be life-threatening. The most severe systemic fungal infections generally afflict people whose host defenses are compromised. Commonly these are patients who have received organ transplants and are on immunosuppressive drug therapy, cancer patients who are immunocompromised as the result of their chemotherapy, and patients with acquired immunodeficiency syndrome (AIDS). In addition, the use of antibiotics, antineoplastics, or immunosuppressants such as corticosteroids may result in colonization of *Candida albicans,* followed by the development of a systemic infection. When this affects the mouth, it is referred to as **oral candidiasis,** or thrush. It is common in newborns and immunocompromised patients. Vaginal candidiasis, commonly called a **yeast infection,** frequently afflicts pregnant women, women with diabetes mellitus, women taking antibiotics, and women taking oral contraceptives. The characteristics of some of the systemic, cutaneous, and superficial mycotic infections are summarized in Table 39-1.

ANTIFUNGAL AGENTS

The drugs used to treat fungal infections are called *antifungal agents.* Systemic mycotic infections and some cutaneous or subcutaneous mycoses are treated with oral or parenteral agents, but these constitute a fairly small group of agents, only three or four of which are commonly used. There are few such agents because the fungi that cause these infections have proved to be very difficult to kill, and research into new and improved agents has occurred at a slow pace, with few important advances yielded so far. One difficulty that has slowed the development of new agents is that frequently the chemical concentrations required for these experimental agents to be effective cannot be tolerated by human beings. Following is a list of those agents that have met with success in the treatment of systemic and severe cutaneous or subcutaneous mycoses:

- amphotericin B
- fluconazole
- flucytosine
- griseofulvin
- itraconazole
- ketoconazole
- miconazole
- nystatin
- terbinafine

Topical antifungal agents are primarily used for the treatment of cutaneous or subcutaneous mycoses and are discussed in detail in Chapter 41 on topical antimicrobials and disinfectants. Following is a list of those topical antifungals approved for clinical use.

- amphotericin B
- butoconazole

Table 39-1 Mycotic Infections

Mycosis	Fungus	Endemic Location	Reservoir	Transmission	Primary Tissue Affected
SYSTEMIC INFECTION					
Blastomycosis	*Blastomyces dermatitidis*	North America	Soil, animal droppings	Inhalation	Lungs
Coccidioidomycosis	*Coccidioides immitis*	Southwestern United States	Soil, dust	Inhalation	Lungs
Cryptococcosis	*Cryptococcus neoformans*	Universal	Soil, pigeon droppings	Inhalation	Lungs/meninges of brain
Histoplasmosis	*Histoplasma capsulatum*	Universal	Soil, bird and chicken droppings	Inhalation	Lungs
CUTANEOUS INFECTION					
Candidiasis	*Candida albicans*	Universal	Humans	Direct contact, nonsusceptible antibiotic overgrowth	Mucous membrane, skin/ disseminated
Dermatophytes, tinea	*Epidermophyton* spp., *Microsporum* spp., *Trichophyton* spp.,	Universal	Humans	Direct and indirect contact with infected persons	Scalp, skin
SUPERFICIAL INFECTION					
Tinea versicolor	*Malassezia furfur*	Universal	Humans	Unknown*	Skin

Malassezia spp. are a usual part of the normal human flora and appear to cause infection in only select individuals.

- ciclopirox
- clioquinol
- clotrimazole
- econazole
- haloprogin
- ketoconazole
- miconazole
- natamycin
- nystatin
- oxiconazole
- sodium thiosulfate
- sulconazole
- terbinafine
- terconazole

Topical antifungals are most commonly used in the treatment of oral, dermatological, and vaginal candidiasis, although occasionally a systemic antifungal is used in the management of severe cases.

Antifungal agents can be broken down into four major groups based on their chemical structures: polyenes (amphotericin B and nystatin), flucytosine, imidazoles (ketoconazole, miconazole, clotrimazole, econazole, and fluconazole), and griseofulvin.

Mechanism of Action

The mechanisms of action of the various antifungal agents differ depending on which of the four groups of agents they belong to. The **polyenes** act by binding to **sterols** in the cell membranes of fungi, the main sterol in fungal membranes being **ergosterol.** Human cell membranes also have sterols in their cell membranes, but in this case it is cholesterol. Polyene antifungals do not bind to human cell membranes, and therefore do not kill human cells, because polyenes have a stronger affinity for ergosterol than for cholesterol. Once the polyene binds to the ergosterol, a channel forms in the fungal cell membrane that allows potassium and magnesium ions to leak out of the cell. This loss of ions causes fungal cellular metabolism to be altered and hence death of the cell.

Flucytosine, also known as *5-fluorocytosine* (5FC), acts in much the same way as the antiviral agents. It is an **antimetabolite,** which is a drug that is taken up into needed cellular metabolic pathways. Once it is taken up into these pathways, it causes the normal pathway to malfunction, and the pathway subsequently shuts down. Flucytosine works by being taken into susceptible fungi, after which it is deaminated by cytosine deaminase to 5-fluorouracil. Because human cells do not have this enzyme, they are not harmed by this antimetabolite. Once the 5-fluorouracil is inside the fungal cell, it interferes with DNA synthesis by incorporating itself into the fungal pathway that produces DNA, with the result that the DNA needed for fungal cell metabolism is lacking and the cell dies.

Imidazoles act as either fungistatic or fungicidal agents, depending on their concentration in the fungus. They are most effective in combating rapidly growing fungi and work by inhibiting a needed enzyme in susceptible fungi. In this case the enzyme is cytochrome P-450, and it is needed to produce ergosterol. When the production of ergosterol is inhibited, another sterol, called *lanosterol,* is made instead. This results in the same problem caused by the polyene antifungals, namely a leaky cell membrane that allows needed potassium to escape. The fungi die because they cannot carry on cellular metabolism.

Griseofulvin works by preventing susceptible fungi from reproducing. It enters the fungal cell through an energy-dependent transport system and inhibits fungal mitosis, or reproduction, by binding to microtubules. This disrupts the cell's mitotic spindle structure, which arrests the metaphase of cell division. It has also been proposed that griseofulvin causes the production of defective DNA, which is then unable to replicate.

Drug Effects

The drug effects of the antifungals are limited to their ability to kill or inhibit the growth of fungi. Some of the fungi susceptible to these agents are the cutaneous, subcutaneous, and systemic mycoses listed in Box 39-1.

Therapeutic Uses

The therapeutic effects of the various antifungals are specific to the individual agents. The side effects of the newer antifungals are fewer and less serious than those of the older agents. However, the agent of choice for the treatment of many severe systemic fungal infections remains one of the oldest antifungals, amphotericin B. Amphotericin B is effective against a wide range of fungi. It is given with flucytosine in the treatment of *Candida* and cryptococcal infections because of the synergy of the two agents. Amphotericin B is also effective for treating aspergillosis, blastomycosis, candidiasis, coccidiodomycosis, cryptococcosis, fungal endocarditis, histoplasmosis, fungal septicemia, and many other systemic fungal infections. The activity of nystatin is similar to that of amphotericin B, but its usefulness is limited because of its toxic effects when given in the doses required to accomplish the same antifungal actions as those of amphotericin B. It is also not available in a parenteral form.

Fluconazole and itraconazole are synthetic imidazole antifungals. Fluconazole can pass into the cerebrospinal

---

BOX 39-1 Fungi Susceptible to Antifungal Agents

CUTANEOUS AND SUBCUTANEOUS MYCOSES
Epidermophyton spp.
Microsporum spp.
Sporothrix spp.
Trichophyton spp.

SYSTEMIC MYCOSES
Asperigillus spp.
Blastomyces dermatitidis
Candida spp.
Coccidioides immitis
Cryptococcus neoformans
Histoplasma capsulatum

fluid (CSF) and inhibit cryptococcal fungi. This makes it effective in the treatment of cryptococcal meningitis. Both drugs are active against oropharyngeal and esophageal *Candida* infections. Itraconazole, on the other hand, is capable of only poor CSF penetration but can be widely distributed throughout other areas of the body. It is indicated for the treatment of fungal infections in immunocompromised and nonimmunocompromised patients with disseminated candidiasis, histoplasmosis, and perhaps invasive aspergillosis. The other systemic imidazole, ketoconazole, inhibits many dermatophytes and fungi that cause systemic mycoses, but it is not active against *Aspergillus* organisms or phycomycetes such as *Mucor* spp. Miconazole, another systemic imidazole antifungal, has a spectrum of activity similar to that of ketoconazole. Of the imidazoles, fluconazole is the most effective one for combating infections with *Candida, Cryptococcus, Blastomyces,* and *Histoplasma* organisms. Fluconazole is very effective against vaginal candidiasis. One day of 150 mg of fluconazole can cure some vaginal candidial infections.

Flucytosine inhibits *Cryptococcus neoformans, Candida albicans,* and many *Cladosporium* and *Phialophora* spp. It does not inhibit *Aspergillus, Sporothrix, Blastomyces,* or *Histoplasma* spp., or *Coccidioides immitis.*

Griseofulvin inhibits dermatophytes of *Microsporum, Trichophyton,* and *Epidermophyton* spp. It has no effect on filamentous fungi such as *Aspergillus,* yeasts such as *Candida* spp., or dimorphoric species such as *Histoplasma.* Terbinafine is a synthetic allylamine derivative used primarily to treat topical fungal infections such as tinea cruris, tinea corporis, and tinea pedis.

Side Effects and Adverse Effects

The major side effects and clinical problems with antifungal agents are encountered most frequently in conjunction with amphotericin treatment. Drug interactions and hepatotoxicity are the primary concerns in patients receiving other antifungal agents, but the IV administration of amphotericin B is associated with a multitude of adverse effects. The most common and problematic of the side effects of the various antifungal agents are listed in Table 39-2.

Interactions

There are many important drug interactions associated with the use of antifungal agents, some of which can be life-threatening. A common underlying source of the problem is the fact that many of the antifungal drugs as well as other agents are metabolized by a highly utilized enzyme system in the liver called the **cytochrome P-450 system.** The result of the coadministration of two agents that are both broken down by this system is that they compete for the limited amount of enzymes, and one of the drugs ends up accumulating. The drugs that interact with the various antifungal agents and the consequences of the interactions are summarized in Table 39-3.

Dosages

For the recommended dosages of selected antifungal agents, see the dosages table on p. 627.

see the dosages table on p. 627.

drug profiles

┅ amphotericin B

As previously mentioned, amphotericin B (Amphocin, Fungizone) remains the agent of choice for the treatment of severe systemic mycoses. It may be given with flucytosine in the treatment of many types of fungal infections because the two agents work synergistically. The main drawback of amphotericin B therapy is that the agent causes many adverse effects. Almost all patients given the agent intravenously experience fever, chills, hypotension, tachycardia, malaise, muscle and joint pain, anorexia, nausea and vomiting, and headache. For this reason, pretreatment with an antipyretic (acetaminophen), antihistamines, and antiemetics may be given to decrease the severity of this infusion-related reaction.

Lipid preparations of amphotericin B have been developed in an attempt to decrease the incidence of its side effects and increase its efficacy. There are currently three lipid preparations of amphotericin B: amphotericin B lipid complex (ABCL or Abelcet), amphotericin B cholesteryl complex (Amphotec), and liposomal amphotericin B (AmBisome). These lipid preparations of amphotericin B are used when patients are intolerant or refractory to non-lipid amphotericin B.

Amphotericin B is a prescription-only drug that is available in both a parenteral and a topical formulation. It is classified as a pregnancy category B agent and is contraindicated in patients who have shown hypersensitivity reactions to it and in those suffering from severe bone marrow suppression. It is available as a 50-mg vial for injection and as a 3% cream, lotion, or ointment for topical application. The lipid preparations of amphotericin B are administered parenterally and are available as a 20-ml single-use vial (Abelcet), 50-mg/20 ml and 100-mg/50-ml vials (Amphotec), and 50-mg vials (AmBisome). Often a 1-mg test dose is given over 20 to 30 minutes to see if the patient will tolerate the amphotericin. It has been used as a local irrigant (bladder irrigation) for the treatment of candidal cystitis and intrapleurally or intraperitoneally for the treatment of fungal infections. The recommended dosages are given in the dosages table on p. 627.

The recommended dosages are given in the dosages table on p. 627.

PHARMACOKINETICS

HALF-LIFE	ONSET	PEAK	DURATION
1-15 days	Variable	1 hr	18-24 hr

Activity

┅ fluconazole

Fluconazole (Diflucan) has proved to represent a significant improvement in the area of antifungal treatment. It has a much better side effect profile than that of amphotericin B, and it also has excellent coverage against many fungi. In fact, it is often

Antifungals: Common Adverse Effects and Cautions

Table 39-2

Body System	Side/Adverse Effects	Caution
AMPHOTERICIN B		Recheck dosage and type of amphotericin B being administered.
Cardiovascular	Cardiac dysrhythmias	
CNS	Neurotoxicity; visual disturbances; hand or feet numbness, tingling, or pain; convulsions	
Kidneys	Renal toxicity, potassium loss, hypomagnesemia	
Pulmonary	Pulmonary infiltrates, other respiratory difficulties	
Other (infusion-related)	Fever, chills, headache, malaise, nausea, occasionally hypotension	
FLUCONAZOLE		Use with caution in patients with renal or hepatic dysfunction.
Gastrointestinal	Nausea, vomiting, diarrhea, stomach pain	
Other	Increased AST and ALT levels	
FLUCYTOSINE		Use with caution in patients with renal dysfunction or bone marrow depression.
CNS	Headache, confusion, dizziness, sedation, vertigo	
Gastrointestinal	Nausea, vomiting, anorexia, diarrhea, abdominal distention, cramps, enterocolitis	
Hematologic	Bone marrow suppression: thrombocytopenia, agranulocytosis, anemia, leukopenia, pancytopenia	
Other	Increased BUN, creatinine, ALT, and AST levels; rash; increased alkaline phosphatase activity	
GRIESEOFULVIN		Avoid during pregnancy.
CNS	Headache, peripheral neuritis, paresthesias, confusion, dizziness, fatigue, insomnia, psychosis	
EENT	Blurred vision, oral candidiasis, furry tongue, transient hearing loss	
Gastrointestinal	Nausea, vomiting, anorexia, diarrhea, cramps, dry mouth, flatulence, increased thirst, dysgeusia	
Genitourinary	Proteinuria, precipitate prophyria	
Hematologic	Leukopenia, granulocytopenia, neutropenia, monocytosis	
Integumentary	Rash, urticaria, photosensitivity, angioedema, systemic lupus erythematosis	
ITRACONAZOLE		Can trigger rare incidences of serious cardiovascular adverse effects.
CNS	Headache, dizziness, insomnia, somnolence, depression	
Gastrointestinal	Nausea, vomiting, anorexia, diarrhea, cramps, abdominal pain, flatulence, gastrointestinal bleeding, hepatotoxicity	
Genitourinary	Gynecomastia, impotence, decreased libido	
Integumentary	Pruritus, fever, rash	
Other	Edema, fatigue, malaise, hypertension, hypokalemia, tinnitus, hypertriglyceridemia, adrenal insufficiency	
KETOCONAZOLE		Avoid contact with eyes.
CNS	Headache, dizziness, somnolence, SIADH	
Gastrointestinal	Nausea, vomiting, anorexia, diarrhea, abdominal pain, hepatotoxicity	
Genitourinary	Gynecomastia, impotence, vaginal burning	
Hematologic	Thrombocytopenia, leukopenia, hemolytic anemia	
Integumentary	Pruritus, fever, chills, photophobia, rash, dermatitis, purpura, urticaria	
Other	Hypoadrenalism, hyperuricemia, hypothyroidism	
MICONAZOLE		Local irritation may occur; avoid contact with eyes.
Cardiovascular	Tachycardia, dysrhythmias	
CNS	Drowsiness, headache, lassitude	
Gastrointestinal	Nausea, vomiting, anorexia, diarrhea, cramps	
Genitourinary	Vulvovaginal burning, itching, pelvic cramps	
Hematologic	Decreased Hct, thrombocytopenia, hyponatremia, hyperlipidemia	
Integumentary	Pruritus, fever, flushing, anaphylaxis, hives	

continued

Table 39-2 Antifungals: Common Adverse Effects and Cautions—cont'd

Body System	Side/Adverse Effects	Caution
NYSTATIN		Local irritation may occur.
Gastrointestinal	Nausea, vomiting, anorexia, diarrhea, cramps	
Integumentary	Rash, urticaria	
TERBINAFINE		Rarely causes irritation.
CNS	Headache, dizziness	
Gastrointestinal	Nausea, vomiting, diarrhea	
Integumentary	Rash, pruritis	
Other	Alopecia, fatigue	

Table 39-3 Antifungal Drugs: Drug Interactions

Drug	Possible Effects
AMPHOTERICIN B	
Digitalis glycosides	Amphotericin B-induced hypokalemia may increase the potential for digitalis toxicity
Nephrotoxic drug	Additive nephrotoxicity
Thiazide diuretics	Severe hypokalemia or decreased adrenal cortex response to corticotropin
FLUCONAZOLE, ITRACONAZOLE, AND MICONAZOLE	
cyclosporine and phenytoin	Increased plasma concentrations of both agents
Oral anticoagulants	Increased effects of anticoagulants seen as increases in PT
Oral hypoglycemics	Reduced metabolism of hypoglycemic agents
GRISEOFULVIN	
Oral anticoagulants	Decreased effects of anticoagulants seen as decreases in PT
Contraceptives and estrogen-containing products	Decreased effectiveness of these agents
KETOCONAZOLE AND MICONAZOLE	
Alcohol and other hepatotoxic drugs	Increased risk of hepatotoxicity
Antacids anticholinergics, H₂ blockers, and omeprazole	Increased gastrointestinal tract pH, which can reduce absorption of ketoconazole
cyclosporine	Increased cyclosporine levels and potential for nephrotoxicity
isoniazid or rifampin	Decreased serum levels of ketoconazole
terfenadine and astemizole	Elevated terfenadine and astemizole levels and cardiotoxicity

PT, Prothrombin time.

preferred to amphotericin B because of these qualities. Oral fluconazole has excellent bioavailability, which means that almost the entire dose administered is absorbed into the circulation. The oral dose and intravenous dose are identical. Fluconazole is a prescription-only antifungal agent that is available in both an oral and a parenteral formulation. It is classified as a pregnancy category B agent and is contraindicated in patients hypersensitive to it. It is available as a 50-, 100-, and 200-mg tablet as well as a 200- and 400-mg IV injection. The recommended dosages are given in the dosages table on p. 627.

PHARMACOKINETICS

HALF-LIFE	ONSET	PEAK	DURATION
22-30 hr	PO: <1 hr	PO: 1-2 hr	Variable

nystatin

Nystatin (Nystat, Nilstat, Mycostatin, Nystex) is a polyene antifungal agent that is often applied topically for the treatment of candidal diaper rash, as prophylaxis against candidal infections during periods of iatrogenic neutropenia in patients receiving immunosuppressive therapy, and for the treatment of oral and vaginal candidiasis. It is not available in a parenteral form but does come in several oral and topical formulations. It is available in a powdered suspension for oral administration in doses of 50, 150, 250, and 500 million U as well as 1, 2, 5, and 10 billion U. It is also available as a nonpowdered suspension in a dose of 100,000 U/ml and as film-coated tablets containing 500,000 U. As a topical preparation it is available in a 100,000-U cream, ointment, powder, spray, and vaginal tablet. Nystatin is classified as a pregnancy category C agent and is contraindicated in patients with a known hypersensitivity to it. The recommended dosages are given in the dosages table on p. 627.

PHARMACOKINETICS

HALF-LIFE	ONSET	PEAK	DURATION
Unknown	2 hr	Unknown	Unknown

DOSAGES Selected Antifungal Agents

agent	pharmacologic class	dosage range	purpose
amphotericin B (Amphocin, Fungizone)	Polyene antifungal antibiotic	*Pediatric/Adult* IV: initial daily dose, 0.25 mg/kg; total daily dose, 1-1.5 mg/kg Topical: apply cream, lotion, or ointment several times a day	Broad spectrum of fungal infections Topical candidiasis
amphotericin B lipid complex (Abelcet, ABLC)	Polyene antifungal	*Pediatric/Adult* IV: 5 mg/kg once daily; infuse at 2.5 mg/kg/hr	Fungal infections
ABCD	Polyene antifungal	*Pediatric/Adult* IV: 3-4 mg/kg; may increase dose to 6 mg/kg	
AmBisone	Polyene antifungal	*Pediatric/Adult* IV: 3 mg/kg; may increase dose to 5 mg/kg	
fluconazole (Diflucan)	Synthetic triazole antifungal	*Adult* IV or PO: 200 mg/day, followed by 100 mg/day for 2-5 wk; doses of 400 mg/day may be required 400 mg/day, followed by 200 mg/day for 4-6 wk 400 mg/day, followed by 200 mg once/day for 10-12 wk after negative CSF cultures	Vaginal candidiasis Oropharyngeal and esophageal candidiasis Systemic candidiasis Cryptococcal meningitis
nystatin (Nystat, Nilstat, Mycostatin, Nystex)	Polyene antifungal antibiotic	*Infant* 200,000 U (oral suspension) in oral cavity qid *Pediatric/Adult* 400,000 U (oral suspension) in oral cavity qid *Adult* PO: 0.5-1 million U (tablet) tid Topical: apply 2-3 times/day Vaginal: Insert 1 vaginal tablet once/day for 2 wk	Oral candidiasis Oral candidiasis Intestinal candidiasis Topical candidiasis Vaginal candidiasis

nursing process

● Assessment

Before administering amphotericin B or any of the other antifungal agents, it is important for the nurse to identify any contraindications to the medication, such as hypersensitivity. Cautious use of these agents is recommended in pregnant or lactating women. Griseofulvin is contraindicated in patients with a hypersensitivity to it or with porphyria, hepatic disease, or lupus. Cautious use is recommended in patients known to be hypersensitive to penicillin and in pregnant women. The contraindications to ketoconazole use are hypersensitivity, pregnancy, lactation, and meningitis, with cautious use recommended in patients who have renal or hepatic disease. Miconazole is contraindicated in patients with a known hypersensitivity to it and should be used cautiously in pregnant women or patients with renal or hepatic disease.

The nurse should also assess the patient's vital signs and check the baseline CBC, Hgb level, Hct value, and RBC. Patients who are to receive ketoconazole should have their liver function assessed because of the hepatotoxicity it can cause. Miconazole use is associated with adverse cardiovascular effects, so pulse, blood pressure, and ECG should be checked and any history of cardiac disease documented. Griseofulvin may pre-cipitate severe blood dyscrasias, so it is important to assess CBC. Baseline renal and liver function and weight should also be assessed before the administration of any of the antifungals.

● Nursing Diagnoses

Nursing diagnoses appropriate to patients receiving antifungals include the following:
- Acute pain related to symptoms of the infectious process.
- Deficient knowledge related to lack of information and experience with the antifungal and any other medication.
- Risk for injury related to side effects of the medication treatment regimen.

● Planning

Goals for patients receiving antifungals include the following:
- Patient states the rationale for compliance with medication therapy.
- Patient states the common side effects of the specific antifungal medication.
- Patient experiences minimal side effects in signs and symptoms of the infection.
- Patient exhibits relief of the symptoms of the fungal infection.
- Patient states the importance of follow-up appointments.

Outcome Criteria

Outcome criteria relevant to patients receiving antifungal agents include the following:

- Patient will be free of the complications or suffer minimal side effects of the antifungal agents such as nausea, vomiting, and gastrointestinal upset.
- Patient will remain compliant with the medication and experience relief of infection and its signs and symptoms related to effective therapy such as normal cultures and no fever.
- Patient will experience improved appetite and energy level after taking the antifungal agents for the prescribed time.
- Patient will return to the physician regularly as recommended by the health care provider for CBC with differential.

Implementation

The nursing interventions appropriate to patients receiving antifungal agents vary depending on the agent. Amphotericin B given intravenously must be diluted properly according to the manufacturer's guidelines. Sterile water or normal saline is recommended for its reconstitution, and normal saline or 5% dextrose in water may be used for infusion, with a test dose of 1 mg per 20 ml of 5% dextrose in water infused over 30 minutes. IV infusion pumps are recommended, the most distal veins should be used.

Fluconazole is administered either orally or intravenously, and when given intravenously, it should be diluted exactly according to the manufacturer's instructions. There are two very different formulations of amphotericin B. One formulation has the detergent deoxycholate (Fungizone). A newer formulation (Amphotec, Abelcet) is associated with less toxicity. However, the dosages differ, with much higher dosages used with the newer formulation than with the deoxycholate-containing formulation. Therefore the nurse must use caution in checking and rechecking doses of the older versus newer formulations. Because of the necrosis that results from extravasation of the agent at the IV site, the nurse should check the site hourly to make sure this has not happened. Griseofulvin must be given carefully and the patient frequently checked during infusions. Oral forms should be given with meals to decrease gastrointestinal upset.

Patients receiving ketoconazole should not take alkaline products or antacids for at least 2 hours before or after dosing, and it should not be taken with coffee, tea, or acidic fruit juices. Just as with any other orally administered antifungal agents, taking it with food helps minimize gastrointestinal upset. Miconazole often causes nausea and vomiting, so use of an antiemetic may be helpful, if ordered, to decrease these problems. Often a physician will order a test dose to be given to the patient so that any untoward reactions can be identified.

It is often necessary to check the vital signs of patients receiving any of the antifungals every 15 to 30 minutes during infusion. In addition, it is important to monitor the intake and output amounts, urinalysis findings, and specific gravity of the urine in patients receiving these medications to identify any deleterious drug effects on the kidneys. It is also important to weigh patients weekly and to document these weights because a gain of more than 2 pounds (1 kg) in a week may indicate medication-induced renal damage.

Patient teaching tips for antifungal agents are presented in the box below.

Evaluation

The therapeutic effects of antifungals include an easing of the symptoms of the infection, with ultimately complete resolution seen in patients who are fully compliant with the therapy. Improved energy levels and normal temperature and other vital signs also indicate a therapeutic response. Side effects for which to monitor in patients receiving these agents are listed in Table 39-2.

---

patient teaching tips

Antifungal Agents

➤ Some patients receiving amphotericin B may need long-term treatment (i.e., weeks to months). If so, its side effects include tinnitus, blurred vision, burning and itching at the infusion site, headache, rash, fever, chills, hypokalemia, gastrointestinal upset, and various anemias. Patients should weigh themselves weekly and notify the physician if they gain more than 2 pounds (1 kg) in a week.

➤ Women taking these medications for the treatment of vaginal infections should abstain from sexual intercourse until the treatment is completed and the infection is resolved. Women should be told to continue to take the medication even if actively menstruating. Patients should notify the physician if symptoms persist past the treatment time period.

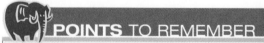

POINTS TO REMEMBER

Fungi

- Very large and diverse group of microorganisms.
- Consist of yeast and molds.
- Yeast are single-celled fungi that may be harmful (causing infections) or helpful (baking and the brewing of beer).

- Molds are multicellular and characterized by long, branching filaments called *hyphae*.

Candidiasis

- An opportunistic fungal infection caused by *Candida albicans*.

- Occurs in patients on broad-spectrum antibiotics, antineoplastics, or immunosuppressants and in immunocompromised persons.
- When occurs in mouth: oral candidiasis or thrush; seen mostly in newborns or immunocompromised persons.
- Vaginal candidiasis: yeast infections; seen mostly in patients with diabetes mellitus, women taking oral contraceptives, and pregnant women.

Antifungals

- Can either be systemically or topically administered.
- Most common systemic antifungals are amphotericin B, fluconazole, itraconazole, and ketoconazole.
- Most common topical antifungals are clotrimazole, miconazole, and nystatin.
- Several chemical categories of both the topical and systemic agents, each with its own unique way of killing fungi.

Nursing Considerations

- Before administering any antifungals, the nurse must thoroughly assess patients to find out whether they have a known hypersensitivity to the medication, what other drugs (prescribed and OTC) are being taken, and what the status of their renal and liver function is.
- Amphotericin B must be properly diluted according to the manufacturer's guidelines and administered using an IV infusion pump
- Tissue extravasation of fluconazole at the IV site leads to tissue necrosis, so site should be checked hourly.
- Therapeutic effects include improved energy levels, normal temperature, and normal vital signs.

REVIEW QUESTIONS

1. Which of the following poses a contraindication to the use of griseofulvin?
   a. Endocrine disease
   b. Hepatic disease
   c. Cardiac disease
   d. Pulmonary disease
2. The nurse should monitor which of the following laboratory parameters in patients receiving amphotericin?
   a. Chloride
   b. Potassium
   c. Hematocrit
   d. Serum creatine
3. Infections caused by fungi, commonly referred to as *mycosis,* can be broken down into those caused by _____ and _____.
   a. yeasts; molds
   b. flat worms; tapeworms
   c. intracellular; extracellular fungi
   d. erythrocytic; exoerythrocytic fungi
4. One of the four classes of antifungals, _____, belongs to the polyenes, which work by binding to a _____ in the cell membranes of fungi. This _____, called _____, is very similar to human _____.
   1. ergosterol
   2. protein

3. amphotericin B
4. ketoconazole
5. fluctyosine
6. cholesterol
7. RNA
8. sterol
   a. 3, 8, 8, 1, and 6
   b. 4, 8, 8, 1, and 6
   c. 3, 2, 2, 6, and 7
   d. 5, 7, 7, 1, and 6
5. The imidazole antifungals, such as _____, work by inhibiting the _____ enzyme system in the fungi, which is required for them to produce a substance needed to make their cell walls.
   1. flucytosine
   2. amphotericin B
   3. fluconazole
   4. acetylcholinesterase
   5. cytochrome P-450
   6. phosphodiesterase
   a. 1 and 5
   b. 2 and 6
   c. 3 and 5
   d. 1 and 4

For Answers see www.harcourthealth.com/MERLIN/Lilley/.

CRITICAL THINKING Activities

1. What laboratory data and other assessment data should be considered before administering any of the systemic antifungals? Specify the data and identify the reason for their importance.
2. One of your patients is to receive Amphotericin B. However, the patient's liver and renal function is somewhat impaired. What laboratory studies are important to monitor, and why is the administration of amphotericin B problematic in this type of patient?
3. What instructions should accompany a prescription of ketoconazole?

For Answers see www.harcourthealth.com/MERLIN/Lilley/.

bibliography

Albanese J, Nutz P: *Mosby's 2001 nursing drug reference and review cards*, St Louis, 2001, Mosby.

American Hospital Formulary Service: *AHFS drug information*, Bethesda, Md, 2000, American Society of Health-System Pharmacists.

Anderson PO, Knoben JE, Troutman WG: *Handbook of clinical drug data 1999-2000*, ed 9, New York, 1999, McGraw-Hill.

Johns Hopkins Hospital, Department of Pediatrics et al: *The Harriet Lane handbook*, ed 15, St Louis, 2000, Mosby.

Keen JH: *Critical care and emergency drug reference*, ed 3, St Louis, 1996, Mosby.

Mosby's GenRx: a comprehensive reference for generic and brand drugs, ed 10, St Louis, 2000, Mosby.

Skidmore-Roth L: *Mosby's 2001 nursing drug reference*, St Louis, 2001, Mosby.

Turkoski BB: *Drug information handbook for nursing 1999-2000: including assessment, administration, monitoring guidelines, and patient education*, ed 2, Cleveland, 1999, Lexi-Comp.

United States Pharmacopeial Convention: *USP DI: drug information for the health care professional. vol. 1*, ed 20, Englewood, Colo, 2000, Micromedex.

Remember to check the **Online Worksheet** for additional learning opportunities: **www.harcourthealth.com/MERLIN/Lilley/**

Activity

Chapter 40

Antimalarial, Antiprotozoal, and Anthelmintic Agents

objectives

www.harcourthealth.com/MERLIN/Lilley/

Look for this symbol for topics covered in the **Online Worksheet**

When you reach the end of this chapter, you should be able to do the following:

1 Identify the various antimalarial, antiprotozoal, and anthelmintic agents.

2 Identify the signs and symptoms of malarial, protozoal, and helminthic infection.

3 Discuss the mechanism of action, indications, cautions, contraindications, side effects, and routes of administration associated with each antimalarial, anthelmintic, and antiprotozoal agent, as well as the relevant nursing interventions for patients receiving them for various infestations.

4 Develop a nursing care plan that includes all phases of the nursing process for patients receiving antimalarial, antiprotozoal, or anthelmintic agents.

---

drug profiles

atovaquone, p. 637
chloroquine, p. 633
diethylcarbamazine, p. 642
iodoquinol, p. 637
○━ mebendazole, p. 643
mefloquine, p. 634
○━ metronidazole, p. 638

niclosamide, p. 643
paromomycin, p. 640
○━ pentamidine, p. 640
praziquantel, p. 643
○━ primaquine, p. 634
pyrantel, p. 644
pyrimethamine, p. 634

○━ Key drug.

---

glossary

4-Aminoquinoline derivatives (ə me′ no kwin′ o len) Antimalarial agents that bind to nucleoproteins and interfere with protein synthesis. (p. 632)

Anthelmintic (an′ ti hel min′ tik) Drug used to treat parasitic worm infections. (p. 641)

Antimalarial (an′ ti mə lar′ e əl) Drug that destroys or prevents the development of plasmodia in human hosts. (p. 632)

Antiprotozoal (an′ ti pro′ tə zo′ əl) Drug that destroys or prevents the development of single-celled microorganisms of the subkingdom protozoa in human hosts. (p. 636)

Erythrocytic phase (e-rith ro-sit′ ik) Phase of the asexual cycle of the parasite that occurs inside the erythrocyte. (p. 632)

Exoerythrocytic phase (ek so-e-rith ro-si′ tik) Phase of the asexual cycle of the parasite that occurs outside the erythrocyte. (p. 632)

Helminthic infection (hel min′ thik) Parasitic worm infection. (p. 640)

Malaria (mə lar′ e ə) Most significant protozoal disease in terms of morbidity and mortality. (p. 631)

Parasite (par′ ə sit) Organism that feeds on another living organism. (p. 635)

Parasitic protozoa (pro′ to zo′ ə) Protozoa that live on or in human beings. (p. 631)

Plasmodium (plaz mo′ de əm) Genus of protozoa that causes malaria. (p. 631)

There are more than 28,000 known types of protozoa. Those that live on or in humans are termed **parasitic protozoa.** Billions of people worldwide are infected with these organisms, and as a result, these infections are considered a serious health problem. Some of the more common protozoal infections are malaria, leishmaniasis, trypanosomiasis, amebiasis, giardiasis, and trichomoniasis. They are relatively uncommon in the United States but are becoming increasingly prevalent among immunocompromised persons, including those with AIDS. Protozoal diseases are especially prevalent among people living in tropical climates because it is easier for protozoa to survive and be transmitted in these year-round warm and humid environments. Even though the population of the United States is relatively free of many of these protozoal infections, international travel and the immigration of people from other countries where such infections are endemic are providing opportunities for increased exposure.

MALARIA

The most significant protozoal disease in terms of morbidity and mortality is **malaria.** In Africa alone it accounts for more than 1 million infant deaths a year. It is caused by a particular genus of protozoa called *Plasmodium,* and there are four species of organisms within this genus, each with its own characteristics and its own ability to resist being killed by antimalarials. Most commonly, malaria is transmitted by the bite of an infected female mosquito. However, malaria can also be transmitted by blood transfusions, congenitally, or through the use of contaminated needles by drug abusers. Despite the combined efforts of many countries to eradicate malaria, it remains the most devastating infectious disease in the world. Many lives are lost, and the cost of treating and preventing the disease imposes a tremendous economic burden on countries, many of which are very poor.

The life cycle of the *Plasmodium* is quite diverse and involves many stages. It has two interdependent life cycles: the sexual cycle, which takes place in the mosquito, and the asexual cycle, which occurs in the human host. In addition, the asexual cycle of the parasite consists of a phase outside the erythrocyte called the **exoerythrocytic phase** and a phase inside the erythrocyte called the **erythrocytic phase.** The malarial parasite undergoes many changes during these two phases (Fig. 40-1).

ANTIMALARIAL DRUGS

Antimalarial agents cannot affect the parasite during the sexual cycle when it resides in the mosquito. However,

during the asexual cycle, which takes place within the human body and is a particularly vulnerable stage, the parasite can be affected by antimalarial drugs. Chloroquine, hydroxychloroquine, quinine, and mefloquine kill the malarial parasite during the erythrocytic stage; primaquine kills the parasite during the exoerythrocytic phase. Often these drugs are given in various combinations to achieve an additive or synergistic protozoacidal effect. Other antibiotics that may be given with these agents are pyrimethamine and sulfadoxine.

Mechanism of Action

The mechanisms of action of the various antimalarial agents differ depending on the chemical family of agents to which they belong. The **4-aminoquinoline derivatives** (chloroquine and hydroxychloroquine) work by binding to nucleoproteins in the organisms and interfering with protein synthesis. They also inhibit DNA and RNA polymerase, an enzyme essential to the production of DNA and RNA. Both of these actions eventuate in the destruction of the parasite by preventing the manufacture of vital parasite-sustaining substances. They are also believed to raise the pH within the parasite, which has the effect of interfering with the parasite's ability to metabolize and utilize erythrocyte hemoglobin and is one reason why

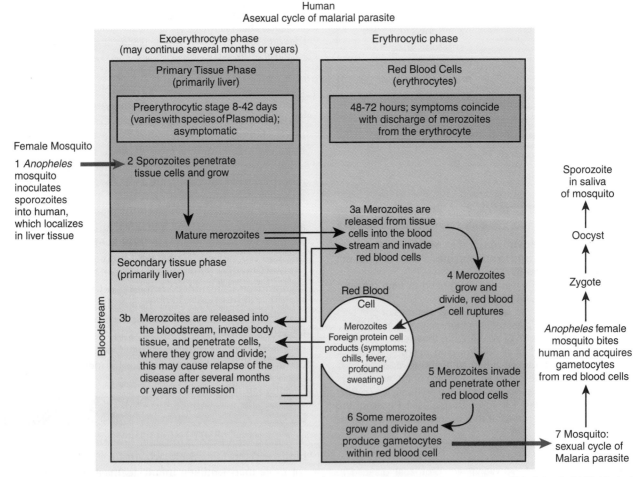

Fig. 40-1 Life cycle of the malarial parasite. (From McKenry LM, Salerno E: *Mosby's pharmacology in nursing,* ed 21, St Louis, 2001, Mosby.)

they are ineffective during the exoerythrocytic phase. Quinine and mefloquine are thought to be similar to the 4-aminoquinoline derivatives in their actions, in that both are believed to raise the pH within the parasite.

The diaminopyrimidines (pyrimethamine and trimethoprim) work by inhibiting dihydrofolate reductase, an enzyme that is needed for the production of certain vital substances in malarial parasites. Specifically, inhibiting this enzyme blocks the synthesis of tetrahydrofolate, a precursor of purines, pyrimidines, and certain amino acids essential for the growth and survival of the parasite. These two agents are also only effective during the erythrocytic phase and are often used with a sulfonamide or sulfone (sulfadoxine or dapsone) because of the resulting synergistic effects exerted by the agents. Together they block sequential steps in the same metabolic pathway for purine, pyrimidines, and amino acid synthesis in plasmodia.

Primaquine has the ability to bind to and alter DNA and is one of the few agents that is effective in the exoerythrocytic phase.

Sulfonamides, tetracyclines, and clindamycin may all be used in combination with some of the antimalarial agents named to further augment the protozoacidal effect.

Drug Effects

The drug effects of the antimalarial agents are mostly limited to their ability to kill parasitic organisms, most of which are *Plasmodium* spp. Some of these agents do, however, have other drug effects. Chloroquine and hydroxychloroquine also have antiinflammatory effects and may be beneficial in the treatment of rheumatoid arthritis and lupus erythematosus. Quinine and quinidine, two plant alkaloids, can also decrease the excitability of both cardiac and skeletal muscles. They also have local anesthetic actions as well as analgesic, antipyretic, and oxytocic effects.

Therapeutic Uses

Antimalarial agents are used to kill *Plasmodium* organisms, the parasites that cause malaria. As already mentioned, different antimalarial agents work during different phases of the parasite's growth inside the human. Those antimalarials exerting the greatest effect on *Plasmodium* organisms during the erythrocytic phase are chloroquine, hydroxychloroquine, and pyrimethamine. Because they are ineffective during the exoerythrocytic phase, however, they cannot prevent infection. Chloroquine and related compounds remain the drugs of choice for the treatment of susceptible strains of malarial parasites. They are highly toxic to all the species of *Plasmodium* except *P. falciparum*, which has proved to be resistant to chloroquine in people with malaria, caused by this species of *Plasmodium*, who live in many areas of the world, including Asia, Africa, and South America.

Quinine, which is available in both an oral and a parenteral form, is only indicated for the treatment of mild attacks, when the oral agent is used, and for the management of acute attacks of multiple-drug—resistant *P. falcip-*

arum, which causes a type of malaria that affects the cerebral hemispheres. A sulfonamide or tetracycline (such as doxycycline) antibacterial agent is always combined with quinine to take advantage of their synergistic protozoacidal effects. The parenteral form of quinine must come from the Centers for Disease Control and Prevention (CDC).

Pyrimethamine is another antimalarial antibiotic that is commonly used in combination with other antibiotics, in most cases a sulfonamide. It is also used in combination with sulfadoxine for the prophylaxis of chloroquine-resistant *P. falciparum* and *P. vivax*. There is a combination product called Fansidar that is a single tablet that contains both sulfadoxine and pyrimethamine. Mefloquine is a newer antimalarial agent that may also be used for the prophylaxis of *falciparum* malaria.

The most effective antimalarial agent for eradicating the parasite during the exoerythrocytic phase is primaquine. Quinacrine, trimethoprim, clindamycin, and dapsone may also be beneficial or work synergistically with these antimalarial agents in the killing of various parasites.

Side Effects and Adverse Effects

Antimalarial agents cause diverse side effects and adverse effects, and these are listed for each drug in Table 40-1.

Interactions

Of the half dozen or so antimalarial agents, only mefloquine and primaquine are associated with any significant drug interactions. These are listed in Table 40-2.

Dosages

For the recommended dosages for selected antimalarial agents, see the dosages table on p. 635.

---

drug profiles

chloroquine

Chloroquine (Aralen) is a synthetic antimalarial agent that is a 4-aminoquinoline derivative. It is also effective against other parasitic infections such as amebiasis and because of its antiinflammatory actions is used in the treatment of rheumatoid arthritis and lupus erythematosus. It is a prescription-only product, and its safety in pregnant women has not been established, although it is generally thought that the drug should be used in pregnant women only when clearly needed. It is classified as a pregnancy category C agent, and hypersensitivity to it, retinal field changes, and porphyria are contraindications to its use. Hydroxychloroquine is also a 4-aminoquinoline derivative with characteristics very similar to those of chloroquine.

Chloroquine is available in both a parenteral and an oral formulation. Chloroquine hydrochloride is

Antimalarial Drugs: Common Adverse Effects

Table 40-1

Body System	Side/Adverse Effect
CHLOROQUINE AND HYDROXYCHLOROQUINE	
Gastrointestinal	Diarrhea, anorexia, nausea, vomiting, abdominal distress
Other	Alopecia, dizziness, increased anxiety, rash, pruritus, headache
MEFLOQUINE	
Central nervous system	Headache, dizziness, insomnia, visual disturbances, increased anxiety, convulsions, depression, psychosis
Gastrointestinal	Stomach pain, anorexia, nausea, vomiting
PRIMAQUINE	
Gastrointestinal	Nausea, vomiting, abdominal distress
Other	Headaches, pruritus, dark discoloration of urine, hemolytic anemia due to G6PD deficiency
PYRIMETHAMINE	
Gastrointestinal	Anorexia; vomiting; taste disturbances; soreness, redness, swelling, or burning of tongue; diarrhea; throat pain; swallowing difficulties; sores, ulcerations, or white spots in mouth; sore throat
Other	Fever, increased bleeding, increased weakness, rash, hemolytic anemia resulting from G6PD deficiency, severe hypersensitivity reactions
QUININE	
Central nervous system	Visual disturbances, dizziness, severe headaches, tinnitus, hearing loss
Gastrointestinal	Diarrhea, nausea, vomiting, abdominal pain or discomfort
Other	Rash, pruritus, hives, respiratory difficulties, wheezing

Activity

used in the parenteral form in a strength of 40 mg/ml for injection. Chloroquine phosphate is used in the oral form as 150- and 300-mg tablets. Commonly recommended dosages are listed in the dosages table on p. 635.

PHARMACOKINETICS

HALF-LIFE	ONSET	PEAK	DURATION
Variable	8-10 hr	2 hr	Variable

primaquine

Primaquine is very similar to both of the 4-aminoquinolines, chloroquine and hydroxychloroquine, but it is an 8-aminoquinolone. It has many of the same characteristics as the 4-aminoquinolines. However, as previously noted, it is one of the few antimalarial agents that can destroy the malarial parasites while they are in their exoerythrocytic phase. It is indicated for the treatment of malaria caused by various species of *Plasmodium: P. falciparum, P. malariae, P. ovale,* and *P. vivax.*

Primaquine is classified as a pregnancy category C agent and is contraindicated in patients with a known hypersensitivity to it, as well as in those with anemia, lupus erythematosus, methemoglobinemia, porphyria, rheumatoid arthritis, methemoglobin reductase deficiency, and G6PD deficiency. It is available as a 15-mg tablet that is administered orally. Commonly recommended dosages are listed in the dosages table on p. 635.

PHARMACOKINETICS

HALF-LIFE	ONSET	PEAK	DURATION
4-7 hr	<2 hr	1-2 hr	24 hr

mefloquine

Mefloquine (Lariam) is an analogue of quinine that is indicated for the management of mild to moderate acute malaria and for the prevention and treatment of chloroquine-resistant malaria and multiple-drug—resistant strains of *P. falciparum,* which as already noted is a very difficult species of *Plasmodium* to kill. Mefloquine is classified as a pregnancy C agent and is contraindicated in patients with a known hypersensitivity to it, a history of epilepsy, or a psychiatric disorder. It is available in 250-mg tablets, taken orally. Commonly recommended dosages are listed in the dosages table on p. 635.

PHARMACOKINETICS

HALF-LIFE	ONSET	PEAK	DURATION
Days to weeks	<24 hr	7-24 hr	Variable

pyrimethamine

Pyrimethamine (Daraprim) is a synthetic antimalarial agent that is structurally related to trimethoprim. These two agents are sometimes referred to as *diaminopyrimidines.* There is a fixed-combination product called *Fansidar* that contains 500 mg of sulfadoxine and 25 mg of pyrimethamine. Pyrimethamine is classified as a pregnancy category C agent and is contraindicated in patients with a known hypersensitivity to it and in those with chloroquine-resistant malaria or with megaloblastic anemia caused by folate deficiency. It is only available in an oral formulation as a 25-mg tablet. Commonly recommended dosages are listed in the dosages table on p. 635.

PHARMACOKINETICS

HALF-LIFE	ONSET	PEAK	DURATION
80-95 hr	<6 hr	1.5-8 hr	Up to 2 wk

Table 40-2 Antimalarial Agents: Drug Interactions

Drug	Mechanism	Result
CHLOROQUINE divalproex, valproic acid	Decreased seizure threshold Decreased serum levels of valproic acid	Increased seizure activity Loss of seizure control
MEFLOQUINE Beta-blockers, calcium-channel blockers, quinidine, quinine	Unknown	Increased risk of dysrhythmia, cardiac arrest, seizures
PRIMAQUINE Other hemolytic agents	Unknown	Increased risk for myelotoxic effects (monitor for muscle weakness)

DOSAGES Selected Antimalarial Agents

agent	pharmacologic class	dosage range	purpose
chloroquine PO$_4$ (Aralen PO$_4$)	Synthetic antimalarial, antiamebic	*Pediatric* PO: 5 mg/kg/wk	Malaria prophylaxis
		Adult PO: 500 mg/wk	Malaria prophylaxis
		Pediatric PO: Total dose of 25 mg/kg administered over 3 days	Malaria treatment
		Adult PO: Total dose of 2.5 g administered over 3 days	Malaria treatment
		Adult PO: 1 g/day for 2 days, followed by 500 mg/day for 2-3 wk	Extraintestinal amebiasis
mefloquine (Lariam)	Synthetic antimalarial	*Adult* PO: 1250 mg as a single dose with 8 oz of H$_2$O PO: 250 mg once weekly	Malaria treatment Malaria prophylaxis
primaquine PO$_4$	Synthetic antimalarial	*Pediatric* PO: 0.5 mg/kg/day for 14 days	Malaria treatment
		Adult PO: 26.3 mg/day for 14 days	Malaria treatment
pyrimethamine (Daraprim)	Folic acid antagonist, antimalarial, antitoxoplasmotic agent	*Pediatric* PO: <4 y/o, 6.25 mg once weekly 4-10 y/o, 12.5 mg once weekly	Malaria prophylaxis
		Adult/Pediatric >10 y/o PO: 25 mg once weekly	Malaria prophylaxis
		Pediatric 4-10 y/o PO: 25 mg for 12 days	Malaria treatment
		Adult PO: 25-50 mg bid for 3 days	Malaria treatment
		Pediatric PO: 1 mg/kg/day in 2 doses for 2-4 days (max 100 mg/day), reduced to one-half for 1 mo with appropriate sulfa drug (max 25 mg/day)	Toxoplasmosis
		Adult PO: 50-75 mg/day with 1-4 g/day of a sulfa drug for 1-3 wk, then 25-50 mg/day for 3-4 wk	Toxoplasmosis
		100 mg qd, then 25 mg qd × 4-5 wk	HIV
		200 mg, then 50-70 mg/day	AIDS

PROTOZOAL INFECTIONS

There are several other common protozoal infections besides malaria. Some of the most common ones are amebiasis, giardiasis, pneumocystosis, toxoplasmosis, and trichomoniasis. Like malaria, these are also more prevalent in tropical regions. The protozoal parasites that cause the most serious infections are *Cryptosporidium* spp., *Isospora belli*, *Pneumocystis carinii*, and *Toxoplasma gondii*.

The protozoa that cause these infections are **parasites,** or organisms that feed on another living organism. They can be transmitted in a number of ways: from person to person, through the ingestion of contaminated water or food, through direct contact with the parasite, or by the bite of an insect (mosquito or tick). Parasitic infections can be classified according to where they occur in the body. They can be systemic and occur almost anywhere in the body; they can affect the gastrointestinal tract, as in the case of amebiasis; or they can affect dermatologic sites, as in the case of lice.

The more common protozoal infections are listed in Table 40-3 along with a brief description of the infection and the antiprotozoal agents commonly used in their treatment. Patients whose immune system is compromised, such as those with leukemia, those with transplanted organs who are on immunosuppressive drugs, and those with acquired immunodeficiency syndrome (AIDS), are at particular risk for acquiring a protozoal infection. Often such infections are fatal in these patients.

ANTIPROTOZOAL AGENTS

The most commonly used **antiprotozoal** agents are as follows:

- iodoquinol, metronidazole, and paromomycin—used for the treatment of intestinal amebiasis
- chloroquine and metronidazole—used for the treatment of extraintestinal amebiasis
- atovaquone, pentamidine, pyrimethamine, and quinacrine—used for the treatment of other infections

Mechanism of Action

The mechanisms of action of the antiprotozoal agents are as different as the agents themselves. The most commonly used of these agents together with a brief description of their mechanisms of action are given in Box 40-1. Pyrimethamine and quinacrine are discussed earlier in this chapter and are therefore not included.

Drug Effects

The drug effects of these antiprotozoal agents are primarily limited to their ability to kill various forms of protozoal parasites, but these differ from agent to agent. The drug effects of the antiprotozoal agents that have not yet been mentioned are summarized in Box 40-2.

Therapeutic Uses

Antiprotozoal agents are used to treat various protozoal infections, ranging from intestinal amebiasis to pneumocystosis. Atovaquone and pentamidine are used for the treatment of *P. carinii* infection. Iodoquinol and paromomycin are effectively able to kill intestinal forms of *E. histolytica* and are used for the treatment of intestinal infections with this parasite. Metronidazole is effective against many forms of bacteria, including anaerobic bacteria, as well as against protozoa and helminths. Infection with the latter is discussed later in this chapter.

Side Effects and Adverse Effects

The side effects and adverse effects of antiprotozoal agents vary greatly depending on the agent, and the ones specific to the common antiprotozoal agents are listed in Table 40-4.

Interactions

The common drug and laboratory test interactions associated with the use of antiprotozoal agents are listed in Table 40-5. Some of these interactions can result in severe toxicities, and it is therefore important to know of them and to understand the mechanism involved.

Dosages

For dosage information on selected antiprotozoal agents, see the dosages table on p. 639.

Table 40-3 Protozoal Infections: Types

Protozoal Infection	Description	Antiprotozoal Agent
Amebiasis	An infection that mainly resides in the large intestine but can also migrate to other parts of the body, such as the liver; it is produced by the protozoal parasite *Entamoeba histolytica*. Usually transmitted in contaminated food or water.	metronidazole, paromomycin, iodoquinol
Giardiasis	Caused by *Giardia lamblia*. It is the most common intestinal protozoal infection, usually residing in the intestinal mucosa (most commonly the duodenum). May cause diarrhea, bloating, and foul-smelling stools. Transmitted by contaminated food or water or by contact with stool from infected persons.	metronidazole, tinidazole
Pneumocytosis	Pneumonias caused by *Pneumocystis carinii* that occur exclusively in immunocompromised people; always fatal if left untreated.	trimethoprim-sulfamethoxazole, dapsone, atovaquone, primaquine pentamidine, clindamycin, trimetrexate.
Toxoplasmosis	Caused by *Toxoplasma gondii;* can produce systemic infection in both immunocompetent and immunocompromised hosts. Domesticated animals, usually cats, serve as intermediate host for parasites, passing infective oocysts in their feces.	sulfonamides with pyrimethamine, clindamycin, metronidazole
Trichomoniasis	A sexually transmitted disease caused by *Trichomonas vaginalis*.	metronidazole

drug profiles

Antiprotozoal agents are used for a number of indications, including *P. carinii* and *T. vaginitis* infections, amebic dysentery, toxoplasmosis, giardiasis, and anaerobic bacterial infections. All are prescription-only drugs because of the potential adverse effects that can arise if they are used inappropriately. These drugs are available in a wide variety of dosage forms, including oral, parenteral, and aerosol preparations. All antiprotozoal agents except for metronidazole are classified as pregnancy category C agents, with metronidazole classified as a category B agent.

atovaquone

Atovaquone (Mepron) is a synthetic antiprotozoal agent indicated for the treatment of mild to moderate *P. carinii* pneumonia in patients who cannot tolerate cotrimoxazole (trimethoprine-sulfamethoxazole). Atovaquone appears to kill protozoa by inhibiting the production of vital substances such as nucleic acids and ATP.

Atovaquone is contraindicated in patients with a hypersensitivity to it and in those who have had a life-threatening allergic reaction to any component of the formulation. It is only available orally as a 750-mg/5 ml suspension. Commonly recommended dosages are given in the dosages table on p. 639. Pregnancy category C.

PHARMACOKINETICS

HALF-LIFE	ONSET	PEAK	DURATION
2-3 days	8-24 hr	24-96 hr	Unknown

iodoquinol

Iodoquinol (Yodoxin, Di-Quinol) is considered a luminal or contact amebicide (killer of intestinal protozoa infections) because it acts primarily in the intestinal lumen. It is indicated for the treatment of intestinal amebiasis.

It is contraindicated in patients with a known hypersensitivity to it or to iodine as well as in those with renal disease, hepatic disease, severe thyroid disease, or a preexisting optic neuropathy. Iodoquinol is available only in an oral preparation of 210- and 650-mg tablets. Commonly recommended dosages are given in the dosages table

---

BOX 40-1　Antiprotozoal Agents: Mechanisms of Action

Antiprotozoal Agent	Mechanism of Action
atovaquone	Protozoal energy is generated in mitochondria; atovaquone selectively inhibits mitochondrial electron transport, resulting in no energy and cell death; it also inhibits pyrimidine synthesis, causing the protozoa to be unable to make life-sustaining substances.
iodoquinol	Called a *luminal* or *contact amebicide* because it acts primarily in the intestinal lumen of the infected host and directly kills the protozoa.
metronidazole	Bactericidal, amebicidal, and trichomonacidal; it can also kill anaerobic bacteria, which it accomplishes by disrupting DNA synthesis as well as inhibiting other nucleic acid synthesis, two substances needed for the survival of many organisms.
paromomycin	Also a luminal or contact amebicide; it is a direct-acting agent and kills by inhibiting protein synthesis in susceptible bacteria by binding to the 30S ribosomal subunit.
pentamidine	Inhibits production of much-needed substances such as DNA and RNA; it can bind to and aggregate ribosomes; it is directly lethal to *P. carinii*, by inhibiting glucose metabolism, protein and RNA synthesis, and intracellular amino acid transport.

BOX 40-2　Antiprotozoal Agents: Drug Effects

Antiprotozoal Agent	Drug Effects
atovaquone	Used for the treatment of acute, mild to moderately severe *P. carinii* pneumonia in patients who cannot tolerate cotrimoxazole.
iodoquinol	Indicated for the treatment of intestinal amebiasis in asymptomatic carriers of *E. histolytica;* it has also been used for the treatment of *G. lamblia* and *T. vaginalis* infections.
metronidazole	An antibacterial (including anaerobes), antiprotozoal, and anthelmintic agent.
pentamidine	Used for the treatment of pneumonia caused by *P. carinii.*
paromomycin	Indicated for the treatment of acute and chronic intestinal amebiasis and as adjunct therapy in management of hepatic coma.

Antiprotozoal Agents: Adverse Effects

40-4

Body System	Side/Adverse Effects
ATOVAQUONE	
Cardiovascular	Hypotension
Hematologic	Anemia, leukemia
Integumentary	Pruritus, urticaria, rash, oral candidiasis
Gastrointestinal	Anorexia, increased AST/ALT, acute pancreatitis, nausea, vomiting, diarrhea, constipation, abdominal pain
CNS	Dizziness, headache, anxiety
Metabolic	Hyperkalemia, hyperglycemia, hyponatremia
Other	Sweating, cough
IODOQUINOL	
Hematologic	Agranulocytosis
Integumentary	Rash; pruritus; discolored skin, hair, nails
CNS	Headache, agitation, peripheral neuropathy
EENT	Blurred vision, sore throat, optic neuritis
Gastrointestinal	Anorexia, gastritis, abdominal cramps, nausea, vomiting, diarrhea, anal itching
Other	Fever, chills, vertigo, weakness, dysesthesia
METRONIDAZOLE	
CNS	Headache, dizziness, confusion, fatigue, convulsions, peripheral neuropathy
EENT	Blurred vision, sore throat, dry mouth, metallic taste, glossitis
Gastrointestinal	Abdominal cramps, pseudomembranous colitis, nausea, vomiting, diarrhea
Genitourinary	Darkened urine, dysuria
Hematologic	Leukopenia, bone marrow depression
Integumentary	Rash, pruritus, urticaria, flushing
PAROMOMYCIN	
Gastrointestinal	Stomach cramps, nausea, vomiting, diarrhea
CNS	Hearing loss, dizziness, tinnitus
PENTAMIDINE	
Cardiovascular	Hypotension, dysrhythmias
Hematologic	Anemia, leukopenia, thrombocytopenia
Integumentary	Pain at injection site, pruritus, urticaria, rash
Genitourinary	Acute renal failure
Gastrointestinal	Increased AST/ALT levels, acute pancreatitis, metallic taste, nausea, vomiting, diarrhea
CNS	Disorientation, hallucinations, dizziness, confusion
Respiratory	Cough, shortness of breath, bronchospasm
Metabolic	Hyperkalemia, hypocalcemia, hypoglycemia followed by hyperglycemia
Other	Fatigue, chills, night sweats

on p. 639. Pregnancy safety information has not been established.

PHARMACOKINETICS

HALF-LIFE	ONSET	PEAK	DURATION
Unknown	Unknown	Unknown	Unknown

metronidazole

Metronidazole (Metric 21, Protostat, Flagyl) is an antiinfective agent that not only has antibacterial activity against microorganisms, which include anaerobic bacteria, but also has antiprotozoal and anthelmintic activity. The therapeutic uses of metronidazole are many and varied and range from the treatment of trichomoniasis, amebiasis, and giardi-

asis to that of anaerobic infections and antibiotic-associated pseudomembranous colitis. It can directly kill intestinal protozoa and kills all other organisms by preventing DNA synthesis.

Contraindications to metronidazole use include hypersensitivity, renal disease, hepatic disease, blood dyscrasias, various CNS disorders, and pregnancy (during first trimester). Thus, it is classified as a pregnancy category B agent. It is available as an oral preparation in the form of 250- and 500-mg tablets and film-coated tablets and parenterally in the form of a 5-mg/ml injection for IV infusion and a 500-mg vial for injection. Commonly recommended dosages are given in the dosages table on p. 639.

Table 40-5 Antiprotozoal Agents: Drug and Laboratory Test Interactions

Antiprotozoal Agent	Mechanism	Result
atovaquone	Compete for binding on protein, resulting in free, active atovaquone	Highly protein-bound drugs; may increase drug concentrations and drug effects
iodoquinol	May interfere with certain thyroid function test results	Increases protein-bound serum iodine concentrations, reflecting a decrease in iodine 131 uptake
metronidazole	Increased plasma acetaldehyde concentration after ingestion of alcohol by decreasing the absorption of vitamin K from the intestines by eliminating the bacteria needed to absorb vitamin K	Alcohol: causes a "disulfiram reaction"; warfarin: may increase action of warfarin
paromomycin	Additive nephrotoxic effects	Use with an aminoglycoside, amphotericin B, colistin, cisplatin, methoxyflurane, polymyxin B, or vancomycin may result in nephrotoxicity
pentamidine	Additive nephrotoxic effects	Use with an aminoglycoside, amphotericin B, colistin, cisplatin, methoxyflurane, polymyxin B, or vancomycin may result in nephrotoxicity

DOSAGES Selected Antiprotozoal Agents

agent	pharmacologic class	dosage range	purpose
atovaquone (Mepron)	Synthetic anti-PCP agent	*Adult* PO: 750 mg with food bid for 21 days	PCP
iodoquinol (Yodoxin, Di-Quinol)	Amebicide	*Pediatric* PO: 40 mg/kg/day in 3 divided doses pc for 20 days (max 1.95 g/day) *Adult* PO: 650 mg tid pc for 20 days (max 2 g/day)	Amebiasis
☞metronidazole (Metric 21, Protostat, Flagyl)	Amebicide, antibacterial, trichomonacide	*Pediatric* PO: 30-50 mg/kg/day in 3 divided doses for 10 days PO: 7.5 mg/kg q6h for 7-10 days (max 4 g/day) IV: 15 mg/kg infused over 1 hr, followed by 7.5 mg/kg infused over 1 hr q6h. IV: 15 mg/kg infused over 30-60 min and completed 1 hr preop and followed by 7.5 mg/kg infused over 30-60 min at 6 and 12 hr after initial dose. *Adult* PO: 250 mg tid × 5-7 days PO: 750 mg tid for 5-10 days PO: 500 mg bid for 7 days or 2 g for 1 day. PO: 500 mg q6-8h (max 4 g/day)	Amebiasis Bacterial infection Surgical bacterial prophylaxis Giardiasis Amebiasis, amoebic liver abscess Trichomoniasis Bacterial infection
paromomycin (Humatin)	Antiamebic and antibacterial aminoglycoside antibiotic	*Pediatric/Adult* PO: 25-35 mg/kg/day in 3 divided doses with meals for 5-10 days *Adult* PO: 4 g/day in 2-4 divided doses for 5-6 days	Amebiasis Hepatic coma
☞pentamidine isethionate (Nebupent, Pentam)	Synthetic anti-PCP agent	*Pediatric/Adult* IM/IV: 4 mg/kg once/day infused over 1 hr for 21 days. *Adult* Inhal: 300 mg in 6 ml sterile water once every 4 wk	PCP PCP prophylaxis

PCP, P. carinii pneumonia.

PHARMACOKINETICS

HALF-LIFE	ONSET	PEAK	DURATION
8-12 hr	<1.5 hr	PO: 1-2 hr	Variable

paromomycin

Paromomycin (Humatin) is an aminoglycoside antibiotic that is used for the treatment of amebiasis and intestinal protozoal infections. It directly kills intestinal protozoa when it comes in contact with them. Its bactericidal activity appears to be related to its ability to inhibit protein synthesis in susceptible organisms by binding to the 30S ribosomal subunit.

The contraindications to its use include hypersensitivity to it, renal disease, and gastrointestinal obstruction. It is only available in an oral formulation as a 250-mg capsule. Commonly recommended dosages are given in the dosages table on p. 639. Pregnancy category C.

PHARMACOKINETICS

HALF-LIFE	ONSET	PEAK	DURATION
Unknown	Unknown	Unknown	Unknown

pentamidine

Pentamidine (Nebupent, Pentam) is an antiprotozoal agent that is used mainly for the management of *P. carinii* pneumonia. It is also effective in combating many other protozoal infections, and it kills these protozoa by inhibiting protein and nucleic acid synthesis. It is used for both the treatment and prophylaxis of *P. carinii* pneumonia in patients at high risk for initial or recurrent infection.

Hypersensitivity to the agent, especially when administered by inhalation, is the sole contraindication to its use. However, it should be used with caution in patients with blood dyscrasias, hepatic or renal disease, diabetes mellitus, cardiac disease, hypocalcemia, or hypertension. Pentamidine is available as a 300-mg oral inhalation solution and also as a 300-mg injection for IV administration. Commonly recommended dosages are given in the dosages table on p. 639. Pregnancy category C.

PHARMACOKINETICS

HALF-LIFE	ONSET	PEAK	DURATION
6-9 hr	0.5-1 hr	<1 hr	Variable

HELMINTHIC INFECTIONS

Parasitic **helminthic infections** (worm infections) are a worldwide problem. No country is spared. It has been estimated that one third of the world's population is infected with these parasites, but those people living in undeveloped countries where sanitary conditions are often poor are by far the most common victims. The incidence of worm infections in the inhabitants of developed countries where sewage treatment is adequate is much lower, and usually only a few select helminthic diseases are the source of the problem. The most prevalent helminthic infection in the United States is enterobiasis.

Helminths that are parasitic in humans are classified in the following way:
1. Platyhelminthes (flatworms)
   • Cestodes (tapeworms)
   • Trematodes (flukes)
2. Nematoda (roundworms)

The characteristics of a few of the most common of the many helminthic infections are summarized in Box 40-3. There are essentially three types of helminths: cestodes (tapeworms), nematodes (roundworms), and trematodes (flukes). These usually reside in the intestines of their host but can also reside in other tissues.

BOX 40-3 **Helminthic Infections**

Infection	Organism and Other Facts
NEMATODA (VARIOUS INTESTINAL AND TISSUE ROUNDWORMS)	
Ascariasis	Caused by *Ascaris lumbricoides* (giant roundworm); resides in small intestine; treated with pyrantel, mebendazole, or albendazole
Enterobiasis	Caused by *Enterobius vermicularis* (pinworm); resides in large intestine; treated with pyrantel, mebendazole, or albendazole
PLATYHELMINTHES (INTESTINAL TAPEWORM OR FLATWORMS)	
Diphyllobothriasis	Caused by *Diaphyllobothrium latum* (fishworm); acquired from fish; treated with niclosamide, paromomycin, praziquantel, or albendazole
Hymenolepiasis	Caused by *Hymenolepis nana* (dwarf tapeworm); treated with niclosamide, paromomycin, praziquantel, or albendazole
Taeniasis	Caused by *Taenia saginata* (beef tapeworm); acquired from beef; treated with niclosamide, paromomycin, praziquantel, or albendazole
	Caused by *Taenia solium* (pork tapeworm); acquired from pork; treated with niclosamide, quinacrine, paromomycin, praziquantel, or albendazole

ANTHELMINTIC AGENTS

Unlike protozoa, helminths are large and have complex cellular structures, and it is by disrupting these structures that **anthelmintic** agents destroy these organisms. The currently available anthelmintic drugs are very specific in the worms they can kill. For this reason the causative worm should be accurately identified before the start of treatment. This can usually be done by analyzing samples of feces, urine, blood, sputum, or tissue from the infected host for the presence of the particular parasite ova or larvae.

There are over a half dozen anthelmintics that are commonly used in the treatment of these infections, and these include the following:

- albendazole (Albenza)
- diethylcarbamazine (Hetrazan)
- ivermectin (Stromectol)
- mebendazole (Vermox)
- niclosamide (Niclocide)
- oxamniquine (Vansil)
- piperazine
- praziquantel (Biltricide)
- pyrantel (Antiminth)
- thiabendazole (Mintezol)

As previously mentioned, anthelmintics are very specific in their actions. Albendazole and mebendazole can be used to treat both tapeworms and roundworms. Oxamniquine and praziquantel are the only agents that can kill flukes (trematodes). The most commonly used anthelmintics and the specific class of worms they are effective in killing are summarized in Table 40-6.

Mechanism of Action

The mechanisms of action of the various anthelmintics vary greatly from agent to agent, although there are some similarities among the agents used to kill similar types of worms. The various anthelmintic agents and their respective mechanisms of action are listed in Box 40-4.

Drug Effects

The drug effects of the anthelmintic agents are limited to their ability to kill various forms of worms and flukes. They have no other drug effects.

Therapeutic Uses

Anthelmintic agents are used to treat infections with roundworms, tapeworms, or flukes. Anthelmintic agents and the particular helminthic infections they are used to treat are listed in Box 40-5.

Side Effects and Adverse Effects

The adverse effects of mebendazole therapy are limited to diarrhea, myelosuppression, and abdominal pain. Those of niclosamide include nausea, vomiting, diarrhea, rectal bleeding, drowsiness, headache, weakness, skin rash, and anal pruritus. Piperazine's adverse effects comprise headache, electroencephalogram (EEG) changes, vertigo, paresthesia, seizures, hives, erythema multiforme, bronchospasm, blurred vision, and cataracts. Pyrantel's adverse effects include headache, dizziness, insomnia, and skin rashes, but more common effects include anorexia, cramps, diarrhea, nausea, and vomiting. Praziquantel's side effect profile includes dizziness, headache, malaise, drowsiness, abdominal pain, and nausea.

Interactions

The concurrent use of pyrantel with piperazine is not recommended, and it should be used cautiously in patients with hepatic impairment.

Dosages

For dosage information for selected anthelmintic agents, see the dosages table on p. 643.

---

drug profiles

Anthelmintics are only available as oral preparations by prescription. The primary anthelmintic agents used to treat infections with intestinal nematodes (roundworms) are pyrantel and mebendazole; diethylcarbamazine is the primary agent used to treat nematode infection in tissue. Thiabendazole and piperazine are used as alternative agents because the indications for their use are limited. Mebendazole and albendazole may be used to treat infection with either cestodes or nematodes, and as previously

---

 Table 40-6 Anthelmintics: Class of Worms Killed

Anthelmintic Drug	Cestodes	Nematodes	Trematodes
		Class of Worms	
albendazole	Yes	Yes	Yes
diethylcarbamazine and thiabendazole	No	Yes (tissue and some intestinal)	No
ivermectin	No	Yes	No
mebendazole	Yes	Yes	No
niclosamide	Yes	No	No
oxamniquine	No	No	Yes
piperazine and pyrantel	No	Yes (giant worm and pin worm)	No
praziquantel	Yes	No	Yes

BOX
40-4

Anthelmintics: Mechanisms of Action

Anthelmintic Drug	Mechanism of Action
albendazole	Intestinal and segmental cells of intestinal larvae and tissue-dwelling larvae are selectively destroyed by degenerating cytoplasmic microtubules; this in turn causes secretory substances to accumulate intracellularly; this leads to impaired cholinesterase secretion and glucose; glycogen becomes depleted leading to decreased ATP production and energy depletion, which immobilizes and kills the worm.
diethylcarbamazine	Inhibits the rate of embryogenesis of nematodes.
ivermectin	Ivermectin potentiates inhibitory signals in the central nervous system of nematodes leading to their paralysis.
mebendazole	Selectively and irreversibly inhibits the uptake of glucose and other nutrients; results in the depletion of endogenous glycogen stores, eventual autolysis of the parasitic worm, and death.
niclosamide	Inhibits mitochondrial oxidative phosphorylation; also decreases generation of ATP by inhibiting the uptake of glucose; cestrodes are then dislodged from the gastrointestinal wall; the worm is digested in the intestine and subsequently expelled from the gastrointestinal tract by normal peristalsis.
oxamniquine and praziquantel	Increase permeability of the cell membrane of susceptible worms to calcium, resulting in the influx of calcium loss; this causes the worms to be dislodged from their usual site of residence in the mesenteric veins to the liver; here they are killed by host tissue reactions; dislodgement of worms is the result of contraction and paralysis of their musculature and subsequent immobilization of their suckers, which causes the worms to detach from the blood vessel wall and be passively dislodged by normal blood flow.
piperazine and pyrantel	Blocks acetylcholine at the neuromuscular junction, resulting in paralysis of the worm; the paralyzed worms are then expelled from the gastrointestinal tract by normal peristalsis.
thiabendazole	Inhibits the helminth-specific enzyme, fumarate reductase.

BOX
40-5

Anthelmintics: Therapeutic Uses

Anthelmintic Drug	Therapeutic Uses
diethylcarbamazine	Bancroft's filariasis, loiasis, onchocerciasis, tropical eosinophilia
albendazole	Neurocysticercosis, Hydatid disease
ivermectin	Nondisseminated intestinal *Stronyloidiasis* (threadworms)
mebendazole	Trichuriasis (whipworm), enterobiasis, ascariasis, *Ancylostoma* infection (common hookworm), *Necator* infection (American hookworm)
niclosamide	*Taenia saginata* infection, diphyllobothriasis, hymenolepiasis
oxamniquine	Schistosomiasis (blood fluke)
piperazine	Enterobiasis, ascariasis
praziquantel	Schistosomiasis, opisthorchiasis (liver fluke), clonorchiasis (Chinese or Oriental liver fluke), fishworm, dwarf tapeworm, neurocysticerosis
pyrantel	Ascariasis, enterobiasis, other helminthic infections
thiabendazole	Cutaneous larva migrans (creeping eruption), strongyloidiasis, trichinosis

mentioned, it is the only agent that can kill organisms in more than one class of helminths. The only other anthelmintic that may be used to treat cestode infection are niclosamide and praziquantel. Paromomycin and quinacrine are alternative agents, the former used in the treatment of either beef or pork tapeworm infection and the latter in the treatment of only infection with pork tapeworm.

diethylcarbamazine

Diethylcarbamazine (Hetrazan, Pec-Dec) is an anthelmintic agent indicated primarily for the treatment of tissue infection with nematodes. It is contraindicated in patients with a known hypersensitivity to it, and its pregnancy safety has not been established. It is generally not recommended for use in pregnant women. It is available in orally administered 50- and 60-mg tablets. Commonly recommended dosages are listed in the dosages table on p. 643.

PHARMACOKINETICS

HALF-LIFE	ONSET	PEAK	DURATION
8 hr	<1 hr	PO: 1-2 hr	Variable

DOSAGES Selected Anthelmintic Agents

agent	pharmacologic class	dosage range	purpose
albendazole	General anthelmintic	PO: 400 mg, repeat in 2 wk 400 mg 200 mg bid × 3 days	Pinworms Hookworms Roundworms (*Ancylostoma brazillense*)
diethylcarbamazine (Hetrazan)	General anthelmintic	*Pediatric* PO: 6-10 mg/kg tid for 7-10 days *Adult* PO: 50 mg day 1, 50 mg tid day 2, 100 mg tid day 3, 2 mg/kg tid days 4-21	Roundworms Roundworms Bancroft's filariasis
mebendazole (Vermox)	Nematode anthelmintic	*Pediatric/Adult* PO: 100 mg once daily 100 mg in AM and PM for 3 days	Enterobiasis Hookworms round- worms, whipworms

niclosamide (Niclocide)	Cestode anthelmintic	*Pediatric*
		PO: 11-34 kg: 1 g as a single dose
		1 g on day 1, then 0.5 g for next 6 days
		>34 kg: 1.5 g as a single dose 1.5 g on day 1, then
		   1 g for next 6 days
		Adult
		PO: 2 g as a single dose (taken as two 1 g doses
		   1 hour apart)
		2 g/day for 7 days
			Beef, fish tapeworm
			Dwarf tapeworm
			
			Beef, fish tapeworms
			
			Dwarf tapeworm

praziquantel (Biltricide)	Trematode anthelmintic	*Pediatric ≥4 y/o/Adult* PO: 60 mg/kg in 3 equally divided doses for 1 day 75 mg/kg in 3 equally divided doses for 1 day	Schistosomiasis Clonorchiasis, opisthorchiasis
pyrantel (Antiminth, Reese's Pinworm Medicine)	Nematode anthelmintic	*Pediatric/Adult* PO: 11 mg/kg as a single dose to max of 1 g	Enterobiasis, roundworms

mebendazole

Mebendazole (Vermox) is a synthetic anthelmintic agent that may be used in the treatment of many types of nematode and a few types of cestode infection. It is classified as a pregnancy category C agent, but it should be used in pregnant women only when the potential benefits justify the possible risks to the fetus. It is contraindicated in patients hypersensitive to it and is only available in an oral formulation as a 100-mg chewable tablet. Commonly recommended dosages are listed in the dosages table above.

PHARMACOKINETICS

HALF-LIFE	ONSET	PEAK	DURATION
6-12 hr	<2 hr	2-4 hr	Variable

niclosamide

Niclosamide (Niclocide) is a synthetic anthelmintic agent that is structurally different from any of the other anthelmintics. It is primarily indicated for the treatment of infection with cestodes (beef, fish, and dwarf tapeworms). It is classified as a pregnancy category B agent and is contraindicated in patients with a known hypersensitivity to it. It is only avail-

able in an oral formulation as a 500-mg chewable tablet. Commonly recommended dosages are listed in the dosages table above.

PHARMACOKINETICS

HALF-LIFE	ONSET	PEAK	DURATION
Unknown	Unknown	Unknown	Unknown

praziquantel

Praziquantel (Biltricide) is one of the primary anthelmintic agents used for the treatment of fluke (trematode) infections, specifically by schistosomiasis, opisthorchiasis, and clonorchiasis. It is also useful against many tapeworm infections. It is classified as a pregnancy category B agent. It is contraindicated in patients who are hypersensitive to it and in lactating women. It is only available in an oral formulation as a 600-mg film-coated tablet. Commonly recommended dosages are listed in the dosages table above.

PHARMACOKINETICS

HALF-LIFE	ONSET	PEAK	DURATION
4-5 hr	<1 hr	1-2 hr	Variable

pyrantel

Pyrantel (Antiminth, Reese's Pinworm Medicine) is a pyrimidine-derived anthelmintic agent that is indicated for the treatment of infection with intestinal nematodes, such as ascariasis, enterobiasis, and other helminthic infections. It is classified as a pregnancy category C agent and is contraindicated in patients who are hypersensitive to it. It is only available in an oral formulation as a 250-mg/5 ml suspension. Commonly recommended dosages are listed in the dosages table on p. 643.

PHARMACOKINETICS

HALF-LIFE	ONSET	PEAK	DURATION
Unknown	<1 hr	1-3 hr	Unknown

nursing process

● Assessment

Before administering an antimalarial agent to a patient, the nurse should take a thorough nursing and medication history and document the findings. Contraindications for which to assess include pregnancy, porphyria, and G6PD deficiency as well as a history of drug allergy to these medications. Baseline vital signs should be checked, and any malarial symptoms (e.g., fever, chills, profound sweating, headache, nausea, joint aching, and fatigue to exhaustion) should be assessed. Signs of malaria include periodic diaphoresis and a remittent fever as high as 104° to 105° F (40° to 40.5° C). Baseline visual status and electrocardiogram (ECG) are also important to assess and the findings documented, as ordered.

It is important to assess patients who are to receive antiprotozoal agents for a history of hypersensitivity to the medications and for the presence of underlying renal, cardiac, thyroid, or liver disease. These and pregnancy are contraindications to the use of these agents. The patient's baseline visual acuity should also be determined and documented.

Before administering any anthelmintic agent, the nurse should assess patients for a history of hypersensitivity and pregnancy because these are contraindications in the use of these agents. Patients' energy levels, activities of daily living, weight, appetite, and other symptoms should be assessed and documented as well.

There are also many drug interactions with these agents that should be assessed and researched before use (see Tables 40-2 and 40-5).

● Nursing Diagnoses

Nursing diagnoses applicable to patients receiving any of the antimalarials, antiprotozoals, or anthelmintics include the following:
- Risk for injury related to medication side effects.

- Imbalanced nutrition, less than body requirements, related to the disease process and side effects of medication.
- Deficient knowledge related to the infection and its treatment.
- Ineffective therapeutic regimen management related to poor compliance to treatment and lack of knowledge about the infection and its treatment.

● Planning

Goals for patients being treated with any of the antiparasitic medications include the following:
- Patient is free of self-injury related to the side effects of medication.
- Patient maintains normal body weight during drug therapy.
- Patient remains compliant with therapy for prescribed length of time.
- Patient experiences minimal body image changes related to disease.
- Patient states side effects of medication as well as symptoms or adverse reactions to report to the physician.

Outcome Criteria

Outcome criteria for patients receiving any of the antiparasitic medications include the following:
- Patient will state measures to take to minimize self-injury related to the side effects of medication such as dosing, time of day, and drug interactions.
- Patient will list foods according to the food guide pyramid to be included in his or her diet to improve overall health.
- Patient will state the symptoms of the infection such as fever, lethargy, loss of appetite.
- Patients will understand the rationale for treatment for prescribed length of time.
- Patient will state the symptoms to report to the physician such as worsening of infection, anorexia, fever.
- Patient will verbalize feelings about altered body image openly with health care professional.
- Patient will state importance of complying with therapy and returning for follow-up visits to the physician to monitor progress and for adverse reactions.

● Implementation

Chloroquine and hydroxychloroquine are administered orally and should be given exactly as prescribed. At the start of the treatment for malaria the patient is given a loading dose, followed by half the dose on the next 2 days. In the prophylaxis of malaria, treatment with these agents is usually started 2 weeks before the person is exposed to the malarious areas and for 8 weeks after the person has left the area; the medication is taken once weekly on the same day of the week during this time span. Mefloquine should be administered once weekly as ordered with at least 8 ounces of water.

Some of these medications, such as thiabendazole, may give the urine an asparagus-like odor or the skin an unusual odor, so patients should be warned of these. Any syrup forms of these agents should be stored in tight and closed containers to prevent chemical changes from occurring in the medication. Quinine sulfate, an antiprotozoal, must be administered intact because it is very irritating to the gastrointestinal mucosa.

Most of the antiprotozoal agents should be given with food when given orally, such as with atovaquone and paromomycin. When administering metronidazole or pentamidine by IM or IV routes, it is important to follow drug company recommendations about dilution and IV infusion rates. Anthelmintic agents should be administered as ordered and for a prescribed length of time.

See the box below for teaching tips in patients receiving any of these antiprotozoal agents.

● Evaluation

The nurse should monitor the patient for the therapeutic effects of the antimalarials, antiprotozoals, and anthelmintic agents, such as the resolution of all symptoms. If prolonged therapy is necessary with antimalarials, CBC and urinalysis should be performed regularly and the patient observed for the signs and symptoms of hemolysis. An ECG may be desirable before and during treatment if the patient has or has had a cardiac disease. An eye examination should be done if the patient experiences visual disturbances. Side effects to watch for consist of visual changes, possible irreversible retinal damage, cardiac dysrhythmias, and thrombocytopenia. These antimalarial medications may precipitate hemolysis in patients with G6PD deficiency (mostly black patients and those of Mediterranean ancestry), so such patients should be closely monitored for its occurrence. With antiprotozoal agents, the patient should be monitored for visual disturbances, gastrointestinal distress, blurred vision, and altered hearing. Patients taking anthelmintics should be monitored for fever, pallor, anorexia, and sudden decrease in RBCs, WBCs, and HgB.

✎ patient teaching tips

Antimalarial, Antiprotozoal, and Anthelmintic Agents

Antimalarials

➤ Patients should take all the medication as prescribed and not stop the medication when they feel as though the symptoms have abated.

➤ The physician or other health care provider should be notified immediately if the patient experiences ringing (tinnitus) in the ears, a hearing decrease, or visual difficulties.

➤ Gastrointestinal upset can be decreased if oral forms are taken with food. The physician should be notified if nausea, vomiting, profuse diarrhea, or abdominal pain occur.

➤ This, and all medications, should be kept out of the reach of children.

➤ Quinidine products may cause dizziness, visual blurring, or yellow discoloration of the skin.

➤ Patients taking medication should exercise caution while driving because of the dizziness the agent can cause.

➤ Alert patients to the possible recurrence of the symptoms of malaria so that they will know to then seek immediate treatment.

➤ Patients should be instructed to take the entire course of the medication and to report any side effects to the physician, such as the symptoms of cinchonism—visual disturbances, dizziness, headache, tinnitus, gastrointestinal distress, blurred vision, and altered auditory acuity.

Antiprotozoals

➤ These agents should be taken exactly as prescribed and the importance of compliance emphasized.

➤ Metronidazole may leave a metallic taste in the mouth, and the patient should be informed of this and that the urine may turn dark.

➤ Metronidazole should not be taken with alcohol.

➤ Most of these agents should be taken with food to avoid gastrointestinal upset.

➤ Atovaquone should be taken with food, and often fatty foods, to increase plasma drug concentration.

Anthelmintics

➤ These agents should be taken exaclty as prescribed and the importance of compliance emphasized.

➤ Patients should also be encouraged to notify the physician immediately if they experience fatigue, fever, pallor, anorexia, darkened urine, and abdominal, leg, or back pain, which could indicate a sudden decrease in RBCs, Hgb, or WBCs.

🐘 POINTS TO REMEMBER

Malaria

- Caused by *Plasmodium*, a particular genus of protozoa.
- Transmitted by the bite of an infected female mosquito.
- Must attack the parasite when it is inside the RBC (erythrocytic phase).
- Primaquine attacks the parasite when it is outside the RBC (exoerythrocytic phase).

Protozoal Infections

- Other common protozoal infections are amebiasis, giardiasis, pneumocytosis, toxoplasmosis, and trichomoniasis.
- The most toxic protozoal infections are those caused by *Cryptosporidium* spp., *Isospora belli*, *Pneumocystis carinii*, and *Toxoplasma gondii*.

- Protozoa are parasites that are transmitted by:
  1. Person-to-person contact
  2. Ingestion of contaminated water or food
  3. Direct contact with the parasite
  4. The bite of an insect (mosquito or tick)

Antiprotozoals

- Atovaquone and pentamidine are used to treat *P. carinii* infections.
- Metronidazole is an antibacterial, antiprotozoal, and anthelmintic.
- Iodoquinol and paromomycin directly kill protozoa such as *Entamoeba histolytica.*

Anthelmintics

- Drugs used to treat parasitic worm infections caused by:
  1. Cestodes (tapeworms)
  2. Nematodes (roundworms)
  3. Trematodes (flukes)

- Important to identify the causative worm—done by finding the parasite ova or larvae in feces, urine, blood, sputum, or tissue.
- Drugs may kill parasite directly or cause it to be expelled from the body.

Nursing Considerations

- Contraindications to the use of antimalarial agents include pregnancy, psoriasis, porphyria, G6PD deficiency, and a history of drug allergy.
- Baseline vital signs should be checked and documented.
- Contraindications to the use of the antiprotozoals include hypersensitivity; underlying renal, cardiac, thyroid, or liver disease; and pregnancy.
- Contraindications to the use of anthelmintics include a history of hypertension; hypersensitivity; visual difficulty; intestinal obstruction; inflammatory bowel disease; malaria; severe hepatic, renal, or cardiac disease; and pregnancy.

REVIEW QUESTIONS

1. Which of the following is the indication for oxamniquine and praziquantel?
   a. Flukes
   b. Pin worms
   c. Tapeworms
   d. Roundworms
2. Which of the following are not appropriate to include in teaching patients about the concurrent use of metronidazole and tinidazole for *Giardia lamblia*?
   a. Urine may turn dark while the patient is on these medications.
   b. Metronidazole may leave a metallic taste in the patient's mouth.
   c. Taking these drugs with food will help minimize gastrointestinal upset.
   d. These agents are taken until the symptoms improve and then discontinued.
3. Which of the following is generally used for treatment of the late stage of HIV with *Pneumocystis carinii*?

   a. Chloroquine
   b. Pentamidine
   c. Mebendazole
   d. Oxamniquine
4. *Entamoeba histolytica* infection has been diagnosed in one of your migrant worker patients, a 25-year-old man. This parasitic protozoal infection of the large intestines is termed:
   a. Amebiasis.
   b. Giardiasis.
   c. Balantidiasis.
   d. Toxoplasmosis.
5. Antimalarial drugs are used to treat patients with infections caused by which genus and species of protozoa?
   a. *Plasmodium* spp.
   b. *Candida albicans*
   c. *Pneumocystis carinii*
   d. *Mycobacterium tuberculosis*

For Answers see www.harcourthealth.com/MERLIN/Lilley/.

CRITICAL THINKING Activities

1. One of your patients has been on the antiprotozoal agent atovaquone (Mepron) for *Pneumocystis carinii* infection. What life-threatening reaction is related to the use of this drug? What can the nurse monitor for in this patient related to the occurrence of this reaction? Why is it also recommended for patients to take Mepron with meals (especially fatty foods)?

2. Your roommate is traveling to a country where there is high risk for malarial infections. She asks you what you think the physician will order for her, if anything at all. After researching this, what would you most likely tell her that the physician will do or suggest?
3. What should be the emphasis of patient teaching to a 21-year-old female who is traveling to a country with high risk of malaria exposure? Explain your answer.

bibliography

Albanese J, Nutz P: *Mosby's 2001 nursing drug reference and review cards*, St Louis, 2001, Mosby.

American Hospital Formulary Service: *AHFS drug information*, Bethesda, Md, 2000, American Society of Health-System Pharmacists.

Anderson PO, Knoben JE, Troutman WG: *Handbook of clinical drug data 1999-2000*, ed 9, New York, 1999, McGraw-Hill.

Compton J: Malaria in the emergency department, *J Emerg Nurs* 23(2):120, 1997.

Johns Hopkins Hospital, Department of Pediatrics et al: *The Harriet Lane handbook*, ed 15, St. Louis, 2000, Mosby.

Keen JH: *Critical care and emergency drug reference*, ed 3, St Louis, 1996, Mosby.

Medical Letter: Drugs for parasitic infections 40(1017):1, January 2, 1998.

Mosby's GenRx: a comprehensive reference for generic and brand drugs, ed 10, St Louis, 2000, Mosby.

Sandford JP: *Guide to antimicrobial therapy*, ed 27, Vienna, Va, 1997, Antimicrobial Therapy.

Skidmore-Roth L: *Mosby's 2001 nursing drug reference*, St Louis, 2001, Mosby.

United States Pharmacopeial Convention: *USP DI: drug information for the health care professional, vol. 1*, ed 20, Englewood, Colo, 2000, Micromedex.

Remember to check the **Online Worksheet** for additional learning opportunities: **www.harcourthealth.com/MERLIN/Lilley/**

Chapter 41

Antiseptic and Disinfectant Agents

objectives

When you reach the end of this chapter, you should be able to do the following:

1 Identify the differences between disinfectants and antiseptics.

2 Identify the most commonly used and prescribed disinfectants and antiseptics.

3 Develop a nursing care plan that includes all phases of the nursing process related to the administration of disinfectants and antiseptics, including patient education guidelines.

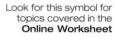

www.harcourthealth.com/MERLIN/Lilley/

Look for this symbol for topics covered in the **Online Worksheet** Activity

---

drug profiles

Acid agents, p. 651	**Iodine compounds,** p. 653
Alcohol agents, p. 652	
Aldehyde agents, p. 652	**Mercurial agents,** p. 653
Biguanide agents, p. 653	**Oxidizing agents,** p. 654
Chlorine compounds, p. 653	**Phenolic compounds,** p. 654
Dyes, p. 653	**Surface-active agents,** p. 654

---

glossary

Acid (as′ id) A compound that yields hydrogen ions when dissociated in solution. (p. 651)

Aldehyde (al′ də hid) Any of a large category of organic compounds derived from a corresponding alcohol by the removal of two hydrogen atoms, as in the conversion of ethyl alcohol to acetaldehyde. (p. 652)

Antiseptic (an′ ti sep′ tik) A substance that inhibits the growth and reproduction of microorganisms without necessarily killing them. (p. 649)

Benzyl (ben′ zəl) A substance used as a topical antiseptic, keratolytic, antiseborrheic, and mild irritant to treat acne. (p. 654)

Community-acquired infection An infection acquired from the environment, including infections acquired indirectly through the use of medications. (p. 648)

Disinfectant (dis′ in fek′ tənt) A chemical applied to nonliving objects to destroy microorganisms. (p. 649)

Hexachlorophene (hek′ sə klor′ o fen) A topical antiinfective and detergent. (p. 654)

Hydrogen peroxide (hi′ dro jən / per ok sid) A topical antiinfective. (p. 654)

Nosocomial infection (nos′ o ko′ me əl) An infection acquired at least 72 hours after hospitalization, often caused by *Candida albicans, Escherichia coli,* hepatitis viruses, herpes zoster virus, *Pseudomonas* organisms, or *Staphylococcus* spp.; also called *hospital-acquired infections.* (p. 648)

Resorcinol (rə sor′ si nol) An antiseptic used as a keratolytic agent in the treatment of dermatoses. It is also used in dyes and pharmaceuticals and as a chemical intermediate. (p. 654)

Topical antimicrobials (tap′ i kəl / an′ ti mi kro′ be əl) A substance applied to any surface that either kills microorganisms or inhibits their growth or replication. (p. 649)

COMMUNITY-ACQUIRED AND NOSOCOMIAL INFECTIONS

Infectious organisms—bacteria, fungi, and viruses—can be acquired from a number of different sources, such as hospitals, workplace, nursing homes, and home. These can, however, be categorized into two main sites of origin: the community and the hospital. **Community-acquired infections** are defined as those infections that are contracted either in the home or in the community. Hospital-acquired infections, more commonly known as **nosocomial infections,** are defined as those that are contracted in a hospital or institutional setting such as a nursing home and that were not present or incubating in the patient upon admission to the hospital. In other words, they are acquired during the hospital stay and from the hospital.

Of the two types of infections, nosocomial infections are much more difficult to treat, and there are several reasons for this. The primary reason is that these microorganisms have been exposed to many strong antibiotics in the past, and those that are left alive in the hospital or institutional setting are the most drug resistant and the most virulent. The particular organisms that cause these infections have changed over time. These various pathogens and the reasons for their prevalence are summarized by the different time periods in Table 41-1.

Nosocomial infections develop in 5% to 10% of hospitalized patients, and the cost of treating them because of the extra hospitalization required amounts to nearly five billion dollars annually. Most of these infections (70% or

Table 41-1 Changing Prevalence of Nosocomial Pathogens

Period	Cause for Change	Pathogen
Before 1940	No antibiotics	Group A streptococci
Mid-1950s	Antibiotic era	Coagulase-positive *Staphylococcus aureus*
Today	New antibiotics	Gram-negative bacilli (*Pseudomonas* spp.), fungi or yeast *(Candida albicans)* herpes virus

Table 41-2 Antiseptics Versus Disinfectants

	Antiseptics	Disinfectants
Where used	Living tissue	Nonliving tissue
Toxic?	No	Yes
Potency	Less	More
Activity against organisms	Primarily inhibits growth (bacteriostatic)	Kills (bactericidal)

Table 41-3 Disinfectants and Antiseptics: Chemical Categories

Agents	Antiseptic	Disinfectant
ACIDS		
Acetic	X	X
Benzoic	X	
Boric	X	
Lactic	X	
ALCOHOLS		
Ethanol	X	X
Isopropanol	X	X
ALDEHYDES		
Formaldehyde		X
Glutaraldehyde		X
BIGUANIDES		
Chlorhexidine gluconate	X	
DYES		
Gentian violet	X	
Carbol-fuchsin	X	
HALOGENS		
Chlorine Compounds		
Sodium hypochlorite	X	X
Halazone		X
Iodine Compounds		
Iodine (tincture and solution)	X	X
Iodophors (povidone)	X	
Mercurials		
Merbromin	X	
Thimerosal	X	
Yellow mercuric oxide	X	
Silver		
Silver nitrate	X	
NITROFURAZONE	X	
OXIDIZING AGENTS		
Benzoyl peroxide	X	
Hydrogen peroxide	X	X
Potassium permanganate	X	
PHENOLIC COMPOUNDS		
Cresol		X
Hexachlorophene	X	
Hexylresorcinol	X	
Resorcinol	X	
SURFACE-ACTIVE AGENTS		
Benzalkonium chloride	X	
Cetylpyridinium chloride	X	

more) consist of urinary tract infections (UTIs) and postoperative wound infections. Often they are acquired from various devices, such as mechanical ventilators, IV infusion lines, catheters, and dialysis equipment. Areas of the hospital where the risk of acquiring a nosocomial infection is particularly high are the critical care, dialysis, oncology, transplant, and burn units. This is because the host defenses of the patients in these areas are typically compromised, making them more vulnerable to infection. It is therefore obvious from the foregoing discussion that it is important for the nurse to be aware of these infections and the methods used to reduce their incidence.

TOPICAL ANTIMICROBIALS

Topical antimicrobials are agents that can be used to reduce the risk of nosocomial infections. They are substances that are applied to any surface for the purpose of either inhibiting or killing as many microorganisms as possible in a given pathogen population. There are two categories of these agents—antiseptics and disinfectants. **Disinfectants** are able to kill organisms and are used only on nonliving objects to destroy organisms that may be present on them. They are sometimes called *cidal agents.* **Antiseptics** can primarily only inhibit the growth of microorganisms but not necessarily kill them and are applied exclusively to living tissue. They are also called *static agents.* Often the terms *disinfectant* and *antiseptic* are used interchangeably and their actions and uses confused. However, as previously noted, not only are these agents not the same from the standpoint of their uses and actions but they can be very harmful if used for the same

purposes. The differences between disinfectants and antiseptics in a clinical sense are summarized in Table 41-2. In chemical terms, some agents differ from disinfectants in their chemical makeup; others may simply be a diluted version of a disinfectant. Table 41-3 contains a list of these agents classified according to their chemical structure.

Table 41-4 Antiseptics and Disinfectants: Mechanism of Action

Agent	Mechanism of Action	Comments
Alcohols	Denature or essentially destroy the microorganism's protein; some may directly lyse the microorganism.	60% to 70% concentration, most effective; >90% or <60% concentration, ↓ bactericidal activity.
Aldehydes	Act via alkylation, inhibiting the formation of the essential amino acid methionine.	Bacteriostatic or bactericidal depending on concentration.
Biguanides	Disrupt bacterial cytoplasmic membranes and inhibit membrane-bound ATPase (inhibit cell wall synthesis).	Chlorhexidine.
Halogens	Precipitate protein and oxidize essential enzymes by binding to and changing structure of proteins.	Iodine compounds: bactericidal; mercurials: bacteriostatic; chlorine compounds: bactericidal.
Oxidizing agents	Attack membrane lipids, DNA, and other essential components of the cell.	3% to 6% concentration: bactericidal and virucidal; 10% to 25% concentration: sporicidal.
Phenolic compounds	Interrupt bacterial electron transport (cellular respiration of microorganisms) and inhibit other membrane-bound enzymes; high concentrations rupture bacterial membranes.	Bacteriostatic or bactericidal dependng on concentration.
Surface-active agents	Denature or essentially destroy the microorganism's protein, cell membrane, and cytoplasm components.	↓ Concentrations: bacteriostatic; ↑ concentrations: bactericidal and fungicidal.

Mechanism of Action

The mechanisms of action of the various antiseptics and disinfectants vary greatly. Some are strong oxidizing or alkylating agents; others work by damaging microbial cell walls. The various mechanisms are discussed by drug class in the drug profiles, but for the purpose of clarity the mechanisms by which the various agents either kill or inhibit the growth of microorganisms are summarized in Table 41-4.

Drug Effects

Antimicrobial agents either inhibit the growth of microorganisms or destroy them, but the extent to which they do this depends on the number and type of microorganisms present, the concentration of the agent, the patient's temperature, and the time of exposure to the agent.

Therapeutic Uses

Living tissue such as skin and mucous membranes cannot be sterilized. However, the risk of infection can be minimized by reducing the number of microorganisms on such tissues. Antiseptics are applied to such living tissues to inhibit the growth of the microorganisms that typically reside there and that can do harm if they get into the body through an incision in the skin or by means of an injection. As a result these agents are contained, for example, in the presurgical scrubs (soaps) used by members of surgical teams to wash their hands in preparation for surgery. They are also applied to the patient's skin before the incision is made. The degerming action is only temporary, however, and limited to the surface. As mentioned in Chapter 36, systemic agents are sometimes administered to surgical patients as prophylaxis against infection caused by microorganisms living in the internal body environment. Besides these soaps and topical solutions, antiseptics are also contained in salves, ointments, mouthwashes, and douches.

Inanimate objects such as tabletops and surgical equipment may be treated with disinfectants as well as autoclaving, radiation, heat, and so on. Disinfectants are also used on instruments and other inanimate objects (fomites) that may harbor pathogens and are therefore a vehicle by which infectious organisms can be introduced into a new host. These instruments acquire these microbes by being placed or inserted into anatomic sites in patients where many organisms naturally dwell (e.g., thermometers, which are placed orally, rectally, or under the axilla, and proctoscopes, which are inserted into the lower gastrointestinal tract to visualize the interior of the structure). Before their use in other patients, the bacteria, fungi, viruses, and spores must be removed from their surfaces to prevent their transmission to others.

The therapeutic effects of the antiseptics and disinfectants vary from class to class. Some agents are very potent and are effective against many types of microorganisms. Others are less potent and have limited activity against only a few microorganisms. The range of microorganisms against which these agents are effective is indicated for the various chemical classes of antimicrobial agents in Table 41-5.

Side Effects and Adverse Effects

Antiseptics and disinfectants are very safe agents, relatively speaking, and when used in the appropriate manner, they are very effective. However, some of them are capable of causing some side effects and adverse effects, mostly comprising topical skin irritations. The others have no known adverse effects but at the very most may cause some skin irritation if used in exceedingly high

41-5 Antiseptics and Disinfectants: Therapeutic Effects

Agent	Bacteria	Tubercle	Therapeutic Effects Fungi	Viruses	Spores
Alcohols	X	X	X	X	
Aldehydes	X	X	X	X	X
Chlorhexidine	X		X		
Chlorine compounds	X	X	X	X	
Dyes	X				
Iodine compounds	X	X	X	X	x
Mercurial compounds	x				
Oxidizing agents	X			X	x
Phenolic compounds	X	X	X	X	
Silver compounds	X				
Surface-active agents	X		X	x	

X, "Static" or "cidal" activity; x, some activity if high concentrations of agent and lengthy exposure.

concentrations. The agents and their side effects and adverse effects are summarized in Table 41-6.

Interactions

There are very few drugs that interact with the antiseptics, although other topical agents that also irritate the skin may produce an additive effect when given in combination with one of them. In addition, a topical agent that augments the systemic absorption of an antiseptic may increase the likelihood of systemic toxicity from these agents. However, because most of these agents are used for short periods, there is very little opportunity for them to interact with other agents. Because disinfectants are not used for direct topical application to patients, there is of course no opportunity for drug interactions to occur.

Dosages

For information on the recommended dosages and concentrations for selected antimicrobial agents, see the dosages table on p. 652.

drug profiles

Following are descriptions of the various chemical categories of antimicrobials.

ACID AGENTS

Acetic (vinegar), benzoic, boric, and lactic acid are all members of the **acid** family of antiseptic and disinfectant agents. It is very commonly used because of its practicality, availability, and low cost. All these acid agents either kill microorganisms or inhibit their growth by creating an acidic environment for organisms that require a neutral or alkaline medium in order to live and grow.

Acetic acid in a 5% solution kills many organisms. In this concentration it is used as a vaginal

Antiseptic and Disinfectant Agents: Adverse Effects
41-6

Body System	Side/Adverse Effects
ALCOHOLS	
Integumentary	Excessive dryness of the skin.
ALDEHYDES	
Integumentary	Burns to skin or mucous membranes.
CHLORHEXIDINE GLUCONATE	
Integumentary	Rarely causes dermatitis, photosensitivity, and irritation of mucosal tissue.
HEXACHLOROPHENE	
Central nervous system	Use as a preoperative scrub or as washes for neonates and burn patients has been stopped because absorption from the skin into systemic circulation has resulted in serious CNS toxicity.
HEXYLRESORCINOL	
Hepatic	Toxicity resulting from systemic absorption from the skin.
Cardiovascular	Myocardial toxicity resulting from systemic absorption from the skin.
Integumentary	May produce burns on skin or mucous membranes.
IODINE COMPOUNDS	
Integumentary	*Iodine* at concentrations >3% may produce skin blistering; burns may appear with *tincture of iodine* when the treated area is covered with an occlusive dressing; it may stain skin and cause irritation and pain at wound sites.
SURFACE-ACTIVE AGENTS	
Integumentary	Chemical burns if left in contact with skin for too long, as in wet packs or occlusive dressings.

DOSAGES Selected Antiseptic and Disinfectant Agents

agent	pharmacologic class	concentration dosage range	purpose
acetic acid (otic: Domeboro, Vosol Otic; irrigation solution)	Antibacterial, antifungal acid antimicrobial	Otic solution 2%; 4-6 gtt 3-4 times a day Irrigation solution: 0.25%; 500-1500 ml/24 hr	Antibacterial, antifungal Bladder irrigation
benzalkonium chloride (Zephiran)	Broad-spectrum cationic detergent, surface-active antimicrobial	Solution concentrate: 17% for preparing dilutions from 1:750 to 1:40,000 Tincture/spray: 1:750	Skin cleanser, antiseptic irrigation solution, instrument storage
carbolic acid (phenol; Chloroseptic)	Phenolic antiseptic	Spray: 0.5% Gargle: 1.4%	Oral antiseptic Local anesthetic
cresol	Phenolic disinfectant	Solution 2%, 5%, 50%	Concurrent/terminal disinfectant
chlorhexidine gluconate (Hibiclens)	Broad-spectrum biguanide antimicrobial	Liquid: 4%	Cleanser, surgical scrub
formaldehyde (formalyde-10, Lazer Formalyde)	Broad-spectrum aldehyde antimicrobial	Solution 37% Solution/spray: 1%	General disinfectant Skin-drying agent
gentian violet (crystal violet)	Antibacterial/antifungal dye	Solution: 1%, 2%; apply 1-2 times/day	Topical antiinfective
hydrogen peroxide	Oxidizing agent	Solution 3%	Wound cleansing, antiseptic
iodine (iodine Topical, Lugol's Solution, Iodine Tincture, Strong Iodine Tincture)	Broad-spectrum iodine antimicrobial	Solution/tincture: 2%, 5%, 7%; apply 1-2 times/day	Topical antiseptic
isopropanol (isopropyl alcohol)	General alcohol antiseptic/ disinfectant/astringent	Solution 70%	Skin astringent, cleansing agent, utensil disinfectant
povidone-iodine (Betadine)	Broad-spectrum iodine antimicrobial	Aerosol: 5%, solution: 10% Mouthwash: 0.5% Surgical scrub: 7.5%	Topical antiseptic
sodium hypochlorite (Dakin's solution)	Broad-spectrum antimicrobial	Solution: 0.25%, 0.5%	Topical antiseptic
thimerosal (Merthiolate)	Organomercurial antiseptic	Solution/spray/tincture: 1:1000; apply 1-3 times/day	Topical antiseptic

douche for antisepsis and as a mild antiseptic-deodorant for the collection containers of indwelling urinary drainage catheters, for bladder irrigation, and for diaper soaks. The 1% solution may be used as a topical antiseptic for certain surgical wounds and burns. See the dosages table above for dosage and concentration information.

ALCOHOL AGENTS

Isopropanol (isopropyl alcohol) and ethanol are both members of the alcohol category of antiseptics. The alcohol solutions are most effective at a concentration of 60% to 70%; at a concentration of more than 95% or less than 60% their "cidal" activity dra-

matically decreases. These agents kill microorganisms by either denaturing their proteins or directly lysing them. Both isopropyl and ethyl alcohol are able to kill bacteria, tubercle bacilli, fungi, and viruses. See the dosages table above for the concentration information on isopropanol.

ALDEHYDE AGENTS

Formaldehyde and glutaraldehyde are members of the **aldehyde** category of agents. These disinfectants act by means of alkylation, inhibiting the formation of the essential amino acid methionine. This either kills organisms or inhibits their growth, depending on the concentration of the solution.

The aldehydes such as formaldehyde and glutaraldehyde are active against all types of microorganisms, including bacteria, tubercle bacilli, fungi, viruses, and spores. Because these agents are somewhat caustic, they can cause burns to the skin or mucous membranes if used as antiseptics. For this reason they are used mostly as disinfectants. Formaldehyde comes as formalin in a 37% concentration, and glutaraldehyde (Cidex) comes in a 2% solution. Both agents are commonly used as disinfectants for instruments. Cidex is used in particular to disinfect and sterilize surgical equipment. See the dosages table on p. 652 for the concentration information for formaldehyde.

BIGUANIDE AGENTS

Chlorhexidine gluconate (Hibiclens) is a biguanide agent with antiseptic activity. Biguanides act by disrupting bacterial cytoplasmic membranes and inhibiting membrane-bound ATPase, which results in the inhibition of cell wall synthesis. Chlorhexidine is active against both gram-positive and gram-negative bacteria. It is used as a bactericidal skin cleansing solution and is useful as a surgical scrub, a hand-washing agent for health care personnel, and as a skin wound cleanser. It may also be used to treat aphthous ulcers of the mouth and for the prevention of dental caries. When used as directed, it causes few side effects. See the dosages table on p. 652 for concentration information.

DYES

Gentian violet, crystal violet, methyl violet, brilliant green, and fuchsin are all rosaniline dyes. These are basic dyes that are currently used only occasionally as antiseptic or antiprotozoal agents. Gentian violet is typically used only topically as a 1% to 2% preparation, and it has both antibacterial and antifungal activity. See the dosages table on p. 652 for dosage information.

CHLORINE COMPOUNDS

Chlorine compounds actively kill bacteria, tubercle bacilli, and viruses but are only partially active against fungi. They have no activity against spores. Sodium hypochlorite (Dakin's solution) is one of the chlorine compounds that is commonly used as a bleaching agent. Its antibacterial action is due to the hypochlorous acid that forms when chlorine reacts with water. Hypochlorous acid is rapidly antibacterial.

Sodium hypochlorite in a 5% solution is commonly used to disinfect utensils, walls, furniture, floors, and swimming pools; in a 0.5% solution it is used on skin surfaces for the treatment of fungous infections such as athletes's foot. The strength of most household bleach solutions is 5.25%. IV drug users who frequently share needles and are at increased risk for acquiring HIV are being given small bottles of bleach to use as a disinfectant for their injection equipment and thus prevent the spread of the virus. See the dosages table on p. 652 for dosage information.

Halazone is a chloramine compound. Chloramines are chlorine-related compounds but are more stable, less irritating, and slower and more prolonged in their action than their chlorine cousins. Halazone is the only chloramine product used in the United States. It is available in tablet form for sanitizing drinking water. Adding 1 or 2 tablets to a liter of water can kill all the pathogens usually found in water within 30 to 60 minutes.

MERCURIAL AGENTS

Topical mercurial antiseptics are relatively weak in their actions. They are primarily bacteriostatic agents whose effectiveness is enhanced by the vehicle in which they are contained. Inorganic mercury compounds such as ammoniated mercury ointment owe their effectiveness primarily to these vehicles, which sustain the bacteriostatic action of the agent. Organic mercurial agents such as thimerosal (Merthiolate) are more bacteriostatic, less irritating, and less toxic than inorganic mercurials. Other examples of mercury compounds that are used as topical antiinfectives are merbromin, yellow mercuric oxide, and triclosan (Septisol).

Mercurial antiseptics probably act by inhibiting bacterial sulfhydryl enzymes, but they may also inhibit tissue enzymes as well, which reduces their usefulness. Ammoniated mercury is used for the treatment of psoriasis, impetigo, dermatomycoses, pediculosis pubis, seborrheic dermatitis, and superficial pyodermas. Skin irritations, as well as hypersensitivity to the agents, have been reported as side effects of these compounds. See the dosages table on p. 652 for the dosage information for thimerosal.

IODINE COMPOUNDS

Iodine (tincture and solution) is a nonmetallic element that readily forms salts when combined with many other elements. Although it is a nonmetallic element, it has a bluish black, metallic luster and a characteristic odor. It is only slightly soluble in water but is completely soluble in alcohol and in aqueous solutions of sodium iodide and potassium iodide. Iodine tincture and solution are both active against and kill all forms of microorganisms—bacteria, tubercle bacilli, fungi, viruses, and spores. Their activity against spores depends on the concentration and the timing of administration. There are actually many forms of iodine, some of which are listed in Table 41-7. See the dosages table on p. 652 for the recommended dosages and concentrations of a few of them.

OXIDIZING AGENTS

Hydrogen peroxide is one of three members of the oxidizing family of antiseptic agents, the other agents being benzoyl peroxide and potassium permanganate. Oxidizing agents work by attacking membrane lipids, DNA, and other essential components of the microorganism's cell. In concentrations of 3% to 6% they are bactericidal and virucidal; at 10% to 25% they are sporicidal.

Hydrogen peroxide is used as a 3% solution to irrigate suppurating wounds and some extensive traumatic wounds. It is used for wound cleansing, before Hickman catheter dressing changes, for the surgical repair of cleft lip, as an irrigation solution for use after some radical head and neck surgeries, for some oral lesions, and for oral cleansing (Peroxyl mouth rinse). **Benzyl** peroxides are used as a topical antiseptic, keratolytic, antiseborrheic, and mild irritant to treat acne.

PHENOLIC COMPOUNDS

Cresol, carbolic acid (phenol), and Lysol are all phenolic compounds that are used only as disinfectants. Because these agents cause burning and possibly blistering, they should not be allowed to come in contact with the skin in concentrations stronger than 2% and never in contact with areas where the skin is broken.

Phenolic compounds work by interrupting bacterial electron transport (cellular respiration of microorganisms) and inhibit other membrane-bound enzymes. At high concentrations they rupture bacterial membranes. Depending on the concentration of the phenolic compound they can be either "static" or "cidal" in their actions. The phenolic compounds are active against bacteria, tubercle, fungi, and viruses, but not spores. See the dosages table on p. 652 for concentration information on cresol and carbolic acid.

Hexachlorophene and **resorcinol** are two other phenolic compounds. Hexachlorophene is available by prescription only and is used as a surgical scrub as well as a bacteriostatic skin cleanser. Resorcinol is bactericidal and fungicidal and is about a third as effective as carbolic acid. It is used to treat acne, ringworm, eczema, psoriasis, seborrheic dermatitis, and similar skin lesions.

SURFACE-ACTIVE AGENTS

Benzalkonium chloride (Zephiran) and cetylpyridinium chloride are surface-active agents. They work by denaturing the microorganism or essentially destroying its protein, cell membrane, and cytoplasm components. At low concentrations they are bacteriostatic and at high concentrations they are bactericidal and fungicidal. These agents are used to treat bacteria, fungi, and some viral topical infections.

Certain substances, when used in combination with surface-acting agents, will absorb the active ingredient and thereby weaken the surface-acting agent. Substances such as organic matter, soaps, anionic detergents, and tap water that contains metallic ions are a few examples. See the dosages table on p. 652 for concentration information on benzalkonium chloride.

table 41-7 Iodine Formulations

Iodine Formulation	Composition	Uses
Aqueous solution	5% iodine and 10% potassium iodide	These forms of iodine are used preoperatively to disinfect the skin. They are applied topically for their antimicrobial effects against bacteria, fungi, viruses, protozoa, and yeasts.
Iodine topical solution	2% iodine	
Iodine tincture	2% iodine in alcohol solution	
Strong iodine solution	5% iodine in water	
Strong iodine tincture	7% iodine in alcohol	
Povidone-iodine (Betadine, Operand, Pharmadine)	Iodine with polyvinylpyrrolidone	Used as a 10% applicator solution or as a 2% scrub, spray, foam, vaginal gel, ointment, mouthwash, perineal wash, or whirlpool concentrate.
Tincture of iodine	2% iodine and 2.4% sodium iodide in 46% ethyl alcohol	For cutaneous infections caused by bacteria and fungi. Even a 1% tincture will kill almost an entire bacterial population in 1.5 min. Three drops in 1 quart (≈1 liter) of drinking water will reduce ameba and bacteria counts in 15 min without impairing palatability.
Iodophors (Betadine, Prepodyne)	Iodine compounds with a carrier that acts as a sustained-release pool of iodine.	Widely used as antiseptics.

nursing process

● Assessment

When any type of topical medication such as an antiseptic is to be administered, the concentration of the medication, length of exposure to the skin, condition of the skin, size of area affected, and hydration status of the skin must be taken into consideration because they have a significant influence on the action of the medication. Before applying any topical medication, it is important for the nurse to find out whether the patient has any drug allergies or has shown any previous sensitivity to antiseptics or other topical agents. If an iodine-based agent such as povidone-iodine is being applied, the nurse should question the patient about allergies to iodine or seafood, because these are contraindications to its use. Patients being treated with peroxide agents should be asked about previous allergies and local reactions to the medication.

The risk of reactions to the antibacterial topical agents is greater because of the sensitivity of patients to antibiotics in different dosage forms. Should a patient have an allergy to a particular type of antibacterial agent, that specific agent should not be used topically, regardless of the dosage form. If a culture and sensitivity test has been ordered, the results should be known before the first application of the antibacterial agent.

● Nursing Diagnoses

Nursing diagnoses appropriate to the use of antiseptics include the following:
- Risk for infection related to compromised skin integrity.
- Risk for infection related to skin trauma or injury resulting from adverse reactions to the topical agent.
- Deficient knowledge related to topical agents and their proper use.

● Planning

Goals related to the administration of antiseptics include the following:
- Patient remains free of adverse reactions to the agent when used for the treatment of skin injury or infection.
- Patient shows evidence of resolution of infection.
- Patient is compliant with the medication regimen.
- Patient experiences minimal to no adverse reactions to medication.
- Patient returns for follow-up visits with physician.

Outcome Criteria

Outcome criteria in patients treated with antiseptics include the following:
- Patient will experience minimal discomfort (such as stinging, itching, burning) resulting from the use of the agent in the treatment of a skin injury or infection.
- Patient will experience maximal therapeutic effects of medication once therapy is complete with resolution of symptoms, such as intact skin, no redness, or no drainage.
- Patient will demonstrate proper technique for applying topical antiseptic with applicator, tongue blade, gloved hand, and proper handwashing technique.
- Patient will state those situations (adverse reactions to medication or worsening of symptoms of infection) when the physician should be notified immediately.

● Implementation

Before applying any topical agent, the nurse should check the physician's order to make sure he or she knows exactly what is required, gather the needed supplies, and wash his or her hands. Standard Precautions should be followed when giving nursing care that entails direct contact with a patient or possible exposure situations. If the skin is intact and it is not otherwise indicated, the nurse should wear nonsterile gloves, but if the skin is not intact or the nurse judges it appropriate, sterile gloves and technique should be used. Often there are specific directions regarding the application of the agent (e.g., the order may specify that the agent be applied with a tongue depressor or that an occlusive dressing be placed). The nurse should follow these directions as well. As with any procedure the nurse should *always* ensure the patient's privacy and comfort. The skin site should be thoroughly cleansed and any other specific directions, such as removing water or alcohol-based topicals with soap and water or normal saline, should be followed. In general, before applying additional doses of a topical medication, the site should be cleansed not only of any debris but of any residual medication.

When using lotions, the nurse should store it under the conditions recommended by the manufacturer and shake it well before using. Creams and ointments are often applied with a sterile cotton-tipped applicator or tongue blade. Any dressings should be applied as ordered and special attention paid to the directions for the application of occlusive, wet, or wet-to-dry dressings. Patient education about the medication and dressings is important to the safe and effective use of these agents. The nurse should make sure to document the site of application and any drainage from the site, whether there is any swelling, the temperature and color of the site, and any painful or other sensations that may occur.

After the medication has been administered, the nurse should wash his or her hands, dispose of contaminated dressings, record the nature of the procedure and findings, and maintain asepsis (surgical asepsis if the wound is open in any way or if the skin is not intact). The nurse should always make sure that the patient is in no danger of causing harm to the site.

Patient teaching tips for antiseptic agents are presented on p. 656.

● Evaluation

When using antiseptics, the patient's therapeutic response may be manifested by improved healing of the affected area, decreased symptoms of inflammation or infection, or even prevention of infection for which the agent was ordered, such as preoperatively. In addition, when using these agents on inanimate objects, be sure to constantly monitor for patient safety from exposure to the agent. It is also important to evaluate patients for any side effects or adverse reactions (see Table 41-6).

patient teaching tips

Administration of Antiseptics

➤ Patients should be instructed to wash their hands before and after applying any topical medication. This is important in preventing the spread of infection and the gross contamination of a wound.

➤ Patients should learn how to properly apply the medication, dressings, and bandage and how to change any dressings so that they can do these things at home after discharge. The instructions the nurse has given and the patients' caregiver's ability to carry them out should also be documented. Patients should also be given written instructions, pamphlets, and other aids that help clarify the procedure and reinforce the importance of doing them correctly.

➤ Make sure patients have all the supplies needed at home to apply the medication, such as tape, gauze dressings and pads, tongue blades, cotton-tipped applicators, and gloves.

➤ Patients should be told to follow the physician's orders regarding the application and use of the topical medication. They should know to apply lotions gently but firmly by tapping the skin surface area. Lotions need to be shaken well before use. A tongue blade or cotton-tipped applicator may be used to apply creams or ointments. Patients should be encouraged to wash their hands before and after applying the medication and to note any unusual color of the skin, odor, or drainage.

POINTS TO REMEMBER

Topical Antimicrobials
- Used to reduce risk of nosocomial infections.
- Applied to topical surfaces to inhibit or kill as many microorganisms as possible.
- Consist of antiseptics and disinfectants.

Disinfectants
- Antimicrobials that are used only on nonliving objects.
- Kill any organisms on these objects.
- They are not the same as antiseptics.

Antiseptics
- Antimicrobials that are used only on living tissues.
- Primarily only inhibit growth and reproduction of microorganisms.

Categories of Antiseptics and Disinfectants
- Categorized by their chemical makeup.
- Alcohols, aldehydes, phenolic compounds, biguanides, surface-active agents, acid agents, dyes, oxidizing agents, chlorine, mercurial, and iodine.

Nursing Considerations
- The nurse should always observe standard precautions whenever applying topical agents.
- Always apply agent to clean, dry skin unless otherwise ordered or specified.
- Instruct patients concerning the proper application technique before their discharge home.

REVIEW QUESTIONS

1. Which of the following statements best describes the difference between disinfectants and antiseptics?
   a. Antiseptics are used to sterilize any plastic surgical equipment.
   b. Antiseptics are used only on nonliving objects to kill microorganisms.
   c. Disinfectants kill organisms and are indicated to be used on nonliving objects.
   d. Disinfectants are used mainly for use on the skin of patients who are being prepared for surgery.

2. Which of the following agents would a patient be allergic to if he states that he has an allergy to seafood or iodine?
   a. Peroxide
   b. Antibiotics
   c. All iodophors
   d. All antiseptics

3. Which of the following is commonly used as a bladder irrigation?
   a. 3% hydrogen peroxide
   b. 10% NS with HCl acid

   c. Acetic acid in 5% solution

   d. 5% bacitracin diluted in NS

4. Which of the following is the safest way to have patients apply their topical antiseptic agent?

   a. Use sterile gloving.

   b. Wash hands and apply vigorously to affected area.

   c. Apply lotions to all affected areas using the same clean hand.

   d. Apply creams or ointments by use of a cotton swab or tongue blade.

5. Which of the following statements about the dermal layer of the skin is correct?

   a. It is the site of the formation of keratin.

   b. It forms a protective covering for the body.

   c. It is the site of the germination of blood cells.

   d. It provides the skin with support because of the blood vessels that it contains.

For Answers see www.harcourthealth.com/MERLIN/Lilley/.

CRITICAL THINKING Activities

1. What is the main purpose of using antiseptics and disinfectants?

2. Can disinfectants and antiseptics be used interchangeably? Why or why not?

3. How would you know that a patient is having a therapeutic response to an antiseptic?

For Answers see www.harcourthealth.com/MERLIN/Lilley/.

bibliography

Albanese J, Nutz P: *Mosby's 2001 nursing drug reference and review cards*, St Louis, 2001, Mosby.

American Hospital Formulary Service: *AHFS drug information*, Bethesda, Md, 2000, American Society of Health-System Pharmacists.

Anderson PO, Knoben JE, Troutman WG: *Handbook of clinical drug data 1999-2000*, ed 9, New York, 1999, McGraw-Hill.

Johns Hopkins Hospital, Department of Pediatrics et al: *The Harriet Lane handbook*, ed 15, St Louis, 2000, Mosby.

Keen JH: *Critical care and emergency drug reference*, ed 3, St Louis, 1996, Mosby.

Mosby's GenRx: a comprehensive reference for generic and brand drugs, ed 10, St Louis, 2000, Mosby.

Skidmore-Roth L: *Mosby's 2001 nursing drug reference*, St Louis, 2001, Mosby.

Thibodeau GA, Patton KT: *Anatomy and physiology*, ed 4, St Louis, 1999, Mosby.

Chapter 42

Antiinflammatory, Antirheumatoid, and Related Agents

objectives

www.harcourthealth.com/MERLIN/Lilley/

When you reach the end of this chapter, you should be able to do the following:

Look for this symbol for topics covered in the **Online Worksheet**

1 Discuss the inflammatory response and the part it plays in the generation of pain.

2 Describe how nonsteroidal antiinflammatory drugs (NSAIDs) and other antiinflammatory agents exert their mechanisms of action.

3 List the various NSAIDs, antigout agents, and antiarthritic agents.

4 Discuss the mechanisms of action, indications, side effects, dosage ranges, cautions, contraindications, and drug interactions associated with the use of NSAIDs, antigout agents, and antiarthritic agents.

5 Develop a comprehensive nursing care plan that includes all phases of the nursing process for the patient receiving NSAIDs, antigout agents, and antiarthritic agents.

drug profiles

○━ **allopurinol**, p. 668
○━ **aspirin**, p. 664
auranofin, p. 669
aurothioglucose and gold sodium thiomalate, p. 669
celecoxib, p. 667
colchicine, p. 668
etanercept, p. 669
○━ **ibuprofen**, p. 665
○━ **indomethacin**, p. 664
ketorolac, p. 666
leflunomide, p. 670
probenecid, p. 668
rofecoxib, p. 667
sulfinpyrazone, p. 669

○━ Key drug.

glossary

Acute salicylate overdose (sal′ i sil′ at) Produces signs and symptoms similar to those of chronic intoxication, but the effects are often more pronounced and occur more quickly. (p. 662)

Chronic salicylate intoxication A toxic condition caused by the ingestion of salicylate, most often in aspirin or oil of wintergreen. (p. 662)

Done nomogram (nom′ o gram) A graph on which a number of variables are plotted so that the value of a dependent variable can be read on the appropriate line when the values of the other variables are given. (p. 663)

Misoprostol (mi so pros′ tol) Used in the prevention of gastric ulcers in patients receiving nonsteroidal antiinflammatory drugs. (p. 662)

Nonsteroidal antiinflammatory drugs A large and chemically diverse group of drugs that possess analgesic, antiinflammatory, and antipyretic activity. (p. 658)

Salicylism (sal′ i sil′ iz əm) A syndrome of salicylate toxicity. (p. 662)

Nonsteroidal antiinflammatory drugs (NSAIDs) are among the most frequently prescribed drugs. Every year approximately 70 million prescriptions are written for these agents. This represents over 5% of all prescriptions. There are now more than 23 different NSAIDs commonly used, plus many more that have limited use. NSAIDs comprise a large and chemically diverse group of drugs that possess analgesic, antiinflammatory, and antipyretic activity. They are also used for the relief of mild to moderate headaches, myalgia, neuralgia, and arthralgia; alleviation of postoperative pain; inhibition of platelet aggregation; relief of the pain associated with arthritic disorders such as rheumatoid arthritis, juvenile arthritis, ankylosing spondylitis, and osteoarthritis; and treatment of gout and hyperuricemia. The list of uses for these versatile drugs is as lengthy as the list of agents.

The use of plants containing salicylates as medicinal agents goes back more than a thousand years. North American Indians used willow bark juice as an antipyretic, and South African Hottentots used a similar mixture as an antirheumatic. Willow and poplar were used as sources of medicinal compounds by both Greek and Roman physicians. Such notable physicians as Hippocrates, Pliny the Elder, and Celsus all chronicled the beneficial effects of these salicylate-containing agents in the treatment of such diverse ailments as gout, fever, sciatica, and earache.

The most common and very first drug in this class was salicylic acid, and it was Hermann Kolbe who devised an economical procedure for the manufacture of a synthetic form of salicylic acid, which made its mass production, and hence availability, possible. Subsequently, in 1899, the most famous descendent of salicylic acid, acetylsalicylic acid

(ASA; aspirin), was marketed, and it rapidly became the most widely used drug in the world. The success of aspirin established the importance of drugs with antipyretic, analgesic, antiinflammatory, and antirheumatic properties—the properties that all NSAIDs share. However, along with aspirin's widespread use came evidence of its potential for causing major toxicologic effects. Gastrointestinal (GI) intolerance, bleeding, and renal impairment became major factors limiting its long-term administration. As a result, efforts were mounted to develop agents that did not have the side effects of aspirin. This led to the discovery of other NSAIDs, which in general are associated with a lower incidence of and less serious toxicities and are also better tolerated than aspirin in patients with chronic diseases.

Before getting into the in-depth discussion of these agents, however, it is first important to explain the arachidonic acid pathway and how it functions because the analgesic and antiinflammatory activity of NSAIDs is thought to result primarily from the inhibition of this pathway.

ARACHIDONIC ACID PATHWAY

When arachidonic acid is released from phospholipids in cell membranes in response to a triggering event (e.g., an injury), it is metabolized by either the prostaglandin pathway or the leukotriene (LT) pathway, both of which are "branches" of the arachidonic acid pathway, as shown in Fig. 42-1. Both of these pathways result in inflammation and pain.

In the prostaglandin pathway, arachidonic acid is converted by cyclooxygenase into various prostaglandins such as prostacyclin (prostaglandin I_2) as well as into thromboxane A_2 (TXA$_2$). Prostaglandins indirectly mediate and perpetuate inflammation by inducing vasodilation and enhancing vasopermeability. These effects in turn potentiate the action of proinflammatory substances, such as histamine and bradykinin, in the production of edema and pain. The LT pathway utilizes lipoxygenases to metabolize the arachidonic acid and convert it into various LTs. Although the actions of these compounds have not been characterized as well as those of prostaglandins, they also appear to be mediators of inflammation. Some LTs promote vasoconstriction, bronchospasms, and vascular permeability.

Pain, headache, fever, and inflammation are all consequences (symptoms) of the activation of the arachidonic acid pathway.

It has been shown that prostaglandins produce headache and pain because, when these substances are injected into test subjects, these are the symptoms that appear. They accomplish this by producing a hyperalgesic state in which the person's nerve endings are sensitized to painful stimuli. Consequently what may not have been a painful stimulus becomes one.

Fever results when prostaglandin E_2 is synthesized in the preoptic hypothalamic region, the area of the brain that regulates temperature.

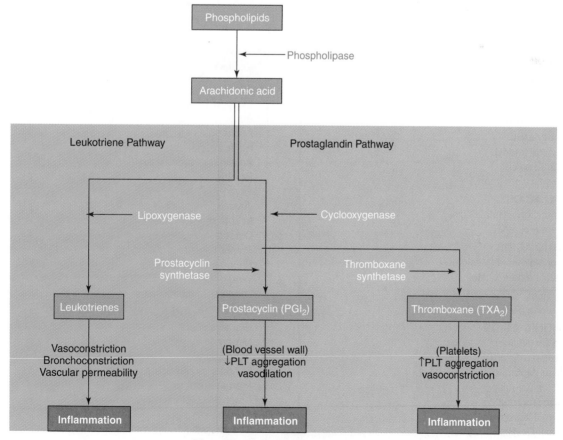

Fig. 42-1 Arachidonic acid pathway.

The inflammatory response is mediated by a host of endogenous compounds, including proteins of the complement system, histamine, serotonin, bradykinin, LTs, and prostaglandins, the latter two being major contributors to the symptoms of inflammation.

NSAIDs

As a single class of agents, NSAIDs constitute an exceptional variety of drugs, and they are used for an equally wide range of indications. Although as many as 70 agents are on the market and new agents are constantly becoming available, they can all be placed into one of six structurally and historically related groups (see Box 42-1). The carboxylic acid agents are more commonly called *salicylates* and, as previously noted, were the first nonsteroidal antiinflammatory agents to be isolated and used therapeutically. They may or may not be included in the NSAID category, however, depending on the particular reference. In this chapter they are included because their chemical and physiologic effects are so similar to those of the agents strictly considered NSAIDs.

Currently, at least one NSAID has been approved for each of the therapeutic indications listed in Box 42-2, and an NSAID is considered the drug of choice for the treatment of most of these conditions. This list of indications will continue to grow as more is learned about the mechanisms by which pain and inflammation are modified. Almost all NSAIDs are used for the treatment of rheumatoid arthritis and degenerative joint disease.

More NSAIDs are becoming available in long-acting sustained-release formulations. Some recent examples are naproxen sodium (Naprelan), diclofenac sodium (Voltaren-XR), and etodolac (Lodine XL). Medication compliance is enhanced with once-a-day medications. This may increase the efficacy of these agents for the treatment of chronic disease states such as osteoarthritis. Other NSAIDs that are not currently marketed but may soon be approved are carprofen (Rimadyl), isoxicam (Maxicam), and proquazone (Anthrex).

Mechanism of Action

NSAIDs relieve *pain* and *headache* by blocking the undesirable effects of prostaglandins. Specifically, aspirin and the other agents inhibit the enzyme cyclooxygenase and thereby prevent the formation of prostaglandins (see Fig. 42-1). This differs from opioids, which relieve pain by interfering with its recognition in the brain.

NSAIDs reduce *fever* by inhibiting prostaglandin E_2, specifically by inhibiting its biosynthesis within the preoptic hypothalamic region, which regulates body temperature.

NSAIDs relieve *inflammation* by inhibiting the LT pathway, the prostaglandin pathway, or both. The lipoxygen-

---

BOX 42-1 NSAIDs and Their Structural Groups

ACETIC ACIDS
diclofenac sodium (Voltaren)
diclofenac potassium (Cataflam)
etodolac (Lodine)
indomethacin (Indocin)
sulindac (Clinoril)
tolmetin (Tolectin)

CARBOXYLIC ACIDS
Acetylated
aspirin (many)
choline magnesium trisalicylate (Trilisate)
diflunisal (Dolobid)

Nonacetylated
salicylamide (many)
salsalate (Disalcid)
sodium salicylate (many)

ENOLIC ACIDS
phenylbutazone (Butazolidin)
piroxicam (Feldene)

FENAMIC ACIDS
meclofenamic acid (Meclomen)
mefenamic acid (Ponstel)

NONACIDIC COMPOUNDS
nabumetone (Relafen)

PROPIONIC ACIDS
fenoprofen (Nalfon)
flurbiprofen (Ansaid)
ibuprofen (Motrin, others)
ketoprofen (Orudis)
ketorolac (Toradol)
naproxen (Naprosyn)
oxaprozin (DayPro)

BOX 42-2 NSAIDs: Indications

FDA-APPROVED INDICATIONS
Acute gout
Acute gouty arthritis
Acute painful shoulder
Ankylosing spondylitis
Bursitis
Fever
Juvenile rheumatoid arthritis
Mild to moderate pain
Osteoarthritis
Primary dysmenorrhea
Rheumatoid arthritis
Tendinitis
Various ophthalmic uses

NON–FDA-APPROVED INDICATIONS
Glomerulonephritis
Nephrotic syndrome
Pericarditis
Periodontal disease
Premature labor
Prophylaxis of migraine headache
Sunscreening
Symptomatic treatment of sunburn

ase (LT) pathway is inhibited by some antiarthritic agents but not by salicylates. Several antiinflammatory drugs block the prostaglandin pathway as well as the LT pathway, whereas others only weakly inhibit cyclooxygenase but primarily inhibit lipoxygenases.

Drug Effects

The drug effects of NSAIDs are wide and varied. There are numerous actions of the drugs within this class. The main drug effects of NSAIDs are those of analgesic, antiinflammatory, and antipyretic effects. Some of the agents in this class of drugs may have all these effects as well as a few others, such as inhibiting platelet aggregation. Although agents may only affect inflammation and pain, NSAIDs are used principally in the symptomatic treatment of mild to moderate pain, fever, inflammatory diseases, and rheumatic fever.

Therapeutic Uses

The therapeutic effects of NSAIDs chiefly stem from their ability to inhibit the arachidonic acid pathway, thus preventing the release of some of the harmful products of this pathway (i.e., prostaglandins and LTs). Some of the more noted therapeutic uses of this broad class of agents are listed in Box 42-3, but they are primarily used for their analgesic, antigout, antiinflammatory, and antipyretic effects; for the relief of vascular headaches; and for platelet inhibition.

NSAIDs are most commonly used for the treatment of rheumatoid arthritis and osteoarthritis, as well as other inflammatory conditions. In this regard, these agents have proved to be highly effective while at the same time do not adversely affect preexisting conditions. They have also proved to be extremely beneficial as adjunctive pain relief medications in patients with chronic syndromes. For the relief of pain they are sometimes combined with an opioid. This can provide pain relief mediated by a mechanism of action different from that of opioids. They also do not cause many of the undesirable effects of opioids, mainly respiratory depression. However, unlike opioids, their effectiveness is limited by a ceiling effect in that any further increase in the dose beyond a certain level increases the risk of adverse effects without a corresponding increase in the therapeutic effect.

Salicylates have further beneficial properties that most NSAIDs do not in that they have potent effects on both the aggregation properties of platelets and the thermoregulatory center in the brain. For this reason they are more commonly used for the treatment of various types of fevers as well as arterial, and possibly venous, thrombosis. Other NSAIDs are commonly used in the treatment of gout, which is caused by the overproduction of uric acid or decreased uric acid secretion, or by both processes. This can often result in hyperuricemia (too much uric acid in the blood), a condition that causes joint pain as a result of the deposition of needlelike crystals of urate precipitate in tissues and the joints.

The appropriate selection of an NSAID calls for a consideration of the patient's history, including any prior medical conditions; the intended use of the agent; the patient's previous experience with NSAIDs; the patient's preference; and the cost. The NSAIDs of choice recommended for use in patients with certain underlying medical conditions are listed in Box 42-3.

Side Effects and Adverse Effects

One of the more common complaints and potentially serious adverse effects of the NSAIDs is GI distress. This can range from mild symptoms such as heartburn to the most severe GI complication—GI bleeding. In fact, the adverse effects of salicylates mainly involve the GI tract and, besides bleeding, include symptomatic GI disturbances and mucosal lesions (e.g., erosive gastritis, gastric ulcer). These problems apparently are more frequently associated with aspirin use than with the use of other NSAIDs. The potential adverse effects of NSAIDs listed in Table 42-1 do not apply to all agents, but they do apply to many of them.

BOX 42-3   NSAIDs Suggested for Patients with Particular Medical Conditions

Medical Condition	Recommended NSAID
Risk for nephrotoxicity	sulindac, nonacetylated salicylate, nabumetone, etodolac, diclofenac, oxaprozin
Hypertension	sulindac, nonacetylated salicylate, ibuprofen, etodolac
Hepatotoxicity	tolmetin, naproxen, ibuprofen, piroxicam, the fenamates
Diabetic neuropathy	sulindac
Dysmenorrhea	fenamates, naproxen, naproxen sodium
Headaches	naproxen, naproxen sodium, ketorolac
Warfarin therapy	sulindac, tolmetin, naproxen, ibuprofen, oxyaprozin
History of aspirin or NSAID allergy	Avoid if possible; if not, consider nonacetylated salicylate
Risk for gastrointestinal toxicity	nonacetylated salicylate, enteric-coated aspirin, diclofenac, nabumetone, etodolac, ibuprofen, oxaprozin
Gout	indomethacin, naproxen, naproxen sodium, sulindac
Ankylosing spondylitis	indomethacin, diclofenac
Osteoarthritis	diclofenac, oxaprozin, indomethacin

NSAIDs: Side Effects and Adverse Effects

Table 42-1

Body System	Side/Adverse Effect
Cardiovascular	Moderate to severe noncardiogenic pulmonary edema
Gastrointestinal	Most frequent: dyspepsia, heartburn, epigastric distress, nausea
	Less frequent: vomiting, anorexia, abdominal pain, GI bleeding, mucosal lesions (erosions or ulcerations)
Hematologic	Altered hemostasis through effects on platelet function
Hepatic	Acute reversible hepatotoxicity
Renal	Reduction in creatinine clearance, acute tubular necrosis with renal failure
Other	Skin eruption, sensitivity reactions, tinnitus, hearing loss

Chronic Salicylate Intoxication: Signs and Symptoms

Table 42-2

Body System	Signs and Symptoms
Cardiovascular	Increased heart rate
Central nervous system	Tinnitus, hearing loss, dimness of vision, headache, dizziness, mental confusion, lassitude, drowsiness
Gastrointestinal	Nausea, vomiting, diarrhea
Metabolic	Sweating, thirst, hyperventilation

Chronic Salicylate Intoxication: Treatment

Box 42-4

Severity	Treatment
Mild	1. Dosage reduction or discontinuation of salicylates.
	2. Symptomatic and supportive therapy.
Severe	1. Discontinuation of salicylates.
	2. Intensive symptomatic and supportive therapy.
	3. Dialysis if: high salicylate levels, unresponsive acidosis (pH <7.1), impaired renal function or renal failure, pulmonary edema, persistent CNS symptoms (e.g., seizures, coma), progressive deterioration despite appropriate therapy.

Many of the side effects and adverse effects of NSAIDs are secondary to their inactivation of protective prostaglandins that help maintain the normal integrity of the stomach lining. When the formation of these beneficial prostaglandins is inhibited, as occurs with NSAIDs, this protective barrier is eliminated. This sets up a perfect environment for ulceration and GI bleeding. To further complicate matters, because NSAIDs prolong bleeding times by inhibiting TXA_2 production, this can exacerbate GI bleeding. However, an agent called **misoprostol** (Cytotec) has proved successful in preventing the gastric ulcers and hence GI bleeding that can occur in patients receiving NSAIDs. It is a synthetic prostaglandin E_1 analogue that potently inhibits gastric acid secretion, which it does by directly inhibiting the function of parietal cells. It also has a cytoprotective component, although the mechanism responsible for this action is unclear. It may prevent disruption of the gastric mucosal barrier, stimulate mucous secretion, stimulate alkaline (bicarbonate) secretion, or enhance mucosal blood flow. It also causes uterine contractions. Because of this it may sometimes be used with other drugs to induce abortion. For women who are able to conceive and do not intend to abort, misoprostol should be avoided.

The kidneys are also dependent to some extent on prostaglandins, especially in the patient who is already renally compromised, because these organs rely on the prostaglandins produced by them for stimulating vasodilation and increased renal blood flow. If NSAIDs inhibit this compensatory mechanism, this may be enough to precipitate acute or chronic renal failure, depending on the patient's current renal function.

Toxicity and Management of Overdose

There are both chronic and acute manifestations of salicylate toxicity. Chronic salicylate intoxication is known as **salicylism** and results from either high doses or prolonged therapy with high doses. The most common signs and symptoms of **chronic salicylate intoxication** are listed in Table 42-2.

The most frequent manifestations of chronic intoxication in adults are tinnitus and hearing loss. Those in children are hyperventilation and central nervous system (CNS) effects such as giddiness, drowsiness, and behavioral changes. These effects usually arise when serum salicylate concentrations exceed 300 μg/ml. Metabolic complications such as metabolic acidosis and respiratory alkalosis are usually present in the setting of chronic intoxication. Metabolic acidosis can also occur in the setting of acute intoxication, but is usually less severe than that in patients with chronic intoxication. Hypoglycemia is also likely to occur and can be life-threatening.

The treatment of chronic intoxication is based on the presenting symptoms. Serum salicylate concentrations may be determined but are not as useful in estimating the severity, because severe intoxication can occur with a concentration as low as 150 μg/ml. The suggested treatment for chronic salicylate intoxication is summarized in Box 42-4.

The signs and symptoms of **acute salicylate overdose** are similar to those of chronic intoxication, but the effects are often more pronounced and occur more quickly. It results from the ingestion of a single toxic dose, and its severity can be estimated based on the estimated amount (in mg/kg of body weight) ingested, as follows:

- Little or no toxicity: <150 mg/kg
- Mild to moderate toxicity: 150-300 mg/kg

BOX 42-5   Chronic Salicylate Intoxication: Treatment Goals

Treatment Goal	Measure
Reduce salicylate absorption	Syrup of ipecac (if patient is alert and awake). Gastric lavage.* Activated charcoal.
Treat fluid and electrolyte imbalance	Appropriate fluid replacement and electrolyte therapy should be implemented promptly, based on fluid, acid-base, and electrolyte status. Therefore arterial pH and blood gases and electrolytes, serum creatine, BUN, and blood glucose should be determined.
Enhance salicylate elimination	Alkaline diuresis: IV administration of sodium bicarbonate to alkalinize the urine to a pH of 7.5 or more with sufficient urine flow. Hemodialysis: the same considerations as those that apply to chronic intoxication.
Provide symptomatic and supportive measures	Hypotension and/or hemorrhagic complications: fluids and transfusions, along with possible vitamin K injections. Respiratory depression: may require assisted pulmonary ventilation and oxygen. Seizures: IV administration of a benzodiazepine or short-acting barbiturate.

*Effective up to 3 to 4 hours after acute ingestion and maybe up to 10 hours after ingestion in the event of massive overdose.

- Severe toxicity: 300-500 mg/kg
- Life-threatening: >500 mg/kg

A serum salicylate concentration measured 6 hours or more after the ingestion may be used in conjunction with the **Done nomogram** to estimate the severity of intoxication and help guide treatment. (This is a graph on which a number of variables are plotted so that the value of a dependent variable can be read on the appropriate line when the other variables are given.) This nomogram is only intended for gauging the severity of acute intoxications, however, and not that of chronic salicylate intoxication.

The pathophysiologic mechanism of salicylate overdose is complex because of the variety of toxic effects produced by salicylates, although the principal ones are extensions of the agents' pharmacologic actions. These are as follows:

- Local GI tract irritation
- Direct CNS stimulation of respiration
- Altered glucose metabolism (stimulation of gluconeogenesis and lipid metabolism)
- Increased tissue glycolysis
- Interference with hemostatic mechanisms

The treatment of acute toxicity stemming from a salicylate overdose involves intensive symptomatic and supportive therapy. The treatment goals should consist of removing salicylate from the GI tract and preventing its further absorption; correcting fluid, electrolyte, and acid-base disturbances; and implementing measures to enhance salicylate elimination. The measures to be taken to achieve these treatment goals are listed in Box 42-5.

An acute overdose of NSAIDs causes effects similar to those of salicylate overdose, but they are generally not as extensive. The symptoms comprise CNS toxicities such as drowsiness, lethargy, mental confusion, paresthesias, numbness, aggressive behavior, disorientation, and seizures and GI toxicities such as nausea, vomiting, and GI bleeding. Intense headache, dizziness, cerebral edema, cardiac arrest, and death have also been known to occur in extreme cases. Treatment should consist of the immediate removal of the ingested agent by inducing emesis with either syrup of ipecac or gastric lavage. This should be followed by the administration of activated charcoal, with supportive and symptomatic treatment initiated thereafter. Hemodialysis appears to be of no value in enhancing the elimination of NSAIDs.

Interactions

The drug interactions associated with the use of salicylates and other NSAIDs can result in significant complications and morbidity. Some of the more common of these are listed in Table 42-3.

These agents can also interfere with laboratory test results. Specifically, salicylates can cause the serum levels of ALT, AST, and alkaline phosphatase to be increased. The hematocrit values, hemoglobin levels, and red blood cell (RBC) counts can all be decreased in patients suffering from GI bleeding stemming from the use of salicylates or other NSAIDs. NSAID use can also cause the serum levels of potassium to be elevated and the serum levels of sodium to be lowered.

Dosages

For the recommended dosages of various NSAIDs, see the dosages table on p. 665.

drug profiles

CARBOXYLIC ACIDS

Salicylates are classified as carboxylic acids and can be either acetylated (aspirin, magnesium cholinesalicylate, and diflunisal) or nonacetylated (salicylamide, salsalate, and sodium salicylate). Although aspirin is the most commonly used of all these agents, the others have many of the same beneficial effects as aspirin. Most salicylates are available

Table 42-3 Salicylates and Other NSAIDs: Drug Interactions

Drug	Mechanism	Result
Alcohol	Additive effect	Increased GI bleeding
Anticoagulants	Platelet inhibition, hypoprothrom- binemia	Increased bleeding tendencies
Aspirin and other salicylates with NSAIDs	Reduce NSAID absorption Additive GI toxicities	Increased GI toxicity with no therapeutic advantage
Corticosteroids and other ulcerogenic agents	Additive toxicities	Increased ulcerogenic effects
cyclosporine	Inhibit renal prostaglandin synthesis	May increase the nephrotoxic effects of cyclosporine
Hypotensive agents and diuretics	Inhibit prostaglandin synthesis	Reduced hypotensive and diuretic effects
Protein-bound drugs	Compete for binding	More pronounced drug actions
Uricosurics	Antagonism	Decreased uric acid excretion

over-the-counter (OTC), the exceptions being choline magnesium trisalicylate (Trilisate), diflunisal (Dolobid), and salsalate (Disalcid). Salicylates are usually available in oral preparations. They are generally rated as pregnancy category C agents, except for aspirin, which is rated as a pregnancy category D agent because it has been shown to be both teratogenic and embryocidal in animals.

aspirin

Aspirin (ASA, and many product names) is known chemically as *acetylsalicylic acid*. It is the prototype salicylate and NSAID and is the most widely used drug in the world. First introduced in the late 1800s, it remains a mainstay of many drug treatment regimens. Aspirin is capable of many beneficial therapeutic effects, including analgesic, antiinflammatory, and antipyretic effects. It has also been shown to have an antithrombotic effect, which is the result of its ability to inhibit platelet aggregation by blocking cyclooxygenase. This action has made it, along with thrombolytics, a primary drug in the treatment of acute myocardial infarction (MI) as well as many other thromboembolic disorders. Aspirin may be used to treat the pain associated with headache, neuralgia, myalgia, and arthralgia, as well as other pain syndromes resulting from inflammation. These include arthritis, pleurisy, and pericarditis. Patients with systemic lupus erythematosus may also benefit from aspirin therapy.

Aspirin is available in many dosage forms: chewing gum, tablets, chewable tablets, delayed-release enteric-coated tablets, extended-release tablets, filmcoated tablets, tablets for solution, capsules, and rectal suppositories. It is also contained in many combination products, some of the more popular combinations being aspirin, acetaminophen, and caffeine combinations (Goody's Headache Powder, Excedrin) and aspirin combined with various ant-

acids (Ascriptin, Bufferin). Aspirin also is available in special dosage forms such as enteric-coated aspirin (Ecotrin). These many dosage formulations and strengths have been developed over the years in response to a need to decrease the GI toxicities associated with aspirin use, to incorporate the beneficial therapeutic effects of aspirin with those of other agents, and to provide the exact dose needed for certain indications.

Aspirin is contraindicated in patients with a known hypersensitivity to salicylates; those with GI bleeding, bleeding disorders, vitamin K deficiency, or a peptic ulcer; children younger than 12 years of age; and children with flulike symptoms. As previously mentioned, it is classified as a pregnancy D agent and its use should be avoided in nursing mothers. Commonly recommended dosages are listed in the dosages table on p. 665.

PHARMACOKINETICS

HALF-LIFE	ONSET	PEAK	DURATION
5-9 hr	15-30 min	1-2 hr	4-6 hr

ACETIC ACIDS

indomethacin

Indomethacin (Indocin) is one of the six commonly used acetic acid NSAIDs, the others being diclofenac sodium, diclofenac potassium, etodolac, sulindac, and tolmetin. All are structurally related. Like the other NSAIDs, indomethacin has analgesic, antiinflammatory, and antipyretic properties. Its therapeutic actions are of particular use in the treatment of rheumatoid arthritis, ankylosing rheumatoid spondylitis, acute gouty arthritis, and the closure of patent ductus arteriosus in premature infants.

Because of its potent actions, indomethacin is available only by prescription. It can be administered by three different routes—orally, rectally, and

DOSAGES Salicylates and Other NSAIDs

agent	pharmacologic class	dosage range	purpose
CARBOXYLIC ACIDS			
aspirin (acetylsalicylic acid [ASA]; many product names)	Salicylate	*Pediatric* PO/rectal: 10-15 mg/kg 4-6 times/day (max 4 g/day) 60-90 mg/kg/day divided q4-6h *Adult* PO/rectal: 325-1000 mg 4-6 times/day (max 4 g/day) 3.2-6 g/day divided 325-650 mg 2-4 times/day PO: 300-325 mg/day	Antipyretic, analgesic Antirheumatic Antipyretic, analgesic Antirheumatic Antithrombotic Post-MI
ACETIC ACIDS			
indomethacin (Indocin)	NSAID	*Infant* <48 hr old; (doses at 12-24 hr intervals) IV: 0.2 mg/kg, followed by 0.1 mg/kg for 2 doses 2-7 days old: IV 0.2 mg/kg for all 3 doses >7 days old: IV: 0.2 mg/kg, followed by 0.25 mg/kg for 2 doses *Pediatric* 1-2 mg/kg/day divided q6-12h (max 4 mg/kg/day) *Adult* 50 mg three times a day and tapered to cessation as soon as possible	Patient ductus arteriosus Antirheumatic Antirheumatic Gout
PROPIONIC ACIDS			
ibuprofen (Motrin, many others)	NSAID	*Pediatric 6 mo-12 yr old* PO: 5 mg/kg if <102.5° F (39.1° C) 10 mg/kg if >102.5° F (39.1° C) q6-5h (max 50 mg/kg/day) *Adult* PO: 200-400 mg q4-6h 400-800 mg 3-4 times/day; do not exceed 3.2 g/day.	Antipyretic Antipyretic, analgesic, dysmenorrhea Antirheumatic
ketorolac (Toradol)	NSAID	*Adult* PO: 20 mg followed by 10 mg q4-6h; do not exceed 40 mg/day or 5 days of therapy* IV/IM: 30-60 mg, followed by 15-30 mg q6h, not to exceed 120 mg/day*	Analgesic
COX-2 INHIBITORS celecoxib (Celebrex)	COX-2 inhibitor	*Adult* PO: 100 to 200 mg once to twice daily	Antirheumatic, analgesic
rofecoxib (Vioxx)	COX-2 inhibitor	*Adult* PO: 12.5 mg to 50 mg daily	Antirheumatic, analgesic

*With ketorolac in patients >65 years of age, <110 lb (50 kg), or with moderately elevated serum creatinine, special dosing considerations are in order for PO, IV, and IM dosing (max 5 days of therapy).

intravenously. The oral dosage forms are a 25- and 50-mg capsule, a 75-mg extended-release capsule, and a 25-mg/5 ml suspension. The rectal suppositories contain 50 mg of the agent, and parenterally, indomethacin is available as a 1-mg injection. Indomethacin is considered as a pregnancy category B agent for women in the first or second trimester of pregnancy, but its use during the last trimester is not recommended because it may inhibit prostaglandin synthesis in the fetus. For the same reason, it is also not recommended for use in nursing women. Hypersensitivity to it, asthma, severe renal and hepatic disease, and ulcer disease are all contraindications to its use. Commonly recommended dosages are listed in the dosages table above.

PHARMACOKINETICS

HALF-LIFE	ONSET	PEAK	DURATION
1.5-2 hr	<30 min	0.5-3 hr	4-6 hr

PROPIONIC ACIDS
ibuprofen

Ibuprofen (Motrin and many others) is the prototype NSAID in the propionic acid category, which also includes fenoprofen, flurbiprofen, ketoprofen, ketorolac, naproxen, and oxaprozin. However, ibuprofen is the most frequently used of the propionic acid agents because of the numerous indications for its use and because of its relatively safe side effect and adverse effect profile. Ibuprofen is also available OTC, either alone or in combination with other agents, of which there are many such products. To reduce toxicity and prevent some of the dose-related side effects of ibuprofen, the maximum strength of the OTC ibuprofen preparations is 200 mg.

Because of the therapeutic actions of ibuprofen, it is an excellent drug for the treatment of rheumatoid arthritis, osteoarthritis, primary dysmenorrhea, gout, dental pain, and musculoskeletal disorders. Ibuprofen is available only in oral formulations: a 40-mg/ml and 100-mg/5 ml suspension; 100-, 200-, 300-, 400-, 600-, and 800-mg film-coated and regular tablets; 50-mg chewable tablets; and a combination product containing 200 mg of ibuprofen and 30 mg of pseudoephedrine. Some of the OTC products are Advil, Midol IB, Motrin IB, and Nuprin.

Ibuprofen is considered a pregnancy category B agent for women in their first or second trimester of pregnancy. It is not recommended for women in the last trimester because it can inhibit prostaglandin synthesis in the fetus. It is also not recommended for nursing women because it can inhibit prostaglandin synthesis in the infant. Hypersensitivity, asthma, and severe renal and hepatic disease are contraindications to its use. Commonly recommended dosages are listed in the dosages table on p. 665.

PHARMACOKINETICS

HALF-LIFE	ONSET	PEAK	DURATION
2-2.5 hr	<30 min	0.6-2 hr	4-6 hr

ketorolac

Ketorolac (Toradol) is another propionic acid NSAID but is unique in that it has very little antiinflammatory action but a very potent analgesic action. As proof of this the analgesic potency of ketorolac is similar to that of opioid analgesics such as morphine and meperidine. It is indicated for the treatment of mild to moderate pain but not for that of osteoarthritis or rheumatoid arthritis because of its limited antiinflammatory effects. A particular advantage of ketorolac is that it may be given parenterally by either the IV or IM route as well as orally and ophthalmically. It is the only NSAID that can be given by all these routes. Ketorolac is available as a 10-mg film-coated tablet; a 15-, 30-, and 60-mg parenteral form; and a 0.5% ophthalmic solution.

Ketorolac is available only by prescription. It is indicated for the short-term (up to 5 days) management of moderately severe acute pain that requires analgesia at the opioid level. It is not indicated for minor or chronic painful conditions. Ketorolac is a very potent NSAID with many contraindications (Box 42-6). Ketorolac is classified as a pregnancy category C agent. Commonly recommended dosages are listed in the dosages table on p. 665.

PHARMACOKINETICS

HALF-LIFE	ONSET	PEAK	DURATION
5-7 hr	0.5-1 hr	1.5-3 hr	6 hr

COX-2 INHIBITORS

Celecoxib (Celebrex), rofecoxib (Vioxx), and meloxicam (Mobic) are NSAIDs that have antiinflammatory, analgesic, and antipyretic activities. They are believed to work by inhibiting prostaglandin synthesis via inhibition of cyclooxygenase-2 (COX-2) but not cyclooxygenase-1 (COX-1). These agents are most commonly referred to as *COX-2 inhibitors*.

The potential advantage of using a COX-2 selective agent is the benefit of decreasing the production of the inflammatory prostaglandins produced by COX-2 without decreasing the production of the prostaglandins produced by COX-1, which are important in regulating other body functions. This COX-2 selectivity allows these agents to control the inflammation and pain while not producing some of the toxicity associated with NSAID therapy.

COX-2 selective inhibitors have little effect on platelet function. These agents were designed, in part, to cause fewer GI adverse effects; however, they are not totally devoid of GI toxicity. Gastritis and upper GI bleeding have been reported with their use. The most common adverse effects include fatigue, dizziness, lower extremity edema, hypertension, dyspepsia, nausea, heartburn, and epigastric discomfort. Potential drug interactions include ACE inhibitors, aspirin, methotrexate, and warfarin.

COX-2 inhibitors are contraindicated in individuals with a hypersensitivity to them and should not be given to patients who have experienced asthma, urticaria, or allergic-type reactions after taking aspirin or other NSAIDs. They are classified as pregnancy category C agents.

BOX 42-6 Contraindications of Ketorolac

Active PUD or history of PUD
Recent GIB or history of GIB
Advanced renal impairment
Labor, delivery, and nursing mothers
Hemorrhagic diathesis
Before any major surgery
Concomitant with NSAIDs
Intrathecal or epidural administration
Suspected or confirmed cerebrovascular bleeding
History of hypersensitivity to ketorolac

celecoxib

Celecoxib (Celebrex) is indicated for the treatment of osteoarthritis and rheumatoid arthritis. It is available as a 100- and 200-mg capsule. Commonly recommended dosages are given in the dosages table on p. 665.

PHARMACOKINETICS

HALF-LIFE	ONSET	PEAK	DURATION
11 hr	0.75-1 hr	3 hr	4-8 hr

rofecoxib

Rofecoxib (Vioxx) is indicated for the relief of the signs and symptoms of osteoarthritis, management of acute pain in adults, and treatment of primary dysmenorrhea. It is available as a 12.5-, 25-, and 50-mg tablet and a 12.5- and 25-mg/5 ml oral suspension. Commonly recommended dosages are listed in the dosages table on p. 665.

PHARMACOKINETICS

HALF-LIFE	ONSET	PEAK	DURATION
17 hr	0.5-1 hr	2-3 hr	6 hr

ENOLIC ACIDS, FENAMIC ACIDS, AND NONACIDIC COMPOUNDS

The last three chemical categories of NSAIDs consist of the smallest number of agents, and the indications for their use are limited. Both phenylbutazone (Butazolidin) and piroxicam (Feldene) belong to the enolic acid family of NSAIDs. These are very potent agents that have been observed to produce severe GI toxicities. They are commonly used in the treatment of mild to moderate osteo-arthritis, rheumatoid arthritis, and gouty arthritis. They are both available only in oral dosage formulations. Phenylbutazone is classified as pregnancy category D agent and piroxicam as a pregnancy category C agent. They both have contraindications similar to those of the other NSAIDs.

Meclofenamic acid (Meclomen) and mefenamic acid (Ponstel) are fenamic acid NSAIDs that are older agents and not used as commonly as the other NSAIDs. They are indicated for the treatment of mild to moderate pain, osteoarthritis, and rheumatoid arthritis. Mefenamic acid is pregnancy category C; meclofenamic acid use is *not* recommended during pregnancy.

Nabumetone (Relafen) is a relatively new NSAID that is better tolerated than some of the other agents by persons intolerant to the other NSAIDs because of the GI tract side effects. It is classified as a nonacidic compound and at present is the only such agent. Currently it is indicated only for the treatment of osteoarthritis and rheumatoid arthritis. It has contraindications similar to those of the other NSAIDs. It is a pregnancy category C agent, and the pregnancy and lactation precautions to nabumeton use are the same as those for ibuprofen use. Commonly recommended dosages for these agents can be found in the dosages table below.

ANTIRHEUMATOID AGENTS

The agents discussed in this section are ones that are not structurally related to NSAIDs but are used to treat some of the same conditions, such as the various forms of arthritis and gout. Acetaminophen is discussed at length in Chapter 9. These agents can be classified broadly as the antigout agents and antiarthritic agents. They have unique characteristics that make them different from NSAIDs and for this reason are discussed separately.

DOSAGES Enolic Acids, Fenamic Acids, and the Nonacidic Compounds

agent	pharmacologic class	dosage range	purpose
meclofenamic acid (Meclomen)	Fenamate NSAID	*Adult* PO: 200-400 mg/day in 3-4 doses	Rheumatoid arthritis, osteoarthritis
		40-100 mg q4-6h	Pain
		100 mg tid	Primary dysmenorrhea
mefenamic acid (Ponstel)	Fenamate NSAID	*Pediatric >14 y/o/Adult* PO: 500 mg, followed by 250 mg q6h with food	Acute pain, dysmenorrhea
nabumetone (Relafen)	Nonacidic NSAID	*Adult* PO: 1000-2000 mg/day	Rheumatoid arthritis, osteoarthritis
phenylbutazone (Butazolidin)	Pyrazolone NSAID	*Adult* PO: 300-600 mg/day in 3-4 divided doses	Rheumatoid arthritis
		400 mg, followed by 100 mg q4h for up to 4-7 days	Gout
piroxicam (Feldene)	NSAID	*Adult* PO: 20 mg/day in a single daily dose; adjust according to response.	Rheumatoid arthritis, osteorthritis

drug profiles

ANTIGOUT AGENTS

Gout is a condition that results from inappropriate uric acid metabolism. People with gout either overproduce or underexcrete uric acid, an end-product of purine metabolism. Purines are part of the normal dietary intake and are used to make the essential nucleoside analogues DNA and RNA. During their metabolism they are converted from hypoxanthine to xanthine and eventually to uric acid. (The normal pathway for the purine metabolism is depicted in Fig. 42-2.) When there is too much uric acid, deposits of uric acid crystals collect in tissues and joints, and this causes the pain of gout because these crystals are like small needles that jab and stick into sensitive tissues and joints.

Antigout agents include such drugs as allopurinol (Zyloprim), colchicine, probenecid (Benemid), and sulfinpyrazone (Anturane). They are targeted at the underlying defect in uric acid metabolism, causing either the underexcretion or overproduction of uric acid.

allopurinol

The beneficial effect of allopurinol (Zyloprim) in the relief of gout is the inhibition of the enzyme xanthine oxidase, which thereby prevents uric acid production. Allopurinol is indicated for patients whose gout is caused by the excess production of uric acid. Oxypurinol, a metabolite of allopurinol, also prevents uric acid production.

Allopurinol is contraindicated in patients with a hypersensitivity to it. Significant adverse effects to the agent include agranulocytosis, aplastic anemia, and serious and potentially fatal skin conditions such as exfoliative dermatitis, Stevens-Johnson syndrome, and toxic epidermal necrolysis. Azathioprine and mercaptopurine both interact with allopurinol, and because of the important interactions that can result, their doses may have to be adjusted.

Allopurinol is available only in oral preparations as a 100- and 300-mg tablet. The recommended adult dosage is 200 to 600 mg per day, to a maximum of 800 mg per day. Allopurinol is a pregnancy category C drug.

colchicine

Colchicine is an antigout medication that has weak antiinflammatory activity, no effect on the urinary excretion of uric acid, and no analgesic activity. It appears to be effective in the treatment of gout by reducing the inflammatory response to the deposits of urate crystals in joint tissue. There are many possible explanations for its ability to do this, but the one favored by most is that it inhibits polymorphonuclear leukocyte metabolism, mobility, and chemotaxis.

Colchicine is a powerful inhibitor of cell mitosis and is extremely toxic, and for this reason it is available by prescription only. It is the drug of choice and primarily limited to the treatment of acute attacks of gout. Colchicine's most common and most severe side effects are GI effects, which can lead to hemorrhagic gastroenteritis. Colchicine can also cause renal failure. There is no specific antidote for colchicine poisoning. Hypersensitivity is the only contraindication to its use. The drug is available parenterally in a 0.5-mg/ml injection. It is also available in 0.5-, 0.6-, or 0.65-mg tablets. The usual adult dosage is an initial dose of 0.6 to 1.2 mg, then 0.6 mg every 1 to 2 hours until the pain disappears or until nausea, vomiting, or diarrhea develops. Colchicine is rated as a pregnancy category D agent.

probenecid

The beneficial effect of probenecid (Benemid) in the treatment of gout is the increased excretion of uric acid in the urine. Drugs that promote this excretion are known as uricosurics. In patients whose gout is due to the underexcretion of uric acid, urate crystals form because uric acid is not being excreted in the urine in sufficient quantities. Instead, most of the uric acid is being resorbed from the renal tubules back into the bloodstream and then conveyed

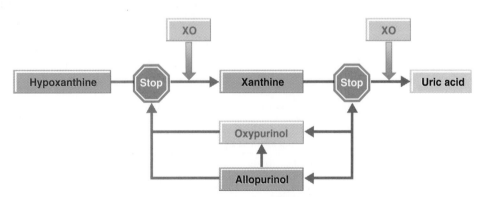

Fig. 42-2 Uric acid production. *XO*, Xanthine oxidase.

throughout the body. Probenecid works by preferentially binding to the special transporter that takes uric acid from the urine and places it back into the blood. The probenecid rather than the uric acid is then resorbed back into the bloodstream while the uric acid remains in the urine and is excreted. Besides its use for the treatment of the hyperuricemia associated with gout and gouty arthritis, it also has the ability to delay the renal excretion of penicillin, thus increasing the serum levels of penicillin and prolonging its effect. Probenecid is available as a 500-mg oral tablet. The usual adult dosage is 250 mg twice a day with food, milk, or antacids for 1 week. After that the dose should be adjusted to maintain normal uric acid levels. ColBenemid is a combination product of colchicine 0.5 mg and 500 mg of probenecid. Probenecid is a pregnancy category B agent.

sulfinpyrazone

Sulfinpyrazone (Anturane) works similarly to probenecid. It is also a uricosuric agent. It is chemically related to the NSAID, phenylbutazone, and, like it, can also cause ulcers. It is therefore contraindicated in patients with peptic ulcer disease. Sulfinpyrazone is available in 100-mg tablets and 200-mg capsules. The usual adult dosage is 100 to 200 mg twice a day for 1 week. The subsequent adjusted maintenance dosage is 200 to 400 mg daily. It is a pregnancy category C agent.

ANTIARTHRITIC AGENTS

Antiarthritic agents suppress arthritic inflammation and are therefore used in the treatment of rheumatoid arthritis. They exhibit antiinflammatory, antiarthritic, and immunomodulating effects and work by inhibiting the movement of various cells into an inflamed, damaged area, such as a joint. These cells (neutrophils, monocytes, and macrophages) are responsible for causing many of the deleterious effects of chronic rheumatoid arthritis. By preventing the accumulation of these cells in the area of the diseased joint, antiarthritic agents prevent progression of the disease. These agents are also believed to be effective in the treatment of such diseases as rheumatoid arthritis by modulating or controlling the involvement of the immune system. The three most commonly used antiarthritic agents are auranofin, aurothioglucose, and gold sodium thiomalate. Antiarthritic agents are available by prescription only and are rated as pregnancy category C agents.

auranofin

Auranofin (Ridaura) is an orally active antiarthritic agent. Twenty-nine percent of it is gold, and like all antiarthritic agents, it has antiinflammatory, antiarthritic, and immunomodulating effects. It is poorly absorbed orally, with only about 25% being absorbed from the GI tract into the blood. Auranofin is contraindicated in patients with a history of gold-induced necrotizing enterocolitis, pulmonary fibrosis, exfoliative dermatitis, bone marrow aplasia, or other types of blood dyscrasia. It is available in 3-mg capsules for oral use. The normal recommended adult dosage is 6 mg once per day or 3 mg twice per day. The dosage can be increased to 9 mg after 6 months if the response is inadequate. Auranofin is a pregnancy category C agent.

aurothioglucose and gold sodium thiomalate

Aurothioglucose (Solganol) and gold sodium thiomalate (Myochrysine) are parenterally administered antiarthritic agents. These products are made by complexing gold with thioglucose and thiomalate via a sulfur atom. Like other antiarthritic agents they have antiinflammatory, antiarthritic, and immunomodulating effects. Aurothioglucose is available as a 50-mg/ml injection; gold sodium thiomalate is available as an injection in strengths of 25 and 50 mg/ml. The normal adult dosage of aurothioglucose is 10 mg per week, increasing to 50 mg per week. The usual maintenance dosage is 25 mg per week. The recommended adult dosage of gold sodium thiomalate is somewhat similar to that of aurothioglucose. It is recommended that it be started at a dose of 10 mg, followed by a second weekly dose of 25 mg. The third and subsequent doses are 50 mg weekly for 14 to 20 weeks. After 0.8 to 1 g has been administered and there is improvement in the patient's condition and no noted toxicity, the maintenance dose should be 50 mg given at 2-week intervals for four doses, followed by 50 mg given monthly. It is a pregnancy category C agent.

etanercept

Etanercept (Enbrel) is a new agent indicated for the treatment of moderately to severely active rheumatoid arthritis in patients who have not responded to one or more disease-modifying antirheumatic drugs (DMARDs). It can be used in combination with methotrexate in patients who do not respond adequately to methotrexate alone. Etanercet works by binding to and neutralizing tumor necrosis factor (TNF). TNF is a known proinflammatory cytokine. Etanercept has been shown to decrease joint swelling, tenderness, and morning stiffness. It has an extremely long half-life (92 hours), which allows for it to be dosed just twice a week. The recommended dose of etanercept is 25 mg subcutaneously. The most common side effect is a mild injection site reaction that typically subsides in 3 to 5 days. Other adverse reactions include mild upper respiratory tract symptoms such as cough, rhinitis, sinusitis, upper respiratory tract infections, and pharyngitis. Etanercept is available as a 25-mg vial for parenteral injection.

leflunomide

Leflunomide (Arava) is a new agent indicated for the treatment of active rheumatoid arthritis. It modulates or alters the immune system's response to rheumatoid arthritis. It has antiproliferative, antiinflammatory, and immunosuppressive activity. Its most common side effects are diarrhea, respiratory tract infection, alopecia, elevated liver function tests, and rash. It is contraindicated in women who are or may become pregnant and should not be used by nursing mothers or those with a hypersensitivity to it. It is classified as a pregnancy category X agent. Leflunomide is most commonly given by a loading dose of 100 mg daily for 3 days, then a maintenance dose of 20 mg daily. Aspirin, NSAIDs, and/or low-dose corticosteroids may be continued during leflunomide therapy. It is available as 10-, 20-, and 100-mg tablets.

nursing process

● Assessment

Before administering NSAIDs, the nurse must assess the patient for the following contraindications to their use: allergies to any of the classes of NSAIDs, GI lesions or peptic ulcer disease, and bleeding disorders. Cautious use, with careful monitoring of the patient for the occurrence of side effects or toxicity, is recommended in pregnant women; patients with renal, cardiac, or hepatic disease; patients with glaucoma (i.e., enolic agents such as phenylbutazone); the elderly; and patients with psychiatric illnesses (i.e., indomethacin, sulindac, tolmetin).

Salicylates in particular are *not* to be given to children under 12 years of age because of the risk of Reye's syndrome (see Pediatric Considerations box). With NSAIDs in pregnant women, careful monitoring is helpful but does not prevent complications. NSAIDs are contraindicated in the third trimester of pregnancy and with lactation. There are also many drug interactions for salicylates and NSAIDs, including alcohol, heparin, phenytoin, anticoagulants, steroids, and sulfonylamides.

A thorough medication history is needed to determine whether the patient is taking any drugs that can interact with NSAIDs. Indole agents (e.g., indomethacin, sulindac) are ulcerogenic and should not be given with corticosteroids and aspirin agents. They should be given cautiously with anticoagulants. Enolic agents (phenylbutazone) enhance the effects of oral anticoagulants, insulin, and oral antidiabetic agents and also inhibit the action of steroids and sex hormones. Phenylpropionic agents (ibuprofen, naproxen) should be used cautiously with anticoagulants, and their concurrent use with aspirin may decrease the antiinflammatory effects of the NSAID.

Ketorolac is indicated only for *short-term use* and for patients experiencing severe acute pain. It is contraindicated in patients with active peptic ulcer disease, recent GI bleeding, a history of peptic ulcer disease or GI bleeding before surgery, or a history of confirmed CVA.

Laboratory tests assessing cardiac, renal, and liver function as well as an RBC, Hgb level, Hct, and platelet count should also be determined and the results documented before the use of NSAIDs. In addition, laboratory studies that assess the status of other diseases (inflammatory-type diseases) may be ordered, such as an evaluation of rheumatoid factors.

Before and during the administration of antiarthritic agents, it is important to assess the patient's respiratory function as dyspnea, wheezing or respiratory problems since the drug may need to be discontinued. Renal status and hepatic function must also be assessed because decreased function of these organs may necessitate a decrease in dosage. Cautions to the use of antiarthritic agents include the elderly, children, pregnant women, and patients with blood dyscrasias. Contraindications to their use include hypersensitivity, lupus erythematosus, uncontrolled diabetes mellitus, congestive heart failure (CHF), renal and liver disease, and hypertension. Drug interactions for which to assess include pencillamine, phenylbutazone, immunosuppressants, antimalarials, and cytotoxic agents, which may all lead to increased occurrence of blood dyscrasias when administered simultaneously with antiarthritic agents. The newer antirheumatics, such as leflunomide and etanercept, carry a high risk of liver toxicity if given with methotrexate or with other agents that are hepatotoxic.

Before administering colchicine it is important to assess the patient for any contraindications, such as allergies, severe GI disorders, renal or hepatic disease, and cardiac diseases. Blood dyscrasias are also a contraindication to the use of this medication. Drug interactions for which to assess include CNS depressants and sympathomimetics. Simultaneous use of these medications with colchicine may lead to increased action of the CNS depressants or the sympathomimetics.

Allopurinol is contraindicated in patients with known allergies to the medication. It should be administered cautiously in patients with renal or hepatic disease. Drug interactions include mercaptopurine and azathiprine (increased bone marrow depression when used with allopurinol) and cyclophosphamide (increased action of the allopurinol).

● Nursing Diagnoses

Nursing diagnoses relevant to the use of NSAIDs and other antiinflammatory agents should always take into

pediatric considerations

Reye's Syndrome

SIGNS AND SYMPTOMS
- Vomiting
- Changes in level of consciousness
- Hypoglycemia
- Altered liver function
- Seizures
- Coma, flaccid paralysis, loss of deep tendon reflexes
- Causes encephalopathy and fatty degeneration of the viscera; occurs primarily in children with peak incidence between 5-15 years of age
- Linked with the use of salicylates and often after a viral illness

MEDICAL MANAGEMENT
- Supportive treatment in an intensive care unit
- Maintain life functions, regain metabolic balance, and control cerebral edema
- IV glucose (10% or higher) for treatment of hypoglycemia
- Monitor blood sugars; insulin may be needed
- Vitamin K for clotting problems
- Fresh-frozen plasma may be needed if there is significant bleeding
- Prophylactic AEDs (antiepileptic drugs)

- Monitor ICP
- Cautious fluid administration
- Osmotic diuretics may be needed with steroids for cerebral edema

NURSING MANAGEMENT
- Critical care setting
- Assess neurologic status, vital signs, and arterial and central venous pressures
- Monitor blood gases and ICP
- Temperature control to prevent elevations and increased O_2 demands
- Elevate HOB
- I & O
- Hyperventilation may be needed with intubation to reduce ICP by lowering CO_2 levels and increasing O_2 levels
- Quiet environment
- Handle gently
- Monitor O_2 for seizure activity
- Family support
- Physical and emotional support for child and family with recovery
- Spiritual care

EDUCATE THE PUBLIC ABOUT REYE'S SO AS TO PREVENT THE PROBLEM!

---

consideration the specific indication for the agents and the patient's medical diagnosis. The following nursing diagnoses may be appropriate:
- Acute pain related to disease process or injury.
- Activity intolerance related to the disorder, condition, or disease process causing the pain.
- Risk for injury to self related to the influence of the disease or treatment.
- Ineffective health maintenance related to lack of knowledge about medication therapy.
- Deficient knowledge related to first-time drug therapy for pain or disease process.

● Planning

Goals pertinent to patients receiving NSAIDs and other antiinflammatory agents include the following:
- Patient is able to describe the use of the medication as it relates to the relief of inflammation and pain.
- Patient experiences pain relief or relief of symptoms within expected period of time.
- Patient uses nonpharmacologic measures to decrease inflammation so that he or she can increase ADLs, including walking.
- Patient reports adverse effects to the physician as indicated.
- Patient remains compliant with medication therapy.

case study **Postoperative Pain**

One of your postoperative abdominal surgery patients is complaining of abdominal pain and nausea as well as breakthrough pain after receiving the pain protocol for Dilaudid PCA and ketorolac tromethamine (Toradol) intramuscularly. She has received Toradol for 5 days in multiple doses. A GI ulcer is now diagnosed and has been attributed to the Toradol. She has a history of ulcer disease.
- *What is the action of Toradol?*
- *What could have been done to prevent the GI bleed and ulcer formation with the Toradol?*

For Answers see www.harcourthealth.com/MERLIN/Lilley/.

Outcome Criteria

Outcome criteria for patients receiving NSAIDs and other antiinflammatory agents include the following:
- Patient will state that pain is characteristic of inflammation, injury, or related disease and will decrease with therapy.
- Patient will identify factors that aggravate or alleviate pain such as movement, activity, noises, and so on.
- Patient will state nonpharmacologic measures to use to promote comfort, such as hot or cold packs, physical therapy, or relaxation therapy, and to increase ADLs, including walking.

- Patient will state side effects of NSAIDs such as GI upset, heartburn, nausea and vomiting, or anorexia.
- Patient will discuss symptoms to report to the physician immediately, such as epigastric distress, nausea and vomiting, abdominal pain, dyspnea, and bleeding or easy bruising.
- Patient will state the importance of correct dosing and of consistency in the self-administration of medication.
- Patient will return for follow-up visits with the physician.

Implementation

The patient should be educated about the various side effects of NSAIDs (see Table 42-1 for those of the most commonly used agents). Should side effects become severe or intolerable or if bleeding or GI pain occur, the physician must be contacted immediately. NSAIDs are often better tolerated if taken with food, milk, or an antacid to avoid irritation. Patients should be watched closely for the occurrence of any unusual bleeding, such as in the stool, because of the risk of GI ulcerations. In addition, it is important to explain to the patient the difference between their onset of action for the relief of acute pain as opposed to their more delayed effect when used for the relief of arthritis pain; in the latter instance the therapeutic effects may not be realized for 3 to 4 weeks. Elderly patients need to be monitored closely for side effects, which may indicate the need for a decreased dose.

Use of ketorolac is only for the short term (intramuscularly or intravenously for 5 days or less). It is critical for safe use that dosing orders be checked carefully and maximum doses not be exceeded per manufacturer's guidelines or physician's orders. Salicylates that are enteric-coated should not be crushed or chewed. Caution patients about the many drug interactions with OTC preparations (discussed further in Chapter 6). Treatment of salicylate overdose is usually by lavage, activated charcoal, and supportive treatment. The newer agents celecoxib, rofecoxib, and meloxicam have specific instructions, such as taking only the prescribed dose; avoiding alcohol (ETOH), aspirin, and OTC agents; and reporting to the physician immediately any stomach pain, unusual bleeding, or blood in vomit or stool. Chest pain, palpitations, and any GI problems should be reported as well.

Antiarthritic agents, such as gold sodium thiomalate, should never be given intravenously and when indicated to be given intramuscularly should be given in deep muscle. After injections, it is important to keep the patient recumbent for at least 10 minutes after the injection. Patient teaching should include instructions about the following:

1. Taking the medication exactly as prescribed, obtaining monthly laboratory work
2. Reporting skin conditions, fatigue, or sores in the mouth since these may indicate the presence of blood dyscrasias
3. Reporting to the physician if there is any blood in the stools or urine and any occurrence of easy bruising or bleeding gums

4. Emphasizing that therapeutic blood levels may take up to 3 to 4 months
5. Emphasizing that sunscreen must be used
6. Emphasizing that contraception is a necessity if taking these agents
7. Forcing fluids (2-3 L/day) unless contraindicated.

Colchicine should be taken on an empty stomach for more complete absorption, which means 1 hour before meals or 2 hours after meals. IV colchicine should be administered as recommended per guidelines and over recommended period of time (such as 1 mg/10-20 ml of NS or sterile water for injections over 2 to 5 minutes). Patients should be instructed to increase their fluid intake (unless contraindicated) up to 3 to 4 liters in 24 hours. Patients must also be instructed to not consume alcohol or OTC cold products that contain alcohol while taking this medication. In addition, patients with gout must be instructed that compliance with the entire medical regimen is critical to the success of its treatment.

Allopurinol should be given with meals to try to prevent the occurrence of GI symptoms (nausea, vomiting, anorexia). If the allopurinol is being administered in conjunction with chemotherapy to try to decrease hyperuricemia associated with the malignancy and treatment, it is recommended that it be given a few days before the antineoplastic therapy. Patients taking allopurinol should be informed to increase fluid intake up to 3 to 4 liters per day, avoid hazardous activities if dizziness or drowsiness occurs with the medication, and to avoid alcohol and caffeine since these drugs will increase uric acid levels and decrease the levels of allopurinol.

See the box on p. 673 for patient teaching tips for the use of NSAIDs.

Evaluation

The therapeutic response to NSAIDs may vary and comprise a decrease in acute pain; a decrease in swelling, pain, stiffness, and tenderness of a joint or muscle area; or a return to normal of such laboratory values as the CBC, RBC, Hgb level, Hct, sedimentation rates, and other arthritis-related laboratory test results. Monitoring for the occurrence of side effects is also essential to their safe and effective use (see Table 42-1).

Evaluating therapeutic responses to antiarthritic agents and other antiinflammatory agents includes monitoring for the increased ability to move joints with less discomfort and an overall increased sense of improvement in the condition. Toxicity to gold products is evident by a decreased hemoglobin (Hgb), WBC count of less than $4000/mm^3$, platelets less than $150,000/mm^3$, hematuria, severe diarrhea, itching, and proteinuria.

A therapeutic response to colchicine includes decreased pain in joints and increased sense of well-being. The patient should be monitored closely for or should report to the physician the occurrence of increased pain, blood in the urine, excessive fatigue and lethargy, and chills or fever.

A therapeutic response to allopurinol would include a decrease in pain in the joints, decrease in uric acid levels, and decrease of stone formation in the kidneys.

patient teaching tips

Use of NSAIDs

➤ Patients should understand that NSAIDs are used for the treatment of pain, an injury, or a disease process and that they work by decreasing the inflammation that leads to pain.

➤ Patients should know the various and most common side effects of the NSAIDs, which are listed below:

- ibuprofen: heartburn, GI upset, ulcers, nausea
- indomethacin: headache, nausea, vomiting, GI upset, ulcers, hemorrhage, hemolytic anemias, epistaxis, blurred vision, rash, leukopenia
- naproxen: vomiting, blurred vision, decreased Hgb level and Hct value.
- piroxicam: GI upset, elevated BUN level, dizziness, vertigo, edema, tinnitus, GI ulcer
- sulindac and tolmetin: GI upset, GI discomfort, ulcers, rash, tinnitus, diarrhea, nausea

➤ Because these agents generally cause GI distress they are often better tolerated if taken with food, milk, or an antacid to avoid GI irritation.

➤ Patients should monitor their stools for bleeding because of the risk of GI ulcerations.

➤ Drug interactions are many, so patients should be given information about the following interactions:

- ibuprofen, naproxen, and fenoprofen: anticoagulants, aspirin, steroids, phenylbutazone
- indomethacin and tolmetin: corticosteroids, phenylbutazone, salicylates, anticoagulants
- meclofenamate sodium: all drugs listed above
- phenylbutazone: oral anticoagulants, oral antidiabetic agents, insulin, penicillin, sulfonamides, barbiturates, sex hormones, steroids
- sulindac: aspirin

POINTS TO REMEMBER

Nonsteroidal Antiinflammatory Drugs (NSAIDs)

- One of the most frequently prescribed categories of drugs.
- First drug in this category to be synthesized was salicylic acid.
- Now more than 70 different NSAIDs, but only 20 are commonly used.

Mechanism of Action

- Work in the arachidonic acid pathway.
- Inhibit cyclooxygenase and/or lipooxygenase, thereby preventing prostaglandin and/or leukotriene synthesis.

Therapeutic Effects

- Analgesic, antiinflammatory, and antipyretic.
- Also used in the treatment of gout, osteoarthritis, juvenile arthritis, rheumatoid arthritis, and dysmenorrhea.

Side Effects

- Three main side effects include:
  1. GI intolerance
  2. Bleeding
  3. Renal impairment
- Misoprostol (Cytotec) may be given to prevent GI intolerance.
- Misoprostol is a prostaglandin analogue.

Nursing Considerations

- Many contraindications to the use of NSAIDs such as GI tract lesions, peptic ulcers, allergies to them, and bleeding disorders.
- Most NSAIDs are better tolerated orally if taken with food to minimize GI upset.
- Patients should be closely monitored for the occurrence of bleeding such as blood in the stools or emesis.
- Therapeutic effects in patients with arthritis usually occur within 3 to 4 weeks.

REVIEW QUESTIONS

1. Which of the following drugs may be given to prevent the gastrointestinal side effects of NSAIDs?
   a. Misoprostol (Cytotec)
   b. Metoprolol (Lopressor)
   c. Metoclopramide (Reglan)
   d. Magnesium sulfate (MgSO$_4$)
2. Which of the following manifestations indicates that your patient is suffering from NSAID toxicity?
   a. Nausea
   b. Anorexia
   c. Dysphagia
   d. Cerebral edema
3. Allopurinol may result in which of the following?
   a. Increased HGB
   b. Elevated WBC counts
   c. Increased polycythemia
   d. Decreased uric acid levels
4. Which of the following statements is inaccurate regarding the administration of colchicine?
   a. Drink only limited amounts of fluid.

b. Do not take alcohol while on this medication.

c. Take this medication on an empty stomach to help with absorption.

d. Increase fluids to at least 3 to 4 liters in 24 hours if not contraindicated.

5. The manifestation of chronic salicylate toxicity in adults includes which of the following?

a. Polyuria

b. Tinnitus

c. Heart block

d. Hyperventilation

For Answers see www.harcourthealth.com/MERLIN/Lilley/.

CRITICAL THINKING Activities

1. Is the following statement true or false? *Acetaminophen is an NSAID and exerts antiinflammatory, antipyretic, analgesic, and antiplatelet effects.* Explain your answer.

2. What are the drug interactions for NSAIDs? What problems may occur if these are used with NSAIDs?

3. Describe the protocol for treating salicylate intoxication of a chronic nature.

For Answers see www.harcourthealth.com/MERLIN/Lilley/.

bibliography

Albanese T, Nutz P: *Mosby's 2001 nursing drug reference and review cards,* St Louis, 2001, Mosby.

Amadio P, Cummings DM, Amadio PB: NSAIDs revisited: selection, monitoring, and safe use, *Postgrad Med* 101(2):257, 1997.

American Hospital Formulary Service: *AHFS drug information,* Bethesda, Md, 2000, American Society of Health-System Pharmacists.

Anderson PO, Knoben JE, Troutman WG: *Handbook of clinical drug data 1999-2000,* ed 9, New York, 1999, McGraw-Hill.

Johns Hopkins Hospital, Department of Pediatrics et al: *The Harriet Lane handbook,* ed 15, St Louis, 2000, Mosby.

Keen JH: *Critical care and emergency drug reference,* ed 3, St Louis, 1996, Mosby.

Mosby's GenRx: a comprehensive reference for generic and brand drugs, ed 10, St Louis, 2000, Mosby.

Skidmore-Roth L: *Mosby's 2001 nursing drug reference,* St Louis, 2001, Mosby.

Turkoski BB: *Drug information handbook for nursing 1999-2000: including assessment, administration, monitoring guidelines, and patient education,* ed 2, Cleveland, 1999, Lexi-Comp.

United States Pharmacopeial Convention: *USP DI: advice for the patient: drug information in lay language, vol. 1I,* ed 20, Englewood, Colo, 2000, Micromedex.

Activity

Remember to check the **Online Worksheet** for additional learning opportunities: **www.harcourthealth.com/MERLIN/Lilley/**

Part eight

Immune and Biologic Modifiers and Chemotherapeutic Agents: Study Skills Tips

- Time Management
- Evaluate Prior Performance
- Anticipate the Test
- Plan for Distributed Study

TIME MANAGEMENT

The first step in preparing for a chapter or part exam is to plan for the time needed. Let us begin by assuming that the next test you have will cover the chapters in Part Eight. First examine the material to determine just how much there is to cover. Look at the objectives, the glossary, and the number of pages of text in each chapter. This will help you determine just how big a task you face. As you are doing this, also consider how much study time you have been devoting to these chapters in the days before the exam. If you have been doing regular study with frequent review sessions, then the demand on your time in the day or two just before the exam will be less than if you have to do a major "cram" session to try to catch up on study that has been put off. The basic question to answer here is a simple one. "How much time do I need to schedule for exam preparation?" The answer varies with each student. Some will need 6, 8, or more hours of preparation time in the 2 to 3 days before the exam. Others will find that 3, 4, or 5 hours will be adequate. You must assess your own learning and prior success to determine what time is necessary for you, but you must set time aside and use it effectively.

There is one thing that should play a major role in helping you determine the time you will need to set aside. Evaluate your performance on prior exams. How have you been doing? How much time have you been spending to achieve that level? If you are not achieving according to your capabilities, then you should certainly consider spending more time preparing for the next exam. If you are achieving at a satisfactory level, then plan on devoting about the same amount of time to test preparation.

The next step in preparing for an exam is to organize the time. Write down what you are going to study and when and how much time you will spend. Consider the following example based on the materials in Chapters 45 and 46:

1. Review Chapter 45 objectives. Monday, 4:00 to 4:30 PM. Note objectives that are unclear for further review.
2. Question and Answer review, Monday, 4:30 to 5:15 PM.
3. Self-test, Chapter 45 glossary. Monday, 6:30 to 7:00 PM. Note terms that need further review for mastery.
4. Review Chapter 46 objectives. Monday, 7:00 to 7:30 PM.
5. Question and Answer review, Monday, 7:30 to 8:00 PM.
6. Self-test, Chapter 46 glossary. Monday, 8:00 to 8:30 PM.

The advantage to this test preparation model is that you now know where you must focus in the days before the exam.

EVALUATE PRIOR PERFORMANCE

As you begin preparing to review for any exam, take some time to look back at previous exams. Evaluate your performance, and use that evaluation to improve on subsequent tests. As you look at prior tests consider the following factors:

What Type of Errors Did I Make?

As students we often find that there are certain question types or forms that are missed consistently. Assess your errors and try to pinpoint any recurring patterns in your mistakes. Did you miss questions that contained an exemption in the multiple choice stem? Question stems that state "all of the following except" and "Which of the following would not be . . ." are exemption questions. Questions like this are often missed because they contain too many apparently correct responses. Remember that an exemption stem means you are looking for the one response choice that is "wrong." The stem asks you to identify the inappropriate response, and it is the best choice.

Did I Have Trouble With Questions That Required Mastery of Terminology?

As part of the evaluation of prior tests, also look at questions that demanded mastery of the terms from the chapters. If you missed more than one or two questions of that type, then you know you need to spend more time in review of terminology.

Did I Miss Concept Questions?

If the question asked you to apply a principle, evaluate a drug response, or in some other way apply knowledge from the course, you are dealing with concepts rather than facts. If you missed a number of concept questions, then you should spend more of your review time studying applications and principles than memorizing facts and terms.

Did I Make Errors Because I Did Not Know the Material?

This question focuses on the quality of your learning. If you miss one or two questions on an exam because you did not learn (or did not remember) the material, it is not a major problem.

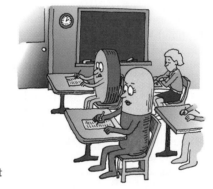

   There will almost always be one or two questions that we do not remember. If you are analyzing past performance and find that there are several questions on which you guessed because you did not recall any information that seemed relevant to the question, it may be necessary to put more time into review. It may be doing more oral rehearsal so that the material is stored in long-term memory. Whatever the cause it is essential that you acknowledge to yourself that you have missed questions because you did not know the material. Once you have acknowledged the problem, take steps to correct it.

ANTICIPATE THE TEST

Do not wait until exam time to find out what you should know. As you do your review try to think like the instructor. Generate questions that you think might be a part of the test. This does not mean you need to try to write multiple choice stems and choices, but you should be trying to focus your review in a way that will facilitate learning and long-term memory.

   Here are some examples of questioning that you might use based on material found in Chapter 46.
   1. What are biologic response modifiers (BRMs)?
   2. What is the role of BRMs in the care of patients with cancer?
   3. What is the role of the immune system in treating cancer?

   The sample questions were drawn from just the first few pages of the chapter. These questions focus on literal comprehension and are relatively easy to generate. Being able to answer them is important, but if all of your questions are literal in nature, it may be difficult to answer questions that require application of principles and concepts. For that reason it is

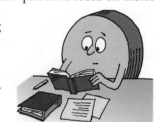

essential that some questions require analysis, synthesis, and/or evaluation of the material. Question 3 is an example of this type of question. Answers to these questions require the learner to put together the literal information and relate the terms to the concepts being explained.

PLAN FOR DISTRIBUTED STUDY

One of the major problems that many students encounter when trying to review for a test is waiting too long to begin the review. This forces students into a review pattern of long hours of intensive study all packed into the last day or two before the exam. This is known as cramming, and although cramming does work to some degree, it is not the most effective way to learn. A better model is to distribute the review over a period of several days with short, 30-minute to 1-hour study sessions several times each day. Distributing practice in this way allows time for you to think about what you have been learning, and it fosters long-term memory.

   One important consideration for review is spending more of the review time doing oral rehearsal (ask and answer sessions) than simply rereading material. Oral rehearsal encourages active learning, which enhances your ability to concentrate, improves comprehension and memory, and thus improves test performance.

Chapter 43

Immunosuppressant Agents

objectives

When you reach the end of this chapter, you should be able to do the following:

1 Discuss the role of immunosuppressive therapy in the treatment of autoimmune diseases.

2 Discuss the mechanisms of action, contraindications, cautions, side effects, and toxicity associated with the most commonly used immunosuppressives.

3 Develop a nursing care plan that includes all phases of the nursing process for the patient receiving immunosuppressants.

4 Discuss the education guidelines for patients receiving an immunosuppressant agent.

www.harcourthealth.com/MERLIN/Lilley/

Look for this symbol for topics covered in the **Online Worksheet** Activity

drug profiles

azathioprine, p. 679
cyclosporine, p. 679
muromonab-CD3, p. 680
sirolimus, p. 680

⊶ Key drug.

glossary

Autoimmune diseases (aw' to i mun') A large group of diseases characterized by the subversion or alteration of the function of the immune system, where the immune response is directed against normal body tissue(s) of the body resulting in pathologic conditions. (p. 677)

Immune-mediated disease A large group of diseases that result when the cells of the immune system react to a variety of situations, such as transplanted organ tissue or drug-altered cell. (p. 677)

Immunosuppressant (im' u no sə pres' ənt) Agent that decreases or prevents an immune response. (p. 677)

Immunosuppressive therapy Drug treatment used to suppress the immune system. (p. 677)

Murine antibodies (mu' rin) Monoclonal immunoglobulins. *Monoclonal* refers to a protein from a single clone of cells, all the molecules of which are the same. *Murine* refers to the family *Muridae*, to which mice belong. An antibody is a protective protein that counters the actions of antigens, substances that cause sensitivity or an allergic response. Thus murine antibodies are protective proteins obtained from mice. Muromonab-CD3 is a murine antibody used to reverse graft rejection. (p. 680)

IMMUNOSUPPRESSANT AGENTS

The human body is under constant attack by invading microorganisms, but it possesses several mechanisms with which to fight off these foreign invaders; one is the immune system. This system defends the body against invading pathogens, foreign antigens, and its own cells that become cancerous or neoplastic. Besides these beneficial functions, however, this highly sophisticated system can also sometimes attack itself and cause what are known as **autoimmune diseases** or **immune-mediated diseases.** It also participates in hypersensitivity, or anaphylactic, reactions, which can be life-threatening. The rejection of kidney, liver, and heart (whole organ) transplants is directed by the immune system as well. From this it is easy to see that the immune system is capable of having many beneficial or detrimental effects.

Agents that decrease or prevent an immune response, and hence suppress the immune system, are known as **immunosuppressants.** Treatment with such drugs is referred to as **immunosuppressive therapy,** and it is used to selectively eradicate certain cell lines that play a major role in the rejection of a transplanted organ. These cell lines must be targeted and selectively altered or suppressed, or organ rejection will occur. The primary immunosuppressant drugs are the corticosteroids (see Chapter 31), cyclophosphamide (see Chapter 45), azathioprine, methotrexate, cyclosporine, muromonab-CD3, and prograf (also known as FK-506). This chapter focuses on azathioprine, cyclosporine, muromonab-CD3, and prograf.

Mechanism of Action

All immunosuppressants have similar mechanisms of action because they all selectively suppress certain lymphocyte cell lines, thereby preventing their involvement in the immune response. This results in a pharmacologically immunocompromised state similar to that in a cancer patient whose bone marrow and immune cells have been destroyed as the result of chemotherapy or that in a patient with acquired immunodeficiency syndrome (AIDS).

Each agent differs in the exact way in which it suppresses certain cell lines involved in an immune response.

The primary mechanism of action of azathioprine in the prevention of organ rejection is its ability to incorporate itself into the normal production pathway for purine nucleotides, which are substances such as DNA and RNA. These substances are vital to the production (synthesis) of such cells as lymphocytes (T-cells). Thus when azathioprine incorporates itself into the normal pathway for the production of DNA and RNA, it creates a faulty end-product that results in a cell that cannot function in the normal immune response. Mycophenolate mofetil (CellCept) is another immunosuppressant agent that works similar to azathioprine. It too is used for prophylaxis of organ rejection concurrently with other immunosuppressant agents such as cyclosporine and corticosteroids.

Cyclosporine and tacrolimus work by inhibiting the release of a substance called *interleukin-2* (IL-2) from specific T-lymphocytes called *CD4 cells* or *T-helper cells*. When IL-2 is released from T-helper cells, it stimulates cytotoxic T-cells, which in turn attack cells that are believed to be foreign cells, such as those of a transplanted organ. They destroy these cells by boring holes through them, resulting in cell lysis and death. These cytotoxic T-cells are believed to be the primary cells responsible for graft rejection. By preventing the release of IL-2 from T-helper cells, cyclosporine and tacrolimus keep these T-cells from being activated and as a result the transplanted organ from being attacked by the immune system.

Sirolimus (Rapamune) is another immunosuppressant agent similar in structure to tacrolimus. Sirolimus has a slightly different mechanism of action. While cyclosporine and tacrolimus inhibit cytokine production by inhibiting the release of IL-2, sirolimus inhibits the body's response to these cytokines. It does this by acting at a later stage in the production of these cellular toxins.

Muromonab-CD3, also known as OKT3, works by binding to the CD3 receptor on mature circulating T-cells, which is located next to the T-cell antigen recognition site. This receptor is involved in the recognition of foreign invaders such as a transplanted organ. By binding to the CD3 receptor, OKT3 therefore prevents the T-cells from being stimulated by foreign antigens and thus inhibits both the generation and function of cytotoxic T-cells, the cells responsible for causing graft rejection. After the initial dose of OKT3, T-cells virtually disappear from the circulation within minutes to hours. Basiliximab (Simulect) and daclizumab (Zenapax) are both monoclonal antibodies. They ultimately have similar mechanism of action to those of OKT3. The difference is that they act as immunosuppressants by binding to and blocking the IL-2 receptor known as CD25 on the surface of activated T-lymphocytes.

Drug Effects

Because of their ability to modify the immune system, immunosuppressants are used in the treatment of organ rejection, rheumatoid arthritis, and other conditions that may have an immunologic cause.

Therapeutic Uses

The therapeutic uses of immunosuppressants are multiple and vary from agent to agent (Box 43-1). They are primarily indicated for the prevention of organ rejection. Only muromonab-CD3 is indicated for treatment of organ rejection once rejection of a transplanted organ is underway. The four newer agents (basiliximab, daclizumab, sirolimus, and mycophenolate mofetil) are all indicated for prophylaxis. Azathioprine is used as an adjunct medication to prevent the rejection of kidney transplants and to ameliorate severe rheumatoid arthritis. Cyclosporine is the primary immunosuppressant agent used in the prevention of kidney, liver, heart, and bone marrow transplant rejection. It may also have beneficial effects in the treatment of other conditions with an immunologic cause such as certain types of arthritis, psoriasis, and irritable bowel disease.

Tacrolimus has many of the same therapeutic effects as cyclosporine, but it is currently indicated only for the prevention of liver transplant rejection, although it has shown promise in preventing the rejection of other transplanted organs as well.

Side Effects and Adverse Effects

Many of the side effects of the immunosuppressants can be devastating to the transplant patient. Although not strictly a side effect, a heightened susceptibility to opportunistic infections is a major risk factor in immunosuppressed patients. Other side effects and adverse effects are limited to the particular agents, and the common effects are listed in Table 43-1.

Activity

Interactions

The drug interactions associated with immunosuppressant use mostly involve cyclosporine. Cyclosporine is capable of many drug interactions, several of which can be very harmful. Drugs that may increase its action are diltiazem, nicardipine, verapamil, fluconazole, itraconazole, clarithromycin, allopurinol, metoclopramide, amphotericin B, cimetidine, and ketoconazole. Drugs that may decrease its effects are nafcillin, carbamazepine, phenobarbital, phenytoin, and rifampin. Although these are the most significant interactions, there are many more of less significance. It is also not recommended that azathioprine be given with allopurinol because allopurinol inhibits azathioprine's metabolism and thereby increases its effects.

Cyclosporine can have a rather profound interaction with grapefruit juice. When they are taken together, there is an increase in the bioavailability of cyclosporine by 20% to 200%. The intentional administration of cyclosporine with grapefruit juice may sometimes be done to achieve therapeutic blood levels of cyclosporine with decreased doses. The manufacturer of cyclosporine does not endorse this.

Dosages

For the recommended dosages of selected immunosuppressant agents, see the dosages table on p. 680.

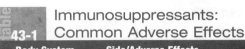

Selected Immunosuppressants: Indications
BOX 43-1

Immunosuppressant	Indications
azathioprine	Adjunct in organ rejection prevention; rheumatoid arthritis
basiliximab	Adjunct in organ rejection prevention
cyclosporine	Organ rejection prevention and treatment; rheumatoid arthritis
daclizumab	Adjunct in organ rejection prevention
muromonab	Organ rejection prevention and treatment
mycophenolate mofetil	Adjunct in organ rejection prevention
sirolimus	Adjunct in organ rejection prevention
tacrolimus	Adjunct in organ rejection prevention

Immunosuppressants: Common Adverse Effects
TABLE 43-1

Body System	Side/Adverse Effects
AZATHIOPRINE	
Hematopoietic	Leukopenia, thrombocytopenia
Hepatic	Hepatotoxicity is a common side effect
CYCLOSPORINE	
Cardiovascular	Moderate hypertension in as many as 50% of patients
Central nervous system	Neurotoxicity including tremors in about 20% of patients
Hepatic	Hepatotoxicity with cholestasis and hyperbilirubinemia
Renal	Nephrotoxicity is common and dose limiting
Other	Hypersensitivity reactions to the vehicle, gingival hyperplasia, and hirsutism
MUROMONAB-CD3	
Cardiovascular	Chest pain
Central nervous system	Pyrexia, chills, tremors
Gastrointestinal	Vomiting, nausea, diarrhea
Respiratory	Dyspnea, wheezing, pulmonary edema
Other	Flulike symptoms, fluid retention

drug profiles

As previously stated, the primary use for immuno-suppressant agents discussed in this chapter is the prevention of organ rejection. Other immunologic disorders may also be treated by these agents. The agents of most importance are azathioprine, cyclosporine, muromonab-CD3, and tacrolimus. These substances are all dispensed by prescription only.

azathioprine

Azathioprine (Imuran) is a chemical analogue of the physiologic purines such as adenine and guanine. Mycophenolate mofetil (CellCept) is another immunosuppressant agent that works similar to azathioprine. It too is used for prophylaxis of organ rejection concurrently with other immunosuppressant agents such as cyclosporine and corticosteroids. It is available in both an oral and parenteral formulation as a 50-mg tablet and a 100-mg injection, respectively. It is classified as a pregnancy category D agent and is contraindicated in patients who have shown a hypersensitivity to it. Commonly recommended dosages are listed in the dosages table on p. 680.

PHARMACOKINETICS

HALF-LIFE	ONSET	PEAK	DURATION
5 hr	2-4 days*	1-2 hr	Unknown

*Onset 6-8 wk for rheumatoid arthritis.

cyclosporine

Cyclosporine (Cyclosporin A, Sandimmune, Neoral) is an immunosuppressant agent that is indicated for the prevention of organ rejection. It is a very potent immunosuppressant and the principal agent in many immunosuppressive drug regimens. Like azathioprine, it may also be used for the treatment of other immunologic disorders, such as various forms of arthritis, psoriasis, and irritable bowel disease.

Cyclosporine is available in two oral formulations. Neoral is an oral formulation that immediately forms a microemulsion in an aqueous environment. This property allows for greater oral bioavailability and more reliable oral absorption than the older formulation of cyclosporine (Sandimmune). Neoral is available as 25-mg and 100-mg soft gelatin capsules (for microemulsion) and an oral solution of 100 mg/ml (also for microemulsion). Sandimmune is available in both oral and parenteral forms. Orally it is available as a 25- and 100-mg liquid-filled capsule and a 100-mg/ml solution. Parenterally it is available as a 50-mg/ml injection. Although these two products contain the same active ingredient (cyclosporine), they cannot be used interchangeably. When changing between Neoral to Sandimmune, dosage adjustments are necessary to account for the greater bioavailability of Neoral. It is recommended that cyclosporine blood concentration be monitored in patients changing from one product to another. Cyclosporine is classified as a pregnancy category C agent and is contraindicated in patients with a known hypersensitivity to it. Commonly recommended dosages are listed in the dosages table on p. 680.

PHARMACOKINETICS

HALF-LIFE	ONSET	PEAK	DURATION
1-2 hr, then 10-27 hr	Unknown	3-5 hr	Unknown

DOSAGES Selected Immunosuppressant Agents

agent	pharmacologic class	dosage range	purpose
azathioprine (Imuran)	Purine antagonist immunosuppressive	*Pediatric/Adult* IV/PO: 3.5 mg/kg/day starting on day of transplant and/or 1-3 days before procedure; usual PO maintenance dose, 1-2 mg/kg/day	Renal transplants
		Adult PO: Start with 1 mg/kg/day as a single dose or divided; may be increased by 0.5 mg/kg/day after 6-8 wk to a max of 2.5 mg/kg/day	Rheumatoid arthritis
cyclosporine (Sandimmune)	Polypeptide antibiotic immunosuppressive	*Pediatric/Adult* PO: 15 mg/kg as a single dose 4-12 hr before surgery; continue initial daily dose (postop) for 1-2 wk, then reduce by 5%/wk to a maintenance dose of 5-10 mg/kg/day IV: Dose is 1/3 PO dose: 5-6 mg/kg as a single dose 4-16 hr before surgery and continued daily postop until patient can be switched to PO dose	Liver, heart, kidney transplant
muromonab-CD3 (Orthoclone) (OKT3)	Immunoglobin (IgG$_{2a}$) immunosuppressive	*Adult* IV: 5 mg/day in a single bolus injection for 10-14 days	Renal transplants, steroid-resistant cardiac and hepatic transplant rejection
sirolimus (Rapamune)	Immunosuppressant	*Adult* PO: loading dose of 6 mg followed by a maintenance dose of 2 mg daily	Organ rejection prophylaxis

muromonab-CD3

Muromonab-CD3 (Orthoclone OKT3) is the only agent indicated for the reversal, and not just the prevention, of graft rejection. It is unique in that it is a monoclonal antibody, and it is very similar to the antibodies naturally produced by the body (immunoglobulin IgG, IgM, IgD, IgA, and IgE). It specifically targets the binding sites on the T-cells that recognize foreign invaders such as a transplanted organ. It differs from human antibodies in that it comes from mice. These types of antibodies are commonly referred to as **murine antibodies,** hence the name *muromonab.* "Muro" stands for *murine;* "mon" for *monoclonal,* which means they come from the same clone; and "ab" for *antibody.* Other monoclonal antibodies used for the prevention of organ rejection are basiliximab (Simulect) and daclizumab (Zenapax).

OKT3 is classified as a pregnancy category C agent and is contraindicated in patients with a hypersensitivity to murine products as well as those who are experiencing fluid overload. It is available only in a parenteral formulation as a 5-mg/5 ml injection. Commonly recommended dosages are listed in the dosages table above.

PHARMACOKINETICS

HALF-LIFE	ONSET	PEAK	DURATION
Unknown	Very rapid	~3 days	Unknown

sirolimus

Sirolimus (Rapamune) is another immunosuppressant agent similar in structure to tacrolimus (Prograf). Sirolimus is a macrocyclic immunosuppressive, antifungal, and antitumor agent produced by fermentation of *Streptomyces hygroscopicus.* Other macrocyclic immunosuppressive agents are cyclosporine and tacrolimus. Sirolimus and tacrolimus are structurally related. Although structurally similar, they have different mechanisms of action. It is available as an oral solution in a 1-mg/ml concentration. It is supplied in unit-of-use pouches containing 1, 2, and 5 ml of solution or 60-and 180-ml glass bottles. Commonly recommended dosages are listed in the dosages table above.

PHARMACOKINETICS

HALF-LIFE	ONSET	PEAK	DURATION
57-68 hr	Unknown	1-3 hr	Unknown

nursing process

● Assessment

Before administering any of the immunosuppressants (azathioprine, cyclosporine, or muromonab-CD3), the nurse should perform a thorough patient assessment and document the findings, including the following data:

- Renal function (BUN and creatinine levels; information about urinary function and normal patterns of elimination)
- Liver function (alkaline phosphatase, AST, ALT, and bilirubin levels; determining whether jaundice, edema, or ascites is present)
- Cardiovascular function (baseline ECG, blood pressure, and pulse; documentation of any cardiovascular disease or history of dysrhythmias, chest pain, or hypertension)
- CNS baseline assessment (motor function and seizure disorders)
- Respiratory assessment (any complaints of dyspnea or wheezing; as documentation of pulmonary disorders or pulmonary edema)

See Table 43-1 for information on other systems affected by the specific agents.

Contraindications to and cautions regarding the use of these agents include the following:

- Cyclosporine is contraindicated in patients with a hypersensitivity to it; cautious use is recommended in patients with severe renal or hepatic disease and in pregnant women.
- Muromonab-CD3 is contraindicated in patients with a hypersensitivity to substances with a murine origin or in patients suffering from fluid overload, cautious use is advised in pregnant women and in children under 2 years of age or who are febrile.

Laboratory studies (e.g., Hgb level, Hct, WBC, and platelet count) should be performed and the results documented before, during (monthly), and after therapy. If the leukocyte count should drop below 3000/mm^3, the drug should be discontinued.

● Nursing Diagnoses

Nursing diagnoses pertinent to patients receiving immunosuppressants include the following:

- Risk of injury related to the physiologic influence of the disease and side effects of immunosuppressants.
- Risk for infection related to altered immune status.
- Acute pain (myalgias and arthralgias) related to side effects of medications.
- Deficient knowledge related to initiation of new treatment regimen.
- Noncompliance related to undesired side effects of drug treatment.

● Planning

Goals in patients receiving immunosuppressants include the following:

- Patient experiences minimal complications during immunosuppressant therapy.
- Patient experiences maximal comfort during drug therapy.

- Patient remains compliant with drug therapy and comes in for follow-up visits with the physician.
- Patient states symptoms of adverse reactions to therapy or of exacerbation of illness to report to physician.

Outcome Criteria

Outcome criteria for patients receiving immunosuppressants include the following:

- Patient will experience minimal problems of immunosuppressant such as myalgias, fever, nephrotoxicity, and hypertension.
- Patient will experience a decrease in disease-related symptoms.
- Patient will be compliant with follow-up visits with physician to monitor therapeutic (decreased symptomology) and adverse reactions to medication (myalgias, arthralgias).
- Patient will notify physician immediately if fever, rash, sore throat, or fatigue develops.
- Patient will state measures to implement to enhance comfort while on immunosuppressant therapy such as use of nonaspirin analgesics, rest, and biofeedback.

● Implementation

When immunosuppressants are being taken orally, it is always important to take them with food to minimize GI upset. It is also important, considering the immunosuppressed state of patients receiving immunosuppressants, that oral forms of the drugs be used whenever possible to decrease the risk of infection associated with IM injections. An oral antifungal medication is usually given with these agents to treat the oral candidiasis common in these patients.

Cyclosporine is now also available in an oral formulation (Neoral). It is important to remember that Sandimmune and Neoral are *not* to be used interchangeably. When given intravenously, cyclosporine should be diluted as recommended in the manufacturer guidelines and given according to the standards of care and institutional policy regarding its administration. Cyclosporine is normally diluted with normal saline or 5% dextrose in water in a concentration of 50 mg of the drug to 20 to 100 ml of diluting solution, which should be infused over 2 to 6 hours using an infusion pump. Intravenously administered muromonab is usually given over 1 minute, and only after the medication is withdrawn through a 0.2 to 0.22 low protein–binding micron filter. A new needle must be used after the medication is withdrawn. It is usually recommended that methylprednisone sodium succinate be administered before and hydrocortisone sodium succinate a half hour after the muromonab injection to minimize reactions to medication. There are several new immunosuppressants on the market used as such and as antifungals and antitumor agents. Both sirolimus and tacrolimus have long half-lives (up to 68 hours), and so toxicity may be a concern.

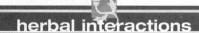

herbal interactions

Echinacea

BENEFIT OF HERB
Prevents colds, stimulates immune system

POTENTIAL INTERACTIONS
May interfere with immunosuppression therapy

CAUTIONS AND NOTES
Contraindicated in patients with compromised immune system (i.e., patients with HIV, AIDS, multiple sclerosis, tuberculosis); long-term use may suppress the immune system

See also the Herbal Interactions box for echinacea, an herbal supplement commonly taken to prevent colds.

Patient teaching tips for immunosuppressants are listed in the box below.

● Evaluation

Therapeutic responses to the immunosuppressants include no rejection of a transplanted organ or graft and no obvious immunosuppression in patients with autoimmune disorders. The nurse should also check the patient for drug-specific side effects and toxicity (see Table 43-1). Blood levels of cyclosporine should be monitored, especially when switching from one product to another.

patient teaching tips

Immunosuppressants

➤ Patients taking any of the immunosuppressants should be encouraged to avoid crowds to minimize the risk of infection. Patients should also be encouraged to report any fever, sore throat, chills, joint pain, or fatigue to the physician because this may indicate severe infection.

➤ It is recommended that women receiving immunosuppressants use some form of contraception during treatment and for up to 12 weeks after the end of therapy.

➤ It may take 3 to 4 months for a therapeutic response to azathioprine to be experienced in patients with rheumatoid arthritis.

➤ Azathioprine interacts with allopurinol, such that the effects of the immunosuppressant are reduced.

➤ Patients who are to undergo transplant surgery and who are receiving cyclosporine should know that several days before surgery they may be told to take it with corticosteroids and they may be also given an oral antifungal as prophylaxis for *Candida* infections.

➤ Patients taking the oral form of cyclosporine should be told to take it with meals or mixed with chocolate milk to prevent GI upset.

➤ Patients taking azathioprine or muromonab-CD3 should be informed that, several days before transplant surgery, they should take all their medication by the oral route, if possible, to avoid its having to be given by IM injections, as this carries the risk of causing infection. They should be told to take the immunosuppressant with food to help decrease the associated GI upset.

➤ Side effects of azathioprine include hepatotoxicity, leukopenia, and thrombocytopenia.

➤ Side effects of cyclosporine include nephrotoxicity, neurotoxicity, and moderate hypertension.

➤ Side effects of muromonab-CD3 include chills, fever, tremors, dyspnea, wheezing, pulmonary edema, chest pain, vomiting, nausea, and diarrhea.

➤ Patients should be made aware that life-long therapy is indicated with organ transplantation.

POINTS TO REMEMBER

Immunosuppressants

- Agents that decrease or prevent the body's immune response.
- Examples are corticosteroids, cyclophosphamide, azathioprine, methotrexate, cyclosporine, muromonab-CD3, and tacrolimus.
- Suppress the action of various cells of the immune system.

Azathioprine

- Suppresses delayed hypersensitivity and antibody responses.
- Antagonizes purine metabolism (DNA, RNA, and protein synthesis).
- Blocks cellular metabolism.
- Inhibits mitosis.

Cyclosporine and Prograf

- Inhibit interleukin-2 release from T-lymphocytes (CD4).
- Used in organ transplant recipients to prevent organ rejection.
- If recipient's immune system cannot recognize the organ as being foreign, it will not mount an immune response against it.

Muromonab-CD3

- Prevents T-cells from recognizing foreign antigens.
- Used in transplant recipients suffering from acute rejection of the donated organ.
- Used to prevent acute rejection.
- Potent immunosuppressant.

Nursing Considerations

- Laboratory studies (e.g., Hgb level, Hct, WBC, and platelet count) should be performed and the results documented before, during (monthly), and after therapy; should the leukocyte count drop below 3000/mm³, the drug should be discontinued.
- Any of these agents being taken orally should always be taken with food to minimize GI upset.

- Because of the immunosuppressed state of the patients receiving immunosuppressants, oral forms of the drugs should be used whenever possible to decrease the risk of infection associated with IM injections.
- Oral antifungals are usually also given with these medications to treat the oral candidiasis common in these patients.
- Patients should be encouraged to report any fever, sore throat, chills, joint pain, or fatigue, which may indicate severe infection.

REVIEW QUESTIONS

1. Which of the following is an appropriate intervention for IV administration of cyclosporine?
   a. It may be undiluted and given IV push.
   b. Dilute with NS or D5W and infuse over 48 hours.
   c. Use NS to dilute the drug and infuse over 2 to 6 hours.
   d. IV administration should only be through a mediport.
2. Which of the following should be assessed before initiation of treatment with muromonab-CD3?
   a. Hct
   b. Hgb
   c. Fluid volume
   d. Electrolyte status
3. Which of the following is a common side effect of azathiprine (Imuran)?
   a. Tremors
   b. Leukopenia

   c. Tachycardia
   d. Fluid retention
4. It is recommended that patients taking immunosuppressants should:
   a. Use oral forms of the agents to prevent the occurrence of oral candidiasis.
   b. Maintain long-term corticosteroid use just as a precaution to prevent drug side effects.
   c. Use some form of contraception during treatment and for up to 12 weeks after the end of therapy.
   d. Be given some other treatment because it may take 6 to 9 months for a therapeutic response to occur.
5. A side effect most commonly associated with the administration of cyclosporine is which of the following?
   a. Hepatoxicity
   b. Neurotoxicity
   c. Polycythemia
   d. Pulmonary fibrosis

For Answers see www.harcourthealth.com/MERLIN/Lilley/.

CRITICAL THINKING Activities

1. K.J. is a 58-year-old heart transplant recipient who is currently taking cyclosporine to prevent his immune system from rejecting his transplanted heart. A cytomegalovirus (CMV) infection has developed, for which he is receiving ganciclovir. How does cyclosporine prevent this patient's immune system from attacking his transplanted heart?

2. What type of medication may be needed with the administration of muromonab-CD3 and why?
3. Your patient is about to undergo a right lung transplant. Why are IM injections to be kept at a minimal during the time before his surgery?
4. What is the patient-teaching emphasis for oral therapy for the patient undergoing a lung transplant who is about to receive an immunosuppressant?

For Answers see www.harcourthealth.com/MERLIN/Lilley/.

bibliography

Albanese J, Nutz P: *Mosby's 2001 nursing drug reference and review cards*, St Louis, 2001, Mosby.

American Hospital Formulary Service: *AHFS drug information*, Bethesda, Md, 2000, American Society of Health-System Pharmacists.

Anderson PO, Knoben JE, Troutman WG: *Handbook of clinical drug data 1999-2000*, ed 9, New York, 1999, McGraw-Hill.

Johns Hopkins Hospital, Department of Pediatrics et al: *The Harriet Lane handbook*, ed 15, St. Louis, 2000, Mosby.

Keen JH: *Critical care and emergency drug reference*, ed 3, St Louis, 1996, Mosby.

Mosby's GenRx: a comprehensive reference for generic and brand drugs, ed 10, St Louis, 2000, Mosby.

Skidmore-Roth L: *Mosby's 2001 nursing drug reference*, St Louis, 2001, Mosby.

Remember to check the **Online Worksheet** for additional learning opportunities: **www.harcourthealth.com/MERLIN/Lilley/**

Chapter 44

Immunizing Agents

objectives

www.harcourthealth.com/MERLIN/Lilley/

When you reach the end of this chapter, you should be able to do the following:

Look for this symbol for topics covered in the **Online Worksheet**

1 Discuss the importance of immunity as it relates to the various immunizing agents.

2 Identify the diseases that are treated with toxoids and vaccines.

3 Compare the mechanisms of action, indications for use, cautions, contraindications, side effects, and routes of administration for various toxoids and vaccines.

4 Develop a nursing care plan that includes all phases of the nursing process related to the administration of immunizing agents.

---

drug profiles

---

glossary

Active immunization (im′ u ni za′ shən) A process that causes a complete and long-lasting immunity to infection to develop through exposure of the body to a relatively harmless form of the antigen. This imprints a memory on the body's immune system and stimulates the body's defenses to fend off any subsequent exposure to the pathogen. (p. 685)

Antibody (an′ ti bod′ e) Molecules used by the cell-mediated immune system to attack and kill all substances foreign to the body. (p. 687)

Antibody titer (ti′ tər) Amount of an antibody needed to react with a specific antigen. (p. 687)

Antigen (an′ ti jən) A substance, usually a protein, that causes the formation of an antibody and reacts specifically with that antibody. (p. 685)

Biological A substance of biologic origin used to prevent, treat, or cure infectious diseases. (p. 685)

Booster shot An antigen, such as a vaccine or toxoid, that is usually administered in an amount smaller than that in the original immunization. It is given to maintain the immune response at an appropriate level. (p. 685)

Cell-mediated immune system Part of the immune system stimulated by active immunizing agents. (p. 687)

Herd immunity Resistance to a disease in an entire community or population because a large proportion of its members are immune to it. (p. 687)

Immunizing biological Toxoid or vaccine targeted against an infectious microorganism. (p. 685)

Immunoglobulin (im′ u no glob′u lin) A glycoprotein used by the cell-mediated immune system to attack and kill all substances foreign to the body. (p. 687)

Passive immunization A process that fights infection but by bypassing the immune system. It involves giving a person serum or concentrated immune globulins obtained directly from humans or animals that directly give that person the means to fight off the invading microorganism. The person's immune system does not have to manufacture them. (p. 685)

Passive immunizing agents Agents containing antibodies that can kill or inactivate pathogens. These are directly injected into a person and provide them with the means to fend off infection, bypassing their own immune system. (p. 687)

Toxoid (tok′ soid) Antigenic (foreign) preparation or gram-positive exotoxin that is detoxified with chemicals or heat. (p. 687)

Vaccine (vak′ sen′) A suspension of live, attenuated, or killed microorganisms that can promote an artificially cultivated active immunity against a particular microorganism. (p. 685)

IMMUNITY AND IMMUNIZATION

Centuries ago it was noticed that people who suffered a certain disease acquired an immune tolerance to it so that, when exposed to it again, they did not suffer a second bout. This basic observation prompted scientists to

Active Versus Passive Immunity

Table 44-1

Differences	Active	Passive
Type of immunization	Toxoid or vaccine	Immune globulin or antitoxin
Mechanism of action	Causes an Ag-Ab response; similar to exposure to natural disease process	Results from direct administration of exogenous Ab; the Ab concentration will decrease over time, so if reexposure is expected, it is wise to continue passive immunizations
Indication	Minimizes or entirely avoids active infection. Provides long-lasting or permanent immunity	For people who are immunodeficient, have a contraindication to active immunization, have been exposed to disease, or anticipate exposure to the disease; it provides temporary protection; it does not stimulate an Ab response in the host

Ab, Antibody; *Ag,* antigen.

investigate ways of artificially producing this tolerance. Along with this came an understanding of the way in which the normal immune system functions, a knowledge important to an understanding of how immunizing agents work. Briefly, when the body first comes in contact with an invading organism **(antigen),** some specific information is imprinted into a memory bank so that the body can effectively repel any later invasion by that same organism. It is because of this process that people rarely suffer twice from certain diseases such as mumps, chickenpox, and measles. Instead they have a complete and long-lasting immunity to those infections.

There are two ways of cultivating this immunity—actively and passively. In **active immunization** the body is exposed to a relatively harmless form of the antigen (foreign invader), which imprints this information on the body's memory bank and stimulates the body's defenses to resist any subsequent exposure, but without actually causing the infection. In **passive immunization,** serum or concentrated immune globulins obtained from humans or animals are injected into a person, directly giving that person the substance needed to fight off the invading microorganism. This type of immunization bypasses the immune system. The major differences between active and passive immunity are summarized in Table 44-1 and discussed in greater depth in the following sections.

ACTIVE IMMUNIZATION

Toxoids and vaccines are known as **immunizing biologicals.** In general, **biologicals** are substances such as antitoxins, serum, toxoids, vaccines, or similar preparations that are used to prevent, treat, or cure infectious diseases. Immunizing biologicals are toxoids or vaccines that target a particular infectious microorganism.

Toxoids

Toxoids are antigenic (foreign) preparations or grampositive exotoxins that are detoxified (attenuated) with chemicals or heat, rendering them nontoxic and unable to revert back to a toxic form, but nonetheless highly anti-

genic. In other words, toxoids are diluted, changed, or altered substances (exotoxins) that are normally secreted from bacteria. When injected into a person, this causes the person's immune system to mount an immune response by producing a specific antibody (an antitoxic antibody) against this antigen, which can then neutralize tissue-destroying bacterial exotoxins that may subsequently be introduced into the body. First developed in 1923 at the Pasteur Institute by Ramon and his associates, the toxoids now available are effective against the toxin-producing diseases diphtheria and tetanus.

Vaccines

Vaccines are suspensions of live, attenuated (weakened), or killed (inactivated) microorganisms that can artificially promote the acquisition of active immunity against the particular organism. These slight alterations in the bacteria and viruses prevent the person injected with the substance from contracting the disease but are able to promote active immunization against the pathogen. People vaccinated with live bacteria or virus enjoy lifelong immunity against that particular disease. Only partial immunity is conferred on those vaccinated with killed bacteria or virus, and for this reason they must be given periodic **booster shots** to maintain the protection of the immune system against infection with this bacteria or virus. One exception to this is the smallpox vaccine because it utilizes live cowpox virus instead of the more virulent smallpox virus.

In fact, some of the first work in the development of vaccines was done in the area of smallpox immunization, starting with Lady Mary Montagu, who in 1718 introduced the Eastern practice of inoculating against the smallpox virus by applying it to the nasal membranes. In 1774 Benjamin Jesty was the first to use cowpox virus inoculations to prevent smallpox. Edward Jenner, an English physician who noticed that milkmaids who had suffered cowpox infections were rarely victims of smallpox, was the first to study the relationship of cowpox to smallpox immunity. This observation led to the development of the smallpox vaccine, which utilizes the cowpox virus. In 1796 he successfully immunized a young boy against smallpox by vaccinating him with cowpox virus obtained from a cowpox vesicle on an infected cow.

With the help of the modern version of this vaccine, smallpox has now been eradicated since 1980. The advent of vaccines in general has dramatically changed the way we deal with public health problems. Today there are more than twenty infectious diseases for which there are vaccines, and the past decade alone has witnessed the appearance of nine new or improved vaccines.

These newer vaccines contain some extract or synthetic extract of the pathogen rather than the actual microbe and are produced by genetic engineering methods. The vaccines yielded are actually viral or bacterial antigenic

BOX 44-1 Available Immunizing Agents

SERUMS
Antivenin (Crotalidae) polyvalent
Antivenin (Lactrodectus mactans)
Antivenin (Micrurus fulvius)
Botulinum antitoxin
Cytomegalovirus immune globulin
Digoxin Immune Fab
Diphtheria antitoxin
Hepatitis B immune globulin
Immune globulin
Rabies immune globulin
Rh$_0$(D) immune globulin
Tetanus immune globulin
Varicella-zoster immune globulin
Widow spider species antivenin

TOXOIDS
Diphtheria and tetanus toxoids
Tetanus and diphtheria toxoids
Tetanus toxoid

VACCINES
BCG vaccine
Cholera vaccine
Haemophilus influenzae type b conjugate vaccine
Hepatitis A virus vaccine inactivated
Hepatitis B virus vaccine inactivated
Influenza virus vaccine
Japanese encehalitis virus vaccine
Lyme disease vaccine
Measles virus vaccine live
Mumps virus vaccine live
Plague vaccine
Pneumococcal vaccine, polyvalent
Poliovirus vaccine live oral
Rabies vaccine
Rubella virus vaccine live
Smallpox vaccine
Typhoid vaccine
Varicella vaccine
Yellow fever vaccine

preparations, and these are the substances that cause the immune system to produce antibodies against them and hence induce immunity. Examples of viral vaccines (antigenic preparations) include hepatitis B and influenza, the latter also possibly containing the whole virus or the split virus particle. Bacterial vaccines against meningitis (meningococcus), *Haemophilus influenzae*, and pneumococcus contain selected bacterial capsular polysaccharides (bacterial particles) that are taken from the respective microbes.

The process of attenuating or killing infectious microbes that are otherwise extremely virulent renders them safe for use in immunizing vaccines by removing that portion of them that causes infection. The advantage to such vaccines is that they have much greater antigenicity and produce more effective and longer-lasting immunity than inactivated vaccines. The attenuating or killing agent is usually a chemical such as formaldehyde or a physical mechanism such as heat. Attenuation may also be accomplished by the repeated passage of the microbe through some medium such as a fertile hen egg or a special tissue culture. The currently available immunizing vaccines are listed in Box 44-1. Besides the individual active immunizing agents, there are several combinations of various vaccines and toxoids, and these are used especially in infants. Examples are the diphtheria and tetanus toxoid with pertussis vaccine (DTP) and the measles, mumps, and rubella vaccine (MMR).

The search for new and better agents will never end. One that is the current focus of worldwide research is the development of a safe and effective vaccine against the human immunodeficiency virus (HIV), which causes acquired immunodeficiency syndrome (AIDS), an endeavor that is proving very difficult and time-consuming. An effective immunizing biological effective against malaria is also being sought. Indeed, an immunizing biological effective against every infectious disease is the ultimate goal.

Activity

PASSIVE IMMUNIZATION

As previously mentioned, passive immunization bypasses the host's immune system and inoculates the person with serum or immune globulins obtained from humans or animals. These substances give the person the means to fight off the invading organism. Passive immunization can occur naturally between a mother and the fetus or the nursing infant when the mother passes maternal antibodies directly either through the placenta to the fetus or through breast milk to the nursing infant. This is called *naturally acquired passive immunity*, but because it can occur only between a mother and the unborn fetus or between the mother and her nursing infant, other ways have had to be found of accomplishing it by artificial means. Such passive immunization is called *artificially acquired passive immunity*. It differs from active immunization in that it is a comparatively transitory (short-lived) immune state.

As noted in Table 44-1, there are specific populations that can benefit from passive immunization but not from active immunization. Such people are those rendered immunodeficient for whatever reason (e.g. drugs, disease) and who therefore cannot develop immunity in response to a toxoid or vaccine injection because their immune systems are too suppressed to do so. People who already have the disease targeted by the passive immunizing agent are also candidates for these agents, especially those with diseases that are rapidly fatal, such as rabies and hepatitis. Because these diseases are so rapidly fatal, the body does not have time to mount an adequate defense against them, with death occurring before it can do so. The passive immunization of these people confers a temporary protection that is usually sufficient to keep the invading organism from killing them, even though it does not stimulate an antibody response.

The passive immunizing agents consist of three groups of agents—antitoxins, immune globulins, and snake and spider antivenins. Antitoxins are purified antiserums that are usually obtained from horses inoculated with the toxin. Immune globulins represent concentrated preparations containing predominantly immunoglobulin G and are harvested from a large pool of blood donors. Antivenins are serums obtained from animals (usually horses) that have been injected with the particular venom. The serum contains immunoglobulins that can neutralize the toxic effects of the venoms.

The currently recommended childhood immunization schedule as recommended by the American Academy of Pediatrics is shown in Fig. 44-1. The annual advisory is a joint effort of the American Academy of Pediatrics (AAP), the CDC's Advisory Committee on Immunization Practices (ACIP), and the American Academy of Family Physicians (AAFP). The 2001 immunization schedule has three major changes: it recommends complete replacement of oral poliovirus vaccine (OPV) with polio vaccine inactivated (IPV); it advises routine childhood hepatitis A virus (HAV) vaccination in 11 states; and it advises continued suspension of rotavirus vaccination.

Activity

IMMUNIZING AGENTS

Mechanism of Action

Active immunizing agents consist of vaccines and toxoids that can be administered either orally or intramuscularly and that work by stimulating that part of the immune system known as the **cell-mediated immune system.** The system makes use of substances called **immunoglobulins,** of which there are five, designated IgM, IgG, IgA, IgE, and IgD, to attack and kill the foreign substances that invade the body. These foreign substances are called *antigens,* and the immunoglobulins are called **antibodies.**

Vaccines contain substances that trigger the formation of these antibodies against specific pathogens. Sometimes these substances are the actual live, attenuated (weakened) pathogen or they are a killed pathogen and the amount of antibodies they cause to be produced can be measured in the blood. The **antibody titer** is the amount

that must be present in the body (blood) to effectively protect the body against the particular pathogen. Sometimes the levels of these antibodies decline over time. When this happens, a second dose of the vaccine is given to restore the antibody titers to a level that can protect the person against the infection. This second dose is referred to as a booster shot.

Toxoids are altered forms of bacterial toxins that stimulate the production of antibodies in the same way as vaccines.

Because both toxoids and vaccines rely on the immunized host to mount an immune response, the host's immune system must be intact. Therefore patients who are immunocompromised, such as those undergoing immunosuppressive chemotherapy, those receiving immunosuppressive therapy to prevent the rejection of transplanted organs, and those with immunosuppressive diseases such as AIDS, and who as a result usually cannot mount an immune response, should not receive vaccines or toxoids.

As previously explained, **passive immunizing agents** are the actual antibodies (immunoglobulins) that can kill or inactivate the pathogen. The process is called "passive" because the person's immune system does not participate in it. However, because of this, immunity acquired in this way generally endures for much less time than that produced by active immunization, lasting only until the injected immunoglobulins are removed from the person's immune system by the reticuloendothelial system.

Drug Effects

Vaccines and toxoids are the active immunizing agents that have been developed for the prevention of many illnesses caused by bacteria and their toxins as well as those caused by various viruses. Antivenins, antitoxins, and immune globulins comprise the passive immunizing agents. Such agents can inactivate spider and snake venom, bacterial toxins (exotoxins), and potentially lethal viruses. A list of the currently available immunizing agents is given in Box 44-1.

Therapeutic Uses

Active immunization is used to prevent infection caused by bacterial toxins or viruses, and as previously noted, it confers long-lasting or permanent immunity. If a person immunized against a particular pathogen is then exposed to that foreign invader, this causes a prompt and significant increase in the person's immunoglobulin (antibody) level. However, there is an interesting phenomenon that occurs in terms of the number of people immunized. The successful immunization of 95% or more of a population confers protection on the entire population. This is called **herd immunity.**

As previously noted, passive immunizing agents consist of antivenins, antitoxins, and immune globulins. Antivenins, also known as *serums,* are used to prevent or minimize the effects of poisoning by the venoms of crotalids (rattlesnakes, copperheads, and cottonmouths), black widow spiders, or coral snakes, some of which can be lethal. Most healthy adults do not die from the bites

Recommended Childhood Immunization Schedule
United States, January - December 2001

Vaccines[1] are listed under routinely recommended ages. [Bars] *indicate range of recommended ages for immunization. Any dose not given at the recommended age should be given as a "catch-up" immunization at any subsequent visit when indicated and feasible.* (Ovals) *indicate vaccines to be given if previously recommended doses were missed or given earlier than the recommended minimum age.*

Information in bold has been added by the American Academy of Family Physicians (AAFP).

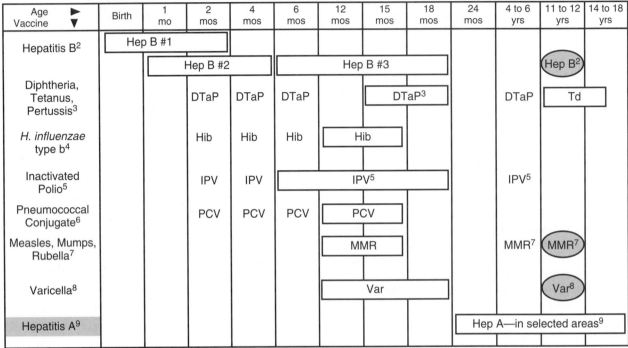

Approved by the Advisory Committee on Immunization Practices (ACIP), the American Academy of Pediatrics (AAP), and the American Academy of Family Physicians (AAFP).

1 This schedule indicates the recommended ages for routine administration of currently licensed childhood vaccines, as of 11/1/00, for children through 18 years of age. Additional vaccines may be licensed and recommended during the year. Licensed combination vaccines may be used whenever any components of the combination are indicated and its other components are not contraindicated. Providers should consult the manufacturers' package inserts for detailed recommendations.

2 <u>Infants born to HBsAg-negative mothers</u> should receive the 1st dose of hepatitis B (Hep B) vaccine by age 2 months. The 2nd dose should be at least one month after the 1st dose. The 3rd dose should be administered at least 4 months after the 1st dose and at least 2 months after the 2nd dose, but not before 6 months of age for infants.
<u>Infants born to HBsAg-positive mothers</u> should receive hepatitis B vaccine and 0.5 mL hepatitis B immune globulin (HBIG) within 12 hours of birth at separate sites. The 2nd dose is recommended at 1-2 months of age and the 3rd dose at 6 months of age.
<u>Infants born to mothers whose HBsAg status is unknown</u> should receive hepatitis B vaccine within 12 hours of birth. Maternal blood should be drawn at the time of delivery to determine the mother's HBsAg status; if the HBsAg test is positive, the infant should receive HBIG as soon as possible (no later than 1 week of age).
<u>All children and adolescents</u> who have not been immunized against hepatitis B should begin the series during any visit. Special efforts should be made to immunize children who were born in or whose parents were born in areas of the world with moderate or high endemicity of hepatitis B virus infection.

3 The 4th dose of DTaP (diphtheria and tetanus toxoids and acellular pertussis vaccine) may be administered as early as 12 months of age, provided 6 months have elapsed since the 3rd dose and the child is unlikely to return at age 15-18 months. Td (tetanus and diphtheria toxoids) is recommended at 11-12 years of age if at least 5 years have elapsed since the last dose of DTP, DTaP, or DT. Subsequent routine Td boosters are recommended every 10 years.

4 Three *Haemophilus influenzae* type b (Hib) conjugate vaccines are licensed for infant use. If PRP-OMP (PedvaxHIB® or ComVax® [Merck]) is administered at 2 and 4 months of age, a dose at 6 months is not required. Because clinical studies in infants have demonstrated that using some combination products may induce a lower immune response to the Hib vaccine component, DTaP/Hib combination products should not be used for primary immunization in infants at 2, 4, or 6 months of age, unless FDA-approved for these ages.

5 An all-IPV schedule is recommended for routine childhood polio vaccination in the United States. All children should receive four doses of IPV at 2 months, 4 months, 6-18 months, and 4-6 years. Oral polio vacccine (OPV) should be used only in selected circumstances. (See MMWR May 19, 2000/49(RR-5);1-22).

6 The heptavalent conjugate pneumococcal vaccine (PCV) is recommended for all children 2-23 months of age. It also is recommended for certain children 24-59 months of age. (See MMWR Oct. 6, 2000/49(RR-9);1-35). **The full AAFP Clinical Policy on Pneumococcal Conjugate Vaccine is available at www.aafp.org/policy/camp/24.html.**

7 The 2nd dose of measles, mumps, and rubella (MMR) vaccine is recommended routinely at 4-6 years of age but may be administered during any visit, provided at least 4 weeks have elapsed since receipt of the 1st dose and that both doses are administered beginning at or after 12 months of age. Those who have not previously received the second dose should complete the schedule by the 11-12 year old visit.

8 Varicella (Var) vaccine is recommended at any visit on or after the first birthday for susceptible children, i.e., those who lack a reliable history of chickenpox (as judged by a health care provider) and who have not been immunized. Susceptible persons 13 years of age or older should receive 2 doses, given at least 4 weeks apart.

9 Hepatitis A (Hep A) is shaded to indicate its recommended use in selected states and or regions, and for certain high risk groups; consult your local public health authority. (See MMWR Oct. 1, 1999/48(RR-12); 1-37).

For additional information about the vaccines listed above, please visit the National Immunization Program Home Page at http://www.cdc.gov/nip/ or call the National Immunization Hotline at 800-232-2522 (English) or 800-232-0233 (Spanish).

Full AAFP immunization policies can be found at the AAFP website www.aafp.org/clinical.

Fig. 44-1 Recommended childhood immunization schedule.

of spiders and snakes if prompt and appropriate treatment (i.e., the administration of the appropriate antivenin) is instituted. However, very young children and elderly people with health problems are particularly susceptible to the effects of the venoms of some of these animals. In either situation an antivenin is needed in order to give the person who has been bitten the substance needed to overcome the effects of the venom.

Certain viruses are very potent and even potentially lethal (e.g., hepatitis B and rabies). They can do major harm very quickly before the infected person can mount an effective immune response against them. The passive immunization of the person with the appropriate immune globulin gives them the antibody needed to fend off the harmful effects of the virus. There are also immune globulins available for protection against some bacterial infections (e.g., pertussis and tetanus).

Antitoxins are used for protection against certain very harmful bacteria such as those that cause botulism and diphtheria.

Side Effects and Adverse Effects

The undesirable effects of the various immunizing agents can range from mild and transient to more serious and even life-threatening ones. The minor and more severe ones are listed in Table 44-2. The minor reactions can be treated with acetaminophen and rest. More severe reactions such as fever higher than 103° F (39.4° C) should be treated with acetaminophen and sponge baths. Serum sickness sometimes occurs after repeated injections of equine-made immunizing agents. The signs and symptoms consist of edema of the face, tongue, and throat; rash; urticaria; arthritis; adenopathy; fever; flushing; itching; cough; dyspnea; cyanosis; vomiting; and cardiovascular collapse. This is best treated with analgesics, antihistamines, epinephrine, or corticosteroids.

The various types of severe reactions that can occur in response to immunizing agents and the time frames involved are summarized in Table 44-3.

Table 44-2 Immunizing Agents: Minor and Severe Adverse Effects

Body System	Side/Adverse Effect
MINOR EFFECTS	
Central nervous system	Fever, adenopathy
Integumentary	Minor rash, soreness at injection site, urticaria, arthritis
SEVERE EFFECTS	
Central nervous system	Fever >103° F (39.4° C), encephalitis, convulsions, peripheral neuropathy, anaphylactic reactions, shock, unconsciousness
Integumentary	Urticaria, rash
Respiratory	Dyspnea
Other	Cyanosis

Interactions

Immunosuppressive agents such as corticosteroids and cancer chemotherapy agents block generation of active immunity. Isoniazid may diminish the response to bacille Calmette-Guérin (BCG) vaccine. Hepatitis B immune globulin has a drug interaction with live vaccines; defer for 3 months after dose of immune globulin.

Dosages

For the recommended dosages of selected immunizing agents, see the dosages table on p. 690.

drug profiles

Some of the more commonly used vaccines, toxoids, and immunoglobulins are described in the following sections. All the available immunizing agents are listed in Box 44-1.

ACTIVE IMMUNIZING AGENTS
bacillus Calmette-Guérin vaccine

BCG vaccine (TICE BCG) is used to promote active immunity to tuberculosis (TB). It is a live, attenuated vaccine derived from a slightly weakened Calmette-Guérin strain of *Mycobacterium bovis*. There are several bacterial strains of this bacteria; the particular strain used in the United States is the Tice substrain. Because this strain is similar to *Mycobacterium tuberculosis*, vaccination with BCG causes a natural infection that promotes cell-mediated immunity against TB through the production of antibodies targeted against this foreign invader. BCG vaccine may also be used as a nonspecific immunotherapeutic agent for the treatment of superficial bladder tumors. When used for this purpose it is directly injected into the bladder (intravesical administration). This process is called *local treatment*. It may also be used for the treatment and possible prevention of recurrent tumors in patients with bladder cancer.

BCG vaccine is available for percutaneous injection using a multiple-puncture device. It is not known whether the vaccine is harmful to the fetus of pregnant women or if it can affect reproduction. It should therefore be used in pregnant women only when absolutely necessary. BCG vaccine is

Table 44-3 Time Frame of Serious Reactions

Reaction	Time Frame
Anaphylaxis	Within 24 hr of immunization
Encephalopathy	Within 7 days of DTP or 15 days of MMR
Death	No time limit

DTP, Diphtheria and tetanus toxoid with pertussis vaccine; *MMR,* measles, mumps, and rubella vaccine.

DOSAGES Selected Immunizing Agents

agent	pharmacologic class	dosage range	purpose
ACTIVE IMMUNIZING AGENTS			
bacillus Calmette-Guérin vaccine (BCG vaccine or TICE BCG)	Live attenuated cow TB vaccine	*Pediatric <1 mo* Half adult dose administered percutaneously multiple puncture disk; WHO recommends administration by intradermal injection *Pediatric >1 mo/Adult* 0.2-0.3 ml on skin by percutaneous administration	TB prophylaxis
diphtheria, tetanus, and acellular pertussis (DtaP)	Mixed toxoid	*Pediatric* IM: One dose q4-8wk × three doses; dose four 6-12 months after the third dose; a booster dose should be given at 4, 5, or 6 years of age (the booster dose is given only if the fourth dose was given before the child's fourth birthday)	Diphtheria, tetanus, and pertusis prophylaxis
Haemophilus influenzae **type b conjugate vaccine (Hib)**	Bacterial capsular antigenic extract vaccine	*Infant 2-6 mo* IM: three 0.5-ml injections about 2 mo apart	*H. influenzae* type b prophylaxis
hepatitis B virus vaccine inactivated (Recombivax HB, Engerix-B)	Viral surface antigen	*Pediatric to 10 y/o* IM: 2.5 or 5 μg doses at birth, then at 1-2 mo and at 6-18 mo of age	Hepatitis B virus prophylaxis
measles, mumps, and rubella virus vaccine live (MMR II)	Live, attenuated viral vaccine	*Pediatric >12 mo/Adult* SC: 0.5 ml and a booster at 4-6 yr	Measles, mumps, rubella prophylaxis
polio vaccine inactivated live oral (Orimune)	Live, attenuated mixed viral vaccine	*Infant* PO: 0.5 ml at 6-12 wk of age, 0.5 ml 6-8 wk later, 0.5 ml at about 12 mo of age	Polio prophylaxis
tetanus and diphtheria toxoids adsorbed (Td = adult)	Mixed toxoid	*Adult* IM: 0.5 ml, followed by 0.5 ml in 4-8 wk and 0.5 ml in 6-12 mo	Diphtheria and tetanus prophylaxis
varicella vaccine (Varivax)	Live, attenuated viral vaccine	*Adult* SC: two 0.5 ml doses given 4-8 wk apart *Pediatric 1 to 12 y/o* SC: one 0.5 ml dose	Varicella (chicken pox and shingles)
PASSIVE IMMUNIZING AGENTS			
hepatitis B immune globulin (H-BIG, Hep-B-Gammagee, HyperHep)	IgG immune globulin	*Infant* IM: 0.5 ml within 12 hr after birth *Adult* IM: 0.06 mg/kg after exposure and repeated in 30 days	Passive hepatitis B prophylaxis
immune globulin IV (Gammagard, Gammar IV, Iveegam, Polygam, Sandoglobulin, Venoglobulin)	Mixed immune globulins	IV: Refer to current manufacturer's dosage recommendations for products not listed Gammagard: 100-400 mg/kg once monthly Sandoglobulin: 200-300 mg/kg once monthly Gammagard: 1 g/kg. Up to 3 doses on alternate days Sandoglobulin: 400 mg/kg on 2-5 consecutive days Gammagard: 400 mg/kg every 3-4 wk	Immune deficiency syndrome Idiopathic thrombocytopenic purpura Infections secondary to B cell lumpho-cytic leukemia
Rh₀ (D) immune globulin (Hyp-Rho-D Mini-Dose, MICRhoGAM, Gamulin)	Immunosuppressant globulin	*Adult/female* IM: inject total contents of a single vial within 72 hr after delivery Micro-dose IM: inject full contents of a single vial after abortion/pregnancy termination up to 12 wk of gestation	Postpartum antibody suppression
tetanus immune globulin-TIG	Immune globulins (Hyper-Tet)	IM: 250 U as a single dose IM: 3000-6000 U	Postexposure passive tetanus prophylaxis Tetanus treatment

contraindicated in patients with a hypersensitivity to it, those showing a significant positive reaction to tuberculin, those who have recently received small-pox immunizations, burn patients, and those with hypogammaglobulinemia, a congenital immuno-deficiency, sarcoidosis, leukemia, lymphoma, a generalized malignant condition, HIV infection, or any other disorder involving an altered natural immune response, such as is the case in patients who are on immunosuppressive therapy. The recommended dosages for the vaccine are given in the dosages table on p. 690.

diphtheria and tetanus toxoids with acellular pertussis vaccine (adsorbed)

Diphtheria, tetanus, and pertussis are very different disorders, but an injection that combines all three vaccines (DTP) has been routinely given to children since the 1940s. Recently, a new vaccine combination called DTaP has been approved. It uses a different form of the pertussis component known as *acellular pertussis*. Acellular pertussis consists of only a single weakened toxoid, whereas previous pertussis vaccines contained multiple toxoids. Experts hope that DTaP will prove to have fewer side effects than DTP, particularly in older patients who are more prone to them, thereby allowing adults to have a pertussis booster.

It has been recommended that children younger than 7 years of age also receive immunization against pertussis. Therefore diphtheria and tetanus toxoids with whole-cell pertussis vaccine adsorbed (DTP) and diphtheria and tetanus toxoids with acellular pertussis vaccine adsorbed (DTaP) are the preferred preparations for primary and booster immunization against these diseases in children 6 weeks to 6 years of age, unless the pertussis component is contraindicated.

Tetanus, diphtheria, and pertussis are prevalent in the populations of many developing countries throughout the world, and as a result, the risk of contracting one of these diseases may be high there. Full immunization against these diseases with DTP or DTaP is recommended for both travelers to these areas as well as the inhabitants. Td is used in persons 7 years of age or older requiring a primary or booster immunization against tetanus for routine wound management. Emergency booster doses of Td (for adult use) are unnecessary when the wound is clean and minor (not tetanus prone) and the patient has received a primary or booster immunization against tetanus within the past 10 years.

These toxoids (DT, Td, DTP, and DTaP) are available only as parenteral preparations to be given as deep IM injections. They are contraindicated in people who have had a prior systemic hypersensitivity

reaction or a neurologic reaction to one of the ingredients. Some manufacturers state that use is contraindicated in the setting of concurrent acute or active infections but not in the setting of minor illness. Although there have been very few, if any, studies documenting the safety of their use in pregnant women, it is generally considered safe to give diphtheria, tetanus, and pertussis toxoids after the first trimester, but optimally during the second or third trimesters. The recommended dosages for these toxoids are given in the dosages table on p. 690.

Diphtheria and tetanus toxoids adsorbed (DT) for pediatric use and tetanus and diphtheria toxoids adsorbed (Td) for adult use are toxoids obtained from the bacteria *Corynebacterium diphtheriae*. To make the agents, diphtheria and tetanus toxins are taken from these bacteria, attenuated into toxoids, and adsorbed onto aluminum hydroxide, aluminum

---

home health/community points

Use of Pertussis Vaccine— Controversy and Community Implications

Since the standard pertussis vaccine was introduced in the 1950s, there has been a decline in the incidence of disease. However, the lack of immunizations over the last decade has led to an increase in the incidence of disease. In addition, some parents have expressed concern over the significant reactions to the pertussis portion of the DPT vaccine, including the possibility of fever, anorexia, vomiting, collapse, and even seizures. Rare and serious acute encephalopathies or status epilepticus has been reported with the administration of the whole-cell pertussis portion of the DTP vaccine. Whether this is a cause or is coincidentally related to the vaccine is hard to determine because of the difficulty in diagnosing serious neurologic-related problems in an infant (i.e., was the neurologic impairment there before the vaccine). The Advisory Committee on Immunization Practices (ACIP) states that DTP vaccines are containdicated in any patient who had an immediate anaphylactoid reaction or encephalopathy within 7 days after the vaccine that is not related to another cause. An acellular vaccine is currently being used, called DTaP, or acellular pertussis vaccine. It holds the same recommendations and schedule as with the whole cell pertussis (at 2 months, 4 months, and 6 months with a booster at 6 months after the initial series and a booster again between 4 and 6 years of age). After the child reaches 7 years of age, the pertussis is no longer advised. DTP vaccines should not be administered to a child if an earlier vaccine caused fever of 105° F or higher, anaphylaxis, or encephalopathy.

Data from Centers for Disease Control and Prevention: Recommended childhood immunization schedule in the United States, *JAMA* 277(5):371, 1997; General Recommendations on Immunization: Recommendations of the Advisory Committee on Immunization Practices, *MMWR* 43(RR-1):1, 1994.

phosphate, or potassium alum. They are given by injection to infants and children (DT) (6 weeks to 6 years old) and older children and adults (Td) (7 years of age and older) with functioning immune systems. They promote immunity to diphtheria and tetanus by inducing the production of specific antitoxins.

Haemophilus influenzae type b conjugate vaccine

H. influenzae type b (Hib) vaccine is a noninfectious, bacteria-derived vaccine. It is made by extracting *H. influenzae* particles that are antigenic (cause an antigen-antibody reaction) and are then attached to a protein carrier. They are given by injection to adults and children considered at high risk of acquiring the *H. influenzae* infection. Conditions that may predispose an individual to Hib infections are septicemia, pneumonia, cellulitis, arthritis, osteomyelitis, pericarditis, sickle cell anemia, an immunodeficiency syndrome, or Hodgkin's disease. Infections caused by Hib are the leading cause of bacterial meningitis in children 3 months to 5 years of age. This form of bacterial meningitis has a mortality rate of 5%. Of those who survive, 20% to 30% suffer serious morbidity in the form of neurologic deficits.

The Hib vaccine may be combined with toxoids to make various combination products. Some examples of these combination products are listed in Box 44-2. All these products are parenteral products that are administered intramuscularly. These vaccines are contraindicated in patients who have had a previous hypersensitivity reaction to any one of the ingredients. It is not known whether the vaccines can cause fetal harm when administered to pregnant women or whether they can affect fertility. As a result, the administration of any of the vaccines during pregnancy is not recommended. The recommended dosages for the vaccine are given in the dosages table on p. 690.

hepatitis B virus vaccine inactivated

Hepatitis B virus vaccine inactivated (Recombivax HB, Engerix-B) is a noninfectious viral vaccine made from yeast fed the genetic code of the hepatitis B surface antigen (HBsAg). The yeast then produces this antigenic substance in mass quantities. After this it is attached to a substance called *alum* and made into the injection that is used to vaccinate people against hepatitis B. This is an example of recombinant DNA technology at work. This antigenic HBsAg is used to promote active immunity to hepatitis B infection in people considered at high risk for potential exposure to the hepatitis B virus or HbsAg-positive materials (e.g., blood, plasma, serum). Health care workers are examples of people considered at high risk.

The vaccine is contraindicated in people who are hypersensitive to yeast. Pregnancy is not considered a contraindication to use. The potential for exposure to hepatitis B infection in a pregnant woman and the potential for the development of chronic infection in the neonate are both good reasons to give the vaccine. The vaccine is administered by IM injection. There are three main formulations designed for three different populations: a *pediatric formulation* for neonates, infants, children, and adolescents; an *adult formulation* for people older than 20 years of age; and a *dialysis formulation* for predialysis and dialysis patients or for other immunocompromised persons. The recommended dosages for this vaccine are given in the dosages table on p. 690.

Activity

influenza virus vaccine

The influenza virus vaccine (FluShield, Fluzone) is the vaccine used to prevent influenza. Each year before the influenza season this vaccine should be administered to high-risk people. It is the single most important influenza control measure.

Each year a new influenza vaccine is made. The influenza vaccine for each new year contains three influenza virus strains (usually two type A and one type B). Of the hundreds of influenza virus strains in our environment, the three that are chosen are the strains that represent the influenza viruses that are likely to circulate in the United States in the upcoming winter. The vaccine is made from highly purified, egg-grown viruses that have been made noninfectious (inactivated).

Influenza illness is characterized by abrupt onset of fever, myalgia, sore throat, and nonproductive cough. Severe malaise may last several days. More severe illness can occur in certain populations. Elderly people and people with underlying health problems are at increased risk for complications of influenza infection. If they become ill with influenza, such members of high-risk groups are

---

more likely than the general population to require hospitalization. Increased mortality results not only from influenza and pneumonia but also from cardiopulmonary and other chronic diseases that can be exacerbated by influenza. More than 90% of the deaths attributed to pneumonia and influenza occur among people 65 years of age or older.

The effectiveness of influenza vaccine in preventing illness varies. Factors that may alter the effectiveness of the influenza vaccine are age and immunocompetence of the vaccine recipient and the degree of similarity between the virus strains included in the vaccine and those that circulate during the influenza season. Healthy people younger than 65 years of age have a 70% chance of preventing illness caused by the influenza virus when there is a good match between vaccine and circulating viruses.

Elderly persons residing in nursing homes can prevent severe illness, secondary complications, and death by taking the influenza vaccine. Among the frail elderly the vaccine can prevent hospitalization and pneumonia up to 50% to 60% of the time and death up to 80% of the time. Achieving a high rate of vaccination among nursing home residents can reduce the spread of infection in a facility, thus preventing disease through herd immunity.

Vaccination with the influenza virus vaccine should be strongly considered in high-risk populations. Such high-risk populations are as follows:

- People 65 years of age or older
- Residents of nursing homes and other chronic-care facilities that house people of any age with chronic medical conditions
- Adults and children with chronic disorders of the pulmonary or cardiovascular systems, including children with asthma
- Adults and children who have required regular medical follow-up or hospitalization during the preceding year because of chronic metabolic diseases (including diabetes mellitus), renal dysfunction, hemoglobinopathies, or immunosuppression (including immunosuppression caused by medications)
- Children and teenagers (6 months to 18 years of age) who are receiving long-term aspirin therapy and therefore might be at risk for developing Reye's syndrome after influenza.

Other populations that require special consideration for vaccination are pregnant women, people infected with HIV, and foreign travelers. These individuals should seek the advice of their physician.

measles, mumps, and rubella virus vaccine live

The measles, mumps, and rubella vaccine (MMR II) is a live, attenuated virus preparation consisting of live measles, mumps, and rubella viruses that are weakened (attenuated). They promote active immunity to measles, mumps, and rubella by inducing the production of virus-specific IgG and IgM antibodies. The antibody response to initial vaccination resembles that caused by primary natural infection.

The measles vaccine or any of the combination products that include the virus are contraindicated in people with a history of anaphylactic, anaphylactoid, or some other immediate reaction to egg ingestion. It is also contraindicated in people who have had an anaphylactic reaction to topically or systemically administered neomycin. These vaccines should not be administered to pregnant women, and pregnancy should be avoided for 3 months after measles virus vaccination and 30 days after vaccination with a rubella-containing (MR or MMR) measles virus vaccine. This precaution is based on the theoretic risk of the live virus vaccine causing a fetal infection.

These vaccines are available only in the parenteral form and should be given only by SC injection. There are several combination products containing the live measles virus vaccine, and these are listed in Box 44-3. The recommended dosages for this vaccine are given in the dosages table on p. 690.

polio vaccine inactivated

The Advisory Committee on Immunization Practices (ACIP) has recently recommended an all-IPV schedule for routine childhood polio vaccination in the United States. This is primarily because poliomyelitis, a severe side effect from the polio vaccine, can be avoided by limiting or eliminating the use of the oral vaccine. Since 1979 the only indigenous cases of poliomyelitis reported in the United States (n = 144) have been associated with use of the live oral poliovirus vaccine (OPV). The current ACIP recommendations are for all children to receive four doses of polio vaccine inactivated (IPV) at ages 2 months, 4 months, 6 to 18 months, and 4 to 6 years. OPV should be reserved for mass vaccination campaigns to control outbreaks of paralytic polio; unvaccinated children who will be traveling in

BOX 44-3	Measles Vaccine Combination Products
Measles Vaccine Combination Products	**Trade Name**
Measles virus vaccine live (more attenuated Enders' line)	Attenuvax
Measles and rubella virus vaccine live	MRVAX II
Measles, mumps, and rubella virus vaccine live	MMR II

fewer than 4 weeks to areas where polio is endemic; and children of parents who do not accept the recommended number of vaccine injections.

IPV is available in a parenteral form as well. Unlike the OPV, which is a live, attenuated virus vaccine, IPV contains an inactivated form of the virus. IPV is administered subcutaneously or intramuscularly. It is classified as pregnancy category B. The recommended dosages for this vaccine are given in the dosages table on p. 690.

OPV (Orimune) is derived from live, attenuated types 1, 2, and 3 poliovirus obtained from monkey kidney tissue cultures. OPV promotes immunity to polio by causing the production of antibodies against the injected live, attenuated virus in the lymphatic tissues surrounding the intestinal tract. This occurs because the vaccine is taken orally. The intestinal tract is the normal portal of entry of poliovirus, and this intestinal immunity may reduce the number of temporary carriers and hence dissemination of the virus.

varicella vaccine

The live attenuated varicella vaccine (Varivax) is the vaccine used to prevent varicella (chicken pox) and herpes zoster (shingles) infections. Varicella primarily occurs in children less than 8 years of age or in individuals with compromised immune systems such as elderly or HIV-infected patients. It is estimated that only 10% of children over 12 years of age are still susceptible to varicella. Only 2% of adults develop varicella infections. However, 50% of the deaths associated with varicella infections are in adults. Half of these are in immunocompromised patients.

The varicella vaccine is attenuated by passage in human and embryonic guinea pig cell cultures. Varicella vaccine must be stored in a freezer. It should not be given to immunodeficient patients, pregnant woman, or to patients who have received high doses of systemic steroids in the previous month. It is also recommended that salicylates be avoided for 6 weeks after vaccination with varicella vaccine because of the possibility of Reye's syndrome. The recommended dosages for this vaccine are given in the dosages table on p. 690.

Activity

PASSIVE IMMUNIZING AGENTS

The currently available antivenins, antitoxins, and immune globulins that comprise the passive immunizing agents are listed in Box 44-1. Those that are more frequently used are described in the following profiles.

hepatitis B immune globulin

Hepatitis B immune globulin (H-BIG$_2$ Hep-B-Gammagee, HyperHep) is used to provide passive immunity to hepatitis B infection in the pro-phylaxis and post-exposure treatment of people exposed to hepatitis B virus or HbsAg-positive materials (e.g., blood, plasma, serum). It is prepared from the plasma of human donors with high titers of antibody to HbsAg. All donors are tested for the antibody to HIV to prevent transmission of the virus.

H-BIG is contraindicated in people who have exhibited hypersensitivity to it. Because of the possible devastating consequences of exposure to hepatitis B infection, pregnancy is not considered a contraindication to the use of H-BIG when there is a clear need for it. H-BIG is available only in a parenteral form that is administered intramuscularly. The recommended dosages for hepatitis B immune globulin are given in the dosages table on p. 690.

immune globulin

Immune globulin (Gammagard, Gammar, Iveegam, Polygam, Sandoglobulin, Venoglobulin) can be administered intramuscularly or intravenously. It is used to provide passive immunity by increasing antibody titer and antigen-antibody reaction potential. The agents are available only parenterally and called *immune globulin IM* (IGIM) and *immune globulin IV* (IGIV), which designates the route of administration. They are given to help prevent certain infectious diseases in susceptible people or to ameliorate the diseases in those already infected with them. Immune globulins are pooled from the blood of at least 1000 human donors. This plasma is prepared by cold alcohol fractionation and usually washed with a detergent to destroy any harmful viruses such as hepatitis or HIV. There are many FDA-approved and non–FDA-approved uses for immune globulins; these are listed in Box 44-4. In recent years there has been a shortage of available immune globulin products. The supply of these agents is dependent upon donors. Immune globulins come from pooled human plasma and are therefore subject to restrictions. Because of fluctuations in supply and the risk-benefit ratio of a human donor, product insurers have restricted reimbursement to force compliance with FDA-approved uses only. "Off-labeled," or non–FDA-approved uses, have been severely curtailed because of this and product shortages.

Immune globulins are contraindicated in patients hypersensitive to them and are classified as pregnancy category C agents. The recommended dosages for the immune globulins are given in the dosages table on p. 690.

Rh$_0$(D) immune globulin

Rh$_0$(D) immune globulin (Rhesonativ, HypRho-D Mini-Dose, MICRhoGAM, Gamulin Rh) is used to suppress the active antibody response and the formation of anti-Rh$_0$(D) in the Rh$_0$(D)-negative person exposed to Rh-positive blood. Because an Rh$_0$(D)-

negative person reacts to Rh-positive blood as if it were a foreign, "non-self" product, an immune response develops against it and an antigen-antibody reaction occurs. This can be fatal, and the administration of this immune globulin helps prevent the reaction, and hence this dire outcome. The most common use of this product is for maternal-fetal Rh incompatibility (postpartum).

$Rh_0(D)$ immune globulin is prepared from the plasma or serum of adults with a high titer of anti-$Rh_0(D)$ antibody to the red blood cell antigen $Rh_0(D)$. This product is available only in a parenteral formulation and is given by IM injection. This immune globulin is contraindicated in people who have been previously immunized with this drug and in $Rh_0(D)$-positive/Du-positive patients. The recommended dosages for $Rh_0(D)$ immune globulin are given in the dosages table on p. 690.

tetanus immune globulin

Tetanus immune globulin (TIG; Hyper-Tet) is a passive immunizing agent effective against tetanus. It contains tetanus antitoxin antibodies that neutralize the exotoxin produced by *Clostridium tetani*, the organism that causes tetanus. TIG is prepared from the plasma of adults hyperimmunized with the tetanus toxoid and is given as prophylaxis to people with tetanus-prone wounds. It may also be used to treat tetanus. Hypersensitivity, active infection, a poliomyelitis outbreak, and immunosuppression are contraindications to its use, and it is classified as a pregnancy category C agent. TIG is available only as a parenteral drug that is given by IM injection. The recommended dosages for TIG are given in the dosages table on p. 690.

varicella zoster immune globulin

Varicella-zoster immune globulin (VZIG) can be used to modify or prevent chickenpox in susceptible individuals who have had recent significant exposure to the disease. Administration of VZIG should be within 96 hours of exposure. Candidates for therapy with VZIG are those at high risk of serious disease or complications if they become infected with the varicella zoster virus (VZV). Some examples are newborn children, premature infants with significant exposure, and immunocompromised adults. Healthy adults, including pregnant women, should be evaluated on a case-by-case basis. The duration of protection against infection VZIG is at least 3 weeks.

VZIG is prepared from plasma of normal blood donors with high antibody titers to VZV. The recommended dose of VZIG is 125 U/kg, up to a maximum of 625 U, given intramuscularly. Higher doses may be considered for immunosuppressed patients. It is important that VZIG be given within 96 hours of exposure, preferably as soon as possible.

BOX 44-4 Uses of Immune Globulins

FDA-APPROVED
Chronic lymphocytic leukemia (CLL)
Hepatitis A
Idiopathic thrombocytopenic purpura (ITP)
IM
Immune deficiencies
IV
Measles
Primary immunodeficiency diseases
Varicella
NON–FDA-APPROVED
AIDS
Asthma
Autoimmune disorders
Cystic fibrosis
Epilepsy
Kawasaki syndrome
Neonatal sepsis
Other viral infections
Respiratory syncytial virus (RSV)

---

nursing process

• Assessment

Before administering a toxoid or vaccine, the nurse should gather complete information about the patient's health history, including information on allergies, the patient's present health status, previous reactions and responses to these agents, any allergy test results, the use of any immunosuppressants, the presence of autoimmune or immunosuppressing disease, infection, and the pregnancy status. In children who are to receive a vaccine or toxoid, the immunization schedule and the dose ordered by the physician must be followed.

Because passive immunizing agents may precipitate serum sickness, patients with chronic illness or who are elderly or debilitated need to be assessed carefully before treatment (i.e., vital signs, intake and output, ECG, and baseline assessment). Contraindications to the use of passive immunizing agents include hypersensitivity to them and patients with active infections or who are immunosuppressed.

Contraindications to the administration of immunizing agents include active infections, febrile illnesses, a history of reactions or serious side effects to the agent, and pregnancy. Patients who are already immunosuppressed (e.g., those with AIDS, elderly patients, patients with chronic diseases or cancer, and neonates) are at increased risk for experiencing serious side effects to toxoids or vaccines, so cautious use of these agents is called for in such patients.

• Nursing Diagnoses

Nursing diagnoses related to the administration of immunizing agents include the following:

• Risk for injury related to possible side effects of or allergic reactions to the immunizing agent.

- Acute pain related to local and/or systemic effects of the injection of a toxoid, vaccine, or passive immunizing agent.
- Deficient knowledge related to the use of toxoids, vaccines, or passive immunizing agents.

● Planning

Goals for patients receiving immunizing agents include the following:
- Patient states side effects of medication.
- Patient manages minimal discomfort stemming from the administration of a toxoid, vaccine, or passive immunizing agent.
- Patient remains compliant with therapy.
- Patient returns for follow-up injections and booster injections and for follow-up visits with the physician.

Outcome Criteria

Outcome criteria related to the use of immunologic agents include the following:
- Patient will experience minimal side effects of or allergic reactions to the immunizing agent such as fever, chills, myalgias, and bronchospasms (allergic).
- Patient will use measures such as nonaspirin analgesics or diphenhydramine (as recommended by physician) to relieve localized discomfort or to alleviate any reactions.
- Patient will remain compliant with therapy for prevention of illness or disease through follow-up visits with physician.
- Patient will state the problems to report immediately to the physician such as fever higher than 101° F, infection, wheezing, or increasing weakness.

● Implementation

When administering immunologic agents, it is always important to recheck the specific protocols concerning their administration and the schedules of administration. In addition, it is always important to check and follow the manufacturer's recommendations concerning how the drug should be stored and administered, routes and site of administration, dosage, precautions pertaining to its use, and contraindications to its use. Parents of young children must be encouraged and told how to maintain an accurate journal of the child's immunization status.

Patient teaching tips are presented in the box below.

● Evaluation

Therapeutic responses in patients receiving immunizing agents are the prevention or amelioration of the disease. Adverse reactions for which to monitor in patients receiving immunizing biologicals include localized swelling, redness, discomfort, and heat. Acetaminophen is recommended for the relief of these side effects in patients of all age groups. Warm compresses on the injection site may also help to ease some of the discomfort. The physician should be notified immediately if fever, rash, itching or shortness of breath occur, because these are the symptoms of an allergic reaction. As immunizing agents improve and newer agents are developed, it is hopeful that, as with DTaP, fewer side effects will occur, resulting in fewer adverse drug events and complications.

---

patient teaching tips

Toxoids and Vaccines

➤ It is not uncommon for patients to experience a localized reaction to the injection of a toxoid, vaccine, or passive immunizing agent. They should be told that they can relieve the discomfort by placing warm compresses on the injection site, resting, and taking acetaminophen. Instructions for the care of infants or children suffering such reactions should be provided by the child's health care provider.

➤ Patients or the parents or caregiver of the child should notify the physician should high or prolonged fever, rash, itching, or shortness of breath occur.

➤ Patients or parents should always keep a double record (two copies kept in separate places) of all the medications being taken.

➤ A vaccine adverse event reporting system is available through the FDA by calling 1-800-822-7967.

POINTS TO REMEMBER

Antibodies and Antigens
- A foreign substance in the body is termed an *antigen*; the body creates a substance called an *antibody* to specifically bind to it.
- The body has cells called *plasma cells* that remember what that particular antigen looks like.
- These plasma cells manufacture the antibodies and will mass produce clones of the antibodies upon reexposure to a particular antigen.

Immunization
- Two types: active and passive.
- Different types of agents used in each.
- Are indicated for use in different patient populations.

Active Immunization
- Utilizes a toxoid or a vaccine.
- Involves exposing the body to a relatively harmless form of the antigen (foreign invader) to imprint mem-

ory and stimulate the body's defenses against any subsequent exposure.
- The person receiving must have an active, functioning immune system.
- Provides long-lasting or permanent immunity.

Passive Immunization
- Utilizes immune globulins, antitoxins, or antivenins.
- Takes serum or concentrated immune globulins obtained from humans or animals.
- Injected into the patient, directly giving him or her the ability to fight off the invading microorganism.
- For patients who are immunocompromised, been exposed to disease, or anticipate exposure to the disease.
- Provides temporary protection.
- Does not stimulate an antibody response in the host.

Nursing Considerations
- Patients who should *not* receive immunizing agents include those with active infections, febrile illnesses, or a history of a previous reaction or serious side effects to the agent. They are also usually contraindicated in pregnant women.
- Patients who are immunosuppressed are at greater risk for suffering serious side effects from immunizing agents.
- Parents should keep updated records of their children's and their own immunizations with any toxoids or vaccines.
- Health care reform and discussions of rationing care necessitates the need to understand the importance of immunizations and their role in preventing disease. However, it is also critical that all risks are addressed.

REVIEW QUESTIONS

1. Which type of immunity occurs when an individual is exposed to relatively harmless forms of antigens to build a defense against subsequent exposures to a specific infection?
   a. Active immunity
   b. Accentuated active immunity
   c. Naturally acquired passive immunity
   d. Artificially acquired passive immunity
2. Severe adverse effects related to immunizing agents include all of the following *except:*
   a. dyspnea.
   b. cyanosis.
   c. adenopathy.
   d. a fever 103° F or above.

3. Which of the following is a severe rare reaction to the influenza vaccine?
   a. Renal failure
   b. Cadiomegaly
   c. Hepatotoxicity
   d. Guillain-Barré syndrome
4. The DTaP or DTP vaccine is first given at what age?
   a. 2 months
   b. 4 months
   c. 8 months
   d. 12 months
5. After given in infancy, the tetanus vaccine should be repeated at what time?
   a. 3 years of age
   b. 6 years of age
   c. 10 years of age
   d. Only as indicated with injury

For Answers see www.harcourthealth.com/MERLIN/Lilley/.

CRITICAL THINKING Activities

1. You are caring for a 56-year-old man who has recently been admitted because he is in a state of acute rejection of his transplanted heart, which he received over a year ago. This patient has been on cyclosporine, azathioprine, and prednisone at home and has now had muromonab (OKT-3) added to help stop the acute rejection. There has been an outbreak of the influenza virus at your hospital. One of your co-workers suggests vaccinating your patient with the flu vaccine that employee health has been administering to the employees. How should you respond to this co-worker in order to express your concern for her statement and its implication to the patient?
2. Describe the schedule currently recommended for immunizations in the United States. What are the implications of not having a child properly immunized?
3. How has health care reform influenced the issue of immunization?

For Answers see www.harcourthealth.com/MERLIN/Lilley/.

bibliography

Albanese J, Nutz P: *Mosby's 2001 nursing drug reference and review cards,* St Louis, 2001, Mosby.

American Academy of Pediatrics: *Immunization protects children: 2001 immunization schedule,* 2001. Available at www.aap.org/family/parents/immunize.htm.

American Hospital Formulary Service: *AHFS drug information,* Bethesda, Md, 2000, American Society of Health-System Pharmacists.

Anderson PO, Knoben JE, Troutman WG: *Handbook of clinical drug data 1999-2000,* ed 9, New York, 1999, McGraw-Hill.

Johns Hopkins Hospital, Department of Pediatrics et al: *The Harriet Lane handbook,* ed 15, St. Louis, 2000, Mosby.

Keen JH: *Critical care and emergency drug reference,* ed 3, St Louis, 1996, Mosby.

Mosby's GenRx: a comprehensive reference for generic and brand drugs, ed 10, St Louis, 2000, Mosby.

Skidmore-Roth L: *Mosby's 2001 nursing drug reference,* St Louis, 2001, Mosby.

United States Department of Health and Human Services: *Healthy children 2000,* Washington, DC, 2000, Health Resources and Services Administration.

United States Pharmacopeial Convention: *USP DI: drug information for the health care professional, vol. 1,* ed 20, Englewood, Colo, 2000, Micromedex.

Remember to check the **Online Worksheet** for additional learning opportunities: **www.harcourthealth.com/MERLIN/Lilley/**

Chapter 45

Antineoplastic Agents

When you reach the end of this chapter, you should be able to do the following:

1 Discuss the purpose of antineoplastic agents in the treatment of cancer.

2 Classify antineoplastic agents and monoclonal antibodies by their mechanisms of action.

3 List the common side effects of and toxic reactions to antineoplastic agents and monoclonal antibodies.

4 Discuss the mechanisms of action, cautions, contraindications, routes of administration, and drug interactions associated with the use of all classes of antineoplastic agents and the monoclonal antibodies.

5 Develop a nursing care plan that includes all phases of the nursing process for the patient receiving antineoplastic agents and monoclonal antibodies.

www.harcourthealth.com/MERLIN/Lilley/

Look for this symbol for topics covered in the **Online Worksheet**

drug profiles

altretamine, p. 722
asparaginase, p. 722
bleomycin, p. 714
carmustine, p. 708
cisplatin, p. 708
cyclophosphamide, p. 708
cytarabine, p. 712
doxorubicin, p. 714
etoposide, p. 717

hydroxyurea, p. 722
mechlorethamine, p. 709
mercaptopurine, p. 712
methotrexate, p. 711
paclitaxel, p. 717
rituximab, p. 720
topotecan, p. 719
trastuzumab, p. 720
vincristine, p. 717

Key drug.

glossary

Alkylation (al′ kə la′ shən) Chemical reaction in which an alkyl group is transferred from an alkylating agent. When such organic reactions occur with a biologically significant cellular constituent such as DNA, they result in interference with mitosis and cell division. (p. 706)

Benign (be nin′) Noncancerous and therefore not an immediate threat to life, even though treatment eventually may be required for health or cosmetic reasons. (p. 700)

Bifunctional Refers to alkylating agents that have two reactive alkyl groups that are able to alkylate two DNA molecules. (p. 706)

Carcinoma (kahr′ si no′ mə) Malignant epithelial neoplasm that tends to invade surrounding tissue and to metastasize to distant regions of the body. (p. 700)

Cell cycle nonspecific Antineoplastic drugs that are cytotoxic in any phase of the cycle. (p. 703)

Cell cycle specific Antineoplastic drugs that are cytotoxic during a specific cell cycle phase. (p. 703)

Dose-limiting side effects Side effects that prevent the antineoplastic agent from being given in higher doses, often limiting the effectiveness of the drug. (p. 704)

Emetic potential (ə me′ tik) Potential of a substance to irritate the cells of the stomach, resulting in nausea and vomiting. (p. 704)

Extravasation (ek stra ve′ ə sa′ shən) Passage or escape into the tissues, usually of blood, serum, or lymph, but in the context of antineoplastic treatment, of the agent. (p. 707)

Growth fraction Percentage of cells in mitosis at any given time. (p. 703)

Leucovorin rescue (loo′ ko vo′ rin) The use of leucovorin to reverse methotrexate-induced toxicity. (p. 710)

Leukemia (loo ke′ me ə) A malignant neoplasm of blood-forming tissues characterized by the diffuse replacement of bone marrow with proliferating leukocyte precursors, abnormal numbers and forms of immature white blood cells in the circulation, and the infiltration of lymph nodes, the spleen, and liver. (p. 701)

Lymphoma (lim fo′ mə) A neoplasm of lymphoid tissue that is usually malignant but in rare cases may be benign. (p. 701)

Malignant (mə lig′ nənt) Tending to worsen and cause death; anaplastic, invasive, and metastatic. (p. 700)

Metastasis (mə tas′ tə sis) The process by which a cancer spreads from the original site of growth to a new and remote part of the body. (p. 700)

Mitosis (mi to′ sis) Process of cell reproduction occurring in somatic cells and resulting in the formation of two genetically identical daughter cells containing the diploid number of chromosomes characteristic of the species. (p. 703)

Mitotic index (mi to′ tik) Number of cells per unit (usually 1000) undergoing mitosis during a given time. (p. 703)

Nadir (na′ dər) Lowest point, such as the blood count after it has been depressed by chemotherapy. Regarding antineoplastic agents, this term refers to the time frame in which they kill bone marrow cells. (p. 705)

Paraneoplastic syndrome (PNS) (par′ ə ne′ o plas′ tik) Signs and symptoms of cancer located at a distance from the tumor or its metastatic sites. (p. 701)

Polyfunctional Refers to the action of alkylating agents that can perform several alkylation reactions. (p. 706)

Sarcoma (sahr′ ko′ mə) A malignant neoplasm of the soft tissues arising in fibrous, fatty, muscular, synovial, vascular, or neural tissue, usually first presenting as a painless swelling. (p. 701)

Tumor (too′ mor) A new growth of tissue characterized by a progressive, uncontrolled proliferation of cells. (p. 700)

Cancer is a broad term embracing a group of diseases that are characterized by uncontrolled cellular growth and possible invasion into surrounding tissue as well as by metastasis to new sites distant from the original body site. This cellular growth differs from normal cell growth in that cancerous cells do not possess a growth control mechanism, and the resulting cell usually has no physiologic function. Cancerous cells will continue to grow and invade adjacent structures, or they may break away from the original tumor mass and travel by means of the blood or lymphatic system to establish a new clone (metastatic lesion) elsewhere in the body.

Metastasis refers to the spreading of a cancer (uncontrolled cell growth) from the original site of growth to a new and remote part of the body (secondary growth). The terms *malignancy, neoplasm,* and *tumor* are often used as synonyms for cancer; however, they all have their own meaning. A neoplasm is a mass of new cells that exhibit uncontrolled cellular reproduction. It is another term for **tumor.** There are two types of neoplasms, or tumors— benign and malignant. A **benign** tumor is of a uniform size and shape and displays no invasive or metastatic properties. The terms *nonmalignant* and *benign* suggest that tumors may be harmless, which is true in most cases. However, a benign tumor can be lethal if it grows in vital tissue and interrupts normal function. **Malignant** neoplasms typically consist of cancerous cells that invade surrounding tissues and metastasize to other tissues and organs where they form metastatic tumor deposits. Some of the various respective characteristics of benign and malignant neoplasms, or tumors, are listed in Table 45-1.

Table 45-1 Tumor Characteristics: Benign and Malignant

Characteristic	Benign	Malignant
Potential to metastasize	No	Yes
Encapsulated	Yes	No
Similar to tissue of origin	Yes	No
Rate of growth	Slow	Unpredictable and unrestrained
Recurrence after surgical removal	Rare	Common

Over 100 types of malignant neoplasms affect humans. They are usually classified by their primary anatomic (organ) location and the type of cell from which the neoplasm develops. Common body sites for malignant neoplasm growth are as follows:

- Bladder and kidney
- Colon
- Prostate gland
- Uterus
- Blood-producing tissue
- Lymphatic system
- Rectum
- Breast
- Lung
- Skin

Tumors are classified according to their tissue of origin, and the various categories are sarcomas, carcinomas, lymphomas, leukemias, and tumors of nervous tissue origin. A list of common malignant tumors and their tissue of origin are provided in Box 45-1. It is important to know the tissue of origin because this determines the type of chemotherapy used, the likely response to therapy, and the prognosis.

Carcinomas arise from epithelial tissue, which is located throughout the body. It covers or lines all body surfaces, both inside and outside the body. Examples are the skin, the mucosal lining of the entire gastrointestinal

Box 45-1 Tumor Classification Based on Specific Tissue of Origin

Tissue of Origin	Malignant Tissue
EPITHELIAL = CARCINOMAS	
Glands or ducts	Adenocarcinomas
Respiratory tract	Small- and large-cell carcinomas
Kidney	Renal cell carcinoma
Skin	Squamous cell, epidermoid, and basal cell carcinoma
CONNECTIVE = SARCOMAS	
Fibrous	Fibrosarcoma
Cartilage	Chondrosarcoma
Bone	Osteogenic sarcoma (Ewing's tumor)
Blood vessels	Kaposi's sarcoma
Peripheral nerve	Neuroblastoma
LYMPHATIC = LYMPHOMAS	
Lymph tissue	Lymphomas (Hodgkin's disease and multiple myeloma)
Synovia	Synoviosarcoma
Mesothelium	Mesothelioma
NERVE	
Glial	Glioma
Adrenal medulla	Pheochromocytoma
BLOOD	
White blood cells	Leukemia

tract, and the bronchial tree (lungs). The purpose of these epithelial tissues is to protect the body's vital organs.

Sarcomas are malignant tumors that arise from connective tissues. This tissue is the most abundant and widely distributed of all tissues and can be found in bone, cartilage, muscle, blood, lymphatic, and vascular tissue. Its purpose is to support and protect other tissues.

Lymphomas arise from the lymphatic tissue, and **leukemias** arise from the various types of leukocytes. These two types of tumors differ from carcinomas and sarcomas in that the cancerous cells do not form solid tumors but are interspersed throughout the lymphatic or circulatory system and interfere with the normal functioning of these systems. The last (fifth) type of tumor is that which originates from neural tissue.

Cancers may produce signs and symptoms caused by changes in tissues remote from the tumor or its site of metastasis. This symptom complex is referred to as the **paraneoplastic syndrome (PNS),** and some of the various disorders produced are listed in Box 45-2. The syndrome is believed to result from the effects of biologically or immunologically active substances secreted by the tumors. Some patients may also exhibit generalized symptoms, such as anorexia, weight loss, fatigue, and fever.

ETIOLOGY OF CANCER

The etiology of cancer remains a mystery for the most part, and cancer researchers have made slow progress toward identifying possible causes. In recent years certain etiologic factors have come to light, however, and some of these and the cancers they cause are listed in Box 45-3. In addition, radiation; oncogenic viruses; and immunologic, ethnic, genetic, and age- and sex-related factors have also been identified.

AGE- AND SEX-RELATED DIFFERENCES

The probability of a neoplastic disease developing generally increases with advancing age, but lymphocytic leukemia and Wilms' tumor are exceptions to this. The incidence of these decreases with age. On the other hand,

lymphocytic and myelocytic leukemia and colon and lung cancer usually develop during middle and old age. These cancers are rare in young children.

With the exception of cancers affecting the reproductive system, few cancers exhibit a sex-related difference in their incidence. Lung and urinary cancers are more common in men than in women, but this may have more to do with exogenous factors such as smoking patterns and exposure to environmental toxins than to sex-related causes. The incidence of colon, rectal, pancreatic, and skin cancers as well as leukemia is almost equal between the sexes.

GENETIC AND ETHNIC FACTORS

Few cancers appear to be inherited on a genetic basis (breast, colon, and stomach cancers are exceptions). Advancements in understanding of tumor biology status have helped guide therapy tremendously. Hormone receptor status (estrogen receptor [ER] and progesterone receptor [PR]) and the presence of certain gene expressions, such as the HER2/neu gene, are a couple of examples. These cancers often show a familial pattern of inheritance. Burkitt's lymphoma is an example of a cancer that shows a racial pattern of inheritance. The disease is more common in young African children and

---

Box 45-2 Paraneoplastic Syndrome Associated with Some Cancers

Paraneoplastic Syndrome	Associated Cancer
Hypercalcemia, sensory neuropathies, SIADH	Lung
Disseminated intravascular coagulation	Leukemia
Cushing's syndrome	Lung, thyroid, testes, adrenal
Addison's syndrome	Adrenal, lymphomas

SIADH, Syndrome of inappropriate antidiuretic hormone secretion.

Box 45-3 Cancer: Proposed Etiologic Factors

Risk Factor	Associated Cancer
ENVIRONMENT	
Radiation (ionizing)	Leukemia, breast, thyroid
Radiation (ultraviolet)	Skin, melanoma
Viruses	Leukemia, lymphoma, nasopharyngeal
FOOD	
Aflatoxin	Liver
Dietary factors	Colon, breast, endometrium, gallbladder
LIFESTYLE	
Alcohol	Esophagus, liver, stomach, larynx
Tobacco	Lung, mouth, esophagus, larynx
MEDICAL DRUGS	
Diethylstilbestrol (DES)	Vaginal in offspring
Estrogens	Endometrial
Alkylating agents	Leukemia, bladder
OCCUPATIONAL	
Asbestos	Lung, mesothelioma
Aniline dye	Bladder
Benzene	Leukemia
Vinyl chloride	Liver
REPRODUCTIVE HISTORY	
Late first pregnancy	Breast
No children	Ovary
Multiple sexual partners	Cervix, uterus

children of African descent than in non-African children. Another example of an ethnic predisposition is the high incidence of nasopharyngeal cancer in people of Chinese extraction.

ONCOGENIC VIRUSES

Extensive research has indicated that there are cancer-causing (oncogenic) viruses that can affect most mammalian species. Examples include the various cat leukemias, the Rous* sarcoma virus in chickens, human papilloma viruses (HPV), and the Shope* papilloma in rabbits.

The herpes viruses are common examples of oncogenic viruses. Epstein-Barr virus, also known as infectious mononucleosis, is associated with the development of Burkitt's lymphoma and nasopharyngeal cancer. There also seems to be a link between the development of cervical cancer and infection with the herpes simplex type 2 virus (herpes genitalis). Other viruses linked to cancers are HPVs, which have been linked to certain bladder cancers.

*Doctors P. Rous and R. Shope were early investigators of oncogenic viruses.

BOX 45-4 Carcinogens

Chemical	Description
Aflatoxins	A group of toxic/carcinogenic products produced by the mold *Aspergillus* which contaminates peanuts and grains; aflatoxins are associated with the development of liver cancers.
Asbestos	Associated with the development of lung cancer and mesothelioma; asbestos is found in pipe and fire insulation, especially in older buildings.
Benzene	Associated with the development of acute myelogenous leukemia
Chimney soot	One of the first carcinogens to be identified (in English chimney sweepers); it is associated with the development of scrotal cancer.
Naphthalene dyes (aniline dyes)	Associated with the development of bladder cancer.
Polyvinyl chloride (PVCs)	Associated with the development of liver sarcomas.
Printer's ink	Associated with the development of liver and bladder cancer.
Smoked fish and meats	Diets rich in smoked food-stuffs is associated with the development of stomach cancer.
Tobacco	Smoking (cigarettes, pipe) and chewing tobacco are associated with the development of respiratory tract cancers.

OCCUPATIONAL AND ENVIRONMENTAL CARCINOGENS

A carcinogen is a physical or chemical agent that can induce the development of a cancer or accelerate its growth. Box 45-4 contains a selected listing of such agents.

DRUGS

Many drugs that were once considered safe have proved to be carcinogenic. For this reason, FDA regulations now mandate that carcinogenic studies be done before any new drug is approved for use. However, no amount of clinical testing can fully reveal all the possible carcinogenic and mutagenic effects. One reason for this is that testing for drug carcinogenic activity is difficult and current test methods are not very satisfactory. Besides this there can be species-related differences in a particular drug (e.g., carcinogenic activity). These effects are not observed in the laboratory animals on which the agent has been tested and only become obvious when used in human subjects. Refer to Box 45-5 for a partial listing of carcinogenic drugs.

RADIATION

Radiation is a well-known and potent carcinogenic agent. In fact, several scientists who studied radiation or who worked on the development of the first atomic bomb* were victims of cancer. There are two basic types of radiation: (1) ionizing, or high-energy, radiation and (2) nonionizing, or low-energy, radiation. Both types can be carcinogenic. Ionizing radiation is very potent and can penetrate deeply into the body. It is called *ionizing* because it causes the formation of ions within living cells.

*Enrico Fermi, a nuclear physicist who worked on the development of the atomic bomb, died of leukemia.

BOX 45-5 Drug Carcinogens

Drug	Associated Carcinogenic Activity
Acetophenetidin (obsolete analgesic also known as phenacetin)	Renal cancer
Anabolic steroids	Liver cancer
Antineoplastics	Leukemia and cancer of the bladder, GI tract, skin
Coal tar preparations	Skin cancer
Diethylstilbestrol (DES)	Vaginal adenocarcinoma in female offspring of mothers who took DES during pregnancy
Estrogens	Vaginal and cervical cancer and postmenopausal endometrial cancer
Reserpine	Possible link to breast cancer

This type of radiation (e.g., x-ray studies, radium implants) is used to treat (irradiate) cancerous tumors. Nonionizing radiation is much less potent and cannot penetrate deeply into the body. Sunlight and ultraviolet light are examples of this type of radiation. Sunlight is a major cause of skin cancer, and ultraviolet light, which was used for the treatment of skin conditions of the head and neck, is known to cause thyroid cancer.

IMMUNOLOGIC FACTORS

The immune system plays an important role in cancer surveillance and the elimination of neoplastic cells. Implication of this can be seen with a variety of patient types. Examples include patients undergoing cancer chemotherapy, organ transplant patients receiving immunosuppressive therapy, patients suffering from immunologic impairment or disease, and patients with acquired immunodeficiency syndrome (AIDS). It has been shown that there is a much higher incidence of cancer in immunocompromised people. It has been suggested that neoplastic cells develop in everyone but that the immune system in healthy people recognizes them as abnormal and eliminates them by means of cell-mediated immunity.

This relationship between cancer and a suppressed immune system has also been noted in cancer patients being treated with immunotherapy consisting of interferon derivatives, the bacillus Calmette-Guérin (BCG) vaccine, and lymphokines.

CELL GROWTH CYCLE

Normal cells in the body divide (proliferate) in a controlled and organized fashion, and this growth is regulated by means of various mechanisms. In contrast, cancer cells lack regulatory mechanisms and they proliferate uncontrollably, though some modulation of cancer cell proliferation may occur if blood flow to the cancer is disrupted. Their growth is usually also constant. Thus an important characteristic of malignant tumors is the time it takes for the tumor to double in size. This doubling time varies greatly for various types of cancers and is directly related to and important in determining the prognosis for a particular patient. Cancer treatment that cannot destroy every neoplastic cell does not retard the regrowth of the tumor, and the time it takes for regrowth to occur depends on the doubling time of the particular cancer. For instance, Burkitt's lymphoma has an extremely short doubling time, whereas multiple myeloma has one of the longest.

The cell growth characteristics for normal and neoplastic cells are similar. Both types of cells go through five distinct growth phase cycles: G_0, the resting phase; G_1, the first growth, or postmitotic, phase; S, the DNA synthesis phase; G_2, the second growth, or premitotic, phase; and M, the **mitosis** phase (cell reproduction). Two identical daughter cells are the final product of this process in one cell. A complete cycle from one mitosis to the next is called the *generation time*, and it is different for all tumors, ranging from hours to days. The cell growth cycle and the events that occur in the various phases are summarized in Box 45-6.

The activity of a mass of tumor cells can also be characterized, and it has an important bearing on the killing power of chemotherapy. The percentage of cells undergoing mitosis at any given time is called the **growth fraction** of the tumor mass. The number of cells that are in the M phase of the cell cycle is called the **mitotic index.** Chemotherapy is most effective when the greatest number of cells are dividing (i.e., when both the growth fraction and mitotic index are high).

Drugs used for chemotherapy are called *antineoplastic agents,* and they can be subdivided into two main groups of agents based on where in the cell cycle they work. Antineoplastic drugs that are cytotoxic in any phase of the cycle are called **cell cycle–nonspecific** (CCNS) agents. Those agents that are cytotoxic during a specific life cycle phase are called **cell cycle–specific** (CCS) agents. CCNS agents are effective against large, slowly growing tumors. CCS agents are effective against rapidly growing tumors. Some examples of CCNS and CCS antineoplastic agents are listed in Box 45-7, and Fig. 45-1 shows where in the general phase of the cell cycle the primary chemotherapeutic agents kill the cancerous cells.

The ultimate goal of any anticancer regimen is to kill every neoplastic cell and produce a cure, but this goal is not achieved in most cases. One reason for this is that

---

Box 45-6 Cell Cycle Phases

Phase		Description
G_0	Resting phase	Most normal human cells exist predominantly in this phase. Cancer cells in this phase are not susceptible to the toxic effects of chemotherapy.
G_1	Postmitotic phase	Enzymes necessary for DNA synthesis are produced.
S	DNA synthesis phase	DNA synthesis takes place, from DNA separation to DNA replication.
G_2	Premitotic phase	RNA and specialized proteins are made.
M	Mitosis phase	Divided into four phases: prophase, metaphase, anaphase, and telophase.

Box 45-7 CCNS and CCS Antineoplastics

Antineoplastic	Cell Cycle Type
Alkylating agent	Cell cycle nonspecific
Antimetabolites	Cell cycle specific in the S phase
Mitotic inhibitors	Cell cycle specific in the M phase

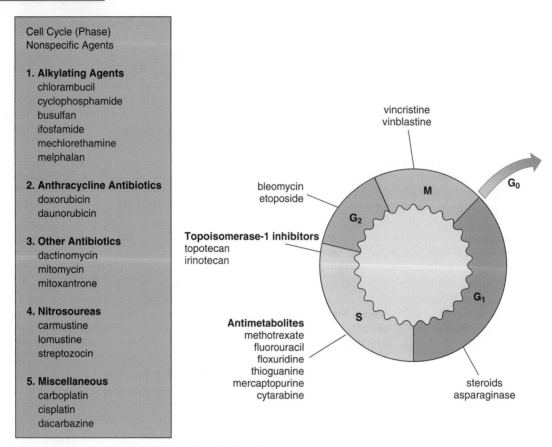

Cell Cycle (Phase)
Nonspecific Agents

1. Alkylating Agents
chlorambucil
cyclophosphamide
busulfan
ifosfamide
mechlorethamine
melphalan

2. Anthracycline Antibiotics
doxorubicin
daunorubicin

3. Other Antibiotics
dactinomycin
mitomycin
mitoxantrone

4. Nitrosoureas
carmustine
lomustine
streptozocin

5. Miscellaneous
carboplatin
cisplatin
dacarbazine

vincristine
vinblastine

bleomycin
etoposide

Topoisomerase-1 inhibitors
topotecan
irinotecan

Antimetabolites
methotrexate
fluorouracil
floxuridine
thioguanine
mercaptopurine
cytarabine

steroids
asparaginase

G_0
M
G_2
G_1
S

Fig. 45-1 Cell cycle specificity of antineoplastics. General phase of the cell cycle with corresponding action of specific antineoplastic agents to produce cancerous cell kill.

antineoplastic agents are usually cytotoxic and not tumoricidal. That is, they can only kill cells while they are dividing, not all the cancer cells regardless of where they are in the cell growth cycle when exposed to the antineoplastic agent. Other factors that affect the chances of cure and the length of survival include the cancer stage at the time of diagnosis, type of neoplasm and its doubling time, efficacy of the cancer treatment, development of drug resistance, and general health of the patient. When total cure is not possible, the primary goal of therapy is then to control the growth of the neoplasm while maintaining the best quality of life for the patient.

No antineoplastic agent is effective against all types of neoplasms, and they also have a low therapeutic index. However, one important discovery yielded by clinical experience is that a combination of agents is usually more effective than single-agent therapy. The reason for this is that, because drug-resistant cells often develop in tumors as the result of the tumor's genetic instability, exposure to multiple drugs with multiple mechanisms and sites of action will destroy more such subpopulations of malignant cells. The delayed onset of resistance to a particular antineoplastic agent is thus a benefit of combination drug therapy. To be most effective, however, the drugs used in such a combination regimen should be those with the following characteristics:

- Effective as sole agents in the treatment of the particular type of cancer

- Different mechanisms of action so that the cytotoxic effect is maximized
- Different cytotoxic properties so that each drug in the combination can be administered in a full therapeutic dose

One major drawback to the use of these agents is that nearly all of them cause side effects and adverse effects. Many of these effects are severe or toxic and stem from the fact that these agents are harmful to all rapidly growing cells—both the harmful cancer cells and beneficial human cells. Three types of such rapidly growing beneficial human cells are hair follicles, gastrointestinal cells, and bone marrow cells. Because the antineoplastic agents cannot differentiate between the cancer cells and these healthy cells, the latter are also killed, with hair loss, nausea and vomiting, and myelosuppression the undesirable consequences, respectively. These effects are called **dose-limiting side effects** because they prevent the antineoplastic agent from being administered in the high doses ideally needed to kill the entire population of cancer cells.

Some antineoplastic agents are more disruptive or harmful to the beneficial cells of the stomach, a property known as the **emetic potential** because it represents the extent to which an agent produces nausea and vomiting. Unfortunately, to prevent these side effects requires that the agent be given in doses that may be relatively ineffective when it comes to destroying the

Antineoplastics: Relative Emetic Potential

HIGH (>90%)
cisplatin
dacarbazine
mechlorethamine
streptozocin
cytarabine*

MODERATELY HIGH (60%-90%)
carmustine
lomustine
cyclophosphamide
actinomycin-D
mithramycin
procarbazine
methotrexate†

MODERATE (30%-60%)
5-fluorouracil
doxorubicin
daunorubicin
L-asparaginase
mitomycin-C

MODERATELY LOW (10%-30%)
bleomycin
hydroxyurea
melphalan
etoposide
teniposide
cytarabine‡
6-mercaptopurine
methotrexate§
thiotepa
vinblastine

LOW (<10%)
busulfan
chlorambucil
6-thioguanine
vincristine
estrogens
progestin
corticosteroids
androgens

*>500 mg/m².
†Doses >200 mg/m².
‡Standard doses.
§Low doses.

legal & ethical principles

Administration of Chemotherapeutic Agents

The law should always be viewed as helpful and as a framework for safe nursing practice. To help maintain safe nursing practice and to adhere to the standards of nursing practice, it is important to look at agents that may be worthy of close attention when performing dosage calculations and in their administration. Chemotherapeutic agents are toxic by their design. Because of their complexity and wide variety of dosing protocols or regimens, we should always be cautious with these medications. To help reduce errors with these groups of medications, it may be necessary to carefully design and implement standardized, preprinted order forms or computerized order sheet sets for all chemotherapeutic agents. The key is to "carefully design" and utilize nursing and pharmacy personnel to look at these issues. One area may be to require two independent calculations for ALL chemotherapy orders to help verify the dosage, an easy intervention to help prevent a possibly life-threatening medication error! ∎

Data from Institute for Safe Medication Practices, 1997.

cancer cells. The emetic potentials of the various antineoplastic drugs are summarized in Box 45-8.

Myelosuppression, or bone marrow suppression (BMS), is another unwanted effect of certain antineoplastics and results from the fact that certain cells in the bone marrow, such as granulocytes, lymphocytes, and platelets, are also destroyed. The specific hematologic disorder resulting from the myelosuppression depends on the particular cell line affected. For instance, if the cells in the bone marrow that make platelets are killed, the patient's platelet count will decrease and he or she will be more susceptible to bleeding. The point at which the bone marrow cells reach their lowest levels is the **nadir.** The time frame within which a patient reaches the nadir may become shorter and the recovery time for the bone marrow may become longer with subsequent courses of antineoplastic treatment.

Activity

ALKYLATING AGENTS

Mustard gas and the derivatives of the nitrogen mustards were the first alkylating agents, with nitrogen mustard (mechlorethamine) the prototypical agent. It was in the 1940s that its antineoplastic activity was discovered, and since that time, many analogues of the agent have been synthesized and introduced into use for the treatment of cancer.

The alkylating agents commonly used in clinical practice in the United States today consist of three categories of agents: classic alkylators; alkylator-like agents, which have a different chemical structure but work by alkyla-

tion; and nitrosoureas, which also have a different chemical structure but work by alkylation. These antineoplastics are generally considered CCNS agents, and they are used to treat a wide spectrum of malignancies, but especially solid tumors and hematologic malignancies. The agents in each category are as follows:

Classic alkylators
• busulfan
• chlorambucil
• cyclophosphamide
• ifosfamide
• mechlorethamine
• melphalan
• thiotepa (triethylene thiophosphoramide)

Alkylator-like agents
• carboplatin
• cisplatin
• dacarbazine
• procarbazine

Nitrosoureas
• carmustine
• lomustine
• streptozocin

Mechanism of Action

Alkylating agents are CCNS antineoplastics that are effective at any stage in the growth cycle of cancer cells and are most effective against rapidly growing cancer cells and normal body cells. These agents work by preventing the cancer cells from reproducing, and they have a unique way of accomplishing this. Specifically, they work by interfering with the chemical structure of the DNA essential to the reproduction of any cell, and they do this by

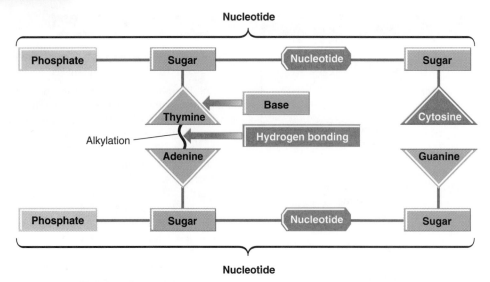

Fig. 45-2 Organization of DNA and site of action of alkylating agents.

Specific Alkylating Agents: Therapeutic Uses

Agent	Type of Cancer
CLASSIC ALKYLATORS	
busulfan	Chronic myelocytic leukemia
chlorambucil	Chronic lymphocytic leukemia, lymphomas, multiple myeloma
cyclophosphamide	Lymphomas, many solid tumors including those of breast, ovaries, and lung
ifosfamide	Germ cell testicular cancer
mechlorethamine	Hodgkin's disease
melphalan	Lymphomas, breast and ovarian carcinomas, multiple myeloma
thiotepa	Superficial bladder cancer, combination therapy for breast cancer
ALKYLATOR-LIKE AGENTS	
carboplatin	Testicular, ovarian, head and neck, and lung cancers
cisplatin	Testicular, ovarian, head and neck, and lung cancers
dacarbazine	Melanomas, Hodgkin's disease, some sarcomas
procarbazine	Hodgkin's disease, other lymphomas, occasionally brain tumors
NITROSOUREAS	
carmustine	Malignant lymphomas, melanomas, gastrointestinal tumors
lomustine	
streptozocin	

transcription can occur, resulting in the creation of a new cell with the same DNA sequence and thus the same characteristics. When these alkyl groups are attached to the DNA, abnormal chemical bonds form between the adjacent DNA molecules, resulting in the formation of defective nucleic acids that cannot then perform the normal cellular reproductive functions mentioned previously.

Alkylating agents can also be characterized by the number of alkyl groups they possess and thus the number of alkylation reactions they can perform. **Bifunctional** alkylating agents have two reactive alkyl groups that are able to alkylate two DNA molecules. There are also **polyfunctional** alkylating agents that can perform several alkylation reactions. The sites on DNA most vulnerable to this reaction are position N7 on guanine, positions 1, 3, and 7 on adenine, and position N3 on cytosine. The alkylating agents that bind to guanine appear to be the most lethal agents. Fig. 45-2 shows the location along the DNA double helix where the alkylating agents work.

Drug Effects

Alkylating agents in most common use today are those that are effective against a wide spectrum of malignancies, including both solid tumors and hematologic malignancies. Alkylating agents are frequently included in combination regimens because of their CCNS killing ability.

Therapeutic Uses

As previously noted, because of their CCNS killing ability, alkylating agents are frequently included in combination regimens and can therefore be used to treat a variety of cancers. The various types of cancer and the different alkylating agents commonly used in their treatment are listed in Box 45-9.

Side Effects and Adverse Effects

Alkylating agents are capable of causing all the dose-limiting side effects described previously. The relative emetic potential of each agent is given in Box 45-8, and the degree of BMS produced by some of these agents,

causing alkyl groups rather than hydrogen atoms to be attached to the nucleic acid. This process is called **alkylation.** Very special bonds are needed for a normal DNA to assume its double-helix form. During the normal process of reproduction the double helix can uncoil and RNA

Alkylating Agents: Bone Marrow Suppression

Table 45-2

Drug	Degree of BMS	Cell Line	Nadir (Days)
busulfan	Moderate-severe	G	21
carboplatin	Moderate	P and G	17
carmustine	Severe	G and P	21
chlorambucil	Moderate-severe	G and L	21
cyclophosphamide	Moderate	G	14
ifosfamide	Moderate	G	10
mechlorethamine	Moderate	G and P	14
melphalan	Moderate	G and P	21
procarbazine	Moderate	G and P	14
thiotepa	Moderate-severe	G and P	21

G, Granulocytes; *L*, lymphocytes; *P*, platelets.

along with the cell line affected and the radius, are summarized in Table 45-2, which includes data only on those agents that cause moderate to severe suppression. There are also major undesirable effects unique to these agents, and these are listed in Table 45-3. These side effects are important because of their severity, but they can be prevented through the use of prophylactic measures. For instance, nephrotoxicity can be prevented by adequately hydrating the patient with intravenously administered fluids, and careful observation and periodic monitoring can prevent pulmonary fibrosis or cardiomyopathy (heart failure).

Management of Extravasation

One of the most devastating consequences of chemotherapy is the loss of a limb or the need for skin grafting because an antineoplastic drug has extravasated into the surrounding tissue during IV administration. Most antineoplastic agents are administered intravenously, and so this is a constant danger in any cancer patient undergoing chemotherapy. Such **extravasation** can result in permanent damage to nerves, tendons, and muscles, with skin grafting and even amputation needed to manage the damage. Good, attentive nursing care can do much to prevent a large proportion of these incidents. If extravasation does occur, timely intervention can prevent the most serious consequences previously mentioned. There are certain basic steps involved in treating the extravasation of any drug, but specific antidotes and additional measures are required when treating the extravasation of antineoplastics.

If extravasation is suspected, administration of the agent must be stopped immediately, but the IV tube should be left in place and any residual drug or blood aspirated from it if possible. The requisite antidote must then be prepared and instilled through the existing IV tube, after which the needle should be removed. If the residual agent cannot be aspirated from the IV tube, the antidote should not be instilled through it. A sterile occlusive dressing that covers the entire area should be placed, and warm or cold compresses applied, depending on the extravasated agent. The affected limb should then be ele-

Alkylating Agents: Severe Adverse Effects

Table 45-3

Alkylating Agent	Severe Side/Adverse Effects
busulfan	Pulmonary fibrosis
carboplatin	Less nephrotoxicity and neuro-toxicity but more BMS
cisplatin	Nephrotoxicity, peripheral neuropathy, ototoxicity
cyclophosphamide	Hemorrhagic cystitis

vated and allowed to rest. The antidotes recommended to reverse the effects of carmustine and mechlorethamine, the methods of administration, and other measures to be instituted are summarized in Box 45-10.

Activity

Interactions

Only a few alkylating agents are capable of causing significant drug interactions. The most important rule of thumb for preventing such drug interactions is to not administer them with any agent capable of causing similar toxicities. For example, a major adverse effect of cisplatin is nephrotoxicity. Therefore it should not be administered with an agent such as an aminoglycoside (gentamicin, tobramycin, or amikacin) because of the resulting additive nephrotoxic effect, and hence increased likelihood of the development of renal failure. Mechlorethamine and cyclophosphamide should not be administered with radiation therapy or with drugs that suppress the bone marrow. These two agents, as well as cisplatin, should also not be given with probenecid or sulfinpyrazone. This combination can result in hyperuricemia or gout because of competition for renal elimination. In addition, cisplatin should not be given with other nephrotoxic or ototoxic drugs. Their additive toxicities increase the risk of nephrotoxicity and ototoxicity.

Dosages

For the recommended dosages of selected alkylating agents, see the dosages table on p. 709.

Alkylating Agent Extravasation: Specific Antidotes

BOX 45-10

Alkylating Agent	Antidote Preparation	Method
carmustine	Mix equal parts of 1 mEq/ml sodium bicarbonate (premixed) with sterile normal saline (1:1 solution); resulting solution is 0.5 mEq/ml.	1. Inject 2-6 ml IV through the existing line with multiple SC injections into the extravasated site. 2. Apply *cold* compresses. 3. Total dose not to exceed 10 ml of 0.5-mEq/ml solution.
mechlorethamine	Mix 4 ml of 10% sodium thiosulfate with 6 ml of sterile water for injection.	1. Inject 5-6 ml IV through the existing line with multiple SC injections into the extravasated site. 2. Repeat SC injections over the next few hours. 3. Apply *cold* compresses. 4. No total dose established.

Activity

drug profiles

carmustine

Carmustine (BCNU, BiCNU) is one of the three currently available nitrosoureas (carmustine, lomustine, and streptozocin). Because they act by alkylation, they are classified as alkylating agents. Carmustine is able to cross the blood-brain barrier and is thus useful in the treatment of primary brain tumors. It may also be used to treat Hodgkin's disease, non-Hodgkin's lymphomas, and multiple myeloma.

A newer approach to the treatment of recurrent glioblastoma multiforme (GBM) is a biodegradable wafer, called a *Gliadel wafer,* that is implanted during surgery. It contains carmustine and polifeprosan and delivers chemotherapy directly to the tumor site, minimizing drug exposure to other areas of the body. The Gliadel wafer is indicated for patients who have operable brain tumors. It complements other standard therapies for brain cancer, such as surgery, radiation, and traditional IV chemotherapy.

Carmustine is classified as a pregnancy category D agent and is contraindicated in patients with a hypersensitivity to it as well as in those suffering from leukopenia or thrombocytopenia. It is available only in a parenteral preparation as a 100-mg vial for IV infusion. Commonly recommended dosages are listed in the dosages table on p. 709.

PHARMACOKINETICS

HALF-LIFE	ONSET	PEAK	DURATION
15 min	Unknown	Several wk	Unknown

cisplatin

Cisplatin (CDDP; Platinol) is an alkylator-like antineoplastic agent that contains platinum. Chemically, cisplatin consists of a platinum atom surrounded by two chloride atoms and two ammonia molecules. It is classified as an alkylator-like antineoplastic agent because it destroys cancer cells in

the same way as the traditional alkylating agents—by forming cross-links with DNA and thereby preventing its replication. It is considered a bifunctional alkylating agent.

Cisplatin is classified as a pregnancy category D agent and is contraindicated within 1 month of radiation therapy or of chemotherapy with another agent. It is also contraindicated in patients with thrombocytopenia and after a recent smallpox vaccination. It is used for the treatment of many solid tumors such as bladder, testicular, and ovarian tumors. It is available only in a parenteral formulation as 10- and 50-mg injections for IV infusion. Commonly recommended dosages are listed in the dosages table on p. 709.

PHARMACOKINETICS

HALF-LIFE	ONSET	PEAK	DURATION
0.3-0.5 hr	Unknown	IV injection immediate	Unknown

cyclophosphamide

Cyclophosphamide (Cytoxan, Neosar, Procytox) is a nitrogen mustard derivative that was discovered during the process of research to improve mechlorethamine. It is a polyfunctional alkylating agent and is used in the treatment of cancers of the bone and lymph as well as solid tumors. Various leukemias, Hodgkin's and non-Hodgkin's lymphomas, multiple myeloma, and some sarcomas may also respond to cyclophosphamide therapy.

It is classified as a pregnancy category D agent and is contraindicated in lactating women. It is available in both oral and parenteral formulations as 25- and 50-mg oral tablets and 100-, 200-, 500-, 1000-, and 2000-mg vials for parenteral injection. Commonly recommended dosages are listed in the dosages table on p. 709.

PHARMACOKINETICS

HALF-LIFE	ONSET	PEAK	DURATION
3-12 hr	Unknown	2-3 hr	Unknown

DOSAGES Selected Alkylating Agents

agent	pharmacologic class	dosage range	purpose
carmustine (BCNU: BiCNU)	Alkylating agent	*Adult* IV: 150-200 mg/m² every 6 wk as a single dose or divided	Brain tumor, Hodgkin's disease, multiple myeloma, non-Hodgkin's lymphoma
cisplatin (DDP; Platinol)	Alkylating agent	*Pediatric/Adult* IV: 20 mg/m²/day for 5 days every 3 wk for 3 courses 100 mg/m² once every 4 wk 50-70 mg/m² every 3-4 wk	Testicular cancer Ovarian cancer Bladder cancer
cyclophosphamide (Cytoxan, Neosar)	Alkylating agent	*Pediatric* PO/IV: loading dose, 2-8 mg/kg/day divided for ≥6 days PO: maintenance, 2.5 mg/kg twice/wk *Adult* PO/IV: loading dose, 1-5 mg/kg/day or 40-50 mg/kg divided for 2-5 days PO: maintenance, 1-5 mg/kg/day IV: maintenance, 10-15 mg/kg every 7-10 days or 3.5 mg/kg twice/wk	Breast cancer; follicular lymphoma; leukemias, including acute lymphoblastic, monocytic, or myelogenous and chronic granulocytic or lymphocytic; malignant lymphomas; malignant lymphomas; lymphocytic lymphosarcoma; multiple myeloma; mycosis fungoides; neuroblastoma; reticulum cell sarcoma; ovarian cancer; retinoblastoma
mechlorethamine (nitrogen mustard; Mustargen)	Alkylating agent	*Adult* IV/interacavitary: 0.4 mg/kg as a single dose or divided for each course	Hodgkin's disease: chronic lymphocytic or myelocytic leukemia; polycythemia vera; bronchogenic carcinoma; pleural, peritoneal, and metastatic cancer; mycosis fungoides

mechlorethamine

Mechlorethamine (Mustine, Mustargen; nitrogen mustard) is a nitrogen analogue of sulfur mustard. It was the very first alkylating antineoplastic drug discovered. Its beneficial effects in the treatment of various cancers were discovered after World War I when the agent, going by the name *mustard gas*, was used for chemical warfare. Some of the cancers for which it is used to treat are Hodgkin's disease, lymphomas, and chronic leukemia. It is the prototypical alkylating agent.

Mechlorethamine is a bifunctional alkylating agent capable of forming cross-linkage between two DNA nucleotides, thereby interfering with RNA transcription and preventing cell division and protein synthesis. Mechlorethamine is available in a parenteral form only to be administered intravenously or by an intracavitary route such as intrapleurally or intraperitoneally. Mechlorethamine is considered a pregnancy category D agent, and hypersensitivity, lactation, myelosuppression, and an acute herpes zoster attack are contraindications to its use. It is available as a 10-mg parenteral injection. Commonly recommended dosages are listed in the dosages table above.

PHARMACOKINETICS

HALF-LIFE	ONSET	PEAK	DURATION
Several min	Several hr	2-3 days	10 wk

ANTIMETABOLITES

Antineoplastic antimetabolites are CCS agents that are structurally similar to normal cellular metabolites and work by mimicking the actions of important natural precursors that are required for the synthesis of DNA and RNA. They are most effective against solid tumors such as colon, rectum, breast, stomach, lung, ovarian, liver, bladder, and pancreas cancer.

Mechanism of Action

Antimetabolites interfere with the biosynthesis of precursors essential to cellular growth by mimicking folic acid, pyrimidines, and purines, thereby interfering with the normal synthesis of nucleic acids in one of two ways: (1) by falsely substituting for purines, pyrimidines, or folic acid or (2) by inhibiting critical enzymes involved in nucleic acid or folic acid synthesis. Thus they affect DNA, RNA, and protein synthesis and, ultimately, cellular replication. Antimetabolites work in the S phase of the cell cycle, during which DNA synthesis occurs. The available antimetabolites and the metabolites they mimic are as follows:

Folic acid antagonist
• methotrexate (MTX)
Purine antagonist
• fludarabine (F-AMP)
• mercaptopurine (6-MP)
• thioguanine (6-TG)

Pyrimidine antagonist
- cytarabine (ARA-C)
- floxuridine (FUDR)
- fluorouracil (5-FU)

Folic Acid Antagonism

The antimetabolite antineoplastic agent methotrexate is an analogue of folic acid and inhibits dihydrofolate reductase, an enzyme responsible for converting folic acid to a reduced folate. This inhibition prevents the formation of the reduced folate that is needed for the synthesis of DNA and hence for cell reproduction. The result is that DNA is not produced and the cell dies.

Purine Antagonism

The purine bases present in DNA and RNA are adenine and guanine, and they are required for the synthesis of the purine nucleotides that are incorporated into the nu-

cleic acid molecules. Mercaptopurine and fludarabine are synthetic analogues of adenine, and thioguanine is a synthetic analogue of guanine. These agents work by incorporating themselves into the metabolic pathway in lieu of these two nucleosides. Once there, they interrupt the synthesis of the DNA and RNA.

Pyrimidine Antagonism

Of the pyrimidine bases, cytosine and thymine make up DNA, and cytosine and uracil make up RNA. These bases are essential for DNA and RNA synthesis. Floxuridine and fluorouracil are synthetic chemical analogues of uracil, and cytarabine is a synthetic analogue of cytosine. These agents act in a way that is very similar to that of the purine antagonist, incorporating themselves into the metabolic pathway for the synthesis of DNA and RNA and thereby interrupting synthesis of the nucleic acids. This stops the formation of the DNA and RNA needed for the cancer cells to live.

Drug Effects

Antimetabolite antineoplastic agents are used for the treatment of a variety of solid tumors as well as some hematologic cancers. They may also be used in combination chemotherapy regimens to enhance the overall cytotoxic effect. Because these agents are available in both oral and topical preparations, they are utilized for low-dose maintenance and palliative cancer therapy.

Therapeutic Uses

Antimetabolites are used for the treatment of a more defined and limited group of cancers. The commonly used agents and their therapeutic uses are listed in Box 45-11.

Side Effects and Adverse Effects

Like all antineoplastic agents, antimetabolites cause hair loss, nausea and vomiting, and myelosuppression. The emetic potentials for some of these agents have already been given in Box 45-8. Those antimetabolites that cause moderate to severe BMS and the cell lines most affected are given in Table 45-4. Major side effects and adverse effects specific to antimetabolite agents are listed in Table 45-5 by the individual agents.

Leucovorin Rescue

High-dose methotrexate therapy can be very toxic to beneficial human cells, but such toxicity can be reversed by what is called **leucovorin rescue.** Chemically, leuco-

---

BOX 45-11 Specific Antimetabolites: Therapeutic Uses

Agent	Type of Cancer
FOLIC ACID ANTAGONISTS	
methotrexate	Solid tumors (breast, head and neck, and lung cancers), acute lymphocytic leukemia, non-Hodgkin's lymphomas
PURINE ANTAGONISTS	
mercaptopurine	Leukemias (acute lymphoblastic and myelogenous and chronic myelocytic)
fludarabine	Chronic lymphocytic leukemia
thioguanine	Leukemias, lymphomas, multiple myelomas, solid tumors
PYRIMIDINE ANTAGONISTS	
capecitabine	Resistant metastatic breast cancer
cytarabine	Leukemias (acute and chronic myelocytic, and acute lymphocytic), non-Hodgkin's lymphomas
floxuridine	Solid tumors (breast, head, neck, liver, brain, gall bladder, and bile duct), GI adenocarcinoma that has metastasized to the liver
fluorouracil	Solid tumors (breast, colon, rectum, stomach, lung, ovarian, liver, bladder, and pancreas)

TABLE 45-4 Antimetabolites: Bone Marrow Suppression

Drug	Degree of BMS	Cell Line	Nadir (Days)
cytarabine	Severe	G and P	10
fludarabine	Moderate-severe	G and L	13
mercaptopurine	Moderate	G and L	10-14

G, Granulocytes; L, lymphocytes; P, platelets.

vorin is a reduced form of folic acid and is involved in the synthesis of purine and pyrimidines into nucleic acids. Because of its ready conversion to other tetrahydrofolic acid derivatives, it is a potent antidote to the toxic effects of folic acid antagonists such as methotrexate. It is believed that, in some cancers, leucovorin works by entering and "rescuing" normal cells, as opposed to cancer cells, from the toxic effects of folic acid antagonists. It is able to do this because of a difference in the membrane transport mechanisms between human and cancer cells.

Interactions

Most of the drug interactions associated with antimetabolite antineoplastic agents can be summarized in one general statement: The coadministration of any other drug that causes a toxicity similar to that of the antimetabolite will result in additive toxicities. Therefore the respective risks and benefits should be carefully weighed before the initiation of therapy with either the antimetabolite or the other agent. Because the concurrent administration of nonsteroidal antiinflammatory drugs (NSAIDs) with methotrexate may result in severe methotrexate toxicity, this combination should be avoided. In addition, cytarabine may decrease the effects of oral digoxin, and the coadministration of mercaptopurine and allopurinol may lead to an additive bone marrow toxicity because both agents are metabolized by xanthine oxidase.

Dosages

For information on the dosages of selected antimetabolite chemotherapeutic agents, see the dosages table on p. 712.

---

drug profiles

FOLATE ANTAGONISTS
○→methotrexate

Methotrexate (Folex PFS, Rheumatrex) is the prototype antimetabolite antineoplastic of the folate antagonist group and is currently the only antineoplastic folate antagonist used clinically. It has proved useful for the treatment of solid tumors such

---

Table 45-5 Antimetabolites: Severe Adverse Effects

Antimetabolite Agent	Severe Side/Adverse Effects
cytarabine	Liver, kidney, lung, stomach, and heart toxicities
floxuridine fludarabine fluorouracil	Kidney and stomach toxicities
mercaptopurine	Liver and kidney toxicities
methotrexate	Liver, kidney, and stomach toxicities
thioguanine	Liver and kidney toxicities

---

as breast, head and neck, and lung cancers as well as for the management of acute lymphocytic leukemia and non-Hodgkin's lymphomas. Methotrexate also has immunosuppressive activity because it can inhibit lymphocyte multiplication. For this reason it may be useful for the treatment of rheumatoid arthritis. Its combined immunosuppressant and antiinflammatory properties may make it useful for the treatment of many other immune-mediated diseases or inflammatory conditions as well.

Methotrexate may also be used in combination with misoprostol as a medical alternative to a surgically induced abortion. An IM injection of methotrexate followed up to 7 days later by intravaginal administration of misoprostol can terminate an early intrauterine pregnancy. Folic acid antagonists like methotrexate have direct cytotoxic effects on trophoblastic tissue. Misoprostol stimlates uterine contractility and expels the products of conception.

Methotrexate is classified as a pregnancy category D agent and is contraindicated in patients who have shown a hypersensitivity to it; those with leukopenia, thrombocytopnia, or anemia; and psoriatic patients with severe renal or hepatic disease. It is

---

research

Where Do Women Receive Their Health Care and How Effective Is the Screening in These Settings?

According to a recent study supported by the Agency for Health Care Policy and Research (HS06910), African-American women are twice as likely as Caucasian women to have breast cancer diagnosed at a later stage, after it has already spread to the lymph nodes. Differences in clinical breast examination or breast self-examination do not explain this racial difference in diagnoses of breast cancer, and dissimilar histories of mammography screening among women accounted for only about 10% of the variation. In a retrospective study at Yale University Medical School, African-American women in the study were nearly twice as likely to have breast cancer diagnosed before 50 years of age and three times as likely to be obese when diagnosed (N = 322). The same study showed that African-American women were significantly more likely than Caucasian women to have never had a mammogram or to have had one in the 3-year period before symptom development or diagnoses. The researchers in this study cite many variables that contribute to effective mammographic screening and the inconsistent quality of such screening documented at the national level. They expressed the need for an evaluation of the settings in which women receive health care to further determine if African-American and Caucasian women benefit equally from this screening technology. ∎

From Jones BA et al: Can mammography screening explain the race difference in stage at diagnoses of breast cancer? CANCER, Vol. 75, No. 8, 1995, p. 2103. Copyright © 1995 American Cancer Society. Reprinted by permission of Wiley-Liss, Inc., a subsidiary of John Wiley & Sons, Inc.

DOSAGES Selected Antimetabolites

agent	pharmacologic class	dosage range	purpose
cytarabine (Ara-C; Cytosar-U, Tarabine PFS)	Pyrimidine antagonist antimetabolite	*Adult/Pediatric* IV: usual combination dose is 100 mg/m²/day as a continuous infusion for days 1-7 or 100 mg/m² q12h for days 1-7 Intrathecal: 5-75 mg/m² administered once a day for 4 days then once every 4 days	Nonlymphocytic leukemia
mercaptopurine (6-MP; Purinethol)	Purine antagonist antimetabolite	*Adult/Pediatric* PO: 2.5-5 mg/kg/day with a maintenance dose of 1.5-2.5 mg/kg/day	Acute lymphatic and myelogenous leukemia, CNS leukemia
methotrexate (MTX Folex, Folex PFS, Rheumatrex)	Folic acid antagonist antimetabolite	*Adult/Pediatric* PO/IM: 15-30 mg/day for 5 days repeated 3-5 times PO/IM: 3.3 mg/m² with prednisone PO: 10-25 mg/m² for 4-8 days for several courses Intrathecal: 12 mg/m² every 2-5 days; max 15 mg PO: 2.5-10 mg for weeks or months	Trophoblastic tumor Lymphoblastic leukemia Lymphoma Meningeal leukemia Mycosis fungoides

available in both oral and parenteral formulations. For oral administration it is available as a 2.5-mg tablet. It is available in a strength of 25 mg/ml for parenteral injection as well as a preservative-free parenteral injection in doses of 20, 50, and 1000 mg or 25 mg/ml. Commonly recommended dosages are given in the dosages table above.

PHARMACOKINETICS

HALF-LIFE	ONSET	PEAK	DURATION
8-10 hr	Unknown	1-4 hr PO serum	Unknown

PURINE ANTAGONISTS

The currently available purine antagonists are fludarabine, mercaptopurine, and thioguanine. Of the three, mercaptopurine and thioguanine are administered orally. Fludarabine is the only purine antagonist that is available in a parenteral formulation.

mercaptopurine

Mercaptopurine (6-MP; Purinethol) is used primarily for the treatment of leukemias (acute lymphoblastic and myelogenous and chronic myelocytic). It is classified as a pregnancy category D agent. It is contraindicated in patients who have shown resistance to the drug as well as in those with leukopenia, thrombocytopenia, or anemia. It is available only in an oral formulation as a 50-mg tablet. Commonly recommended dosages are given in the dosages table above.

PHARMACOKINETICS

HALF-LIFE	ONSET	PEAK	DURATION
21-47 min	Unknown	2 hr serum	Unknown

PYRIMIDINE ANTAGONISTS

The currently available antimetabolite antineoplastics that are members of the pyrimidine antagonist family are cytarabine, floxuridine, fluorouracil, and gemcitabine. They are available only in parenteral formulations. Floxuridine and fluorouracil are classified as pregnancy category D agents and cytarabine as a category C agent.

cytarabine

Cytarabine (Ara-C; Cytosar-U) is primarily used in the treatment of leukemias (acute myelocytic and lymphocytic and chronic myelocytic) and non-Hodgkin's lymphomas. As previously noted, it is available only as a parenteral agent as 20-, 100-, 500-, 1000-, and 2000-mg/ml vials to be given either by intrathecal or SC injection. Commonly recommended dosages are given in the dosages table above. Cytarabine is a pregnancy category D agent.

Gemcitabine (Gemzar) is an antineoplastic agent structurally related to cytarabine. Gemcitabine is believed to have a superior antitumor activity to that of cytarabine. It has shown activity in a variety of tumors, including breast, non-small cell lung, and ovarian cancers. Gemcitabine has been approved by the FDA as first-line therapy for locally advanced or metastatic cancer of the pancreas.

PHARMACOKINETICS

HALF-LIFE	ONSET	PEAK	DURATION
10 min, then 1-3 hr	Unknown	20-60 min serum	Unknown

CYTOTOXIC ANTIBIOTICS

Cytotoxic antibiotics consist of natural antibiotics produced by the mold *Streptomyces* as well as two synthetic cytotoxic antibiotics not produced by this mold. They are used only for the treatment of cancer because they are too toxic for the treatment of infections. Cytotoxic antibiotics differ in the toxicities they cause, but they all produce BMS, with the exception of bleomycin, which causes pulmonary toxicity (pulmonary fibrosis and pneumonitis). Other severe toxicities associated with the use of cytotoxic antineoplastics are congestive heart failure (CHF) (daunorubicin) and rare acute left ventricular failure (doxorubicin). The available cytotoxic antibiotics according to the specific subclass to which they belong are as follows:

Anthracyclines
- daunorubicin
- doxorubicin
- idarubicin

Other cytotoxic antibiotics
- bleomycin
- dactinomycin
- mitomycin
- mitoxantrone
- pentostatin
- plicamycin

Mechanism of Action

Cytotoxic antibiotic antineoplastic agents are CCNS agents, although some, such as daunorubicin, are more active in the S phase. In most cases, however, the agents are active during all phases of the cell cycle. By virtue of their source of origin (i.e., the *Streptomyces* mold), they all also have antibacterial activity and can kill certain bacteria; some may even kill viruses. Most act either by the process of alkylation, which was previously explained for the alkylating agents, or by a process called *intercalation*, which involves the insertion of the drug molecule between the two strands of DNA, a process that is very similar to the way in which antimetabolites work in that ultimately DNA synthesis is blocked. Specifically, it involves the binding of the agent to the nucleotide pairs of the DNA helix, causing the shape of the DNA helix to change and in turn making it unstable so that it begins to unwind. The result is the blockade of DNA, RNA, and protein synthesis. Some cytotoxic antibiotic agents can do all three, but others affect DNA synthesis only. Agents such as anthracyclines work by intercalation.

Drug Effects

Cytotoxic antibiotic antineoplastic agents are used to treat a variety of solid tumors as well as some hematologic malignancies. They may also be used in combination chemotherapy regimens to enhance the overall cytotoxic effect.

Therapeutic Uses

Cytotoxic antibiotic antineoplastics are used to treat a wide variety of cancers, and these and the agents used to treat them are given in Box 45-12.

BOX 45-12 Specific Cytotoxic Antibiotics: Therapeutic Uses

Agent	Type of Cancer
ANTHRACYCLINES	
daunorubicin	Myelogenous monocytic and acute nonlymphocytic leukemia, Ewing's sarcoma, Wilms' tumor, neuroblastoma, rhabdomyosarcoma
doxorubicin	Solid tumors (of every major organ), Wilms' tumor, neuroblastomas, lymphomas, sarcomas, Hodgkin's disease, lymphoblastic leukemia
idarubicin	Acute myelocytic leukemia (in combinations of antineoplastics)
OTHER CYTOTOXIC ANTIBIOTICS	
bleomycin	Solid tumors (head, neck, penis, cervix, and vulva of squamous cell origin), Hodgkin's disease, sarcomas (lymphosarcoma, reticulum cell, and testicular)
dactinomycin	Sarcomas, melanomas, trophoblastic tumors in women, testicular cancer, Wilms' tumor, rhabdomyosarcoma
mitomycin	Solid tumors (pancreas, stomach, head and neck, breast)
mitoxantrone	Leukemias (acute nonlymphocytic and relapsed leukemia), breast cancer
pentostatin	Alpha-interferon-refractory hairy cell leukemia
plicamycin	Testicular cancer, hypercalcemia, hypercalciuria; symptomatic treatment of advanced neoplasms

---

BOX 45-13 Cytotoxic Antibiotics: Bone Marrow Suppression

Drug	Degree of BMS	Cell Line	Nadir (Days)
dactinomycin	Severe	G and P	10
daunorubicin	Severe	G and P	10
doxorubicin	Moderate	G	14
idarubicin	Severe	G and P	10
mitomycin	Moderate	G and P	28
mitoxantrone	Moderate-severe	G and P	12
pentostatin	Moderate-severe	G and L	15

G, Granulocytes; *L*, lymphocytes; *P*, platelets.

Side Effects and Adverse Effects

As with all the antineoplastic agents, cytotoxic agents have the undesirable effect of causing hair loss, nausea and vomiting, and myelosuppression. The emetic potentials of the various agents in this category are given in Box 45-8, and those cytotoxic agents that cause moderate to severe BMS and the cell lines most affected are listed in Box 45-13. Major side effects specific to these agents are given in Table 45-6.

| Table 45-6 | Cytotoxic Antibiotics: Severe Adverse Effects |

Cytotoxic Antibiotic Agent	Severe Side/Adverse Effects
bleomycin	Pulmonary fibrosis, pneumonitis
dactinomycin	Liver toxicities, extravasation
daunorubicin	Liver toxicities, extravasation
doxorubicin	Liver and cardiovascular toxicities
idarubicin	Liver and cardiovascular toxicities
mitomycin	Liver, kidney, and lung toxicities
mitoxantrone	Cardiovascular toxicities
plicamycin	Extravasation

Box 45-14 Antidote for Doxorubicin Extravasation

1. Cool site to patient tolerance for 24 hr.
2. Elevate and rest extremity for 24-48 hr, then have patient resume normal activity as tolerated.
3. If pain, erythema, or swelling persists beyond 48 hr, discuss with the physician the need for surgical intervention.

Toxicity and Management of Overdose

Because all cytotoxic antibiotic antineoplastics are administered intravenously, extravasation of the agent with its devastating consequences is a constant danger. The basic steps involved in the treatment of extravasation were discussed in the section on alkylating agents. The specific antidote for mitomycin extravasation is that used for mechlorethamine (see p. 709). Box 45-14 outlines management of the extravasation of doxorubicin. Some of the severe cardiac toxicities (e.g., cardiomyopathy) of the cytoxic antineoplastic agents can be prevented by the prophylactic use of dexrazoxane (Zinecard). It has been shown to reduce the incidence and severity of cardiomyopathy associated with doxorubicin. Routine monitoring of cardiac ejection fraction with multiple gated acquisition (MUGA) scans, cumulative dose limitations for some of the cytoxic antineoplastic agents, and the use of cytoprotectant agents such as dexrazoxane can decrease the chances of this devastating toxicity.

Interactions

The cytotoxic antibiotics that are used as chemotherapeutic agents interact with many drugs. They all tend to produce increased toxicities when used in combination with other chemotherapeutic agents or with irradiation. Some agents, most notably bleomycin and doxorubicin, have been known to cause the serum digoxin levels to increase.

Dosages

For recommended dosages of selected cytotoxic agents, see the dosages table on p. 715.

drug profiles

ANTHRACYCLINE CYTOTOXIC ANTIBIOTICS

Three of the older cytotoxic antibiotics are the anthracycline antibiotics doxorubicin, daunorubicin, and idarubicin. They all have similar pharmacologic actions in that they all work through the process of in-

tercalation. In addition, they are effective in all phases of the cell growth cycle. These agents are used for the treatment of a wide range of cancers but are available only in parenteral formulations. All are classified as pregnancy category D agents.

doxorubicin

Doxorubicin (Adriamycin RDF, Adriamycin PFS, Rubex) is a very potent and effective chemotherapeutic agent, and for this reason, it is used in many combination chemotherapy regimens. It is contraindicated in patients with a known hypersensitivity to it, lactating women, and patients with systemic infections (pregnancy [first trimester] category D). It is available only in 10-, 20-, 50-, 100-, and 150-mg vials as well as in a 2-mg/ml strength for injection.

Doxarubicin is now available in a liposomal drug delivery system. Doxil (liposomal doxorubicin) is doxorubicin encapsulated in a lipid bilayer called a *liposome.* The advantage to liposomal encapsulation is decreased systemic toxicity and increased duration of action. Liposomal encapsulation extends the biologic half-life of doxorubicin to 50 to 60 hours and increases its affinity for cancer. Doxil is currently indicated for Kaposi's sarcoma, which primarily affects individuals afflicted with the virus that causes AIDS. Commonly used dosages are given in the dosages table on p. 715.

PHARMACOKINETICS

HALF-LIFE	ONSET	PEAK	DURATION
Up to 36 hr	Unknown	Very rapid	Unknown

OTHER CYTOTOXIC ANTIBIOTICS

The other cytotoxic antibiotics have characteristics similar to those of anthracyclines. They are also CCNS agents that are effective against a wide range of cancers. All are available only in parenteral formulations. There are currently six agents in this class: bleomycin, dactinomycin, mitomycin, mitoxantrone, pentostatin, and plicamycin.

bleomycin

Bleomycin (Blenoxane) is active against both gram-positive and gram-negative bacteria as well as

DOSAGES Selected Cytotoxic Antibiotics

agent	pharmacologic class	dosage range	purpose
bleomycin (BLM; Blenoxane)	Antineoplastic cytotoxic antibiotic	*Adult* IM/IV/SC: 0.25-0.5 U/kg 1-2 times/wk	Hodgkin's disease, lymphosarcoma, recticulum cell sarcoma, squamous cell cancer, testicular cancer
doxorubicin (ADR, Adriamycin RDF, Adriamycin PSF, Rubex, Doxil)	Antineoplastic cytotoxic antibiotic	*Adult* IV: 60-75 mg/m² every 21 days or 30 m² for 3 days, then either repeat every 4 wk or give 20 mg/m²/wk IV: 20 mg/m² over at least 30 min, once every 3 wk	Breast, bladder, ovarian, thyroid, bronchogenic cancers; Hodgkin's and non-Hodgkin's lymphomas; acute lymphoblastic/ myeloblastic leukemia; neuroblastoma; soft-tissue/bone sarcoma; Wilms' tumor; Kaposi's sarcoma

fungi, but because of its cytotoxicity its use as an antibiotic is prohibited. It kills cancer cells in all phases of the cell cycle in much the same way as the alkylating agents do—by inhibiting the incorporation of a nucleotide base, thymidine, into DNA. The result is that cancer cells cannot produce the needed DNA and protein, and they die.

Bleomycin is used to treat a variety of cancers. However, it is very toxic, one of its most harmful toxicities being its effect on the lungs. Pulmonary fibrosis and pneumonitis are the consequences. It is classified as a pregnancy category D agent and is contraindicated in patients with a hypersensitivity to it. The doses are measured in units as opposed to milligrams. It is available as 15- and 30-U vials, which are administered subcutaneously, intravenously, or intramuscularly. Commonly used dosages are given in the dosages table above.

PHARMACOKINETICS

HALF-LIFE	ONSET	PEAK	DURATION
2 hr	Unknown	30-60 min	Unknown

IM: time to reach peak serum levels.

MITOTIC INHIBITORS

Mitotic inhibitors consist of natural products obtained from the periwinkle plant (*Catharenthus roseus,* formerly called *Vinca rosea*) and of semisynthetic agents obtained from the mandrake plant (May apple). The periwinkle plant yields antineoplastic alkaloids. These are vinblastine (VLB), vincristine (VCR), and vinorelbine. They are known as *vinca alkaloids.* Etoposide (VP-16) and teniposide (ETP) are semisynthetic derivatives of podophyllotoxin, which is obtained from the resinous extract of the mandrake plant. A new agent has been discovered recently that also comes from a plant source and affects mitosis. This is paclitaxel (Taxol), and it comes from the bark of the slow-growing Western (Pacific) yew.

Docetaxel is a semisynthetic taxoid produced from the needles of the European yew tree. It is pharmacologically similar to paclitaxel. These agents and their plant sources are listed below:

Vinca alkaloids (periwinkle)
- vinblastine
- vincristine
- vinorelbine

Podophyllotoxin derivatives (may apply)
- etoposide
- teniposide

Yew tree
- doxetaxel
- paclitaxel
- taxotere

Mechanism of Action

The plant alkaloids vary in their site of action in the cell cycle. They all affect the cell cycle shortly before or during mitosis. This entire family of antineoplastics prevents mitosis from occurring in an unknown way and thus stops the cell cycle by disrupting the mitotic spindles crucial to the success of metaphase. It is for this reason that they are called *mitotic inhibitors.*

The vinca alkaloids (vincristine, vinblastine, and vinorelbine) kill cancer cells by binding to tubulin during the metaphase of mitosis (M phase). This prevents the assembly of microtubules, which results in the dissolution of the mitotic spindle. Without these mitotic spindles, dividing cells cannot then multiply and divide appropriately. This causes cell division and DNA, RNA, and protein synthesis to be inhibited. Without these substances, all cells, including cancer cells, die.

The podophyllotoxin derivatives (etoposide and teniposide) exert their cytotoxic effects by damaging DNA and thereby inhibiting or altering DNA synthesis. They have also been shown to directly induce single- and double-stranded DNA breaks. These agents are considered CCS agents because they appear to kill during the late S phase and the G_2 phase of the cell cycle.

The Pacific yew tree derivative (paclitaxel) works in the late G_2 phase and M phase of the cell cycle. It is therefore a CCS agent and works by causing the formation of a nonfunctional microtubule. These microtubules are needed for mitotic spindles to function properly. Therefore paclitaxel halts mitosis in metaphase.

Drug Effects

Mitotic inhibitors are CCS agents that are used to treat a variety of solid tumors as well as some hematologic malignancies. Depending on the particular agent, they can work in any phase of the cell cycle (late S phase, throughout G_2 phase, and M phase), but they work primarily in metaphase during mitosis. Mitotic inhibitors may also be used in combination chemotherapy regimens to enhance the overall cytotoxic effect.

Therapeutic Uses

The commonly used mitotic inhibitor antineoplastic agents and their therapeutic uses are listed in Box 45-15.

Side Effects and Adverse Effects

As is the case for all the antineoplastic agents, mitotic inhibitor antineoplastic agents cause hair loss, nausea and vomiting, and myelosuppression. The emetic potentials of some of the agents are given in Box 45-8, and those agents that cause moderate to severe BMS and the cell lines most affected are listed in Box 45-16. Major side effects specific to these agents are summarized in Table 45-7.

Toxicity and Management of Overdose

All of the mitotic inhibitor antineoplastics are administered intravenously, making extravasation of the agents and its serious consequences a constant threat. The basic steps to be taken in the treatment of the extravasation of any drug have already been discussed in the section on alkylating agents. Specific antidotes and additional measures to be taken for the treatment of the extravasation of the mitotic inhibitors are given in Box 45-17.

Interactions

Many notable drug interactions are associated with the mitotic inhibitors. Etoposide competes for protein binding with warfarin and can result in increased prothrombin time and INRs. When paclitaxel is given with cisplatin, it can result in increased myelosuppression due to additive toxicities. When paclitaxel is given with ketoconazole, it can result in decreased metabolism of paclitaxel and lead to its accumulation. When teniposide is given with methotrexate, it causes increased methotrexate clearance, resulting in decreased methotrexate duration. When vinblastine is given with methotrexate or bleomycin, it increases the action of these two agents. Vinblastine and phenytoin coadministration can result in decreased absorption and/or increased metabolism, resulting in decreased phenytoin levels.

Dosages

For the recommended dosages of selected mitotic inhibitors, see the dosages table on p. 718.

Box 45-15 Specific Mitotic Inhibitors: Therapeutic Uses

Agent	Type of Cancer
VINCA ALKALOIDS	
vinblastine	Lymphomas, including Hodgkin's and non-Hodgkin's lymphomas; neuroblastoma; Kaposi's sarcoma; mycosis fungoides; histiocytosis; solid tumors (breast and testicular cancers)
vincristine	Lymphomas, Hodgkin's disease, neuroblastoma, leukemias; rhabdomyosarcoma, osteogenic, and other sarcomas; solid tumors (breast and lung cancers); Wilms' tumor
PODOPHYLLOTOXIN DERIVATIVES	
etoposide	Leukemias, lymphomas, neuroblastoma, melanoma, solid tumors (lung, testicular, and ovarian cancer)
teniposide	Childhood acute lymphoblastic leukemia
PACIFIC YEW TREE DERIVATIVE	
paclitaxel	Metastatic ovarian cancer not responsive to other chemotherapy; ever-expanding therapeutic uses

---

Box 45-16 Mitotic Inhibitors: Bone Marrow Suppression

Drug	Degree of BMS	Cell Line	Nadir (Days)
paclitaxel	Severe	G, P, and L	10-14
teniposide	Moderate	G and P	14
vinblastine	Moderate-severe	G and P	10

G, Granulocytes; L, lymphocytes; P, platelets.

Table 45-7 Mitotic Inhibitors: Severe Adverse Effects

Antibiotic Agent	Severe Side/Adverse Effects
etoposide	Liver and kidney toxicities
teniposide	Liver toxicities
vinblastine	Liver, kidney, and lung toxicities, convulsions
vincristine	Liver toxicities, convulsions

drug profiles

Mitotic inhibitors consist of three groups of agents that are derived from plant sources: vinca alkaloids (periwinkle), podophyllotoxin derivatives (May apple), and the Pacific yew tree. They are all available in a parenteral form and are all classified as pregnancy category D agents. Etoposide is the only agent available in an oral formulation as well.

etoposide

Etoposide (VP-16, VePesid) is a semisynthetic podophyllotoxin derivative with a structure, mechanism of action, and side effect profile similar to those of teniposide. As previously noted, it is believed to kill cancer cells in the late S phase and the G_2 phase of the cell cycle. It is indicated for the treatment of small-cell lung cancer and testicular cancer.

Hypersensitivity, bone marrow depression, severe hepatic or renal disease, and bacterial infection are the contraindications to its use. It is available in an oral formulation as a 50-mg liquid-filled capsule and as a 20-mg/ml injection for IV infusion. Commonly recommended dosages are listed in the dosages table on p. 718. Pregnancy category D.

PHARMACOKINETICS

HALF-LIFE	ONSET	PEAK	DURATION
0.2-19 hr	Unknown	1-1.5 hr*	Unknown

*PO: time to reach peak serum levels.

paclitaxel

Paclitaxel (Taxol) is a natural mitotic inhibitor that is obtained from the bark of the Pacific yew tree. The same tree is the source for another mitotic inhibitor known as docetaxel (Taxotere). Docetaxel is made from the renewable needle biomass of this yew tree. Paclitaxel is currently approved for the treatment of advanced ovarian cancer, metastatic ovarian cancer that is not responsive to other chemotherapy (usually platinum-containing regimens), breast cancer, non–small-cell lung cancer, and Kaposi's sarcoma. However, because of its excellent clinical effectiveness, it is also being used for the treatment of many other types of cancers. Paclitaxel is extremely water insoluble (hydrophobic), and for this reason, it is put into a solution containing oil rather than water. The particular oil is a type of castor oil called Cremophor EL, the same oil in which cyclosporin is mixed and which many patients cannot tolerate, showing hypersensitivity reactions similar to anaphylactic reactions. For this reason, before patients receive paclitaxel they are premedicated with a steroid, antihistamine, and an H_2 antagonist (cimetidine, ranitidine, famotidine, or nizatidine).

Paclitaxel is contraindicated in patients with a hypersensitivity to either it or the castor oil base. It is available only in a parenteral formulation as a 6-mg/ml, 5-ml, or 16.7-ml vial. Common dosage recommendations are listed in the dosages table on p. 718. Pregnancy category D.

PHARMACOKINETICS

HALF-LIFE	ONSET	PEAK	DURATION
13.1-52.7 hr	Unknown	Variable	7-8 mo

vincristine

Vincristine (VCR; Oncovin, Vincasar PFS) is an alkaloid isolated from the periwinkle plant that is indicated for the treatment of lymphomas, Hodgkin's disease, neuroblastoma, leukemias, rhabdomyosarcoma, osteogenic and other sarcomas, solid tumors (breast and lung), and Wilms' tumor. It is contraindicated in patients with a hypersensitivity to it and in infants. It is available only in a parenteral formulation as a 1-mg/ml injection. Common dosage recommendation are listed in the dosages table on p. 718. Pregnancy category D.

PHARMACOKINETICS

HALF-LIFE	ONSET	PEAK	DURATION
10-155 hr	Unknown	Rapid	Unknown

BOX 45-17   Mitotic Inhibitor Extravasation: Specific Antidotes

Mitotic Inhibitor Agent	Antidote Preparation	Method
etoposide teniposide vinblastine vincristine	Hyaluronidase (Wydase) 150 U/ml: add 1 ml NaCl (150 U/ml)	1. Inject 1-6 ml into the extravasated site with multiple SC injections. 2. Repeat SC dosing over the next few hours. 3. Apply *warm* compresses.* 4. No total dose established.

*Important: corticosteroids and topical cooling appear to worsen toxicity.

DOSAGES Selected Mitotic Inhibitors

agent	pharmacologic class	dosage range		purpose
etoposide (VP-16; VePesid)	Mitotic inhibitor	**Adult** IV: 50-100 mg/m²/day on days 1-5 to 100 mg/m²/day on days 1, 3, and 5		Testicular cancer
		IV: 35 mg/m²/day for 4 days to 50 mg/m²/day for 5 days PO: twice the IV dose rounded to the nearest 50 mg		Small-cell lung cancer
paclitaxel (Taxol)	Mitotic inhibitor	**Adult** IV: 135 mg/m² or 175 mg/m² over 3 hr, repeated every 3 wk		Carcinoma of the ovary
		IV: 175 mg/m² over 3 hr, repeated every 3 wk		Carcinoma of the breast
vincristine (LCR, VCR; Oncovin, Vincasar PFS)	Mitotic inhibitor	**Pediatric** IV: 2 mg/m² at weekly intervals; max 2 mg **Adult** IV: 1.4 mg/m² at weekly intervals; max 2 mg		Acute leukemia, Hodgkin's disease, lymphosarcoma, rectiulum cell sarcoma, rhabdomyosarcoma, neuroblastoma, Wilms' tumor

TOPOISOMERASE-1 INHIBITORS

Topoisomerase-1 inhibitors are a new class of chemotherapy agents isolated from the bush *Camptothecus accuminata*. The two currently available are topotecan (Hycamptin) and irinotecan (CPT-11, Camptosar). These agents have shown significant activity against a broad range of tumors. Topotecan is currently approved for treatment of metastatic ovarian cancer after failure of initial or subsequent chemotherapy as well as small-cell lung cancer. Irinotecan is currently approved for metastatic colorectal cancer that has recurred or progressed after standard therapy with the antineoplastic agent fluorouracil. These new agents are considered CCS antineoplastics. They work by inhibiting the enzyme topoisomerase-1 causing reversible single-strand DNA breaks during the S-phase of the cell cycle.

Mechanism of Action

Topoisomerase-1 inhibitors are CCS agents. They kill cells when they are in the S-phase of the cell cycle. They inhibit cell replication by inhibiting the enzyme topoisomerase-1. Interference with this enzyme results in single-strand DNA breaks, which inhibits the replication of DNA essential for the replication of cancer cells.

Drug Effects

Topoisomerase-1 inhibitors are used to treat ovarian and colorectal cancer. Because of their potency and effectiveness in cancers resistant to other antineoplastic agents, they may also be used to treat other cancers in the future.

Therapeutic Uses

The two currently available topoisomerase-1 inhibitors are used to treat ovarian and colorectal cancer. Topotecan has been shown to be very effective in treating ovarian cancer. It has even been effective after platinum-containing regimens and paclitaxel have failed. Irinotecan has been shown to have significant activity against a broad range of tumor types, including colorectal, non–small-cell lung, cervical, ovarian, and non-Hodgkin's lymphoma.

Side Effects and Adverse Effects

As with many cancer chemotherapeutic agents, the main side effect demonstrated by topotecan is suppression of blood cells produced in the bone marrow. This bone marrow suppression is predictable, noncumulative, reversible, and manageable. Topotecan should not be given to patients with baseline neutrophil counts of less than 1500. The most frequent nonhematologic side effects are gastrointestinal. These are moderate nausea and vomiting as well as mild to moderate diarrhea.

Irinotecan has been associated with severe diarrhea. This diarrhea is called *cholinergic diarrhea* and may occur during irinotecan infusion. It is recommended to be treated with atropine unless contraindicated. Delayed diarrhea may occur 2 to 10 days after infusion of irinotecan. This diarrhea can be severe and even life threatening. It should be treated aggressively with loperamide. Severe myelosuppression and nausea and vomiting are also possible.

Toxicity and Management of Overdose

Little information is available on overdose of these agents. However, it would be expected that the adverse events seen with recommended dosages would be seen in overdose. There are no antidotes for overdose of these agents. Maximum supportive care should be instituted to prevent dehydration caused by diarrhea with irinotecan as well as large aggressive dosing of loperamide. Bone marrow suppression caused by topotecan and irinotecan can be lessened with the use of colony-stimulating factors such as sargramostim and filgrastim.

Interactions

Other antineoplastics that have similar side-effect profiles should not be given concurrently with topoisomerase-1

agent	pharmacologic class	dosage range	purpose
irinotecan (CPT-11, Camptosar)	Topoisomerase-1 Inhibitor	Adult IV: 125 mg/m² once weekly for 4 wk followed by a 2 wk rest period	Recurrent colorectal cancer that failed to respond to fluorouracil
topotecan (Hycamptin)	Topoisomerase-1 Inhibitor	Adult IV: 1.5 mg/m² daily for 5 days, starting day one of a 21 day course of treatment	Metastatic ovarian cancer that failed initial or subsequent chemotherapy

inhibitors. Laxatives and diuretucs should not be given concomitantly with irinotecan because of the potential to worsen the dehydration resulting from the severe diarrhea that can be caused with irinotecan.

Dosages

For recommended dosages of selected topoisomerase-1 inhibitors, see the dosages table above.

drug profiles

Topoisomerase-1 inhibitors are a new class of chemotherapy agents isolated from the bush *Camptothecus accuminata*. They are semisynthetic derivatives of camptothecin (CPT), an alkaloid extract from plants such as the one just mentioned. The two currently available are topotecan (Hycamptin) and irinotecan (CPT-11), Camptosar. These agents have shown significant activity against a broad range of tumors from colorectal to ovarian cancers. These new agents are cell-cycle specific antineoplastics. They are both classified as pregnancy category D agents. They are contraindicated in patients who have a history of hypersensitivity reaction to them or to any of their ingredients.

topotecan

Topotecan (Hycamptin) is a very effective antineoplastic agent. After initial therapy with other antineoplastics, cancer cells frequently become resistant to their effects. Topotecan produced responses even after such agents as platinum-containing regimens and paclitaxel have failed. Topotecan has been extensively studied in the treatment of ovarian cancer and small-cell lung cancer. It is available only in 4-mg single-dose vials for injection. Commonly used dosages are given in the dosages table above.

PHARMACOKINETICS

HALF-LIFE	ONSET	PEAK	DURATION
2-3 hr	Variable	Unknown	7-11 days

MONOCLONAL ANTIBODIES

Monoclonal antibodies are quickly becoming standards of therapy in many areas of medicine. Monoclonal antibodies have advantages over traditional antineoplastics in that they can target specific cancer cells with great accuracy. This prevents the destruction of good cells and avoids many of the side effects traditionally associated with antineoplastics. Trastuzumab (Herceptin) and rituximab (Rituxan) are two monoclonal antibodies used to treat malignancies.

Mechanism of Action

Trastuzumab works by inhibiting the proliferation of human tumor cells that overexpress human epidermal growth factor receptor 2 protein (HER2). This HER2 protein is overexpressed in 25% to 30% of cases of primary breast cancer. It is an adverse prognostic factor for early-stage breast cancer. Trastuzumab is a mediator of antibody-dependent cellular cytotoxicity (ADCC).

Rituximab specifically binds to antigen CD20. This antigen is a protein on the membranes of B-cells found in patients with non-Hodgkins lymphoma. Antigen CD20 is expressed on greater than 90% of B-cell non-Hodgkin's lymphomas. Once rituximab binds to these B-cells, a host immune response causes lysis of these cells.

Drug Effects

The drug effects of the monoclonal antibodies are very specific and focus on the particular cell that they consider an antigen. Trastuzumab is an antibody to certain tumor cells that release a specific protein, whereas rituximab is an antibody to certain B-cells. Their drug effects are specific and narrow. They are beginning to be used with traditional antineoplastic agents to enhance the overall cytotoxic effects.

Therapeutic Uses

Trastuzumab is used for the treatment of patients with metastatic breast cancer. Metastatic breast cancer tumors that overexpress the HER2 protein are the only types of breast cancer for which trastuzumab should be used. It is generally reserved for patients who have received one or more chemotherapy regimens for their metastatic disease. Trastuzumab has been used in combination with paclitaxel and has been shown to have great success against metastatic breast cancer. Trastuzumab should only be used in patients who have tumors that overexpress the HER2 protein.

Rituximab is used for the treatment of non-Hodgkin's lymphoma. The specific type of non-Hodgkins lymphoma is relapsed or refractory low-grade of follicular, antigen CD20-positive, B-cell non-Hodgkin's lymphoma.

Side Effects and Adverse Effects

The side effects of trastuzumab and rituximab are listed in Table 45-8. The most frequently reported side effects (>20%) for trastuzumab include fever, chills, headache, infection, nausea, vomiting, and diarrhea. Fever, chills, and headache are also frequently reported with the use of rituximab.

Potentially fatal infusion-related events can occur with rituximab. Severe bronchospasm, dyspnea, hypotension, and/or angioedema preceded death in most cases. Severe respiratory events, including hypoxia, pulmonary infiltrates, and adult respiratory distress syndrome, contributed to six of the eight reported deaths. This reaction is termed *cytokine release syndrome*.

Dosages

For information on the recommended dosages of the antineoplastic monoclonal antibodies trastuzumab and rituximab, see the dosages table below.

Table 45-8 Monoclonal Antibodies: Adverse Effects

Body System	Side/Adverse Effects
Cardiovascular	Angioedema, hypotension, tachycardia, congestive heart failure
Central nervous system	Fever, chills, headache, asthenia, dizziness, pain, insomnia, depression
Gastrointestinal	Nausea, abdominal pain, vomiting, anorexia
Hematologic	Neutropenia, anemia
Respiratory	Bronchospasm, cough
Musculoskeletal	Myalgia, bone pain, arthralgia
Miscellaneous	Throat irritation, infection

drug profiles

The addition of the antineoplastic monoclonal antibodies has revolutionized the way that certain cancers are currently treated. They are extremely specific agents that target certain tumor cells and bypass normal cells. However, they are very expensive and can be very toxic. They are used alone as well as with other traditional antineoplastic agents.

rituximab

Rituximab (Rituxan) is one of the two currently available antineoplastic monoclonal antibodies. It binds to malignant cells, allowing the body's immune system to recognize and eliminate these cells. Rituximab has become a standard agent to treat patients with follicular low-grade non-Hodgkin's lymphoma who have failed previous therapy.

It is available as a 10-mg/ml and 50-mg/ml injection. It is recommended to premedicate with acetaminophen and diphenhydramine before each infusion of the drug to reduce potential infusion-related side effects. Safety and efficacy of rituximab in children has not been established. Rituximab is a pregnancy category C agent. Common dosage recommendations are listed in the dosages table below.

PHARMACOKINETICS

HALF-LIFE	ONSET	PEAK	DURATION
59-174 hr*	First 3 days or within 14 days*	Unknown†	6-9 mo*

*Depends on indication.
†Depends on values of numbers of circulating CD20-positive B-cells and measures of disease burden.

trastuzumab

Trastuzumab (Herceptin) is one of the two currently available antineoplastic monoclonal antibodies. Trastuzumab kills tumor cells by mediating antibody-dependent cellular cytotoxicity. This is accomplished by inhibiting proliferation of human tumor cells that overexpress HER2 protein. This overexpression of the HER2 gene has been established as an adverse prognostic factor for early-stage breast cancer. Because of the relatively selective expression of HER2 on cancer cells, it has been an appealing target for antineoplastic therapy. The combination of trastuzumab and pac-

DOSAGES Antineoplastic Monoclonal Antibodies

agent	pharmacologic class	dosage range	purpose
rituximab (Rituxan)	Monoclonal antibody	*Adult* IV: 375 mg/m² once weekly for 4 weeks	Non-Hodgkin's lymphoma
trastuzumab (Herceptin)	Monoclonal antibody	*Adult* IV: 4 mg/kg as a 90-min infusion on day 1, followed by 2 mg/kg as 30-min infusions weekly	Metastatic breast cancer

litaxel has produced encouraging results. Researchers are now investigating the combination of trastuzumab with vinorelbine (Navelbine) with study results showing a 71% response rate.

Trastuzumab has a boxed warning that administration can result in the development of ventricular dysfunction and CHF. Patients should be monitored for signs and symptoms of CHF and ventricular dysfunction before and during treatment. There have been over 60 postmarketing reports of serious adverse events. Hypersensitivity reactions, infusion reactions, and pulmonary events associated with the use of trastuzumab have been fatal. Trastuzumab is considered a pregnancy category B agent with no contraindications to its use. It is available only as a 440-mg powder for injection. Common dosage recommendations are listed in the dosages table on p. 720.

PHARMACOKINETICS

HALF-LIFE	ONSET	PEAK	DURATION
2-12 days	Unknown	16-32 wk*	Unknown

*Depends on dose.

MISCELLANEOUS ANTINEOPLASTICS

The miscellaneous antineoplastic agents are those that, because of their unique structure and mechanisms of action, cannot be classified into the previously described categories. These agents are as follows:
- altretamine
- asparaginase
- cladribine
- hydroxyurea
- mitotane
- Hormonal agents

Mechanism of Action

The antineoplastic drugs that fall into the miscellaneous category are a very diverse group of agents that kill cancer cells by a variety of mechanisms. The proposed mechanisms of action of these various agents are given in Table 45-9.

Drug Effects

The miscellaneous antineoplastics cited consist of both CCS and CCNS agents, and depending on the particular agent, they can work in any phase of the cell cycle. They are used to treat a variety of solid tumors as well as some hematologic malignancies and may also be used in combination chemotherapy regimens to enhance the overall cytotoxic effect.

Therapeutic Uses

The miscellaneous antineoplastics are used for the treatment of a wide variety of cancers. The agents and their therapeutic uses are listed in Box 45-18.

Side Effects and Adverse Effects

Like all antineoplastic agents, the miscellaneous agents also cause hair loss, nausea and vomiting, and myelosuppression. The emetic potentials of some of these agents are given in Box 45-8. The only agent that causes BMS in the moderate to severe range is hydroxyurea, and the characteristics of the BMS it causes are summarized in Box 45-19. Major side effects specific to these agents are given in Table 45-10.

Interactions

Some important drug interactions with the miscellaneous antineoplastics are important to note. Asparaginase, when coadministered with mercaptopurine or methotrexate, can have additive hepatotoxic effects. Prednisone coadministration with asparaginase can result in additive effects on the pancreas, resulting in hyperglycemia. Mitotane coadministered with barbiturates, warfarin, or phenytoin can result in increased metabolism of mitotane. This can lead to decreased mitotane levels and effectiveness. CNS depressants given with mitotane will result in additive CNS depression.

Miscellaneous Antineoplastics: Mechanisms of Action

Agent	Cell Cycle	Mechanism of Action
altretamine	CCNS	Inactivates DNA.
asparaginase	CCS (G₁ phase)	Catalyzes the conversion of the amino acid asparagine to aspartic acid and ammonia; some leukemic cells are unable to produce the asparagine that is required for the synthesis of DNA and essential proteins and survival of the cells.
cladribine	CCNS	Inhibits DNA synthesis and repair in a way similar to that of antimetabolites but has cytotoxic effects on resting as well as proliferating lymphocytes.
hydroxyurea	CCS (S phase)	Interferes with DNA synthesis by inhibiting the incorporation of thymidine into DNA.
mitotane	CCNS	Covalently bonds to mitochondrial proteins, causing a direct cytotoxic effect and resulting in the inhibition of adrenocortical function; it is an adrenocortical cytotoxic agent.

Specific Miscellaneous Antineoplastics: Therapeutic Uses
45-18

Agent	Type of Cancer
altretamine	Palliative treatment of recurrent, persistent ovarian cancer
asparaginase	Acute lymphocytic leukemia
cladribine	Active hairy cell leukemia, chronic lymphocytic leukemia, non-Hodgkin's lymphomas, acute myeloid leukemia, autoimmune hemolytic anemia
hydroxyurea	Chronic myelocytic leukemia, recurrent or metastatic ovarian cancer, squamous cell carcinoma of the head and neck
mitotane	Adrenocortical carcinoma

Miscellaneous Antineoplastics: Bone Marrow Suppression
45-19

Drug	Degree of BMS	Cell Line	Nadir (Days)
Hydroxyurea	Severe	G	7

G, Granulocytes.

Dosages

For information on recommended dosages of the agents in the miscellaneous category, see the dosages table on p. 723.

drug profiles

The various agents in the miscellaneous category of antineoplastics are used to treat a wide range of neoplasms, ranging from recurrent, persistent ovarian cancer and hairy cell leukemia to adrenocortical carcinoma. Altretamine and hydroxyurea are administered orally, and asparaginase, cladribine, and mitotane are available only in parenteral preparations.

altretamine

Altretamine (Hexalen) is a CCNS agent that is used for the palliative treatment of recurrent, persistent ovarian cancer after the completion of first-line treatment with cisplatin or alkylating agent–based combination therapy. Its mechanism of action appears to be the production of metabolites that bind to precursors of DNA, thus preventing its formation and leading to cell death.

It is contraindicated in patients with a hypersensitivity to it and in those suffering from either severe BMS or severe neurologic toxicity. Altretamine is available only in an oral formulation as a 50-mg

Miscellaneous Agents: Severe Adverse Effects
45-10

Antineoplastic Agent	Severe Side/Adverse Effects
altretamine	Liver and CNS toxicities
asparaginase	Liver, kidney, lung, and CNS toxicities
cladribine	Hematologic toxicities
hydroxyurea	CNS toxicities
mitotane	Genitourinary and lung toxicities

capsules. Common dosage recommendations are listed in the dosages table on p. 723. Pregnancy category D.

PHARMACOKINETICS

HALF-LIFE	ONSET	PEAK	DURATION
4.7-10.2 hr	Unknown	0.5-3 hr*	2-36 mo

*In plasma.

asparaginase

Asparaginase (Elspar) is used for the treatment of acute lymphocytic leukemia. Its mechanism of action is slightly different from that of traditional antineoplastics in that it is an enzyme which catalyzes the conversion of the amino acid asparagine to aspartic acid and ammonia. Leukemic cells are then unable to synthesize the asparagine required for them to synthesize DNA and other essential proteins necessary for cell survival.

Asparaginase is contraindicated in patients who are hypersensitive to it, as well as in infants, lactating women, and patients with pancreatitis. It is available only in a parenteral form as a 10,000-IU dosage for injection. Common dosage recommendations are listed in the dosages table on p. 723. Pregnancy category C.

PHARMACOKINETICS

HALF-LIFE	ONSET	PEAK	DURATION
8-30 hr	Unknown	Several days plasma	23-33 days

hydroxyurea

Hydroxyurea (Hydrea) most closely resembles the antimetabolite antineoplastics in its actions. It interferes with the synthesis of DNA by inhibiting the incorporation of thymidine into DNA. It works in the S phase of the cell cycle, making it a CCS agent.

Hypersensitivity, leukopenia, thrombocytopenia, and anemia are the contraindications to its use. It is a potent inhibitor of bone marrow cell production, and thus causes severe BMS. Its maximum destruction of granulocyte cell lines (nadir) occurs about 1 week after the start of therapy. Hydroxyurea is

DOSAGES Selected Miscellaneous Antineoplastic Agents

agent	pharmacologic class	dosage range	purpose
altretamine (Hexalen)	Cytotoxic antineoplastic	*Adult* PO: 260 mg/m²/day in 4 divided doses PC and HS for 14 to 21 days in a 28-day treatment cycle	Ovarian cancer
asparaginase (Elspar)	Antineoplastic enzyme	*Adult/Pediatric* IV: 200 IU/kg/day for 28 days	Acute lymphocytic leukemia
hydroxyurea (Hydrea)	Urea-derived antineoplastic	*Adult* PO: 20-30 mg/kg/day as a single dose or 80 mg/kg as a single dose every third day 20-30 mg/kg/day as a single dose	Solid tumors Chronic myelocytic leukemia

available only in an oral formulation as a 500-mg capsules. Common dosage recommendations are listed in the dosages table above.

PHARMACOKINETICS

HALF-LIFE	ONSET	PEAK	DURATION
~7.5 hr	Unknown	2 hr serum	Unknown

HORMONAL AGENTS

Hormonal agents are used in the treatment of a variety of neoplasms in both males and females. These agents are used most commonly as palliative and adjuvant therapy. With certain types of cancer they may also be used as drugs of first choice. Some of the more common hormonal agents for female specific neoplasmas such as breast are tamoxifen (Nolvadex), megestrol (Megace), toremifene (Fareston), medroxyprogesterone (Provera), aminoglutethimide (Cytadren), and fluoxymesterone (Halotestin). For male-specific neoplasms such as prostate, the following agents are used: flutamide (Eulexin), leuprolide (Lupron), anastrazole (Arimidex), goserelin (Zoladex), estramustine (Emcyt), and bicalutamide (Casodex).

nursing process

Discussion of the nursing process applicable to patients receiving antineoplastic agents is broken down according to the different classes of agents. The nursing actions appropriate to treatment with each antineoplastic agent are presented in Box 45-20.

• Assessment

A patient should be thoroughly assessed before administration of any antineoplastic agent. Various blood counts, x-ray examination, CEA levels, and other studies may be necessary. The patient's mucous membrane status also needs to be assessed. Each antineoplastic agent has several drug interactions, and this should be assessed carefully before drug administration. Antimetabolite agents such as flurouracil are contraindicated in patients who have recently had or been exposed to chickenpox or herpes zoster because they may exacerbate the subsequent or residual symptoms of these diseases. Fluorouracil and other agents that cause bone marrow suppression should be used cautiously in patients with renal, cardiac, or hepatic dysfunction; bone marrow dysfunction; or infiltration of the malignancy to the bone marrow. Baseline vital signs and the patient's overall health status, renal and liver function, intake and output, and weight should all be assesed and the findings recorded before any agent is administered.

Before administering methotrexate, another antimetabolite, the nurse should check the patient to make sure he or she does not have ascites, pleural effusion, or renal dysfunction, since these are contraindications to its use. Cautious use is recommended in patients suffering from BMS, infection, stomatitis, peptic ulcer disease, or ulcerative colitis. If the patient has had or has been exposed to chickenpox, exposure to methotrexate may cause the subsequent or residual disease process to become more generalized. It can also further increase the hyperuricemia that occurs in patients with gout or renal stones. Cautious use is recommended as well in patients who are receiving other cytotoxic agents or irradiation plus in elderly, debilitated, or very young patients. It is important to get a list of the current medications the patient is taking so the drug interactions can be avoided (see earlier discussion of the drugs that interact with antimetabolites).

Cautious use of mechlorethamine is recommended in patients who are pregnant or breastfeeding. Cautious use is also recommended in patients suffering from BMS, infection, herpetic infections, or chickenpox; those with a history of gout or renal stones; and those who have had previous chemotherapy or radiotherapy because of the compounding of adverse reactions that can occur. It is important to obtain and document the baseline blood urea nitrogen (BUN) level, urinalysis findings, renal function study results, CBC, and the results of audiometric

Nursing Implications: Antineoplastics*

box 45-20

Antineoplastic Agent	Classification	Nursing Implications
asparaginase, hydroxyurea	Miscellaneous	Administer asparaginase IV after dilution with recommended fluids (i.e., 10,000 IU/5 ml sterile H_2O or 0.9% NaCl with no preservatives). Administer hydroxyurea orally with extra fluids and an antiemetic 30-60 min before.
carmustine and lomustine	Nitrosoureas	Give IV after proper dilutional guidelines have been followed, usually diluting 100 mg of drug into 3 ml of ethyl alcohol (usually provided that way); then further dilute in 27 ml of sterile water for injection followed by further dilution in 100-500 ml of 0.9% NaCl or D5W; give over 1 hr or more; discontinue infusion if discomfort occurs. Antiemetic use 30-60 min before infusion. Increase fluids up to 3 liters per day, unless contraindicated, to prevent urate deposits from forming in urine. Follow guidelines for mouth care. Apply warm compresses to IV site to relieve inflammation, and reduce flow rate if burning sensation occurs; monitor site continuously.
cisplatin (CAUTION: Do not confuse this agent's name with carboplatin; they are in the same class of agents but have very different doses.)	Alkylating agent	Administer IV after diluting 10 mg/10 ml or 50 mg/50 ml sterile water for injection, then withdraw dose and dilute ½ dose with 1000 ml D_5 0.2 NaCl or D_5 ½ NaCl with 37.5 g mannitol. IV INF is administered usually over 3-4 hr with a 0.45 μm filter. Check site for infiltration. Do not use aluminum equipment. Hydrate patient with 1-2 L over 8-12 hr before treatment.
cyclophosphamide	Alkylating agent	Follow instructions for mechlorethamine. Administer IV or PO with forced fluid intake because adequate hydration is needed to prevent hemorrhagic cystitis. Allopurinol may also be needed to maintain normal uric acid levels and prevent alkalinization of the urine. Administer IV after diluting to a concentration of 100 mg/5 ml of sterile water; shake and let stand until clear then may dilute more in up to 250 ml of D5W or NS; give via Y-tube or three-way stopcock at ≤100 mg/min. Always check IV site for extravasation and use 21-, 23-, or 25-gauge needle. Give as early in the morning as possible so can be eliminated before bedtime. Maintain diet low in purine, high in iron and vitamins.
fluorouracil	Antimetabolite	Administer IV undiluted through a stopcock or Y-tube; give over 1-3 min or dilute in NS or D5W and give over 2-8 hr in an IV infusion. Administer antiemetic therapy 30 min to 1 hr before therapy (as ordered) to prevent nausea. Antibiotics may be needed to prevent infection. Antispasmodic may be needed to manage diarrhea. Use strict asepsis with patients. Increase fluids up to 3 liters per day, unless contraindicated, to prevent dehydration. Change IV site q48h. Perform mouth care with water and club soda or with soft-bristle toothbrush or cotton-tipped applicator. Encourage diet high in iron and vitamins, low in fiber, and including few dairy products, especially if patient also undergoing irradiation.
mechlorethamine	Alkylating agent	Use guidelines for administering cytotoxic agent and give IV after diluting with 10 mg/10 ml of sterile water or NaCl; leave needle in the vial and withdraw dose; give through stopcock or Y-tube. Slow IV infusion is often done using 21-, 23-, or 25-gauge needle; constant monitoring of IV site is necessary to prevent extravasation and the resulting necrosis.

*This box lists major classifications with examples; for additional agents in the same class, refer to specific manufacturer guidelines or discussion in chapter text.

Nursing Implications: Antineoplastics—cont'd

Antineoplastic Agent	Classification	Nursing Implications
mechlorethamine—cont'd		With extravasation, it is important to discontinue solution, leave needle in place, infuse with isotonic sodium thiosulfate, and apply ice pack for 6-12 hr or follow hospital policy guidelines.
		Encourage fluid intake of up to 3 liters per day to prevent formation of urate deposits in the urine; also encourage adequate diet, special skin and mouth care, and diet low in purines, organ meats, and dried beans.
methotrexate	Folic acid antagonist	Administer after diluting in sterile water for injection at a concentration of 5 mg/2 ml and give through a Y-tube or three-way stopcock at a rate of ≤10 mg/1 min.
		Antacids given before oral agent may help minimize GI upset.
		Give antiemetic 30-60 min before therapy.
		Allopurinol may be ordered to help control serum uric acid levels.
		Encourage intake of up to 3 liters of fluids per day, unless contraindicated.
		Leucovorin rescue is ordered within 12 hr to prevent tissue damage and severe side effects of MTX.
paclitaxel	Mitotic inhibitor	Monitor VS during the first hour of IV infiltration, and monitor the site for infiltration.
		IV solutions should follow proper dilutional guidelines and generally include 0.9% NaCl, 5% dextrose, and D_5LR to a concentration of 0.3-1.2 mg/ml.
		Use of an in-line filter <0.22 μm is recommended.
		Use only glass bottles, polypropylene, polyolefen bags, and administration sets; do NOT use PVC bags or sets.
		Premedication often includes dexamethasone, diphenhydramine, cimetidine, or ranitidine.
vincristine and related agents	Mitotic inhibitor	Administer antacids before oral dose to minimize GI upset.
		Administer IV only after diluting 10 mg/10 ml NaCl and follow administration guidelines.
		Administer antiemetics 30-60 min before (as ordered).

testing so that other problems or complications of therapy can be watched for and prevented.

Paclitaxel is contraindicated in allergic patients, pregnant women, patients with polyoxyethylated costoril, or if neutropenia is present ($<1800\text{-}2000/mm^3$). It should be given cautiously to children and to people lactating or having CNS disorders or cardiovascular disease. Always assess for drug and IV incompatibilities.

Cyclophosphamide is contraindicated in lactating women, and nitrosoureas are contraindicated in patients with leukopenia and thrombocytopenia. Cautious use of cyclophosphamide and nitrosoureas is recommended in pregnant or lactating women and in patients with renal or hepatic dysfunction, BMS, infection, or tumors infiltrating the bone marrow.

The cautions applicable to cyclophosphamide treatment also pertain to cisplatin therapy. If the patient has recently had chickenpox, shingles, or infection with a live virus, caution is indicated. In addition to the routine baseline assessment, the patient's audiometric and neurologic status should also be tested and the findings documented. The contraindications and cautions that apply to doxorubicin use are the same as those that apply to cyclophosphamide therapy.

Topotecan and irinotecan are newer topoisomerase inhibitors. These agents are contraindicated in patients with a history of allergies to either drug. Drug interactions include laxatives and diuretics.

Mitotic inhibitors such as vinblastine and vincristine are contraindicated in patients who have had chickenpox or shingles. Doxorubicin, an antineoplastic antibiotic, is contraindicated during pregnancy, allergic reactions, lactation, and systemic infections. It should be given cautiously to patients with compromised renal, hepatic, cardiac, or bone marrow function.

With monoclonal antibodies such as trastuzumab and rituximab, it is important to understand that contraindications include hypersensitivity to the agent. Cautious use is necessary for patients with CHF, stroke, or any disabling cardiac failure disease. In addition, it may be discontinued in the patient with a clinically significant decreased ejection fraction. Extreme caution should be used with all patients with preexisting cardiac disease and advanced age because this may predispose the patient to cardiac toxicity. Drug interactions include paclitaxel. Rituximab is contraindicated in patients who are hypersensitive to the drug and to murine proteins found in the drug. Cautious use is important in patients with respiratory or cardiac disease.

NURSING CARE PLAN Chemotherapy

You have just initiated paclitaxel (Taxol) chemotherapy on a 44-year-old patient who has been recently diagnosed with ovarian cancer. Family members are asking many questions about paclitaxel, including what side effects to expect, how long the treatment regimen will last, and what they need to be aware of when she returns home, including problems to report to the oncologist.

assessment	**Nursing Diagnosis**	Risk for injury (bleeding, easy bruising, infection) related to side effects of medication
	Subjective Data	"What is paclitaxel?"
		"How does it work?"
		"What side effects can I expect with it?"
		"What is the usual treatment plan?"
	Objective Data	Newly-diagnosed patient with ovarian cancer
		Paclitaxel infusion to begin immediately
		Supportive family
		Patient and family inquire about the drug and treatment plan
planning and outcome criteria	**Goals**	Patient and family will verbalize an understanding of paclitaxel before therapy is initiated
	Outcome Criteria	Patient and family will report or verbalize the following during treatment:
		• Side effects that should be reported to health care provider
		• Action of paclitaxel
		• Treatment plan
implementation		Patient and family teaching session to include the following information:
		• Paclitaxel helps prevent the rapid division and growth of malignant cells by affecting certain specific structures within the cancer cell.
		• Treatment usually consists of IV infusion given over 24 hours every 3 weeks for a time specified for you by the oncologist.
		• Common side effects include bradycardia (pulse <60), hypotension (low blood pressure), nausea, vomiting, diarrhea, mucositis (sores in mouth and mucous membranes), abnormal lab values (Hgb, Hct, WBCs, platelets) (which we will monitor closely), low white blood cell counts, low platelets, anemias (we also monitor for these), hair loss, joint pain, numbing and tingling of extremities.
		• Contraceptive measures are recommended during treatment and up to 4 months after treatment because of adverse effects on a fetus.
		• Avoid use of aspirin, NSAIDs (ibuprofen), straight razors for shaving, or commercial mouthwashes (alcohol content) because bleeding may occur.
		• Report any abnormal bleeding from anywhere, such as in the stool, urine, easy bruising.
		• Report fatigue, headache, irritability, shortness of breath, and dizziness because these may indicate anemia.
		• You may want to go ahead and select a wig matching your hairstyle and color now, so as you lose hair, your wig will be available. Your hair may be a different color and texture when it grows back.
		• You should not receive any vaccinations while on chemotherapy.
evaluation		Positive therapeutic outcomes include the following:
		• Increased response of tumor cells to the chemotherapy
		• Prevention of rapid division of malignant cells
		• Minimal side effects

● Nursing Diagnoses

General nursing diagnoses pertinent to patients receiving antineoplastic agents and monoclonal antibodies, regardless of the class, include the following:
• Risk for impaired skin integrity and oral mucous membranes related to stomatitis from drug therapy.

• Acute pain related to neoplastic process and GI side effects such as anorexia, nausea, and vomiting.
• Impaired skin integrity related to effects of antineoplastic therapy.
• Risk for injury, weakness, and falls related to effects of BMS.

- Disturbed body image related to alopecia or other effects of the antineoplastic agent and the neoplasm.
- Diarrhea related to effects of the antineoplastic agents.
- Risk for infection related to BMS and resultant neutropenia.

Following are the diagnoses specific to the use of various agents:

Methotrexate
- Impaired skin integrity related to dermatologic side effects of the drug, with resultant vasculitis or photosensitivity.

Mechlorethamine
- Disturbed sensory perception related to the effects of the antineoplastic.
- Impaired skin integrity resulting from extravasation.

Cyclophosphamide and nitrosoureas
- Disturbed body image related to disturbed gonadal functioning and growth, alopecia, and darkened skin.
- Decreased cardiac output related to toxicity of medication.
- Impaired urinary elimination (hemorrhagic cystitis, nephrotoxicity) related to cyclophosphamide use.

Cisplatin
- Impaired physical mobility related to anemia-induced fatigue.
- Disturbed sensory perception (hearing loss, optic neuritis) related to ototoxicity.
- Risk for injury related to loss of reflexes and numbness of hands and feet and ataxia stemming from neurotoxicity.

Doxorubicin
- Decreased cardiac output related to cardiotoxicity of chemotherapy agent.

Vinblastine and vincristine
- Impaired urinary elimination related to hyperuremia, uric acid nephropathy, and neurotoxicity with joint and back pain.

Trastuzumab and rituximab
- Decreased cardiac output related to the adverse effects of the monoclonal antibodies.
- Acute pain related to the side effects of monoclonal antibodies such as fever and headache.

- Risk for injury related to general overall weakness caused by side effects of monoclonal antibodies.

Planning

Goals related to the administration of antineoplastic agents, regardless of the class, include the following:
- Patient regains normal or prechemotherapy level of oral mucosa integrity with minimal discomfort and problems stemming from stomatitis.
- Patient experiences increased comfort levels during antineoplastic therapy.
- Patient experiences minimal breaks in skin integrity during antineoplastic therapy.
- Patient experiences minimal to no self-injury during antineoplastic therapy.
- Patient maintains a positive self-concept during antineoplastic therapy.
- Patient regains normal or prechemotherapy bowel elimination patterns.
- Patient has minimal problems with infection during chemotherapy.

Following are the goals specific to the use of various antineoplastic agents:

Methotrexate
- Patient's skin remains intact while receiving antineoplastic agents.

Mechlorethamine

- Patient experiences minimal sensory-perceptual loss (hearing loss) resulting from the effects of the antineoplastic therapy.
- Patient states measures to minimize side effects and adverse effects to chemotherapy.

Cyclophosphamide and nitrosourea

- Patient verbalizes feelings frequently.
- Patient regains prechemotherapy activity and energy levels.
- Patient experiences minimal alterations in urinary elimination patterns.

Cisplatin

- Patient maintains energy levels or near normal energy levels.
- Patient experiences minimal problems associated with possible neurotoxicity.

Doxorubicin

- Patient remains free of or has minimal cardiac difficulties.

Vinblastine and vincristine

- Patient maintains normal fluid volume status during chemotherapy.

Trastuzumab and rituximab

- Patient maintains normal cardiac status during therapy.
- Patient remains free from injury during therapy.

Outcome Criteria

Outcome criteria pertinent to patients receiving antineoplastic agents or monoclonal antibodies, regardless of the class, include the following:

- Patient will use measures to minimize alterations in mucous membranes caused by stomatitis such as frequent mouthcare with toothettes and/or use of alcohol-based mouthwash.
- Patient will use nonpharmacologic and pharmacologic methods such as relaxation therapy, music therapy, and biofeedback to control pain related to neoplastic processes and to manage the GI side effects such as anorexia, nausea, and vomiting.
- Patient will use measures to enhance skin integrity while undergoing antineoplastic therapy such as keeping skin clean, dry, and lubricated.
- Patient will state methods to use to minimize risk for self-injury related to effects of BMS such as avoiding crowds (e.g., patients with leukopenia), straight razors, venipuncture, and injections, if possible (e.g., patients with decreased platelets).
- Patient will verbalize openly his or her concerns and fears regarding any self-concept disturbances related to alopecia and other effects of the antineoplastic therapy and the neoplasm.
- Patient will use nonpharmacologic methods (diet, fluids, exercise) and pharmacologic methods (e.g., bulk-forming laxatives) to regain normal or prechemotherapy bowel elimination patterns.
- Patient will minimize risk for infection by adhering to methods of preventing infection such as consuming a high-protein diet and avoiding crowds while blood counts are decreased.

Following are outcome criteria specific to the use of various antineoplastic agents:

Methotrexate

- Patient will use sunscreen and other skin protection to avoid skin injury while experiencing the dermatologic side effects of the drug, with resultant vasculitis or photosensitivity.

Mechlorethamine

- Patient will report any changes in hearing ability stemming from the effects of the antineoplastic therapy to the physician immediately.
- Patient will immediately report any unusual changes in the skin surrounding the IV insertion site in order to prevent impaired skin integrity related to extravasation.

Cyclophosphamide and nitrosourea

- Patient will verbalize feelings openly about any disturbance of self-concept related to disturbed gonadal functioning and growth, alopecia, and darkened skin.
- Patient will adhere to activity restrictions because of the altered cardiac output related to the toxicity of the medication but maintain some approximation of normal activity or of the prechemotherapy level of activity.
- Patient will state measures to take to prevent or minimize hemorrhagic cystitis or nephrotoxicity related to cyclophosphamide use, such as forcing liquids (2000 ml/day) before, during, and after chemotherapy.

Cisplatin

- Patient will conserve energy throughout the day when experiencing anemia-induced fatigue but maintain ADLs during chemotherapy.
- Patient will state ways to prevent or minimize the loss of reflexes, the numbness of the hands and feet, and the ataxia related to neurotoxicity.

Doxorubicin

- Patient will report any cardiac difficulty such as shortness of breath, dysrhythmias, or chest pain resulting from possible cardiotoxicity.

Vinblastine and vincristine

- Patient will force fluids (at least 2000 ml/day) within the restrictions specified by the physician to prevent or minimize hyperemia, uric acid nephropathy, or neurotoxicity with joint and back pain.

Trastuzumab and rituximab

- Patient will state symptoms to report to the physician immediately, such as chest pain, palpitations, dizziness, and shortness of breath.
- Patient states ways to maximize overall strength and well-being during treatment such as nutritional supplementation, changing positions slowly, accommodating ADLs to weakended state, and asking for assistance.

● **Implementation**

The respective drug interactions and side effects associated with the various agents are described in the section that discusses individual classes of agents in the first part of this chapter and in Box 45-20.

NURSING CARE PLAN Breast Cancer

Mrs. E.S., a 65-year-old woman with a recent diagnosis of estrogen receptor positive breast tumor, has begun life-long chemotherapy with tamoxifen citrate therapy as an adjunct to surgical therapy with a modified radical mastectomy of the left breast. Vital parameters are as follows: Hgb and Hct within normal limits, WBC 4500, platelets 100,000, vital signs within normal limits. Other data pertinent to Mrs. E.S. include complaints of metallic taste, some nausea, and decreased energy levels with a problem some days of taking in only very minimal amounts of food. No antiemetics, antacids, vitamins, iron supplements, or nutritional supplements are being taken.

assessment	*Nursing Diagnosis*	Imbalanced nutrition, less than body requirements, related to adverse and toxic effects of chemotherapy
	Subjective Data	"I just hate these hot flashes." "Everything tastes so metallic." "Do I really have to take this all the time?" "I just don't feel like eating most of the time . . . nothing tastes good anymore . . "
	Objective Data	Breast cancer diagnosed 2 mo ago 65 yr in otherwise good health Estrogen receptor positive breast tumor WBC 4500 Platelets 100,000 No weight loss Takes tamoxifen citrate 10 mg bid Decreased energy level but able to carry out ADLs
planning and outcome criteria	*Goals*	Patient will maintain diet of six frequent feedings with Ensure snacks within 2 wk
	Outcome Criteria	Patient will show improved appetite as evidenced by: • Energy level • Intake of foods within the basic food groups • No weight loss • Decreased complaints of diminished appetite
implementation		• Encourage use of antiemetic 30-60 min before dosing of tamoxifen, as ordered, to prevent nausea and vomiting if a problem. • Weekly weights at home. • Antacid before medication, with physician's order, and give PM dose of medication after evening meal unless contraindicated. • Encourage patient to try cola, Jell-O, dry toast, or crackers if unable to tolerate other regular food products until nausea subsides. • Encourage fluid intake of at least 2-3 L/day to prevent dehydration unless contraindicated. • Encourage and give sample menus of a diet high in iron and vitamins such as green leafy vegetables, organ meats, nutritional supplements such as Ensure, and iron or vitamin supplements as ordered. • Encourage increased activity, as tolerated, to help increase appetite. • Encourage patient to keep daily journal of meals and nutritional intake. • Patient should call the physician should dietary intake decrease and nausea and vomiting occur.
evaluation		Patient will show improved nutritional status as evidenced by: • Energy level • No weight loss • Normal lab values such as Hgb, Hct, BUN, protein levels • Nausea and vomiting • Dietary intake with nutritional supplements • Improved appetite, fewer complaints of poor taste • Little to no nausea and vomiting

For the monoclonal antibodies, trastuzumab is generally given over 30 to 90 minutes, but all protocols should be followed. Adverse reactions such as chills, fever, headache, nausea, or vomiting should be reported immediately. Weakness and dizziness are expected, so monitor the patient carefully and make sure proper precautions are taken if the patient is at home. Any persistent GI side effects, back or joint pain, palpitations, shortness of breath, edema, and unusual weight gain should be reported immediately to the health care provider. Rituximab is not to be given IV push or bolus and should only be given per protocol. Premedication may be needed with acetaminophen and diphenhydramine before infusion of the drug. Withholding of any antihypertensive medications may need to be considered up to 12 hours before drug infusion because of transient hypotension with the administration of rituximab. Symptomatic treatment may be needed with bronchodilators as well. The patient should report or you should contact the physician immediately if the patient experiences high fever, chills, difficulty breathing, or congestion during the treatment. In addition, persistent dizziness, edema, unusual weight gain, shortness of breath, chest pain, fatigue, and fever should also be reported.

Patient teaching tips for antineoplastic agents are listed in the box below.

● Evaluation

Therapeutic responses to antineoplastic and monoclonal antibiotic therapy include a decrease in the tumor size and in the spread of malignancy, as well as improved energy levels, ADLs, and quality of life after chemotherapy. Laboratory studies, CEAs, blood counts, x-ray examinations, CT scans, and MRIs may be used to monitor tumor response (at intervals) to the chemotherapy. It is also important to monitor patients for bleeding tendencies and the signs and symptoms of infection or anemia during and after therapy. The oral mucosa should be examined daily to identify dryness, sores, ulcerations, white patches, and bleeding of the gums. Other problems to watch for include oral discomfort and difficulty swallowing. Abnormal changes should be reported to the physician. Yellowing of the skin, abdominal pain, fever, sore throat, decreased urine production, dehydration, rapid respirations, poor skin turgor, loss of weight and appetite, skin lesions, rashes, and restlessness should also be reported immediately to the physician. Side effects of each agent are listed earlier in this chapter and in the patient teaching tips box.

✎ patient teaching tips

Antineoplastic Agents

➤ Patients should report black tarry stools, chills, fever, sore throat, or shortness of breath to the physician immediately.

➤ Patients receiving 5-fluorouracil should be told about the importance of observing protective isolation and of eating foods high in iron and vitamins. They should avoid consuming foods high in fiber as well as foods containing citric acid, foods that are hot or cold, and foods that have a rough texture. Patients should be told to report the symptoms of stomatitis, which consist of bleeding, white spots or patches, and ulcerations of the mouth. Patients should be told to examine their mouths daily and to report any problems immediately to the nurse or physician. They should also know to report headache, fatigue, faintness, shortness of breath (anemia), bleeding and easy bruising (drop in platelet count), and sore throat and fever (infection) at the first sign of these symptoms. Women will need an alternative form of nondrug contraception during therapy. Patients should also be told to avoid taking aspirin or aspirin-containing products as well as products containing ibuprofen.

➤ Patients receiving antineoplastics may want to purchase or rent a wig or hairpiece because of the hair loss that occurs during treatment. The hair loss is temporary, however. The American Cancer Society often has some wigs available and usually at no cost, so patients should be told to contact the local chapter for information on

this. Patients should avoid using alcohol and aspirin, razors, and commercial mouthwash during treatment with MTX and most antineoplastic agents.

➤ Sterility and amenorrhea may occur in patients on mechlorethamine or cyclophosphamide therapy, but these are reversible once therapy is discontinued. Patients taking these agents should know to report the usual symptoms of infection, anemia, and bleeding, as already mentioned. Hair loss is possible, so patients may wish to wear a wig or hairpiece.

➤ Patients receiving carmustine or lomustine should follow the guidelines already given concerning protective isolation and mouth care, and they should know to report bleeding and the signs or symptoms of anemia or infection. They should also be told to avoid using aspirin, ibuprofen, alcohol, commercial mouthwashes, and razors.

➤ Patients receiving etoposide or teniposide, as well as their family members, should be warned about the possible complications of therapy, such as infection, anemia, and bleeding disorders, and told to report any complaints, side effects, or changes in breathing to the physician. Hair loss is expected, so patients should consider getting hairpieces or wigs before the start of therapy. Patients should be told to change positions slowly because of the hypotension that can occur.

➤ Doxorubicin is available in a liposomal drug delivery system, and directions for its use must be followed closely. Patients receiving any form of doxorubicin may experience thrombocytopenia, nausea, vomiting, leukopenia, anorexia, stomatitis, hypertension, sinus tachycardia, impotence, and amenorrhea.

➤ A Gliadel wafer is also being used as an implanted wafer and delivers chemotherapy directly to the tumor site. This agent contains carmustine and polifeprosan. See above for patient teaching tips on carmustine.

➤ Patients may be encouraged to increase fluids, if not contraindicated, to help prevent constipation. Foods high in fiber are usually avoided because diarrhea is a side effect of chemotherapy.

POINTS TO REMEMBER

Cancer

- A group of diseases that are characterized by uncontrolled cellular growth.
- Can invade into surrounding tissue and metastasize to new sites distant from the original body site.
- Metastasis is the spreading of a cancer from the original site of growth.
- A neoplasm or tumor is a mass of new cells that exhibit uncontrolled cellular reproduction.
- Paraneoplastic syndromes consist of signs and symptoms that arise at a distance from the tumor or its sites of metastasis.

Benign Tumors

- Tumors that are characterized by uniform size and shape.
- Show no invasiveness or metastatic properties.

Malignant Tumors

- *Malignancy* specifically refers to a neoplasm that is malignant as opposed to benign.
- Typically composed of cancerous cells.
- They invade surrounding tissues, metastasize, and migrate to other tissues and organs, where they form metastatic tumor deposits.

Tumor Classification by Tissue of Origin

- Epithelial = carcinoma
  Connective = sarcoma
  Lymphatic = lymphoma
  Blood = leukemia

Antineoplastics

- Cell cycle-specific (CCS) and cell cycle-nonspecific (CCNS) agents.

- CCS agents kill cancer cells during specific phases of the cell growth cycle.
- CCNS agents kill cancer cells during any phase of their cell growth cycle.

Nursing Considerations

- Chemotherapy may be used in many situations and requires very astute and prudent nursing care as well as critical decisions concerning its administration.
- Assessment of baseline vital signs, complete blood counts, and assessment of overall health status, renal and liver function, intake and output, and weights should be performed and the findings recorded before the start of any chemotherapy.
- The hair that regrows after alopecia may be a different color and consistency than it was originally, and the patient should be warned about this and other possible side effects before the start of therapy.
- Oral hygiene should be performed at least once every 8 hours, sometimes more frequently, to prevent stomatitis.
- A holistic approach to the care of the cancer patient must focus on the patient's strengths and minimize the weaknesses at this time in his or her life.
- Patients receiving cisplatin are at risk for suffering seizures, reduced urinary output, nephrotoxicity, and neurotoxicity and require frequent monitoring and astute nursing care to prevent or treat these problems in a timely fashion.
- Antimetabolite agents such as fluorouracil are contraindicated in patients with a recent history of or recent exposure to chickenpox or herpes zoster because of the risk of exacerbation of the subsequent or residual symptoms of the disease.

REVIEW QUESTIONS

1. A patient is in danger of contracting an infection if her absolute granulocyte count declines to less than:
   a. 100 cells/mm^3.
   b. 1000 cells/mm^3.
   c. 10,000 cells/mm^3.
   d. 100,000 cells/mm^3.

2. Which of the following should be included in patient teaching regarding stomatitis as a side effect of 5-fluorouracil therapy?
   a. Use full-strength hydrogen peroxide for prevention.
   b. NSAIDs or aspirin may help the pain and is encouraged qid.

c. Lemon glyceride swabs should be used long term to prevent oral thrush or bleeding.

d. Examine the mouth daily for bleeding, white spots, and ulcers on the back of the throat.

3. Your patient is suffering from GI side effects from chemotherapy, including anorexia and nausea. Which of the following would you recommend to her?

a. Remain NPO during the acute phase of treatment.

b. Eat large meals four times daily with high fiber and protein to help prevent weight loss.

c. Normal eating patterns will return within 48 hours after the chemotherapy has stopped.

d. Eat six small feedings with nutritional supplementation, and an antiemetic may be needed.

4. Leucovorin rescue is recommended for which of the following agents?

a. Cisplatin

b. Cyclosporin

c. Methotrexate

d. Mercaptopurine

5. The patient receiving cyclophosphamide must:

a. Attain adequate hydration before the start of therapy.

b. Be adequately anesthetized before infusion of the drug.

c. Have his or her ECG and arterial line pressures monitored during therapy.

d. Receive instructions about the life-threatening complications stemming from the neurotoxicity it can cause.

6. Side effects of mechlorethamine include which of the following?

a. Darkened skin

b. Sensory-perceptual loss (hearing loss)

c. Chronic inflammatory bowel disorders

d. Disturbed gonadal function and growth

For Answers see www.harcourthealth.com/MERLIN/Lilley/.

CRITICAL THINKING Activities

1. Two broad categories of drugs used to treat cancer are cell cycle–specific agents and cell cycle–nonspecific agents. Explain the difference between the two categories of drugs based on their mechanisms of action.

2. G.B. is a 45-year-old woman who has just been diagnosed with breast cancer. She has agreed to undergo chemotherapy and will begin a course of combination chemotherapy consisting of a CMF regimen, as follows:
Cyclophosphamide, 100 mg/m^2: PO days 1-14
Methotrexate, 40 mg/m^2: IVB days 1 and 8
Fluorouracil, 600 mg/m^2: IVB days 1 and 8
Repeat cycle every 28 days.

She weighs 135 pounds and is 5 feet, 4 inches tall. From the body surface area (BSA) nomogram in the appendix, calculate what doses of cyclophosphamide, methotrexate, and fluorouracil she should receive.

3. Your patient is experiencing stomatitis and is taking cisplatin. What kinds of food would you encourage her to avoid? Explain your answer.

For Answers see www.harcourthealth.com/MERLIN/Lilley/.

bibliography

Albanese J, Nutz P: *Mosby's 2001 nursing drug reference and review cards*, St Louis, 2001, Mosby.

American Hospital Formulary Service: *AHFS drug information*, Bethesda, Md, 2000, American Society of Health-System Pharmacists.

Anderson PO, Knoben JE, Troutman WG: *Handbook of clinical drug data 1999-2000*, ed 9, New York, 1999, McGraw-Hill.

Johns Hopkins Hospital, Department of Pediatrics et al: *The Harriet Lane handbook*, ed 15, St Louis, 2000, Mosby.

Keen JH: *Critical care and emergency drug reference*, ed 3, St Louis, 1996, Mosby.

Madeya M: Oral complications from cancer therapy, *Oncol Nurs Forum* 23(5):801, 1996.

McKenry LM, Salerno E: *Mosby's pharmacology in nursing*, ed 21, St Louis, 20001, Mosby.

Methotrexate and misoprostol for abortion, *Med Lett* 38(973):39, 1996.

Mosby's GenRx: a comprehensive reference for generic and brand drugs, ed 10, St Louis, 2000, Mosby.

Skidmore-Roth L: *Mosby's 2001 nursing drug reference*, St Louis, 2001, Mosby.

Activity

Remember to check the **Online Worksheet** for additional learning opportunities: **www.harcourthealth.com/MERLIN/Lilley/**

Chapter 46

Biologic Response Modifiers

objectives

When you reach the end of this chapter, you should be able to do the following:

www.harcourthealth.com/MERLIN/Lilley/

Look for this symbol for topics covered in the **Online Worksheet**

1 List the side effects, adverse reactions, and toxic effects associated with the biologic response modifiers.

2 Classify the biologic response modifiers by specific classification grouping.

3 Discuss the use of biologic response modifiers in the treatment of neoplasms.

4 Discuss the mechanisms of action, cautions, contraindications, routes of administration, and drug interactions associated with biologic response modifiers.

drug profiles

- **aldesleukin,** p. 740
- **epoetin alfa,** p. 741
- **filgrastim,** p. 742
- **interferon alfa-2a,** p. 737
- **interferon alfa-2b,** p. 737
- **interferon alfa-n3,** p. 737
- **interferon beta-1a,** p. 737
- **interferon beta-1b,** p. 737
- **interferon gamma-1b,** p. 738
- **oprelvekin,** p. 740
- **sargramostim,** p. 742

Key drug.

glossary

Antibody (an' ti bod' e) An immunoglobulin that binds to antigens to form an antibody-antigen complex. (p. 734)

Antigen (an' ti jen) Substance that is foreign to the human body. (p. 734)

B-cells Cells of the humoral immune system that attack foreign invaders; synonymous with lymphocytes. (p. 734)

Biologic response modifiers (BRMs) Agents whose primary site of action is the immune system. (p. 734)

Cellular immunity One of the two major components of the immune system; acts in accordance with humoral immunity to recognize and destroy foreign particles and cells. (p. 734)

Colony-stimulating factors (CSFs) Cytokines that regulate the growth, differentiation, and function of bone marrow stem cells. (p. 735)

Cytokines (si' to kin) Immune system protein that directs the actions and communications between the cellular and humoral divisions of the immune system and augments or enhances the immune response. (p. 736)

Cytotoxic T-cells (si to tok' sik) Cells that directly kill their target cells without the help of other immune system cells. (p. 735)

Humoral immunity (hu' mər əl) One of the two major components of the immune system; acts in accordance with cellular immunity to recognize and destroy foreign particles and cells. (p. 734)

Interferon (in tər fer' on) Biologic response modifier that enhances the activity of macrophages and natural killer cells. (p. 735)

Lymphokine-activated killer (LAK) cell Cell resulting from the multiplication of T-cells that recognizes cancer cells and ignores normal cells. (p. 739)

Memory cells Cells involved in the humoral immune system that remember the exact characteristics of a particular foreign invader or antigen. (p. 734)

Monoclonal (mon o klon' əl) A group of identical cells or organisms derived from a single cell. (p. 734)

Plasma cells Lymphoid or lymphocyte-like cells found in the bone marrow, connective tissue, and sometimes blood; they produce antibodies. (p. 734)

Stem cells Precursors of mature blood cells; they bind to specific receptors and direct the growth and differentiation of distinct cell lines. (p. 741)

T-helper cells Cells that direct the actions of most of the other cells of the immune system. (p. 735)

T-lymphocytes Workhorses of the cellular immune system that are differentiated by their function in the immune system. (p. 734)

T-suppressor cells Cells that regulate and limit the immune response; opposite of T-helper cells. (p. 735)

Tumor antigens Chemical compounds expressed on the surfaces of tumor cells; they tell the immune system that these cells do not belong in the body, labeling the tumor cells as foreign. (p. 734)

In the past, care of patients with cancer required an understanding of three treatment modalities: surgery, radiation, and chemotherapy. Although these are highly sophisticated methods of cancer treatment, many cancer patients still are not cured. Surgery and radiation therapy are, at best, local or regional treatments. As discussed in the preceding chapter, adjuvant therapy is needed to destroy undetected distant micrometastases. The advantage of cytotoxic chemotherapy with antineoplastics is that these agents attack tumor cells throughout the body. However, this advantage is also the greatest limitation because all normal cells are exposed to the cytotoxic drug effects as well. Toxicity to normal cells may cause the administration of many other drugs to correct antineoplastic-induced side effects, or chemotherapy doses may have to be reduced to decrease side effects. This will simultaneously reduce their effectiveness.

Over the last two decades medical technology has developed a group of agents whose primary site of action is the immune system. These agents are collectively known as **biologic response modifiers (BRMs).** BRMs make up the fourth type of cancer therapy. The current modalities available to treat cancer are surgery, radiation, chemotherapy, and BRMs. BRMs are also used to treat autoimmune diseases.

BRMs can be broadly defined as agents that modify the body's own immune system (biologic response) so that it can destroy bacteria, viruses, and cancerous cells. The immune system is thought of primarily as our defense system against disease-carrying bacteria and viruses, but it is also an effective antitumor defense system. An intact immune system can identify cells as malignant and destroy them. In contrast to chemotherapy, the immune system can distinguish between tumor cells and normal body tissues. Normal cells are recognized as "self" and are not destroyed.

There are three major mechanisms by which BRMs work. The first mechanism augments, restores, or modifies the host defenses against the tumor. The second mechanism uses agents that are directly toxic to tumors (kill tumors). The third mechanism modifies the tumor's biology. To better understand this important class of anticancer drugs, a quick review of the immune system is beneficial.

IMMUNE SYSTEM

The immune system is an intricate biologic defense network of cells that are capable of distinguishing an unlimited variety of substances as being either foreign ("nonself") or being our own ("self"). When one of these foreign substances such as a bacteria or virus enters the body, the cells of the immune system recognize it as being nonself and eliminate or neutralize the invader. Tumors are not truly foreign substances because they arise from cells of normal tissues that have undergone uncontrolled growth. However, tumor cells do express chemical compounds on their surfaces that signal the immune system that these cells do not belong in the body. These chemical markers, called **tumor antigens** (Ag), label the tumor cells as abnormal cells.

The two major components of the body's immune system are **humoral immunity** and **cellular immunity.** These two systems act together to recognize and destroy humoral foreign particles and cells. Communication be-

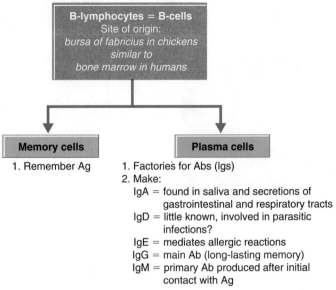

Fig. 46-1 Cells of the humoral immune system. *Ab,* Antibody; *Ag,* antigen; *Ig,* immunoglobin.

tween these two divisions is vital to the success of the immune system. Attack of tumor cells by **antibodies** produced by the humoral immune system prepares those tumor cells for destruction by the white blood cells (WBCs) of the cellular immune system. This is just one example of the effective way these two divisions of the immune system function and communicate.

Humoral Immune System

The specific "soldiers," or cells, of the humoral immune system that attack foreign invaders are lymphocytes. They are also called **B-cells** because they originate from the bone marrow and the bursa. B-cells (B-lymphocytes) are cells that are specific for production of antibodies. They remain dormant until that particular foreign substance antigen is detected.

B-lymphocytes are transformed in several steps into plasma cells. **Plasma cells** can be considered factories for the production of antibodies. Antibodies (Ab) are also known as immunoglobulins (Ig). They belong to and are made by the body. These cells bind to **antigens** to form an antibody-antigen complex. The antibodies that a particular plasma cell makes are all identical; therefore they are called **monoclonal.** They are made specifically to kill or neutralize the particular foreign antigen that the B-cell initially recognizes as being nonself. There are five major types of immunoglobulins: IgA, IgD, IgE, IgG, and IgM. These unique types have different structures and functions and are found in various areas of the body. As the B-lymphocytes are transformed to plasma cells, some become memory cells. **Memory cells** "remember" the exact characteristics of the particular foreign invader or antigen. The cells of the humoral immune system are shown in Fig. 46-1.

Cellular Immune System

The workhorses of the cellular immune system are the **T-lymphocytes,** also called *T-cells.* They are referred to as

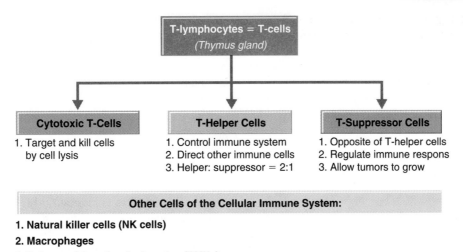

Fig. 46-2 Cells of the cellular immune system.

T-cells because one of their sites of origin is the thymus gland. There are three distinct populations of T-cells: **cytotoxic T-cells, T-helper cells,** and **T-suppressor cells.** They can be differentiated by the function they perform. Cytotoxic T-cells directly kill their targets by causing cell lysis. This is accomplished without the help of other immune system cells. T-helper cells are considered the master controllers of the immune system. These cells direct the actions of most of the other cells of the immune system, such as lymphokines (interferons [IFNs], interleukins, tumor necrosis factor, and monoclonal antibodies). T-suppressor cells have the opposite effect on the immune system, by regulating or limiting the immune response. They have the most important negative influence on antitumor actions of the immune system. Overactive T-suppressor cells may be responsible for and permit tumor growth. A healthy immune system has about twice as many T-helper cells as T-suppressor cells at any one time.

The cells of the cellular immune system are believed to be the major cells involved in the destruction of cancer cells. The cancer-killing cells that make up the cellular immune system are macrophages, several types of T-cells, natural killer (NK) cells, and polymorphonuclear leukocytes. Fig. 46-2 shows the components of the cellular immune system.

Therapy with BRMs combines the knowledge of several disciplines, including biology, genetics, immunology, pharmacology, medicine, and nursing. The therapeutic effects of BRMs are as follows:

- Regulation or augmentation of the immune response
- Cytotoxic or cytostatic activity directed toward cancer cells
- Inhibition of metastases, prevention of cell division, or inhibition of cell maturation

Box 46-1 lists the currently available BRMs that are used in the treatment of cancer or as adjunctive agents for patients receiving chemotherapy. They are classified according to biologic effects. There are many other types of BRMs, but those listed are the ones that are most commonly used in clinical practice.

BOX 46-1

Biologic Response Modifiers

INTERFERONS (IFNS)
Interferon-alpha
Interferon-beta
Interferon-gamma

INTERLEUKINS (ILS)
Interleukin-2 (IL-2)

VACCINES
Bacillus Calmette-Guérin vaccine (BCG)

COLONY-STIMULATING FACTORS (CSFS)
Granulocyte CSF (G-CSF)
Granulocyte-macrophage CSF (GM-CSF)
Erythrocyte CSF (EPO)

INTERFERONS

Before the commercial use of **colony-stimulating factors (CSFs),** IFNs were the best studied and most widely used BRMs. **Interferons** (IFNs) are BRMs that enhance the activity of macrophages and NK cells. These are the cells of the immune system that kill cancer cells. They are proteins that have three basic properties: antiviral, immune-modulating, and antitumor. Chemically they are glycoproteins (glyco = sugar and protein = amino acids). There are three different groups of IFNs, each with its own antigenic and biologic activity. They can be separated into alpha (α), beta (β), and gamma (γ) interferons. They are most commonly used in the treatment of hematologic malignancies or cancers. They can be manufactured from genetically modified *Escherichia coli* bacteria (*E. coli*) by recombinant DNA (rDNA) technology. In addition, IFNs are also obtained from pooled human leukocytes that have been stimulated (challenged) with various natural and synthetic inducers (antigens). Box 46-2 lists the available IFN preparations.

box 46-2

Interferon Preparations

INTERFERON-α
IFN alfa-2a (recombinant)*
IFN alfa-2b (recombinant)*
IFN alfa-n3†

INTERFERON-β
IFN beta-1a (recombinant)*
IFN beta-1b (recombinant)*

INTERFERON-γ
IFN gamma-1b (recombinant)*

*Recombinant refers to the origin (e.g., made by rDNA technology).
†The agent has been made with pooled human leukocytes.

Mechanism of Action

IFNs possess both antiviral and antineoplastic effects. Their effects on cancer cells are believed to be a combination of direct inhibitory effects on DNA and protein synthesis and multiple effects on the host's immune system. IFNs increase the cytotoxic activity of NK cells and the phagocytic ability of macrophages. It is important to note that these characteristics of IFNs are ineffective at high doses. Unlike that of conventional cytotoxic antineoplastics, the optimal biologic dose of IFNs is not necessarily the maximum dose tolerated by the patient. IFNs are also believed to increase the expression of cancer cell antigens on the cell surface, which enables the immune system to recognize them more easily.

Drug Effects

IFNs are recombinantly made natural substances that are identical to the IFNs that are present within our own bodies. Therefore they have the same properties of the IFNs in our own immune system. They protect our cells from virus attack by enabling our own cells to produce proteins (enzymes) that stop virus replication and prevent viruses from penetrating healthy cells. They prevent cancer cells from dividing and replicating and increase the activity of other cells in the immune system such as macrophages, monocytes, and NK cells. IFNs have three different effects on the immune system. They can (1) restore its function if it is impaired, (2) augment (amplify) the immune system's ability to function as the body's defense, and (3) inhibit the immune system from working. This is especially useful if the immune system has become dysfunctional, such as in an autoimmune disorder like systemic lupus erythematosis (SLE). Inhibiting the dysfunctional immune system prevents further damage to the body.

Therapeutic Uses

The beneficial actions of IFNs (antiviral, antineoplastic, and immunomodulatory) make them excellent agents for the treatment of viral infections, various cancers, and some autoimmune disorders. Box 46-3 lists the currently accepted indications for the use of interferons.

Side Effects and Adverse Effects

The most common side effects and adverse effects can be broadly classified as flulike effects: fever, chills, headache, malaise, myalgia, and fatigue. The major dose-limiting side effect of IFNs is fatigue. In high doses, patients become so exhausted that they are essentially confined to bed. Other side effects and adverse effects that can be seen with IFNs include anorexia, dizziness, nausea, vomiting, and diarrhea (Table 46-1).

Interactions

Drug interactions are seen with both IFN-α products (2a and 2b) when used with drugs such as aminophylline that are metabolized in the liver via the cytochrome P-450 enzyme system. The combination results in decreased metabolism and increased accumulation of these drugs, which leads to toxicity. There is also some evidence that concomitant use of IFNs and antiviral agents such as zidovudine enhances the activity of both. IFN-γ products can produce additive toxic effects to the bone marrow when used with other myelosuppressive agents.

Dosages

For recommended dosages, see the dosages table on p. 738.

drug profiles

The three major classes of IFNs (IFN-α, IFN-β, and IFN-γ) vary in their antigenic makeup, biologic actions, and pharmacologic properties. The best known IFN class is IFN-α. These drugs can be made recombinantly with *E. coli* or collected from pooled human leukocytes.

IFN products are biologic response modifiers that can be broadly classified as cytokines. **Cytokines** are immune system proteins that serve two essential functions. Cytokines direct the actions and communication between the cellular and humoral divisions of the immune system and augment or enhance the immune response. Other cytokines are tumor necrosis factor, interleukins, CSFs, and transfer factor. In 1957 they were found to have antiviral activity; their beneficial effects in treating cancer were discovered much later.

With the exception of the CSFs, IFNs are the most well studied and most widely used of the BRMs. There are three IFN-αs, two IFN-βs, and one IFN-γ.

BOX 46-3 Interferon: Therapeutic Uses

ANTIVIRAL USES
Rhinovirus
Papillovirus
Retrovirus
Hepatitis
Condyloma

ANTINEOPLASTIC USES
Hairy cell leukemia
Kaposi's sarcoma
Multiple myeloma
T-cell lymphoma
Chronic myeloid leukemia
Renal cell carcinoma
Melanoma
Bladder cancer

IMMUNOMODULATORY USES
Multiple sclerosis
Other autoimmune disorders

INTERFERON-α PRODUCTS
interferon alfa-2a, interferon alfa-2b, interferon alfa-n3

The most widely used IFN products are from the IFN-α class. They are also referred to as *leukocyte interferons* because they are produced from human leukocytes. IFN alfa-2a (Roferon-A) and IFN alfa-2b (Intron A) are pure clones of single alpha subtypes manufactured by recombinant DNA technology. This means that they are consistent from lot to lot. These two products differ in the sequence of two amino acids. IFN alfa-n3 (Alferon N) is a polyclonal mixture of all alpha subtypes. It is the product of pooled human leukocytes.

IFNs are classified as pregnancy category C agents and are contraindicated in hypersensitivity. They are most commonly given by either IM or SC routes of administration. However, IFNs have been given by IV and intraperitoneal routes as well. Alpha interferons are available only parenterally as 3-, 6-, 10-, and 36-million U/ml solutions (Roferon-A); 3-, 5-, 10-, 18-, 25-, and 50-million U/ml solutions (Intron A); and a 5-million U/ml solution (Alferon-N). Commonly recommended dosages are listed in dosages table on p. 738.

PHARMACOKINETICS

HALF-LIFE	ONSET	PEAK	DURATION
2a: 3.7-8.5 hr	3-4 hr	IM: 3.8-7.3 hr	24 hr
2b: 2-3 hr	3 hr	IM: 3 hr	Variable

INTERFERON-β PRODUCTS
interferon beta-1a

IFN beta-1a (Avonex) is one of the two currently available interferon-β products. It interacts with specific cell receptors found on the surface of human cells and possesses antiviral and immunoregulatory activity. It is indicated for the treatment of relapsing multiple sclerosis to slow progression of physical disability and decrease frequency of clinical exacerbations. It may also be used for the treatment of AIDS, AIDS-related Kaposi's sarcoma, re-

TABLE 46-1 Interferons: Adverse Effects

Body System	Side/Adverse Effect
Cardiovascular	Tachycardia, cyanosis, ECG changes, rare MI, orthostatic hypotension
Central nervous system	Mild confusion, somnolence, irritability, poor concentration, seizures, hallucinations, paranoid psychoses
Gastrointestinal	Nausea, diarrhea, vomiting, anorexia, taste alterations, dry mouth
Hematopoietic	Neurtropenia, thrombocytopenia
Renal/hepatic	Increased BUN, creatinine, proteinuria, liver function tests (transaminases)

nal cell carcinoma, malignant melanoma, and acute non-A, non-B hepatitis.

It is available as a 33-μg (6.6 million unit) powder for injection. It is contraindicated in patients with a history of hypersensitivity to natural or recombinant interferon-β, human albumin, or any other component of the formulation. It is considered a pregnancy category C agent. Common dosage recommendations are listed in the dosages table on p. 738.

PHARMACOKINETICS

HALF-LIFE	ONSET	PEAK	DURATION
10 hr	12 hr	3-15 hr	4 days

interferon beta-1b

IFN beta-1b (Betaseron) is manufactured from cultures of *E. coli* by means of recombinant DNA technology and is identical to the body's IFN-β. The *E. coli* has been modified to include a plasmid that incorporates the gene for human IFN-β. The *E. coli* then mass produces the exact genetic sequence for IFN beta-1b. As with the other IFNs it has antiviral, antineoplastic, and immunomodulating activities. IFN beta-1b is indicated to reduce the frequency

DOSAGES Selected Interferons

agent	pharmacologic class	dosage range	purpose
INTERFERON-α PRODUCTS			
interferon alfa-2a (Roferon-A, Intron A, Alferon N)	Immunomodulator	IM/SC: 3 million IU/day for 16-24 wk; maintenance dose 3 million IU 3 times/wk	Hairy cell leukemia
		IM/SC: 36 million IU/day for 10-12 wk; maintenance dose 36 million IU 3 times/wk	Kaposi's sarcoma (AIDS-related)
interferon alfa-2b (Intron A)	Immunomodulator antineoplastic antiviral	*Adult* IM/SC: 3 million IU 3 times/wk for up to 6 mo	Chronic hepatitis non-A, non-B, non-C
		IM/SC: 30-35 million IU/wk as 5 million IU/day or 10 million IU 3 times/wk for 16 wk	Chronic hepatitis B
		IM/SC: 2 million IU/m² 3 times/wk	Hairy cell leukemia
		IM/SC: 30 million IU/m² 3 times/wk	Kaposi's sarcoma (AIDS-related)
		IM/SC: 1 million IU into each wart (lesion) 3 times/wk PM	Condylomata acuminata (genital/perianal warts)
interferon alfa-n3 (Alferon N)	Immunomodulator antiviral	*Adult* IM/SC: 250,000 IU/wart twice/wk for up to 8 wk; do *not* exceed 2.5 million IU/treatment session	Condylomata acuminata
INTERFERON-β PRODUCTS			
interferon beta-1a (Avonex)	Immunomodulator	*Adult* IM: 30 mg once a week	Multiple sclerosis
interferon beta-1b (Betaseron)	Immunomodulator	SC: 0.25 mg (8 million IU) qod	Multiple sclerosis
INTERFERON-γ PRODUCTS			
interferon-gamma-1b (Actimmune)	Immunomodulator	SC: Body surface area >0.5 m²: 50 μg/m² 3 times/wk Body surface area <0.5 m²: 1.5 μg/kg 3 times/wk	Reducing frequency/ severity of infections associated with chronic granulomatous disease

of neurologic exacerbations of relapsing-remitting multiple sclerosis and is classified as a pregnancy category B agent. It is available only parenterally as a 9.6 million-U vial for SC injection. Commonly recommended dosages are listed in the dosages table above.

PHARMACOKINETICS

HALF-LIFE	ONSET	PEAK	DURATION
Up to 4.3 hr	3-4 hr	1-8 hr	Variable

INTERFERON-γ PRODUCTS
interferon gamma-1b

IFN gamma-1b (Actimmune) is the last of the currently available IFN products. It was approved by the FDA in 1991 for the treatment of serious infections associated with chronic granulomatous disease. Its use in the treatment of cancer has not been approved. It is similar in its characteristics to other members of the IFN family of BRMs. It is produced by rDNA technology. IFN gamma-1b is available parenterally only as a 3 million-U single-dose vial for SC injection. Commonly rec-

ommended dosages are listed in the dosages table above.

PHARMACOKINETICS

HALF-LIFE	ONSET	PEAK	DURATION
IM: 2.9 hr	4 hr	4 hr	24 hr

INTERLEUKINS

Interleukins are classified in the immune system as lymphokines. Lymphokines are soluble proteins that are released from activated lymphocytes (particularly from T-cells and NK cells). There are many interleukins (IL-2, IL-3, IL-4, IL-5, IL-6, and IL-11), and more are being identified as we increase our knowledge of the immune system.

The two interleukins currently available are interleukin-2 (IL-2 or aldesleukin) and interleukin-11 (IL-11 or oprelvekin). Aldesleukin is produced by activated T-cells in response to macrophage-"processed" antigens and secreted interleukin-1 (IL-1). Aldesleukin was formerly called *T-cell growth factor* because, among other actions, it aids in the growth and differentiation of T-lymphocytes. Aldesleukin is not directly toxic but acts primarily as an

BOX 46-4 Interleukin-2: Drug Effects

MODULATING EFFECTS	ENHANCING EFFECTS
Proliferation of T-cells	Killer T-cell activity
Synthesis and secretion of cytokines	Amplifies effects of these cytokines
Increases production of B-cells (Abs)	Enhances the cytotoxic actions of NK cells and LAK cells
Proliferation and activation of NK cells	
Proliferation and activation of LAK cells	

NK, Natural killer, *LAK,* lymphokine-activated killer.

BOX 46-5 Interleukin-2: Therapeutic Uses

NUMEROUS STUDIES	LIMITED STUDIES
Metastatic renal cell carcinoma	Glial tumors
Malignant melanoma	Non-Hodgkin's lymphomas
Colorectal adenocarcinoma	Hodgkin's disease
	Lung carcinoma
	Head and neck cancer
	Ovarian cancer
	Breast carcinoma

immunomodulator and immunorestorer. Oprelvekin is an endogenous substance produced by bone marrow cells. Oprelvekin (Neumega) is a recombinant DNA product produced from *E. coli.*

Mechanism of Action

Interleukins cause multiple effects and actions within the immune system, one of which is beneficial antitumor action. Aldesleukin binds to receptor sites on certain WBCs called T-cells, causing the T-cells to multiply. One type of cell that results from this multiplication is the **lymphokine-activated killer (LAK) cell.** The LAK cells recognize cancer cells and ignore normal cells (avoiding the toxic effects of antineoplastics). When the LAK cells come into contact with cancer cells, the cancer cells are destroyed.

Oprelvekin is a thrombopoietic growth factor. Although it is an interleukin like aldesleukin, it shares more similarities with the CSFs. Oprelvekin directly stimulates the proliferation of hematopoietic stem cells and megakaryocyte progenitor cells. This results in megakaryocyte maturation, which in turn results in increased platelet production. The similarities between G-CSF, GM-CSF, and oprelvekin are that G-CSF stimulates granulocyte production, GM-CSF stimulates granulocytes and macrophages, and oprelvekin stimulates platelet production. They all stimulate the production of a necessary cell line for normal health.

Drug Effects

The drug effects of aldesleukin are multiple. The lymphokine aldesleukin directs and enhances the function of the immune system and its cells. It is therefore said to be an immunomodulator and an immunorestorer. The drug effects of aldesleukin are listed in Box 46-4.

The drug effects of oprelvekin are primarily limited to proliferation of hematopoietic stem cells and megakaryocyte progenitor cells. The resulting drug effect of stimulating these two different types of early cell lines is increased production of platelets.

Therapeutic Uses

The best documented clinical activity is that seen in the treatment of melanomas and renal cell carcinomas. Other cancers that have shown varying degrees of response to therapy with aldesleukin are listed in Box 46-5. Oprelvekin is used for the prevention of severe thrombocytopenia and the reduction of the need for platelet transfusions after myelosuppressive chemotherapy in patients with nomyeloid malignancies who are at high risk for severe thrombocytopenia.

Side Effects and Adverse Effects

Unfortunately, therapy with aldesleukin is frequently complicated by severe toxicity. A syndrome known as capillary leak syndrome is responsible for the severe toxicities of aldesleukin. As the name implies, capillary leak syndrome refers to the condition induced by interleukin therapy in which the capillaries lose their ability to retain vital colloids such as albumin, protein, and other essential components of blood vessels. Because the capillaries are "leaky," these substances migrate into the surrounding tissues. This results in massive fluid retention (20 to 30 pounds), which can lead to the following life-threatening problems: respiratory distress, congestive heart failure (CHF), dysrhythmias, and myocardial infarction (MI). The positive side to this is that these are all reversible after discontinuation of the interleukin therapy. Close patient monitoring and vigorous supportive care are essential in the patient receiving aldesleukin therapy. Other side effects and adverse effects that may be associated with IL-2 therapy are fever, chills, rash, fatigue, hepatotoxicity, myalgias, headaches, and eosinophilia.

Oprelvekin's primary side effects are edema, fever, headache, rash, tachycardia, vasodilation, nausea and vomiting, diarrhea, and dyspnea. Most adverse events with oprelvekin are mild or moderate in severity and reversible after discontinuation of oprelvekin dosing.

Interactions

Aldesleukin, when given with antihypertensives, can have additive hypotensive effects. Corticosteroids coadministered with aldesleukin can reduce antitumor effectiveness. The toxic effects of aldesleukin are increased when it is administered with aminoglycosteroids, indomethacin, cytotoxic chemotherapy, methotrexate, asparaginase, and doxorubicin.

Dosages

For recommended dosages, see the dosages table on p. 742.

drug profiles

Aldesleukin is a human IL-2 derivative that is made by recombinant DNA technology. It is a cytokine that is produced by lymphocytes and therefore belongs to the lymphokine family of BRMs. Aldesleukin is currently FDA-approved only for the treatment of metastatic renal cell carcinoma, despite its activity in other cancers. It is recommended by the manufacturer to be administered only in a hospital setting under the supervision of a qualified physician experienced in the use of antineoplastic agents and only when the benefits are thought to outweigh the possible risks.

⊶ aldesleukin

Aldesleukin (IL-2; Proleukin) is a BRM that kills cancer cells by causing the production of LAK cells, which recognize and destroy cancer cells. Although many interleukins have been identified, aldesleukin is one of only two currently available interleukins. Aldesleukin is classified as a pregnancy category C agent and is contraindicated in patients with hypersensitivity, abnormal thallium stress test or pulmonary function tests, and organ allografts. It is available only in parenteral form as a 22 million-U vial for IV infusion. Although it is recommended to be given over 15 minutes by IV infusion, it has been given by IV bolus, continuous infusion, and SC, perilesional, intraperitoneal, intrahepatic, and intrathecal routes. Commonly recommended dosages are listed in the dosages table on p. 742.

PHARMACOKINETICS

HALF-LIFE	ONSET	PEAK	DURATION
85 min	< or = 4 wk*	Unknown	< or = 12 mo

*To reach therapeutic onset.

oprelvekin

Oprelvekin (Neumega) is one of the two currently available interleukins. It works and is used more like a CSF in that it primarly produces a particular cell line, the platelets. It is currently indicated to prevent severe thrombocytopenia, the need for platelet transfusions after chemotherapy, which would wipe out a patient's platelets.

It is available as a 5-mg powder for injection. It is contraindicated in patients with a history of hypersensitivity to it or any other component of the formulation. It is considered a pregnancy category C agent. Common dosage recommendations are listed in the dosages table on p. 742.

PHARMACOKINETICS

HALF-LIFE	ONSET	PEAK	DURATION
7 hr	5-9 days*	3 hr†	14 days

Activity

*Platelet counts begin to increase.
†Peak serum concentrations.

COLONY-STIMULATING FACTORS

CSFs are cytokines that regulate the growth, differentiation, and function of bone marrow stem cells. **Stem cells** are the precursors of mature blood cells such as platelets, granulocytes, and macrophages. They include the kidney-derived protein erythropoietin (EPO), granulocyte CSF (G-CSF), granulocyte-macrophage CSF (GM-CSF), macrophage CSF (M-CSF), and interleukin-3 (IL-3). Each binds to specific receptors and directs the growth and differentiation of distinct cell lines. The survival of the mature cells and regulation of their biologic activity is also a consequence of CSF binding. Box 46-6 lists the CSFs and the cell lines that they stimulate.

CSFs are not directly toxic to cancer cells, but they do have beneficial effects in the treatment of cancer. CSFs decrease the duration of chemotherapy-induced neutropenia, enable higher doses of chemotherapy to be given, decrease bone marrow recovery time after bone marrow transplants or radiation, and stimulate other cells in the immune system to destroy or inhibit the growth of cancer and viral- or fungal-infected cells.

Mechanism of Action

The same mechanism of action applies to all five CSFs (EPO, IL-3, G-CSF, GM-CSF, and M-CSF). These agents are produced by recombinant DNA technology and thus are identical to endogenously produced CSFs. These substances work by binding to receptors on the surface of cells in the bone marrow. These particular cells are called *progenitor cells* and are responsible for the production of particular cell lines (red blood cells [RBCs], WBCs, platelets, etc.). When a CSF binds to the surface, the progenitor cell is stimulated to make new cells, mature, and become functionally active. The principal effects on the progenitor cells are proliferation, differentiation, and activation. They may also enhance certain functions of mature cell lines.

Drug Effects

CSFs have many potential effects. They can decrease the duration of neutropenia or low neutrophil counts. This is typically seen after chemotherapy because the cytotoxic effects of the antineoplastic agents are not only directed at the cancer cells but also kill the bone marrow cells. CSFs also limit the severity of this toxic chemotherapy-induced effect by preventing decrease of neutrophil counts.

Another beneficial drug effect of CSFs is the stimulation of certain immune cells (macrophages and granulocytes) to destroy or inhibit the growth of tumor cells and viral- or fungal-infected cells. They enhance the immune system's ability to kill off cancer cells, viruses, and fungi.

Therapeutic Uses

There are many beneficial therapeutic uses of CSFs. Because they decrease the duration of low neutrophil

box 46-6

Colony-Stimulating Factors: Target Cell Lines

CSF	Cell Line Stimulated
EPO (erythropoietin)	Erythrocytes (RBCs)
IL-3 (interleukin-3)	Pluripotent stem cells*
G-CSF (granulocyte CSF)	Granulocytes
GM-CSF (granulocyte-macrophage CSF)	Granulocytes and macrophages
M-CSF (macrophage CSF)	Macrophages

*The first cell involved in the production of cells that arise from the bone marrow.

Colony-Stimulating Factors: Common Adverse Effects

Body System	Side/Adverse Effect
Cardiovascular	Hypertension (EPO) and edema
Gastrointestinal	Anorexia, nausea, vomiting, diarrhea
Integumentary	Alopecia and rash
Respiratory	Cough, dyspnea, sore throat
Other	Fever, blood dyscrasias, headache, bone pain

table 46-2

EPO, Erythropoetin.

counts (WBCs), they reduce the incidence and the duration of infections. These infections normally appear in patients who have experienced destruction of bone marrow cells as a result of cytotoxic chemotherapy. CSFs stimulate these cells to grow and mature and thus directly oppose the detrimental bone marrow actions of chemotherapy.

Because of CSFs' effect on the cells of the bone marrow, higher doses of chemotherapy can be given, resulting in the destruction of a greater number of cancer cells.

The effect of CSFs on the bone marrow cells also results in a decrease of the recovery time of bone marrow cells after bone marrow transplants and radiation therapy. Both bone marrow transplantation and radiation therapy are toxic to the bone marrow. When a CSF is administered, bone marrow cells return to normal counts in a drastically shortened time.

CSFs also enhance the cells of the immune system, such as macrophages and granulocytes. This results in an enhanced ability to kill cancer cells and inhibition of both viral- and fungal-infected cells.

Side Effects and Adverse Effects

Side effects and adverse effects associated with the use of CSFs are mild. The most common are fever, muscle aches, bone pain, and flushing. The common side effects and adverse effects associated with CSFs are listed in Table 46-2.

Interactions

Of the currently available BRMs, G-CSF (filgrastim) and GM-CSF (sargramostim) are the only two agents that have any significant drug interactions. The most significant drug interaction with these two agents occurs when myelosuppressive antineoplastic agents given with them. G-CSF and GM-CSF are given to enhance the production of bone marrow cells; therefore when myelosuppressive antineoplastics are given with them, they directly antagonize each other. Typically these BRMs are given once myelosuppressive antineoplastics have reached their nadirs.

Dosages

For recommended dosages, see the dosages table on p. 742.

drug profiles

CSFs are cytokines that regulate the growth, differentiation, and function of bone marrow stem cells. **Stem cells** are the precursors of mature blood cells such as platelets, granulocytes, and macrophages. They include the kidney-derived protein EPO, G-CSF, GM-CSF, M-CSF, and IL-3. Each binds to specific receptors and directs the growth and differentiation of distinct cell lines. The survival of the mature cells and regulation of their biologic activity is also a consequence of CSF binding. Only three of the five CSFs are currently available—EPO, G-CSF, and GM-CSF.

epoetin alfa

Epoetin alfa (EPO recombinant, Epogen, and Procrit) is a biosynthetic form of the natural hormone EPO, which is normally secreted from the kidneys in response to a decrease in RBCs and many other stimuli. Epoetin is a CSF that is primarily responsible for erythropoiesis (formation of RBCs). It is made by means of rDNA technology, resulting in the production of mass quantities of identical EPO alfa.

Epoetin is used to correct deficiencies of endogenous EPO production. These conditions are common in patients with anemia resulting from end-stage renal disease, HIV infection, and cancer. Its use is associated with two potential serious adverse effects that should be closely monitored. Epoetin causes the progenitor cells in the bone marrow to manufacture more RBCs and mature these immature RBCs more quickly. If therapy is not stopped when the hemoglobin and hematocrit (H/H) reach a certain level or if the H/H rises too quickly, hypertension and seizures can result.

EPO should be used during pregnancy only when the potential benefits justify the possible risks to the fetus. As such it is classified as a pregnancy category C agent. It is contraindicated in hypersensitivity. EPO is available only in a parenteral form as 2000-, 3000-, 4000-, and 10,000-U vials for IV or

DOSAGES Selected Interleukins and Colony-Stimulating Factors

agent	pharmacologic class	dosage range	purpose
INTERLEUKINS			
aldesleukin (Proleukin)	Lymphokine antineoplastic	*Adult* IV: 600,000 IU/kg dose by a 15 m infusion q8h for 14 doses; repeated following a 9-day period	Selected metastatic renal cell carcinoma
oprelvekin (IL-11, Neumega)	Platelet growth factor	*Adult* SQ: 50 μg/kg daily *Pediatric* SQ: 75-100 μg/kg daily	Prevent thrombocytopenia
COLONY-STIMULATING FACTORS			
epoetin alfa (Erythropoietin recombinent, Epgen, Procrit)	Erythropoietic agent	*Adult* IV/SC: 50-100 U/kg 3 times/wk, and adjust dose when the hematocrit is close to 36% IV/SC: 100 U/kg 3 times/wk for 8-12 wk SC: 150 U/kg 3 times/wk for 8 wk	Anemia associated with chronic renal failure Zidovudine associated anemia Chemotherapy-associated anemia
filgrastim (Neupogen)	Granulocyte colony-stimulating factor (G-CSF)	IV/SC: Usual dose of 5 ug/kg as a single daily injection with a range of 0.6-120 μg/kg/day IV/SC: 10 μg/kg/day SC: 5 μg/kg/day SC: 6 μg/kg twice day	Chemotherapy-induced neutropenia Bone marrow transplantation Cyclic/diopathic neutropenia Congenital neutropenia
sargramostim (Leukine)	Granulocyte-macrophage colony-stimulating factor (GM-CSF)	IV: 250 μg/m²/day in 2-hr infusion for 14 days; may be repeated in 7 days; a third course of 500 μg/m²/day for 14 days may be required IV: 250 μg/m²/day in a 2-hr infusion starting 2-4 hr after transplant infusion for 21 days	Bone marrow transplantation delay/failure Myeloid recovery

SC injection. Commonly recommended dosages are found in the table above.

PHARMACOKINETICS

HALF-LIFE	ONSET	PEAK	DURATION
4-13 hr	7-10 days	5-24 hr (serum)	Variable

filgrastim

Filgrastim (G-CSF, Neupogen) is a human G-CSF. G-CSF stimulates the cells in the bone marrow that are precursors to granulocytes. Granulocytes are basophils, eosinophils, and neutrophils. These are more commonly referred to as WBCs and are the body's primary defense against bacterial and fungal infections. Filgrastim has the same pharmacologic effects as endogenous human G-CSF. It affects the proliferation, differentiation, and activation of the cells that make neutrophils.

Filgrastim is indicated to decrease infections (febrile neutropenia) in patients receiving myelosuppressive antineoplastics for nonmyeloid malignancies. Filgrastim is classified as a pregnancy category C agent and is contraindicated in hy-

persensitivity and excessive myeloid blast cells (10% in the blood or bone marrow). Filgrastim is available only in a parenteral form as 300- and 480-μg vials for IV or SC injection. Commonly recommended dosages are found in the table above.

PHARMACOKINETICS

HALF-LIFE	ONSET	PEAK	DURATION
3-5 hr*	1 hr	2-6 hr	12-24 hr

*Highly variable.

sargramostim

Sargramostim (GM-CSF, Leukine) is a human GM-CSF. GM-CSF stimulates the cells in the bone marrow that are precursors to granulocytes and macrophages. Sargramostim has the same pharmacologic effects as endogenous human GM-CSF. It affects the proliferation, differentiation, and activation of the cells that make granulocytes and macrophages.

Sargramostim is indicated for use in bone marrow transplantation patients for myeloid recovery

Activity

(bone marrow recovery) after autologous bone marrow transplantation in Hodgkin's and non-Hodgkin's lymphomas and acute lymphoblastic leukemia. Sargramostim is classified as a pregnancy category C agent and is contraindicated in hypersensitivity and excessive myeloid blast cells (10% in the blood or bone marrow). Sargramstim is available only in a parenteral form as 250- and 500-µg vials for IV or SC injection. Commonly recommended dosages are found in the table on p. 742.

PHARMACOKINETICS

HALF-LIFE	ONSET	PEAK	DURATION
2 hr	4 hr*	SC: 2 hr	10 days*

*Therapeutic effect.

nursing process

● Assessment

Before administering any of the IFN agents, it is important for the nurse to rule out any of the contraindications to its use, such as hypersensitivity to the drug, egg proteins, IgG, or neomycin. Cautious use with close monitoring is recommended during pregnancy, during lactation, in children, and in patients with cardiac disease, angina, CHF, COPD, diabetes mellitus, bleeding disorders (hemophilia, thrombophlebitis), bone marrow depression, and convulsive disorders. In addition, baseline vital signs and an assessment of infection, CBC, level of consciousness, mental status, and any confusion should be obtained and documented.

IL-1 and IL-2 are lymphokines that are commonly ordered BRMs. Before administering these agents, you should assess the patient for underlying diseases, such as cardiac conditions, because cautious use is recommended in these situations. Contraindications to its use include hypersensitivity to the drug and to proteins of *E. coli*. These interleukins are *not* to be given with antineoplastics. Serum laboratory values such as CBC, platelet levels, BUN, creatinine, urinalysis, aspartate transaminase (AST), and alkaline phosphatase should be checked before treatment and twice weekly during therapy. Neutrophil counts must also be obtained and documented.

● Nursing Diagnoses

Nursing diagnoses are as follows:
- Acute pain related to the side effects of immunomodulators.
- Imbalanced nutrition, less than body requirements, related to GI side effects of BRMs.
- Impaired skin integrity (rash) related to side effects of BRMs.
- Risk for injury (falls) related to weakness and fatigue from BRMs.
- Impaired gas exchange related to side effects of BRMs.

● Planning

Goals related to administration of the BRMs include the following:
- Patient regains prechemotherapy (and as near normal as possible) nutritional status.
- Patient experiences minimal weight loss during therapy.
- Patient maintains or regains normal GI/GU patterns.
- Patient's mucous membranes regain and/or maintain intactness during therapy.
- Patient is free of self-injury related to drug therapy.

Outcome Criteria

Outcome criteria related to the administration of immunomodulators are as follows:
- Patient will describe nutritional needs and a menu to follow according to the food guide pyramid and other dietary changes, as prescribed (e.g., high calorie, low residue).
- Patient will state measures to minimize GI side effects such as small, frequent meals and avoiding spicy foods.
- Patient will be without injured tissue during therapy because of good mouth and oral hygiene daily and as needed.
- Patient will state ways to minimize self-injury related to weakness and fatigue from BRMs such as assistive devices, grab bars or rails, and help at home.

● Implementation

IFN agents are usually given subcutaneously or intramuscularly and should be given at bedtime to minimize CNS side effects. Acetaminophen may be needed for the commonly occurring side effects of headache, fever, and joint aches. Fluids should be increased while patients are taking these medications.

GM-CSF and other CSFs are immunomodulators, and response to the medication in patients who receive these should be closely monitored. Sargramstim should be administered after reconstitution with 1 ml of sterile water without preservatives for injection, and the vial should not be shaken. For IV infusions, you should

NURSING CARE PLAN Neutropenia

Mr. J.L., a 73-year-old retired fireman, presents to the oncologist's office with complaints of fever, fatigue, and cough. Upon examination of the patient and a look at his WBC levels (3200/mm³), the physician orders an injection of filgrastim (Neupogen). The patient asks many questions about the injection, including what to expect and if it will really help. His wife, a retired public health nurse in excellent health, is eager to help in any way, and asks you, the oncology nurse, for some information.

assessment	**Nursing Diagnosis**	Acute pain related to side effects of neutropenia (joint pain, nausea and vomiting, sores in mouth)
	Subjective Data	"I've been coughing for 2 days."
		"I feel so tired and like I have the flu."
		"What is this drug?"
	Objective Data	WBC at 3200/mm³
		Temperature 101.4°
		P110 R34
		Status post 2 rounds of chemotherapy
		Diagnosis of liver cancer
planning and outcome criteria	**Goals**	Patient and wife will verbalize instructions and side effects before leaving the oncologist's office.
	Outcome Criteria	Before the end of this office visit, patient and wife will report or verbalize the following:
		• Side effects of filgrastim
		• Symptoms that should be reported to the health care provider
		• Importance of return visits for laboratory studies
implementation		Patient education with written *and* verbal instructions including the following points:
		• Side effects you may experience and nausea, vomiting, diarrhea, sores in mouth, and pain in your joints and bones.
		• Call us at any time if your bone or joint pain is not responding to rest and low doses of acetaminophen; we may need to order a stronger pain pill.
		• We will be monitoring your CBC and platelet counts today and about two times each week, and we may continue filgrastim treatment until the oncologist thinks your WBCs are at a safer level.
		• If you require frequent injections, we may teach you and your wife how to give the SC injection, if you are willing to learn the technique.
evaluation		Positive therapeutic outcomes include the following:
		• Absence of symptoms and side effects of infection
		• Return of WBC to acceptable levels
		• Minimal side effects of filgrastim
		• Increased ADLs
		• Improved overall well-being

dilute the medication in 0.9% NaCl. If the final concentration is >10 μg/ml, you should add human albumin to the NaCl to make a final concentration of 0.1% before adding the sargramstim. This agent is to be given within 6 hours after reconstitution.

Interleukins, such as filgrastim (G-CSF), should be given with single-use vials only. This agent is generally given until absolute neutrophil count (ANC) is approximately 10,000/mm³ after the expected chemotherapy neutrophil nadir, which is usually a 2-week period. The vial should not be shaken when withdrawing solution. Aldesleukin,

another interleukin, should be administered by IV infusion every 8 hours as ordered.

See the patient teaching tips for BRMs on p. 745.

● Evaluation

Therapeutic responses to BRMs include a decrease in the growth of the lesion or mass, decreased tumor size, and ease in breathing. Other therapeutic responses include improved or even maintained blood counts and absence of infection, anemias, and hemorrhage. Possible side effects are presented in Table 46-2.

patient teaching tips

Biologic Response Modifiers

➤ Patients should avoid hazardous tasks because of CNS changes. Fatigue is a common side effect. Patients should report signs of infection such as sore throat, fever, diarrhea, and vomiting. Pregnancy is discouraged while the patient is taking BRMs.

➤ Interleukins can be self-administered, so patients should learn self-injection technique and proper disposal of equipment such as needles and syringes. A corresponding instruction sheet should be provided for the patient.

➤ Bone pain and flulike symptoms often occur with some of the CSFs and may require the use of non-narcotic analgesics. Patients should report any side effects (hair loss, fever, joint pain, chills, diarrhea, edema, anemia, anorexia, fatigue, hypotension, thrombocytopenia) to their physician immediately so that dosage can be changed, corrected, or reconsidered.

POINTS TO REMEMBER

Cancer Treatments

- Traditional involved surgery, radiation, and chemotherapy.
- These are at best local or regional therapy.
- Often adjuvant therapy is needed to destroy undetected distant micrometastases.
- Fourth type of cancer therapy is collectively known as biologic response modifiers (BRMs).

Biologic Response Modifiers

- Modify a person's own immune system (biologic response) to foreign invaders.
- Body's own immune system is exploited to destroy cancerous cells.
- Can either augment, restore, or modify the host defenses against the tumor.
- May be directly toxic to tumors.
- May modify the tumor's biology.

Immune System

- Humoral and cellular immune system act together to recognize and destroy foreign particles and cells.
- Humoral immune system is composed of lymphocytes known as B-cells until they are transformed into plasma cells when they come in contact with an antigen (foreign substance).
- Plasma cells then manufacture antibodies to that antigen.
- There are five antibodies known as immunoglobulins (IgA, IgD, IgE, IgG, and IgM).
- Cellular immune system is composed of T-lymphocytes and T-cells.
- Cytotoxic, helper, and suppressor T-cells.

Interferons

- BRMs that enhance the activity of macrophages and natural killer cells.
- Have three basic properties: antiviral, immune-modulating, and antitumor actions.
- Different from interleukins, which are lymphokines.
- Lymphokines are substances that are released from activated lymphocytes (T-cells and natural killer cells).

Colony-Stimulating Factors

- Substances that regulate the growth, differentiation, and function of bone marrow stem cells, which are the precursors of mature blood cells (platelets, granulocytes, and macrophages).

Nursing Considerations

- Nursing management associated with the administration of BRMs focuses on careful asepsis, proper nutrition, oral hygiene, and the prevention of infection.
- Nursing care of patients receiving BRMs often focuses on comfort because of the flulike symptoms associated with these agents.
- BRMs have the ability to alter the immunologic relationship between a tumor and the patient with cancer to provide a potentially therapeutic response.
- Interferons, monoclonal antibodies, lymphokines, and cytokines are examples of BRMs.
- Side effects common to BRMs include fatigue, flulike symptoms, leukopenia, nausea, and vomiting.

REVIEW QUESTIONS

1. Which of the following best describes the action of interferons in the management of malignant tumors?
   a. Interferons increase the production of specific anti-cancer enzymes.
   b. Interferons have antiviral and antitumor properties and strengthen the immune system.
   c. Interferons stimulate the production and activation of T-lymphocytes and cytotoxic T-cells.

d. Interferons are retrieved from healthy donors and help improve the cell-killing action of T-cells.

2. Capillary leak syndrome while a patient is experiencing interleukin treatment may result in all of the following except:
   a. Dehydration.
   b. Fluid retention.
   c. Myocardial infarction.
   d. Congestive heart failure.

3. Which of the following is an appropriate nursing intervention for the patient receiving sargramstin?
   a. Reconstitute wih only 10% dextrose.
   b. Give the agent within 6 hours of reconstitution.
   c. Shake the solution after mixing, and administer up to 24 hours.

d. Administer the agent without concern for dilution or type of solution.

4. Colony-stimulating factors may result in which of the following?
   a. Gynecomastia
   b. Hypertrichosis
   c. Prevention of decrease of neutrophils
   d. Prevention of occurrence of polycythemia

5. Which of the following would not be an appropriate nursing intervention for patients receiving interferon?
   a. Increase fluids.
   b. Avoid NSAIDs.
   c. Limit fluid intake.
   d. Administer acetaminophen for aching.

For Answers see www.harcourthealth.com/MERLIN/Lilley/.

CRITICAL THINKING Activities

1. C.F. is to receive Neupogen after a course of carmustine and radiation for a brain tumor. C.F. weighs 132 pounds. The protocol that the oncologist has given you states that the G-CSF should be dosed at 5 μg/kg. What dose should the patient receive, and what vial should be used so as to waste as little drug as possible?

2. What is so important about the timing of the dosage of colony-stimulating factor in treatment of neoplasms?

3. Many medications, especially chemotherapy, may lead to the adverse effect of bone marrow suppression of various blood cell components. What symptoms would you expect to see if your patient had diminished production of platelets? Red blood cells? White blood cells? Explain your answers.

For Answers see www.harcourthealth.com/MERLIN/Lilley/.

bibliography

Albanese J, Nutz P: *Mosby's 2001 nursing drug reference and review cards,* St Louis, 2001, Mosby.

American Hospital Formulary Service: *AHFS drug information,* Bethesda, Md, 2000, American Society of Health-System Pharmacists.

Anderson PO, Knoben JE, Troutman WG: *Handbook of clinical drug data 1999-2000,* ed 9, New York, 1999, McGraw-Hill.

Johns Hopkins Hospital, Department of Pediatrics et al: *The Harriet Lane handbook,* ed 15, St Louis, 2000, Mosby.

Keen JH: *Critical care and emergency drug reference,* ed 3, St Louis, 1996, Mosby.

McKenry LM, Salerno E: *Mosby's pharmacology in nursing,* ed 21, St Louis, 2001, Mosby.

Mosby's GenRx: a comprehensive reference for generic and brand drugs, ed 10, St Louis, 2000, Mosby.

Skidmore-Roth L: *Mosby's 2001 nursing drug reference,* St Louis, 2001, Mosby.

Straw L, Conrad K: Patient education resources related to biotherapy and the immune system, *Oncol Nurs Forum* 21(7):1223, 1994.

Wolf BA: Overview of therapeutic drug monitoring and biotechnologic drugs, *Therapeutic Drug Monitoring* 18:402, 1996.

Activity

Remember to check the **Online Worksheet** for additional learning opportunities: **www.harcourthealth.com/MERLIN/Lilley/**

Drugs Affecting the Gastrointestinal System and Nutrition: Study Skills Tips

- Active Questioning
- What are the Right Questions?
- Kinds of Questions
- Questioning Applications

ACTIVE QUESTIONING

There is one technique for study that cannot be overemphasized: active questioning. In the PURR study model it is critical to be able to generate questions in the Plan, Rehearsal, and Review steps. The questions you generate when applying PURR are essential in helping you maintain concentration as you study, improving your comprehension as you read assigned material, and developing long-term memory. Active questioning is a strategy that you must practice continuously. It is a strategy that develops with practice.

WHAT ARE THE RIGHT QUESTIONS?

Some questions generated during the Plan step will be useful and will focus on exactly the right issues for maximum learning. On the other hand, sometimes the questions generated by looking at the chapter outline or accented material in the body of 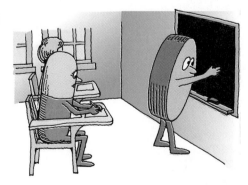 the text will be inappropriate. These questions seem logical and important when you are working with the limited amount of information available using the Plan step, but as you read the chapter you will find that they miss the mark. Do not worry about whether each question you ask is perfectly focused. As you read, rehearse, and review the material, you can and should revise questions based on your growing understanding of the material. The important point is to ask many questions to help you maintain active involvement in the learning process and anticipate questions that will appear on exams. The more questions you ask, the more effective you will become both as an active questioner and as an active learner.

KINDS OF QUESTIONS

First, you must realize that there is more than one kind of question to be asked. Over the years there have been many questioning hierarchies proposed by educators and scholars. The different kinds of questions vary from three or four to as many as seven or eight. Following is a simple approach that focuses on two types of questions.

Literal Questions

Literal questions are those that are answered directly and specifically by the text. When you were reading a story in elementary school and the teacher asked, "What did Sally do when she lost her movie money?" you were able to answer easily because the question asked for specific information that was stated clearly and directly in the story. If you were reading an American history text and found a topic heading, "The First President," an obvious question would be: "Who was the first president?" The answer is one that would be stated clearly and directly in the body of this topic heading. These are examples of literal questions. A literal question usually has a single correct response. The answer is stated directly in the text, and every reader will find that same information.

Interpretive Questions

Interpretive questions are more challenging questions that require the reader to interpret, synthesize, evaluate, and analyze the material. Interpretive questions require knowledge of the literal information in addition to understanding the reading material well enough to be able to select several different pieces or bits of data and put them together to formulate a response that demonstrates your understanding. In the American History example about the first president, an interpretive question might be, "Why was George Washington considered to be such an exemplary model as the first president of the new nation?" This question requires that you know not only the literal facts about Washington, but also that you are able to evaluate and judge

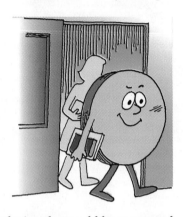

those facts to reach a conclusion that could be supported by the literal information. Even though a question is interpretive in nature, it is possible that there will be only one correct response. However, it is equally possible that there is more than one correct response to an interpretive question. The literal information can be evaluated in a number of different ways in responding to the question, and the answers derived by different readers will vary. Both kinds of questions are essential in the learning process.

QUESTIONING APPLICATION

On the second page of Chapter 50 you will see the italicized phrase, *excessive need or excessive loss.* Italicization is used to gain the reader's attention and to indicate that the italicized material is especially noteworthy. Accented material should always be considered as a potential source of questions. What is excessive need? What is excessive loss? Again, we can begin the questioning with simple, literal questions, but it is essential that interpretive questions also be asked. What do excessive need and loss have to do with the care of the patient? How can we determine if there is excessive need and/or loss? What should be done to remedy excessive need or loss? These questions require that you read for broader general understanding and not just focus on the "facts."

At the end of each chapter there is a section entitled "Critical Thinking Activities." Even though this information is stated in question form, you should consider generating additional questions of your own. The first question in Chapter 50 is, "Explain why patients with a cardiac history need a baseline ECG and serum calcium assessment performed before initiation of calcium supplemental therapy." In answering it, some additional questions will help you focus your learning. What is serum calcium? How does calcium affect cardiac patients? Why? Is calcium supplemental therapy inappropriate for all cardiac patients? If not, what are the circumstances that might rule out supplemental calcium? Of what signs and symptoms should the caregiver be aware if calcium supplemental therapy is being administered to a cardiac patient?

The more active you become as a questioner the easier it will become to ask the kinds of questions that are necessary for your own learning.

Chapter 47

Antacids and Acid Controllers

www.harcourthealth.com/MERLIN/Lilley/

objectives

Look for this symbol for topics covered in the **Online Worksheet**

When you reach the end of this chapter, you should be able to do the following:

1 Discuss the physiologic influence of various gastrointestinal diseases, specifically peptic ulcer disease, gastritis, spastic colon, gastroesophageal reflux disease (GERD), and hyperacidic states.

2 Identify the various agents used to treat gastric disorders, including antacids, H$_2$ histamine-blocking agents, and proton pump inhibitors.

3 Describe the mechanisms of action, indications, cautions, contraindications, side effects, and dosages associated with the use of various antacids and acid controllers.

4 Discuss the patient education guidelines associated with the use of antacids, H$_2$ histamine-blocking agents, and proton pump inhibitors.

5 Develop a nursing care plan that includes all phases of the nursing process related to the administration of antacids and acid controllers.

drug profiles

aluminum-containing **antacids**, p. 753

calcium-containing **antacids**, p. 753

○━**cimetidine**, p. 756

famotidine, p. 756

magnesium-containing **antacids**, p. 754

○━**misoprostol**, p. 759

○━**omeprazole**, p. 758

pantoprazole, p. 758

○━**sucralfate**, p. 760

○━Key drug.

Mucoid cell (mu′ koid) Cell whose function is to secrete mucus that serves as a protective mucous coat against the digestive properties of hydrochloric acid (also called surface epithelia cells). (p. 750)

Parietal cells (pə ri′ ə təl) Cell responsible for producing and secreting hydrochloric acid; the primary site of action for many of the drugs used to treat acid-related disorders. (p. 750)

Pepsin (pep′ sin) Proteolytic enzyme responsible for breaking down proteins. (p. 750)

Simethicone (si meth′ i kon) Substance that alters the elasticity of mucus-coated bubbles causing them to break. (p. 753)

glossary

Activated charcoal Substance that appears to be effective in reducing breath H$_2$ and intestinal complaints caused by ingestion of indigestible carbohydrates. (p. 754)

Antacids (ant a′ sid) Large group of prescription and over-the-counter drugs used to correct too much acid production and hyperacidity of the stomach. (p. 749)

Antiflatulents (an′ ti flatí u lənt) Agents used to relieve the painful symptoms associated with gas by binding to or altering intestinal gas. (p. 749)

Chief cells Cells that secrete the enzyme pepsinogen. (p. 750)

Gastric gland (gas′ trik) Highly specialized secretory gland composed of many different types of cells: parietal, chief, mucus, endocrine, and enterochromaffin. (p. 750)

Gastric hyperacidity (gas′ trik \ hi′ pər ə sid′ i te) Overproduction of stomach acid. (p. 749)

Hydrochloric acid (HCl) (hi′ dro klor′ ik) Acid secreted by the parietal cells in the lining of the stomach that maintains the environment of the stomach at a pH of 1 to 4. (p. 751)

One of the conditions of the stomach requiring drug therapy is hyperacidity, or too much acid production. Left untreated this condition can lead to such serious conditions as ulcer disease and gastric reflux. **Antacids** are a large group of prescription and over-the-counter (OTC) drugs that may be used to correct this condition. Overproduction of stomach acid is also referred to as **gastric hyperacidity.**

Another condition or disorder of the gastrointestinal (GI) tract is gas. Gas can appear in the GI tract as a consequence of the normal digestive process and air swallowing, or it can result from disorders such as diverticulitis, dyspepsia, peptic ulcers, postoperative gaseous distention, and spastic or irritable colon. **Antiflatulents** are agents that are used to relieve the painful symptoms associated with gas. Other drugs and their role in the treatment of GI-related disorders are also discussed.

ACID-RELATED PATHOPHYSIOLOGY

For a more complete understanding of the large family of drugs used to treat acid-related disorders of the stomach, a brief overview of GI system function and the role of hydrochloric acid (HCl) in digestion is beneficial. The stomach secretes many substances:

- HCl
- Bicarbonate
- Pepsinogen
- Intrinsic factor
- Mucus
- Prostaglandins

Each one of these substances has a specific role in the digestive process.

The stomach, although one structure, can be divided into three functional areas. Each area has specific glands with which it is associated. These glands are composed of different cells, and these cells secrete different substances. Figure 47-1 shows three functional areas of the stomach and the distribution of the three different stomach glands.

The three primary glands in the stomach are the cardiac, pyloric, and gastric glands. These glands are named for their position in the stomach. The cardiac glands are located around the cardiac orifice; the gastric glands are in the fundus, over the greater part of the body of the stomach; and the pyloric glands are in the pyloric region and in the transitional zone between the pyloric and the fundic zones. The gastric glands are the largest in number and are of primary importance when discussing acid-related disorders and drug therapy.

The **gastric gland** is a highly specialized secretory gland composed of many different types of cells: parietal, chief, mucus, endocrine, and enterochromaffin. Each cell secretes a specific substance. The three primary cells are mucoid cells, chief cells, and parietal cells. These cells are depicted in Figure 47-1.

Parietal cells are responsible for producing and secreting HCl. They are the primary site of action for many of the drugs used to treat acid-related disorders. **Chief cells** secrete pepsinogen. Pepsinogen is a proenzyme that becomes pepsin when activated by exposure to acid. **Pepsin** breaks down proteins and is referred to as a *proteolytic enzyme*. **Mucoid cells** are mucus-secreting cells that are also

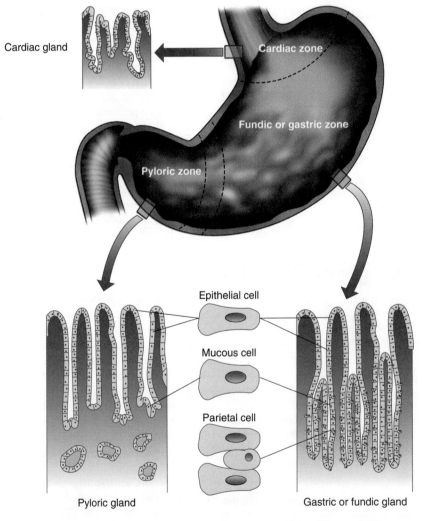

Fig. 47-1 The three specific zones of the stomach and the different glands.

called *surface epithelia cells.* The secreted mucus serves as a protective mucous coat against the digestive properties of HCl. Table 47-1 lists the cells of the gastric glands and their functions.

The three cells of the gastric gland (chief, mucoid, and parietal) play an important role in the digestive process. When the balance of these three cells and their secretions is impaired, acid-related diseases occur. The most harmful of these disorders is peptic ulcer disease (PUD); the most common is hyperacidity. Many lay terms (e.g., indigestion, sour stomach, heartburn, acid stomach) have been used to describe this condition of overproduction of HCl by the parietal cells.

HCl is an acid that is secreted by the parietal cells in the lining of the stomach. It is the primary substance secreted in the stomach that maintains the environment of the stomach at a pH of 1 to 4. There are many stimulants of HCl secretion by the parietal cells. Some of these stimulants are normal and good. Others, such as large, fatty meals; consumption of excessive amounts of alcohol; and emotional stress, may result in hyperproduction of HCl from the parietal cells and disorders such as PUD.

Because the parietal cell is the source of HCl production, it is the primary target for many of the most effective drugs for the treatment of acid-related disorders. A closer look at how the parietal cell receives signals to produce and secrete HCl will enhance the understanding of the mechanism of action of many of the drugs used to treat acid-related disorders.

The wall of the parietal cell has three types of receptors: acetylcholine (Ach), histamine, and gastrin. When any one of these is occupied, the parietal cell will produce and secrete HCl. Figure 47-2 shows the parietal cell with its three receptors. Once these receptors have become occupied, a

Table 47-1	Three Cells of the Gastric Gland	
Cell Type	**Function**
Chief	Secretes pepsinogen → pepsin
	Breaks down proteins in the diet
Mucoid	Secretes mucus
	Provides a protective mucous coat to protect stomach from digestion of itself from hydrochloric acid
Parietal	Secretes hydrocloric acid
	Keeps the pH of the stomach between 1 and 4 so as to properly digest food

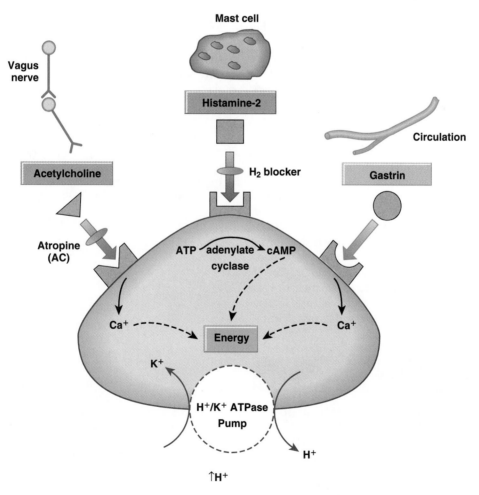

Fig. 47-2 Parietal cell stimulation and secretion.

second messenger is sent. In the case of histamine receptors, occupation results in the production of adenylate cyclase. Adenylate cyclase converts adenosine triphosphate (ATP) to cylic adenosine monophosphate (cAMP), which provides energy for the proton pump. The proton pump is a pump for hydrogen ions located in the parietal cell. The pump requires energy to work. If energy is present, the hydrogen potassium ATPase system will be activated and the pump will be able to produce hydrogen ions needed for the production of HCl.

Ranitidine, famotidine, nizatidine, and cimetidine block hydrogen ion secretion from the parietal cells by binding to these receptors. Anticholinergic (see Chapter 19) drugs such as atropine block ACh receptors, resulting in decreased hydrogen ion secretion from the parietal cells. Proton pump inhibitors bind to the H^+/K^+ ATPase pump and irreversibly inhibit this enzyme, resulting in a total inhibition of hydrogen ion secretion from the parietal cells.

ANTACIDS

Antacids have been used for centuries in the treatment of patients with acid-related disorders. The ancient Greeks used crushed coral (calcium carbonate) in the first century AD to treat patients with dyspepsia. They were the principal anti-ucler treatment until the availability of the H_2-receptor blockers in the late 1970s. For decades the classic treatment for acid-related disorders was a combination anticholinergic/antacid regimen. With the introduction of H_2 blockers as well as proton pump inhibitors (H^+/K^+ ATPase inhibitors), protective agents and mucus-producing prostaglandins are rapidly replacing the anticholinergics for acid-related GI disease. However, the antacids are still extensively used, especially on the OTC market. They are available in a variety of dosage preparations as sole antacid preparations or in multiple antacid formulations. In addition, many antacid preparations contain the antiflatulent agent simethicone, which reduces gas and bloating.

There are basically three forms of antacids: aluminum, magnesium, and calcium based. Many aluminum-based formulations combine magnesium, which contributes to the acid-neutralizing capacity and counteracts the constipating effects of aluminum. There are multiple salts of calcium. Calcium carbonate is the most commonly used salt of calcium when calcium is used as an antacid. It is not used as often as the other antacids because its use may result in kidney stones and increased gastric acid se-

cretion. Sodium bicarbonate is a highly soluble antacid form with a quick onset but a short duration of action. It may also cause metabolic alkalosis.

Some of the available aluminum, magnesium, and calcium salts that are used in many of the antacid formulations are listed in Box 47-1. There are far too many individual antacid products to mention all formulations. The OTC antacid formulations are available as capsules, chewable tablets, effervescent granules and tablets, powders, suspensions, and tablets.

Mechanism of Action

As the name implies, antacids were originally believed to work by neutralization of gastric acidity. They do nothing to prevent the overproduction of acid but neutralize it once it is in the stomach. It is now believed that, especially at low doses, antacids promote gastric mucosal defensive mechanisms. They do this by stimulating mucus, prostaglandin, and bicarbonate secretion from the cells inside the gastric glands. Mucus serves as a protective barrier against the destructive properties of HCl. Bicarbonate helps buffer the acidic properties of HCl. Prostaglandins prevent histamine from stimulating adenylate cyclase. Without adenylate cyclase, no cAMP is formed and no second messenger is available to activate the proton pump.

Drug Effects

The primary drug effect of antacids is the reduction of the symptoms associated with various acid-related disorders such as PUD and hyperacidity disorders. By raising the pH of the stomach from 1.3 to 1.6 (only 0.3 points), acid in the gastric juices will be 50% neutralized; if the pH is raised an entire point from 1.3 to 2.3, a 90% reduc-

Antacids: Drug-Interacting Mechanisms 47-2	
Mechanism	**Description**
Chelation	A chemical binding or inactivation of another drug to the antacid reducing the absorption of the other durg into the bloodstream.
Altered stomach pH	Drugs that are ionized will have reduced absorption into the bloodstream; increasing the pH of the stomach with an antacid will cause drugs that are acid salts (HCl salts) to be more ionized and less absorbed and drugs that are basic salts (sulfate salts) to be less ionized and more readily absorbed into the bloodstream.
Altered urinary pH	The same alteration in absorption in the stomach will affect excretion of basic and acidic drugs in the urine because the urinary pH will be elevated and acidic drugs will be more ionized, less absorbed, and more excreted.

Aluminum, Calcium, and Magnesium Salts in Antacids 47-1		
ALUMINUM SALTS	**CALCIUM SALTS**	**MAGNESIUM SALTS**
Carbonate	Carbonate	Carbonate
Hydroxide		Hydroxide
Phosphate		Oxide
		Trisilicate

tion of acid will occur. This causes the pain reduction associated with acid-related disorders.

The ability of antacids to reduce the pain associated with acid-related disorders is thought to be a result of inhibition of the protein-digesting ability of pepsin, an increase in the resistance of the stomach lining to irritation, and an increase in the tone of the lower esophageal sphincter.

Therapeutic Uses

Antacids are selected for their potential acid-neutralizing capacity and their onset of action. Antacids are indicated for the relief of symptoms associated with hyperacidity related to peptic ulcer, gastritis, gastric hyperacidity, and heartburn.

Side Effects and Adverse Effects

The side effects and adverse effects of the antacids are limited. The magnesium preparations, especially milk of magnesia (MOM), can cause diarrhea. They should also be used with caution or not at all in patients with renal failure. Magnesium ions cannot be excreted in renal failure patients. Magnesium accumulates and leads to toxicity. The aluminum- and calcium-containing formulations can result in constipation. For this reason many combination antacids have been formulated with agents that have counteracting side effects in an attempt to ameliorate the effects. Excessive use of these agents can result in systemic alkalosis. This is more common with sodium bicarbonate. Another adverse effect that is more common with the calcium-containing products is rebound hyperacidity, or acid rebound, in which the patient experiences hyperacidity on discontinuation of the antacid. Long-term self-medication with antacids may mask symptoms of serious underlying diseases such as bleeding ulcers.

Interactions

Antacids are capable of causing several drug interactions when administered with other drugs. There are four basic mechanisms by which antacids cause these interactions. Understanding these mechanisms enhances the knowledge of interactions with antacids. These mechanisms include adsorption (chelation) of other drugs to antacids, which reduces the ability of the other drug to be absorbed into the body; chemical inactivation, which produces insoluble complexes; increased stomach pH, which increases the absorption of basic drugs and decreases the absorption of acidic drugs; and increased urinary pH, which increases the excretion of acidic drugs and decreases the excretion of basic drugs. These mechanisms are further explained in Table 47-2.

Dosages

For information on dosages for selected antacid agents, see the dosages table below.

drug profiles

There are many antacids and antacid combinations. One way to categorize the large family of antacid drugs is separation by the type of metal they contain: aluminum, calcium, or magnesium. Antacids are generally considered safe for use in pregnancy if prolonged or high doses are avoided. The pregnancy category is not established. Most antacids are OTC drugs.

aluminum-containing antacids

The amount of antacid necessary to neutralize HCl depends on the patient, the condition being treated, and the buffering capacity of the preparation used. The acid-neutralizing property of antacids varies. Examples of aluminum-containing antacids and aluminum-magnesium combination products are listed in Box 47-2.

calcium-containing antacids

Calcium-containing antacids are currently being advertised as an extra source of calcium. Calcium carbonate neutralization will produce gas and possibly belching. For this reason it may be combined with an antiflatulent type of drug such as **simethicone.**

DOSAGES Selected Antacid Agents

agent	pharmacologic class	dosage range	purpose
ALUMINUM-CONTAINING ANTACIDS			
aluminum-carbonate (Basaljel)	Antacid	*Adult* PO: 800 mg q2h prn, up to 12 times/day	Hyperacidity
CALCIUM-CONTAINING ANTACIDS		*Adult*	
calcium carbonate (Tums)	Antacid	PO: 0.5-1.25 g prn	Hyperacidity
MAGNESIUM-CONTAINING ANTACIDS		*Adult*	
magnesium hydroxide (MOM)	Antacid	PO: 0.65-1.3 g prn, up to 4 times/day; pediatric dose is 1/4 to 1/2 adult dose	Hyperacidity
COMBINATION PRODUCTS		*Adult*	
aluminum and magnesium (Maalox, Mylanta)	Antacid	PO: 500-1800 mg 3-6 times/day between meals and bedtime	Hyperacidity

Aluminum-Containing Antacids

CARBONATE SALT	HYDROXIDE SALT	PHOSPHATE SALT	COMBINATION PRODUCTS
Basaljel	AlternaGel	Phosphajel	Gaviscon
	Amphojel		Maalox
			Mylanta

Magnesium-Containing Antacids

CARBONATE SALT	HYDROXIDE SALT	OXIDE SALT	TRISILICATE
Bisodol powder	Milk of magnesia (MOM)	Mag-Ox	Gaviscon
Alkets			

Calcium-containing products have a long duration of acid action, which can cause hyperacidity rebound. One example of a calcium-containing antacid is calcium carbonate (Tums).

magnesium-containing antacids

Magnesium-containing antacids commonly cause a laxative effect, and frequent administration of these antacids alone often cannot be tolerated. The administration of magnesium-containing antacids is dangerous in patients with renal failure because the failing kidney cannot excrete the extra magnesium and accumulation may occur. Examples of magnesium-containing antacids are listed in Box 47-3.

Other agents that may be added in antacid combination products are antiflatulents. Flatulence is the passage of gas via the rectum, a disturbing symptom for many patients but rarely an indicator of serious disease. Gas in the upper GI tract is composed of swallowed air and is thus largely nitrogen. It is usually expelled from the body by belching. However, the composition of flatulence is determined largely by dietary intake of carbohydrates and the metabolic activity of the bacteria in the intestines. These bacteria, anaerobic bacteria, produce fermentation with the production of hydrogen (H_2), carbon dioxide (CO_2), and in some patients, methane (CH_4).

Several agents have been used to bind or alter intestinal gas. **Activated charcoal** and simethicone are OTC antiflatulents and may be added to many antacid products. They are also available as sole agents. Activated charcoal appears to be effective in reducing breath H_2 and intestinal complaints caused by ingestion of indigestible carbohydrates. Simethicone alters the elasticity of mucus-coated bubbles, which causes the bubbles to break. Although simethicone is frequently used, limited data support its effectiveness.

H₂ ANTAGONISTS

Histamine type 2 receptor (H_2) antagonists are the prototypical acid secretory antagonists. These agents reduce but do not abolish stimulated acid secretion. They have become the most popular drugs for the treatment of many acid-related disorders, including PUD. This can be attributed to their efficacy, patient acceptance, and excellent safety profile. There are presently four FDA approved H_2 antagonists. They are listed in Box 47-4.

There is little difference among the four available H_2 blockers from an efficacy standpoint. Their relative potencies differ, but increased potency does not necessarily confer a therapeutic advantage, provided the drugs can be administered in equipotent doses without toxicity. All four available H_2 antagonists are available OTC.

Mechanism of Action

The efficacy of the H_2 blockers is related to their ability to competitively block the H_2 receptor of acid-producing parietal cells, thus rendering the cells less responsive not only to histamine but also to the stimulation of ACh and gastrin. This is shown in Fig. 47-2. Up to 90% inhibition of vagal-stimulated and gastrin-stimulated acid secretion occurs by histamine blockers. However, complete inhibition has not been shown.

Drug Effects

The drug effects of the H_2 blockers are limited to specific blocking actions on the parietal cells of the gastric glands in the stomach. The parietal cells are responsible for the production of hydrogen ions and ultimately HCl. The H_2 blockers compete with histamine for binding sites on the surface of parietal cells. The drug effects of H_2 blockers are decreased hydrogen ion production from the parietal cells, which results in an increase in the pH of the stomach, and relief of many of the symptoms associated with hyperacid-secreting conditions.

Therapeutic Uses

H_2 blockers have many therapeutic effects related to their ability to suppress acid production in the stomach. The

Box 47-4 Currently Available H₂ Blockers

cimetidine (Tagamet, Tagamet HB*)
famotidine (Pepcid, Pepcid AC*)
nizatidine (Axid, Axid AR*)
ranitidine (Zantac)

Box 47-5 H₂ Antagonists: Indications

SHOWN TO BE EFFECTIVE
Gastric ulcer
Gastroesophageal reflux disease
Hypersecretory conditions (e.g., Zollinger-Ellison syndrome)
Duodenal ulcer (with or without evidence of *H. pylori*)
Upper GI bleeding

MAY BE EFFECTIVE
Stress ulcers
Prevention and management of allergic condition in combination with H₁ blockers (e.g., urticaria and anaphylactic reactions)
Peptic esophagitis

four currently available agents have identical mechanisms of action but vary in potency and side effect profile. Although they may differ in their formal FDA-approved indications, they all suppress acid secretion in the stomach. Some of the indications for H₂ blockers are listed in Box 47-5.

Side Effects and Adverse Effects

H₂ antagonists have a remarkably low incidence of side effects (less than 3%). The four available blockers are similar in many respects but have some differences in side effect profiles. Table 47-3 lists the side effects and adverse effects seen with these agents. CNS side effects occur in less than 1% of patients taking H₂ antagonists. Cimetidine may induce impotence and gynecomastia. This is the result of cimetidine inhibiting estradiol metabolism and displacement of dihydrotestosterone from peripheral androgen-binding sites. All four H₂ agonists may increase the secretion of prolactin from the anterior pituitary.

Interactions

Besides the different side effect profiles of the four H₂ antagonists, differences in the drug interactions of H₂ antagonists exist. These may be of potential clinical importance. Cimetidine binds the hepatic cytochrome P-450 microsomal oxidase system. This is a group of enzymes in the liver that metabolize many different drugs by oxidation. By inhibiting oxidation of drugs metabolized via this pathway, cimetidine may raise the blood concentrations of these drugs. Ranitidine has only 10% to 20% of the binding action of cimetidine on the P-450 system, and nizatidine and famotidine have essentially no effect. This interaction has little clinical significance for most drugs, but problems occur with medications with a narrow therapeutic-to-toxic ratio, such as theophylline, warfarin, lidocaine, and phenytoin. All H₂ antagonists may inhibit the absorption of certain drugs, such as ketoconazole, that require an acidic GI environment for gastric absorption. The absorption of H₂ antagonists may be impaired in individuals who smoke. Smoking has been shown to decrease the effectiveness of H₂ blockers. For optimal results, the H₂ antagonist should be taken 1 hour before antacids.

Dosages

For dosage information for the H₂ antagonists, see the dosages table on p. 756.

Table 47-3 H₂ Blockers: Adverse Effects

Body System	Side/Adverse Effect
Central nervous system	Headache, lethargy, confusion, depression, halluincations (<1% total), slurred speech
Endocrine	Impotence, increased prolactin, gynecomastia (with cimetidine)
Gastrointestinal	Diarrhea, abdominal cramps, jaundice
Genitourinary	Increased BUN, liver function tests, creatinine
Hematopoietic	Agranulocytosis, thrombocytopenia, neutropenia, aplastic anemia
Integumentary	Urticaria, rash, alopecia, sweating, flushing, exfoliative dermatitis

drug profiles

H₂ antagonists are the prototypical acid secretory antagonists. These agents reduce but do not abolish stimulated acid secretion. They are among the most frequently used drugs in the world. This can be attributed to their efficacy, patient acceptance, and excellent safety profile. As previously mentioned, except for relative potencies, there are only minor differences among the four currently available H₂ antagonists, which are cimetidine (Tagamet), famotidine (Pepcid), nizatidine (Axid), and ranitidine (Zantac). Potency and equipotent dosages of the four available H₂ antagonists are listed in Table 47-4.

All H₂ antagonists are currently available by prescription and OTC. Each agent is available orally, and all except nizatidine are also available parenterally. H₂ antagonists are classified as pregnancy category B agents and are contraindicated in hypersensitivity.

DOSAGES Selected H₂ Antagonists

agent	pharmacologic class	dosage range		purpose
cimetidine (Tagamet, Tagamet HB)	H₂ antagonist	*Adult* PO: 200 mg bid		Dyspepsia, heartburn
		PO: 300 or 400 mg qid with meals and hs or 800 mg hs		Ulcers
		PO: 1600 mg/day divided		GERD
		PO/IM/IV: 300 mg or higher qid with meals and hs; do not exceed 2400 mg/day		Pathologic hypersecretion
famotidine (Pepcid, Pepcid AC)	H₂ antagonist	*Adult* PO: 10 mg bid		Dyspepsia, heartburn
		PO: 40 mg/day hs or 20 mg bid		Ulcers
		PO: 20-160 mg qh		Pathologic hypersecretion
		PO: 20 mg bid		GERD
		IV: 20 mg q12h		Pathologic hypersecretion
nizatidine (Axid, Axid AR)	H₂ antagonist	*Adult* PO: 75 mg bid		Dyspepsia, heartburn
		PO: 300 mg hs or 150 mg bid		Ulcers
		PO: 150 mg bid		GERD
ranitidine (Zantac)	H₂ antagonist	*Adult* PO: 75 mg bid		Dyspepsia, heartburn
		PO: 150 mg bid or 300 mg hs		Ulcers
		PO: 150 mg bid		Pathologic hypersecretion, GERD
		PO: 150 mg qid		Erosive esophagitis
		IM/IV: 50 mg q6-8h		Any indications

GERD, Gastroesophageal reflux disease.

Table 47-4 H₂ Angatonists: Potency and Equipotent Dosages

	Cimetidine	Rantidine	Nizatidine	Famotidine
Relative potency	1	4–8	4–8	20–50
Equivalent dose (mg)	1600	300	300	40

cimetidine

In 1977 cimetidine (Tagamet) was the first agent in this class to be released on the market. It is the prototypical H₂ antagonist. Cimetidine may be given orally and intravenously either by injection or continuous IV infusion. Cimetidine is available as 200-, 300-, 400-, and 800-mg tablets and a 300-mg/5 ml oral solution. The parenteral form of cimetidine is a 150-mg/ml injection. Common dosage recommendations are listed in the dosages table above.

PHARMACOKINETICS

HALF-LIFE	ONSET	PEAK	DURATION
2 hr	15-60 min	1-2 hr	4-5 hr

famotidine

Famotidine (Pepcid, Pepcid AC) is another commonly used H₂ blocker. It can be given orally or intravenously. Famotidine is available as 10-, 20-,

and 40-mg tablets; 10-mg chewable tablets; a 40-mg/5 ml suspension; a 10-mg/ml injection; and a 20-mg/50 ml NaCl infusion. Common dosage recommendations are listed in the dosages table above.

PHARMACOKINETICS

HALF-LIFE	ONSET	PEAK	DURATION
2.5-3.5 hr	15-60 min	1-2 hr	6-8 hr

PROTON PUMP INHIBITORS

The newest drugs introduced for the treatment of acid-related disorders are the proton pump inhibitors lansoprazole (Prevacid), omeprazole (Prilosec), rabeprazole (Aciphex), and pantoprazole (Protonix). Omeprazole was the first agent in this class of antisecretory drugs. The enzyme H⁺/K⁺ ATPase is the final common step in the acid-secretory process of the parietal cell (see Fig. 47-2).

Table 47-5 Current FDA-Approved Regimens for Eradicating *H. pylori*

Drug	Dosage	Frequency	Duration (wk)
omeprazole (Prilosec)	20 mg	bid	2
clarithromycin (Biaxin)	500 mg	tid	2
Followed by omeprazole	20 mg	qid	2
ranitidine bismuth citrate (Tritec)	400 mg	bid	4
and			
clarithromycin	500 mg	tid	2
lansoprazole	30 mg	bid	2
clarithromycin	500 mg	bid	2
amoxicillin	1 g	bid	2
bismuth subsalicylate (Pepto-Bismol)	525 mg	qid	2
metronidazole (Flagyl)	250 mg	qid	2
tetracycline	500 mg	qid	2
(This regimen is sold as the Helidac Kit by Procter & Gamble)			

If there is energy present to run the pump, it will release hydrogen ions out of the parietal cell. Because hydrogen ions are protons (positively charged substances) the pump may also be called the proton pump. Anticholinergics and antihistamines (H_2 blockers) do not stop the action of the pump. Other substances are able to stimulate the pump even in the presence of these drugs. They are thus unable to totally inhibit acid production.

Mechanism of Action

Proton pump inhibitors irreversibly bind to H^+/K^+ ATPase. The binding of this enzyme prevents the movement of hydrogen ions out of the parietal cell into the stomach, thereby blocking all gastric acid secretion. Although H_2 blockers may block close to 90% of all acid secretion, proton pump inhibitors effectively block all acid secretion. Because proton pump inhibitors stop over 90% of 24-hour acid secretion, it makes most patients achlorhydric (without acid). For acid secretion to return to normal after a proton pump inhibitor has been stopped, the parietal cell must synthesize new H^+/K^+ ATPase.

Drug Effects

Proton pump inhibitors are almost the ideal drugs for hypersecretion of acid. Their drug effects are confined to the parietal cell and specifically to the H^+/K^+ ATPase enzyme. Although there are other proton pumps in the body, the H^+/K^+ ATPase is distinct structurally and mechanically from other H^+-transporting enzymes and appears to exist only in the parietal cell. Thus the action of proton pump inhibitors is limited to total inhibition of gastric acid secretion.

Activity

Therapeutic Uses

The ability to totally inhibit the production of acid from the parietal cells in the stomach gives the proton pump inhibitors many beneficial therapeutic effects. Some con-

cerns have been expressed regarding their stability in the prohibition of acid secretion. Most of these concerns stem from long-term use of these agents in humans. Some have shown that this may produce enterochromaffin-like (ECL) cells and carcinoid tumors. The initial concern about the carcinogenic potential of omeprazole and lansoprazole has subsided. Now these agents are FDA approved for GERD maintenance therapy. These agents are currently indicated as first-line therapy for erosive esophagitis, for symptomatic GERD that is poorly responsive to customary medical treatment, and for short-term treatment of active duodenal ulcers and active benign gastric ulcers. The only chronic therapeutic use for these agents is maintenance of healing of erosive esophagitis and pathologic hypersecretory conditions, including Zollinger-Ellison Syndrome.

Omeprazole and lansoprazole have been approved for the treatment of patients with *Helicobacter pylori* infections. Many treatment regimens have emerged to cure *H. pylori*-induced ulcers; these are listed in Table 47-5. *H. pylori* eradication has been shown to reduce the risk of duodenal ulcer recurrence as well.

Side Effects and Adverse Effects

Omeprazole and lansoprazole appear to be remarkably safe for short-term therapy. The frequency of adverse effects has been similar to that of placebo or H_2 antagonists. Some of the other less common side effects and adverse effects seen with proton pump inhibitors are listed in Table 47-6.

Interactions

There are few drug interactions with proton pump inhibitors. There is the possibility that proton pump inhibitors may increase serum levels of diazepam and phenytoin. There is also the possibility that there may be an increased chance for bleeding in patients who are on both a proton pump inhibitor and warfarin. Other

Proton Pump Inhibitors: Adverse Effects

47-6

Body System	Side/Adverse Effect
Central nervous system	Headache, dizziness
Gastrointestinal	Diarrhea, abdominal pain, vomiting, nausea, anorexia
Genitourinary	Proteinuria, hematuria, glycosuria
Hematopoietic	Pancytopenia, thrombocytopenia, neutropenia, leukocytosis, anemia
Integumentary	Rash, dry skin, urticaria, pruritis, alopecia
Respiratory	Upper respiratory infections, cough
Other	Back pain, fever, fatigue

possible interactions include interference with keto-conazole, ampicillin, iron salts, and digoxin absorption. Sucralfate may delay absorption of these agents. To avoid this, give the proton pump inhibitor 30 minutes before giving sucralfate.

Dosages

For recommended dosages, see the dosages table on p. 759.

---

drug profiles

omeprazole

Omeprazole (Prilosec) is one of four proton pump inhibitors. A fifth proton pump inhibitor may be soon on the market; it is esomeprazole (Nexium), a single-isomer version of omeprazole. The proton pump inhibitors bind to and inhibit the enzyme H^+/K^+ ATPase, which is the final common step in the acid-secretory process of the parietal cell.

The ability of omeprazole to totally prohibit the production of acid from the parietal cells in the stomach gives it many beneficial therapeutic effects. As mentioned in the section on therapeutic uses, omeprazole is currently approved only for acute treatment of severe GERD unresponsive to conventional therapy, endoscopically proven erosive esophagitis, and the chronic treatment of Zollinger-Ellison syndrome.

Omeprazole is available only in an oral formulation as a 10-, 20-, and 40-mg sustained-release capsule. It is classified as a pregnancy category C agent and is contraindicated in hypersensitivity. Common dosage recommendations are listed in the dosages table on p. 759.

PHARMACOKINETICS

HALF-LIFE	ONSET	PEAK	DURATION
Variable	2 hr*	0.5-3.5 hr	24 hr

*50%-86% acid secretion reduction.

pantoprazole

Pantoprazole (Protonix) is currently the only proton pump inhibitor that is available in an oral and an intravenous preparation. It is indicated for the short-term treatment (up to 8 weeks) in the healing and symptomatic relief of erosive esophagitis associated with GERD. The other currently available proton pump inhibitors have more indications than pantoprazole; however, pantoprazole is the only parenterally available proton pump inhibitor. This distinction will provide expanded use of proton pump inhibitors in patients who are unable to tolerate oral medications, such as intensive care patients who are intubated. Pantoprazole is available as a 40-mg oral tablet and a 40-mg/ml injection. It is contraindicated in patients with a known hypersensitivity to it and is considered a pregnancy category C agent. Common recommended dosages are listed in the dosages table on p. 759.

PHARMACOKINETICS

HALF-LIFE	ONSET	PEAK	DURATION
1 hr	24 hr*	2.5 hr	Unknown

*50% decrease in acid secretion 1 day after initiation.

OTHER DRUGS

Antacids, antiflatulents, H_2 antagonists, and proton pump inhibitors are some of the many commonly used drugs to treat acid-related disorders. Some of the other drugs that may be used to treat acid-related and other disorders are sucralfate, misoprostol, bismuth, anticholinergics, and tricyclic antidepressants (TCAs). Some of these agents, such as anticholinergics and TCAs, are mentioned in other chapters. Sucralfate and misoprostol are discussed here.

SUCRALFATE

Sucralfate (Carafate) is an agent used as an acute cytoprotective agent in the treatment of stress ulcerations and chronically in PUD. It works in a manner that is totally different from that of the antacids, H_2 antagonists, and proton pump inhibitors. A closer look at sucralfate's chemical structure provides insight into its many actions.

Mechanism of Action

Sucralfate has as its basic structure a sugar, sucrose. Sulfates and aluminum hydroxide groups are attached to that sugar in the place where there are normally hydroxyl groups. Once sucralfate comes into contact with the acid of the stomach, it begins to dissociate into aluminum hy-

DOSAGES Omeprazole, Sucralfate, and Misoprostol

agent	pharmacologic class	dosage range	purpose
misoprostol (Cytotec)	Antisecretory	*Adult* PO: 200 μg qid with meals and hs for duration of NSAID therapy	Gastric ulcer prophylaxis during NSAID therapy
omeprazole (Prilosec)	Proton pump inhibitor	*Adult* PO: 20 mg/day for 4-8 wk PO: 60-360 mg/day divided	Esophagitis, duodenal ulcer Hypersecretory conditions
pantoprazole (Protonix)	Proton pump inhibitor	*Adult* PO/IV: 40 mg qd	GERD
sucralfate (Carafate)	Antiulcer agent	*Adult* PO: 1 g qid ac	Duodenal ulcers

droxide and sulfate anions. Sucralfate is sometimes referred to as a *cytoprotective agent.* The sulfated sucrose molecules of sucralfate are attracted to and bind to the base of ulcers and erosions, forming a protective barrier over the base of this area. By binding to the exposed proteins of ulcers and erosions, sucralfate limits access of pepsin, which normally breaks down proteins, either causing ulcers or making them worse. This is believed to be the primary mechanism by which sucralfate heals ulcers and protects erosions. It has a multitude of other effects that may also explain its mechanism of action.

Drug Effects

The drug effects of sucralfate are numerous. This can be attributed to its unique structure, which contains sucrose (a sugar), sulfate anions (negatively charged particles), and aluminum hydroxide (an antacid). The many drug effects of sucralfate are listed in Table 47-7.

Therapeutic Uses

Sucralfate has many attractive characteristics that make it a beneficial agent for the treatment of such disorders as stress ulcers, erosions, and PUD.

Side Effects and Adverse Effects

Sucralfate has little absorption from the gut into the blood and is chemically inert. These characteristics make it virtually devoid of systemic toxicity. The most common side effects are constipation and nausea, which appear 2% to 3% of the time. Dry mouth may also be seen.

Interactions

Sucralfate may impair the absorption of certain drugs, particularly tetracycline. This can be avoided by the administration of sucralfate without any other medications. This binding property of sucralfate may be used therapeutically. Sucralfate binds phosphates in the GI tract and has been used as a phosphate binder in patients with chronic renal failure.

Dosages

For recommended dosages of sucralfate, see the dosages table above.

Table 47-7 Sucralfate: Drug Effects

Characteristic	Drug Effect
Sulfate anions	Binds to positively charged tissue proteins that are exposed at the tissue surface of an ulcer or an erosion.
Weak base	Buffers the acidic pH of the stomach.
Epidermal growth factor	Binds and concentrates epidermal growth factor (EGF), which accelerates the healing process.
Prostaglandin synthesis	Stimulates gastric mucosal prostaglandin E_2 synthesis.
Stimulation of mucus and bicarbonate	The aluminum salt stimulates the secretion of mucus and bicarbonate from the cells of the stomach to counteract the actions of hydrochloric acid.

drug profiles

misoprostol

Misoprostol (Cytotec) is a synthetic prostaglandin analogue. Prostaglandins have a wide variety of biologic activities. They are believed to inhibit gastric acid secretion and exhibit "cytoprotective" activity. They are believed to protect the gastric mucosa from injury, possibly by enhancing the local production of mucus or bicarbonate, by promoting local cell regeneration, or possibly by maintaining mucosal blood flow.

Because of their inhibitory effects on gastric acid secretion and their cytoprotective properties, synthetic analogues of prostaglandins (of the E class) have been produced. They were made with the expectation that they might be useful agents for the treatment of PUD. Misoprostol, an E analogue, has been shown to be effective in reducing the incidence of gastric ulcers in patients taking non-steroidal antiinflammatory drugs (NSAIDs). The drug has been approved by the FDA for this prophylactic use.

Misoprostol may also be used in combination with methotrexate as a medical alternative to a surgically induced abortion. An IM injection of methotrexate followed up to 7 days later by intra-vaginal administration of misoprostol can terminate an early intrauterine pregnancy. Misoprostol stimlates uterine contractility and expels the products of conception. Misoprostol is used in combination with another prostaglandin (RU 486 [Mifeprex]) to induce abortion in early pregnancy.

Although some studies show that synthetic analogues of prostaglandins promote the healing of duodenal ulcers, they must be used in doses that usually produce more disturbing side effects, such as abdominal cramps and diarrhea. Thus they are not believed to be as effective as the H_2 blockers for this indication. Pregnancy category X.

Activity

sucralfate

Sucralfate is available only with a prescription in an oral formulation as a 1-g oral tablet and as a 1-g/10 ml oral solution. Sucralfate is classified as a pregnancy category B agent and is contraindicated in hypersensitivity. Common dosage recommendation for sucralfate is 1 g four times a day.

PHARMACOKINETICS

HALF-LIFE	ONSET	PEAK	DURATION
6-20 hr	1 hr	2-4 hr	3-6 hr

nursing process

● Assessment

Before administering an antacid agent, the nurse should assess the patient and gather information regarding the following: presence of CHF, hypertension, sodium restrictions, and other cardiac diseases, especially if the antacid is high in sodium content; fluid imbalances; dehydration; GI obstruction; renal disease; and pregnancy. (Patients with CHF or hypertension should use low-sodium antacids such as Riopan, Maalox, or Mylanta II.) Under these conditions, antacids, must be used cautiously. Contraindications to the use of aluminum-containing antacids include hypersensitivity to the drug.

Magnesium antacids should be used cautiously in patients who have a history of renal insufficiency and also in pregnant or lactating patients. Contraindications to the use of magnesium antacids include hypersensitivity to the medication. Calcium-containing antacids are used frequently, especially as a source of calcium. However, they carry the risk of rebound hyperacidity, milk-alkali syn-drome, and changes in systemic pH, especially if the patient has abnormal renal functioning. Milk-alkali syndrome and rebound hyperacidity are also problematic with the administration of antacids containing sodium bicarbonate. Sodium bicarbonate is generally not recommended as an antacid because of the high risk of systemic electrolyte disturbances and alkalosis. Sodium content in sodium bicarbonate is high and can be problematic for patients who have hypertension, CHF, or renal insufficiency.

There are many drug interactions with antacids because of the effect on absorption of the medication that is given concurrently with the antacid. Some of the medications whose effects are increased by the use of antacids include quinidine (antidysrhythmic), pseudoephedrine (decongestant), levodopa (antiparkinson agent), valproic acid (anticonvulsant), and dicumarol (anticoagulant). Medications with decreased effects when used simultaneously with antacids include digoxin (cardiac glycoside), corticosteroids, cimetadine and ranitidine (H_2 receptor-blocking agents), iron preparations, phenothiazines (antiemetics and tranquilizer), salicylates (aspirin), and isoniazid (INH, antituberculin agent). See Table 47-2 for further information on drug interactions.

H_2 receptor antagonists are contraindicated in patients with known drug allergy or who have impaired renal function or liver disease. Cautious use is recommended in patients who are confused, disoriented, or elderly. Omeprazole has several drug interactions, including diazepam, phenytoin, and warfarin.

Proton pump inhibitors are contraindicated in patients who are allergic to the drug, and it should be used cautiously with patients who are pregnant or lactating and with children. Hepatic enzymes (AST [SGOT], ALT [SGPT]), and alkaline phosphatase should be monitored before and during treatment. There are also several drug incompatibilities, especially in a syringe, and these should always be checked before administration. Other drug interactions include anticoagulants, sulfonylureas, antacids, diazepam, anticholinergics, and metoclopramide. Sucralfate may also delay absorption of oral forms.

● Nursing Diagnoses

Nursing diagnoses related to the administration of antacids include the following:

- Acute pain related to gastric hyperacidity and other GI disorders.
- Constipation related to side effects of aluminum-containing antacids and other drugs used for hyperacidity.
- Diarrhea related to side effects of magnesium-containing antacids and other drugs used for hyperacidity.
- Deficient knowledge related to lack of information about antacids, H_2 receptor antagonists, or proton pump inhibitors, their use, and potential side effects.

● Planning

Goals are as follows:

- Patient has minimal to no pain during therapy with antacids or other acid-controlling agents.

NURSING CARE PLAN Peptic Ulcer

Dr. K.T., a 46-year-old college professor, has been diagnosed with gastritis and a small peptic ulcer after having an endoscopy today. Serum electrolytes were within normal limits; however, gastrin levels were elevated. The physician has encouraged a regular exercise program, stress management, eating a regular diet high in fiber and vegetables, and avoiding alcohol and nicotine (he is a nonsmoker and only drinks occasionally). Along with his discharge care instructions for postendoscopy, he also received a prescription for omeprazole (Prilosec).

assessment		

Nursing Diagnosis — Acute pain, epigastric, related to diagnosis of reflux and peptic ulcer

Subjective Data — Complaint of heartburn and gastric reflux with pain waking him at night
Snacks on junkfood frequently to "soak up" acid

Objective Data — High stress job
No alcohol and does not smoke
Heartburn × 6 mo
Takes antacids daily
Recent endoscopy with diagnosis of reflux and peptic ulcer with prescription for omeprazole

planning and outcome criteria

Goals — Patient will experience more comfort from relief of reflux and ulcer pain within 1 wk of treatment with medications

Outcome Criteria — Patient will state the following ways to minimize discomfort associated with reflux and PUD:
• Take medications as prescribed
• Follow a proper diet
• Decrease stress
• Eliminate other factors that elevate gastric acid production

implementation

Patient teaching should include the following:
• Always take medication as prescribed and take before meals. Do not open, chew, or crush capsule.
• Report any severe diarrhea to the physician.
• Follow diet as recommended by physician and limit gas-producing foods and those that are acidic such as orange juice, and avoid highly spicy foods.
• Decrease food intake before bedtime to avoid reflux at night.
• Sleep with head of bed slightly elevated.
• Avoid alcohol, nicotine, and caffeine.
• Exercise regularly at least 3 times/wk to help decrease stress.
• Participate in relaxing activities and attend stress-reducing seminars at the hospital this month.
• Follow diet high in fiber and drink at least 2-3 liters of fluid a day.
• Avoid snacking, especially at bedtime.
• Eat a balanced diet with all four food groups represented.
• Follow-up with physician as ordered.
• Contact physician should gastric pain increase.

evaluation

Patient shows a therapeutic response such as:
• Absence of epigastric pain
• Less belching
• Absence of abdominal fullness and swelling
• Normal stool patterns
• Less GI upset
• Changes in lifestyle that are positive in decreasing stress
• Changes in diet
• Better sleeping patterns
• Taking medication as prescribed

- Patient experiences minimal side effects while using antacids or acid-controlling agents.
- Patient remains compliant to therapy.

Outcome Criteria

Outcome criteria related to the administration of antacids include the following:

- Patient will experience increased comfort as related to the use of these GI agents.
- Patient will state expected side effects such as constipation or diarrhea and when to seek further assistance regarding their management.
- Patient will state the importance of compliance and following administration guidelines associated with the use of antacids or acid controllers to help decrease manifestations of disease or disorder.

Implementation

When giving antacids, always be sure that chewable tablets are well-chewed and liquid forms are thoroughly shaken before administration. Administer all antacid agents with at least 8 ounces of water to enhance absorption of the antacid in the stomach, except for newer forms that are "rapid-dissolve" agents. Should constipation or diarrhea occur with single agents, suggest a combination aluminum and magnesium product. It is also recommended that when you administer an antacid as ordered, do not administer it within 1 to 2 hours of other medications because of the effect of antacids on the absorption of medications in the stomach.

Since so many H_2 receptor antagonists are now available OTC, it is critical to patient safety that patients are still educated regarding proper use and administration. For example, cimetidine should be given with meals, and antacids (if also given) should be given 1 hour before or after the cimetidine. Patient education should be emphasized regarding drug interactions (e.g., oral anticoagulants are just one of many), side effects, and other OTC products to avoid.

Ranitidine should be given with meals and antacids should be taken 1 hour before or after, if also ordered; 50 mg may be diluted in 50-100 ml of 0.9% NaCl, D_5W, LR, or $D_{10}W$ and given over 15 to 20 minutes. IV forms should be diluted 50 mg/20 ml NS, D_5W, or LR and given at 50 mg or less/5 minutes or more. Refer to

For Answers see www.harcourthealth.com/MERLIN/Lilley/.

case study ### Gastroesophageal Reflux Disease

A 47-year-old attorney has just undergone an endoscopy to rule out gastroesophageal reflux disease (GERD) and gastritis secondary to stress-induced hyperacidity. The physician has placed him on sucralfate (Carafate) three times a day and at bedtime, as well as omeprazole (Prilosec) 20 mg once a day.

- *What laboratory studies are indicated for patients receiving omeprazole? Explain the significance of these studies. How long is therapy with this proton pump inhibitor indicated?*
- *What is the rationale for use of sucralfate in GERD?*

appropriate sources for information on other specific agents and their IV administration.

Omeprazole should be taken before meals, and the entire capsule should be taken whole, not crushed, opened, or chewed. Omeprazole may also be given with antacids, if ordered. Like omeprazole, most of the proton pump inhibitors are given short term, which should be emphasized to patients. Always double-check the names and dosages of these drugs because of similar sounding agents.

Patient teaching tips for these agents are presented in the box below.

Evaluation

Therapeutic response to the administration of antacids, antisecretory compounds, or histamine H_2 receptor antagonists includes relief of symptoms associated with the hyperacidity related to the diagnosis of peptic ulcer, gastritis, esophagitis, gastric hyperacidity, or hiatal hernia (i.e., decrease in epigastric pain, fullness, and abdominal swelling). Side effects for which to check in patients on antacids or antiflatulents include nausea, vomiting, abdominal pain, and diarrhea. Constipation, milk-alkali syndrome, and acid rebound are complications associated with sodium bicarbonate and calcium antacids. Therapeutic response to proton pump inhibitors is similar to those listed for administration of antacids. In addition, the patient should report decreased use of any OTC agents.

patient teaching tips

Antacids and Other Acid Controllers (H_2 Receptor Antagonists and Proton Pump Inhibitors)

➤ Patients should not take any other medications within 1 to 2 hours after taking an antacid. The antacid will affect the absorption of many medications in the stomach, so it is better to take antacids without any other medications.

➤ Patients should contact the physician immediately if they experience constipation, diarrhea, an increase in abdominal pain, or any change in symptomatology.

➤ If patients are taking enteric-coated medications, it is important for them to know that antacids may promote premature dissolving of the enteric coating. Enteric coatings are used to diminish stomach upset in irritating medications, and if the coating is destroyed early in the stomach, GI upset may occur.

➤ Patients should take antiflatulents such as simethicone as recommended by manufacturer directions. Chewable forms must always be chewed thoroughly; liquid preparations should be shaken thoroughly before administration.

➤ Patients should take histamine H₂ receptor antagonists exactly as prescribed.

➤ Omeprazole should be taken before meals, and the entire capsule should be taken whole and not crushed, chewed, or opened; it can be taken with antacids.

➤ Sucralfate should be taken on an empty stomach, and antacids, if indicated, should be avoided

unless ½ hour before or 1 hour after sucralfate administration.

➤ Patients requiring these medications should avoid caffeine, alcohol, harsh spices, and black pepper, because these may aggravate the underlying condition.

➤ All OTC GI medications should be taken as ordered. The patient should contact his or her health care provider if symptoms are not relieved as indicated on directions.

POINTS TO REMEMBER

Acid Physiology

- The stomach secretes many substances (hydrochloric acid, pepsinogen, mucus, bicarbonate, intrinsic factor, and prostaglandins).
- The parietal cell is responsible for the production of acid.
- In acid-related disorders there is an impairment in the balance between these substances.
- The most common impairment is hyperacidity or the overproduction of acid.
- The most harmful is peptic ulcer disease (PUD).

Drug Therapy

- Antacids have been used for centuries and were the mainstays of antiulcer therapy until the 1970s.
- In the 1970s the H₂ antagonists arrived on the scene.
- Later came the proton pump inhibitors.
- Other agents are sucralfate and misoprostol.

H₂ Antagonists

- Histamine type 2 blockers bind to and block histamine receptors located on parietal cells.
- This blockade renders these cells less responsive to stimuli and thus acid secretion.
- Up to 90% inhibition can be achieved with these agents.

Proton Pump Inhibitors

- Block the final step in the acid production pathway-H⁺/K⁺ ATPase.
- This energy-requiring pump is needed to pump out H⁺ ions or protons.
- Block all acid secretion.

Other Drug Therapy

- Sucralfate is a cytoprotective agent for stress ulcerations and PUD.
- Binds to exposed proteins of ulcers and thus limits pepsin's proteolytic action.
- Misoprostol is a synthetic prostaglandin analogue.

- Inhibits gastric acid secretion, enhances local production of mucus or bicarbonate.
- Also helps maintain mucosal blood flow.

Nursing Considerations

- Cautious use of antacids is recommended in patients with congestive heart failure, hypertension, sodium restrictions, and other cardiac diseases, especially if the antacid is high in sodium content.
- Other cautions to antacid use include fluid imbalances, dehydration, GI obstruction, renal disease, and pregnancy.
- Contraindications to the use of aluminum-containing antacids include hypersensitivity.
- There are many drug interactions with antacids because of the effect on absorption of the medication that is given concurrently with the antacid, so always check for interactions before giving the medication.
- It is best *not* to administer other medications within 1 to 2 hours after giving an antacid; but contact the physician if medication time needs to be rescheduled.
- If taking enteric-coated medications, it is important to know that antacids may result in premature dissolving of the enteric coating, and stomach upset may occur.
- Antacids containing magnesium are contraindicated in patients with renal failure; aluminum-containing antacids must be used cautiously in patients with renal failure. The recommended dosage of most antacids is usually 15 to 60 ml with water every 1 to 3 hours after meals and at bedtime.
- Antiflatulents are useful in the management of conditions associated with excessive gas production, such as postoperative flatus and bloating, diverticulitis, irritable or spastic colon, air swallowing associated with anxiety, and PUD.
- H₂ histamine antagonists are used in the management of PUD by elevating the gastric pH to help neutralize the effects of hyperacidic or hypersecretory states in the GI tract.

REVIEW QUESTIONS

1. One of your patients, a 30-year-old business executive, is taking simethicone for excessive flatus associated with diverticulitus. Which of the following best describes the mechanism of action by which simethicone reduces flatus?
   a. It neutralizes gastric pH, thereby preventing gas.
   b. It buffers the effects of pepsin on the gastric wall.
   c. It decreases gastric acid secretion and minimizes flatus.
   d. It disperses and prevents gas formation in the stomach.
2. H_2 antagonists would most likely adversely interact with which of the following?
   a. Codeine
   b. NSAIDs
   c. Ketoconazole
   d. Acetaminophen
3. Digoxin preparations and adsorbers should not be given simultaneously. As a nurse, you are aware that if these agents are given simultaneously, which of the following will occur?
   a. Increased absorption of the digoxin
   b. Decreased absorption of the digoxin
   c. Increased absorption of the adsorbent
   d. Decreased absorption of the adsorbent
4. When used with hyperacidic disorders of the stomach, antacids are given to elevate the gastric pH to:
   a. 2.0.
   b. 4.0.
   c. 6.0.
   d. Greater than 8.0.
5. One of your patients is receiving digitalis orally and is also to receive an antacid at the same time. Your most appropriate action, based on the pharamacokinetics of antacids, is to:
   a. Delay the digitalis for 1 to 2 hours until the antacid is absorbed.
   b. Give the antacid at least 2 to 4 hours before administering the digitalis.
   c. Administer both medications as ordered and document in nurses' notes.
   d. Contact the physician regarding the drug interaction and request a change in the time of dosing of the drugs.

For Answers see www.harcourthealth.com/MERLIN/Lilley/.

CRITICAL THINKING Activities

1. What is the purpose of adding simethicone to GI agents?
2. Are there any concerns regarding the use of antacids in patients with decreased renal functioning? Explain your answer.
3. Is the following statement true or false? Explain your answer. *Antacids coat the stomach, and are therefore beneficial to patients with ulcers.*

For Answers see www.harcourthealth.com/MERLIN/Lilley/.

bibliography

Albanese J, Nutz P: *Mosby's 2001 nursing drug reference and review cards,* St Louis, 2001, Mosby.

American Hospital Formulary Service: *AHFS drug information,* Bethesda, Md, 2000, American Society of Health-System Pharmacists.

Anderson PO, Knoben JE, Troutman WG: *Handbook of clinical drug data 1999-2000,* ed 9, New York, 1999, McGraw-Hill.

Johns Hopkins Hospital, Department of Pediatrics et al: *The Harriet Lane handbook,* ed 15, St. Louis, 2000, Mosby.

Keen JH: *Critical care and emergency drug reference,* ed 3, St Louis, 1996, Mosby.

Mosby's GenRx: a comprehensive reference for generic and brand drugs, ed 10, St Louis, 2000, Mosby.

Skidmore-Roth L: *Mosby's 2001 nursing drug reference,* St Louis, 2001, Mosby.

United States Pharmacopeial Convention: *USP DI: drug information for the health care professional, vol. 1,* ed 20, Englewood, Colo, 2000, Micromedex.

Activity

Remember to check the **Online Worksheet** for additional learning opportunities: **www.harcourthealth.com/MERLIN/Lilley/**

Chapter 48

Antidiarrheals and Laxatives

objectives

When you reach the end of this chapter, you should be able to do the following:

1 Identify the various agents used as antidiarrheals and laxatives.

2 Define the terms *antidiarrheal, cathartic,* and *laxative.*

3 Discuss the mechanisms of action, indications, cautions, contraindications, side effects, and dosages associated with the use of antidiarrheals, laxatives, and cathartics.

4 Develop a nursing care plan that includes all phases of the nursing process in the administration of antidiarrheals, cathartics, and laxatives.

www.harcourthealth.com/MERLIN/Lilley/

Look for this symbol for topics covered in the **Online Worksheet**

drug profiles

attapulgite, p. 769

belladonna-alkaloid combinations, p. 769

bismuth subsalicylate, p. 769

diphenoxylate and atropine, p. 770

○━docusate salts, p. 776

glycerin, p. 776

Lactobacillus acidophilus, p. 770

lactulose, p. 776

○━loperamide, p. 770

magnesium salts, p. 777

○━methylcellulose, p. 774

mineral oil, p. 774

polyethylene glycol, p. 776

psyllium, p. 774

senna, p. 777

○━ Key drug.

glossary

Acute diarrhea (ə kut′ \ di′ ə re′ə) Diarrhea that is sudden in onset in a previously healthy individual, lasting from 3 days to 2 weeks. (p. 766)

Adsorbent (ad sor′ bənt) Antidiarrheal agent that acts by coating the walls of the gastrointestinal tract, absorbing the bacteria or toxins causing the diarrhea, and eliminating them with the stools. (p. 766)

Anticholinergic (an′ ti ko′ lin ər′ jik) Antidiarrheal agent that acts by decreasing the muscular tone of the intestine and thus decreasing peristalsis. (p. 766)

Bulk-forming laxatives Agents that absorb water into the intestine, which increases bulk, distending the bowel to initiate reflex bowel activity and promoting a bowel movement. Bulk-forming laxatives act in a manner similar to that of fiber naturally contained in the diet. (p. 772)

Chronic diarrhea Diarrhea that lasts for over 3 to 4 weeks, associated with recurring passage of diarrheal stools, fever, loss of appetite, nausea, vomiting, weight reduction, and chronic weakness. (p. 766)

Constipation (kon′ sti pa′ shən) A condition of abnormally infrequent and difficult passage of feces through the lower gastrointestinal tract. (p. 770)

Diarrhea (di′ ə re′ ə) Abnormal frequent passage of loose stools. (p. 766)

Emollient laxatives (e mol′ e ənt) Agents often referred to as *stool softeners* and *lubricant laxatives.* The fecal softeners work by lowering the surface tension of fluids resulting in more water and fat being absorbed into the stool and the intestines. The lubricant type of emollient laxatives work by lubricating the fecal material and the intestinal walls. This prevents water from leaking out of the intestines and softens and expands the stool. (p. 772)

Hyperosmotic laxatives Agents that produce their laxative effects by increasing fecal water content, which results in distention, increased peristalsis, and evacuation. (p. 773)

Intestinal flora modifiers (flor′ ə) Product obtained from bacterial cultures, most commonly *Lactobacillus* organisms. (p. 767)

Laxative (lak′ sə tiv) Agent that promotes bowel evacuation by increasing the bulk of the feces, softening the stool, or lubricating the intestinal wall. (p. 771)

Opiate (o′ pe ət) Antidiarrheal agent that acts by decreasing motility of the bowel, causing constipation and sedation, and often reducing pain associated with diarrhea. (p. 767)

Saline laxative (sa′ len) Agent that works primarily in the small intestines by preventing water from being absorbed. (p. 773)

Stimulant laxative Agent that stimulates movement of the intestines by stimulating the nerves that innervate the intestines, resulting in increased peristalsis activity in the intestinal tract. (p. 773)

Diarrhea and the diseases commonly associated with it are among the leading causes of death and morbidity in underdeveloped nations, accounting for 5 to 8 million deaths per year in infants and small children. Diarrheal disorders also have a financial impact on our society. Outpatient costs and loss of time from work because of acute infectious diarrhea have been estimated to cost $23 billion per year, or $106 per person, in the United States. To the gastroenterologist, the "big three" symptoms of gastrointestinal (GI) disease are abdominal pain, nausea and/or vomiting, and diarrhea.

Diarrhea is defined as the abnormal frequent passage of loose stools or, more specifically, the abnormal passage of stools with increased frequency, fluidity, and weight, or with increased stool water excretion. **Acute diarrhea** refers to diarrhea that is sudden in onset in a previously healthy individual. It lasts anywhere from 3 days to 2 weeks and is self-limiting, resolving without sequelae. **Chronic diarrhea** lasts for over 3 to 4 weeks and is associated with recurring passage of diarrheal stools, fever, loss of appetite, nausea, vomiting, weight reduction, and chronic weakness.

The probable cause of diarrhea should be taken into consideration when designing a drug regimen to treat it. Some causes of acute diarrhea are bacterial, drug-induced, viral, nutritional, and protozoal. Some causes of chronic diarrhea include tumors, diabetes mellitus, hyperthyroidism, Addison's disease, and irritable bowel syndrome. Nonspecific treatment is directed at the cessation of the increased stool frequency associated with diarrhea, alleviation of abdominal cramps, and prevention of dehydration from fluid and electrolyte loss and weight loss and nutritional deficits from malabsorption.

ANTIDIARRHEALS

The agents used to treat diarrhea are called *antidiarrheals;* they are divided into different groups based on specific mechanisms of action: adsorbents, antimotility drugs (anticholinergics and opiates), bacterial replacement drugs (intestinal flora modifiers), antisecretory drugs, and enzymes. The specific classes and the agents in each are listed in Table 48-1.

Mechanism of Action

Antidiarrheal agents have varying mechanisms of action. It is important to know the specific mechanism of an agent to ensure that the appropriate agent is being used (treating the underlying cause).

Adsorbents act by coating the walls of the GI tract; they remain in the intestine, bind to the causative bacteria or toxin, and eliminate it from the body through the stool.

Anticholinergics work by decreasing peristalsis (rhythmic contractions of the GI tract) and the muscular tone of the intestine, thus slowing the movement of substances through the GI tract. They are often used in

Table 48-1 Antidiarrheals: Drug Categories and Selected Agents

Category	Antidiarrheal Agents
Adsorbents	Activated charcoal, aluminum hydroxide, attapulgite, bismuth subsalicylate, cholestyramine, kaolin-pectin, polycarbophil
Anticholinergics	Atropine, hyoscyamine, hyoscine
Opiates	Opium tincture, paregoric, codeine, diphenoxylate, loperamide
Intestinal flora modifiers	*Lactobacillus acidophilus*

Box 48-1 Antidiarrheals: Therapeutic Effects

Agent	Therapeutic Effect
ADSORBENTS Activated charcoal, aluminum hydroxide, attapulgite, bismuth subsalicylate, cholestyramine, kaolin-pectin, and polycarbophil	Of the adsorbents, kaolin-pectin, bismuth salts, attapulgite, and aluminum hydroxide are the most commonly used. These agents act by coating the walls of the GI tract, absorbing the bacteria or toxins causing the diarrhea, and eliminating them with the stools, thus removing the substances that are actually causing the diarrhea.
ANTICHOLINERGICS atropine, hyoscyamine, and hyoscine	Anticholinergics decrease intestinal muscle tone and peristalsis, thereby slowing the movement of fecal matter through the GI tract. They are often combined with other antidiarrheals to increase their effectiveness.
INTESTINAL FLORA MODIFIERS *Lactobacillus acidophilus*	Intestinal flora modifiers suppress the growth of diarrhea-causing bacteria and help reestablish the normal intestinal flora that has been depleted by the diarrhea.
OPIATES Opium tincture, paregoric, codeine, diphenoxylate, and loperamide	Opiates are used in the treatment of diarrhea because of their constipating effects and their therapeutic pain-relieving effects. They cause constipation by lowering the motility of the bowel and relieving rectal spasms. By slowing the time it takes to pass food through the intestines, water and electrolytes have a greater chance of being absorbed, which reduces stool frequency and volume.

combination with adsorbents and opiates. Anticholinergics are discussed in detail in Chapter 19.

Intestinal flora modifiers are products obtained from bacterial cultures, most commonly *Lactobacillus* organisms. They make up the majority of the body's normal bacterial flora and are the organisms that are most commonly destroyed by antibiotics. Exogenously supplying these bacteria helps restore the balance of normal flora and suppress the growth of diarrhea-causing bacteria.

The primary action of **opiates** is to decrease bowel motility. Secondary mechanisms of action that make opiates beneficial in the treatment of diarrhea include reducing the pain associated with diarrhea and relieving rectal spasms. Because they decrease the transit time of food, they permit longer contact of the intestinal contents with the absorptive surface of the bowel, increasing the reabsorption of water and electrolytes from the stool and reducing stool frequency and net volume.

Drug Effects

Although all classes of antidiarrheal agents counteract diarrhea, other drug effects vary depending upon the drug class and its specific mechanism of action. Within the class of adsorbents, bismuth subsalicylate is a form of aspirin, or acetylsalicylic acid, and therefore it has many of the same drug effects as aspirin (see Chapter 42). Activated charcoal is not only helpful in coating the walls of the GI tract and adsorbing bacteria, but it is also useful in cases of overdose because of its drug-binding properties. Colestipol and cholestyramine are anion exchange resins that are prescription antidiarrheals and lipid-lowering agents. Besides binding to diarrhea-causing toxins, they have the additional benefit of decreasing cholesterol levels.

Anticholinergics have many drug effects beyond those of diarrhea relief (see Chapter 19). Some of the antidiarrheals in the opiate family are used solely for their therapeutic effects in treating diarrhea, whereas others have analgesic properties and may be used to treat various types of pain. The drug effects of intestinal flora modifiers are limited to their antidiarrheal influence.

Therapeutic Uses

All four antidiarrheal drug families effectively combat diarrhea, although the therapeutic effects vary slightly from family to family. Because diarrhea has various causes, it is useful to know that antidiarrheals have different mechanisms of action that allow the caregiver to pick an agent that is specific to the underlying cause of the diarrhea. Box 48-1 lists the four families of antidiarrheal drugs and their specific therapeutic effects.

Side Effects and Adverse Effects

The side effects and adverse effects of the antidiarrheals are also specific to each drug family. Most of these potential effects are minor and not life threatening. The major side effects of specific agents in each drug class are listed in Table 48-2.

Interactions

Many drugs are absorbed from the intestines into the bloodstream, where they are delivered to their respective sites of action. Many of the antidiarrheals have the potential to alter this normal process, either by increasing or decreasing the absorption of these other drugs.

The adsorbents, when given with many agents, can decrease their effectiveness primarily by decreasing their absorption. Examples include digoxin, clindamycin,

Table 48-2 Selected Antidiarrheals: Adverse Effects

Agent	Body System	Side/Adverse Effect
ADSORBENTS		
bismuth subsalicylate	Hematopoietic	Increased bleeding time
	Gastrointestinal	Constipation, dark stools
	Central nervous system	Confusion, twitching
	Other	Hearing loss, tinnitus, metallic taste, blue gums
ANTICHOLINERGICS		
atropine, hyoscyamine, hyoscine	Genitourinary	Urinary retention and hesitancy, impotence
	Central nervous system	Headache, dizziness, confusion, anxiety, drowsiness
	Cardiovascular	Hypotension, hypertension, bradycardia, tachycardia
	Integumentary	Dry skin, rash, flushing
	Eye, ear, nose, throat	Blurred vision, photophobia, increased pressure in the eye
OPIATES		
codeine	Central nervous system	Drowsiness, sedation, dizziness, lethargy
	Gastrointestinal	Nausea, vomiting, anorexia, constipation
	Respiratory	Respiratory depression
	Cardiovascular	Bradycardia, palpitations, hypotension
	Genitourinary	Urinary retention
	Integumentary	Flushing, rash, urticaria

quinidine, probenecid, and hypoglycemic agents. Oral anticoagulants are more likely to cause increased bleeding times or bruising when they are coadministered with adsorbents. This is thought to be primarily because the adsorbents may bind to vitamin K, which is needed to make certain clotting factors. The toxic effects of methotrexate are more likely to occur when it is given with adsorbents.

The therapeutic effects of the anticholinergic antidiarrheals can be decreased by coadministration with antacids. Amantadine, tricyclic antidepressants (TCAs), monoamine oxidase inhibitors (MAOIs), and antihistamines, when given with anticholinergics, can result in increased anticholinergic effects. The opiate antidiarrheals will have additive CNS depressant effects if they are given with CNS depressants, alcohol, narcotics, sedative-hypnotics, antipsychotics, and skeletal muscle relaxants.

Bismuth subsalicylate can increase bleeding times and bruising when administered with oral anticoagulants. Cholestyramine, when administered with glipizide, can result in decreased hypoglycemic effects.

Dosages

For the recommended dosages of antidiarrheal agents, see the dosages table below.

drug profiles

Drug therapy for diarrhea is dependent upon the cause of the diarrhea and the antidiarrheal that will best combat it. All antidiarrheals are orally administered agents available as suspensions, tablets, or capsules. Some antidiarrheals are over-the-

DOSAGES Selected Antidiarrheal Agents

agent	pharmacologic class	dosage range	purpose
attapulgite (Kaopectate)	Adsorbent antidiarrheal	*Chewable tablets* *Pediatric* PO: 3-6 y/o: 1 tablet after each BM 6-12 y/o: 2 tablets after each BM (up to 7 doses/day) *Adult* PO: 4 tablets after each BM *Concentrated liquid* *Pediatric* PO: 3-6 y/o: 7.5 ml after ach BM 6-12 y/o: 15 ml after each BM *Adult* PO: 30 ml after each BM *Maximum strength tablet* *Pediatric* PO: 6-12 y/o: 1 tablet after each BM *Adult* PO: 2 tablets after each BM	Diarrhea
belladonna alkaloids (Donnatal, Donnatal Extentabs, Kinesed)	Fixed-combination anticholinergic	*Adult* PO: 5-10 ml or 1-2 capsules or tablets 3-4 times/day or 1 tablet q12h (Donnatal Extentabs)	Decreased intestinal motility
bismuth subsalicylate (Pepto-Bismol)	Antimicrobial, antisecretory, antidiarrheal	*Pediatric* (repeated q30-60 min not to exceed 8 doses/day) PO: 3-6 y/o: 5 ml or $1/_3$ tablet 6-9 y/o: 10 ml or $2/_3$ tablet 9-12 y/o: 15 ml or 1 tablet *Adult* PO: 30 ml or 2 tablets q30-60 min (not to exceed 8 doses/day)	Diarrhea
Lactobacillus acidophilus (Bacid, Lactinex)	Intestinal flora modifier	*Bacid:* PO: 2 capsules 2-4 times/day *Lactinex:* PO: 1 granule packet with liquids or food 3-4 times/day 4 tablets 3-4 times/day with liquid	Diarrhea
loperamide hydrochloride (Imodium, Imodium A-D, Pepto-Diarrhea Control)	Opiate antidiarrheal	*Pediatric* PO: 2-5 y/o: 1 mg tid PO: 6-8 y/o: 2 mg bid PO: 8-12 y/o: 2 mg tid *Adult* PO: 4 mg followed by 2 mg after each BM (not to exceed 16 mg/day)	Decreased intestinal motility

BM, Bowel movement.

counter (OTC) medications, whereas others require a prescription.

ADSORBENTS

As mentioned previously, adsorbents bind to the diarrhea-causing bacteria and pass them out with the stool. Of the adsorbent antidiarrheals, bismuth subsalicylate, attapulgite, aluminum hydroxide, and kaolin-pectin are the most commonly used. These agents are all OTC medications and are classified in different pregnancy categories. They are contraindicated in children under 3 years of age.

bismuth subsalicylate

Bismuth subsalicylate (Pepto-Bismol) is a salicylate by chemical structure; therefore it should be used with caution in children and teenagers who have or are recovering from chicken pox or flu because of the attendant risk of Reye's syndrome. It can also cause all the side effects and adverse effects that are associated with an aspirin-based product. Two alarming but harmless side effects are temporary darkening of the tongue and/or stool. It is a pregnancy category C agent. Bismuth subsalicylate is available OTC as a 262-mg chewable tablet and caplet or a 262- and 524-mg/15 ml suspension. Commonly recommended dosages are listed in the dosages table on p. 768.

PHARMACOKINETICS

HALF-LIFE	ONSET	PEAK	DURATION
24-33 hr*	0.5-2 hr	2-5 hr	Variable

*For bismuth.

attapulgite

Attapulgite (Kaopectate) has replaced the use of kaolin-pectin in this preparation. Kaolin is a naturally hydrated aluminum compound that is now rarely used as an antidiarrheal agent. However, pectin, which is extracted from apples or citrus fruit, is used in many combination products. Attapulgite is also an OTC antidiarrheal and is a pregnancy category C agent. It is available as 300- and 600-mg chewable tablets and caplets, 750-mg maximum-strength tablets, and a 600- and 750-mg/15 ml solution. Commonly recommended dosages are listed in the dosages table on p. 768.

PHARMACOKINETICS

HALF-LIFE	ONSET	PEAK	DURATION
Unknown	12 hr	14-20 hr	Unknown

ANTICHOLINERGICS

The anticholinergics atropine, hyoscyamine, and hyoscine are used either alone or in combination with other antidiarrheals because they slow GI tract motility. These agents are commonly referred to as *belladonna alkaloids* and are discussed in Chapter 18. Their safety margin is not as broad as that of many of the other antidiarrheals because they can cause serious adverse effects if used inappropriately. For this reason they are available only by prescription.

belladonna-alkaloid combinations

Belladonna alkaloids (Donnatal, Donnatal Extentabs) are used to treat many GI disorders, including diarrhea. Of the belladonna-alkaloid combination products, Donnatal is the most commonly used.

The belladonna-alkaloid preparations are classified as pregnancy category C agents and are contraindicated in patients who have shown a hypersensitivity to anticholinergics and in patients with narrow-angle glaucoma, GI obstruction, myasthenia gravis, paralytic ileus, and toxic megacolon. Donnatal tablets contain a combination of four different alkaloids: atropine (0.0194 mg), hyoscyamine (0.1037 mg), phenobarbital (16.2 mg), and scopolamine (0.0065 mg). There are many dosage forms of this combination: oral capsules, elixir, tablets, and extended-release tablets. Donnatal Extentabs contain 48.6 mg of phenobarbital and increased amounts of all the other above-mentioned alkaloids. Commonly recommended dosages are listed in the dosages table on p. 768.

pediatric considerations

Antidiarrheal Preparations

- Always check with the physician or pediatrician before administering antidiarrheal preparations to a child at home, and report the symptoms in case further assessment or medical management is needed.
- Dehydration and electrolyte loss occur very rapidly in the pediatric patient.
- Always contact the physician for proper dosage of antidiarrheals for any child under 6 years of age or if you have any doubt regarding the amount to administer. Dosages are usually calculated by body weight, and the guidelines or directions provided for most OTC medications are for averaged-sized children over 12 years of age. *Never hesitate* to contact the physician with any concern or question regarding a pediatric patient.
- Abdominal distention, firm abdomen, painful abdomen, and worsening or no improvement in the diarrhea 24 to 48 hours after medication administration should be reported to the physician immediately. Measuring amounts of diarrhea by the number of diapers or number of stools per day provides important information.
- Bloody diarrhea or a sluggish, lethargic, or confused patient should always be reported immediately to a physician.

PHARMACOKINETICS

HALF-LIFE	ONSET	PEAK	DURATION
Unknown	1-2 hr*	2-3 hr*	6-8 hr*

*Anticholinergic effects.

OPIATES

There are five opiate-related antidiarrheal agents: codeine, diphenoxylate with atropine, loperamide, paregoric, and tincture of opium. The only opiate-related antidiarrheal that is available as an OTC medication is loperamide; all others are prescription-only drugs because of the risks of respiratory depression and dependency associated with opiate use.

diphenoxylate and atropine

Diphenoxylate (Logen, Lomenate, Lofene, Lomotil) is a synthetic opiate agonist that is structurally related to meperidine (Demerol). It acts on smooth muscle of the intestinal tract, inhibiting GI motility and excessive GI propulsion. It has little or no analgesic activity. Diphenoxylate has been combined with subtherapeutic quantities of atropine to prevent deliberate overdosage. The amount of atropine present in the combination is too small to interfere with the constipating effect of diphenoxylate. However, when taken in large doses, the combination results in extreme anticholinergic effects (e.g., dry mouth, abdominal pain, tachycardia, and blurred vision).

The combination of diphenoxylate and atropine is classified as a pregnancy category C agent. It is contraindicated in patients who have shown a hypersensitivity reaction to it and in patients suffering from diarrhea associated with pseudomembranous colitis or toxigenic/enterotoxin bacteria. This combination antidiarrheal is available only as oral agents in a solution or tablets. The solution form of Lomotil contains 2.5 mg/5 ml of diphenoxylate and 0.025 mg/5 ml of atropine; the tablets contain 2.5 mg of diphenoxylate and 0.025 mg of atropine.

PHARMACOKINETICS

HALF-LIFE	ONSET	PEAK	DURATION
2.5-4 hr*	40-60 min*	2-3 hr*	3-4 hr*

*Diphenoxylate component.

loperamide

Loperamide (Imodium, Imodium A-D) is a synthetic antidiarrheal that is similar to diphenoxylate. It inhibits both peristalsis in the intestinal wall and intestinal secretion, thereby decreasing the number of stools and the water content. Although the drug exhibits many characteristics of the opiate class, physical dependence on loperamide has not been reported. Because of its safety profile it is the only opiate antidiarrheal agent that is available as an OTC medication.

Loperamide is classified as a pregnancy category B agent and is contraindicated in patients who have shown a hypersensitivity reaction to it. It is also contraindicated in patients with severe ulcerative colitis, pseudomembranous colitis, and acute diarrhea associated with *E. coli.* Loperamide is available only in oral form as 2-mg capsules or tablets and a 1-mg/5 ml solution. Commonly recommended dosages are listed in the dosages table on p. 768.

PHARMACOKINETICS

HALF-LIFE	ONSET	PEAK	DURATION
7-15 hr	1-3 hr	4 hr	40-50 hr

INTESTINAL FLORA MODIFIERS

Intestinal flora modifiers suppress the growth of diarrhea-causing bacteria and reestablish the normal florae that reside in the intestine. They are bacterial cultures that have been obtained from *Lactobacillus* organisms. Currently available agents are discussed as follows.

Lactobacillus acidophilus

Lactobacillus acidophilus (Bacid, Intestinex, Lactinex) is an acid-producing bacteria prepared in a concentrated, dried culture for oral administration. It is a normal inhabitant of the GI tract, where it creates an unfavorable environment for the overgrowth of harmful fungi and bacteria through the fermentation of carbohydrates, which produces lactic acid. *Lactobacillus acidophilus* has been used for more than 75 years in the treatment of uncomplicated diarrhea, particularly that caused by antibiotic treatment that destroys normal intestinal florae. It is available as an OTC medication in the following oral forms: a capsule (Bacid and Intestinex), an enteric-coated capsule (Enterodophilus), a 1-g powder (Lactinex granules), and tablets (Lactinex). Commonly recommended dosages are listed in the table on p. 768.

PHARMACOKINETICS

HALF-LIFE	ONSET	PEAK	DURATION
Unknown	Unknown	Unknown	Unknown

LAXATIVES

Laxatives are used for the treatment of **constipation,** which is defined as a condition of abnormally infrequent and difficult passage of feces through the lower GI tract. Individuals may complain of constipation if they think they defecate too infrequently or with too much effort, if their stools are too hard or too small, if defecation is painful, or if they have a sense of incomplete evacuation. Constipation is a symptom, not a disease; it is a disorder of movement through the colon and/or rectum that can be caused by a variety of diseases or drugs. Some of the more common causes of constipation are noted in Box 48-2.

Box 48-2   Causes of Constipation

Causes	Examples
Metabolic and endocrine disorders	Diabetes mellitus, hypothyroidism, pregnancy, hypercalcemia, hypokalemia
Neurogenic disorders	Autonomic neuropathy, intestinal pseudo-obstruction, multiple sclerosis, spinal cord lesions, Parkinson's disease, cerebrovascular accident
Adverse drug effects	Analgesics, anticholinergics, iron supplements, aluminum antacids, calcium antacids, opiates, calcium channel blockers, Vinca alkaloids
Lifestyle	*Poor bowel movement habits:* Voluntary refusal to defecate resulting in constipation
	Diet: Poor fluid intake and/or low-residue (roughage) diets or excessive consumption of dairy products
	Physical inactivity: Lack of proper exercise, especially in elderly individuals
	Psychologic: Anxiety, stress, hypochondria

The GI tract is responsible for the digestive process that involves (1) ingestion of dietary intake, (2) digestion of dietary intake into basic nutrients, (3) absorption of basic nutrients, and (4) storage and removal of fecal material via defecation.

Ingestion→Digestion→Absorption→Storage and removal

The usual time span between ingestion and defecation is 24 to 36 hours.

The last segment of the GI tract, the large intestine (colon) is responsible for (1) forming the stool by removing excess water from the fecal material, (2) temporarily storing the stool until defecation, and (3) extracting essential vitamins from the intestinal bacteria (especially vitamin K).

The colon is 120 to 150 cm in length and is separated from the small intestine by the ileocecal valve. The colon extends into its last segment, the rectum, which terminates at the anus. The rectum is the temporary storage site for the stool, which is composed of water and unabsorbed and indigestible material. Evacuation of the rectal contents is accomplished by bowel movements.

A bowel movement (defecation) is a reflex act that involves both smooth and skeletal muscles. The entry of feces into the rectum stimulates mass peristaltic movement that results in a bowel movement. However, voluntary initiation or inhibition of defecation is also possible via skeletal muscle pathways.

Treatment of constipation must involve an understanding of the whole patient, with special attention given to the underlying causes for the constipation. Treatment should be individualized, taking into consideration the patient's age, concerns, and expectations; duration and severity of constipation; and potential contributing factors. Treatment can be either surgical or nonsurgical; nonsurgical treatment can be separated into three broad categories of approach: dietary (e.g., fiber supplementation), behavioral (e.g., increased physical activity), and pharmacologic. The focus in this chapter is pharmacologic treatment.

Laxatives promote bowel movements by (1) affecting fecal consistency, (2) increasing fecal movement through the colon, and (3) removing stool from the rectum. Laxatives are useful in relieving constipation, in preparing for some medical procedures, and in removing unwanted substances from the body. Some of the more common indications for laxative use are listed as follows:

- Removal of intestinal parasites
- Inactive colon
- Reduction of ammonia absorption in hepatic encephalopathic conditions
- Treatment of drug-induced constipation
- Pregnancy and/or postobstetric period
- Poor physical activity
- Removal of toxic substances from the body
- Poor dietary habits
- Megacolon
- Preparation for colonic diagnostic procedures or surgery
- Facilitation of bowel movements with reduced pain in anorectal disorders

Of the OTC medications, laxatives are some of the most misused. Chronic and often inappropriate use of laxatives may result in laxative dependence, produce damage to the bowel, or lead to previously nonexistent problems. With the exception of the bulk-forming type, laxatives should not be used for long periods of time. All laxatives share the same general contraindications and precautions, including cautious use in the presence of acute surgical abdomen; appendicitis symptoms such as abdominal pain, nausea, and vomiting; fecal impaction (mineral oil enemas excepted); intestinal obstructions; and undiagnosed abdominal pain. They are also contraindicated in patients who have shown a hypersensitivity reaction to them.

Laxatives are divided into five major groups based on mechanism of action: bulk-forming, emollient, hyperosmotic, saline, and stimulant laxatives. Table 48-3 lists the currently available laxative agents by their respective drug family.

Mechanism of Action

All laxatives promote bowel movements, but each class of laxative has a different mechanism of action. They may act by (1) affecting fecal consistency, (2) increasing fecal movement through the colon, and/or (3) removing stool

Laxatives: Drug Categories and Selected Agents

Table 48-3

Category	Laxative Agents
Bulk-forming	psyllium, polycarbophil, methylcellulose
Emollient	docusate salts, mineral oil
Hyperosmotic	polyethylene glycol, lactulose, sorbitol, glycerine
Saline	magnesium sulfate, magnesium phosphate, magnesium citrate
Stimulant	castor oil, senna, anthraquinones

from the rectum. **Bulk-forming laxatives** act in a manner similar to that of the fiber naturally contained in the diet. They absorb water into the intestine, which increases bulk and distends the bowel to initiate reflex bowel activity, thus promoting a bowel movement.

Emollient laxatives are also referred to as *stool softeners* (docusate salts) and *lubricant laxatives* (mineral oil). Fecal softeners work by lowering the surface tension of GI fluids, resulting in more water and fat being absorbed into the stool and the intestines. The lubricant type of emollient laxatives work by lubricating the fecal material and the intestinal wall, preventing water from leaking out of the intestines, which softens and expands the stool.

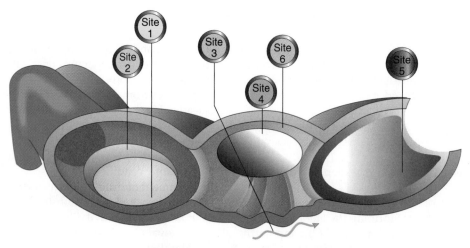

Site 1 Stool softener
Example: Docusate
Mechanism: Wetting agent used to soften fecal mass
Onset of action: 1 to 3 days
Precaution: Liquid dosage form may cause throat irritation; dilute in fruit juice or milk before administration.

Site 2 Bulk forming (high fiber)
Example: Psyllium hydrophilic
Mechanism: Absorbs water to increase bulk, distending bowel to initiate reflex bowel activity
Onset of action: 12 hours to 3 days
Precaution: Contraindicated in patients with dysphagia because esophageal obstruction may result. Avoid in dehydrated persons or individuals with limited or restricted fluid intake.

Site 3 Stimulant
Example: Senna
Mechanism: Increase peristalsis via nerve stimulation in colon
Onset of action: 6 to 12 hours
Precaution: May cause discoloration of feces and urine (alkaline urine from pink, red to brown; acid urine from yellow to brown)

Site 4 Osmotic saline
Example: Magnesium citrate
Mechanism: Increases water content of feces, resulting in distention, peristalsis, and evacuation. Laxation may be enhanced by release of cholecystokinin.
Onset of action: 1 to 3 hours
Precaution: Avoid use in patients who are dehydrated or whose renal function is impaired and in those with a colostomy or ileostomy. Ensure adequate fluid intake of at least 8 ounces of fluid with each dose to prevent dehydration.

Site 5 Lubricant
Example: Mineral oil
Mechanism: Coats surface of feces and colon to ease passage of stool; also softens fecal mass.
Onset of action: 6 to 8 hours
Precaution: Avoid administration within 2 hours of meals because it may reduce absorption of vitamins A, D, E, and K. Avoid use in dysphagic and bedridden patients because aspiration of mineral oil may result in lipid pneumonitis.

Site 6 Combination of stool softener and stimulant
Example: Docusate and senna
Mechanism: Stool softener and stimulant
Onset of action: 6 to 12 hours
Precaution: As noted for individual laxatives

Fig. 48-1 Site and mechanism of action of laxatives within the intestines.

Hyperosmotic laxatives work by increasing fecal water content, which results in distention, increased peristalsis, and evacuation. Their site of action is limited to the large intestine.

Saline laxatives increase osmotic pressure in the small intestine by inhibiting absorption and increasing water and electrolyte secretions, resulting in a watery stool; the increased distention promotes peristalsis and evacuation. Rectal enemas of sodium phosphate, a saline laxative, produce defecation 2 to 5 minutes after administration.

As the name implies, **stimulant laxatives** stimulate the nerves that innervate the intestines, resulting in increased peristalsis. They also increase fluid in the colon, which increases bulk and softens the stool. See Figure 48-1 for a brief explanation of how and where in the intestine the various laxatives work.

Drug Effects

The drug effects of laxatives are numerous, although their action is primarily limited to the site of the intestines, and thus they have few, if any, systemic effects. Table 48-4 lists the specific drug effects of the different laxatives.

Therapeutic Uses

The various therapeutic uses for laxatives range from common constipation to bowel preparation before surgery. The therapeutic effects vary by category. See Table 48-5 for specific therapeutic indications for each laxative drug class.

Side Effects and Adverse Effects

As is true for the drug and therapeutic effects of laxatives, the side effects and adverse effects of the various agents are specific to the laxative group. Most of the side effects from laxatives are confined to the site of the intestines; however, the overuse and misuse of laxatives lead to many unwanted effects that are not expected or designed to occur with appropriate use. The major side effects and adverse effects of the laxative agents are listed in Table 48-6.

Interactions

Many drugs are absorbed in some part of the intestine. Since laxatives alter intestinal function, they can interact with other drugs quite readily. Bulk-forming laxatives can decrease absorption of antibiotics, digoxin,

Table 48-4 Laxatives: Drug Effects

Drug Effect	Bulk	Emollient	Hyperosmotic	Saline	Stimulant
Increases peristalsis	Y	Y	Y	Y	Y
Causes increased secretion of water and electrolytes in small bowel	Y	Y	N	Y	Y
Inhibits absorption of water in small bowel	Y	Y	N	Y	Y
Increases wall permeability in small bowel	N	Y	N	N	Y
Causes wall damage in small bowel	N	Y	N	N	Y
Acts only in large bowel	N	N	Y	N	N
Increases fecal mass water	Y	Y	Y	Y	Y
Softens fecal mass	Y	Y	Y	Y	Y

Y, Yes; N, no

Table 48-5 Laxatives: Therapeutic Uses

Laxative Group	Therapeutic Use
Bulk-forming	Acute and chronic constipation, irritable bowel syndrome, diverticulosis
Emollient	Acute and chronic constipation, softening of fecal impacts, facilitation of bowel movements in anorectal conditions
Hyperosmotic	Chronic constipation, diagnostic and surgical preparations
Saline	Constipation, removal of helminths and parasites, diagnostic and surgical preparations
Stimulant	Acute constipation, diagnostic and surgical bowel preparations

Table 48-6 Laxatives: Adverse Effects

Laxative Group	Side/Adverse Effect
Bulk-forming	Impaction above strictures, fluid overload, electrolyte imbalances, gas formation, esophageal blockage, allergic reaction
Emollient	Skin rashes, decreased absorption of vitamins, lipid pneumonia, electrolyte imbalances
Hyperosmotic	Abdominal bloating, rectal irritation, electrolyte imbalances
Saline	Magnesium toxicity (with renal insufficiency), electrolyte imbalances, cramping, diarrhea, increased thirst
Stimulant	Nutrient malabsorption, skin rashes, gastric irritation, electrolyte imbalances, discolored urine, rectal irritation

nitrofurantoin, salicylates, tetracyclines, and oral anticoagulants. Mineral oil can decrease the absorption of fat-soluble vitamins (A, D, E, and K). Hyperosmotic laxatives can cause increased CNS depression if they are given with barbiturates, general anesthetics, opioids, and antipsychotics. Oral antibiotics can decrease the effects of lactulose. Stimulant laxatives decrease absorption of antibiotics, digoxin, nitrofurantoin, salicylates, tetracyclines, and oral anticoagulants.

Dosages

For the recommended dosages of selected laxatives, see the dosages table on p. 775.

drug profiles

As mentioned previously, laxatives are used for the treatment of constipation; such treatment must involve an understanding of the whole patient. Of the five major groups of laxatives many are available as OTC medications, whereas others require a prescription for use. The following are prototypical agents from each of the laxative groups.

BULK-FORMING LAXATIVES

Bulk-forming laxatives are composed of water-retaining (hydrophilic) natural and synthetic cellulose derivatives. Psyllium is an example of a natural bulk-forming laxative, and methylcellulose is an example of a synthetic cellulose derivative. Other bulk-forming laxatives are malt-soup–extract preparations and polycarbophil preparations. Bulk-forming agents increase water absorption, resulting in greater total volume (bulk) of the intestinal contents. Unlike some of the other laxatives, bulk-forming laxatives tend to produce normal, formed stools. Their site of action is limited to the GI tract so there are few, if any, systemic effects. However, they should be taken with liberal amounts of water to prevent esophageal obstruction and/or fecal impaction. These laxatives are OTC medications and are classified as pregnancy category C agents. The bulk-forming laxatives are among the safest available and the only ones that are recommended for long-term use.

⊶ methylcellulose

Methylcellulose (Citrucel) is a synthetic bulk-forming laxative that attracts water into the intestine and absorbs excess water into the stool, stimulating the intestines and increasing peristalsis. It is contraindicated in patients who have shown a hypersensitivity reaction to it and in those with GI obstruction or hepatitis. Methylcellulose is an oral agent available as 105-mg and 364-mg powders and 500-mg tablets. Commonly recommended dosages are listed in the dosages table on p. 775.

PHARMACOKINETICS

HALF-LIFE	ONSET	PEAK	DURATION
Unknown	12-24 hr	Unknown	Unknown

psyllium

Psyllium (Metamucil, Fiberall, Peridem) is a natural bulk-forming laxative obtained from the dried seed of the *Plantago psyllium* plant. It has many of the characteristics of methylcellulose. Psyllium is contraindicated in patients who have shown a hypersensitivity reaction to it and in those with intestinal obstruction or fecal impaction. Its use is also contraindicated in patients experiencing abdominal pain and/or nausea and vomiting. Psyllium is available as 1.7-g and 3.4-g chewable wafers and as a variety of powdered products with strengths ranging from 309 mg to 1000 mg. There is also a psyllium combination product combining 542 mg of psyllium and 123 mg of senna. Commonly recommended dosages are listed in the dosages table on p. 775.

PHARMACOKINETICS

HALF-LIFE	ONSET	PEAK	DURATION
Unknown	12-24 hr	Unknown	Unknown

EMOLLIENT LAXATIVES

Emollient laxatives either directly lubricate the stool and the intestines, as with mineral oil, or they act as fecal softeners. By lubricating the fecal material and the intestinal walls, lubricant emollient laxatives prevent water from leaking out of the intestines, which softens and expands the stool. Stool softeners (docusate salts) work by lowering the surface tension of fluids, allowing more water and fat to be absorbed into the stool and the intestines.

mineral oil

Mineral oil (Agoral Plain, Fleet Mineral Oil Enema, Kondremul, Zymenol) eases passage of stool by preventing water from escaping the stool and lubricating the intestines. Mineral oil is the only lubricant laxative in the emollient category; it is a mixture of liquid hydrocarbons derived from petroleum. It is most commonly used to treat constipation associated with hard stools or fecal impaction.

Mineral oil is classified as a pregnancy category C agent and is contraindicated in patients who have shown a hypersensitivity reaction to it. Its use is also contraindicated in patients with intestinal obstruction, abdominal pain, and nausea and vomiting. Mineral oil agents are available as enemas or as 1.4-, 2.75-, and 4.75-g/5 ml oral suspensions. There are also many combination products that contain mineral oil such as Haley's M-O, which is a mixture of 1 mg/5 ml of mineral oil and 4 mg/5 ml of milk of magnesia. Commonly recommended dosages are listed in the dosages table on p. 775.

DOSAGES Selected Laxative Agents

agent	pharmacologic class	dosage range	purpose
docusate sodium (calcium, potassium, and sodium salts)	Fecal softener	*Pediatric <3 y/o* PO: 10-40 mg/day (qd-qid) *Pediatric 3-6 y/o* PO: 20-60 mg/day (qd-qid) *Pediatric 6-12 y/o* PO: 40-150 mg/day (qd-qid) *Adult/Pediatric ≥12 y/o* PO: 50-500 mg/day (qd-qid)	Stool softener
glycerin (Fleet Babylax, Glycerin, Sani-Supp)	Hyperosmotic laxative	*Rectal:* Insert one adult, child, or infant suppository into rectum qd-bid prn	Constipation
lactulose (Chronulac, Constilac, Duphalac, Cephulac)	Disaccharide laxative	*Adult* PO: 15-30 ml/day	Constipation
magnesium salts	Saline laxative	*Citrate—Adult/Pediatric* *<6 y/o* PO: 2-4 ml/kg/day (qd-bid) *6-12 y/o* PO: 100-150 ml/day (qd-bid) *>12 y/o* PO: 150-300 ml/day (qd-bid) *Sulfate—Adult/Pediatric* PO: ≥ 12 y/o: 10-30 g/day 6-11 y/o: 5-10 g/day 2-5 y/o: 2.5-5 g/day	Constipation
methylcellulose (Citrucel)	Bulk-forming laxative	*Adult/Pediatric >12 y/o* PO: 1 Tbsp in 8 oz of water 1-3 times/day *Pediatric 6 to ≤ 12 y/o* PO: ½ adult dose in 4 oz of water 1-3 times/day	Constipation
mineral oil (Agoral Plain, Mineral Oil Enema, Kondremul, Zymenol)	Emollient laxative	*Pediatric ≤ 12 y/o* PO: 15-45 ml as a single daily dose *Pediatric 6-11 y/o* PO: 5-15 ml/day at bedtime *Adult/Pediatric ≥12 y/o* PO: 5-45 ml as a single daily dose at bedtime *Pediatric 2-11 y/o* PO: 30-60 ml/day	Constipation Enema
polyethylene glycol (CoLyte, GoLytely, OCL)	Bowel evacuant	*Adult* PO: 4 L daily administered in 240-ml doses q10min	Bowel cleansing before examination
psyllium (Metamucil, Fiberall)	Bulk-forming laxative	*Adult/Pediatric ≥ 12 y/o* PO: 1-2 tsp in 8 oz of water 1-3 times/day *Pediatric 6 to ≤12 y/o* PO: ½ the adult dose in 4 oz of water 1-3 times/day	Constipation
senna (Black Draught, Dr. Caldwell Senna Laxative, Fetcher's Castoria, Senokot, Senolax)	Stimulant/irritant laxative	*Pediatric* PO: 10-20 mg/kg/dose (qhs) *1 mo-1 y/o* PO: 55-109 mg qhs to max 218 mg/day *1-5 y/o* PO: 109-218 mg qhs to max 436 mg/day *5-15 y/o* PO: 218-436 mg qhs to max 872 g/day PR: children >27 kg: 326 mg (1/2 supp) qhs *Adults* PO: granules: 1 tsp qhs; max dose 2 tsp bid	Constipation

PHARMACOKINETICS

HALF-LIFE	ONSET	PEAK	DURATION
Unknown	6-8 hr	Unknown	Unknown

⊶docusate salts

Docusate salts (calcium, potassium, and sodium) are fecal softening emollient laxatives that facilitate the passage of water and lipids (fats) into the fecal mass, softening the stool. The currently available agents in each salt form are as follows:

- Calcium salt (docusate calcium)
- Pro-Cal-Sof capsules
- Surfak capsules
- Potassium salt (docusate potassium)
- Diocto-K capsules
- Kasof capsules
- Sodium salt (docusate sodium)
- Colace capsules, liquid, syrup
- Dialose capsules, tablets
- D.S.S. capsules
- Modane Soft capsules
- Regutol tablets

These agents are used to treat constipation, soften fecal impacts, and facilitate easy bowel movements in patients with hemorrhoids and other painful anorectal conditions. In addition to the above-mentioned docusate-salt formulations, there are also combination products available. Docusate is classified as a pregnancy category C agent and is contraindicated in patients who have shown a hypersensitivity reaction to it and in those with intestinal obstruction, fecal impaction, and nausea and vomiting. Commonly recommended dosages are listed in the dosages table on p. 775.

PHARMACOKINETICS

HALF-LIFE	ONSET	PEAK	DURATION
Unknown	1-3 days	Unknown	1-3 days

HYPEROSMOTIC LAXATIVES

The hyperosmotic laxatives polyethylene glycol (PEG), lactulose sorbitol, and glycerine relieve constipation by increasing the water content of feces, resulting in distention, peristalsis, and evacuation. They are most commonly used to treat constipation and to evacuate the bowels before diagnostic and surgical procedures.

polyethylene glycol

PEG (CoLyte, GoLytely, OCL) is most commonly used before diagnostic or surgical bowel procedures because it is a very potent laxative that induces total cleansing of the bowel. PEG is contraindicated in patients with GI obstruction, gastric retention, bowel perforation, toxic colitis, toxic megalocolon, or ileus. It is classified as a pregnancy category C agent. The particular PEG that is used in

the products mentioned is PEG-3350; its composition is as follows (in g/L):

- PEG 3350 60
- Sodium chloride 1.46
- Potassium chloride 0.745
- Sodium bicarbonate 1.68
- Sodium sulfate 5.68

An oral solution of PEG-3350 and electrolytes is available for GI lavage. Diarrhea usually occurs within 30 to 60 minutes after ingestion; complete evacuation and cleansing of the bowel is accomplished within 4 hours. Commonly recommended dosages are listed in the dosages table on p. 775.

PHARMACOKINETICS

HALF-LIFE	ONSET	PEAK	DURATION
Unknown	1 hr	2-4 hr	4 hr

lactulose

Lactulose (Chronulac, Duphalac, Enulose) is a disaccharide sugar containing one molecule of galactose and one molecule of fructose (two types of sugar molecules). It is a synthetic derivative of the natural sugar lactose, which is not digested in the stomach or absorbed in the small bowel. Instead it is passed unchanged into the large intestine where it is metabolized. This process produces lactic acid, formic acid, and acetic acid, creating a hyperosmotic environment that draws water into the colon and produces a laxative effect. This drug-induced acidic environment also reduces blood ammonia levels by forcing ammonia from the blood into the colon. This has proved helpful in treating patients with systemic encephalopathy.

Lactulose is classified as a pregnancy category B agent and is contraindicated in patients who have shown a hypersensitivity reaction to it and in patients on a low galactose diet. It is available as either a 3.33-g/5 ml oral or rectal solution. Commonly recommended dosages are listed in the dosages table on p. 775.

PHARMACOKINETICS

HALF-LIFE	ONSET	PEAK	DURATION
Unknown	24 hr	24-48 hr	Variable

Activity

glycerin

Glycerin (Fleet Babylax, Glycerin, Sani-Supp) promotes bowel movements by increasing osmotic pressure in the intestine, which draws fluid into the colon. Because it is a very mild laxative, it is often used in children. Sorbitol, another hyperosmotic laxative, has similar properties. Glycerin is classified as a pregnancy category C agent and is contraindicated in patients who have shown a hypersensitivity reaction to it. It is available as a 4 ml per applicator rectal solution and as a suppository.

Commonly recommended dosages are listed in the dosages table on p. 775.

PHARMACOKINETICS

HALF-LIFE	ONSET	PEAK	DURATION
30-45 min	16-36 min	1 hr	2-4 hr

SALINE LAXATIVES

Saline laxatives consist of various magnesium and sodium salts. They increase osmotic pressure and draw water into the colon, producing a watery stool usually within 3 to 6 hours of ingestion. The currently available magnesium and sodium salt agents are listed in Box 48-3.

magnesium salts

The magnesium saline laxatives magnesium citrate, Milk of Magnesia, and Epsom salts are commonly used, unpleasant tasting OTC laxative preparations. They should be used with caution or not at all in patients with renal insufficiency because they can be absorbed into the systemic circulation, causing hypermagnesemia. They are most commonly used for rapid evacuation of the bowel in preparation for endoscopic examination and to help remove unabsorbed poisons from the GI tract.

They are classified as pregnancy category B agents and are contraindicated in patients who have shown a hypersensitivity reaction to them. Their use is also contraindicated in patients with renal diseases, abdominal pain, nausea and vomiting, obstruction, acute surgical abdomen, and rectal bleeding. Magnesium hydroxide is available as a 77.5-mg/ml suspension, a concentrated milk of magnesia preparation, and 300- and 500-mg tablets. It is also used in a variety of combination products such as Haley's M-O. Other magnesium products are listed in the discussion of saline laxatives. Commonly recommended dosages are listed in the dosages table on p. 775.

PHARMACOKINETICS

HALF-LIFE	ONSET	PEAK	DURATION
Unknown	0.5-3 hr	3 hr	Variable

STIMULANT LAXATIVES

Stimulant laxatives, consisting of natural plant products and synthetic chemical agents, induce intestinal peristalsis. Plant-derived stimulant laxatives include bisacodyl, disacodyl tannex, and phenolphthalein (white and yellow). The anthraquinones make up another subgroup of the stimulant laxatives, including agents such as cascara sagrada, senna, aloe (casanthrol), and danthron. Their site of action includes the entire GI tract. The action of the stimulant laxatives is proportional to the dose. They are the most likely of all the laxative classes to cause dependence.

BOX 48-3 Magnesium and Salt Agents

MAGNESIUM LAXATIVES

Sulfate
Epsom salt

Hydroxide
Milk of magnesia
Phillip's Milk of Magnesia
Haley's M-O

Citrate
Citrate of Magnesia

SODIUM LAXATIVES

Phosphate
Fleet Phospho-Soda
Fleet Enema

---

senna

Senna (Black Draught, Dr. Caldwell Senna Laxative, Fetcher's Castoria, Senokot, Senolax) is an example of a commonly used OTC stimulant laxative. Senna can be obtained from the dried leaves of the *Cassia acutifolia* plant. It may be used for acute constipation or bowel preparation for surgery or examination. Because it stimulates the GI tract, it may cause abdominal pain. It can produce complete bowel evacuation in 6 to 12 hours. It is available in a variety of dosages in the forms of suppositories, tablets, syrup, and granules.

PHARMACOKINETICS

HALF-LIFE	ONSET	PEAK	DURATION
Variable	6-24 hr	24 hr	24-36 hr

---

nursing process

● Assessment

Before administering antidiarrheal preparations, the nurse should obtain and document a thorough history of bowel patterns, general state of health, and recent history of illness or dietary changes. The adsorbent bismuth subsalicylate should not be given to children under 16 years of age or teenagers with chicken pox because of the risk of Reye's syndrome. It should also not be given to patients who are allergic to either of the chemical ingredients (bismuth or salicylates). Caution and careful monitoring are required with the use of adsorbents in patients who are elderly or who have a history of decreased bleeding time, clotting disorders, recent bowel surgery, or confusion.

Anticholinergics should not be administered to a patient who has a history of allergy to such medications or to patients with glaucoma, benign prostatic hypertrophy, urinary retention, recent bladder surgery, or cardiac history. Other contraindications to use include myasthenia

Mr. J.C., an 83-year-old truck assembly line supervisor, has been retired for 15 years. He continues to enjoy reasonably good health and rides his bicycle approximately 5 miles each day. He has a history of BPH and constipation secondary to polyps of the colon and a low-fiber diet. He has just met with the gastroenterologist and is now asking you for information on how to manage his constipation. In your assessment, you discover he is taking a laxative containing senna, drinks 3 to 4 glasses of water each day, eats small amounts of grain products, and—except for an occasional (once per month) "pot of country greens"—has poor fiber intake.

Develop a comprehensive teaching guide for Mr. J.C. that includes specific instructions on the following:

- *Consider nonpharmacologic measures for management of constipation, including recommended fluid intake, amount of fiber, and what foods to consume and other dietary suggestions.*
- *If OTC drug therapy is used, make some safe recommendations with rationales for their use.*

A patient whom you follow with home health has been taking psyllium (Metamucil) for complaints of constipation. When you arrive today to help her with her morning care and medication administration, she complains that the Metamucil gets "stuck in her throat," so she went back to taking her old Ex-Lax.

- *What important patient education points should you emphasize with this patient?*

- Patients is free from self-injury related to possible weakness and dizziness or from side effects of either groups of medications.
- Patient remains compliant to medication and nonpharmacologic measures.

Outcome Criteria

Outcome criteria for the patient receiving antidiarrheals, laxatives, and cathartics include, but are not limited to, the following:

- Patient will report the signs and symptoms of fluid and electrolyte loss such as weakness, lethargy, decreased urinary output, and dizziness.
- Patient will state measures to avoid side effects and injuries related to change in bowel patterns, changes in fluid and electrolyte status, or treatment such as changing positions slowly.
- Patient will state methods of administration that enhance effective and safe use of antidiarrheals, laxatives, or cathartics such as taking as prescribed.
- Patient will state nonpharmacologic measures to relieve constipation, flatus, and diarrhea such as forcing fluids, increasing fiber or bulk, or withdrawing irritating food sources from diet.

● Implementation

Antidiarrheals should be taken exactly as prescribed, with strict adherence to the recommended dosage. Make sure that patients are aware of their fluid intake and any dietary changes. Patients should also be aware of the precipitating factors of the diarrhea and, if symptoms persist, they should know to contact a physician immediately. Documentation of bowel pattern changes, weight, fluid volume status, intake and output, and mucous membrane status should be done before, during, and after the initiation of treatment.

Bulk-forming laxatives, such as psyllium and methylcellulose, must be administered as specified by package inserts, which is usually in the morning and evening. They should be given alone (i.e., not with food) and mixed with at least 6 to 8 ounces of fluid and drunk immediately to prevent possible obstruction. Instructions for administering mineral oil agents are similar to those for other laxatives with the additional concern of preventing aspiration in the elderly patient. Bisa-

gravis, paralytic ileus, and toxic megacolon. Cautious use is recommended in patients with a history of confusion, dizziness, hypotension, hypertension, bradycardia, tachycardia, or blurred vision.

Bulk-forming laxatives, such as psyllium preparations, are often used to treat chronic constipation and have few side effects. A thorough history of presenting symptoms and elimination patterns must be completed and documented before administering the medication to ensure patient safety. In addition, the patient's intake and output ratio and electrolytes should be assessed and documented before initiating therapy to establish baseline values for later comparison.

● Nursing Diagnoses

Nursing diagnoses associated with the use of antidiarrheals, laxatives, and cathartics include, but are not limited to, the following:

- Diarrhea related to various GI disorders.
- Deficient fluid volume related to excessive loss of water and electrolytes through stool with diarrhea.
- Risk for injury related to weakness and dizziness from possible excessive loss of fluid and electrolytes through stool.
- Deficient knowledge related to possible chronic laxative abuse, side effects of laxatives and cathartics, and nonpharmacologic measures to relieve constipation.

● Planning

Goals related to the administration of antidiarrheals, laxatives, and cathartics include the following:

- Patient remains free of fluid and electrolyte disturbances related to changes in bowel patterns.

codyl and cascara sagrada should be given with water only because of interactions with milk, antacids, and H₂ blockers.

Patient education is important to compliance and safe, effective use of laxatives or cathartics. See the box below for the patient teaching tips.

• Evaluation

Therapeutic responses to antidiarrheals, laxatives, and cathartics include an improvement in the GI-related signs and symptoms reported by the patient as well as improvement in bowel sounds and no abnormal findings from an assessment of the abdomen and bowel patterns. Side effects for which to monitor in patients vary according to drug classification group.

---

patient teaching tips

Laxatives, Cathartics, and Antidiarrheals

➤ Patients should swallow all laxative tablets whole with at least 6 to 8 oz of water. Make sure patients do not crush or chew tablets, especially if they are enteric coated.

➤ If taking a bulk-forming laxative such as psyllium or methylcellulose (Metamucil), patients should be sure to take it as directed by the manufacturer with at least 240 ml (8 oz) of water.

➤ Long-term use of laxatives or cathartics often results in decreased bowel tone and may lead to dependency.

➤ Patients should be honest with their physician, nurse, or any other health care provider regarding their dietary habits, fiber and fluid intake, and elimination patterns. A normal bowel pattern does not necessarily mean a bowel movement everyday.

➤ Patients should not take a laxative or cathartic if they are experiencing nausea, vomiting, and/or abdominal pain.

➤ Patients should contact their physician if they experience severe abdominal pain, muscle weakness, cramps, and/or dizziness, which may indicate possible fluid or electrolyte loss.

➤ Patients should take antidiarrheals exactly as prescribed. Stool frequency, consistency, and amount should be recorded for comparison and evaluation.

➤ A healthy, high-fiber diet and increased fluid intake should always be encouraged as an alternative to laxative use.

POINTS TO REMEMBER

Diarrhea

- Leading cause of morbidity and mortality in underdeveloped countries.
- Between 5 and 8 million deaths per year in infants and children.
- Loss of time and productivity at work has an enormous financial impact with an estimated cost of $23 billion per year or $106 per person per year in the United States.
- Acute and chronic types.

Drug Therapy

- Adsorbents, anticholinergics, opiates, and intestinal flora modifiers.
- Most acute diarrhea is self-limiting, subsiding in 3 days to 2 weeks.
- Fluid and electrolyte replacement is vital.
- Encourage patients to check and recheck dosage instructions before taking medication and note any drug-food or drug-drug interactions.

Anticholinergics

- Decrease muscle tone of GI tract and decrease peristalsis.
- Can cause urinary retention, headache, confusion, dry skin, rash, and blurred vision.
- Belladonna alkaloids (Donnatal) are common anticholinergic antidiarrheals.

Adsorbents

- Coat walls of GI tract, absorbing bacteria or toxins causing diarrhea, and eliminating them with stool.
- May increase bleeding, cause constipation, dark stools, and black tongue.
- Bismuth subsalicylate and attapulgite (Kaopectate) are common adsorbents.

Intestinal Flora Modifiers

- Bacterial cultures of *Lactobacillus*.
- Supply normal intestinal florae destroyed by infection or antibiotics.
- Suppress the growth of diarrhea-causing bacteria.

Opiates

- Decrease bowel motility and thus permit longer contact of intestinal contents with absorptive surface of the bowel.
- Reduce pain associated with rectal spasms.

Laxatives

- Laxatives and cathartics may cause side effects that precipitate problems in volume.
- Patients must be made aware of abuse potential and the problems associated with the misuse of laxatives.
- Encourage patient to keep a log of daily elimination patterns and any problems related to laxative use.

Nursing Considerations

- Keep these medications, as well as all other medications, out of the reach of children because they may be very toxic to a child.
- Report abdominal distention, firm abdomen, pain and worsening (or no improvement) of diarrhea, and

GI-related signs and symptoms to the physician immediately.
- Long-term use may lead to laxative dependence. Bulk-forming laxatives are not habit-forming.
- Always check for possible drug-drug and drug-food interactions with antidiarrheals and laxatives.

REVIEW QUESTIONS

1. Which of the following is most commonly done before a diagnostic colonoscopy for total bowel cleansing?
   a. Fleet enema three times
   b. GoLytely 24 hours before the procedure
   c. 24 to 48 ounces of mineral oil the night before
   d. Soap suds enema twice daily for 48 hours before procedure
2. What is the major concern regarding the administration of oral methylcellulose?
   a. Dehydration
   b. Polycythemia
   c. Inducing CHF
   d. Possible obstruction
3. Which of the following medications is not to be taken with digoxin?
   a. NSAIDs
   b. Furosemide
   c. Pepto-Bismol
   d. Acetaminophen

4. The classification of methylcellulose is:
   a. Potent laxative.
   b. Glycerin osmotic.
   c. Hypertonic osmotic.
   d. Bulk-forming laxative.
5. Which of the following is a good patient teaching tip for patients taking laxatives?
   a. Crush any capsules or enteric tablets.
   b. Take the laxative tablets with at least 6 to 8 ounces of water.
   c. Bisacodyl should be given with milk and antacids to decrease GI upset.
   d. If one dose works, then doubling up is recommended for bad constipation.
6. Which of the following is a side effect associated with loperamide (Imodium)?
   a. Dysphagia
   b. Epigastric pain
   c. Excessive salivation
   d. CNS overstimulation

For Answers see www.harcourthealth.com/MERLIN/Lilley/.

CRITICAL THINKING Activities

1. You need to explain to a group of elderly patients the importance of seeking treatment for diarrhea. During your discussion with the group, the following questions were posed to you:
   - "What are some non-drug therapies I can use once I have begun to recover from diarrhea caused by a virus or the flu?"
   - "If I have eaten something 'bad,' does it matter if I take something to stop the diarrhea?"

Answer these questions for the elderly population and provide rationales for your responses.
2. Your pediatric patient's mother calls the clinic because her 4-month-old daughter has had diarrhea for about 8 hours. What would you recommend over the phone and why?
3. Why is it important that elderly patients are monitored closely while taking GoLytely in preparation for bowel procedures or diagnostic studies? Explain your answer.

For Answers see www.harcourthealth.com/MERLIN/Lilley/.

bibliography

Albanese J, Nutz P: *Mosby's 2001 nursing drug reference and review cards,* St Louis, 2001, Mosby.
American Hospital Formulary Services: *AHFS drug information,* Bethesda, Md, 2000, American Society of Health-System Pharmacists.

Anderson PO, Knoben JE, Troutman WG: *Handbook of clinical drug data 1999-2000,* ed 9, New York, 1999, McGraw-Hill.
Johns Hopkins Hospital, Department of Pediatrics et al: *The Harriet Lane handbook,* ed 15, St. Louis, 2000, Mosby.

Keen JH: *Critical care and emergency drug reference,* ed 3, St Louis, 1996, Mosby.

Mosby's GenRx: a comprehensive reference for generic and brand drugs, ed 10, St Louis, 2000, Mosby.

Skidmore-Roth L: *Mosby's 2001 nursing drug reference,* St Louis, 2001, Mosby.

Tierney LM, McPhee SJ, Papadakis MA: *Current medical diagnosis and treatment 1998,* ed 37, Norwalk, Conn, 1997, Appleton & Lange.

United States Pharmacopeial Convention: *USP DI: drug information for the health care professional, vol. 1,* ed 20, Englewood, Colo, 2000, Micromedex.

MERLIN Activity

Remember to check the **Online Worksheet** for additional learning opportunities: **www.harcourthealth.com/MERLIN/Lilley/**

Chapter 49

Antiemetic (Antinausea) Agents

www.harcourthealth.com/MERLIN/Lilley/

Look for this symbol for
topics covered in the
Online Worksheet
Activity

objectives

When you reach the end of this chapter, you should be able to do the following:

1 Discuss the pathophysiology of nausea and vomiting.

2 Identify the neurotransmitters involved in the process of nausea and vomiting.

3 Identify the antiemetic drugs and their drug classification grouping.

4 Identify the mechanisms of action, indications for use, contraindications, cautions, and drug interactions associated with the various types of antiemetic agents.

5 Develop a nursing care plan that includes all phases of the nursing process related to the administration of antiemetic agents.

6 Cite the patient teaching guidelines for patients receiving antiemetics.

drug profiles

dronabinol, p. 788	**ondansetron,** p. 788
meclizine, p. 786	⊶ **prochlorperazine,** p. 786
⊶ **metoclopramide,** p. 788	⊶ **scopolamine,** p. 786

⊶ Key drug.

glossary

Anticholinergic (an′ ti ko′ lin ər′ jik) Drug given to treat motion sickness. (p. 783)

Antiemetic agent (an′ te ə met′ ik) Drug given to relieve nausea and vomiting. (p. 783)

Antihistamine (an′ ti his′ tə men) Agent that works by inhibiting vestibular stimulation. (p. 784)

Chemoreceptor trigger zone (CTZ) The area in the brain that is involved with the sensation of nausea and vomiting. (p. 783)

Emesis (em′ ə sis) The forcible emptying or expulsion of gastric and, occasionally, intestinal contents through the mouth; also called *vomiting*. (p. 782)

Nausea Sensation often leading to the urge to vomit. (p. 782)

Neuroleptic agent (nur′ o lep′ tik) Drug that prevents nausea and vomiting by blocking dopamine receptors on the chemoreceptor trigger zone. (p. 784)

Prokinetic agent (pro ki net′ ik) Drug that prevents nausea and vomiting by blocking dopamine in the chemoreceptor trigger zone, making the zone less sensitive to impulses sent to it from the gastrointestinal tract. (p. 784)

Serotonin blocker (ser′ o to′ nin) Agent that prevents vomiting and nausea by blocking serotonin receptors located in the gastrointestinal tract, the chemoreceptor trigger zone, and the vomiting center. (p. 784)

Tetrahydrocannabinoid (tet′ rə hi′ dro kə nab′ i noid) The major psychoactive substance in marijuana. Nonintoxicating doses have been used experimentally to treat glaucoma and to relieve nausea and increase the appetite in patients receiving cancer chemotherapy. (p. 784)

Vomiting The forcible emptying or expulsion of gastric and, occasionally, intestinal contents through the mouth; also called *emesis*. (p. 782)

Vomiting center (VC) The area in the brain that is involved in stimulating the physioloigc events that lead to nausea and vomiting. (p. 782)

NAUSEA AND VOMITING

Nausea and vomiting are two gastrointestinal (GI) disorders that can be not only extremely unpleasant but also lead to more serious complications if not treated promptly. **Nausea** is an unpleasant feeling that often precedes vomiting. If it does not subside spontaneously or is not relieved by medication, it can lead to vomiting. **Vomiting,** which is also called **emesis,** is the forcible emptying or expulsion of gastric and, occasionally, intestinal contents through the mouth. There is a variety of stimuli that can induce nausea and vomiting, including foul odors or tastes, irritation of the stomach or intestines, and certain drugs (ipecac or antineoplastic agents).

Much research into the nature of nausea and vomiting has been done over the past decade, resulting in a better understanding of the physiology of these phenomena. This improved understanding has included the concept of a **vomiting center (VC)** in the brain that is responsible for initiating the necessary physiologic events that lead to nausea and eventually vomiting. There are in turn several pathways that transmit stimuli to the VC and the **chemoreceptor trigger zone (CTZ),** another area in the brain involved in the causation of nausea and vomiting. These pathways communicate with the CTZ and VC by means of neurotransmitters, and thereby alert these areas of the brain to the existence of nauseating substances (nauseous stimuli) that need to be expelled from the body. Once the VC and CTZ are stimulated, they initiate the events that stimulate the vomiting reflex. The neurotransmitters involved in this process and their respective receptors are listed in Table 49-1. The various pathways and the areas of the body that send the signals to the VC via these pathways are illustrated in Figure 49-1.

ANTIEMETIC AGENTS

The drugs used to relieve nausea and vomiting are called **antiemetic agents.** The discovery of new agents coupled with a better understanding of the way in which the older drugs work has had a dramatic impact on the way in which nausea and vomiting are now treated. All of these agents work at some site in the vomiting pathway, and there are six categories of such agents. By combining agents from these various categories, the antiemetic effectiveness of the resulting agent is increased because it can then block more than just one of the pathways in the overall vomiting pathway. Some of the more commonly used antiemetics in the different categories are listed in Table 49-2, and the sites where they work in the vomiting pathway are shown in Figure 49-2.

Mechanism of Action

The numerous drugs used to prevent or treat nausea and vomiting have many different mechanisms of action. Most work by blocking one of the pathways in the vomiting pathway, as shown in Figure 49-2, and in doing so block the stimulus that induces vomiting. The mechanisms of action of the drugs in the six antiemetic drug categories are summarized in Table 49-3.

Anticholinergics act by binding to and blocking acetylcholine (ACh) receptors on the vestibular nuclei, which are located in the labyrinth. By preventing ACh from binding to these receptors, nauseous stimuli originating from this area cannot be transmitted to the CTZ. Anticholinergics also block receptors located in the reticular formation and by doing so prevent ACh from binding to

Table 49-1 Neurotransmitters Involved in Nausea and Vomiting

Neurotransmitter	Site in the Vomiting Pathway
Acetylcholine (ACh)	Vestibular, vomiting center, and labyrinth pathways
Dopamine (D_2)	GI tract and CTZ
Histamine (H_1)	Vestibular, vomiting center, and labyrinth pathways
Prostaglandins (PG)	GI tract
Serotonin (5 HT_3)	GI tract, CTZ, and vomiting center

GI, Gastrointestinal; *CTZ,* chemoreceptor trigger zone.

Table 49-2 Antiemetics: Common Drug Categories

Antiemetic Category	Antiemetic Agents
Anticholinergic agents (acetylcholine blockers)	scopolamine
Antihistamine agents (H_1 receptor blockers)	promethazine, meclizine, dimenhydrinate, diphenhydramine
Neuroleptic agents	chlorpromazine, perphenazine, prochlorperazine, promethazine, thiethylperazine, triflupromazine, trimeprazine
Prokinetic agents	metoclopramide, cisapride
Serotonin blockers	granisetron, ondansetron, dolasetron
Tetrahydrocannabinoids	dronabinol

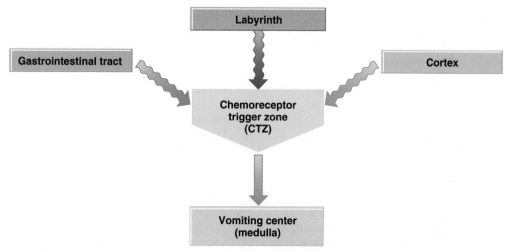

Fig. 49-1 The various pathways and areas in the body sending signals to the vomiting center.

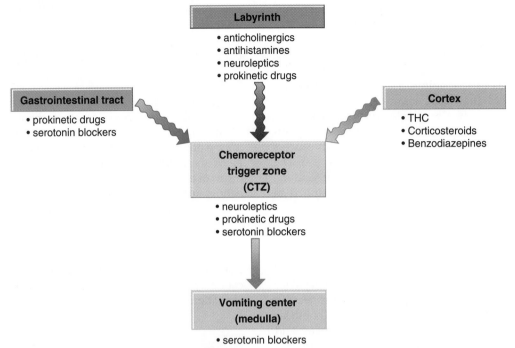

Fig. 49-2 Sites of action of selected antiemetics.

Antiemetics: Mechanisms of Action

Table 49-3

Antiemetic Category	Mechanism of Action
Anticholinergic agents	Block acetylcholine receptors in the vestibular nuclei and reticular formation.
Antihistamine agents	Block histamine₁ receptors, thereby preventing acetylcholine from binding to receptors in the vestibular nuclei.
Neuroleptic agents	Block dopamine in the CTZ and may also block acetylcholine.
Prokinetic agents	Block dopamine in the CTZ or stimulate acetylcholine receptors in the GI tract.
Serotonin blockers	Block serotonin receptors in the GI tract, CTZ, and VC.
Tetrahydro-cannabinoid	Has inhibitory effects on the reticular formation, thalamus, and cerebral cortex.

CTZ, Chemoreceptor trigger zone; *GI*, gastrointestinal; *VC*, vomiting center.

these receptors so that nauseous stimuli originating from this area cannot be transmitted to the VC.

Antihistamines (H₁ receptor blockers) act by inhibiting vestibular stimulation in a manner that is very similar to the way in which anticholinergics work. They inhibit ACh by binding to histamine₁ receptors, which thereby prevent cholinergic stimulation in both the vestibular and reticular systems. Nausea and vomiting occur when these areas of the brain are stimulated.

Neuroleptic agents prevent nausea and vomiting by blocking dopamine receptors on the CTZ. Many of the neuroleptics also have anticholinergic actions similar to those of the anticholinergics.

Prokinetic agents, in particular metoclopramide, act by blocking dopamine in the CTZ, which causes it to be desensitized to the impulses it receives from the GI tract.

Serotonin blockers work by blocking serotonin receptors located in the GI tract, the CTZ, and VC. There are many subtypes of serotonin receptors, and these various receptors are located throughout the body (CNS, smooth muscles, platelets, and GI tract). The subtype of receptor involved in the mediation of nausea and vomiting is the 5-HT₃ receptor. These receptors are the site of action for the serotonin blockers such as ondansetron and granisetron.

Tetrahydrocannabinoid (THC) is the major psychoactive substance in marijuana. In the form of the drug dronabinol (Marinol), it is occasionally used as an antiemetic because of its inhibitory effects on the reticular formation, thalamus, and cerebral cortex. These effects cause an alteration in mood and the body's perception of its surroundings, which may be beneficial in relieving nausea and vomiting. Although this particular category of antiemetics is used very rarely, there are occasionally

Table 49-4 Antiemetics: Therapeutic Uses

Antiemetic Category	Therapeutic Effects
Anticholinergic agents	Motion sickness, secretion reduction before surgery, nausea and vomiting
Antihistamine agents	Motion sickness, nonproductive cough, sedation, rhinitis, allergy symptoms, nausea and vomiting
Neuroleptic agents	Psychotic disorders (mania, schizophrenia, anxiety), intractable hiccups, nausea and vomiting
Prokinetic agents	Delayed gastric emptying, gastroesophageal reflux, nausea and vomiting
Serotonin blockers	Nausea and vomiting associated with cancer chemotherapy, postoperative nausea and vomiting
Tetrahydro-cannabinoids	Nausea and vomiting associated with cancer chemotherapy anorexia associated with weight loss in AIDS patients

Table 49-5 Antiemetics: Adverse Effects

Body System	Side/Adverse Effects
ANTICHOLINERGICS	
CNS	Dizziness, drowsiness, disorientation
EENT	Blurred vision, dilated pupils, dry mouth
Genitourinary	Difficult urination, constipation
Integumentary	Rash, erythema
ANTIHISTAMINES	
CNS	Dizziness, drowsiness, confusion
EENT	Blurred vision, dilated pupils, dry mouth
Genitourinary	Urinary retention
NEUROLEPTIC AGENTS	
Cardiovascular	Orthostatic hypotension, ECG changes, tachycardia
CNS	Extrapyramidal symptoms, pseudoparkinsonism, akathisia, dystonia, tardive dyskinesia, headache
EENT	Blurred vision, dry eyes
Genitourinary	Urinary retention
GI	Dry mouth, nausea, vomiting, anorexia, constipation
PROKINETIC AGENTS	
Cardiovascular	Hypotension, supraventricular tachycardia
CNS	Sedation, fatigue, restlessness, headache, dystonia
GI	Dry mouth, nausea and vomiting, diarrhea
SEROTONIN BLOCKERS	
CNS	Headache
GI	Diarrhea, transient increased AST and ALT levels
Other	Rash, bronchospasm
TETRAHYDROCANNABINOIDS	
CNS	Drowsiness, dizziness, anxiety, confusion, euphoria
EENT	Visual disturbances
GI	Dry mouth

unusual cases of nausea and vomiting that respond well to THCs.

Drug Effects

The drug effects of the antiemetic agents are related to their mechanisms of action. As previously explained, these agents act by blocking receptors that, when occupied by neurotransmitters, stimulate various vomiting pathways. These receptors are also located in areas throughout the CNS as well as in other areas of the body. For this reason, antiemetics may have drug effects other than antiemetic ones. For instance, by blocking ACh and histamine receptors throughout the CNS and the GI tract, anticholinergic drugs and antihistamines may also cause drowsiness, drying of secretions, and prevention of smooth muscle spasms. In addition, neuroleptic agents calm the CNS, an effect beneficial in treating the symptoms of various psychotic disorders (anxiety, tension, and agitation).

Therapeutic Uses

The therapeutic uses of the antiemetic agents vary depending on the category of agents. There are, however, many indications for drugs in each category. These agents have a variety of therapeutic uses because of the wide distribution of dopamine, ACh, and serotonin receptors throughout the body. Most antiemetics act on these receptors to produce a specific physiologic response. The specific therapeutic effects of each class of antiemetic agents are listed in Table 49-4.

Side Effects and Adverse Effects

Most of the side effects and adverse effects of the antiemetics stem from their nonselective blockade of receptors. For example, antihistamines not only bind to histamine₁ receptors and prevent ACh from binding to receptors in the vestibular nuclei, but they also bind to histamine receptors located elsewhere in the body, thus, for instance, causing secretions to become dry. Some of the more common side effects associated with the various categories of antiemetics are listed in Table 49-5.

Activity

Interactions

The drug interactions associated with the antiemetic agents are also specific to the individual categories of agents. Anticholinergic antiemetics will have additive drying effects if given with antihistamines and antidepressants. Antihistamine antiemetics, when given with barbiturates, opioids, hypnotics, tricyclic antidepressants (TCAs), and alcohol, can increase CNS depression. Neuroleptic antiemetics, when given with levodopa, may cancel the beneficial effects of levodopa. Increased CNS depression can be seen when alcohol or other CNS depressants are given with neuroleptic agents. Qunidine and neuroleptic agents may result in increased adverse cardiac effects. Prokinetic agents, when given with alcohol, can result in additive CNS depression. Anticholinergics and analgesics can block the motility effects of metoclopramide. Serotonin blockers and THCs have no significant drug interactions and are therefore not mentioned in the table.

Dosages

For the recommended dosages of selected antiemetic agents, see the dosages table on p. 787.

---

drug profiles

The various antiemetics have many different therapeutic uses, but the ultimate goals of such therapy are to minimize or prevent fluid and electrolyte disturbances, minimize deterioration in the nutritional status, and blunt the memory of the nausea and vomiting experience. Most of the antiemetics act by blocking receptors within the CNS, but some work directly in the GI tract. As previously noted, there are six main classes of antiemetic agents. However, there are other agents that may also be used to treat nausea and vomiting. These are corticosteroids (dexamethasone) and anxiolytics (lorazepam). When used in combination therapies, these latter agents plus the THCs are very beneficial in preventing the nausea and vomiting caused by cancer chemotherapy. Chemotherapy-induced nausea and vomiting (CINV) and postoperative nausea and vomiting (PONV) can be especially difficult to treat and result in devastating adverse effects. The serotonin blockers have proven to be very effective in preventing CINV and PONV.

ANTICHOLINERGICS

scopolamine

Scopolamine (Transderm-Scop) is the primary anticholinergic drug used as an antiemetic. It has potent effects on the vestibular nuclei, which are located in the inner ear and represent the area of the brain that controls balance. It works by blocking the binding of ACh to the cholinergic receptors in this region, thereby correcting an imbalance between the two neurotransmitters ACh and norepinephrine. These effects make scopolamine one of the most commonly used drugs for the treatment and prevention of the nausea and vomiting associated with motion sickness.

Scopolamine is classified as a pregnancy category C agent. It is contraindicated in patients with a known hypersensitivity to it and in patients with glaucoma. Scopolamine is available in many dosage formulations. The most commonly used formulation is the 72-hour transdermal patch, which releases a total of 0.5 mg of the agent. It is also available as 0.3-, 0.4-, 0.86-, and 1-mg/ml parenteral injections as well as a hydrobromide salt that is used for ophthalmic purposes.

PHARMACOKINETICS

HALF-LIFE	ONSET	PEAK	DURATION
Unknown	1-2 hr	6-8 hr	8 hr

ANTIHISTAMINES

Antihistamine antiemetics are some of the most commonly used and most safe antiemetics, some of the popular ones being promethazine, meclizine, dimenhydrinate, and diphenhydramine. Many of them are available over-the-counter (OTC).

meclizine

Meclizine (Antivert, Bonine, Dizmiss, Ru-Vert-M) is available in several oral formulations as 12.5-, 25-, and 50-mg tablets; 25-mg chewable tablets; 25-mg film-coated tablets; and 15- and 25-mg capsules. It is most commonly used to treat the dizziness, vertigo, and nausea and vomiting associated with motion sickness. It is classified as a pregnancy category B agent, and hypersensitivity, shock, and lactation are contraindications to its use. Commonly recommended dosages are listed in the dosages table on p. 787.

PHARMACOKINETICS

HALF-LIFE	ONSET	PEAK	DURATION
6 hr	1 hr	Variable	8-24 hr

Activity

NEUROLEPTIC AGENTS

Prochlorperazine, chlorpromazine, perphenazine, promethazine, thiethylperazine, triflupromazine, and trimeprazine are antiemetics in the neuroleptic class. Many of these agents are used to treat psychotic disorders such as mania and schizophrenia, the associated anxiety, and intractable hiccups and nausea and vomiting.

prochlorperazine

Prochlorperazine (Compazine) is classified as a pregnancy category C agent and is contraindicated in patients with a hypersensitivity to phenothiazines, those in a coma, and those suffering from seizures, encephalopathy, or bone marrow depression. It is available in many dosage formulations:

DOSAGES Selected Antiemetic Agents

agent	pharmacologic class	dosage range	purpose
ANTICHOLINERGIC AGENTS scopolamine (Transderm-Scop)	Anticholinergic solanaceous alkaloid	Apply one patch to hairless area behind ear every 3 days	Motion sickness prophylaxis
ANTIHISTAMINE AGENTS meclizine (Antivert, Bonine, Dizmiss, Ru-Vert-M)	Anticholinergic antihistamine	*Adult* PO: 25-50 mg 1 hr before travel and repeated once daily during travel 25-100 mg/day	Motion sickness prophylaxis Vertigo
NEUROLEPTIC AGENTS prochlorperazine (Compazine)	Phenothiazine	*Pediatric* PO/rectal: 20-29 lb (9-13 kg): 2.5 mg 1-2 times/day; 30-39 lb (13.5-17.5 kg): 2.5 mg 2-3 times/day; 40-85 lb (18-38 kg), 2.5 mg tid or 5 mg bid IM: 0.132 mg/kg *Adult* PO: 5-10 mg 3-4 times/day IM: 5-10 mg q3-4h (max 40 mg/day) Rectal: 25 mg bid	Antiemetic
PROKINETIC AGENTS metoclopramide (Maxolon, Octamide, Reglan)	Dopamine antagonist antiemetic	*Adult* IV: 1-2 mg/kg (30 min before chemo and q2-4h) IV: 10-20 mg	Chemotherapy antiemetic Barium removal, intubation-associated emesis, postoperative nausea
SEROTONIN BLOCKERS ondansetron (Zofran)	Antiserotonergic antiemetic	*Pediatric 4-12 y/o* PO: 4 mg tid, with first dose administered 30 min before chemotherapy, repeated 4 and 8 hr after first dose *Child 4-18 y/o* IV: 3 doses of 0.15 mg/kg, with first dose infused over 15 min and given 30 min before chemotherapy, repeated 4 and 8 hr after first dose *Adult* PO: 8 mg tid, with first dose administered 30 min before chemotherapy, repeated 4 and 8 hr after first dose, followed by 8 mg q8h for 1-2 days after completion of chemotherapy IV: 3 doses of 0.15 mg/kg, with first dose infused over 15 min and administered 30 min before chemotherapy, repeated 4 and 8 hr after first dose, *or* 32 mg infused over 15 min and administered 30 min before chemotherapy IV: 4 mg over 2-5 min	Chemotherapy antiemetic Postoperative nausea
TETRAHYDRO-CANNABINOIDS dronabinol (Marinol)	Marijuana-derived antiemetic	*Adult* PO: Initially, 5 mg/m^2/dose 4-6 doses/day; if needed, the dose may be increased by 2.5 mg/m^2 increments to a max of 15 mg/m^2/dose	Chemotherapy antiemetic

Activity

2.5-, 5-, and 25-mg suppositories; a 5-mg/5 ml oral solution; a 5-mg/ml parenteral injection; 10-, 15-, and 30-mg extended-release capsules; and 5-, 10-, and 25-mg film-coated tablets. Commonly used dosages are listed in the dosages table on p. 787.

PHARMACOKINETICS

HALF-LIFE	ONSET	PEAK	DURATION
6-8 hr*	30-40 min*	2-4 hr*	3-4 hr*

*Immediate-release products.

PROKINETIC AGENTS

Prokinetic agents promote the movement of substances through the GI tract and increase GI motility. The prokinetic agent used to prevent nausea and vomiting is metoclopramide. Janssen Pharmaceutica stopped marketing cisapride in the United States as of July 14, 2000. As of December 31, 1999 the use of cisapride has been associated with 341 reports of heart rhythm abnormalities, including 80 reports of deaths.

metoclopramide

Metoclopramide (Maxolon, Octamide, Reglan) is the oldest and most commonly used prokinetic agent. It is available only by prescription because it can cause some severe side effects if not used correctly. Metoclopramide is also used for the treatment of delayed gastric emptying and gastroesophageal reflux. It is classified as a pregnancy category B agent and is contraindicated in patients with a seizure disorder, pheochromocytoma, breast cancer, or GI obstruction, and also in patients with a hypersensitivity to it, procaine, or procainamide.

Metoclopramide is available in both oral and parenteral formulations as 5-mg/5 ml oral solutions, 5- and 10-mg tablets, and a 5-mg/ml parenteral injection. Commonly used dosages are listed in the dosages table on p. 787.

PHARMACOKINETICS

HALF-LIFE	ONSET	PEAK	DURATION
PO: 2.5-5 hr	PO: 20-60 min	PO: 1-2 hr	PO: 3-4 hr

SEROTONIN BLOCKERS

The serotonin blockers are also called *5-HT3 receptor blockers* because they block the 5-HT3 receptors in the GI tract, CTZ, and VC. Because of their specific actions, they cause few adverse effects. They are indicated for the prevention of nausea and vomiting associated with cancer chemotherapy and also for the prevention of postoperative radiation-induced nausea and vomiting.

Currently there are three agents in this category: dolasetron (Anzemet), granisetron (Kytril), and ondansetron (Zofran). The three agents are primarily used for the prevention of nausea or vomiting.

ondansetron

Ondansetron (Zofran, Zofran ODT) is a commonly used serotonin blocker. It is a prescription-only drug available orally or intravenously. Ondansetron is classified as a pregnancy category B agent. The only contraindication to its use is hypersensitivity. Ondansetron is available as a 2-mg/ml parenteral injection, a 32-mg/50 ml (premixed) parenteral solution, 4- and 8-mg tablets, a 4-mg/5 ml oral solution, and 4- and 8-mg oral disintegrating tablets (ODT). Commonly used dosages are listed in the dosages table on p. 787.

PHARMACOKINETICS

HALF-LIFE	ONSET	PEAK	DURATION
3-5.5 hr*	15-30 min*	1-1.5 hr*	6-12 hr*

*Zofran IV.

TETRAHYDROCANNABINOIDS
dronabinol

Dronabinol (Marinol) is the only currently available THC, and it is a synthetic derivative of the major active substance in marijuana. Dronabinol was approved by the FDA in 1985 for the treatment of the nausea and vomiting related to cancer chemotherapy. It is generally used as a second-line agent after treatment with other antiemetics has failed. Dronabinol is classified as a pregnancy category B agent and is contraindicated in patients with hypersensitivity to dronabinol and in the treatment of nausea and vomiting stemming from any cause other than cancer chemotherapy. It is available as 2.5-, 5-, and 10-mg capsules. Commonly used dosages are listed in the dosages table on p. 787.

PHARMACOKINETICS

HALF-LIFE	ONSET	PEAK	DURATION
25-36 hr	30-60 min	1-3 hr	4-6 hr

nursing process

• Assessment

Before administering any antiemetic agent, the nurse should perform a thorough nursing assessment of the patient, obtain a complete history concerning the nausea and vomiting, and document the findings. Precipitating factors, weight loss, baseline vital signs, and laboratory findings such as electrolyte levels and fluid volume status should also be assessed and the findings documented regardless of the antiemetic agent being used.

The anticholinergic agent scopolamine is contraindicated in patients with a hypersensitivity to it and in those with glaucoma. Cautious use with careful and close monitoring is recommended in patients suffering from blurred vision, dizziness, or benign prostatic hyperplasia (BPH). The effects of antihistamines and antidepressants are enhanced when these agents are used with anticholinergic antiemetics, so the nurse should find out whether the patient is taking these other agents.

Antihistamines such as meclizine are often the most commonly used and safest antiemetics. Meclizine is contraindicated in patients with a hypersensitivity to it, those in shock, and lactating women. Cautious use is recommended in patients suffering from BPH, dizziness, confusion, or blurred vision. Barbiturates, opioids, hypnotics, TCAs, and alcohol cause increased CNS depression when used with antihistamines, so the patient should be asked about the use of these agents and about alcohol consumption.

Neuroleptic agents such as prochlorperazine are contraindicated in patients with a hypersensitivity to them and in those suffering from coma, seizures, encephalopathy, or bone marrow depression. Cautious use is encouraged in patients with hypotension, cardiac dysrhythmias, BPH, or a CNS disorder. The effect of levodopa is decreased or absent in patients with Parkinson's disease taking neuroleptic agents. An increase in adverse cardiac effects occurs when quinidine and neuroleptic agents are taken simultaneously.

Prokinetic agents such as metoclopramide are often reserved for the treatment of the nausea and vomiting associated with chemotherapy and radiation therapy. Contraindications to its use include hypersensitivity to it or to procaine or procainamide, seizure disorders, pheochromocytoma, breast cancer, and GI obstruction. Cautious use is recommended in pregnant or lactating women and in patients with congestive heart failure (CHF) or GI hemorrhage. The action of metoclopramide is decreased when it is used with anticholinergics or opiates. Increased sedation occurs when prokinetic agents are used with alcohol and other CNS depressants.

Ondansetron, a serotonin blocker, increases tolerance to chemotherapy because of its very effective antiemetic properties. It is contraindicated in patients with a hypersensitivity to it, and cautious use is recommended in pregnant or lactating women, children, and the elderly. Before its use, the patient should be asked about the nature of the nausea and vomiting caused by chemotherapy and the findings documented.

The THC agent dronabinol is used only in patients who are undergoing chemotherapy and experiencing the attendant nausea and vomiting. Documentation of the nature of the nausea and vomiting is essential. A thorough nursing history and assessment must also be done before the start of therapy.

Nursing Diagnoses

Nursing diagnoses appropriate to patients receiving antiemetics include the following:
- Risk for injury related to side effects of the medication.
- Risk for injury (falls) related to weakness from vomiting.

---

case study **Chemotherapy**

Ms. V.S., a 68-year-old retired seamstress, has begun outpatient chemotherapy for a recent diagnosis of breast cancer. She has recovered well from a right modified mastectomy with well-healed incisions and is now physically and emotionally ready for her 3-month regimen of chemotherapy. Her premeds consist of a variety of medications, including granisetron (Kytril).

Her home medication list includes oral ondansetron (Zofran).
- *What is the mechanism of action of granisetron that makes it effective in the management of chemo-induced nausea and vomiting?*
- *What important patient teaching points should you emphasize to Ms. V.S. about ondansetron?*

For Answers see www.harcourthealth.com/MERLIN/Lilley/.

- Impaired physical mobility related to weakness from fluid and electrolyte disturbances secondary to vomiting.

Planning

Goals for patients receiving antiemetics include the following:
- Patient remains free of injury from nausea, vomiting, or medication therapy.
- Patient manages the side effects or identifies when to seek medical care for them.
- Patient regains normal fluid volume status and electrolyte levels.
- Patient regains normal levels of activity.

Outcome Criteria

Outcome criteria for patients receiving antiemetics include the following:
- Patient will state measures to implement to prevent injury such as assistance while ill, rising slowly, and changing positions slowly.
- Patient will state side effects of the medication to report to the physician such as severe sedation, confusion, or lethargy.
- Patient will state measures to implement in order to prevent further fluid volume deficits such as use of oral fluids, clear liquids, or chilled gelatin.
- Patient will increase activity day by day by 10 to 15 minutes.
- Time frame for goals and outcome criteria must be individualized with all patients.

Implementation

It is important to administer IV undiluted forms of diphenhydramine at a rate of 25-mg/min. IM forms should be administered in large muscles, such as the gluteus maximus, and the sites should be rotated. Antiemetics such as prochlorperazine maleate, thiethylperazine maleate, and metoclopramide that are used to prevent nausea and vomiting in patients undergoing chemotherapy should be administered before the chemotherapy.

When metochlopramide is given orally, it should be given 30 minutes before meals and at bedtime. If given intravenously, it should be given slowly over 1 to 2 minutes. Parenteral infusions should not be given over less than 15 minutes. In addition, solutions for parenteral dosage should be kept for only 48 hours and protected from light. This agent should not be given in combination with any other medications, such as phenothiazines, which together would cause extrapyramidal reactions.

Diphenidol hydrochloride, an antiemetic used mainly for the treatment of Ménière's disease, should be administered with food, water, or milk to decrease GI upset and should not be used with alcohol or other CNS depressants.

Thiethylperazine maleate is used for preventing the nausea and vomiting associated with surgery, radiation therapy, and chemotherapy. It should not be given intravenously because of the severe hypotension it can cause when given by this route. Trimethobenzamide may also produce hypotension, so it should be administered carefully, especially when given with other CNS depressants. IM injections should be given deep in the upper outer quadrant of the gluteal muscle to prevent site irritation. The scopolamine transdermal patch should be applied behind the ear at least 4 hours before the antiemetic effect is desired. The area behind the ear should be cleansed and dried before its application.

Ondansetron should be diluted in 50 ml of either 5% dextrose in water or 0.9% NaCl solution, or in amounts specified by hospital policy or in the manufacturer's guidelines. If three doses are to be given, the individual doses should be infused over 15 minutes. Granisetron, a newer antiemetic, provides 24-hour protection against chemotherapy-induced nausea and vomiting. In adult patients the agent is administered intravenously over 5 minutes, starting ½ hour before the chemotherapy session. Dronabinol should be administered 1 to 3 hours before chemotherapy, even if the agent is given at home before the appointment at the oncologist's office.

Patient teaching tips for antiemetic agents are presented in the box below.

● Evaluation

The therapeutic effects of antiemetics range from a decrease in to no complaints of nausea and vomiting and no complications, such as fluid and electrolyte imbalances and weight loss. The patient should also be monitored for adverse effects such as GI upset, drowsiness, lethargy, weakness, extrapyramidal reactions, and orthostatic hypotension.

---

patient teaching tips

Antiemetic Administration

➤ Patients taking any of the antiemetics should be warned about the drowsiness they can cause, and as a result, told to avoid performing any hazardous tasks or driving. Patients should also be cautioned about taking antiemetics with alcohol and other CNS depressants because of the possible toxicity and CNS depression that can occur.

➤ Ondansetron hydrochloride may cause headache that can be relieved with a simple analgesic.

➤ Patients taking dronabinol should be reminded to change positions slowly to prevent the syncope or dizziness resulting from the hypotensive effects of the agent. They should also avoid taking any other CNS depressants with this antiemetic and be cautious when engaging in activities that require mental alertness.

➤ Transderm scopolamine patches should be rotated and applied to nonirritated areas behind the ear; hands should be washed thoroughly before and after application.

POINTS TO REMEMBER

Antiemetics

• Vomiting, or emesis, is the forcible emptying or expulsion of gastric and occasionally intestinal contents through the mouth.

• Antiemetics are the drugs that relieve or prevent nausea and vomiting.

• The various categories of agents are anticholinergics, antihistamines, neuroleptic agents, prokinetic agents, serotonin blockers, and tetrahydrocannabinoids.

• Used to prevent motion sickness, to reduce secretions before surgery, to treat delayed gastric emptying, and to prevent postoperative nausea and vomiting, as well as in the management of many other conditions.

Anticholinergics and Antihistamines

• Anticholinergics work by blocking ACh receptors in the vestibular nuclei and reticular formation.

• This blockade prevents areas in the brain from being stimulated by nauseous stimuli.

• Antihistamines work by blocking histamine$_1$ receptors, which has the same effect as the anticholinergics.

Neuroleptics and Prokinetics

• Neuroleptics block dopamine in the CTZ and may also block ACh.

• Prokinetic agents also block dopamine receptors.

Serotonin blockers

• Highly effective antiemetics, most commonly used for the prevention of chemotherapy-induced nausea and vomiting.

• Work by blocking serotonin (5-HT3) receptors in the GI tract, CTZ, and the VC.

Nursing Considerations

- Nausea and vomiting may be treated very effectively with antiemetics and prudent nursing care.
- Antiemetics in general should be given before a chemotherapy agent is administered, often ½ to 3 hours before treatment.
- Most antiemetics cause drowsiness.
- Ondansetron and granisetron are newer antiemetics that are making chemotherapy much more bearable for patients.

- Dronabinol therapy is used to prevent chemotherapy-induced nausea and vomiting and is associated with postural hypotension.
- Caution patients taking antiemetics that drowsiness and hypotension may occur, so they should avoid driving and using heavy machinery during use.
- Monitor parameters reflecting hydration status such as input and output, skin turgor, and vital signs

REVIEW QUESTIONS

1. Which of the following are side effects of a ondansetron (Zofran)?
   a. Polyuria
   b. Syncope
   c. Headache
   d. Hemorrhage
2. Which of the following agents works by blocking dopamine in the chemoreceptor trigger zone (CTZ) in the medulla for antiemetic properties?
   a. Prokinetic agents
   b. Serotonin blockers
   c. Histamine blockers
   d. Chemosensitive agents
3. Antiemetics used with chemotherapy are generally:
   a. always given IV push.
   b. very sedating for up to 48 hours.
   c. well tolerated without dizziness or sedation.
   d. given 30 minutes or even 3 hours before the chemotherapy.
4. As a nurse practitioner, when trying to suggest a protocol for motion sickness prevention on a cruise, which of the following agents would be used?
   a. ondansetron
   b. prednisolone
   c. transdermal scopolamine
   d. metoclopramide ointment
5. What is the mechanism of action of ondansetron and granisetron?
   a. Block serotonin.
   b. Inhibit acetylcholine.
   c. Block dopamine receptors.
   d. Inhibit effects on reticular formation, thalamus, and cerebral cortex.

For Answers see www.harcourthealth.com/MERLIN/Lilley/.

CRITICAL THINKING Activities

1. Explain how ondansetron (Zofran) decreases the nausea and vomiting associated with chemotherapy. Compare its effectiveness to prochlorperazine for treatment of chemotherapy-induced nausea and vomiting.

2. Explain the mechanism(s) behind chemotherapy-induced nausea and vomiting.
3. Which of the following agents would *not* be given IV, and explain your answer: diphenydramine, thiethylperazine maleate, ondansetron, and granisetron.

For Answers see www.harcourthealth.com/MERLIN/Lilley/.

bibliography

Albanese J, Nutz P: *Mosby's 2001 nursing drug reference and review cards*, St Louis, 2001, Mosby.

Anderson PO, Knoben JE, Troutman WG: *Handbook of clinical drug data 1999-2000*, ed 9, New York, 1999, McGraw-Hill.

Dershwitz M: Advances in antiemetic therapy, *Anesth Clin North Am* 12(1):PAGE, 1995.

Johns Hopkins Hospital, Department of Pediatrics et al: *The Harriet Lane handbook*, ed 15, St Louis, 2000, Mosby.

Keen JH: *Critical care and emergency drug reference*, ed 3, St Louis, 1996, Mosby.

Koda-Kimble M, Young L, editors: *Applied therapeutics: the clinical use of drugs*, Vancouver, Wash, 1995, Applied Therapeutics, Inc.

McEvoy GK: *AHFS drug information*, Bethesda, Md, 1998, American Society of Hospital Pharmacists.

Mosby's GenRx: a comprehensive reference for generic and brand drugs, ed 10, St Louis, 2000, Mosby.

Skidmore-Roth L: *Mosby's 2001 nursing drug reference*, St Louis, 2001, Mosby.

United States Pharmacopeial Convention: *USP DI: drug information for the health care professional, vol. 1*, ed 20, Englewood, Colo, 2000, Micromedex.

Activity

Remember to check the **Online Worksheet** for additional learning opportunities: **www.harcourthealth.com/MERLIN/Lilley/**

Chapter 50

Vitamins and Minerals

objectives

www.harcourthealth.com/MERLIN/Lilley/

Look for this symbol for topics covered in the **Online Worksheet** Activity

When you reach the end of this chapter, you should be able to do the following:

1 Discuss the importance of the various vitamins and minerals to the functioning of the human body.

2 Describe the nutritional states and diseases caused by vitamin and mineral imbalances.

3 Discuss the treatment of the various vitamin or mineral imbalances.

4 Discuss the mechanisms of action, indications, cautions, contraindications, dosages, recommended daily allowances (RDAs), and associated measures to decrease side effects of each vitamin or mineral supplement.

5 Discuss the nursing process as related to the administration of vitamins and minerals.

drug profiles

ascorbic acid, p. 807
calcifediol, p. 798
calcitriol, p. 799
calcium, p. 810
cyanocobalamin, p. 806
dihydrotachysterol,
  p. 799
ergocalciferol, p. 799
magnesium, p. 811

niacin, p. 804
phosphorus, p. 811
pyridoxine, p. 805
riboflavin, p. 802
thiamine, p. 802
vitamin A, p. 797
vitamin E, p. 800
vitamin K₁, p. 801

glossary

Beriberi (ber′ e ber′ e) A disease of the peripheral nerves caused by an inability to assimilate thiamine. Symptoms are fatigue, diarrhea, appetite and weight loss, and disturbed nerve function, causing paralysis and wasting of limbs, edema, and heart failure. (p. 801)

Coenzyme (ko en′ zim) A nonprotein substance that combines with a protein molecule to form the active enzyme. (p. 793)

Enzymes (en′ zim) Specialized proteins that catalyze chemical reactions in organic matter. (p. 793)

Fat-soluble vitamins (sol′ u bəl) Vitamins that can be dissolved (i.e., are soluble) in fat. These vitamins can be stored in large amounts in the liver and fatty tissues, thus daily ingestion of these vitamins is not necessary to maintain good health. (p. 793)

Minerals (min′ ər əlz) Inorganic substances that are ingested and attach to enzymes or other organic molecules. Minerals play a vital role in regulating many body functions. (p. 793)

Pellagra (pə lag′ rə) A disease resulting from a niacin or tryptophan deficiency or a metabolic defect that interferes with

the conversion of tryptophan to niacin. It is characterized by scaly dermatitis, glossitis, inflammation of the mucous membranes, diarrhea, and mental disturbances. (p. 803)

Rhodopsin (ro dop′ sin) The purple pigmented compound in the rods of the retina, formed by a protein, opsin, and a derivative of vitamin A, retinol. (p. 794)

Rickets (rik′ əts) A condition caused by a vitamin D deficiency. Symptoms include soft, pliable bones, causing such deformities as bowlegs and knock knees; nodular enlargement on the ends and sides of the bones; muscle pain; enlarged skull; chest deformities; spinal curvature; enlargement of the liver and spleen; profuse sweating; and general tenderness of the body when touched. (p. 798)

Scurvy (skur′ ve) A condition resulting from an ascorbic acid deficiency. It is characterized by weakness, anemia, edema, spongy gums, mucocutaneous hemorrhages, and hardening of leg muscles. (p. 806)

Tocopherols (to kof′ ər olz) Biologically active chemicals that make up vitamin E compounds. (p. 799)

Vitamins (vi′ tə minz) An organic compound essential in small quantities for normal physiologic and metabolic functioning of the body. (p. 793)

Water-soluble vitamins (sol′ u bəl) Vitamins that can be dissolved (i.e., are soluble) in water. Because water-soluble vitamins are not stored in the body for long periods, daily ingestion of these vitamins is necessary for good health. (p. 793)

Vitamins and minerals are essential in our lives whether we are conscientious in our food choices or consume whatever we desire. The importance that the United States as a nation places on vitamins and minerals is evidenced by the nutritional information available on any packaged food product. Under most circumstances, daily requirements of vitamins and minerals are met by ingestion of fluids and regular, balanced meals. Ingesting food helps us maintain adequate stores of essential vitamins and minerals and serves to preserve the intestinal mass and structure, secrete hormones and enzymes, and prevent harmful overgrowth of bacteria.

Various life events can occur that create *excessive need* or *excessive loss* of nutrients, vitamins, minerals, electrolytes, and fluids, requiring replacement or supplementation. Excessive vitamin and mineral needs can occur with almost any illness and are typically seen in burn victims and AIDS patients. Excessive loss of vitamins and minerals may be the result of poor dietary intake, an inability to swallow after cancer chemotherapy or radiation, or mental disorders such as anorexia nervosa. Poor dietary absorption attributable to many types of gastrointestinal (GI) disorders or alcoholism can also contribute to inadequate intake that may require vitamin and mineral supplementation.

For the body to heal and repair itself it needs the essential building blocks provided by carbohydrates, fats, and proteins. Vitamins and minerals are needed to efficiently utilize them. **Vitamins** are *organic* molecules needed in small quantities for normal metabolism and other biochemical functions such as growth or repair of tissue. They attach to enzymes or coenzymes and help them activate metabolic or building processes in the body. Minerals are as important as vitamins. **Minerals** are *inorganic* elements or salts found naturally in the earth. Like vitamins, mineral ions bind with enzymes or other organic molecules and help regulate many body functions. The collagen, hormone, and enzyme synthesis that is needed to heal wounds requires vitamins and minerals.

Although vitamins and minerals are essential to life, there are instances when we are unable to acquire these essential compounds through diet or when a normal diet cannot meet the increased demand for them. In such cases vitamin and mineral supplementation is necessary. This chapter discusses both vitamins and minerals and their therapeutic effects.

VITAMINS

As mentioned previously, vitamins are organic molecules needed in small amounts to carry on normal metabolism in the body. **Enzymes** are proteins secreted by cells; they act as catalysts to induce chemical changes in other substances, but they themselves remain chemically unchanged by the process. A **coenzyme** is a substance that enhances or is necessary for the action of enzymes. Vitamins function primarily as coenzymes in various metabolic pathways throughout the body. Many enzymes are totally useless without the appropriate vitamins to bind with to cause them to function properly. For example, coenzyme A (CoA) is an important carrier molecule associated with the citric acid cycle. However, it requires pantothenic acid (vitamin B_5) to complete its function in the citric acid cycle.

All known vitamins or their precursors (provitamins) are synthesized by plants. The human body requires vitamins in specific amounts on a daily basis and obtains them from plant foods and, to a lesser extent, from animal food sources. Nondietary supplemental amounts of vita-

min B complex and vitamin K are obtained from intestinal microbial synthesis. In addition, vitamin D can be synthesized by the skin with the proper precursors when exposed to sunlight. An insufficient diet will cause various nutrition-related vitamin deficiencies. As a result of extensive study, the National Academy of Science has compiled a chart of vitamins and minerals. Table 50-1 lists the recommended daily allowances (RDAs) suggested for the maintenance of good nutrition.

Vitamins are classified as either fat or water soluble. **Water-soluble vitamins** can be dissolved in water; **fat-soluble vitamins** are dissolvable in fat. Because water-soluble vitamins (B-complex group and vitamin C) cannot be stored in the body in large amounts over long periods of time, daily intake is required to prevent the development of deficiencies. Conversely, fat-soluble vitamins (A, D, E, and K) do not need to be taken daily because they are stored in the liver and fatty tissues in large amounts. Deficiency in these vitamins occurs only after prolonged deprivation from an adequate supply or from disorders that prevent their absorption. Table 50-2 lists the fat-soluble and water-soluble vitamins.

FAT-SOLUBLE VITAMINS

The fat-soluble vitamins are A, D, E, and K. As a group they share the following characteristics:

- Present in both plant and animal foods
- Stored primarily in the liver
- Exhibit slow metabolism or breakdown
- Excreted via the feces
- Can become toxic if excessive amounts are consumed

VITAMIN A

Vitamin A (retinol) is derived from animal fats such as those found in dairy products (butter and milk), eggs, meat, liver, and fish liver oils. The vitamin A stored in animal tissues was derived from carotenes, which are found in plants (green and yellow vegetables and yellow fruits). Carotenes or carotenoids are precursors to vitamin A and are thus called *provitamin A carotenoids*. They must be converted to vitamin A by enzymes in the intestinal mucosa. When beta-carotene, a major precursor of vitamin A, is consumed, it is broken down to form two molecules of vitamin A. The sources of vitamin A as discussed are outlined as follows:

Vitamin A → animal source → dairy products, meat, liver
Provitamin A (carotene) → plant source →
                          green and yellow vegetables, yellow fruit

Mechanism of Action

Vitamin A is an exogenous substance because it must be obtained from either plants or animals. Vitamin A is required for the growth and development of bones and teeth and is also necessary for maintaining other processes, including reproduction, integrity of mucosal and epithelial surfaces, and cholesterol and steroid synthesis. It is essential for

Table 50-1 Recommended Daily Dietary Allowances (designed for the maintenance of good nutrition of practically all healthy people in the United States)*

	Age (yr)	Weight		Height		Protein (g)	Fat-Soluble Vitamins		
		kg	lb	cm	in		Vitamin A (μg RE)†	Vitamin D (μg)‡	Vitamin E (mg α TE)§
Infants	0-0.5	6	13	60	24	13	375	7.5	3
	0.5-1.0	9	20	71	28	14	375	10	4
Children	1-3	13	29	90	35	16	400	10	6
	4-6	20	44	112	44	24	500	10	7
	7-10	28	62	132	52	28	700	10	7
Males	11-14	45	99	157	62	45	1000	10	10
	15-18	66	145	176	69	59	1000	10	10
	19-24	72	160	177	70	58	1000	10	10
	25-50	79	174	176	70	63	1000	5	10
	51+	77	170	173	68	63	1000	5	10
Females	11-14	46	101	157	62	46	800	10	8
	15-18	55	120	163	64	44	800	10	8
	19-24	58	128	164	65	46	800	10	8
	25-50	63	138	163	64	50	800	5	8
	51+	65	143	160	63	50	800	5	8
Pregnant						60	800	10	10
Lactating	0-6 mo					65	1300	10	12

From McKenry LM, Salerno E: *Mosby's pharmacology in nursing,* ed 19, St Louis, 1995, Mosby.
*The allowances are intended to provide for individual variations among most people as they live in the United States under usual environmental stresses. Diets should be based on a variety of common foods in order to provide other nutrients for which human requirements have been less well defined.
†Retinol equivalents 1 Retinol equivalent = μg retinol or 6 μg β carotene.
‡As cholecalciferol, 10 μg cholecalciferol = 400 IU vitamin D.
§α-Tocopherol equivalents. 1 mg d-α-tocopherol = 1 α TE.
‖NE (niacin equivalent) is equal to 1 mg of niacin or 60 mg of dietary tryptophan.

Table 50-2 Fat- and Water-Soluble Vitamins

Fat-Soluble		Water-Soluble	
Designation	Name	Vitamins	Name
vitamin A	retinol	vitamin B$_1$	thiamine
vitamin D	D$_3$, cholecalciferol	vitamin B$_2$	riboflavin
	D$_2$, ergocalciferol	vitamin B$_3$	niacin
vitamin E	tocopherols	vitamin B$_5$	pantothenic acid
vitamin K	K$_1$, phytonadione	vitamin B$_6$	pyridoxine
	K$_2$, menaquinone	vitamin B$_{12}$	cyanocobalamin
		Biotin	
		Folic acid	
		vitamin C	ascorbic acid

night vision and for normal vision because it is part of one of the major retinal pigments called *rhodopsin.* Vitamin A is converted to the aldehyde, *cis* retinal, which combines with opsin to form **rhodopsin,** the visual pigment that is required for normal "rod vision" in the retina.

Drug Effects

The drug effects of vitamin A are diverse. It may be used as a supplement to satisfy normal body requirements or an increased demand such as in infants and pregnant and

nursing women. Vitamin A may also be used to treat and correct the result of a long-term deficiency that leads to such conditions as hyperkeratosis of the skin, night blindness, retarded infant growth, and xerophthalmia. Vitamin A is also used to treat various forms of acne.

Therapeutic Uses

Therapeutic uses for vitamin A are listed in Box 50-1. As it indicates, vitamin A is primarily utilized as a dietary supplement and for treatment of deficiency states and

Water-Soluble Vitamins							Minerals					
Vitamin C (mg)	Thiamine (mg)	Ribo-Flavin (mg)	Niacin (mg NE)‖	Vitamin B₆ (mg)	Folic Acid (μg)	Vitamin B₁₂ (μg)	Calcium (mg)	Phos-Phorus (mg)	Mag-Nesium (mg)	Iron (mg)	Zinc (mg)	Iodine (μg)
30	0.3	0.4	5	0.3	25	0.3	400	300	40	6	5	40
35	0.4	0.5	6	0.6	35	0.5	600	500	60	10	5	50
40	0.7	0.8	9	1.0	50	0.7	800	800	80	10	10	70
45	0.9	1.1	12	1.1	75	1.0	800	800	120	10	10	90
45	1.0	1.2	13	1.4	100	1.4	800	800	170	10	10	120
50	1.3	1.5	17	1.7	150	2	1200	1200	270	12	15	150
60	1.5	1.8	20	2	200	2	1200	1200	400	12	15	150
60	1.5	1.7	19	2	200	2	1200	1200	350	10	15	150
60	1.5	1.7	19	2	200	2	800	800	350	10	15	150
60	1.2	1.4	15	2	200	2	800	800	350	10	15	150
50	1.1	1.3	15	1.4	150	2	1200	1200	280	15	12	150
60	1.1	1.3	15	1.5	180	2	1200	1200	300	15	12	150
60	1.1	1.3	15	1.6	180	2	1200	1200	280	15	12	150
60	1.1	1.3	15	1.6	180	2	800	800	280	15	12	150
60	1.0	1.2	13	1.6	180	2	800	800	280	10	12	150
70	1.5	1.6	17	2.2	400	2.2	1200	1200	320	30	15	175
95	1.6	1.8	20	2.1	280	2.6	1200	1200	355	15	19	200

Box 50-1 Vitamin A: Indications

DIETARY SUPPLEMENT
Infants
Pregnant women
Nursing women

DEFICIENCY STATES
Hyperkeratosis of the skin
Night blindness
Retarded infant growth
Xerophthalmia

SKIN CONDITIONS
Acne (vitamin A derivatives)
Keratosis follicularis
Psoriasis

Table 50-3 Vitamin A: Adverse Effects

Body System	Side/Adverse Effect
Central nervous system	Headache, increased intracranial pressure, lethargy, malaise
Gastrointestinal	Nausea, vomiting, anorexia, abdominal pain, jaundice
Integumentary	Drying of skin, pruritis, increased pigmentation, night sweats
Metabolic	Hypomenorrhea, hypercalcemia
Musculoskeletal	Arthralgia, retarded growth

Activity

ticed in bones, mucous membranes, the liver, and skin. Table 50-3 lists some of the symptoms of long-term, excessive ingestion of vitamin A.

skin conditions. A normal diet should provide adequate amounts of vitamin A, but in cases of excessive need or inadequate dietary intake, vitamin A supplementation is indicated to avoid problems associated with deficiency. Symptoms of vitamin A deficiency include night blindness, xerophthalmia, keratomalacia, hyperkeratosis, retarded growth, weakness, and increased susceptibility of mucous membranes to infection.

Side Effects and Adverse Effects

There are very few acute side effects and adverse effects associated with normal vitamin A ingestion. Only after long-term, excessive ingestion of vitamin A do symptoms appear. Side effects and adverse effects are usually no-

Toxicity and Management of Overdose

The major toxic effects of vitamin A result from ingestion of excessive amounts, which occurs most commonly in children. A few hours after administration of an excess dose of vitamin A (>25,000 U/kg) irritability, drowsiness, vertigo, delirium, coma, vomiting, and/or diarrhea may occur. In infants, excessive amounts of vitamin A can cause an increase in cranial pressure, resulting in symptoms such as bulging fontanelles, headache, papilledema, exophthalmos, and visual disturbances. Over several weeks a generalized peeling of the skin and erythemia may occur. These symptoms seem to disappear a few days after discontinuation of the drug, which is the only treatment necessary in situations of overdose.

DOSAGES Selected Vitamins

agent	pharmacologic class	dosage range	purpose
A (Aquasol A and Del-Vi-A)	Fat-soluble	*Adult* PO: 25,000-50,000 IU/day *Pediatric* ≥*12 months* PO: 200,000 as single dose; repeat next day and 4 weeks later *6-12 months* PO: 100,000 IU as single dose; repeat next day and 4 weeks later	Deficiency
B$_2$ (riboflavin)	Water-soluble B-complex group	*Adult* PO: 5-30 mg/day *Pediatric* PO: 3-10 mg/day	Deficiency
B$_3$ (niacin)	Water-soluble B-complex group	*Adult* PO: 300-500 mg/day PO: Initially, 100 mg 3 times/day, increase by 300 mg/day at 4- to 7-day intervals; maintenance: 1-2 g 3 times/day; max 8 g/day *Pediatric* PO: ≤300 mg/day	Deficiency Hyperlipoproteinemia
B$_6$ (pyridoxine)	Water-soluble B-complex group	*Adult* PO: 10-20 mg/day for 3 weeks, followed by 2-5 mg/day as maintenance therapy *Pediatric* PO: 5-25 mg/day for 3 weeks, followed by 1.5-2.5 mg/day as maintenance therapy	Deficiency
B$_{12}$ (cyanocobalamin)	Water-soluble B-complex group	*Adult* IM/SC: 100 μg/day *Pediatric* IM/SC: 30-50 μg/day	Deficiency
C (ascorbic acid)	Water-soluble	*Adult* IM/PO: 100-250 mg qd-bid for at least 2 weeks *Pediatric* IM/IV/SC/PO: 100-300 mg/day, divided qd-bid for at least 2 weeks	Deficiency
calcifediol (Calderol)	Fat-soluble	*Adult/Pediatric >10 y/o* PO: 50-100 μg/day *Pediatric 2-10 y/o* PO: 50 μg/day *Pediatric ≤2 y/o* PO: 20 μg/day	Deficiency
calcitriol (Calcijex and Rocaltrol)	Fat-soluble	*Adult* PO: 0.25 μg/dose qd-qod, then every 4-8 weeks with usual maintenance dose being 0.5-1 μg/day IV: 0.5 μg/day given 3 times a week; usual dose 0.5-3 μg/day *Pediatric* *>12 months* PO: 200,000 as single dose; repeat next day and 4 weeks later *6-12 months* PO: 100,000 IU as single dose; repeat next day and 4 weeks later	Deficiency
dihydrotachysterol (DHT and Hytakerol)	Fat-soluble D analogue	*Adult/Child (>12 y/o)* PO: 0.75-2.5 mg/day for 4 days, then 0.2-1.5 mg/day *Pediatric* PO: 1-5 mg/day for 4 days, then 0.5-1.5 mg/day *Neonatal* PO: 0.05-0.1 mg/day	Hypoparathyroidism

DOSAGES Selected Vitamins—cont'd

agent	pharmacologic class	dosage range	purpose
D₂ (ergocalciferol)	Fat-soluble	*Adult/Pediatric* PO: 2000-5000 IU/day for 6-12 weeks	Nutritional rickets
		Adult PO: 25,000-200,000 IU/day *Pediatric* PO: 50,000-200,000 IU/day	Hypoparathroidism
		Adult PO: 10,000-60,000 IU/day *Pediatric* PO: 400,000-800,000 IU/day; increased by 10,000-20,000 IU every 3-4 months if needed	Vitamin D–resistant rickets
E (tocopherol)	Fat-soluble	*Adult* PO: 60-75 U/day	Deficiency
		Premature Neonatal PO: 15-30 U/day	Retinopathy prophylaxis

Interactions

Vitamin A is absorbed to a lesser extent with the simultaneous use of lubricant laxatives and cholestyramine. In addition, the use of isotretinoin with vitamin A can result in additive effects and possibly toxicity.

Dosages

For the RDAs of vitamin A, see Table 50-1. For the recommended dosages of vitamin A, see the dosages table on p. 796.

drug profiles

There are three forms of vitamin A: retinol, retinyl palmitate, and retinyl acetate. Medications containing vitamin A may require a prescription, but many OTC products such as multivitamins are also available. All vitamin A products are classified as pregnancy category A agents and are contraindicated in patients who have a hypersensitivity to vitamin A and in those with oral malabsorption syndromes.

vitamin A

Vitamin A (Aquasol A) is available orally as 10,000-, 25,000-, and 50,000-U capsules; 10,000-U tablets; and a 50,000-U/ml solution. It is also available parenterally as an injection. Doses for vitamin A can be expressed in USP units or microgram retinol equivalents (RE). A microgram RE can be calculated if the number of USP units of vitamin A is known: (1 USP 5 0.3 μg RE). Current RDAs are listed in Table 50-1.

PHARMACOKINETICS

HALF-LIFE	ONSET	PEAK	DURATION
13 days*	42 days†	Unknown	Unknown

*First order, three compartment model, the delta half-life.
†Follicular hyperkeratosis resolution with 300 μg/day of retinol.

VITAMIN D

Vitamin D, also called the *sunshine vitamin*, is responsible for the proper utilization of calcium and phosphorus in the body. The term *vitamin D* designates a group of analogue steroid structural chemicals with vitamin D activity. The two most important members of the vitamin D family are vitamin D₂ (ergocalciferol) and vitamin D₃ (cholecalciferol). They have different sites of origin but similar functions in the body. Ergocalciferol (vitamin D₂) is plant vitamin D and is therefore obtained through dietary sources. The natural form of vitamin D produced in the skin by ultraviolet irradiation (sun), 7-dehydrocholesterol, is referred to as *cholecalciferol* (vitamin D₃). This endogenous synthesis of vitamin D₃ usually produces sufficient amounts to meet daily requirements. Chemically the two vitamin D compounds are different, but physiologically they produce the same effect.

Vitamin D₂ → ergocalciferol → plant vitamin D
Vitamin D₃ → cholecalciferol → human vitamin D

Vitamin D then is obtained through endogenous synthesis and through vitamin D₂-containing foods such as fish oils, salmon, sardines, and herring; fortified milk, bread, and cereals; and animal livers, tuna fish, eggs, and butter.

Mechanism of Action

The basic function of vitamin D is to regulate the absorption and subsequent utilization of calcium and phosphorus. It is also necessary for the normal calcification of bone. Vitamin D in coordination with parathyroid hormone and calcitonin regulates serum calcium levels by increasing absorption from the small intestine and extracting calcium from the bone when needed. As ergocalciferol and cholecalciferol, vitamin D is inactive and requires transformation into active metabolites for biologic activity. Both vitamin D₂ and vitamin D₃ are biotransformed primarily in the liver by the actions of the parathyroid hormone. The resulting calcifediol is then transported to the kidney where it is converted to calcitriol, which is believed to be the most active vitamin D analogue. Calcitriol promotes the intestinal absorption of calcium and phosphorus and the deposition of calcium and phosphorus in the teeth and bones.

Drug Effects

The drug effects of vitamin D are very similar to those of vitamin A and essentially all vitamin and mineral compounds. It is used as a supplement to satisfy normal daily requirements or an increased demand as in infants and pregnant and nursing women. Vitamin D may also be used to treat and correct the result of a long-term deficiency that leads to such conditions as infantile **rickets,** tetany, and osteomalacia. Vitamin D can also help promote the absorption of phosphorus and calcium. Because of vitamin D's role in the regulation of calcium and phosphorus, it may be used to correct deficiencies of these two elements.

Therapeutic Uses

Vitamin D can be used either to supplement the present daily intake of vitamin D or to treat a deficiency of vitamin D. In the case of supplementation it is given as a prophylactic measure to prevent deficiency-related problems. Vitamin D is also used therapeutically to treat conditions resulting from long-term insufficiency. Box 50-2 lists the therapeutic indications for vitamin D.

Side Effects and Adverse Effects

As with vitamin A, very few acute side effects and adverse effects are associated with normal vitamin D ingestion. Only after long-term, excessive ingestion of vitamin D do symptoms appear. Such effects are usually noticed in the GI tract or CNS and are listed in Table 50-4.

Toxicity and Management of Overdose

The major toxic effects from ingesting excessive amounts of vitamin D occur most commonly in children. Discontinuation of vitamin D and reduced calcium intake reverse the toxic state. The amount of vitamin D considered to be too much varies considerably among individuals, but is generally thought to be

1.25 to 2.5 mg of ergocalciferol daily in adults and 25 μg daily in infants and children.

The toxic effects of vitamin D are those associated with hypertension, such as weakness, fatigue, headache, anorexia, dry mouth, metallic taste, nausea, vomiting, abdominal cramps, ataxia, and bone pain. If not recognized and treated, these symptoms can progress to impairment of renal function and osteoporosis.

Interactions

Reduced absorption of vitamin D occurs with the simultaneous use of lubricant laxatives and cholestyramine. Patients taking digitalis preparations can develop cardiac dysrhythmias as a result of vitamin D intake.

Dosages

For the RDAs of vitamin D, see Table 50-1. For the recommended dosages of vitamin D, see the dosages table on p. 796.

---

drug profiles

There are three forms of vitamin D: calcifediol, calcitriol, and dihydrotachysterol. Vitamin D is available in OTC medications, such as a multivitamin product, or by prescription. All vitamin D products are classified as pregnancy category A agents and are contraindicated in patients who have shown a hypersensitivity reaction to them and in patients with hypercalcemia, renal dysfunction, or hyperphosphatemia.

calcifediol

Calcifediol (Calderol) is the 25-hydroxylated form of cholecalciferol (vitamin D_3). It is a vitamin D analogue primarily used for the management of hypocalcemia in patients with chronic renal failure who are undergoing hemodialysis. Calcifediol is also used for histologic signs of hyperparathyroid disease. It is available only as 20- and 50-μg capsules. Commonly recommended dosages are listed in the dosages table on p. 796.

BOX 50-2

Vitamin D: Therapeutic Indications

Dietary supplement
Hypocalcemia
Hypoparathyroidism
Hypophosphatemia
Osteodystrophy
Osteomalacia
Osteoporosis
Pseudohypoparathyroidism
Rickets

TABLE 50-4

Vitamin D: Adverse Effects

Body System	Side/Advere Effect
Cardiovascular	Hypertension, dysrhythmias
Central nervous system	Fatigue, weakness, drowsiness, headache
Gastrointestinal	Nausea, vomiting, anorexia, cramps, metallic taste, dry mouth, constipation
Genitourinary	Polyuria, albuminuria, increased BUN
Musculoskeletal	Decreased bone growth bone pain, muscle pain

Activit

PHARMACOKINETICS

HALF-LIFE	ONSET	PEAK	DURATION
16 days	Variable	Unknown	Unknown

calcitriol

Calcitriol (Rocaltrol, Calcijex) is the 1,25-dihydroxy-lated form of cholecalciferol (vitamin D_3). It is a vitamin D analogue used for the management of hypocalcemia in patients with chronic renal failure who are undergoing hemodialysis. It is also used in the treatment of hypoparathyroidism and pseudohy-poparathyroidism, vitamin D–dependent rickets, hypophosphatemia, and hypocalcemia in premature infants. It is available orally as 0.25- and 0.5-μg capsules and 1 μg/ml oral solution and parenterally as a 1- and 2-μg/ml injection. Commonly recommended dosages are listed in the dosages table on p. 796.

PHARMACOKINETICS

HALF-LIFE	ONSET	PEAK	DURATION
3-6 hr	<3 hr	3-6 hr	3-5 days

dihydrotachysterol

Dihydrotachysterol (Hytakerol) is a vitamin D analogue that is administered orally once daily for the treatment of any of the above mentioned conditions. Intramuscular use is indicated for patients with GI, liver, or biliary disease associated with malabsorption of vitamin D analogues. It is available orally as 1.25-mg capsules; 0.125-, 0.2-, and 0.4-mg tablets; and 0.2 mg/ml and 0.25 mg/ml solutions. It is considered a pregnancy category C agent. Common recommended dosages are listed in the dosages table on p. 796.

PHARMACOKINETICS

HALF-LIFE	ONSET	PEAK	DURATION
Unknown	Unknown	Unknown	Unknown

ergocalciferol

Ergocalciferol (Drisdol, Calciferol) is vitamin D_2. Its use is indicated for patients with GI, liver, or biliary disease associated with malabsorption of vitamin D analogues. It is available orally and parenterally. Oral agents include 1.25-mg (50,000 U) capsules, 1.25-mg (50,000 U) tablets, and a 200-μg (8000 U)/ml solution. A 12.5-mg/ml parenteral injection is available for intramuscular use. It is considered a pregnancy category C agent. Common recommended dosage are listed in the dosages table on p. 796.

PHARMACOKINETICS

HALF-LIFE	ONSET	PEAK	DURATION
19 days*	30 days†	Unknown	Months to years

*Biologic half-life.
†therapeutic effects.

VITAMIN E

Four biologically active chemicals called **tocopherols** (alpha, beta, gamma, and delta) make up the vitamin E compounds. Alpha-tocopherol is the most biologically active natural form of vitamin E. Dietary plant sources of vitamin E are fruits, grains, cereals, vegetables, oils, and wheat germ. Animal sources include eggs, chicken, and meats. The exact biologic function of vitamin E is unknown, but it is believed to act as an antioxidant.

Mechanism of Action

Although vitamin E is a powerful biologic antioxidant and an essential component of the diet, its exact nutritional function has not been fully demonstrated. The only significant deficiency syndrome for vitamin E has been recognized in premature infants. In this situation vitamin E deficiency may result in irritability, edema, thrombosis, and hemolytic anemia.

Drug Effects

The drug effects of vitamin E are not as well defined as those of the other fat-soluble vitamins. It is believed to protect polyunsaturated fatty acids, a component of cellular membranes. It has also been shown to hinder the deterioration of substances such as vitamin A and ascorbic acid (vitamin C), two substances that are highly oxygen sensitive and readily oxidized, thus acting as an antioxidant.

Therapeutic Uses

Vitamin E is most commonly used as a dietary supplement to augment present daily intake or to treat a deficiency. Those at greatest risk of complications from vitamin E deficiency are premature infants. As previously mentioned, vitamin E has recently received much attention as an antioxidant. Preventing the oxidation of various substances prevents the formation of toxic chemicals within the body, some of which are believed to cause cancer. There is a popular but unproved theory that vitamin E has beneficial effects for patients with cancer, heart disease, premenstrual syndrome (PMS), and sexual dysfunction.

Side Effects and Adverse Effects

As with vitamin D, very few acute side effects and adverse effects are associated with normal vitamin E ingestion because it is relatively nontoxic. Side effects and adverse effects are usually noticed in the GI tract or CNS and are listed in Table 50-5.

Table 50-5 Vitamin E: Adverse Effects

Body System	Side/Adverse Effect
Central nervous system	Fatigue, headache, blurred vision
Gastrointestinal	Nausea, diarrhea, flatulence
Genitourinary	Increased BUN
Musculoskeletal	Weakness

Activity

Dosages

For the RDAs of vitamin E, see Table 50-1. For the recommended dosages of vitamin E, see the dosages table on p. 796.

---

drug profiles

Vitamin E is available as an OTC medication. It has four forms—alpha-, beta-, gamma-, and delta-tocopherol. It is available in many multivitamin preparations and is also available by prescription. All vitamin E products are classified as pregnancy category A agents and are contraindicated in patients who have shown a hypersensitivity reaction to them.

vitamin E

Vitamin E (Aquasol E,) activity is generally expressed in USP or international units. One unit of vitamin E equals the biologic activity of 1 mg of dl-alpha-tocopheryl acetate, 1.12 mg of dl-alpha-tocopheryl acid succinate, 910 μg of dl-alpha-tocopherol, 735 μg of d-alpha-tocopheryl acetate, 830 μg of d-alpha-tocopheryl acid succinate, and 670 μg of d-alpha-tocopherol. Vitamin E is available only in an oral formulation as regular and water-miscible capsules, an oil solution, and regular and chewable tablets. Current RDAs for vitamin E are listed in Table 50-1. Commonly recommended dosages for vitamin E are listed in the dosages table on p. 796.

PHARMACOKINETICS

HALF-LIFE	ONSET	PEAK	DURATION
Variable	Unknown	Unknown	Variable

VITAMIN K

Vitamin K is the last of the four fat-soluble vitamins (A, D, E, and K). There are three types of vitamin K—phytonadione (vitamin K_1), menaquinone (vitamin K_2), and menadione (vitamin K_3). The primary dietary sources of vitamin K_1 are green leafy vegetables (e.g., cabbage, spinach), meats, and milk. The body does not store large amounts of vitamin K; however, vitamin K_2 is synthesized by the intestinal flora, thus providing an endogenous supply.

Vitamin $K_1 \rightarrow$ phytonadione $\rightarrow$
          green leafy vegetables (exogenous)
Vitamin $K_2 \rightarrow$ menaquinone $\rightarrow$
          intestinal flora (endogenous)

Vitamin K is essential for the synthesis of blood coagulation factors, which takes place in the liver. Vitamin K–dependent blood coagulation factors are factors II, VII, IX, and X. Other names for these clotting factors are as follows:

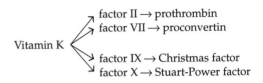

Vitamin K
factor II $\rightarrow$ prothrombin
factor VII $\rightarrow$ proconvertin
factor IX $\rightarrow$ Christmas factor
factor X $\rightarrow$ Stuart-Power factor

Mechanism of Action

As mentioned previously, vitamin K activity is essential for effective blood clotting because it facilitates the hepatic biosynthesis of factor II (prothrombin), factor VII (convertin), factor IX (Christmas factor), and factor X (Stuart-Power factor). Vitamin K deficiency results in coagulation disorders caused by hypoprothrombinemia.

Drug Effects

The drug effects of vitamin K are limited to its action on the vitamin K–dependent clotting factors produced in the liver (II, VII, IX, and X). Coagulation defects affecting these clotting factors can be corrected with administration of vitamin K. Vitamin K deficiencies are rare because intestinal flora are able to synthesize sufficient amounts. If a deficiency develops, it can be corrected with vitamin K supplementation.

Therapeutic Uses

Vitamin K is indicated for dietary supplementation and for treating deficiency states. Although rare, deficiency states can develop with inadequate dietary intake or broad-spectrum inhibition of the intestinal flora, resulting from administration of broad-spectrum antibiotics. Deficiency states can also be seen in newborns because of malabsorption attributable to inadequate amounts of bile or selected drugs, and as a result of the administration of specific anticoagulants that inhibit hepatic vitamin K activity. Coumarin- and indanedione-derivative anticoagulants thin the blood by inhibiting vitamin K–dependent clotting factors in the liver. Administration of vitamin K will override the mechanism by which the anticoagulants inhibit production of vitamin K–dependent clotting factors.

Side Effects and Adverse Effects

Vitamin K is relatively nontoxic and thus causes very few side effects and adverse effects. Severe reactions limited to hypersensitivity or anaphylaxis have occurred rarely during or immediately after IV administration. Side effects and adverse effects are usually related to injection site reactions and hypersensitivity. See Table 50-6 for a list of such major effects by body system.

Toxicity and Management of Overdose

Toxicity is primarily limited to use in the newborn. Hemolysis of red blood cells (RBCs) can occur, especially in infants with low levels of glucose-6-phosphate dehydrogenase (G6PD). In this case, replacement with blood products is indicated.

Table 50-6 Vitamin K: Adverse Effects

Body System	Side/Adverse Effect
Central nervous system	Headache, brain damage (large doses)
Gastrointestinal	Nausea, decreased liver function tests
Hematopoietic	Hemolytic anemia, hemoglobinuria, hyperbilirubinemia
Integumentary	Rash, urticaria

Box 50-3 Water-Soluble Vitamins: Alternate Names

Vitamin B complex	Vitamin B_1 → thiamine
	Vitamin B_2 → riboflavin
	Vitamin B_3 → niacin
	Vitamin B_5 → pantothenic acid
	Vitamin B_6 → pyridoxine
	Vitamin B_9 → folic acid
	Vitamin B_{12} → cyanocobalamin
Vitamin C	→ ascorbic acid

Dosages

The RDA for vitamin K is 5 to 30 μg for infants and children, 45 to 65 μg for women, and 45 to 80 μg for men. The dose of phytonadione (AquaMEPHYTON, Konakion, Mephyton) is 0.5 to 1 mg as a single IM dose for infants within 1 hour after delivery and 2.5 to 10 mg administered orally or parenterally as an IM or SC injection for adults.

drug profiles

The most frequently used form of vitamin K is phytonadione (vitamin K_1). Both phytonadione and menadione (vitamin K_3) are available by prescription only in oral and parenteral forms. Menadione is classified as a pregnancy category X agent, whereas phytonadione is a category C agent. They are both contraindicated in patients who have shown a hypersensitivity reaction to them. Their use is also contraindicated during the last few weeks of pregnancy and in patients with severe hepatic disease.

vitamin K_1

Vitamin K_1 (Phytonadione, Mephyton, Aqua-MEPHTYON) is available orally as a 5-mg tablet and parenterally as 1- and 10-mg IV or IM injections.

PHARMACOKINETICS

HALF-LIFE	ONSET	PEAK	DURATION
Unknown	Variable	1-2 hr	Unknown

WATER-SOLUBLE VITAMINS

The water-soluble vitamins include the vitamin-B-complex group and vitamin C (ascorbic acid). They are present in a variety of plant and animal food sources. The vitamin B complex is a group of 10 vitamins that are often found together in food, although they are chemically dissimilar and have different metabolic functions. Because the B vitamins were discovered in sequential order, they were grouped together as B complex vitamins. The most commonly used B complex and C vitamins are listed in Box 50-3.

Water-soluble vitamins are a chemically diverse group sharing only the characteristic of being dissolvable in water. Like fat-soluble vitamins, they act primarily as coenzymes or oxidation-reduction agents in important metabolic pathways. Unlike fat-soluble vitamins, water-soluble vitamins are not stored in the body in appreciable amounts. Therefore dietary intake must be adequate and regular or deficiency states will develop. Because these vitamins are water-soluble, excess amounts are excreted in the urine. The body excretes what it does not need, which makes toxic reactions to water-soluble vitamins very rare.

VITAMIN B_1

Vitamin B_1 (thiamine) is present in a wide variety of foods, especially whole grains, liver, and beans. When it is combined with adenosine triphosphate (ATP) the result is thiamine pyrophosphate coenzyme, which is required for carbohydrate metabolism. A deficiency of vitamin B_1 results in the classic disease **beriberi** or Wernicke's encephalopathy (cerebral beriberi). Common findings in beriberi include brain lesions, polyneuropathy of peripheral nerves, serous effusions, and cardiac anatomic changes. Vitamin deficiency can result from poor diet, extended fever, hyperthyroidism, liver disease, alcoholism, malabsorption, and pregnancy and breast feeding.

Mechanism of Action

As mentioned previously, thiamine is an essential precursor for the formation of thiamine pyrophosphate. In addition to carbohydrate metabolism, several other metabolic pathways require thiamine to function, including the Krebs cycle.

Drug Effects

The drug effects of vitamin B_1 are multiple. The integrity of the peripheral nervous system, cardiovascular system, and the GI tract are all heavily dependent upon thiamine.

Therapeutic Uses

The beneficial drug effects and the essential role of thiamine in so many metabolic pathways make it useful in treating a variety of disorders, including thiamine deficiency and metabolic disorders. It is also used as a dietary supplement and an oral insect repellent. Some of the deficiency states treated by thiamine are beriberi,

Wernicke's encephalopathy syndrome, and peripheral neuritis associated with pellagra or neuritis of pregnancy.

Thiamine is used as a dietary supplement in cases of malabsorption such as those induced by alcoholism, cirrhosis, or GI disease. Thiamine may be useful in preventing deficiency in patients with these diseases. Some metabolic disorders that benefit from thiamine treatment are subacute necrotizing encephalomyelopathy, maple syrup urine disease, and lactic acidosis associated with pyruvate carboxylase deficiency and hyper-β-alaninemia.

Other areas in which thiamine may have therapeutic value are the management of poor appetite, ulcerative colitis, chronic diarrhea, and cerebellar syndrome.

Side Effects and Adverse Effects

Adverse effects are rare but include hypersensitivity reactions, nausea, restlessness, pulmonary edema, pruritus, urticaria, weakness, sweating, angioedema, cyanosis, and cardiovascular collapse. Administration by IM injection can produce local tenderness, and IV injections can produce anaphylaxis.

Interactions

Thiamine is incompatible with alkaline- and sulfite-containing solutions.

Dosages

The RDAs for thiamine are 0.3 to 1 mg for infants and children, 1.1 mg for women, and 1.2 to 1.5 mg for men. In addition, ingestion of raw fish, a high carbohydrate diet, and heavy exercise are situations in which a higher intake of thiamine is required. The usual dose for treating beriberi is 10 to 20 mg intramuscularly three times daily for 2 weeks, with the addition of a multivitamin with 5 to 10 mg of thiamine for 1 month. See also Table 50-1.

drug profiles

thiamine

Thiamine is classified as a pregnancy category A agent and is contraindicated only in individuals with a history of a hypersensitivity reaction. Thiamine is available orally as 50-, 100-, 250-, and 500-mg tablets and parenterally as a 100-mg/ml injection.

PHARMACOKINETICS

HALF-LIFE	ONSET	PEAK	DURATION
Unknown	Unknown	Unknown	24 hr

VITAMIN B$_2$

Vitamin B$_2$ (riboflavin) is found in leafy green vegetables, eggs, nuts, meats, and yeast. Riboflavin serves several important functions. In the body, riboflavin is converted into two coenzymes (flavin mononucleotide [FMN] and flavin adenine dinucleotide [FAD]) that are essential for tissue respiration. Another B vitamin, vitamin B$_6$ (pyridoxine), requires riboflavin for activation. It is also needed to convert tryptophan into niacin and to maintain erythrocyte integrity. A deficiency of riboflavin results in cutaneous, oral, and corneal changes that include cheilosis, seborrheic dermatitis, and keratitis. Alcoholism is a major cause of riboflavin deficiency.

Mechanism of Action

As mentioned previously, vitamin B$_2$ is an important precursor for the synthesis of FMN and FAD that are required in tissue respiration pathways. Riboflavin also plays an important part in transfer reactions, especially in carbohydrate catabolism.

Drug Effects

The drug effects of riboflavin are mainly limited to replacement therapy for deficiency states. Deficiency is rare and does not usually occur in healthy people. However, deficiency may occur as a result of malnutrition or intestinal malabsorption or because of alcoholism or other diseases or infections.

Therapeutic Uses

Riboflavin is primarily used as a dietary supplement and to treat deficiency states. Although few disorders result because of a deficiency of riboflavin, supplementation is sufficient treatment for those disorders. Patients who may suffer from riboflavin deficiency are those with long-standing infections, liver disease, alcoholism, or malignancy and those taking probenecid. Riboflavin supplementation may be beneficial in treating microcytic anemia, acne, migraine headache, congenital methemoglobinemia, muscle cramps, and burning feet syndrome.

Side Effects and Adverse Effects

Riboflavin is a very safe and effective vitamin; to date, no side effects or toxic effects have been reported. In large doses riboflavin will discolor urine to a yellow-orange.

Dosages

For the RDAs of riboflavin, see Table 50-1. For commonly recommended dosages of riboflavin, see the dosages table on p. 796.

drug profiles

riboflavin

Riboflavin (vitamin B$_2$) is needed for normal respiratory reactions. It is a safe, nontoxic water-soluble vitamin with almost no adverse effects; it is classified as a pregnancy category A agent. It is available only orally as 25-, 50-, and 100-mg tablets. Commonly recommended dosages of riboflavin are listed in the dosages table on p. 796.

PHARMACOKINETICS

HALF-LIFE	ONSET	PEAK	DURATION
66-84 min	Unknown	Unknown	24 hr

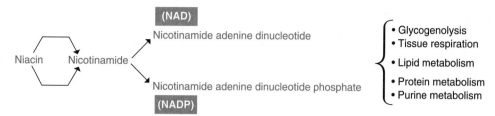

Fig. 50-1 Niacin, once in the body, is converted to NAD and NADP, which are coenzymes needed for many metabolic processes.

VITAMIN B₃

Vitamin B₃ (niacin) can be synthesized from tryptophan, an essential amino acid obtained from protein digestion. Niacin is present in meats, beans, yeast, liver, and wheat germ. Once in the body, niacin is converted to niacinamide, which is then converted into two coenzymes, nicotinamide adenine dinucleotide (NAD) and nicotinamide adenine dinucleotide phosphate (NADP). These coenzymes are needed for glycogenolysis, tissue respiration, and lipid, protein, and purine metabolism (Fig. 50-1).

A dietary deficiency of niacin will produce the classic symptoms of **pellagra** as follows:

- *Mental:* Various psychotic symptoms
- *Neurologic:* Neurasthenic syndrome
- *Cutaneous:* Crusting, erythema, and desquamation
- *Mucous membrane:* Oral, vaginal, and urethral lesions
- *Gastrointestinal:* Diarrhea or bloody diarrhea

Niacin is also an antihyperlipidemic agent. Niacin lowers serum cholesterol and triglyceride levels by reducing very-low-density lipoprotein (VLDL) synthesis. The principal carrier of cholesterol in the blood is low-density lipoprotein (LDL). Since VLDL is the precursor to LDL, reducing VLDL will result in reduction of LDL and, consequently, harmful plaque-forming, artery-narrowing cholesterol.

Mechanism of Action

The actions of vitamin B₃ are not due to niacin in the ingested form but rather to the metabolic product of niacin, niacinamide (except in the function of reducing serum cholesterol). The body may also utilize dietary tryptophan to produce niacinamide by oxidizing niacin and then converting it to niacinamide. As mentioned previously, niacinamide is required for lipid metabolism, tissue respiration, and glycogenolysis (Fig. 50-2).

Drug Effects

The drug effects of niacin result from the production of NAD and NADP, which are necessary for glycogenolysis (the breakdown of stored glycogen to usable glucose). As explained previously, it is also necessary for tissue respiration and lipid, protein, and purine metabolism, and it also acts as a cholesterol- and triglyceride-lowering agent by reducing VLDL synthesis.

Therapeutic Uses

Niacin is indicated for the prevention and treatment of pellagra, a condition caused by a deficiency of vitamin B₃ that is most commonly the result of malabsorption. As

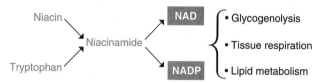

Fig. 50-2 Niacin and tryptophan combine to make niacinamide, a needed component for NAD and NADP, which are needed for many body processes.

Table 50-7	Niacin: Adverse Effects
Body System	**Side/Adverse Effect**
Cardiovascular	Postural hypotension, dysrhythmias, atrial fibrillation
Central nervous system	Headache, dizziness, anxiety, sensation of warmth
Gastrointestinal	Nausea, vomiting, diarrhea, peptic ulcer
Genitourinary	Hyperuricemia
Hepatic	Abnormal liver function tests, hepatitis
Integumentary	Flushing, dry skin, rash, pruritis, keratosis
Metabolic	Decreased glucose tolerance

stated previously, niacin is also an antihyperlipidemic agent that reduces VLDL synthesis, resulting in lower serum cholesterol and triglyceride levels.

Side Effects and Adverse Effects

The most frequent side effects associated with the use of niacin are flushing, pruritis, and gastrointestinal distress. These usually subside with continual use. They are most frequently seen when larger doses of niacin are used in the treatment of hyperlipidemia. Table 50-7 lists side effects and adverse effects by body system.

Dosages

For the RDAs of niacin, see Table 50-1. Commonly recommended dosages of niacin are listed in the dosages table on p. 796.

drug profiles

Niacin (vitamin B₃) is used to treat pellagra, hyperlipidemias, and peripheral vascular disease. It is classified as a pregnancy category C agent and is contraindicated in patients who are pregnant and those who have diabetes, gout, hepatic dysfunction, and an active peptic ulcer. Its use should be monitored closely in patients who have a history of coronary artery disease, gallbladder disease, jaundice, liver disease, or arterial bleeding.

niacin

Niacin (Nicobid, Nia-Bid, Nico-400, Nicotinex, Niacor, Slo-Niacin) is available orally as 125-, 250-, 300-, 400-, and 500-mg extended-release capsules; 150-, 250-, 500-, and 750-mg extended-release tablets; 25-, 50-, 100-, 250-, 500-mg regular-strength tablets; a 50-mg/5 ml elixir; and a 100-mg/ml injection. For the RDAs of niacin see Table 50-1. Commonly recommended dosages of niacin are listed in the dosages table on p. 796.

PHARMACOKINETICS

HALF-LIFE	ONSET	PEAK	DURATION
45 min	Variable	Serum: 45 min	Variable

VITAMIN B_6

Vitamin B_6 (pyridoxine) is composed of three compounds—pyridoxine, pyridoxal, and pyridoxamine. Plant sources that contain pyridoxine include whole grains, wheat germ, nuts, and yeast. Fish and organ meats contain both pyridoxal and pyridoxamine.

Pyridoxine is taken up by RBCs where it is converted into the coenzyme pyridoxal phosphate, which is necessary for many metabolic functions such as protein, carbohydrate, and lipid utilization in the body. It also plays an important part in the conversion of tryptophan to niacin or serotonin.

Deficiency of vitamin B_6 can lead to sideroblastic anemia, neurologic disturbances, seborrheic dermatitis, cheilosis, and xanthurenic aciduria. It may also result in epileptiform convulsions, especially in neonates and infants; hypochromic microcytic anemia; and glossitis and stomatitis. Inadequate intake or poor absorption of pyridoxine causes the development of these conditions. Vitamin B_6 deficiency may occur as a result of uremia, alcoholism, cirrhosis, hyperthyroidism, malabsorption syndromes, and congestive heart failure (CHF). It may also be induced by various drugs, such as isoniazid (INH), cycloserine, ethionamide, hydralazine, penicillamine, or pyrazinamide.

Mechanism of Action

Pyridoxine, pyridoxal, and pyridoxamine are all converted to the active forms of vitamin B_6, *pyridoxal phosphate* and *pyridoxamine phosphate*. They act as coenzymes in a wide variety of reactions, including the transamination of amino acids and the conversion of tryptophan to niacin. They are also essential in the synthesis of gamma-aminobutyric acid (GABA), an inhibitory neurotransmitter in the CNS. They are important in the synthesis of heme and the mainte-

nance of the hematopoietic system. Pyridoxine deficiency principally affects the peripheral nerves, skin, mucous membranes, and the hematopoietic system.

Drug Effects

The drug effects of pyridoxine are the result of the two coenzymes pyridoxal phosphate and pyridoxamine phosphate. As mentioned previously, pyridoxine is necessary for the integrity of the peripheral nerves, skin, mucous membranes, and the hematopoietic system.

Therapeutic Uses

Pyridoxine is used to prevent and treat vitamin B_6 deficiency. Although deficiency of vitamin B_6 is rare, it can occur in conditions of inadequate intake or poor absorption of pyridoxine. The situations in which this may occur were explained in a previous section. Seizures that are unresponsive to usual therapy, morning sickness during pregnancy, and various metabolic disorders may respond to pyridoxine therapy. Pyridoxine is also used to treat premenstrual syndrome (PMS) and hyperoxaluria.

Side Effects and Adverse Effects

Side effects and adverse effects with pyridoxine are rare and usually do not occur with normal doses; high doses and chronic usage may produce side effects and adverse effects as listed in Table 50-8. Toxic effects are a result of very large doses sustained for several months. Neurotoxicity is the most likely result, but this will subside upon discontinuation of the pyridoxine.

Interactions

Pyridoxine exhibits several significant interactions with selected drugs. Pyridoxine will reduce the activity of levodopa, so vitamin formulations containing B_6 should be avoided. Drugs that have an antivitamin effect on pyridoxine include cycloserine, ethionamide, INH, pyrazinamide, and oral contraceptives.

Dosages

For the RDAs of vitamin B_6, see Table 50-1. For the commonly recommended dosages of vitamin B_6, see the dosages table on p. 796.

drug profiles

Pyridoxine is a water-soluble B complex vitamin composed of three components: pyridoxine, pyridoxal, and pyridoxamine. It has several vital roles

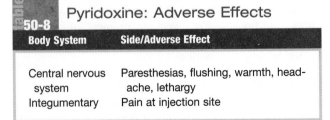

Pyridoxine: Adverse Effects

TABLE 50-8

Body System	Side/Adverse Effect
Central nervous system	Paresthesias, flushing, warmth, headache, lethargy
Integumentary	Pain at injection site

in the body but is primarily responsible for the integrity of peripheral nerves, skin, mucous membranes, and the hematopoietic system.

pyridoxine

Pyridoxine is classified as a pregnancy category A agent and is contraindicated in patients who have shown a hypersensitivity reaction to it. It is available orally as 25-, 50-, and 100-mg tablets; 100-mg time-released tablets; and a 100-mg/ml injection. For the RDAs of vitamin B_6, see Table 50-1. Commonly recommended dosages of vitamin B_6 are listed in the dosages table on p. 796.

PHARMACOKINETICS

HALF-LIFE	ONSET	PEAK	DURATION
15-20 days	Unknown	Unknown	Unknown

VITAMIN B₁₂

Vitamin B_{12} (cyanocobalamin) is a cobalt-containing, water-soluble B complex vitamin. It is synthesized by microorganisms and is present in the body as two different coenzymes, adenosylcobalamin and methylcobalamin. Cyanocobalamin is a required coenzyme for many metabolic pathways, including fat and carbohydrate metabolism and protein synthesis. It is also required for growth, cell replication, hematopoiesis, and nucleoprotein and myelin synthesis (Fig. 50-3).

Cyanocobalamin is present in foods of animal origin, particularly liver, kidney, fish and shellfish, meat, and dairy foods. Plants contain only minimal amounts. Vitamin B_{12} deficiency will result in GI lesions, neurologic symptoms that can result in degenerative CNS lesions, and megaloblastic anemia. The major cause of cyanocobalamin deficiency is malabsorption. Other possible but less likely causes are poor diet, chronic alcoholism, and chronic hemorrhage.

Mechanism of Action

Humans must have an exogenous source of cyanocobalamin because it is required for nucleoprotein and myelin synthesis, cell reproduction, normal growth, and the maintenance of normal erythropoiesis. The cells that have the greatest requirement for vitamin B_{12} are those that divide rapidly such as epithelial cells, bone marrow, and myeloid cells.

Reduced sulfhydryl (SH) groups are required to metabolize fats and carbohydrates and to synthesize protein.

Cyanocobalamin is involved in maintaining SH groups in the reduced form that is required by many SH-activated enzyme systems. Cyanocobalamin deficiency can lead to neurologic damage that begins with an inability to produce myelin and is followed by gradual degeneration of the axon and nerve head.

Cyanocobalamin has biologic activity that is identical to that of the antipernicious factor present in liver extract called the *extrinsic factor* and *Castle's factor.* The oral absorption of cyanocobalamin (extrinsic factor) requires the presence of the intrinsic factor (gastric intrinsic factor), which is a glycoprotein secreted by gastric parietal cells. A complex is formed between the two factors and is then absorbed by the intestines. This is depicted in Fig. 50-4.

Drug Effects

The drug effects of cyanocobalamin are very much like those of the other water-soluble vitamins. It is used to treat or prevent vitamin B_{12} deficiency caused by malabsorption or strict vegetarianism. If not treated, this condition can lead to megaloblastic anemia and irreversible neurologic damage. Cyanocobalamin is also useful in the treatment of pernicious anemia caused by a endogenous lack of intrinsic factor.

Therapeutic Uses

Cyanocobalamin is used to treat deficiency states that develop because of an insufficient intake of the vitamin. As mentioned previously, this is most often the result of malabsorption or poor dietary intake. Poor dietary intake is most common in vegetarians because the primary source of cyanocobalamin is foods of animal origin. Cyanocobalamin is used to treat vitamin B_{12} deficiency states, especially pernicious anemia. It is also included in a multivitamin formulation that is used as a dietary supplement.

The use of vitamin B_{12} to treat pernicious anemia and other megaloblastic anemias results in a rapid conversion of a megaloblastic bone marrow to a normoblastic bone marrow. The preferred route of administration of vitamin B_{12} in treating megaloblastic anemias is by deep IM injection.

Side Effects and Adverse Effects

Vitamin B_{12} is nontoxic and large doses must be ingested to produce adverse effects, which include itching, transitory diarrhea, and fever. Other side effects and adverse effects are listed by body system in the Table 50-9.

Interactions

Use with anticonvulsants, aminoglycoside antibiotics, and long-acting potassium preparations will decrease the

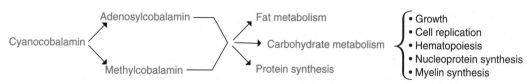

Fig. 50-3 Cyanocobalamin is a required coenzyme for many body processes.

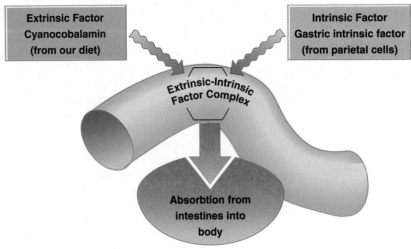

Fig. 50-4 The oral absorption of cyanocobalamin requires the presence of the intrinsic factor secreted by gastric parietal cells.

Cyanocobalamin: Adverse Effects

Table 50-9

Body System	Side/Adverse Effect
Cardiovascular	Congestive heart failure, peripheral vascular thrombosis, pulmonary edema
Central nervous system	Flushing, optic nerve atrophy
Gastrointestinal	Diarrhea
Integumentary	Itching, rash, pain at injection site
Metabolic	Hypokalemia

oral absorption of vitamin B_{12}. In addition it has been suggested that chloramphenicol will antagonize the hematologic response of vitamin B_{12}.

Dosages

For RDAs of vitamin B_{12}, see Table 50-1. Commonly recommended dosages of vitamin B_{12} are listed in the dosages table on p. 796.

drug profiles

Cyanocobalamin is a water-soluble B complex vitamin required for maintaining body fat and carbohydrate metabolism and protein synthesis. It is also needed for growth, cell replication, blood cell production, and the integrity of normal nerve function.

cyanocobalamin

Cyanocobalamin (Cyanoject) is available both as OTC preparations and by prescription. Most of the OTC cyanocobalamin-containing products are multivitamin preparations, whereas many of the sole cyanocobalamin-containing products contain large doses for parenteral injection and are available by prescription only. Cyanocobalamin is classified as a pregnancy category A agent and is contraindicated in patients who have shown a hypersensitivity reaction to it and in those with optic nerve atrophy.

Cyanocobalamin is available orally as 25-, 50-, 100-, 250-, 500-, and 1000-μg tablets; parenterally as 100-, and 1000-μg/ml injections; and as a 500-μg/spray nasal gel. Commonly recommended dosages for vitamin B_{12} are listed in the dosages table on p. 796.

PHARMACOKINETICS

HALF-LIFE	ONSET	PEAK	DURATION
6 days	Unknown	Plasma: 8-12 hr	Unknown

VITAMIN C

Vitamin C (ascorbic acid) is a water-soluble vitamin present in citrus fruits and juices, tomatoes, cabbage, cherries, and liver. It can be synthesized for use as a drug and is used in many therapeutic situations. Prolonged ascorbic acid deficiency results in the nutritional disease **scurvy**, which is characterized by gingivitis and bleeding gums, loss of teeth, anemia, subcutaneous hemorrhage, bone lesions, and delayed healing of soft tissues and bones. It was recognized for several centuries, especially among sailors; in 1795 the British navy ordered the eating of limes to prevent the disease.

Mechanism of Action

Vitamin C is reversibly oxidized to dehydroascorbic acid in the body, and it acts in oxidation-reduction reactions. It is required for several important metabolic activities, including collagen synthesis and the maintenance of connective tissue; tissue repair; maintenance of bone, teeth, and capillaries; and folic acid metabolism (specifically, the conversion of folic acid into its active metabolite). Accordingly, it is essential for erythropoiesis. Vitamin C enhances the absorption of iron and is required for the synthesis of lipids, proteins, and steroids. It has also been shown to aid in cellular respiration and resistance to infections.

Drug Effects

The drug effects of vitamin C are the prevention of scurvy and dietary supplementation. Because vitamin C is an acid, it can also be used as a urinary acidifier. In larger doses vitamin C is also believed to lessen the severity of and prevent the common cold. This use of vitamin C is controversial and not well supported with clinical data.

Therapeutic Uses

Vitamin C is used to treat diseases associated with vitamin C deficiency and as a dietary supplement. It is most beneficial in patients who require larger daily requirements because of pregnancy, lactation, hyperthyroidism, fever, stress, infection, trauma, burns, smoking, and cold exposure and the consumption of certain drugs (e.g., estrogens, oral contraceptives, barbiturates, tetracyclines, and salicylates). The benefits of other uses of vitamin C are less well documented. For example it is a common practice to take vitamin C to prevent or treat the common cold. However, most large controlled studies have shown that ascorbic acid has little or no value as a prophylactic for colds.

Side Effects and Adverse Effects

Vitamin C is usually nontoxic unless excessive dosages are consumed. Megadoses can produce nausea, vomiting, headache, and abdominal cramps and will acidify the urine, resulting in the formation of cystine, oxalate, and urate renal stones. Furthermore, individuals who discontinue taking excessive daily doses of ascorbic acid can suffer from scurvy-like symptoms.

Interactions

Ascorbic acid has the potential to interact with many classes of drugs. However, clinical experience concerning many interactions is inconclusive. For example, it has been reported that ascorbic acid can decrease the effectiveness of oral anticoagulants. This does not always happen, but practitioners should be aware of this possibility. Coadministration with acid-labile drugs such as penicillin G or erythromycin should be avoided. As mentioned previously, megadoses of vitamin C can acidify the urine, which can enhance the excretion of basic drugs and delay the excretion of acidic drugs.

Dosages

The RDAs of vitamin C are listed in Table 50-1. For the commonly recommended dosages of vitamin C, see the dosages table on p. 796.

drug profiles

Ascorbic acid is a water-soluble vitamin required in the prevention and treatment of scurvy. As explained previously, it is required for erythropoiesis and the synthesis of lipids, protein, and steroids.

ascorbic acid

Ascorbic acid (Ascorbicap, Cebid Timecelles, Ce-Vi-Sol, Cecon) is available in OTC preparations such as multivitamin products and by prescription. It is classified as a pregnancy category C agent and has no contraindications.

Ascorbic acid is available orally as a 60-mg lozenge; 60-, 100-, and 500-mg/ml solutions; a 500-mg extended-release capsule; 50-, 100-, 250-, 500-, and 1000-mg tablets; 100-, 250-, 500-, and 1000-mg chewable tablets; and 500-, 1000-, and 1500-mg extended-release tablets. It is also available parenterally as 100-, 250-, and 500-mg/ml injections. See Table 50-1 for the RDAs for vitamin C. Commonly recommended dosages are listed in the dosages table on p. 796.

PHARMACOKINETICS

HALF-LIFE	ONSET	PEAK	DURATION
Unknown	Unknown	Unknown	Unknown

MINERALS

Minerals are essential nutrients that are classified as inorganic compounds. They act as building blocks for many body structures and thus are necessary for a variety of physiologic functions. They are also needed for intracellular and extracellular body fluid electrolytes. Iron is essential for the production of hemoglobin, which is necessary for oxygen transport throughout the body. Minerals are required for muscle contraction, nerve transmission, and the makeup of essential enzymes.

Mineral compounds are composed of various metallic and nonmetallic elements that are chemically combined with ionic bonds. When these compounds are dissolved in water they separate (dissociate) into positively charged metallic cations and electrolytes or negatively charged nonmetallic anions and electrolytes (Fig. 50-5).

Ingestion of mineral nutrients provides essential elements necessary for vital bodily functions. Elements that are required in larger amounts are called *macrominerals;* those required in smaller amounts are called *microminerals* or *trace elements.* Table 50-10 lists the classification of nutrient elements as either macrominerals or microminerals and as metal or nonmetal.

CALCIUM

Calcium is the most abundant mineral element in the human body, accounting for approximately 2% of the total body weight. The highest concentration of calcium is in bones and teeth. Calcium is widely distributed in many foods, especially milk and dairy products. Calcium requirements are high for growing children and for women who are pregnant or breastfeeding. The efficient absorption of calcium requires adequate amounts of vitamin D.

Calcium deficiency results in hypocalcemia and affects many bodily functions. Causes of calcium deficiency include inadequate calcium intake and/or insufficient vitamin D to facilitate absorption, hypoparathyroidism, and malabsorption syndrome, especially in older people. Calcium deficiency–related disorders include infantile rickets, adult osteomalacia, muscle cramps, osteoporosis (especially in postmenopausal females), hypothyroidism, and renal dysfunction. Table 50-11 lists the possible causes of calcium deficiency and the resulting disorders.

Calcium is essential for the normal maintenance and function of the nervous, muscular, and skeletal systems

as well as cell membrane and capillary permeability. It is an important catalyst in many enzymatic reactions and is essential in many physiologic processes, including transmission of nerve impulses; contraction of cardiac, smooth, and skeletal muscles; renal function; respiration; and blood coagulation. Calcium also plays a regulatory role in the release and storage of neurotransmitters and hormones, in white blood cell (WBC) and hormone activity, in the uptake and binding of amino acids, and in intestinal absorption of cyanocobalamin (vitamin B_{12}) and gastrin secretion. The roles of calcium in normal physiologic processes are summarized in Table 50-12.

Mechanism of Action

Calcium participates in a variety of essential physiologic functions and is a building block for body structures. Specifically calcium is involved with the proper development and maintenance of teeth and skeletal bones. It is an important catalyst in many of the coagulation pathways in the blood. Calcium acts as a cofactor in clotting reactions involving the intrinsic and extrinsic pathways of thromboplastin. It is also a cofactor in the conversion of prothrombin to thrombin by thromboplastin and the conversion of fibrinogen to fibrin.

Drug Effects

Calcium salts are used as a source of calcium cations for the treatment or prevention of calcium depletion in patients for whom dietary measures are inadequate. Many conditions may be associated with calcium deficiency:

- Hypoparathyroidism
- Vitamin D deficiency
- Premenstrual syndrome

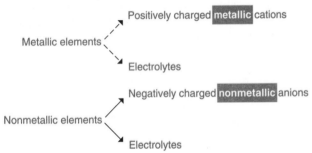

Fig. 50-5 When mineral compounds are dissolved in water, they separate into positively-charged metabolic cations or negatively-charged nonmetallic anions and electrolytes.

Mineral Elements

Table 50-10

Element	Symbol	Type	Ionic/Electrolyte Form
MACROMINERALS			
Calcium*	Ca	Metal	Ca^{+2} calcium cation
Chlorine	Cl	Nonmetal	Cl^{-1} chloride anion
Magnesium*	Mg	Metal	Mg^{+2} magnesium cation
Phosphorus*	P	Nonmetal	PO_4^{-3} phosphate anion
Potassium	K	Metal	K^{+1} potassium cation
Sodium	Na	Metal	Na^{+1} sodium cation
Sulfur	S	Nonmetal	SO_4^{-2} sulfate anion
MICROMINERALS			
Chromium	Cr	Metal	Cr^{+3} chromium cation
Cobalt	Co	Metal	Co^{+2} cobalt cation
Copper	Cu	Metal	Cu^{+2} copper cation
Fluorine	F	Nonmetal	F^{-1} fluoride anion
Iodine*	I	Nonmetal	I^{-1} iodide anion
Iron*	Fe	Metal	Fe^{+2} ferrous cation
Manganese	Mn	Metal	Mn^{+2} manganese cation
Molybdenum	Mo	Metal	Mo^{+6} molybdenum cation
Selenium*	Se	Metal	Se^{+4} selenium cation
Zinc*	Zn	Metal	Zn^{+2} zinc cation

*Mineral elements that have a current RDA.

- Pregnancy and lactation
- Renal failure
- Achlorhydria
- Steatorrhea
- Menopause
- Alkalosis
- Chronic diarrhea
- Sprue
- Pancreatitis
- Hyperphosphatemia

Therapeutic Uses

Calcium is used to treat various manifestations of deficiency states, including adult osteomalacia, hypothyroidism, infantile rickets or tetany, muscle cramps, osteoporosis, and renal insufficiency. In addition, calcium is used as a dietary supplement for women during pregnancy and lactation.

There are over 12 different selected calcium salts available for treatment or nutritional supplementation. Each calcium salt contains a different amount of elemental calcium per gram of calcium salt. Table 50-13 lists the available salts and their associated calcium contents.

Table 50-11 Calcium Deficiency: Causes and Disorders

Cause	Disorder
Inadequate intake	Infantile rickets
Insufficient vitamin D	Adult osteomalacia
Hypoparathyroidism	Muscle cramps
Malabsorption syndrome	Osteoporosis

Table 50-12 Physiologic Processes Requiring Calcium

Role	Physiologic Influence
Normal maintenance and function	Nervous system
	Muscular system
	Skeletal system
	Cell membranes
	Capillary permeability
Physiologic processes	Transmission of nerve impulses
	Contraction of cardiac, smooth, and skeletal muscles
	Renal function
	Respiration
	Blood coagulation
Regulatory	Release and storage of neurotransmitters and hormones
	Uptake and binding of amino acids
	Cyanocobalamin (vitamin B_{12}) absorption
	Gastrin secretion

Side Effects and Adverse Effects

Although adverse effects and toxicity are rare, hypercalcemia can occur; symptoms include anorexia, nausea, vomiting, and constipation. In addition when calcium salts are administered by IM or SC injection, mild to severe local reactions, including burning, necrosis and sloughing of tissue, cellulitis, and soft tissue calcification, may occur. Venous irritation may occur with IV administration. Other side effects and adverse effects associated with both oral and parenteral use of calcium salts are listed in Table 50-14.

Toxicity and Management of Overdose

Chronic and excessive calcium intake can result in severe hypercalcemia, which can cause cardiac irregularities, delirium, and coma. Management of acute hypercalcemia may require hemodialysis, whereas milder cases will respond to discontinuation of calcium intake.

Interactions

Calcium salts will chelate (bind) with tetracyclines to produce an insoluble complex. If hypercalcemia is present in patients taking digitalis preparations, serious cardiac dysrhythmias can occur.

Dosages

For the RDAs of calcium, see Table 50-1.

Table 50-13 Calcium Salts: Calcium Content

Calcium Salt	Ca Content (per gram)
Phosphate tribasic	400 mg (20 mEq)
Carbonate	400 mg (20 mEq)
Phosphate dibasic anhydrous	290 mg (14.5 mEq)
Chloride	270 mg (13.5 mEq)
Acetate	253 mg (12.7 mEq)
Phosphate dibasic dihydrate	230 mg (11.5 mEq)
Citrate	211 mg (10.6 mEq)
Glycerophosphate	191 mg (9.6 mEq)
Lactate	130 mg (6.5 mEq)
Gluconate	90 mg (4.5 mEq)
Gluceptate	82 mg (4.1 mEq)
Glubionate	64 mg (3.2 mEq)

Table 50-14 Calcium Salts: Adverse Effects

Body System	Side/Adverse Effect
Cardiovascular	Hemorrhage, rebound hypertension
Gastrointestinal	Constipation, obstruction, nausea, vomiting, flatulence
Genitourinary	Renal dysfunction, renal stones, renal failure
Metabolic	Hypercalcemia, metabolic alkalosis

drug profiles

calcium

Calcium salts are minerals that are primarily used in the treatment or prevention of calcium depletion in patients in whom dietary measures are inadequate. Many calcium salts are available, all with a different content of elemental calcium per gram of salt. Calcium is available in both oral and parenteral forms.

The calcium salts are classified as pregnancy category C agents and are contraindicated in patients who have shown a hypersensitivity reaction to them and in patients with hypercalcemia, hyperparathyroidism, and bone tumors. There are numerous dosages and names of calcium preparations. Consult manufacturer instructions for recommended dosages. The calcium salts are available in liquid-filled capsules, powders, oral suspensions, tablets, chewable tablets, film-coated tablets, oral solutions, and parenteral injections. For the RDAs of calcium, see Table 50-1.

PHARMACOKINETICS

HALF-LIFE	ONSET	PEAK	DURATION
Unknown	Unknown	Unknown	Unknown

---

case study — Magnesium Sulfate Therapy

D.C., a 68-year-old female, was admitted to CCU 2 days ago for exacerbation of CHF. After 2 days of diuretic treatment with furosemide (Lasix), the physician orders serum potassium and magnesium levels, which come back with serum magnesium at 0.9 mEq/L. The physician orders magnesium sulfate 16 mEq q6h for two doses with the first dose now. The night supervisor has to retrieve the medication because the pharmacy is closed and returns to your unit with the medication. You are aware of many medication errors with magnesium sulfate, so you are extra cautious in checking and double checking the order. However, you notice that the vials are labeled 16 grams, which is equal to 130 mEq versus the 16 mEq.

- *What are the normal serum levels for magnesium?*
- *What are some of the indications for magnesium sulfate as a medication:*
  a. *Anticonvulsant*
  b. *Tocolytic*
  c. *Antidysrhythmic*
  d. *Electrolyte replacement agent*
- *Think back to your basic anatomy and physiology education and provide a rationale for the use of magnesium sulfate in patients with CHF.*
- *What are some manifestations of overdosage with magnesium sulfate?*

For Answers see www.harcourthealth.com/MERLIN/Lilley/.

MAGNESIUM

Magnesium is one of the principal cations present in the intracellular fluid. It is an essential part of many enzyme systems associated with energy metabolism. Magnesium deficiency (hypomagnesia) is usually caused by (1) malabsorption, especially in the presence of high calcium intake; (2) alcoholism; (3) long-term IV feeding; (4) diuretics; and (5) metabolic disorders, including hyperthyroidism and diabetic ketoacidosis. Symptoms associated with hypomagnesia include cardiovascular disturbances, neuromuscular impairment, and mental disturbances.

Dietary intake from vegetables and other foods will usually prevent magnesium deficiency. However, magnesium is required in greater amounts in individuals with diets high in protein-rich foods, calcium, and phosphorus.

Mechanism of Action

The precise mechanism for magnesium has not been fully determined. Magnesium is a known cofactor for many enzyme systems. It is required for muscle contraction and nerve physiology. Magnesium produces an anticonvulsant effect by inhibiting neuromuscular transmission for selected convulsive states.

Therapeutic Uses

Magnesium is used to treat magnesium deficiency and as a nutritional supplement in total parenteral nutrition (TPN) and multivitamin preparations. It is used as an anticonvulsant in magnesium deficiency, preeclampsia, and eclampsia.

Side Effects and Adverse Effects

Adverse effects of magnesium are due to hypermagnesia, which results in tendon reflex loss, difficult bowel movements, CNS depression, respiratory distress and heart block, and hypothermia.

Toxicity and Management of Overdose

Toxic effects are extensions of symptoms caused by hypermagnesia, a major cause of which is the long-term use of magnesium products (especially antacids in patients with renal dysfunction). Severe hypermagnesia is treated with a calcium salt administered intravenously in doses up to 10 mEq.

Interactions

Use of magnesium with neuromuscular blocking agents and CNS depressants produces additive effects.

Dosages

The RDA for magnesium is 6 to 10 mg for infants and children, 10 to 15 mg for women, and 10 to 12 mg for men. The usual dose of magnesium for treating convulsant conditions is 4 to 5 g intravenously or intramuscularly, repeated as required. For the RDAs of magnesium, see Table 50-1.

drug profiles

magnesium

Magnesium is a mineral that has a variety of dosage forms and uses. Magnesium is an essential part of many enzyme systems. When absent or diminished in the body, cardiovascular, neuromuscular, and mental disturbances can occur.

Magnesium sulfate is the most common form of magnesium used as a mineral replacement. It is classified as a pregnancy category C agent and is contraindicated in hypersensitivity and renal disease. It is available in the parenteral form as a 4%, 8%, 10%, 12.5%, and 50% injection. For the RDA of magnesium, see Table 50-1.

PHOSPHORUS

Phosphorus is widely distributed in foods, and thus a dietary deficiency is rare. Deficiency states are usually nondietary and are primarily due to malabsorption, extensive diarrhea or vomiting, hyperthyroidism, hepatic disease, and long-term use of aluminum or calcium antacids.

Mechanism of Action

Phosphorus in the form of the phosphate group and/or anion (PO_4^{-3}) is a required precursor for the synthesis of essential body chemicals. In addition, the mineral is an important building block for body structures. Phosphorus is required as a structural unit for the synthesis of nucleic acid and the adenosine-phosphate compounds (adenosine monophosphate [AMP], adenosine disphosphate [ADP], and adenosine triphosphate [ATP]) responsible for cellular energy transfer. It is also necessary for the development and maintenance of the skeletal system and teeth. The skeletal bones contain up to 85% of the phosphorus content of the body. In addition, magnesium is required for the proper utilization of many B-complex vitamins, and it is an essential component of physiologic buffering systems.

Therapeutic Uses

Phosphorus is used to treat deficiency states and as a dietary supplement in many multivitamin formulations.

Side Effects and Adverse Effects

Adverse effects are usually associated with phosphorus replacement products. Effects include diarrhea, nausea, vomiting, and other GI disturbances. Other side effects include confusion, weakness, and breathing difficulties.

Toxicity and Management of Overdose

Toxic reactions to phosphorus are extremely rare and are usually restricted to the ingestion of the pure element.

Interactions

Antacids can reduce the oral absorption of phosphorus.

Dosages

The RDA for phosphorus is 800 to 1200 mg for infants and children and 300 to 800 mg for adults. For the RDAs of phosphorus, see Table 50-1.

drug profiles

phosphorus

Phosphorus is a very essential mineral to our well-being. It is needed to make energy in the form of ADP and ATP for all our bodily processes. Fortunately it is present in a variety of foods and drinks, and a true dietary deficiency is rare. Phosphorus is present in a large number of drug formulations and appears as a phosphate salt (PO_4).

Phosphorus is classified as a pregnancy category C agent and should be used with caution in patients with renal impairment. It is available in both oral and parenteral formulations. Oral phosphorus is available as capsules and tablets. The capsules are available as sodium phosphate and contain 250 μg of phosphorus combined with 7 mEq of sodium and 7 mEq of potassium and as potassium phosphate that contains 250 μg of phosphorus combined with 14.25 mEq of potassium. The parenteral form contains 94 μg of phosphorus with 4 mEq of sodium per milliliter. Recommended dosages vary depending on the indication. The RDA is listed in Table 50-1.

nursing process

● Assessment

Before administering vitamins, the nurse must assess patients for nutritional disorders with an evaluation of baseline hemoglobin (Hgb), hematocrit (Hct), WBC and RBC counts, and protein and albumin levels. A daily journal of dietary intake and a history of dietary patterns and meals must also be documented. To test for vitamin A deficiency a baseline assessment of the patient's vision, including night vision, and an examination of the appearance of the skin and mucous membranes must be done. Serum laboratory values of vitamin A less than 20 μg/dl in adults and 10 μg/dl in children indicate a deficiency. Interactions of vitamin A with the drug isotretinoin may lead to toxicity, with manifestations such as headache, nausea, vomiting, elevated liver enzymes, and dry, cracked skin.

Vitamin D is contraindicated in patients with hypercalcemia or hypervitaminosis D. Cautious use is recommended, with close and careful monitoring in patients with arteriosclerosis, hyperphosphatemia, renal or cardiac dysfunction, and hypersensitivity to vitamin D. Baseline assessment should include a status assessment of the patient's skeletal formation and a baseline serum calcium level. Serum calcium levels under

NURSING CARE PLAN Magnesium Sulfate Therapy

D.G. is a 49-year-old CHF patient on the cardiac care unit who has been admitted for exacerbation of the disease. After initial treatment with Lasix IV and digoxin, the physician orders serum potassium and magnesium levels. D.G.'s magnesium levels come back low, and the physician orders magnesium sulfate 16 mEq IV for two doses.

assessment	*Nursing Diagnosis*	Risk for injury related to potential side effects of CNS depressants
	Subjective Data	"The physician says my magnesium levels are low. What type of drug am I going to receive, and what are its side effects?"
		"I rarely take any medications. Is this a safe medication?"
		"What will it do to me?"
	Objective Data	Patient admitted for diagnosis or exacerbation of CHF
		Low serum magnesium levels upon admission to CCU
		IV therapy ordered with infusion of magnesium
		Asking questions about magnesium sulfate therapy
		Anxious about treatment and not used to taking medications
planning and outcome criteria	*Goals*	At the end of the teaching session, patient will verbalize an understanding of treatment with magnesium sulfate.
	Outcome Criteria	Patient will verbalize the following during teaching session:
		• Reason for use of magnesium
		• Common side effects
		• Nursing monitoring of patient (to decrease patient's anxiety) during magnesium infusion
implementation		Inform patient of the following:
		• Magnesium sulfate therapy is used to return magnesium to within normal levels and to prevent problems with heart conduction and impulse formation, but also to prevent seizures in certain patients.
		• Common side effects include sweating; depressed, deep reflexes; flushing; drop in blood pressure; and decreased respiratory functioning.
		• The patient will be monitored closely for the following:
		— Vital signs every 15 min after IV dosing with a check of temperature, pulse, blood pressure, and respirations
		— Input and output every 4 hr with at least 120 ml/4 hr with at least 30 ml/hr; if less the physician will be contacted
		— Mental status
		— Respiratory status with a focus on respiratory rate, character, and rhythm
		— Hypermagnesemia (too much magnesium), which is manifested by depressed patellar (knee jerk) reflex, flushing, confusion, weakness, drop in body temperature, and shortness of breath
		• Calcium gluconate will be on hand should toxicity occur because this will help reverse the symptoms.
evaluation		Positive therapeutic outcome: elevated magnesium levels to within normal limits

7.5 mg/dl indicate possible vitamin D deficiency. In addition, it would be advisable to monitor baseline levels of inorganic phosphorus and serum citrate. Drug interactions may occur with antacids, high doses of calcium preparations, thiazide diuretics, and products high in vitamin D.

Before administering vitamin E, patients should be assessed for hypoprothrombinemia secondary to vitamin E deficiency. Vitamin E will aggravate this condition and result in hematologic problems such as bleeding. Baseline assessment data include a check of skin integrity and determination of the presence or absence of edema and any muscle weakness.

Vitamin B_1 (thiamine) hypersensitivity may cause skin rash and wheezing. Since it is rare that only one vitamin B_1 deficiency occurs, deficiencies of all forms of vitamin B_1 must be ruled out. Baseline assessments of vital signs, mental status, and urinary thiamine levels must be done. For adults, less than 27 μg/dl indicates deficiency.

Vitamin C is contraindicated in patients with cystinuria, oxalosis, or a history of gout or urate kidney stones. In patients with sickle cell anemia, large doses of vitamin C may precipitate a sickle cell crisis. Diabetic patients may experience abnormal glucose levels when taking large doses of vitamin C.

There are few contraindications to the administration of trace elements. However, baseline assessments of nutritional status and specific nutrition-related laboratory studies (Hgb, Hct, RBC and WBC counts, trace elemental laboratory values) should be ordered by the physician and documented before initiation of therapy. Trace elements should be administered as ordered and only after the element or mineral, reviewed laboratory studies, and specific manufacturer guidelines for administration have been researched. Cautious use is recommended in any patient with liver or biliary disease.

Before administering calcium and magnesium the patients' current levels should be obtained and recorded. Calcium is contraindicated in patients who are hypercalcemic and have digitalis toxicity, ventricular fibrillation, or renal calculi. Cautious use is recommended in patients who are pregnant or breastfeeding, in children, in patients with renal or respiratory disease or failure, and in patients taking digitalis. Calcium interacts with digitalis, calcium channel blockers, amphotericin, cephalothin, digoxin, digitoxin, epinephrine, tetracycline, sodium warfarin, phosphate, and sodium bicarbonate. Baseline ECGs are often necessary in patients who have cardiac disease. If decreased QT and T wave inversion are observed, calcium is often discontinued or given in reduced dosages.

Magnesium is contraindicated in patients with hypersensitivity to it, and cautious use is recommended in patients with severe renal disease, GI bleeding, diarrhea, and possible intestinal obstruction. Magnesium interacts with tetracyclines, anticholinergics, iron salts, cimetadine, corticosteroids, and chlordiazepoxide.

● Nursing Diagnoses

Nursing diagnoses include, but are not limited to, the following:

Vitamin A therapy
- Disturbed sensory perception (visual) related to night blindness from vitamin A deficiency.

Vitamin D therapy
- Acute pain related to bone or skeletal deformities resulting from vitamin D deficiency.
- Impaired physical mobility related to poorly developed muscles from vitamin D deficiency.

Vitamin E
- Impaired physical mobility related to vitamin E deficiency.
- Diarrhea related to vitamin E side effects.

Vitamin B$_1$ (thiamine) deficiency
- Disturbed thought processes related to vitamin B$_1$ deficiency.

Other vitamin B forms
- Impaired physical mobility related to fatigue from poor nutrition.

Vitamin C (ascorbic acid)
- Acute pain in joints related to disease from vitamin deficiencies.
- Impaired tissue integrity related to lack of vitamin C.

● Planning

Goals related to the use of vitamins and minerals are as follows:
- Patient maintains sensory and perceptual integrity during therapy.
- Patient experiences minimal complaints related to vitamin and mineral therapy.
- Patient's skin integrity remains intact.
- Patient regains and maintains activity level considered normal for him or her.

Outcome Criteria

Outcome criteria related to the above goals include the following:
- Patient will openly verbalize fears and anxieties about possible visual changes.
- Patient will keep skin clean, dry to moist (as needed), to maintain skin intactness and prevent infection.
- Patient will increase ADLs as warranted and as tolerated.
- Patient will return to pre-illness levels of function.

● Implementation

Before administering vitamin A, the nurse should check and document the patient's diet and signs and symptoms of hypervitaminosis and hypercarotenemia (excess vitamin A). Vitamin D should be given with concurrent evaluations of renal function and serum calcium levels, especially at the beginning of therapy. The nurse should monitor growth measurements before the beginning of therapy in children, and all patients should be assessed for signs of toxicity such as constipation, anorexia, nausea, vomiting, metallic taste, and dry mouth.

The water-miscible forms of vitamin E are more rapidly absorbed, and patients should always be encouraged to obtain adequate vitamin intake through diet. Vitamin B$_1$ (thiamine) therapy is usually administered in an oral preparation, but parenteral forms are also available. Niacin should be administered with milk or food to decrease GI upset. Oral forms of niacin are preferred. If administered intravenously, pyridoxine should be given at a rate of 50 mg/min and may be given with most IV fluids. Cyanocobalamin should be administered orally with meals to increase its absorption. Ascorbic acid should be administered orally, if possible; if administered intravenously it should be given at a rate no greater than 100 mg/min. The oral effervescent forms should be dissolved in at least 6 oz of fluid such as water or juice.

When vitamin C is prescribed for acidification of the urine, it is important to frequently assess urinary pH. If vitamin C is administered intravenously, it should be given as a continuous infusion (not to exceed 100 mg/min) as an additive to IV solutions. Oral effervescent tablets should be dissolved thoroughly in water before administration.

Because of venous irritation, calcium should be given via an IV infusion pump when given intravenously. The nurse should also monitor closely for hypercalcemia. Calcium should be given slowly intravenously (<1 ml/min for adults) to avoid cardiac dysrhythmias and cardiac arrest, and the patient should be kept recumbent for 15 minutes after the infusion. Should extravasation occur, you should discontinue the infusion immediately. The physician may order infusion with 1% procaine or other antidote to reduce vasospasm and dilute the effects of calcium on surrounding tissue. Follow institutional guidelines regarding treatment of calcium extravasation. Oral calcium supplements should be given 1 to 3 hours after meals.

Magnesium should be administered according to manufacturer guidelines and as ordered. Because different dosages result in different effects, always recheck the order, dosage, and intended use and therapeutic effects.

For patient teaching tips related to vitamins, minerals, and trace elements, see the box below.

● Evaluation

Therapeutic responses to vitamin A therapy include restoration of normal vision and intact skin. Side effects include lethargy, night blindness, skin and corneal changes, and in infancy, failure to thrive. Therapeutic response to vitamin D include improved bone growth and formation and an intact skeleton with decreased or no pain. Side effects include constipation, anorexia, metallic taste, and dry mouth.

Therapeutic responses to vitamin E include improved muscle strength, more intact skin, and alpha-tocopherol levels within normal limits. Side effects include blurred vision, dizziness, drowsiness, breast enlargement, and flulike symptoms. Therapeutic response to vitamin B_1 (thiamine) includes improved mental status with less confusion. Therapeutic responses to riboflavin, niacin, pyridoxine, and cyanocobalamin include improved skin integrity, normal vision, improved mental status, and normal RBC, Hgb, and Hct levels. Therapeutic responses to vitamin C include improved capillary intactness, skin and mucous membrane integrity, healing, and energy and mental state. An adverse reaction associated with vitamin C is precipitate formation in the urine with possible stone formation. Side effects for the B vitamins and ascorbic acid are included in the discussion and tables pertinent to each vitamin.

Therapeutic responses to trace elements include resolution of the deficient state and associated signs and symptoms, depending on the specific element or mineral.

patient teaching tips

Vitamins, Minerals, and Trace Elements

➤ Patients should be provided with information and counseling about the best sources of dietary vitamin A, such as egg yolks, butter, milk, liver, kidney, cream, cheese, and fortified margarine. Carotene, the precursor to vitamin A, is found in leafy green vegetables and yellow and orange fruits and vegetables.

➤ Patients taking vitamin D should be closely monitored and should maintain regular visits to the physician for review of diet and calcium therapy. Patients should be instructed about foods high in vitamin D such as egg yolks, vitamin D–fortified milk, fish liver oils, whole grain cereals, wheat germ, liver, and vegetable oils. Unless medically contraindicated, careful exposure to the sun should be encouraged.

➤ Patients should be provided with information and counseling about necessary foods to include in their diet. Examples of such information follow.

  ➤ Foods high in vitamin E include vegetable oils, wheat germ, whole grain cereals, egg yolks, and liver.

➤ Vitamin B is found in many different foods. Thiamine is found in enriched cereals or whole grains, pork, nuts, fish, organ and muscle meats, poultry, rice bran, and green vegetables. Riboflavin is found in milk and other dairy products, meats, eggs, fish, poultry, and enriched grains and cereals.

➤ Niacin is found in meats, eggs, whole grain and enriched cereals, breads, flour, milk, and other dairy products. Pyridoxine is found in meats, poultry, fish, eggs, whole grains, sweet potatoes, lima beans, and bananas.

➤ Patients who have had a gastrectomy or ileal resection or who have pernicious anemia should be informed of the necessity for cyanocobalamin in their diet.

➤ Patients taking up to 600 mg/day of vitamin C should be informed that they may experience a slight increase in daily urination patterns and that more than 1 g per day may lead to diarrhea. They should also be informed of foods high in ascorbic acid such as citrus fruits, tomatoes, strawberries, cantaloupe, and raw peppers.

➤ Patients taking trace elements (e.g., zinc, copper, magnesium, iodine, chromium) must take medication as prescribed. They should also know to call the physician if any unusual reactions occur.

➤ Patients who are trying to increase calcium intake should be informed of foods high in calcium, such as milk and other dairy products, shellfish, and dark green leafy vegetables. Patients taking calcium supplements should be told to limit foods high in oxalate and zinc such as nuts, legumes, chocolate, spinach, and soy products and to avoid bran because these foods decrease the absorption of oral calcium supplementation. Patients should also know that calcium products chelate or bind with tetracyclines and thus decrease or negate their effects.

POINTS TO REMEMBER

Nursing Considerations

- Over-the-counter use of vitamins and minerals may lead to serious problems and side effects; therefore a physician should be consulted before supplementation.
- Nurses must incorporate the nutritional status of each patient into the nursing care plan to provide "comprehensive" care during medication therapy.
- The nurse's participation in health promotion and wellness includes providing information about dietary needs and the body's need for vitamins and minerals.

- Patient education as related to vitamin and mineral replacement must focus on dietary sources of the specific nutrient, drug and food interactions, and side effects. Patients must be instructed about when it is necessary to contact the physician.
- Vitamins and minerals can be dangerous to the patient if given without concern and caution for the patient's overall condition and underlying disease processes.
- Never assume that because the drug is a vitamin or a mineral it does not have adverse reactions or toxicity—most of them can become toxic.

REVIEW QUESTIONS

1. Which of the following may occur if IV calcium is given too rapidly?
   a. Ototoxicity
   b. Liver failure
   c. Renal shutdown
   d. Cardiac dysrhythmias
2. Which of the following should be avoided if calcium supplements are taken for osteoporosis?
   a. Vitamin D decreases the absorption and excretion of calcium.
   b. Penicillin antibiotics enhance the toxicity of calcium in the body.
   c. Tetracyclines, in newer form, do not bind with calcium as previously thought.
   d. Foods high in oxalate and zinc may decrease the absorption of calcium supplements.

3. Which of the following indicates vitamin D toxicity?
   a. Diarrhea
   b. Urticaria
   c. Metallic taste
   d. Increased appetite
4. Which of the following nursing diagnosis is most appropriate for a patient with deficient levels of vitamin A?
   a. Diarrhea
   b. Urinary retention
   c. Altered skin integrity
   d. Sensory/perceptual deficit (visual)
5. Vitamin C has the normal functioning of:
   a. Erythropoiesis.
   b. Glycogenolysis.
   c. Maintaining renal performance.
   d. Enhancing cardiac contractility.

For Answers see www.harcourthealth.com/MERLIN/Lilley/.

CRITICAL THINKING Activities

1. Explain why patients with a cardiac history need a baseline ECG and serum calcium assessment performed before initiation of calcium supplemental therapy.
2. Your patient is experiencing constipation and abdominal pain since beginning calcium therapy. Your assessment reveals a distended abdomen and diminished bowel sounds. What could be occurring, and what should your nursing actions be at this time?
3. Ms. Wall takes 2500 mg calcium carbonate daily in the form of an OTC calcium supplement. How much elemental calcium is Ms. Wall actually taking?

bibliography

Albanese J, Nutz P: *Mosby's 2001 nursing drug reference and review cards,* St Louis, 2001, Mosby.

American Hospital Formulary Service: *AHFS drug information,* Bethesda, Md, 2000, American Society of Health-System Pharmacists.

Anderson PO, Knoben JE, Troutman WG: *Handbook of clinical drug data 1999-2000,* ed 9, New York, 1999, McGraw-Hill.

Johns Hopkins Hospital, Department of Pediatrics et al: *The Harriet Lane handbook,* ed 15, St Louis, 2000, Mosby.

Keen JH: *Critical care and emergency drug reference,* ed 3, St Louis, 1996, Mosby.

LaChance P: Overview of key nutrients: micronutrient aspects, *Nutr Rev* 56 (4 Pt 2):534, 1998.

McEvoy GK: *AHFS drug information,* Bethesda, Md, 1998, American Society of Hospital Pharmacists.

McKenry LM, Salerno E: *Mosby's pharmacology in nursing,* ed 21, St Louis, 2001, Mosby.

Mosby's GenRx: a comprehensive reference for generic and brand drugs, ed 10, St Louis, 2000, Mosby.

Skidmore-Roth L: *Mosby's 2001 nursing drug reference,* St Louis, 2001, Mosby.

Remember to check the **Online Worksheet** for additional learning opportunities: **www.harcourthealth.com/MERLIN/Lilley/**

Chapter 51

Nutritional Supplements

objectives

When you reach the end of this chapter, you should be able to do the following:

1 Discuss the anatomy and physiology of the gastrointestinal system.

2 List the various enteral and parenteral supplements with their ingredients.

3 Describe the process of initiating and maintaining continuous and intermittent enteral feedings, and total parenteral nutrition (TPN).

4 Compare the various enteral feeding tubes.

5 Discuss the mechanisms of action, cautions, contraindications, and nursing implications associated with enteral and parenteral nutritional supplements.

6 Develop a nursing care plan that includes all phases of the nursing process for patients receiving enteral and parenteral supplemental feedings.

7 Identify home health care needs for patients receiving enteral or parenteral nutritional feedings.

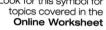
www.harcourthealth.com/MERLIN/Lilley/

Look for this symbol for
topics covered in the
Online Worksheet Activity

---

drug profiles

amino acids, p. 823	**fats**, p. 823
carbohydrate formulation, p. 820	**lipid emulsions**, p. 823
carbohydrates, p. 823	**protein formulation**, p. 821
fat formulation, p. 820	

---

glossary

Anabolism (ə nab'ə liz' əm) Constructive metabolism characterized by the conversion of simple substances into the more complex compounds of living matter. (p. 822)

Catabolism (kə tab' o liz əm) A complex metabolic process in which energy is liberated for use in work, energy storage, or heat production by the destruction of complex substances by living cells to form simple compounds. (p. 822)

Enteral nutrition (en' ter əl) The provision of food or nutrients via the gastrointestinal tract. (p. 818)

Essential amino acids Those amino acids that cannot be manufactured by the body. (p. 823)

Essential fatty acid deficiency A condition that develops if fatty acids that the body cannot produce are not present in dietary or nutritional supplements. (p. 823)

Hyperalimentation (hi'pər al' i men ta' shən) Same as *parenteral nutrition.* (p. 821)

Malnutrition (mal' noo trish' ən) Any disorder of nutrition. (p. 817)

Multivitamin infusion (MVI) Vitamins and minerals added, depending on the patient's needs. (p. 824)

Nonessential amino acids Those amino acids that the body can produce without extracting from dietary intake. (p. 822)

Nutrient (noo' tre ənt) A substance that provides nourishment and affects the nutritive and metabolic processes of the body. (p. 817)

Nutritional supplements Means of providing adequate nutritional support to meet the body's nutritional needs. (p. 818)

Nutritional support Support for the body's nutritional needs. (p. 817)

Parenteral nutrition (pə ren' tər əl) The administration of nutrients by a route other than through the alimentary canal, such as intravenously. (p. 818)

Semiessential amino acids Those that can be produced by the body but not in sufficient amounts in infants and children. (p. 823)

Total parenteral nutrition Same as *parenteral nutrition.* (p. 821)

The integrity and normal function of all cells within the body require a constant supply of nutrients. **Nutrients** are dietary products that undergo chemical changes when ingested (metabolism) and cause tissue to be enhanced and energy to be liberated. Nutrients are required for cell growth and division, enzyme activity, protein-carbohydrate-fat synthesis, muscle contraction, neurohumoral secretion, wound repair, immune competence, gut integrity, and numerous other essential cellular functions. Providing for these nutritional needs is known as **nutritional support.** Adequate nutritional support is needed to prevent the breakdown of proteins for use as energy to sustain essential organ systems. **Malnutrition** can decrease organ size and impair the function of organ systems (cardiac, respiratory, gastrointestinal [GI], hepatic, renal, and so on). **Nutritional supplements** are a means of providing adequate nutritional support to meet the body's nutritional needs.

Malnutrition is a condition in which the body's essential need for nutrients is not met by nutrient intake. The purpose of nutritional support is the successful prevention, recognition, and management of malnutrition. Nutritional supplements are dietary products used to provide nutritional support. Many nutritional supplement products can be administered to patients in a variety of ways. Nutritional supplements vary in the amounts and chemical complexity of carbohydrate, protein, and fat. The electrolyte, vitamin, mineral, and osmolality of the specific product can vary as well. These nutrients may be given in a digested form, a partially digested form, or an undigested form. Nutritional supplements can also be tailored for specific disease states.

A wide variety of nutritional supplements is needed because of the wide variety of conditions for which pa-

tients require nutritional support. Patients' nutrient requirements vary according to age, gender, size or weight, physical activity, preexisting medical conditions, and current medical or surgical treatment. Nutritional supplements are classified according to the method of administration. They can be classified as either enteral or parenteral. **Enteral nutrition** is the provision of food or nutrients with the GI tract as the route of administration. Nutritional supplements may also be administered parenterally. **Parenteral nutrition** differs from enteral nutrition in the route of administration. Nutritional supplements are delivered directly into the circulation by means of IV infusion. The selection of either enteral nutrition or parenteral nutrition and the specific nutritional composition of the product depends on the specific patient profile and the clinical situation.

Nutritional support
- Enteral nutrition → Gastrointestinal tract
- Parenteral nutrition → Circulation

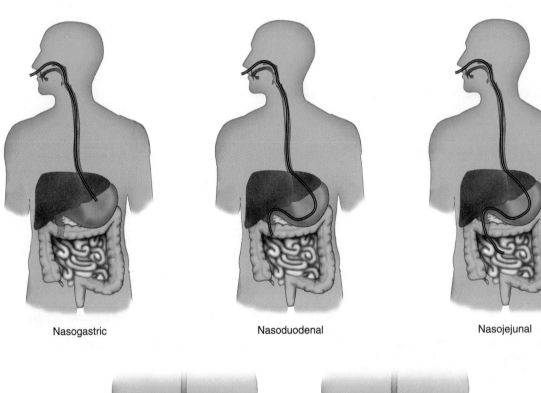

Nasogastric   Nasoduodenal   Nasojejunal

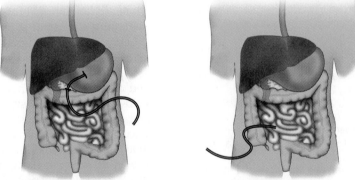

Gastrostomy   Jejunostomy

Fig. 51-1 Tube feeding routes. (From Beare PG, Myers JL: *Adult health nursing*, St Louis, 1998, Mosby.)

ENTERAL NUTRITION

Enteral nutrition is the provision of food or nutrients through the GI tract. The most common and least invasive route of administration is oral consumption. A feeding tube is used in the other five routes (Fig. 51-1). The six routes of enteral nutrition delivery are listed in Box 51-1. Patients who may benefit from feeding tube delivery of nutritional supplements include those with abnormal esophageal or stomach peristalsis, altered anatomy secondary to surgery, depressed consciousness, or impaired digestive capacity. Nutrients may be administered via the enteral or parenteral routes depending on the clinical situation. Many processes occur from the beginning of the digestive system in the mouth to the end of the digestive system in the anus. These processes have evolved over time to most effectively digest dietary nutrients. The enteral route is considered to be the superior route of administration of nutritional supplements.

Approximately 100 different enteral formulations are available. The enteral supplements have been divided into basic groups according to the basic characteristics of the individual formulations. The four enteral formulation groups are elemental, polymeric, modular, and altered amino acid. These are described in Box 51-2.

Mechanism of Action

The enteral formula groups provide the basic building blocks for anabolism. Different combinations and amounts of these agents are used based on the individual patient's anabolic needs. After the body receives and absorbs these nutrients, it must process them into living matter.

Drug Effects

Enteral nutrition can be used to supplement an oral diet that is currently insufficient for a patient's nutrient needs or used solely to meet all the patient's nutrient needs.

Therapeutic Uses

Enteral nutrition supplies complete dietary needs through the GI tract by the normal oral route or by feeding tube.

It is used for patients who are unable to consume or digest normal foods, have accelerated catabolic status, or are undernourished because of disease. Box 51-3 lists the main types of enteral nutrition supplements and their indications.

Side Effects and Adverse Effects

The most common side effect and adverse effect from the nutritional supplements is GI intolerance. The most common result of this intolerance is diarrhea. Infant nutritional formulations are most commonly associated with allergies and digestive intolerance. The other nutritional supplements are most commonly associated with osmotic diarrhea. Rapid feeding or bolus doses can result

---

BOX 51-1 Routes of Enteral Nutrition Delivery

Route	Description
Gastrostomy	Feeding tube surgically inserted directly into the stomach
Jejunostomy	Feeding tube surgically inserted into the jejunum
Nasoduodenal	Feeding tube placed from the nose to the duodenum
Nasojejunal	Feeding tube placed from the nose to the jejunum
Nasogastric	Feeding tube placed from the nose to the stomach
Oral	Nutritional supplements delivered by mouth

BOX 51-2 Enteral Formulations

ALTERED AMINO ACID FORMULATIONS

Amin-Aid
Hepatic-Aid
Lonalac
Stresstein
Travasorb Renal
Traum-Aid HBC

Contents: varying amounts of specific amino acids

Indications: patients with genetically altered metabolism problems

ELEMENTAL FORMULATIONS

Peptamen
Vital HN
Vivonex Plus
Vivonex TEN

Contents: dipeptides, tripeptides, or crystalline amino acids, glucose oligosaccharides, and vegetable oil or medium-chain triglycerides

Comments: minimum digestion; residue is minimal

Indications: partial bowel obstruction, irritable bowel disease, radiation enteritis, bowel fistulas, and short bowel syndrome

MODULAR FORMULATIONS

Carbohydrate
Moducal
Polycose

Fat
MCT Oil
Microlipid

Protein
Casec
Promod
Propac
Stresstein

Contents: single nutrient formulas (protein, carbohydrate, or fat)

Indications: can be added to a monomeric or polymeric formulation to provide a more individual specialized nutrient formulation

POLYMERIC FORMULATIONS

Complete
Ensure
Ensure-Plus
Isocal
Osmolite
Portagen
Precision LR
Sustacal

Contents: complex nutrients (proteins, carbohydrates, and fat)

Indications: preferred over elemental for patients with fully functional GI tracts and few specialized nutrient requirements; preferred because hyperosmolarity of elemental formulas causes more GI problems

BOX 51-3 **Enteral Nutrition Supplements: Therapeutic Effects**

COMPLETE NUTRITIONAL FORMULATIONS
1. Unable to consume or digest normal foods
2. Accelerated catabolic status
3. Undernourished because of disease

INCOMPLETE NUTRITIONAL FORMULATIONS
1. Genetic metabolic enzyme deficiency
2. Hepatic or renal impairment

INFANT NUTRITIONAL FORMULATIONS
1. Sole nutritional intake for premature and full-term infants
2. Supplemental nutritional intake for older infants receiving solid foods
3. Supplemental nutrition for breast-fed infants

in dumping syndrome, which produces intestinal disturbances. In addition, tube feeding can often result in aspiration.

Interactions

Various nutrients can interact with drugs to produce significant food-drug interactions. With some exceptions, food usually delays the absorption of drugs when administered simultaneously. Chemical inactivation with high gastric acid content or prolonged emptying time can result in decreased effects of cephalosporins, erythromycin, and penicillins when given with nutritional supplements. An increased absorption rate resulting in increased therapeutic effects can be seen when adrenal steroids or vitamins A and D are given with nutritional supplements. Decreased antibiotic effects of tetracycline are seen when it is given with nutritional supplements as a result of chemical inactivation that occurs when they complex with calcium.

Dosages

Because nutrient requirements vary greatly, dosages are individualized according to patient needs.

drug profiles

Enteral nutrition can be provided by a variety of supplements. The individual patient characteristics determine the appropriate enteral supplement. There are four basic types of enteral formulations: elemental, polymeric, modular, and altered amino acid.

ELEMENTAL FORMULATIONS

Elemental formulations are enteral supplements that contain dipeptides, tripeptides, or crystalline amino acids. Because of the composition of elemental formulation supplements, minimal digestion is required. These agents are indicated in patients

with partial bowel obstruction, irritable bowel disease, radiation enteritis, bowel fistulas, and short bowel syndrome. They are contraindicated in patients who have had hypersensitivity reactions to them. Elemental formulation supplements are available without a prescription and have no pregnancy category.

POLYMERIC FORMULATIONS

Polymeric formulations are enteral supplements that contain complex nutrients derived from proteins, carbohydrates, and fat. The polymeric formulations are some of the most commonly used enteral formulations because they most closely resemble normal dietary intake. They are preferred over elemental formulations in patients with fully functional GI tracts and have no specialized nutrient needs. They are also less hyperosmolar than elemental formulations and therefore cause fewer GI problems. They are contraindicated in patients who have had hypersensitivity reactions to them. They are available without a prescription and have no pregnancy category.

Ensure is a commonly used enteral supplement from the polymeric formulation category of enteral nutrition products. It is lactose free and also is available in a higher caloric formula called Ensure-Plus. Other polymeric formulations are Complete-B, Isocal, Magnacal, Meritene, Osmolite, Portagen, Precision LR, and Sustacal. These agents contain complex nutrients such as casein and soy protein as protein, corn syrup and maltodextrins as carbohydrates, and vegetable oil or milk fat for fat. They are available in liquid formulations only.

MODULAR FORMULATIONS
carbohydrate formulation

Moducal and Polycose are examples of commonly used enteral supplements from the carbohydrate modular formulation category. They are carbohydrate supplements that supply carbohydrates only. They are intended to be used as an addition to monomeric or polymeric formulations to provide a more individual specialized nutrient formulation. These products are available without a prescription, have no pregnancy category, and are contraindicated only if a patient has had a hypersensitivity reaction to them. They are available in liquid formulations only.

fat formulation

Microlipid and MCT Oil are the formulations available in the fat category. Microlipid is a fat supplement supplying solely fats. It is a concentrated source of calories and contains 4.5 calories per ml. These agents are used to help individualize nutrient formulations. They may be used in malabsorption

Peripheral and Central Parenteral Nutrition: Characteristics

51-1

Considerations	Characteristics	
	Peripheral	**Central**
Goal of nutritional therapy (total versus supplemental)	Supplemental (total if moderate to low needs)	Total
Length of therapy	Short (<2 wk)	Long (>7-10 days)
Osmolarity	Isotonic (<600 mosm/L)	Hypertonic (2000 + mosm/L)
Fluid tolerance	Must be high	Can be fluid restricted
Dextrose	<5% to 12.5%	10% to 50%
Amino acids	3% to 5%	3% to 7%
Fats	10% to 20%	10% to 20%
Calories/day	<2000 kcal/day	>2000 kcal/day

and other GI disorders or in patients with pancreatitis. These products are available without a prescription, have no pregnancy category, and are contraindicated only if a patient has had a hypersensitivity reaction to them. They are available in liquid formulations only.

protein formulation

Casec, Promod, and Propac are examples of protein modular formulations They are used to increase and provide additional proteins to enhance patients' protein intake. They are derived from a variety of sources such as whey caseine, egg whites, and amino acids. All of the available products are dried powders that have to be reconstituted with water. They may sometimes be reconstituted by placing them in enteral feedings that are already in liquid form. They are indicated in patients with increased protein needs. They are contraindicated in patients who have had hypersensitivity reactions to them. Protein formulation supplements are available without a prescription and have no pregnancy category.

ALTERED AMINO ACID FORMULATIONS

Amin-Aid is one of the many amino acid formulation nutritional supplements available. Many of the nutritional supplements in this category are also listed as modular formulations because they can be used as both single-nutrient formulas and as nutrition formulations for patients with genetic errors of metabolism. Amino acid formulations are used most commonly in patients who have metabolic disorders such as phenylketonuria, homocystinuria, and maple syrup urine disease. They are also used to supply nutritional support to patients with such illnesses as renal impairment, eclampsia, congestive heart failure (CHF), or liver failure.

PARENTERAL NUTRITION

Parenteral nutritional supplementation (IV administration) is the preferred method for patients who are unable to tolerate and maintain adequate enteral or oral intake. Instead of administering partially digested nutrients into the GI tract, totally digested vitamins, minerals, amino acids, dextrose, and so on are administered intravenously directly into the circulatory system. This effectively bypasses the entire GI system, eliminating the need for absorption, metabolism, and excretion. Parenteral nutrition is also called **total parenteral nutrition** (TPN) or **hyperalimentation.**

TPN can supply all the calories, carbohydrates, amino acids, fats, trace elements, and other essential nutrients needed for growth, weight gain, wound healing, convalescence, immunocompetence, and other health-sustaining functions.

Parenteral nutrition can be administered either through a peripheral vein or a central vein. Each route of delivery of parenteral nutrition has specific requirements and limitations. It is generally accepted that parenteral nutrition should be considered only when oral or enteral support is impossible or when the GI absorptive or functional capacity is not sufficient to meet the nutritional needs of the patient. Some of the conditions that must be considered in the decision to place a patient on peripheral versus central hyperalimentation are listed in Table 51-1.

Activity

PERIPHERAL TPN

Peripheral TPN is one route of administration of parenteral nutrition. A peripheral vein is used to deliver nutrients to the patient's circulatory system. It is usually a temporary method of administration. The long-term administration of nutritional supplements via a peripheral vein may lead to phlebitis and ultimately the loss of a limb. There is a variety of indications for peripheral TPN. Peripheral TPN should be considered a temporary measure to provide adequate nutrient needs in patients with mild deficits or who are restricted from oral intake and have slightly elevated metabolic rates.

Peripheral TPN is most valuable in patients who do not have large nutritional needs, can tolerate moderately large fluid loads, and need nutritional supplements only temporarily. Peripheral TPN may be used alone or in combination with oral nutritional supplements to provide the necessary fat, carbohydrate, and protein needed by the patient to maintain health.

Mechanism of Action

Peripheral TPN provides the basic building blocks for anabolism. Different combinations and amounts of these agents are used based on the individual patient's anabolic needs. After the body receives these nutrients, it must process them into living matter.

Drug Effects

Peripheral TPN is used to administer nutrients to patients who need more nutrients than present oral intake can provide or to provide entire daily nutrition. Peripheral TPN is meant only as a temporary means (less than 2 weeks) of delivering TPN.

Therapeutic Uses

Conditions in which patients may benefit from the delivery of peripheral TPN are as follows:
- Procedures that restrict oral feedings
- Anorexia caused by radiation or cancer chemotherapy
- GI illnesses that prevent oral food ingestion
- After any type of surgery
- When nutritional deficits are minimal, but oral nutrition will not be started for more than 5 days

Side Effects and Adverse Effects

The most devastating adverse effect of peripheral TPN is phlebitis, which is a vein irritation or inflammation of a

vein. If severe enough and not treated appropriately, phlebitis can lead to the loss of a limb. However, this is rare. Another potential adverse effect is fluid overload. Peripheral TPN is limited to lower dextrose-concentrated solutions, generally less than 10%, to avoid sclerosing vein. Larger amounts of nutritional supplements are needed with lower concentrated solutions to meet a patient's daily nutritional requirements. Some patients, such as those with renal failure or CHF, cannot tolerate large fluid volume. In these patients peripheral TPN may be contraindicated or used cautiously only if absolutely necessary.

Dosages

Dosage requirements vary from patient to patient. Age, gender, weight, and numerous other factors must be considered for proper administration of TPN. Guidelines for amino acids appear in Table 51-2.

drug profiles

The individual components of peripheral and central TPN are the same. The difference lies in the concentrations and amounts of the components delivered per volume of nutritional supplement. The four basic components of peripheral or central TPN are amino acid, carbohydrate, lipid, and trace elements and electrolytes. Most of the electrolyte components are discussed in Chapter 25.

AMINO ACIDS

Amino acids have many roles in the maintenance of normal nutritional status. The primary role is protein production, or **anabolism.** Adequate amino acids in nutritional supplements reduce the breakdown of proteins **(catabolism)** and also help promote normal growth and wound healing.

Amino acids are commonly classified as essential or nonessential according to whether they can or cannot be produced by the body. **Nonessential amino acids** are those that the body produces and are therefore not needed in dietary intake. The body

Table 51-2 Amino Acids: Recommended Dosage Guidelines

Healthy		Undernourished or Traumatized
Adult	Infant/Child	
0.9 g/kg	1.4 to 2.2 g/kg	3 g/kg or more

Box 51-4 Amino Acids: Classification

ESSENTIAL	NONESSENTIAL	SEMIESSENTIAL
Isoleucine	Alanine	Arginine
Leucine	Asparagine	Histidine
Lysine	Aspartic acid	
Methionine	Cysteine	
Phenylalanine	Glutamine	
Threonine	Glutamic acid	
Tryptophan	Glycine	
Valine	Proline	
	Serine	
	Tyrosine	

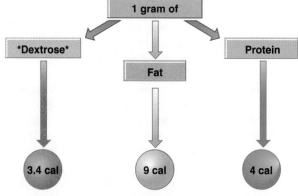

Fig. 51-2 One gram of dextrose, fat, or protein will provide varying amounts of energy as calories.

is able to manufacture from nitrogen sources all but eight of the available amino acids. **Essential amino acids** are those amino acids that cannot be produced by the body. Therefore they must be included in daily dietary intake. Amino acids are used as building blocks for protein that is needed for normal growth and development. Two amino acids, histidine and arginine, are not manufactured by the body in large enough quantities during rapid growth periods such as infancy or childhood. Thus they are referred to as **semiessential amino acids.** Box 51-4 lists the amino acids according to their categories.

amino acids

Amino acid crystalline solutions (Aminosyn 3%, 5%, and 10% and Free-Amine III 8.5% and 10%) can be used in either peripheral or central hyperalimentation. The two currently available amino acid solutions differ only in their respective concentrations. These drugs have no restrictions regarding pregnancy and have no contraindications to use. The dosage of these solutions varies depending on the patient's weight and requirements. Recommended dosages for healthy and traumatized patients are listed in Table 51-2.

carbohydrates

In nutritional support, carbohydrates are usually supplied to patients through dextrose. Under normal circumstances both carbohydrates and lipids are used as calorie sources (Fig. 51-2). Concentrations of dextrose in TPN are important considerations. In peripheral TPN, dextrose concentrations are kept below 10% to decrease the possibility of phlebitis. In central TPN, dextrose concentrations can range from 10% to 50% but are commonly 25% to 35%. Because dextrose is a sugar, supplemental insulin may be given simultaneously in nutritional supplements. A balanced nutritional supplement that contains dextrose and lipids for caloric sources decreases the need for large amounts of insulin.

fats

The average North American diet consists of 40% fat. The ideal diet should contain 30% fat. Of the total calories supplied, 40% to 50% of the calories are obtained through fat grams. Intravenous fat emulsions serve two functions: they supply essential

fatty acids and they are a source of energy or calories. As with the amino acids, certain fatty acids are essential because the body cannot produce them. Linoleic acid cannot be synthesized by the body. It is needed to produce linolenic and arachidonic acid. If these fatty acids are not present in dietary or nutritional supplements, an essential fatty acid deficiency may develop. Clinical signs of **essential fatty acid deficiency** are hair loss, scaly dermatitis, growth retardation, reduced wound healing, decreased platelets, and fatty liver (Fig. 51-3).

lipid emulsions

The currently available lipid emulsions, Intralipid and Liposyn, are available as either 10% or 20% emulsions. They differ in fat origin. Liposyn is made from safflower oil, and Intralipid is made from soybean oil (Fig. 51-4).

Fat emulsions should be calibrated to deliver no more than 60% of the total daily caloric intake. Fat emulsions are beneficial when combined with dextrose solutions. The use of fat to meet caloric needs prevents potentially harmful conditions, such as hyperglycemia, hyperinsulinemia, and hyperosmolarity, that can occur when a patient's entire caloric needs are being met solely by dextrose. A normal diet should contain 30% fat, 40% protein, and 30% carbohydrate.

Activity

TRACE ELEMENTS

Trace element solutions are available individually or in many different combinations. The following are considered trace elements:
- Zinc
- Chromium
- Copper

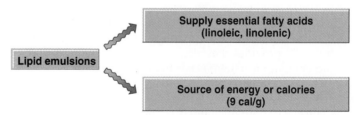

Fig. 51-3 Lipid emulsions supply essential fatty acids and energy.

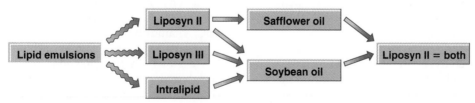

Fig. 51-4 Liposyn II is made from safflower oil and soybean oil; Intralipid and Liposyn III are made from soybean oil.

Trace Element Formulations

BOX 51-5

TRACE ELEMENT COMBINATIONS	TRACE ELEMENTS WITH ELECTROLYTES (SMALL VOLUME)
M.T.E. 4	Tracelyte
M.T.E. 5	Tracelyte
M.T.E. 6	(with double electrolytes)
Others	

- Selenium
- Manganese
- Iodine
- Molybdenum

Other combination trace element formulations are listed in Box 51-5. Specific dosages and frequencies depend on the individual patient's requirements. Vitamins and minerals may also be added accordingly. A common multivitamin combination is **multivitamin infusion (MVI).**

CENTRAL TPN

In central TPN a large central vein is used to deliver nutrients directly into the patient's circulation. Usually the subclavian or internal jugular vein is used. Central TPN is generally indicated for patients who require nutritional supplements for prolonged periods of time, usually more than 7 to 10 days. It can also be used in the home care setting. There is a variety of indications for central TPN. The disadvantages of central TPN are the risks associated with insertion, use, and maintenance of the central vein. There is a greater potential for infection, more serious catheter-induced trauma and related events, metabolic alterations, and other technical or mechanical problems than with TPN.

Central TPN works by delivering essential nutrients directly into the circulation via a central vein. It is most valuable in patients who have large nutritional needs, who cannot tolerate large fluid loads, and who need nutritional supplements for prolonged periods of time. Central TPN provides the necessary fat, carbohydrate, and protein that the patient needs to maintain health.

Mechanism of Action

Central TPN provides the basic building blocks for anabolism. Different combinations and amounts of these agents are used based on the individual patient's anabolic needs. After the body receives these nutrients, it must process them into living matter.

Drug Effects

Central TPN is used to supply nutrients to patients who cannot ingest nutrients by mouth and cannot meet required daily nutritional needs by the enteral or peripheral parenteral routes. Central TPN can safely provide nutritional needs for extended periods of time.

Therapeutic Uses

Central TPN delivers total dietary nutrients to patients who require nutritional supplementation. Patients who may benefit from the delivery of central TPN include the following:
- Patients having large nutritional requirements (metabolic stress or hypermetabolism)
- Patients needing nutritional support for prolonged periods (more than 7 to 10 days)

Side Effects and Adverse Effects

The most common side effects and adverse effects of central TPN are those surrounding the use of the central vein for delivery of the TPN. The risks associated with insertion of the infusion line, as well as the use and maintenance of the central vein for administration of TPN, can create some complications. There is a greater potential for infection, more serious catheter-induced trauma and related events, and other technical or mechanical problems than with peripheral TPN. There are larger and more concentrated volumes of nutritional supplements being delivered with central TPN and therefore a greater chance for metabolic complications such as hyperglycemia.

Dosages

Administration is individualized according to patient needs.

Activity

---

drug profiles

The same formulations used in peripheral TPN are used in central TPN. Often the concentrations of fluids administered through the central vein are much higher than those used in peripheral nutrition supplements. Besides these minor differences the nutritional supplements used are identical.

---

nursing process

● Assessment

The nurse should conduct a thorough nutritional assessment with a dietary history, weekly and daily food intakes, and weight and height before any nutritional supplementation. Consultation with a registered dietician is crucial to identification of the nutrients that are missing in a particular patient's diet. After an assessment, the physician may need to be contacted about the need for a consult on either an inpatient or outpatient basis. Laboratory studies including total protein, albumin, BUN, RBC, WBC, vitamin B_{12}, cholesterol, and Hgb will be needed. Other laboratory studies may include cholesterol, electrolytes, total lymphocyte count, serum transferrin, iron levels, urine creatinine clearance, lipid profile, and urinalysis (to assess protein loss). Anthropometric measurements and weights also provide much-needed data. The data collected will help the physician and other members

NURSING CARE PLAN | Total Parenteral Nutrition

Ms. J.D. is about to receive TPN with fat emulsions of Intralipid 10% for management of weight loss and cachexia related to long-term treatment of breast cancer. This is her first treatment with TPN, and she has many questions, expecially about the "fat emulsions." She asks, "Are these safe to go into my circulation?" and "Are you sure these won't hurt me?"

assessment	**Nursing Diagnosis**	Deficient knowledge (teaching) related to new experience with treatment regimen
	Subjective Data	Patient reports the following: • Weight loss >10 lb in 3 wk • Decreased appetite and energy • Increased fatigue
	Objective Data	Diagnosis of breast cancer Treatment with chemotherapy (long-term) Weight loss
planning and outcome criteria	**Goals**	Patient will verbalize understanding of purpose of TPN— especially Intralipid therapy—by the end of one treatment.
	Outcome Criteria	Before the end of the infusion, patient will do the following: • State the purpose of Intralipid treatment • Verbalize the side effects of the treatment • State the therapeutic benefit of treatment with Intralipid
implementation		Patient education will include the following information about Intralipid 10%: • The action of this fat emulsion is that it provides neutral triglycerides, primarily unsaturated fatty acids, that are needed for energy and heat production. • It is used for increasing caloric intake and to prevent fatty acid deficiency. • Side effects that may occur include headache, drowsiness, nausea, vomiting, high lipid levels, dyspnea, and altered liver function. • The therapeutic effects of this treatment include higher fatty acid levels, weight gain, and more energy.
evaluation		Positive therapeutic outcomes include the following: • Increase in weight • Fatty acids at adequate levels • Increased energy levels

of the health care team select the appropriate nutritional supplements for the patient.

Before beginning enteral nutritional supplements of elemental formulation, such as Vivonex, it must be determined if the patient has a history of allergic reaction to its contents. Polymeric formulations, such as Ensure, are contraindicated in patients with a hypersensitivity to any of its ingredients. Modular formulations such as Centrality, fat formulations such as Microlipid, and protein formulations such as Hepatic-Aid are also contraindicated in patients with known hypersensitivity. Altered amino acid formulas are contraindicated in patients who have a known hypersensitivity to the formulation. Enteral feedings are generally contraindicated in patients who are capable of oral intake or who have intestinal obstruction, severe vomiting, or esophageal fistulas.

Casec, Promod, and Propac are protein formulations that are reconstituted with water for enteral feedings. They are contraindicated in patients with allergies to whey, egg whites, and the product.

● Nursing Diagnoses

Nursing diagnoses appropriate for the patient receiving enteral or parenteral nutritional supplementation are as follows:
• Diarrhea related to the enteral feedings.
• Ineffective airway clearance related to possible aspiration of enteral feedings.
• Deficient fluid volume related to nutritional status.
• Risk for infection related to parenteral infusions and the break in skin integrity.
• Ineffective individual therapeutic management related to lack of information.

● Planning

Goals related to nutritional supplements are as follows:
• Patient remains free of complications associated with enteral feedings.
• Patient regains near-normal to normal bowel patterns.
• Patient remains free of injury during nutritional support.
• Patient remains free of infection.

- Patient regains normal fluid volume status.
- Patient remains compliant and makes return visits to the physician as needed.

Outcome Criteria

Outcome criteria are as follows:
- Patient (or caregiver) will state method of administration of enteral feedings through the tube feedings and subsequent nursing care, such as checking enteral tube placement.
- Patient will identify measures to decrease diarrhea such as use of drug and nondrug therapies.
- Patient (or caregiver) will demonstrate adequate technique for enteral tube feedings to decrease risk of aspiration with emphasis on elevated head of bed and checking tube placement.
- Patient will state measures to minimize risk of infection at TPN site such as making sure site is changed as ordered and assessed for redness, swelling, or drainage.
- Patient will begin to show adequate fluid volume status with improved turgor, improved urinary output, and a return to normal lab values.
- Patient will state symptoms to report to the physician such as increased lethargy, fever, shortness of breath, etc.

● Implementation

In general, monitoring the status of the patient during and after enteral feedings is crucial to safe and prudent nursing care. Tinting tube feedings with blue food coloring helps assist the nurse in detection of aspiration in the tube-feeding substance. Gastric residual volumes should be obtained and documented before each feeding and before each medication is administered. Stop the tube feeding and aspirate stomach contents to detect any residual. If the volume is more than that from 2 hours of continuous feeding, return the aspirate, hold the feeding, and contact the physician.

For intermittent bolus feedings, if the residual amount is greater than 50% of the volume previously infused, return the aspirate, withhold the feeding, and contact the physician. Reduced feeding volume will probably be ordered by the physician. Always remember that the head of the bed should remain elevated during tube feedings to decrease the risk of aspiration. The process of tube feedings is presented in Chapter 8.

Newer tubes for nasogastric and enteral feeding are less thick and hard and are thinner (Nos. 5 through 10 French) and more pliable for better patient tolerance. However, the smaller-diameter tubes make checking for gastric aspiration more difficult. If the attempt is unsuccessful, instill air and auscultate over the gastric area. Air sound in the stomach denotes accurate placement. Place the end of the tube in water to test for air bubbles, which signify incorrect placement.

To prevent clogging of the feeding tube with formula, it is often helpful to flush the tube with 30 ml of cranberry juice (per policy) followed by 10 ml of water. The juice may help break up the formula residue and unclog certain tubes.

Physician-ordered enteral feeding infusion rates and concentration should be followed carefully. Usually the initial rate is 50 ml/hr at one-half strength but can be increased per patient tolerance to a rate of 25 ml/hr at three-fourth strength concentration. Although more rapid feeding increases the risk of hyperglycemia or dumping syndrome, nurses should continue to increase the patient's intake because 1000 ml to 2000 ml of the milk-based formula (1 kcal/ml) is needed to provide adequate calories and recommended daily allowances (RDAs) for vitamins and minerals. Tube-feeding formulas should always be at room temperature. If all the necessary steps to decrease or prevent diarrhea have failed, antidiarrheal medications may be needed.

Lactose-free solutions are also available and should be used when individuals are lactose intolerant. Patients who suffer from this condition experience cramping, diarrhea, abdominal bloating, and flatulence with the ingestion of lactose.

Infusions of TPN should be assessed every hour. The entire system as well as the condition of the patient should be included in this assessment. It is good practice to examine the patient first and then check the TPN insertion site and the tubing at the site of connection to the infusion pump. Patency should be assessed every hour as well.

Tubing should be changed every 24 hours to prevent infection. It is recommended that tubing changes occur daily with the beginning of each new infusion. A 0.22-μm filter is used to trap bacteria, including *Pseudomonas* species. The patient's temperature should be recorded every 4 hours. Any increased temperature should be reported to the physician immediately because it may be the first sign of infection. The patient should also be checked frequently for signs and symptoms of hyperglycemia, such as headache, dehydration, and weakness. IV rates should never be accelerated to increase reduced volume because this may precipitate hyperglycemia. Insulin replacement may be needed, so glucometer readings are important for immediate recognition and treatment of hyperglycemia.

Hypoglycemia is manifested by cold, clammy skin, dizziness, tachycardia, and tingling of the extremities. Hypoglycemia associated with TPN may be prevented by gradual reduction of the IV rate to allow the pancreas time to adapt to the changing blood glucose levels. If TPN is discontinued abruptly, rebound hypoglycemia may occur. This can be prevented with infusion of 5% to 10% glucose in situations in which TPN must be discontinued immediately.

Fluid overload may occur with TPN, manifested by weak pulse, hypertension, tachycardia, confusion, decreased urine output, and pitting edema. This can be prevented by maintaining IV rates and assessing the IV infusion every hour. If signs of overload occur, the nurse should slow the infusion rate, remain with the patient, and contact the physician immediately. A continual assessment of the patient and vital signs is also necessary at this time.

Patient teaching tips for nutritional supplements are found in the box below.

● Evaluation

Therapeutic responses to nutritional supplementation include improved well-being, energy, strength, and performance of activities of daily living; an increase in weight; and laboratory studies that reflect a more positive nutritional status. Besides evaluation of outcome criteria, evaluation of the patient and family input and participation in care are important because the patient should always be encouraged to participate in the planning and evaluation of care.

Activity

---

patient teaching tips

Nutritional Supplements

➤ Because patients often go home with tube feedings, the patient and family should begin preparation for this procedure at least 1 week before discharge. Individualized patient teaching about the procedure and care of the tube requires at least 6 hours. More instructional time is needed if the tube is to be inserted and removed at night only.

➤ Incorrect placement is characterized by coughing, choking, difficulty in speaking, and cyanosis.

➤ The patient should have written and verbal instructions. Ross Laboratories (Tel: 800-227-5767) is an excellent contact for questions and explanations.

➤ Physician phone numbers and those for other resources should be kept at the patient's home for immediate use when needed.

➤ The physician should be contacted if diarrhea, nausea, vomiting, fever, or any other unusual symptoms occur.

➤ Patients on home parenteral nutrition will need some support from home health care. Practice is critical to acquisition of skill by the patient and family. All procedures for storage; cleansing of site; care of site; dressing changes; irrigation of the catheter; pump function and care; and changing of the bag, filters, and tubing should also be demonstrated and practiced well before the patient is discharged.

➤ Patients on TPN should be weighed daily at the same time wearing the same clothing. Intake and output volumes should be noted and recorded.

➤ Glucose levels should be checked at home. Procedures for use of glucometers and periodically checking urine glucose should be demonstrated and practiced.

➤ Potential complications of TPN are manifested by fever, cough, chest pains, dyspnea, and chills and may indicate adverse reactions to lipid infusions. Chest pain and coughing may indicate air embolism. Restlessness, nervousness, fainting, and tachycardia are associated with hypoglycemia. Nausea, vomiting, polyuria, polydipsia, and elevated glucose levels may indicate hyperglycemia. If any of these occur, the patient should discontinue the infusion and contact the physician immediately.

POINTS TO REMEMBER

Nursing Considerations

● A thorough nutritional assessment and possible consultation with a registered dietitian or nutritionist are essential for adequate intervention for the malnourished patient.

● There are various enteral feedings with different nutritional content, including some that are lactose free.

● Enteral feedings may result in complications such as hyperglycemia, dumping syndrome, and aspiration of feeding.

● Parenteral nutrition is often administered through a central vein catheter because of the hyperosmolarity of substances used.

● Parenteral feedings may result in air embolism, hyperglycemia, or hypoglycemia. If discontinued abruptly, infection and fluid volume overload may result.

● Cautious and astute nursing care with enteral or parenteral nutritional supplementation may prevent or decrease the occurrence of associated complications.

REVIEW QUESTIONS

1. What would occur if a patient who had been receiving TPN was suddenly taken off the infusion after several days of therapy?
   a. Dysphagia
   b. Hyperkalemia
   c. Fluid overload
   d. Rebound hypoglycemia

2. Which of the following supplements provides the best overall enteral nutrition?
   a. Ensure
   b. Lonalac
   c. Vital HN
   d. Stresstein

3. TPN is associated with which of the following adverse effects?
   a. Hyperglycemia
   b. Fluid hydration
   c. GI hypoperistalsis
   d. Dumping syndrome
4. One of your patients is a newly diagnosed cancer patient who is scheduled to have radiation and chemotherapy. What type of therapy may be ordered to help with the anticipated severe anorexia and the extra nutritional support she may need?

   a. Peripheral TPN with 15% glucose
   b. Oral Ensure qid and at hour of sleep
   c. Nasogastric tube feedings around the clock
   d. Parenteral TPN, especially if a central line is present
5. Which of the following is the most common side effect from nutritional supplementation?
   a. Diarrhea
   b. GI bleeding
   c. Polymalagia
   d. Diabetes insipidus

For Answers see www.harcourthealth.com/MERLIN/Lilley/.

CRITICAL THINKING Activities

1. Which nursing actions will help address the nursing diagnosis of diarrhea or diarrhea as related to enteral feedings?

2. What outcome criteria will address the nursing diagnosis of fluid volume deficit related to nutritional deficit?
3. What is the concern for abrupt withdrawal of a 10% glucose TPN solution? Explain your answer.

For Answers see www.harcourthealth.com/MERLIN/Lilley/.

bibliography

Albanese J, Nutz P: *Mosby's 2001 nursing drug reference and review cards,* St Louis, 2001, Mosby.

Anderson PO, Knoben JE, Troutman WG: *Handbook of clinical drug data 1999-2000,* ed 9, New York, 1999, McGraw-Hill.

Heinburger DC: *Handbook of clinical nutrition,* ed 3, St Louis, 1997, Mosby.

Johns Hopkins Hospital, Department of Pediatrics et al: *The Harriet Lane handbook,* ed 15, St Louis, 2000, Mosby.

Keen JH: *Critical care and emergency drug reference,* ed 3, St Louis, 1996, Mosby.

McEvoy GK: *AHFS drug information,* Bethesda, Md, 1998, American Society of Hospital Pharmacists.

Mosby's GenRx: a comprehensive reference for generic and brand drugs, ed 10, St Louis, 2000, Mosby.

Skidmore-Roth L: *Mosby's 2001 nursing drug reference,* St Louis, 2001, Mosby.

Activity

Remember to check the **Online Worksheet** for additional learning opportunities: **www.harcourthealth.com/MERLIN/Lilley/**

Miscellaneous Therapeutics: Hematologic, Dermatologic, Ophthalmic, and Otic Agents: Study Skills Tips

- Time Management
- PURR
- Repeat the Steps

TIME MANAGEMENT

As you plan your study time for Part Ten, it should be very clear that Chapter 54 will take significantly more time to complete than the other chapters. Do not let the length of the chapter overwhelm you. Apply the principles of time management to this chapter and you will succeed. The most important aspect of time management to apply to this chapter is the use of clear goal statements and action plan steps to help you achieve the goals.

Goal Statements

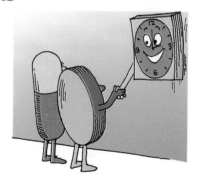

Remember the criteria for goal statements. First, they must be realistic. The statements must be things you know you can accomplish. Second, they must be specific to the task. "I will study the chapter" is not a very specific goal. Specify what you expect to accomplish. "I will master the 24 terms in the chapter glossary" is a more specific goal statement. Third, there must be a time limit. How long will you spend in achieving this goal? Set a time limit for the completion of each activity for the quantity of time to be spent in each learning activity. Finally, goal statements must be measurable. In the example about studying the glossary, including the number of terms contained in Chapter 54 helps clarify the goal.

Action Planning

The second segment of time management is the use of action planning. An action plan is a series of smaller, specific activities that you will accomplish to meet your goal statements. Your goal is to master the 24 terms. What will you do to meet that goal?

Action Steps Example

1. I will spend 1 hour making vocabulary drill cards for the terms found in the glossary in Chapter 54 from 3:00 to 4:00 PM on Monday.
2. I will spend 15 minutes in rehearsal and review of these cards every day until the exam on this chapter is over.
3. Each time I cannot define and explain a term I will put an "x" on the card to identify it as a term needing more review.
4. I will spend 1 hour the night before the exam doing a comprehensive review of the terms in Chapter 54, with special emphasis on those cards that have one or more x marks.

Action steps help ensure that you are spending your study time actively focusing on what you need to learn.

PURR
Prepare Example

Chapter 54, Objective 4: "Discuss the mechanisms of action, cautions, side effects, and contraindications of ophthalmic preparations and associated nursing implications."
- Question 1. What does *ophthalmic* mean? (Literal question [LQ])

- Question 2. What are ophthalmic preparations? (LQ)
- Question 3. What is the mechanism of action of ophthalmic preparations? (LQ)
- Question 4. Is there more than one mechanism of action? (LQ)
- Question 5. If there is more than one mechanism of action, how are the mechanisms similar and how are they different? (Interpretive Question)

These questions are only suggestions of generated questions based on the chapter objectives. Many more questions can be asked about Objective 4. These questions are an essential part of the study process. Questions help make you an active reader and an active learner. The more questions you generate the easier it will be to understand the chapter.

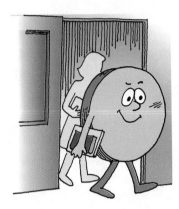

Outline Example

1. *Looking through the chapter, decide how much material is appropriate.* The section that begins with "Antiglaucoma Drugs" is probably too much material. Looking at the chapter headings, this section could be broken down into five blocks of material. Block one would cover the material under the heading "Parasympathomimetics." Block two would be the material under the heading "Sympathomimetics." The next three blocks would be "Beta-adrenergic blockers," "Carbonic anhydrase inhibitors," and "Osmotic diuretics."

2. *Apply the Prepare step to each block.* Beginning with "Parasympathomimetics," generate some questions to guide your reading. Remember that it is important to ask questions that will focus on both literal information and questions that will help you interpret, evaluate, and analyze when you read.

3. *Read the material.* As soon as you have completed the self-questioning over the first block of material, read the material in the chapter. It is important that the reading be done immediately. Read for understanding, and as you read remember the questions you generated. This approach will help your concentration and comprehension.

4. *Take a short break.* Once you have completed the reading of this section of the chapter, give your mind a chance to reflect and consolidate the learning. Limit the time you allow for a break and use the time for something pleasurable. Give yourself 5 or 10 minutes to read the newspaper, get a snack, or just take a short walk.

5. *Rehearse.* Before going on to the next section of the chapter it is important to spend a few minutes in rehearsal. Using the questions from Step 2, go back over the material you read and try to respond to those questions. When you find yourself unable to answer a question, put a mark in the text beside the heading that caused the difficulty and move on. The mark will serve as a reminder for future review. At this point, the objective is not complete mastery of the material. The objective is to see what you have learned so that you can move smoothly into the next section. Breaking a chapter into blocks is useful, but it is imperative that the links between sections be made as you study.

6. *Review.* After completing two or three major sections of the chapter, it is time to review. Start at the beginning of the chapter. Ask your questions. Try to answer them. If you cannot formulate a clear answer, then some rereading is necessary. Also, pay attention to the marks made during the rehearsal step. Those marks indicate areas that you have already identified as needing review. When rereading, remember that the object is to read only as much of the material as needed to be able to respond to self-generated questions. There simply is not enough time to read the entire chapter a second or third time.

REPEAT THE STEPS

Prepare, read for understanding, take a short break, and then rehearse the material just read. It may seem that this process takes an excessive amount of time and involves a lot of repetition, but in the long run this process will produce better learning. The time spent in Prepare, Understand, and Rehearsal will reduce the time needed to review. Frequent review as you move through the chapter will make the final review at exam time proceed more quickly and enable you to achieve mastery of the material.

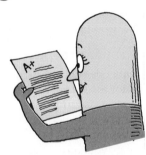

Chapter 52

Blood-Forming Agents

www.harcourthealth.com/MERLIN/Lilley/

objectives

When you reach the end of this chapter, you should be able to do the following:

1 Discuss the importance of iron, vitamin B$_{12}$, and folic acid.

2 Discuss the various conditions when blood-forming agents may be indicated.

3 Discuss the mechanisms of action, cautions, contraindications, uses, dosages, special administration techniques, and measures to enhance the effectiveness of and and decrease side effects related to the various blood-forming agents.

4 Develop a comprehensive nursing care plan that includes all phases of the nursing process related to the administration of blood-forming agents.

Look for this symbol for topics covered in the **Online Worksheet**

drug profiles

ferrous fumarate, p. 834
folic acid, p. 836
○━ **iron dextran,** p. 835

○━ Key drug.

glossary

Cytoplasmic maturation (si′ to plaz′ mik \ mach′ u ra′ shən) A type of defect that accounts for anemias secondary to maturation defects. (p. 832)

Erythrocyte (ə rith′ ro sit) Another name for red blood cell. (p. 831)

Erythropoiesis (ə rith′ ro poi e′ sis) The process of erythrocyte production involving the maturation of a nucleated precursor into a hemoglobin-filled, nucleus-free erythrocyte that is regulated by erythropoietin, a hormone produced by the kidney. (p. 836)

Fragmented (frag′ mənt ed) Composed of and resembling fragments or pieces. (p. 832)

Globin (glo′ bin) A protein chain of which there are four structural different chains: alpha-1 and alpha-2 and beta-1 and beta-2. (p. 832)

Hematopoeisis (hem′ ə to poi e′ sis) The normal formation and development of all blood cell types in the bone marrow. (p. 831)

Heme (hem) The pigmented, iron-containing, nonprotein portion of the hemoglobin molecule. (p. 832)

Hemoglobin (he′ mo glo′ ben) A complex protein-iron compound in the blood that carries oxygen to the cells from the lungs and carbon dioxide away from the cells to the lungs. (p. 832)

Hypochromic (hi′ po kro′ mik) Pertaining to less than normal color. The term usually describes a red blood cell and helps further characterize anemias associated with decreased synthesis of hemoglobin. (p. 832)

Microcytic (mi krə ′sit ik) Pertaining to smaller-than-normal cells. (p. 832)

Pernicious anemia (pər nish′ əs ə nē mē ə) A blood disorder characterized by a low number of RBCs. (p. 836)

Reticulocytes (rə tik′ u lo sitz′) An immature erythrocyte characterized by a meshlike pattern of threads and particles at the former site of the nucleus. (p. 831)

Spherocytes (sfer o′ sitz) Small, globular, completely hemoglobinated erythrocytes without the usual central pallor. (p. 832)

HEMATOPOIESIS

The formation of new blood cells is one of the primary functions of bones. Bones are also responsible for support, protection, movement, and mineral storage. They provide a framework for the body that acts as a support and also serves to protect delicate internal organs. Bones in coordination with muscles help the body move, and major reservoirs of minerals, such as calcium and phosphorus, are stored in bone. However, the process of red blood cell (RBC), or **erythrocyte,** formation is the focus of this chapter. **Hematopoiesis,** the process of blood cell formation (RBCs, WBCs, and platelets), takes place in the myeloid tissue. This specialized tissue is located primarily in the ends or epiphyses of certain long bones, in the flat bones of the skull, in the pelvis, and in the sternum and ribs.

When RBCs are manufactured in the bone marrow by myeloid tissue, they are released into the circulation as immature RBCs called **reticulocytes.** Once in the circulation, reticulocytes undergo a 24- to 36-hour maturation process to become mature, fully functional RBCs. Once in the circulation they have a life span of about 120 days.

It is important to know the structural components of the RBC in order to understand how anemia develops and why certain drugs are used to correct it. Over one-third of an RBC is made of **hemoglobin.** Hemoglobin is composed of two parts heme and globin. **Heme** is a red pigment; each molecule of heme contains one atom of iron. **Globin** is a protein chain that consists of four structurally different parts or globulins: alpha$_1$ and alpha$_2$ and beta$_1$ and beta$_2$ ($\alpha_1 + \alpha_2$ and $\beta_1 + \beta_2$). Together one molecule of heme and one protein chain of globin make one hemoglobin molecule (Fig. 52-1).

TYPES OF ANEMIA

Anemias are classified into four main types based on underlying causes. Knowledge of the etiologies of anemias will help you to understand the therapies used to treat them. Anemias can be caused by maturation defects, or they can be secondary to increased destruction. Two types of maturation defects cause anemias: cytoplasmic maturation defects and nuclear maturation defects. Factors responsible for increased destruction can be either intrinsic or extrinsic (Fig. 52-2). Some common causes of iron-deficiency anemia are blood loss, surgery, childbirth, GI bleeding, and hemorrhoids.

RBCs in anemias associated with **cytoplasmic maturation** defects appear **hypochromic** (lighter red than normal) and **microcytic** (smaller than normal) on blood smear. All cytoplasmic maturation anemias occur as a result of abnormal hemoglobin synthesis. Since hemoglobin is synthesized from both iron and globin, a deficiency in either one can lead to a hemoglobin deficiency (Fig. 52-3).

Anemias associated with immature RBC nuclear maturation defects occur secondary to defects in DNA or protein synthesis problems. DNA and protein require vitamin B$_{12}$ and folate to be present in normal amounts for their proper production. If either of these two vitamins is absent or deficient, anemias secondary to nuclear maturation defects may develop (Fig. 52-4). RBCs in such anemias appear to be *normochromic* (normal in color) and *macrocytic* (larger than normal) on blood smear.

Anemias secondary to increased RBC destruction can occur because of abnormalities in the RBCs themselves (intrinsic factors) as a result of factors outside (extrinsic) the RBCs. The erythrocytes in anemias attributable to intrinsic or extrinsic factors have **spherocytes** and appear to be **fragmented** when observed on blood smear. Intrinsic RBC abnormalities are usually the result of a genetic defect. Some examples are sickle cell anemia, hereditary spherocytosis, and glucose-6-phosphate dehydrogenase (G6PD) deficiency. Extrinsic mechanisms for increased RBC destruction are not attributable to abnormalities in the RBC itself. Examples of extrinsic mechanisms are drug-induced antibodies that target and destroy RBCs, septic shock that produces disseminated intravascular coagulation (DIC), and mechanical forces such as intra-aortic balloon pumps and ventricular assist devices that directly damage RBCs (Fig. 52-5).

IRON

Iron is an essential mineral for the proper function of all biologic systems in the body. It is an oxygen carrier in hemoglobin and myoglobin, is used for tissue respiration, and is used in many enzyme reactions in the body. Although iron is stored in many sites throughout the body (liver, spleen, and bone marrow), it is the principal nutritional deficiency in the United States, resulting in anemia. Individuals who require the greatest amount of iron are women, especially pregnant women, and children. They are also the individuals who are most likely to develop iron-deficiency anemia.

Dietary sources for iron are meats and certain vegetables and grains. This form of iron must be converted by

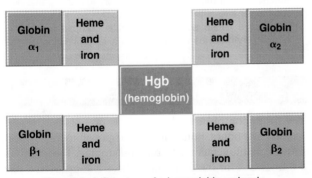

Fig. 52-1 Structure of a hemoglobin molecule.

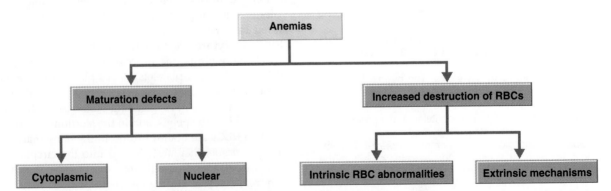

Fig. 52-2 Underlying causes of anemia are maturation defects and factors secondary to increased destruction. *RBC*, Red blood cell.

gastric juices before it can actually be absorbed. Other foods such as orange juice, veal, fish, and ascorbic acid may help with iron absorption. Conversely, eggs, corn, beans, and many cereal products containing phytates may impair iron absorption.

Supplemental iron contained in multivitamins plus iron or iron supplements alone are indicated for the treatment of iron-deficiency anemia. Iron preparations are available as ferrous salts. See Table 52-1 for a list of the currently available iron salts and their respective iron content.

Mechanism of Action

Iron is a required component of a number of enzyme systems in the body and is necessary for energy transfer in the cytochrome oxidase and xanthine oxidase enzyme systems. It is present in hemoglobin and myoglobin,

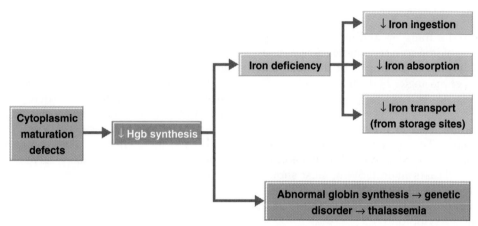

Fig. 52-3 A schematic showing the forms of abnormal hemoglobin synthesis in cytoplasmic maturation anemia.

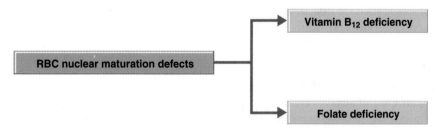

Fig. 52-4 Red blood cell (RBC) nuclear maturation defects occur because of vitamin B$_{12}$ or folate deficiencies.

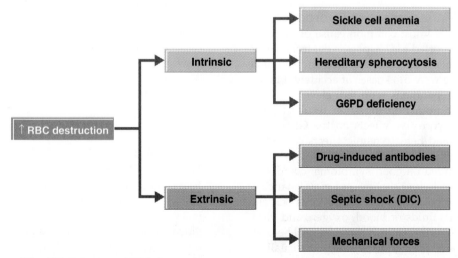

Fig. 52-5 Increased RBC destruction occurs as a result of intrinsic and extrinsic factors.

Table 52-1	Ferrous Salts: Iron Content
Ferrous Salts	**Iron Content**
Ferrous fumarate	33% iron or 330 mg/g
Ferrous gluconate	12% iron or 120 mg/g
Ferrous sulfate	20% iron or 200 mg/g
Ferrous sulfate (dessicated, dried, or exsiccated)	30% iron or 300 mg/g

Table 52-2	Iron Preparations: Adverse Effects
Body System	**Side/Adverse Effect**
Gastrointestinal	Nausea, constipation, epigastric pain, black and red tarry stools, vomiting, diarrhea
Integumentary	Temporarily discolored tooth enamel and eyes, pain upon injection

which are necessary for transport and utilization of oxygen. Administration of iron corrects iron-deficiency states such as anemia, dysphagia, dystrophy of the nails and skin, and fissuring of the angles of the lips.

Drug Effects

Iron preparations are used to prevent and treat iron-deficiency syndromes. The symptoms associated with iron-deficiency anemia can be alleviated by the administration of iron. In all cases an underlying cause should be identified. After identification of the cause, treatment should attempt to correct the cause rather than simply alleviating the symptoms.

Therapeutic Uses

As mentioned previously, iron preparations are used to prevent and treat iron-deficiency syndromes because the agents replenish iron stores needed for RBC development and energy and oxygen transport and utilization. Iron supplementation is also used in epoetin therapy. It is essential for the production of RBCs.

Side Effects and Adverse Effects

The most frequent side effects and adverse effects associated with iron preparations are nausea, vomiting, diarrhea, constipation, stomach cramps, and stomach pain. Excess iron intake can lead to accumulation and iron toxicity. See Table 52-2 for a more complete listing of the undesirable effects seen with iron preparations.

Toxicity and Management of Overdose

Iron overdose is the most common cause of pediatric poisoning deaths reported to U.S. poison control centers. Many iron supplements are enteric coated and resemble candy. In 1991, there were 5144 cases of accidental ingestion of oral iron preparations reported; eleven of these were fatal. Toxicity from iron ingestion results from a combination of the corrosive effects on the GI mucosa and the metabolic and hemodynamic effects caused by the presence of excessive elemental iron.

Treatment is founded on good symptomatic and supportive measures, including suction and maintenance of airway, correction of acidosis, and control of shock and dehydration with IV fluids or blood, oxygen, and vasopressor. Abdominal radiographs may be helpful because iron preparations are radiopaque and may be visualized on x-ray film. Serum iron concentrations may be helpful

in establishing severity of ingestion. A serum iron concentration >300 μg/dl places the patient at serious risk of toxicity. The stomach should be emptied immediately with syrup of ipecac–induced emesis or by lavage. Since many of the iron products are extended-release formulations that release contents in the intestines rather than the stomach, whole gut lavage is generally believed to be superior and more effective. This should be followed by a saline cathartic or possible surgical removal of intake iron tablets. In patients with severe symptoms of iron intoxication such as coma, shock, or seizures, chelation therapy with deferoxamine should be initiated.

Interactions

The absorption of iron can be enhanced when it is given with ascorbic acid or decreased when given with antacids. Iron preparations can decrease the absorption of thyroid drugs, tetracyclines, and quinolone antibiotics.

Dosages

For the recommended dosages of iron preparations, see the dosages table on p. 835.

Activity

drug profiles

Iron preparations are available by prescription and as OTC medications. They are classified as pregnancy category A agents except iron dextran, which is a pregnancy category C agent. They are contraindicated in patients who have shown a hypersensitivity reaction to them. Their use is also contraindicated in patients with ulcerative colitis and regional enteritis, hemosiderosis and hemochromatosis, peptic ulcer disease, hemolytic anemia, cirrhosis, gastritis, and esophagitis. At the initiation of and throughout therapy, hemoglobin and hematocrit should be monitored. These laboratory values, as well as patient's symptomatic response, should help guide therapy.

ferrous fumarate

The ferrous fumarate iron salts (Femiron, Feostat, Hemocyte, and Span-FF) contain the largest amount of iron per gram of salt consumed. Ferrous fumarate is 33% elemental iron. Ferrous sulfate and ferrous gluconate are two other forms of iron that are commonly used. Therefore a 325-mg tablet of ferrous fu-

DOSAGES — Selected Iron Preparations and Folic Acid

agent	pharmacologic class	dosage range	purpose
ferrous fumarate (Femiron, Feostat, Hemocyte, Span-FF)	Oral iron salt	Expressed in mg of elemental iron *Pediatric* PO: 4-6 mg/kg/day in 3 divided doses *Adult* PO: 50-200 mg/bid	Iron deficiency
folic acid	Vitamin B-complex group	*Adult/Pediatric* PO: 0.25-1 mg/day 3-15 mg/day	Folate deficiency Tropical sprue
	Water soluble B-vitamin	*Pediatric/Adult* PO: 0.25 mg to 1 mg daily, until desired hematologic response PO: 100 μg to 1 mg daily, according to individual requirements *Adult* PO: 3 to 15 mg daily PO: 1 mg daily	Deficiency Nutritional supplement Tropical sprue Pregnancy
iron dextran (INFeD)	Parenteral iron salt	Expressed in mg of elemental iron. Dosages must be calculated for each patient according to manufacturer's tables. *Pediatric* IM: <5 kg: 25 mg (0.5 ml)/day <10 kg: 50 mg (1 ml)/day All other patients: 100 mg (2 ml/day)	Iron deficiency when oral iron is unsatisfactory

marate provides 107 mg of elemental iron. Ferrous fumarate is available only as an oral preparation in the following forms: a 325-mg extended-release capsule; a 45-mg/0.6 ml suspension drop and a 100-mg/5 ml suspension; a 60-, 195-, 200-, 300, 324-, and 325-mg tablet; and a 100-mg chewable tablet. Commonly recommended dosages for iron salts are listed in the dosages table above.

PHARMACOKINETICS

HALF-LIFE	ONSET	PEAK	DURATION
6 hr	3-10 days*	Unknown	Variable

*Increased reticulocyte values.

iron dextran

Iron dextran (INFeD) is a colloidal solution of iron (as ferric hydroxide) and dextran. Ferrlecit is another parenteral formulation of iron that has recently been approved for iron-deficiency anemia. It is intended for IV or IM use. Anaphylactic reactions to iron dextran, including fatal anaphylaxis, have been reported in only 0.2% to 0.3% of patients. Because of this, a test dose of 25 mg of iron dextran should be administered by the chosen route and appropriate method of administration before injection. Although anaphylactic reactions usually occur within a few moments after the test dose, it is recommended that a period of at least 1 hour elapse before the remaining portion of the initial dose is given. Individual doses of 2 ml or less may be given on a daily basis until the calculated total amount required has been reached. INFeD is

geriatric considerations

Iron Agents

- Instructions on how to take oral forms of iron are crucial to safe administration. Patients should not make changes in the medication regimen such as doubling doses or discontinuing without a physician's order.
- Elderly patients should be instructed on food sources high in iron and how to include them in their menu planning. Instructions on how to steam vegetables and not overcook foods would also be helpful to ensure that foods do not lose folic acid compounds.
- Patients should be instructed to take oral iron with meals to help buffer and minimize GI distress.
- Encourage elderly patients to use community resources and provide lists to them of resources for meals, such as churches in the community that have elderly care programs or agencies such as Meals on Wheels. This may help improve nutritional intake.

given undiluted at a gradual rate not to exceed 50 mg (1 ml) per minute. Iron dextran is available as a 50 mg/ml parenteral injection for either IV or IM use. Commonly recommended dosages for iron salts are listed in the dosages table above.

PHARMACOKINETICS

HALF-LIFE	ONSET	PEAK	DURATION
5-20 hr	Unknown	IM: 24-48 hr	≤3 wk

FOLIC ACID

Folic acid is a water-soluble B complex vitamin. It is converted to tetrahydrofolic acid in the body, which is then used for normal **erythropoiesis** and to produce nucleoproteins such as DNA and RNA. The human body requires oral intake of folic acid. Dietary sources of folic acid are dried beans, peas, oranges, and green vegetables.

Folic acid is primarily used to prevent and treat folic acid deficiency. Folic acid should not be used to treat anemias until the underlying cause and type of anemia have been determined. The potential risk involved in administering folic acid without first determining the cause is that folic acid will correct the hematologic changes of anemia but mask pernicious anemia symptoms. Pernicious anemia requires specific treatment other than folic acid. If the pernicious anemia is masked, underlying neurologic damage progresses. **Pernicious anemia** is a blood disorder characterized by a low number of RBCs. It is sometimes the result of a dietary deficiency of vitamin B_{12} used in the formation of new RBCs. In many cases, pernicious anemia results from the failure of the stomach lining to produce intrinsic factor. Intrinsic factor allows vitamin B_{12} to be absorbed. Several conditions can lead to folic acid deficiency; however, since folic acid is absorbed in the upper duodenum, malabsorption syndromes are the most common cause of deficiency.

Mechanism of Action

Dietary ingestion of folate is required for the production of nucleoproteins such as DNA and RNA. It is also essential for normal erythropoiesis. Folic acid is not active in the ingested form. It must first be converted to tetrahydrofolic acid, which is a cofactor for reactions in the biosynthesis of purines and thymidylates of nucleic acids.

Drug Effects

Folic acid is used primarily for the treatment of megaloblastic anemia resulting from folate deficiency. It is indicated in the treatment of nutritional macrocytic anemia; megaloblastic anemias of pregnancy, infancy, and childhood; and megaloblastic anemia associated with primary liver disease, alcoholism and alcoholic cirrhosis, intestinal strictures, anastomoses, or tropical sprue. Other types of folate deficiency that may respond to therapy with folic acid are those that result from renal dialysis or the administration of drugs such as phenytoin, primidone, barbiturates, oral contraceptives, or nitrofurantoin. Folic acid may be used in large doses in the treatment of tropical sprue. The prophylactic use of folic acid in the prevention of fetal neural tube defects is another possible use. Currently all prenatal vitamins contain folic acid for this reason.

Therapeutic Uses

Anemias caused by folic acid deficiency can be treated by exogenous supplementation of folic acid. There is also much evidence to support the use of folic acid in the prevention of neural tube defects such as spina bifida, anencephaly, and encephalocele. It is recommended that ad-

ministration begin at least 1 month before pregnancy and through early pregnancy to reduce the risk of fetal neural tube defects. Indications for folic acid are as follows:

- Megaloblastic anemia
- Tropical sprue
- Prophylaxis of neural tube defects

Megaloblastic anemia is most often due to poor dietary intake and is most frequently seen in infancy, childhood, and pregnancy.

Side Effects and Adverse Effects

Side effects and adverse effects associated with folic acid are rare. Allergic reaction or yellow discoloration of urine may occur.

Interactions

No significant drug interactions are reported with folic acid.

Dosages

For recommended dosages of folic acid, see the dosages table on p. 835.

---

drug profiles

Folic acid is a water-soluble B complex vitamin that is used primarily in the treatment and prevention of folic acid deficiency and anemias caused by folic acid deficiency. It is essential in the body for the production of normal RBCs and nucleoproteins such as DNA and RNA.

folic acid

Folic acid is available as an OTC medication in multivitamin preparations and by prescription as a single agent. It is classified as a pregnancy category A agent and is contraindicated in patients who have shown a hypersensitivity reaction to it and in patients with anemias other than megaloblastic/macrocytic anemia, vitamin B_{12} deficiency anemia, and uncorrected pernicious anemia. Folic acid is available as an oral formulation in 0.4-, 0.8-, and 1-mg tablets and as 5- and 10-mg/ml parenteral injections. Commonly recommended dosages for folic acid are listed in the dosages table on p. 835.

PHARMACOKINETICS

HALF-LIFE	ONSET	PEAK	DURATION
Unknown	Unknown	60-90 min	Unknown

OTHER BLOOD-FORMING AGENTS

Other agents that may be used in the prevention and treatment of anemia are cyanocobalamin (vitamin B_{12}) and erythropoietin (Epogen or Procrit). Cyanocobalamin is discussed in detail in Chapter 50, and erythropoietin is discussed in Chapter 46.

nursing process

• Assessment

Before the nurse administers any of the iron products, it is important to assess for contraindications to use such as hypersensitivity reactions, colitis, enteritis, hemochromatosis, peptic ulcer disease, hemolytic anemia, and cirrhosis. Long-term use of hemopoietic agents for treatment of anemia should be approached cautiously. Laboratory studies such as hemoglobin (Hgb), hematocrit (Hct), reticulocytes, and bilirubin levels should be obtained and documented before initiation of drug treatment. A nutritional assessment should also be performed with concentration on the amount of iron intake in the patient's diet (a nutritional consult may be necessary).

Folic acid has the major contraindication of hypersensitivity to it or any derivative of it. Drug interactions with folic acid include chloramphenicol, phenobarbital, hydantoins, and methotrexate unless leucovorin rescue is possible. It is incompatible with calcium, chlorpromazine, iron sulfate, vitamin B complex with vitamin C in solution or syringe, and dextrose 40% concentrations. Hgb, Hct, and reticulocyte counts as well as baseline levels of folate should be assessed before initiation of therapy.

Iron dextran is contraindicated in hypersensitivity and all anemias with the exception of iron-deficiency anemia. It is also contraindicated in patients with liver disease. Cautious use and careful monitoring is recommended in patients with acute renal disease, asthma, and rheumatoid arthritis; pregnant or lactating women; infants under 4 months of age; and children. Iron dextran must not be mixed with other medications in syringe or solution, and it interacts with chloramphenicol and oral iron (increased toxicity).

Before the nurse administers vitamin B_{12}, it is important to obtain data about drug allergies to it. In addition, the vitamin interacts with alcohol, colchicine (an antigout drug), paraaminosalicylic acid, and some antibiotics. Treatment of vitamin B_{12} deficiencies is critical in prevention of possibly irreversible neurologic damage. Therefore assessment of underlying symptoms before initiating drug therapy is essential for effective treatment. A thorough dietary history is important, and patients should be questioned about their intake of foods high in vitamin B_{12}, such as organ meats, clams, oysters, seafood, nonfat dry milk, and fermented cheeses. Inadequate intake of these foods may contribute to the deficiency.

Ferrous salts are contraindicated in patients with ulcerative colitis and other GI disorders, peptic ulcer disease, and liver disease (such as cirrhosis). Drug interactions include levodopa, methyldopa, penicillamine, and tetracycline, all of which lead to a decreased absorption of each of these agents. Vitamin C increases ferrous fumarate's absorption.

Folic acid is contraindicated in patients with anemias other than megaloblastic or macrocytic anemia and with

vitamin B_{12} deficiency–related anemias. Drug interactions include methotrexate, triamterene, and sulfonamides (all of which lead to decreased action of the folic acid), as well as phenytoin, estrogens, and glucocorticoids (all of which lead to increased need for folic acid).

Activity

• Nursing Diagnoses

Nursing diagnoses associated with the use of blood-forming agents include, but are not limited to, the following:
- Activity intolerance related to fatigue and lethargy associated with anemias.
- Risk for injury related to side effects of iron products.
- Deficient knowledge related to limited exposure to use of medication.
- Imbalanced nutrition, less than body requirements, related to disease process.

• Planning

Goals for the patient receiving blood-forming agents include, but are not limited to, the following:
- Patient maintains normal level of activity as ordered.
- Patient remains free of self-injury related to anemia or use of iron products.
- Patient discusses rationale for use, side effects, and patient education guidelines related to use of blood-forming agents.
- Patient attains normal nutritional status through use of pharmacologic and nonpharmacologic measures.

Outcome Criteria

Outcome criteria related to the administration of blood-forming agents include the following:
- Patient will be able to tolerate gradual increase in activity as ordered while taking blood-forming agents such as ADLs to walking 10 minutes per day with increases as tolerated.
- Patient will use measures to minimize occurrence of side effects of blood-forming agents such as taking with food.
- Patient will take the medication exactly as prescribed to enhance efficacy of medication.
- Patient will state symptoms to report associated with increased symptomatology related to disease process or to adverse reactions to medications such as abdominal distention, cramping, nausea, and vomiting.
- Patients will keep daily journal of dietary intake to share with health care provider every week.
- Patient will use examples of a balanced diet for daily menu planning.

• Implementation

Liquid oral forms of iron products should be taken through a plastic straw to avoid discoloration of tooth enamel and should be diluted adequately per manufacturer's guidelines. Oral forms should also be given with juice (but not antacids or milk) between meals for maximal absorption. Should GI distress occur, the iron should be taken with meals.

Iron dextran should be administered only after all oral iron preparations have been discontinued and only after a test dose of iron dextran has been ordered (usually 25 mg by preferred route with remaining dose given 1 hour later). IM iron should be administered deep in a large muscle mass using a Z-track method and a 19- to 20-gauge, 2- to 3-inch needle that is long enough to administer the drug deep in the muscle mass. IV iron dextran should be given after the IV line is flushed with 10 ml of normal saline. IV iron dextran may be given undiluted or with 50 to 250 ml of normal saline. You should always check the label on the IV bottle to be sure that the vial is *without* preservatives and that IV administration is verified on the label. Epinephrine and resuscitative equipment should be available in case of an anaphylactic reaction. In addition, it may be necessary for the patient to remain recumbent 30 minutes after the IV injection to prevent orthostatic hypotension. Iron dextran is never to be mixed with other drugs in the syringe or with 5% glucose in distilled water.

Ferrous salts, if given to infants, should be administered only with vitamin E to prevent the possible occurrence of hemolytic anemia. It is best to give the medication between meals for maximal absorption. The patient should be informed to not take the medication with antacids or milk (or at least 1 hour before or after administration) because it will interfere with its absorption. The medication should be stored in a light-resistant, air-tight container. Patients should be cautioned to not lie down or remain in a reclining position for 15 or 30 minutes to avoid esophageal irritation or corrosion. It is also important to remind patients that any iron product will cause the stools to turn black or dark green.

Folic acid should be given with food. If ordered to be given intravenously, it may be administered undiluted if 5 mg or less and over 1 minute. Folic acid is often added to total parenteral nutrition solutions and other IV solutions, so compatibility should be checked before mixing the solutions with the medication.

Patient teaching tips for blood-forming agents are presented in the box below.

● Evaluation

Therapeutic responses to iron products include increased nutritional status, increased weight, increased activity tolerance and well-being, and absence of fatigue. Side effects include nausea, constipation, epigastric pain, black and tarry stools, and vomiting. Toxic signs include nausea, diarrhea (green, tarry stools), hematemesis, pallor, cyanosis, shock, and coma.

Therapeutic effects of vitamin B_{12} include decreased anorexia, dyspnea on exertion, palpitations, tachycardia, psychosis, and visual disturbances. With use of vitamin B_{12}, patients who have congestive heart failure (CHF) or cardiac disorders should be closely monitored for worsening of CHF or pulmonary edema.

---

patient teaching tips

Blood-Forming Agents

➤ Patients taking iron products should be informed of potential poisoning if medication is increased beyond recommended levels.

➤ Patients should be informed that iron products should not be crushed and that the tablets should be swallowed whole.

➤ All medications should be kept away and out of the reach of children.

➤ Patients should be informed that one iron product cannot be substituted for another. Each product contains different forms of the iron salt in different amounts.

➤ Patients taking iron products should avoid reclining positions for 15 to 30 minutes after taking the drug to avoid esophageal irritation or corrosion.

➤ Patients should be encouraged to continue to eat foods high in iron such as meat, dark green leafy vegetables, dried beans, dried fruits, and eggs.

➤ Patients should be informed to take oral forms of vitamin B_{12} with fruit juice and/or with meals to help disguise the taste.

➤ Patients should be informed that IM vitamin B_{12} is used to treat pernicious anemia and must be taken for life.

➤ Patients taking vitamin B_{12} should be encouraged to eat a well-balanced diet, including foods high in vitamin B_{12} such as egg yolks, fish, organ meats, oysters, dairy products, and clams. They should also avoid persons with infections because of a compromised immune system.

 ## POINTS TO REMEMBER

Nursing Considerations

• Iron and vitamin B_{12} are very important in the treatment of many disorders and diseases, such as malignancies, to achieve RBC and Hgb formation that is as adequate as possible, and to help prevent nutritional deficits that can affect all body systems, especially the immune system.

• Blood-forming agents are often used in the treatment of pernicious anemias, malabsorption syndromes, hemolytic anemias, hemorrhage, and renal and liver diseases.

• The patient must have a thorough assessment, including a head-to-toe nursing assessment, dietary history, and list of medications (including OTC agents) to rule

out any major nutritional deficits. Baseline values in nutritional disorders should also be documented.
- Iron dextran, if given intramuscularly, should be administered by Z-track method.
- A doctor should be consulted before any vitamin B_{12} or iron products are administered.
- Oral iron products are not interchangeable.

- Oral iron products may lead to GI and esophageal irritation.
- Lifelong vitamin B_{12} injections (IM) are needed for treatment of pernicious anemias unless contraindicated.
- Foods high in vitamin B_{12} include egg yolks, fish, organ meats, dairy products, and oysters; foods high in iron include dark green vegetables, dried beans, and dried fruits.

REVIEW QUESTIONS

1. Which of the following needs to be administered concurrently with ferrous fumarate in infants to prevent the possibility of hemolytic anemia?
   a. KCl
   b. NaCl
   c. Vitamin C
   d. Vitamin E
2. Which of the following is considered a contraindication to the use of iron supplements?
   a. Diabetes
   b. Weakness
   c. Hemolytic anemia
   d. Poor nutritional state
3. Oral iron may result in which of the following?
   a. Anuria
   b. Decreased Hgb
   c. Black and tarry stools
   d. Yellow and red discoloration to the urine

4. Which of the following statements is *most* appropriate for the individual needing teaching about his or her iron supplement?
   a. Do not take with meals.
   b. The iron should be taken at least qid.
   c. Make sure to take oral iron with milk and or an antacid.
   d. Eat foods that are high in iron such as dark-green, leafy vegetables.
5. In the evaluation of the therapeutic regimen for a patient on iron supplements for about 1 month to 6 weeks, which of the following would indicate a therapeutic response for the treatment of anemia?
   a. Elevated glucose
   b. Increased fatigue
   c. Decreased palpitations
   d. Increased visual disturbances

For Answers see www.harcourthealth.com/MERLIN/Lilley/.

CRITICAL THINKING Activities

1. In your clinical area, take a 24-hour dietary intake history of any of your assigned patients. Analyze their intake, while hospitalized, for iron content. In addition, note the medications ordered to identify any supplemental vitamins or iron tablets and to identify any drug interactions. Also note any laboratory values, such as RBC, Hgb, Hct, bilirubin levels, and reticulocyte levels.

2. Discuss the importance of monitoring reticulocyte counts, Hgb, and Hct levels once oral iron therapy has been initiated.
3. Discuss tips you should share with a patient who is taking oral iron supplements.

For Answers see www.harcourthealth.com/MERLIN/Lilley/.

bibliography

Albanese J, Nutz P: *Mosby's 2001 nursing drug reference and review cards,* St Louis, 2001, Mosby.
Anderson PO, Knoben JE, Troutman WG: *Handbook of clinical drug data 1999-2000,* ed 9, New York, 1999, McGraw-Hill.
Dipiro JT et al: *Pharmacotherapy: a pathophysiologic approach,* ed 4, New York, 1999, McGraw-Hill.
Fauci AS: *Harrison's principles of internal medicine,* ed 14, New York, 1998, McGraw-Hill.

Johns Hopkins Hospital, Department of Pediatrics et al: *The Harriet Lane handbook,* ed 15, St Louis, 2000, Mosby.
Keen JH: *Critical care and emergency drug reference,* ed 3, St Louis, 1996, Mosby.
McEvoy GK: *AHFS drug information,* Bethesda, Md, 2000, American Society of Hospital Pharmacists.
Mosby's GenRx: a comprehensive reference for generic and brand drugs, ed 10, St Louis, 2000, Mosby.
Skidmore-Roth L: *Mosby's 2001 nursing drug reference,* St Louis, 2001, Mosby.

Remember to check the **Online Worksheet** for additional learning opportunities: www.harcourthealth.com/MERLIN/Lilley/

Chapter 53

Dermatologic Agents

objectives

www.harcourthealth.com/MERLIN/Lilley/

Look for this symbol for
topics covered in the
Online Worksheet

When you reach the end of this chapter, you should be able to do the following:

1 Discuss the normal anatomy, physiology, and functions of the skin.

2 Describe the different skin disorders, infections, and conditions commonly affecting the skin.

3 Identify the various dermatologic agents used in treatment of skin disorders, infections, or infestations, and describe their classifications.

4 Discuss the mechanisms of action, indications, contraindications, cautions, and side effects associated with dermatologic agents.

5 Develop a nursing care plan that includes all phases of the nursing process for the patient receiving any of the various dermatologic agents, including thorough patient teaching.

drug profiles

bacitracin, p. 842
benzoyl peroxide, p. 843
clotrimazole, p. 845
⊶erythromycin, p. 843
isotretinoin, p. 844
⊶lindane, p. 847

⊶miconazole, p. 846
minoxidil, p. 848
silver sulfadiazine, p. 848
tretinoin, p. 844

⊶Key drug.

Scabies (ska′ bez) A contagious disease caused by *Sarcoptes scabiei*, the itch mite, characterized by intense itching of the skin and injury to the skin (excoriation) resulting from scratching. (p. 847)

Tinea (tin′ e ə) A group of fungal skin diseases caused by dermatophytes of several kinds and characterized by itching, scaling, and, sometimes, painful lesions. *Tinea* is a general term for infections of various causes that occur on several sites. Also called *ringworm*. (p. 844)

glossary

Actinic keratosis (ak tin′ ik ker′ ə to′ sis) A slowly developing, localized thickening of the outer layers of the skin resulting from long-term, prolonged exposure to the sun. Also called *solar keratosis*. (p. 848)

Dermatologic agent (dər′ mə to loj′ ik) Drug used to treat reactions or disorders of the skin. (p. 842)

Dermis (dər′ mis) The layer of the skin just below the epidermis, consisting of papillary and reticular layers and containing blood and lymphatic vessels, nerves and nerve endings, glands, and hair follicles. (p. 841)

Epidermis (ep′ i dər′ mis) The superficial, avascular layers of the skin, made up of an outer, dead, cornified portion and a deeper, living, cellular portion. (p. 841)

Keratolytic (ker′ ə to lit′ ik) A drug that promotes loosening and shedding of the outer layer of the skin. (p. 843)

Pediculicides (pə dik′ u li sidz) A drug that kills lice. (p. 847)

Pediculosis (pə dik u lo′ sis) An infestation with bloodsucking lice. (p. 847)

Scabicide (ska′ bi sid) Any one of a large group of drugs that destroy the itch mite *Sarcoptes scabiei*. They are used with caution in children. (p. 847)

SKIN

The largest organ of the body is the skin. It covers the body and serves several functions, many of which we take for granted. It serves as a protective barrier for the internal organs. Without skin, harmful external forces such as microorganisms and chemicals would gain access to and damage or destroy many of our delicate internal organs. Part of this protection includes its ability to maintain a surface pH of 4.5 to 5.5. This weakly acidic environment discourages the growth of microorganisms that grow at a more alkaline pH of 6 to 7.5, explaining why infected skin usually has a higher pH. The skin also has the ability to sense changes in temperature (hot or cold), pressure, or pain, information that is then transmitted to nerve endings. The temperature of the environment around us changes constantly and can be extremely hot or cold. Despite this, our body maintains an almost constant internal temperature in any environment thanks in large part to the skin, which plays a

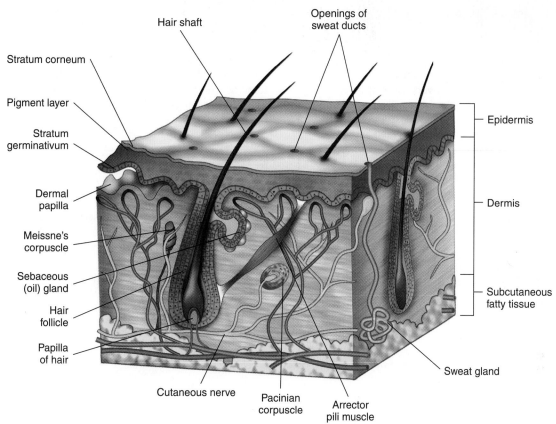

Fig. 53-1 A microscopic view of the skin. The epidermis, shown in longitudinal section, is raised at one corner to reveal the ridges in the dermis. (Modified from Thibodeau GA, Patton KT: *Anatomy and physiology,* ed 4, St Louis, 1999, Mosby.)

major role in the regulation of body temperature. Heat loss and conservation are regulated in coordination with the blood vessels that supply blood to the skin and by means of perspiration. The skin is also able to excrete fluid and electrolytes through sweat glands. In addition, it can store fat, synthesize vitamin D, and provide a site for drug absorption.

The skin is made up of two layers—the **dermis** and the **epidermis** (Fig. 53-1). The outer skin layer, or epidermis, is composed of four layers. Going from the outermost to innermost layer, these are the stratum corneum, stratum lucidum, stratum granulosum, and the stratum germinativum. The respective functions of these layers are described in Box 53-1. None of these layers has a direct blood supply of their own. Instead, their nourishment is provided through diffusion.

The dermis lies between the epidermis and subcutaneous fat and differs from the epidermis in many ways. It is approximately 40 times thicker than the epidermis. Traversing the dermis is a rich supply of blood vessels, nerves, lymphatic tissue, elastic tissue, and connective tissue, which provide extra support and nourishment to the skin. Also contained in this layer are the exocrine glands—eccrine, apocrine, and sebaceous glands—and the hair follicles. The functions of the various types of exocrine glands are explained in Box 53-2.

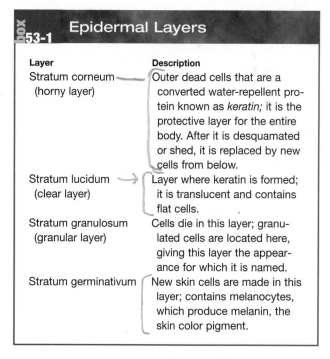

Epidermal Layers

BOX 53-1

Layer	Description
Stratum corneum (horny layer)	Outer dead cells that are a converted water-repellent protein known as *keratin;* it is the protective layer for the entire body. After it is desquamated or shed, it is replaced by new cells from below.
Stratum lucidum (clear layer)	Layer where keratin is formed; it is translucent and contains flat cells.
Stratum granulosum (granular layer)	Cells die in this layer; granulated cells are located here, giving this layer the appearance for which it is named.
Stratum germinativum	New skin cells are made in this layer; contains melanocytes, which produce melanin, the skin color pigment.

Below the dermis is a layer of loose connective tissue called the *hypodermis.* It helps make the skin flexible. It is also here that the subcutaneous fat tissue is located, which provides thermal insulation and cushioning or padding. It is also the source of nutrition for the skin.

Exocrine Glands of the Skin

Gland	Function
Sebaceous	Large lipid-containing cells that produce oil or film that covers the epidermis; it protects and lubricates skin and is water repellent and antiseptic.
Eccrine	Sweat glands that are located throughout the skin surface; help regulate body temperature and prevent skin dryness.
Apocrine	Mainly in axilla, genital organs, and breast areas; emit an odor; believed to be scent or sex glands.

Start

DERMATOLOGIC AGENTS

Reactions or disorders of the skin are common and numerous. The drugs used to treat these disorders can be administered directly to the site and are called **dermatologic agents.** There are many such agents available in a multitude of formulations, some of the more common of which are as follows:

- Ointment
- Gel/jelly
- Oil
- Cream
- Aerosol spray
- Paste
- Aerosol foam
- Tape
- Lotion
- Powder

Each formulation has certain characteristics that make it suitable for specific indications. The formulations, their characteristics, and examples of each are summarized in Table 53-1.

There are also several categories of dermatologic agents:

- Antibacterial agents
- Emollients
- Antiinflammatory agents
- Antifungal agents
- Keratolytics
- Local anesthetics
- Antiviral agents
- Debriding agents
- Antipruritic agents
- Antineoplastics
- Burn drugs
- Topical vasodilators

TOPICAL ANTIINFECTIVES

Topical antiinfectives consist of antibacterial, acne, antifungal, and antiviral drugs that, as the name implies, are applied topically. The systemically administered antiinfective agents are discussed in detail in Part Seven, where their specific pharmacologic characteristics are also de-

scribed. Their topical uses are discussed here, as are any characteristics specific to this use. Although they have many of the same properties as the systemic forms, there are some differences in terms of their toxicities and side effects. The drugs used to treat dermatologic parasitic infections, the pediculicides and scabicides, as well as the drugs commonly used to treat acne, are also covered in this section.

drug profiles

ANTIBACTERIAL AGENTS

Common skin disorders caused by various bacteria are folliculitis, impetigo, furuncles, carbuncles, and cellulitis. The bacteria responsible are most commonly *Streptococcus pyogenes* and *Staphylococcus aureus.* Dermatologic antibacterial agents are used to treat or prevent these skin infections, the most commonly used ones being bacitracin, polymyxin, and neomycin.

bacitracin

Bacitracin (Baciguent) is a polypeptide antibiotic that is applied topically for the treatment or prevention of local skin infections caused by susceptible aerobic and anaerobic gram-positive organisms such as staphylococci, streptococci, anaerobic cocci, corynebacteria, and clostridia. It works by inhibiting bacterial cell wall synthesis, which leads to cell death. It can be either bactericidal or bacteriostatic, depending on the causative organism.

Bacitracin is active against many gram-positive organisms such as staphylococci, streptococci, anaerobic cocci, corynebacteria, and clostridia. Its antimicrobial spectrum is broadened when it is used in combination with other topical antibiotics, and there are several such combination products available. Most contain neomycin and polymyxin B. Bacitracin has a low order of toxicity when applied topically. Rash and allergic anaphylactoid reactions have occurred. If itching, burning, inflammation, or other signs of sensitivity occur, bacitracin should be discontinued. Ointment formulations of the agent are the ones most frequently used, but powders and aerosols are also available. As a single-agent product, bacitracin is available as a 500-U/g ointment and a powder that is applied to the affected area one to three times daily.

ACNE AGENTS

Other antibacterial agents are used to treat acne, the skin infection commonly caused by *Propionibacterium acnes.* These agents include benzoyl peroxide, clindamycin, erythromycin, meclocycline, tetracycline, isotretinoin, and the vitamin A acid called *retinoic acid.* Many other agents are also used in the treatment and prevention of acne.

Activity

Table 53-1 Dermatologic Formulations: Characteristics and Examples

Formulation	Characteristics	Examples
Aerosol foam	Can cover large area Useful for drug delivery into a body cavity (e.g., vagina or rectum) or hairy areas	Proctofoam, Epifoam, contraceptive foams
Aerosol spray	Spreads thin liquid or powder film Covers large areas Useful when skin is tender to touch (e.g., burns)	Solarcaine, Desenex, Kenalog
Cream	Contains water and can be removed with water Not greasy or occlusive Usually white semisolid Good for moist areas	Hydrocortisone cream, Benadryl cream
Gel/jelly	Contains water and possibly alcohol Easily removed and good lubricator Usually clear, semisolid substance Useful when lubricant properties are desirable	K-Y jelly, Saligel, Surgilube
Lotion	Contains water, alcohol, and solvents May be a suspension, emulsion, or solution Good for large or hairy areas	Calamine lotion, Lubriderm lotion, Kwell lotion
Oil	Contains very little if any water Occlusive, liquid Not removable with water Excellent emollient properties	Lubriderm bath oil
Ointment	Contains no water and is not removable with water Is occlusive, greasy, and semisolid Desirable for dry lesions because of occlusiveness	Petrolatum (Vaseline), zinc oxide ointment, A & D ointment
Paste	Similar properties to those of the ointments Contains more powder than ointments Excellent protectant properties	Zinc oxide paste
Powder	Slight lubricating properties May be shaken on affected area Promotes drying of area where applied	Tinactin powder, Desenex powder
Tape	Most occlusive formulation Consistent topical drug delivery Useful when small, straight areas require drug application	Cordran tape

benzoyl peroxide

The microorganism that most commonly causes acne, *Propionibacterium acnes,* is an anaerobic bacteria that needs an environment poor in oxygen to grow. Benzoyl peroxide is effective in combating such infection because it slowly and continuously liberates active oxygen, causing antibacterial, antiseptic, drying, and keratolytic actions. These actions create an environment unfavorable for the continued growth of the *P. acnes* bacteria, and they soon die. Such drugs as benzoyl peroxide that soften scales and loosen the outer horny layer of the skin are referred to as **keratolytics.**

Benzoyl peroxide generally produces signs of improvement within 4 to 6 weeks. Side effects are infrequent and rarely a problem. Most are confined to the skin and involve peeling skin, red skin, or a sensation of warmth. Blistering or swelling of the skin is generally considered an allergic reaction to the product and is an indication to stop treatment.

Benzoyl peroxide is available as a 2.5%, 5%, or 10% lotion and a 2.5% cream that is usually applied topically one to four times a day. It also is available as a cleansing bar that is used two or three times daily and as a cream or cleansing lotion that is applied one to two times daily. Benzoyl peroxide is rated as a pregnancy category C agent. Benzoyl peroxide is also available as a soap, gel, and cream.

erythromycin

Erythromycin (A/T/S, EryDerm, T-Stat, Erygel) is a macrolide antibiotic used for the topical treatment of acne vulgaris, a common form of acne. It usually only stops the growth of the acne-causing bacteria (bacteriostatic), but it may kill bacteria either when given in high concentrations or when the organisms are highly susceptible. It exerts its antibacterial effects by inhibiting protein synthesis in susceptible organisms.

Erythromycin topical preparations are applied to the cleansed affected areas each morning and evening. Skin reactions are the most common side effect and consist of erythema, desquamation, tenderness, dryness, pruritus, burning, oiliness, and acne. Erythromycin is available as a 1.5% or 2% solution, a 2% gel, or a 2% ointment and is classified as a pregnancy category C agent. It is contraindicated in patients with known hypersensitivity to it.

isotretinoin

Isotretinoin (Accutane) is an oral and topical product indicated for the treatment of severe recalcitrant cystic acne. Isotretinoin inhibits sebaceous gland activity and has antikeratinizing and antiinflammatory effects. Isotretinoin is classified as a pregnancy category X agent. It is available as 10-, 20-, and 40-mg capsules and a topical product. It is contraindicated in patients who are pregnant or have hypersensitivity to it.

tretinoin

Tretinoin (retinoic acid, vitamin A acid, Renova, Retin-A) is a derivative of vitamin A that is used to treat acne and ameliorate the dermatologic changes (e.g., fine wrinkling, mottled hyperpigmentation, roughness) associated with photodamage. The drug appears to act as an irritant on the skin, in particular the follicular epithelium. Specifically, it stimulates the turnover of epidermal cells, which results in skin peeling. While this is occurring, the free fatty acid levels are reduced and horny cells cannot then adhere to one another. Without fatty acids and horny cells, acne and its comedo, or pimple, cannot exist.

Topically administered tretinoin has been shown to enhance the repair of skin damaged by ultraviolet radiation or sunlight. It does this by increasing the formation of fibroblasts and collagen, both of which are needed to rebuild skin. The drug also may reduce collagen degradation by inhibiting the enzyme collagenase that breaks down collagen.

As with erythromycin, tretinoin's main side effects are local inflammatory reactions, which are reversible when therapy is discontinued. Some of the most common side effects are excessively red and edematous blisters, crusted skin, and temporary alterations in skin pigmentation. Tretinoin is available in many topical formulations: a topical powder; a 0.025%, 0.05%, and 0.1% topical cream; a 0.01% and 0.025% topical gel; and a 0.05% topical solution. Because of its potential to cause severe irritation and peeling, it may initially be applied once every 2 or 3 days, preferably using the lower-concentration cream or gel. Tretinoin is a pregnancy category C agent.

Retin-A Micro has been approved for the treatment of acne vulgaris. This newer acne treatment entraps tretinoin in a synthetic polymer called a *Microsponge system.* This system is made of round microscopic particles of synthetic polymer. These microspheres act as a reservoir for tretinoin, allowing the skin to absorb small amounts of tretinoin over time. Retin-A Micro is available as a gel.

Another agent in the retinoid family is tazaroten (Tazorac). Tazaroten is a receptor-selective retinoid. It is thought to normalize epidermal differentiation, reducing the influx of inflammatory cells into the skin. Synthetic retinoids are vitamin A analogues and are thought to play a role in skin cell differentiation and proliferation. It is available as a 0.05% and 0.1% gel and is approved for the treatment of stable plaque psoriasis and mild to moderately severe facial acne vulgaris. Tazarone is a pregnancy category X agent.

Activity

ANTIFUNGAL AGENTS

A few fungi produce keratinolytic enzymes, which allows them to live on the skin. Topical fungal infections are primarily caused by *Candida* spp. (candidiasis), dermatophytes, and *Malassezia furfur* (tinea versicolor). These fungi exist in moist, warm environments, preferably in dark areas such as the feet or groin.

Candidal infections are most commonly caused by *Candida albicans,* a yeastlike opportunistic fungus present in the normal flora of the mouth, vagina, and intestinal tract. Two significant factors that commonly predispose a person to a candidal infection are broad-spectrum antibiotic therapy, which promotes an overgrowth of nonsusceptible organism in the natural body florae, and immunodeficiency disorders such as those that occur in patients with cancer, AIDS, or organ transplants. Because these infections favor warm, moist areas of the skin and mucous membranes, they most frequently occur orally (a form commonly seen in infants called *thrush*), vaginally, and cutaneously in such sites as beneath the breasts and in diaper areas. They may also cause nail infections.

Dermatophytes are a group of three closely related genera consisting of *Epidermophyton* spp., *Microsporum* spp., and *Trichophyton* spp. that utilize the keratin found on the skin for their growth. They pro-

research

Dermatologic Preparations

Read two nursing research articles published within the past 5 years about tretinoin, and answer the following questions:

- What is the controversy concerning the use of tretinoin in pregnant women?
- What are the pros and cons of topical tretinoin therapy for sun-induced aged skin disorders?
- Why are some insurers not covering tretinoin in middle-age women?

duce superficial mycotic (fungal) infections of keratinized tissue (hair, skin, and nails). Infections caused by dermatophytes are collectively called **tinea,** or ringworm, infections. The name *ringworm* comes from the fact that the infection often assumes a circular pattern at the site of infection. The tinea infections are further identified by the body location where they occur: tinea pedis (foot), tinea crusis (groin), tinea corporis (body), and tinea capitis (scalp). Tinea infections are also known as *athlete's foot* or *jock itch.*

Fungi usually invade the stratum corneum, which is the dead layer of desquamated cells. Inflammation occurs when the fungi invade this layer; sensitivity occurs when they penetrate the epidermis and dermis.

Many of the fungi that cause topical infections are very difficult to eradicate. They are very slow growing, and antifungal therapy may be required for periods ranging from several weeks to as long as a year. However, many topical antifungal drugs are available for the treatment of both dermatophyte infections and those caused by yeast and yeastlike fungi. Some of these agents, their dosage forms, and their uses are listed in Table 53-2.

The most commonly reported side effects of topical antifungals include local irritation, pruritus, a burning sensation, and scaling. Ciclopirox, clotrimazole, miconazole, and haloprogin are classified as pregnancy category B agents, and econazole and ketoconazole are classified as pregnancy category C agents. Hypersensitivity is the one contraindication to the use of any of these agents.

clotrimazole

Clotrimazole (Mycelex troche, Lotrimin, Mycelex-G) is available over-the-counter (OTC) as well as with

Topical Antifungal Agents

Table 53-2

Drug	Trade Names	Dosage Forms	Use	Legal Status
amphotericin B	Fungizone	3% cream, 3% lotion, 3% ointment	Candidiasis	Rx
butenafine	Mentax	1% cream	Tinea pedis	Rx
butoconazole	Femstat	2% vaginal cream	Candidiasis	Rx
ciclopirox olamine	Loprox	1% cream, 1% lotion	Candidiasis, dermatophytoses, tinea versicolor	Rx
clioquinol	Vioform	3% cream, ointment	Dermatophytoses	OTC
clotrimazole	Gyne-Lotrimin	1% cream, 100- and 500-mg vaginal tablets	Candidiasis	OTC
	Lotrimin	1% cream, 1% lotion, 1% solution	Candidiasis, tinea versicolor	Rx
	Lotrimin AF	1% cream, 1% lotion, 1% solution	Dermatophytoses	OTC
	Mycelex	1% cream, 1% solution	Dermatophytoses	Rx
	Mycelex	10-mg troches	Oropharyngeal candidiasis	
	Mycelex-7	1% vaginal cream, 100-mg vaginal tablets	Candidiasis	OTC
	Mycelex G	500-mg vaginal tablets	Candidiasis	Rx
econazole nitrate	Spectazole	1% cream	Candidiasis, dermatophytoses	Rx
haloprogin	Halotex	1% cream, 1% solution	Dermatophytoses, tinea versicolor	Rx
ketoconazole	Nizoral	2% cream, 2% shampoo	Candidiasis, dermatophytoses, tinea versicolor	Rx
		1% cream		OTC
miconazole nitrate	Micotin	2% cream, 2% powder, 2% spray	Dermatophytoses	OTC
	Monistat Derm	2% cream	Candidiasis, dermatophytoses, tinea versicolor	Rx
		1% cream		
naftifine HCl	Naftin	1% cream, 1% gel	Dermatophytoses	Rx
natamycin	Natacyn	5% ophthalmic suspension	Ocular fungal infections	Rx
nystatin	Nilstat/Mycostatin	Cream, ointment, powder	Candidiasis	Rx
oxiconazole nitrate	Oxistat	1% cream, 1% lotion	Dermatophytoses	Rx
sodium thiosulfate	None	25% solution	Tinea versicolor	OTC
sulconazole	Exelderm	1% cream, 1% solution	Dermatophytoses	Rx
terbinafine HCl	Lamisil	1% cream	Dermatophytoses	Rx
tolnaftate	NP = 27	1% cream, 1% solution	Dermatophytoses	OTC
	Tinactin	1% cream, 1% solution		

Rx, Prescription only; *OTC,* over the counter.

a prescription. It is available as a lozenge for the treatment of oropharyngeal candidiasis, commonly known as *thrush*. It also is available as a cream, lotion, or solution for the treatment of dermatophytoses, superficial mycoses, and cutaneous candidiasis. Such topical preparations are also available for intravaginal administration in the treatment of vulvovaginal candidiasis, commonly called a *yeast infection*, and vaginal trichomoniasis.

Clotrimazole is available in many topical formulations: a powder; a 10-mg oral topical lozenge; a 1% cream, lotion, and solution; a 1% vaginal cream; and a 100- and a 500-mg vaginal tablet. Different dosages and the different dosage forms are used for the treatment of the various fungal infections.

⌖ miconazole

Miconazole (Monistat, Micotin, Monistat 7) is a topical antifungal agent that is available in several OTC and prescription products. It inhibits the growth of several fungi, including dermatophytes and yeast, as well as gram-positive bacteria and is commonly used to treat dermatophytoses, superficial mycoses, cutaneous candidiasis, and vulvovaginal candidiasis. It is in many OTC remedies for athlete's foot, jock itch, and yeast infections.

For the treatment of athlete's foot, jock itch, ringworm, and other susceptible fungal infections, miconazole should be applied sparingly to the cleansed, dry, infected area twice daily, in the morning and evening. For the treatment of yeast infections, one 200-mg suppository should be inserted in the vagina once daily at bedtime for 3 consecutive days or 100 mg (one suppository or 5 g of the 2% cream) should be administered intravaginally once daily at bedtime for 7 days.

The most common side effects of topically administered miconazole are vulvovaginal burning and itching, pelvic cramps and rash, urticaria, stinging, burning, and contact dermatitis. It is available in a variety of topical formulations: a 2% aerosol spray and powder, a 2% powder, a 2% cream, a 2% vaginal cream, and a 100- and 500-mg vaginal suppository.

Activity

ANTIVIRAL AGENTS

As noted in the chapter on antiviral agents, viral infections are very difficult to treat because they live in the body's own healthy cells and use their cell mechanisms to reproduce. The same holds true for topical viral infections. Infections caused by herpes simplex types 1 and 2 are particularly serious and are becoming more common. The only antiviral agents currently available to treat such topical viral infections are acyclovir and penciclovir.

Acyclovir and penciclovir work by inhibiting the viral enzymes necessary for DNA synthesis. They are applied topically for the treatment of initial and recurrent her-

pes simplex infections in immunocompromised patients. However, often these topical infections can be prevented or treated more efficaciously with systemically administered antiviral agents. Topically applied acyclovir does not cure viral skin infections but does appear to decrease the healing time and associated pain.

Acyclovir and penciclovir are available as a 1% topical ointment that is applied every 3 hours, or six times daily, for 1 week. A finger cot or rubber glove should be worn for the application of the ointment to prevent the spread of infection. The most common side effects are stinging, itching, and rash. Acyclovir and penciclovir are classified as pregnancy category C agents and are contraindicated in patients with hypersensitivity to them.

Activity

TOPICAL ANESTHETIC, ANTIPRURITIC, AND ANTIINFLAMMATORY AGENTS

Topical anesthetic agents are drugs that are used to numb the skin. They accomplish this by inhibiting the conduction of nerve impulses from sensory nerves, thereby reducing or eliminating the pain or pruritus associated with insect bites, sunburn, and plant allergies such as poison ivy, as well as many other uncomfortable skin disorders. They are also used to numb the skin before giving a person a painful injection. Topical anesthetics are available as ointments, creams, sprays, liquids, and jellies, and have been discussed in Chapter 10.

Topical antipruritic agents contain antihistamines or corticosteroids. Many exert a combined anesthetic and antipruritic action when applied topically. The antihistamines and their therapeutic effects are covered in Chapter 34. New recommendations for the use of topical antihistamines state that they should not be used in the following situations because of systemic absorption and subsequent toxicity: chickenpox, widespread poison ivy, and large body-surface-area inducement.

Topical antiinflammatory agents are most commonly corticosteroids, and they are generally indicated for the relief of inflammatory and pruritic dermatoses. By administering them topically, many of the undesirable systemic side effects associated with the use of the systemically administered corticosteroids are averted. The beneficial drug effects of the corticosteroids are their antiinflammatory, antipruritic, and vasoconstrictor actions.

Topical corticosteroids have many acquired properties that have the effect of altering their relative potency and hence the conditions they are used to treat. For instance, corticosteroids that are fluorinated are used for the treatment of dermatologic disorders such as psoriasis. The vehicle in which the corticosteroid is contained also has the effect of altering their vasoconstrictor property and therapeutic efficacy. Ointments are generally the most penetrating, followed next by gels, creams, and lotions. Propylene glycol also enhances the penetration of the corticosteroid and its vasoconstrictor effects. Most corticosteroids are available in many topical formulations, thus offering a variety of options. The currently available topical corticosteroids along with their respective potencies are listed in Box 53-3.

Side effects of the agents include skin reactions such as acne eruptions, allergic contact dermatitis, burning sensations, dryness, itching, hypopigmentation, purpura, hirsutism (usually facial), folliculitis, round and swollen face, and alopecia (usually of scalp). An overgrowth of a bacteria, fungus, or virus and immunosuppression are others. The usual adult dosage of these drugs is one or two applications daily, as directed. Less potent topical corticosteroids are used in children but following the same schedule. Corticosteroids are classified as pregnancy category C agents and are contraindicated in patients with hypersensitivity to them. Since many of these products are available orally as well as topically, there is the potential to administer both simultaneously. This is not recommended and potentially harmful. The combined use of topical and oral preparations of the same drug can lead to toxicity.

MISCELLANEOUS DERMATOLOGIC AGENTS

There are many other topically applied drugs. Those discussed here are the topical ectoparasiticidal (scabicides and pediculicides), hair growth, antineoplastic, and antiinfective drugs. Many of these agents are available both OTC and by prescription.

BOX 53-3	**Topical Corticosteroids**
Range of Potency	**Corticosteroid**
Most potent	Betamethasone dipropionate (cream and ointment), clobetasol propionate, halobetasol propionate, and diflorasone diacetate
Very potent	Amcinonide, betamethasone dipropionate (lotion), desoximethasone (cream and ointment, 0.25%), fluocinolone, halcinonide, triamcinolone acetonide (cream and ointment, 0.5%), mometasone furoate
Potent	Betamethasone, betamethasone valerate (0.1% cream, ointment, and lotion), desoximethasone (0.5% gel), fluocinolone acetonide, flurandrenolide, halcinonide, and triamcinolone acetonide.
Less potent	Betamethasone valerate (reduced strength cream, 0.01%), clocortolone, desonide, fluocinolone acetonide, flurandrenolide, hydrocortisone valerate, triamcinolone acetonide (cream, ointment, and lotion, 0.1%)
Least potent	Dexamethasone, hydrocortisone, methylprednisolone

Skin penetration and thus potency is enhanced by the vehicle containing the steroid. In decreasing order of effectiveness are ointments, gels, creams, and lotions.

---

drug profiles

TOPICAL ECTOPARASITICIDAL DRUGS

Ectoparasites are insects that live on the outer surface of the body, and the drugs that are used to kill them are called *ectoparasiticidal drugs.*

Lice are transmitted from person to person by close contact with infested people, clothing, combs, or towels. A parasitic infestation on the skin with lice is called **pediculosis,** and such infestations go by one of three different names, depending on the location of the infestation:

- Pediculosis pubis → pubic louse or "crabs," caused by *Phthirus pubis*
- Pediculosis corporis → body louse, caused by *Pediculus humanus corporis*
- Pediculosis capitis → head louse, caused by *Pediculus humanus capitis*

Common findings in infested people include itching, eggs of the lice on the hair shafts (called nits), lice on the skin or clothes, and in the case of pubic lice, sky blue macules on the inner thighs or lower abdomen. Pediculoses are treated with a class of drugs called **pediculicides,** the most commonly used one being lindane.

A second common parasitic skin infection is that caused by the itch mite *Sarcoptes scabiei,* commonly known as *scabies.* **Scabies** is transmitted from person to person by close contact, such as sleeping next to an infested person. The scabies mite causes irritation and itching by boring into the horny layers of skin located in cracks and folds. Itching seems to be most common in the evening. The drugs used to treat these infestations are called **scabicides.**

Treatment of these parasitic infestations should begin with identification of the source of infestation in order to prevent reinfestation. Next, the clothing and personal articles of the infested person should be decontaminated. This is best accomplished by washing them in hot, soapy water or by dry cleaning. All close contacts of the person should be treated as well, also to prevent reinfestation. Besides lindane, malathion (Prioderm), crotamiton (Eurax), and permethrin (Nix, Elimite) are other ectoparasiticidal drugs.

lindane

Lindane (Kwell, Scabene) is a chlorinated hydrocarbon originally developed as an agricultural insecticide. It is both a scabicide and a pediculicide because it is effective in treating both scabies and pediculosis. It is available in three topical formulations: a 1% cream, lotion, and shampoo.

For the treatment of pubic or body lice, the cream or lotion is applied in a sufficient quantity to cover the skin and hair of the infested and surrounding areas. It is left on for 12 hours and then thoroughly washed off. A second application is seldom needed. Head lice can be treated with lindane shampoo, which should be worked into the hair and left on for 4 minutes. The hair should then be rinsed and dried, after which the nits (eggs) should be combed from the hair shafts. The treatment for scabies is similar. It involves the application of lindane over the entire body, from the neck down. It is left on for 8 to 12 hours and washed off. Side effects of lindane are an eczematous skin rash and rarely CNS toxicity. The latter is more common in young children and in cases of overuse. The FDA has recently recommended labeling changes that encourage lindane use only after other agents have been tried.

TOPICAL HAIR GROWTH DRUGS
minoxidil

Minoxidil (Rogaine) is a vasodilating drug that is administered systemically to control hypertension. Topically it has the same vasodilating effect, but when used in this way, it is applied to the scalp to stimulate hair growth. The vasodilation it causes is one possible explanation for how it stimulates hair growth. It may also act at the level of the hair follicle, possibly stimulating hair follicle growth directly.

It can be used in both men and women suffering from baldness or hair thinning. Treatment consists of administering the agent to the affected (balding and anticipated balding) area twice daily, usually morning and evening. It generally takes 4 months before results are seen, however. Systemic absorption of the topically applied minoxidil is possible. Therefore the side effects of topically applied minoxidil are systemic ones, such as tachycardia, fluid retention, and weight gain. Topically administered minoxidil is available as 2% and 5% solutions. Each metered dose delivers 1 ml or 20 mg of the agent.

Activity

TOPICAL ANTINEOPLASTIC DRUGS

Various premalignant skin lesions and basal cell carcinomas may be treated with the topically applied antineoplastic drug fluorouracil (Efudex, Fluoroplex). It acts by destroying rapidly growing cells such as premalignant and malignant cells. It is also used topically in the treatment of solar or **actinic keratosis** and basal cell carcinomas of the skin when surgical and other techniques are impractical or unfeasible.

The adverse effects associated with the topical use of this antineoplastic are much different from those seen in association with the systemic administration of the agent. Such effects are minimal and generally limited to local inflammatory reactions such as dermatitis, stomatitis, and photosensitivity. Major adverse effects of fluorouracil topical therapy are swelling, scaling, pain, pruritus, burning, soreness, tenderness, suppuration, scarring, and hyperpigmentation.

Fluorouracil is available as a 1% and 5% topical cream and a 1%, 2%, and 5% topical solution. It can be applied with a nonmetallic applicator, clean fingertips, or gloved fingers. If the fingers are used, they should be washed thoroughly immediately after application. Either a 1% or 2% fluorouracil solution should be used for the treatment of multiple actinic keratoses of the head and neck. It should be applied twice daily to the lesions. Superficial basal cell carcinoma may be treated with 5% fluorouracil, administered twice daily for at least 3 to 6 weeks.

TOPICAL ANTIINFECTIVE DRUGS
silver sulfadiazine

One of the concerns in burn victims is infection at the burn site, but there are two problems posed by the use of either topically or systemically administered antiinfective agents in this setting. Because of the systemic absorption of a drug that can occur in compromised skin areas such as burns, the agent cannot be so toxic, or the quantities absorbed so toxic, that if absorbed into the circulation this leads to untoward effects. On the other hand, the blood supply to burned areas is often drastically reduced, such that systemically administered antibiotics either cannot reach the site or do so only in quantities too low to be effective. Therefore the only way of applying these agents to ensure that they reach the burn site is to do so topically. Some of the commonly used agents that have proved both effective and safe in the prevention or treatment of infections in burns are silver sulfadiazine (Silvadene), mafenide (Sulfamylon), and nitrofurazone (Furacin).

Silver sulfadiazine is a synthetic antiinfective agent produced when silver nitrate reacts with sulfadiazine. It appears to act on the cell membrane and cell wall of susceptible bacteria and is used as an adjunct in the prevention and treatment of infection in second- and third-degree burns. The side effects of silver sulfadiazine are similar to those of other topical drugs and include pain, burning, or itching. It is available as a 1% cream and should be applied topically to cleansed, debrided, burned areas once or twice daily using a sterile-gloved hand.

nursing process

● Assessment

Before using any of the dermatologic preparations, the nurse should rule out the presence of the many conditions and problems that may be a contraindication to its use, one being known hypersensitivity to any of the agents. It is important for the nurse to always check to make sure the patient has no drug allergies and has shown no previous sensitivity to antimicrobials or any of the other topical agents. Patients who are to be treated with benzoyl peroxide agents should be checked for allergies and previous local reactions to the medication. Antibacterial topical agents are associated with a broader risk of reactions because of the generalized sensitivity of patients to the same antibiotic in its different dosage forms. Therefore should a patient have an allergy to a particular antibacterial agent, that agent should not be used topically either. Always be sure that if culture and sensitivity testing has been ordered, the specimen has been collected before the first application of the antibacterial agent.

When administering any type of topical medication, such as an antimicrobial, steroid, or antiacne agent, the concentration of the medication, length of exposure to the skin, condition of the skin, size of the area affected, and hydration status of the skin should all be taken into consideration because all have a significant effect on the action of the medication.

The skin, and in particular the area affected, must be inspected thoroughly under an adequate light source and the area palpated with a gloved hand, especially in dark-skinned patients because often an erythematous area may not be visible but may be palpated as an area of warmth. Conditions that aggravate the problem should also be noted. With oral tretinoin, liver function studies should be assessed. With lindane, it is important to assess and identify the source of scabies infection. Ototoxicity and nephrotoxicity should be assessed with the use of silver sulfadiazine. All findings should be thoroughly documented and reflect a systematic and bilateral assessment of all areas.

The patient's overall health status and hygiene practices should also be assessed, including whether the patient has suffered any trauma or whether his or her immune system is suppressed. Exudate or drainage material should also be obtained for culture studies before therapy is initiated but with a physician's order. The nurse should also remember that the skin of the very young and the very old is often more permeable to some of the dermatologic preparations such as corticosteroids. Often, inflammation of the skin, abrasions, or breaks in the skin are contraindications to the use of some of the topical agents.

● Nursing Diagnoses

Nursing diagnoses pertinent to the use of dermatologic preparations include the following:
- Impaired skin integrity related to disease or disorder causing break in skin barrier.
- Acute pain related to the skin condition or adverse reactions to the topical preparation.
- Deficient knowledge related to lack of experience with and exposure to use of topical agents.
- Ineffective therapeutic regimen related to lack of information about importance of compliance.

● Planning

Goals related to the administration of dermatologic preparations include the following:
- Patient's skin remains intact and healed in appearance and integrity.
- Patient remains compliant with therapy.
- Patient remains free of injury to skin while on therapy.
- Patient experiences minimal to no complications of therapy.

Outcome Criteria

Outcome criteria related to the administration of dermatologic agents include the following:
- Patient's skin will improve daily (i.e., there will be less redness, drainage, discomfort, itching, rash, etc.).
- Patient will have fewer complaints about localized skin discomfort (e.g., pain, itching).
- Patient will demonstrate how to apply medication as prescribed and to follow physician's orders in its application.
- Patient will state the rationale for treatment, the side effects of the dermatologic preparation, and symptoms to report associated with the dermatologic therapy.
- Patient will remain compliant with the medication therapy with resultant improved condition.

● Implementation

Generally speaking, before applying any more topical medication, the nurse should cleanse thoroughly the site of any debris as well as any residual medication, making sure to follow any specific directions, such as removing water or alcohol-based topicals with soap and water.

Standard precautions should be maintained. The nurse should wear gloves, not only to prevent contamination from secretions but also to prevent absorption of the medication through his or her skin. If using lotions, they should be stored according to the manufacturer's recommendations and shaken well before using. Creams and ointments are often applied with a sterile cotton-tipped applicator or tongue blade. Any dressings should be applied as ordered, and special attention should be paid to directions concerning occlusive, wet, or wet-to-dry dressings. Information about the site of application; drainage, swelling, temperature, color, and painful or other sensations; and the type of treatment rendered and response should all be documented.

The manufacturer's guidelines regarding the use of any of the dermatologic preparations should always be followed because often each medication has a different type of base solution and specific application procedures are required for different dosage forms. In addition, it is

Dermatologic Agents: Nursing Implications

53-3

Classification	Specific Agents	Nursing Implications
Antiinfectives and antibiotics	bacitracin, neomycin, clindamycin, erythromycin, tetracycline	• Bacitracin is odorless and nonstaining. • Neomycin may cause sensitization and photosensitivity when used with topical gentamicin. • Apply thin film of clindamycin and assess for allergy to drug and other antibiotics. • Erythromycin is applied with fingertips and hands each morning and evening. • Tetracycline is applied until area is moistened, but avoid eyes and mucous membranes because of alcohol content. • Allergic reactions noted by burning, redness, swelling, and stinging.
Antiinflammatories	betamethasone benzoate, dexamethasone, fluocinolone acetonide, fluocinonide, hydrocortisone, methylprednisolone	• All of these help stabilize cell membranes, and the ointment bases and glycol enhance the penetration of the agent into the skin. They usually are applied two times a day, and application technique depends on site. Monitor serum cortisol levels every other month until discharge in patients receiving long term. Be careful with occlusive dressings because this can lead to follicle infections, heat retention, or systemic effects, but occlusive dressings are often ordered. • Avoid sunlight on affected areas because burns may occur.
Antiparasitics	lindane, malathion	• With lindane, leave shampoo on for 4 minutes, then rinse and use nit comb to remove nits (eggs) from the hair shafts. Cream and lotions are usually left on for 12 hours, then washed off. Pubic lice is treated by applying for 12 hours, then washing off. • With malathion, there must be much care because it is flammable. Avoid open flames and hair dryers. Apply to hair and wash off after 8 to 12 hours.
Acne products (keratolytics)	benzoyl peroxide, tretinoin	• With benzoyl peroxide, effects are seen in 4 to 6 weeks; applied by lotion, bar, or cream sparingly. • Tretinoin to be applied each night at bedtime; apply after cleansing and allow 30 minutes to dry. If applied to wet skin, there may be increased redness or drying. Avoid ultraviolet light, weather extremes, or sunlight. Avoid abrasive cleansers and other keratolytic products because of possible toxicity to the skin. Wear sunscreen during therapy. • Follow directions closely when using the new Micro-sponge System with Retin-A Micro.
Burn products	silver sulfadiazine	• Apply as a 1% cream only to clean, debrided wounds and with gloved hands; apply ¹⁄₁₆ inch thick; keep continuously covered. Daily cleansing and debriding are important. Hemolysis may occur in patients with G6PD deficiency. If applied to extensive areas, adverse systemic reactions may occur similar to those seen for sulfonamide.
Antivirals	acylovir, penciclovir	• To be applied using a finger cot or gloved hand to prevent autocontamination; avoid contact with eyes. With genital lesions, loose covering or clothing over lesion is recommended to prevent further irritation to site. Avoid sexual activity if active lesions; can be transmitted even if the person is asymptomatic; condom use is encouraged depending on location of lesion. Apply a half-inch (1.25-cm) ribbon of ointment to about a 4-inch (10 cm) area. • Begin treatment when symptoms arise.
Antifungals	amphotericin B, clotrimazole, haloprogin, ketoconazole, nystatin, miconazole	• Can apply any of these very liberally to a clean, dry, affected skin area. Occlusive dressings are not recommended unless ordered. Avoid contact with eyes. Encourage good hygiene; keep area dry and clean; keep dry with powders to prevent maceration; keep area exposed to air and keep dry. Avoid alcohol use, since nausea, vomiting, or hypertension may occur because of some systemic absorption. Notify health care provider if sore throat, fever, or skin rash occurs (may indicate overgrowth of organisms).

important to follow any instructions or orders regarding adjuvant therapy. Often an occlusive or wet dressing may be needed, and medicated areas may need to be protected from exposure to air or sunlight. Strict adherence to the proper method of application and dosage of any dermatologic preparation is important to its effectiveness; however, doubling-up on dosing if a dose is missed is not recommended.

After completing the application procedure, the nurse should wash his or her hands, dispose of contaminated dressings, chart the procedure and findings, and maintain asepsis (surgical asepsis if the wound is open in any way or the skin is not intact). The privacy, comfort, and safety of the patient must be maintained, as it would be for any procedure. See Table 53-3 for the nursing implications pertinent to each group of dermatologic agents.

Patient teaching tips for dermatologic agents are presented in the box at right.

● Evaluation

Therapeutic responses to the various dermatologic preparations include improved condition of skin and healing of lesions or wounds; a decrease in the size of the lesions with eventual resolution of the lesions; and a decrease in swelling, redness, weeping, itching, and burning of the area. The physician should be notified if a therapeutic response is not noted within an appropriate time (for some agents, possibly 48 to 72 hours; for acne agents, often no response is seen for 1 to 2 months). Side effects for which to monitor include an increased severity of symptoms such as redness, swelling, pain, and drainage; fever; or any other unusual adverse reactions. Side effects may range from slight irritation of the site where the topical agent has been applied to an allergic reaction to toxic systemic effects. Always research each agent thoroughly so side effects and toxic effects can be understood and monitored for during therapy.

patient teaching tips
Dermatologic Preparations

➤ Instruct patients to keep their skin clean and dry and to maintain adequate general hygiene and diet during therapy for skin disorder.
➤ Patients should apply medication only as ordered and follow instructions carefully.
➤ Patients should be told to avoid exposure to sunlight, unless it is indicated.
➤ Patients should apply dressings to the area after the medication has been applied, as ordered or per the manufacturer's guidelines.
➤ Patients should be instructed to notify the physician of any unusual or adverse reactions.
➤ Patients must know that compliance with therapy is crucial to the therapeutic effectiveness of dermatologic preparations.
➤ Antifungals should be administered as ordered and consistently because fungal infections are very difficult to treat and often require prolonged therapy.
➤ Have patients demonstrate the application technique because this is important to ensuring effective therapy and compliance.

POINTS TO REMEMBER

Pharmacologic Principles
● Dermatologic agents are used to treat topical infections.
● Common skin disorders caused by bacteria: folliculitis, impetigo, furuncles, carbuncles, cellulitis.
● The bacteria most frequently responsible for acne is *Propionibacterium acnes.*
● The fungi that are responsible for causing topical fungal infections are *Candida,* dermatophytes, and *Malassezia furfur.*
● The most common topical fungal infections are candidal infections such as yeast infections.
● One of the most common topical viral infections is herpes simplex types 1 and 2.

Topical Anesthetics
● Used topically to numb the skin.
● Some indications include insect bites, burns (sunburn), poison ivy, and before painful injections.

Topical Antiinflammatory Agents
● Most commonly used are corticosteroids.
● Indicated for relief of topical inflammatory and pruritic disorders.

● Beneficial effects of corticosteroids include antiinflammatory, antipruritic, vasoconstrictor actions.

Topical Antineoplastics
● Used to treat various skin lesions that are believed to be premalignant, as well as basal cell carcinomas.
● Commonly used agent: fluorouracil.

Nursing Considerations
● Adverse and toxic reactions to dermatologic agents *can* and *do* happen, so cautious administration, per physician's orders and manufacturer's guidelines, is critical to ensure safe and effective treatment.
● Adequate and correct application of these agents by the nurse is also critical to ensure safe and effective treatment.
● Patient education about the medication, its administration, and effectiveness is important to ensure compliance.
● The effectiveness of the therapy is determined by whether the lesions or affected areas heal or resolve without adverse reactions.

REVIEW QUESTIONS

1. Tretinoin has been ordered for a young adolescent at the clinic. Which of the following are important to discuss with him regarding this medication?
   a. Avoid foods high in sodium and water.
   b. Extreme weather and sunshine pose no problem for him.
   c. Avoid ultraviolet light, weather extremes, and abrasive cleaners.
   d. The drug may cause a pallor discoloration around the chin and eyes.

2. Silver sulfadiazine has been ordered for the patient's second-degree hand burns. Which of the following statements should be shared with the patient about this drug?
   a. Apply to the area, even if debris or pus is apparent on the burn.
   b. Apply with a gloved hand, keep the area covered, and follow directions.
   c. It should be generously applied and vigorously rubbed into the area.
   d. Keeping the area exposed after application is important to the healing.

3. Minoxidil is used topically to treat:
   a. Petechia.
   b. Hair loss.
   c. Gynecomastia.
   d. Varicose veins.

4. Patient teaching about minoxidil for hair loss should include which of the following statements?
   a. Apply at least ½ of the tube twice daily for best results.
   b. Therapeutic results may take up to 4 months after treatments begin.
   c. Systemic absorption is not a concern with this type of hair-loss treatment.
   d. Avoid massaging into the scalp to prevent systemic absorption and resultant hypertensive episodes.

5. Which of the following topical forms of a corticosteroid medication usually result in better penetration to the skin?
   a. Gels
   b. Creams
   c. Lotions
   d. Ointments

For Answers see www.harcourthealth.com/MERLIN/Lilley/.

CRITICAL THINKING Activities

1. Develop a teaching plan for a 29-year-old mother who has a 6-year-old child newly diagnosed with head lice. Include an emphasis on how to prevent contaminating others and preventing future episodes.

2. Do you consider tretinoin therapy beneficial for all patients? Why or why not? Support your answer.

3. Discuss the major functions of the epidermis that make its intactness so important to homeostasis.

For Answers see www.harcourthealth.com/MERLIN/Lilley/.

bibliography

Albanese J, Nutz P: *Mosby's 2001 nursing drug reference and review cards*, St Louis, 2001, Mosby.

American Hospital Formulary Service: *AHFS drug information*, Bethesda, Md, 2000, American Society of Health-System Pharmacists.

Anderson PO, Knoben JE, Troutman WG: *Handbook of clinical drug data 1999-2000*, ed 9, New York, 1999, McGraw-Hill.

Habif TP: *Clinical dermatology: a color guide to diagnosis and therapy*, ed 3, St Louis, 1996, Mosby.

Johns Hopkins Hospital, Department of Pediatrics et al: *The Harriet Lane handbook*, ed 15, St Louis, 2000, Mosby.

Keen JH: *Critical care and emergency drug reference*, ed 3, St Louis, 1996, Mosby.

McEvoy GK: *AHFS drug information*, Bethesda, Md, 2000, American Society of Hospital Pharmacists.

McKenry LM, Salerno E: *Mosby's pharmacology in nursing*, ed 21, St Louis, 2001, Mosby.

Mosby's GenRx: a comprehensive reference for generic and brand drugs, ed 10, St Louis, 2000, Mosby.

Skidmore-Roth L: *Mosby's 2001 nursing drug reference*, St Louis, 2001, Mosby.

United States Pharmacopeial Convention: *USP DI: drug information for the health care professional, vol. 1*, ed 20, Englewood, Colo, 2000, Micromedex.

Activity

Remember to check the **Online Worksheet** for additional learning opportunities: **www.harcourthealth.com/MERLIN/Lilley/**

Chapter 54

Ophthalmic Agents

objectives

www.harcourthealth.com/MERLIN/Lilley/

Look for this symbol for topics covered in the **Online Worksheet** Activity

When you reach the end of this chapter, you should be able to do the following:

1 Discuss the anatomy and physiology of the structures of the eye.

2 List the various ophthalmic agents used within their classifications.

3 Describe the process of instilling eye drops or eye ointments.

4 Discuss the mechanisms of action, cautions, side effects, and contraindications of ophthalmic preparations and associated nursing implications.

5 Develop a comprehensive nursing care plan that includes education for patients receiving ophthalmic agents.

drug profiles

acetazolamide, p. 866
acetylcholine, p. 860
apraclonidine, p. 863
artificial tears, p. 876
○━ atropine sulfate, p. 876
bacitracin, p. 871
betaxolol, p. 864
chloramphenicol, p. 872
chymotrypsin, p. 876
○━ ciprofloxacin, p. 871
○━ cromolyn, p. 876
cyclopentolate, p. 876
dexamethasone, p. 874
dipivefrin, p. 863
echothiophate and isoflurophate, p. 861
○━ erythromycin, p. 870

flurbiprofen, p. 874
○━ fluorescein, p. 876
○━ gentamicin, p. 870
glycerin, p. 867
hyperosmolar sodium chloride, p. 876
ketorolac, p. 874
mannitol, p. 867
natamycin, p. 870
○━ physostigmine, p. 861
○━ pilocarpine, p. 860
silver nitrate, p. 872
sulfacetamide, p. 871
tetracaine, p. 876
tetracycline, p. 872
timolol, p. 864
vidarabine, p. 872

○━ Key drug.

glossary

Accommodation (ə kom′ ə da′ shən) The state or process of adapting or adjusting one thing or set of things to another. In ophthalmology, *accommodation* refers to the adjustment of the eye to variation in distance; the elasticity of the lens allows it to change shape and focusing power. (p. 856)

Acute (congestive) angle-closure glaucoma (glow ko′ mə) Glaucoma that occurs if the pupil in an eye with a narrow angle between the iris and cornea dilates markedly, causing the folded iris to block the exit of aqueous humor. Also called *angle-closure glaucoma.* (p. 858)

Aqueous humor (a′ kwe əs \ hu′mər) The clear, watery fluid circulating in the anterior and posterior chambers of the eye. (p. 855)

Bactericidal (bak ter′ i si′ dəl) Kills bacteria. (p. 868)

Bacteriostatic (bak ter′ e o stat′ ik) Stops the growth of bacteria. (p. 869)

Canal of Schlemm A tiny vein at the angle of the anterior chamber of the eye that connects with the pectinate villi, draining the aqueous humor and funneling it into the bloodstream. Also called *Schlemm's canal.* (p. 856)

Cataract (kat′ ə rakt) An abnormal progressive condition of the lens of the eye, characterized by loss of transparency. A gray-white opacity can be seen within the lens. If cataracts are untreated, sight is eventually lost. At onset vision is blurred; then bright lights glare diffusely, and distortion and double vision may develop. (p. 856)

Cones Photoreceptive cells in the retina of the eye that enable a person to visualize colors. (p. 856)

Cornea (kor′ ne ə) The convex, transparent, anterior part of the eye. It is nonvascular and allows light to pass through it to the lens. (p. 855)

Cycloplegia (si′ klo ple′ je ə) Paralysis of the ciliary muscles, which prevents the accommodation of the lens to variations in distance. Certain ophthalmic drugs are used to induce cycloplegia to allow examination of the eye. (p. 856)

Cycloplegics (si′ klo ple′ jikz) Drugs that paralyze the ciliary muscles of the eye. (p. 856)

Dilatator muscle (dil′ ə ta′ tər) A muscle that contracts the iris of the eye and dilates the pupil. It is composed of radiating fibers, like spokes of a wheel, that converge from the circumference of the iris toward the center. The sympathetic nervous system controls this muscle. Also called *dilatator pupillae.* (p. 855)

Glaucoma (glaw ko' mə) An abnormal condition of elevated pressure within an eye because of obstruction of the outflow of aqueous humor. (p. 857)

Lens (lenz) The transparent, crystalline, curved structure of the eye that is located directly behind the iris and the pupil and attached to the ciliary body by ligaments. (p. 856)

Lysozyme (li' so som) An enzyme with antiseptic actions that destroys some foreign organisms. It is normally present in tears, saliva, sweat, and breast milk. (p. 855)

Miotics (mi ot' iks) Drugs that constrict the pupil. (p. 856)

Open-angle glaucoma (glaw ko' mə) A type of glaucoma that is often bilateral, develops slowly, and is genetically determined. The obstruction that prevents outflow of aqueous humor is believed to be within the canal of Schlemm. It occurs more commonly than closed-angle glaucoma. Open-angle glaucoma is also called *chronic glaucoma.* (p. 858)

Ophthalmoscopic examinations (of thal mə skop' ik) An eye examination using an ophthalmoscope. An ophthalmoscope is a device used to examine the interior of the eye. It includes a light, a mirror with a single hole through which the examiner may look, and a dial holding several lenses of varying strengths. (p. 858)

Pupil (pu' pil) A circular opening in the iris of the eye, located slightly to the nasal side of the center of the iris. The pupil lies behind the anterior chamber of the eye and the cornea and in front of the lens. Its diameter changes with contraction and relaxation of the muscular fibers of the iris as the eye responds to changes in light, emotional states, and other kinds of stimulation. The pupil is the window of the eye through which light passes to the lens and the retina. (p. 855)

Rod One of the tiny cylindric photoreceptive elements arranged perpendicularly to the surface of the retina. Rods are especially sensitive in low-intensity light and are responsible for black and white vision. (p. 856)

Sphincter muscle (sfingk' tər) A circular band of muscle fibers that constricts a passage or closes a natural opening in the body, such as the *sphincter pupillae.* The sphincter pupillae is a muscle that expands the iris, narrowing the diameter of the pupil of the eye. The parasympathetic nervous system controls this muscle. (p. 855)

Tears Watery saline or alkaline fluid secreted by the lacrimal glands to moisten the conjunctiva. It is isotonic and contains an enzyme called *lysozyme.* Tears are also called *dacrya.* (p. 855)

Uvea (u' ve ə) The fibrous tunic beneath the sclera that includes the iris, the ciliary body, and the choroid of the eye. Also called *tunica vasculosa bulbi* or *uveal tract.* (p. 855)

Vitreous humor (vit' re əs) A transparent, semigelatinous substance contained in a thin membrane filling the cavity behind the crystalline lens of the eye. Also called *corpus vitreum* or *vitreous body.* (p. 856)

STRUCTURE OF THE EYE

To thoroughly understand the agents used to treat disorders of the eye, it is necessary to understand the structure and normal function of the eye. The eye is the organ responsible for the sense of sight. Figure 54-1 illustrates the structures of the eye, all of which are needed for accurate eyesight. Each eyeball is nearly spherical and approximately 1 inch in diameter. Each eye is recessed into a

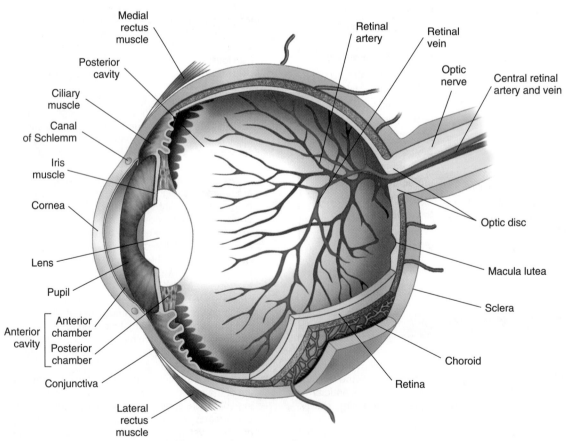

Fig. 54-1 A horizontal section through the left eyeball, looking from the top down. (Modified from Thibodeau GA, Patton KT: *Anatomy and physiology,* ed 4, St Louis, 1999, Mosby.)

skull cavity in the frontal orbit of the skull. The exposed anterior (front) portion is covered by three layers: the protective external layer (cornea and sclera), middle layer (choroid, iris, and ciliary body), and light-sensitive retina. All of these layers are protected by the eyelid, an external protection device.

The eye is held in place and moved by several sets of muscles that are controlled by cranial nerves. These muscles include the rectus and oblique muscles. There are four types of rectus muscles: inferior, superior, medial, and lateral. There are two types of oblique muscles: inferior and superior. These muscles are shown in Figure 54-2. In addition to the structures associated with the sight organ, there are several accessory structures. The structure and purpose of each are as follows:

- *Eyebrow:* Rows of short hair above (superior) the upper eyelids. The eyebrow protects the eye from direct light, falling dust or other small particles, and perspiration coming from the forehead.
- *Eyelid:* Layer of muscle and skin lined by the conjunctiva. The eyelid is moveable and can open or close. It protects the eye when closed and allows for vision when open.
- *Eyelashes:* Two or three rows of hairs that are located on the edge (margin) of the eyelids. They help prevent small particles from falling into the eye when it is open.
- *Palpebral fissure:* The space between the upper and lower eyelids when the eyelids are open.
- *Sclera:* A tough white coat of fibrous tissue that surrounds the entire eyeball except for the cornea. Commonly called the *white of the eye.*
- *Conjunctiva:* Mucous membrane that lines the eyelids and covers the exposed surface of the eyeball.
- *Iris:* Colored (pigmented) muscular apparatus behind the cornea.
- *Pupil:* The variable-sized opening in the center of the iris that allows light to enter into the eyeball when the eyelids are open.
- *Medial canthus:* The site of union near the nose for the upper and lower eyelids.
- *Lacrimal caruncle:* A small and rounded elevation covered by modified skin at the medial palpebral commissure.
- *Lateral canthus:* The site of union away from the nose for the upper and lower eyelids.

LACRIMAL GLANDS

The eye is kept moist and healthy by an intricate network of connected canals, ducts, and sacs. They work together to keep the eye moist. The lacrimal glands produce tears that bathe and cleanse the exposed anterior portion of the eye. **Tears** are composed of an isotonic, aqueous solution that contains an enzyme called **lysozyme,** which acts as an antibacterial to help prevent eye infections.

LAYERS OF THE EYE

The fibrous outer layer of the eye has two parts—the sclera and the cornea. The sclera is a tough, fibrous layer that protects and maintains the shape of the eye. The **cornea** is a nonvascular transparent portion of the outer layer that allows light to enter the eye. It is pain sensitive and obtains nutrition from the **aqueous humor,** the clear watery fluid that circulates in the anterior and posterior chambers of the eye.

The vascular middle layer of the eye is composed of the anterior iris, ciliary body, and posterior choroid. These three structures are collectively called the **uvea.** The *iris* gives color to the eye and has an adjustable-sized opening in the center called the **pupil.** The main function of the iris is to regulate the amount of light that enters the eye by causing the size of the pupil to vary. Pupil size is controlled by a circular smooth muscle called the **sphincter muscle** and radial smooth muscle called the **dilatator muscle.** The circular muscles decrease pupil size, and the radial muscles increase pupil size. The parasympathetic nervous system (PSNS) innervates the sphincter muscles, whereas the sympathetic nervous system (SNS) controls the dilatator muscles (Fig. 54-3).

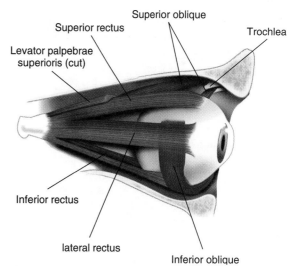

Fig. 54-2 Extrinsic muscles of the right eye. Lateral view. (Modified from Thibodeau GA, Patton KT: *Anatomy and physiology,* ed 4, St Louis, 1999, Mosby.)

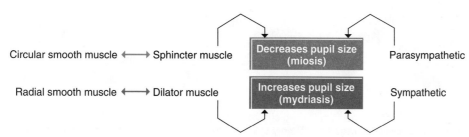

Fig. 54-3 Different nervous systems control pupil size.

The anterior portion of the sclera becomes the *ciliary body,* which produces aqueous humor. The aqueous humor is removed from the anterior chamber via the **canal of Schlemm.** The *choroid* is a thin dark layer that lines most of the internal side of the sclera. The function of the choroid is to absorb light and prevent its reflection out of the eye.

The **lens** is the transparent crystalline structure of the eye, located directly behind the iris and the pupil. It is held in place by ligaments that are attached to the ciliary body. Accordingly the lens divides the interior of the eyeball into posterior (back) and anterior (forward) chambers. The larger chamber behind the lens is filled with a jelly-like fluid called the **vitreous humor** that is constantly being formed by the ciliary body.

The transparent lens is composed of uniform layers of protein fibers that are encased by a clear connective tissue capsule. A loss of lens transparency results in a visual condition called **cataracts.** Before light images reach the retina, they are focused into a sharp image by the biconvex lens of the eye. The elasticity of the lens enables it to change its shape and focusing power. This process is called **accommodation** and is facilitated by the ciliary body. Paralysis of accommodation is called **cycloplegia.**

Mydriatics are drugs that dilate the pupil; those agents that constrict the pupil are called **miotics** (e.g., acetylcholine, physostigmine, and pilocarpine). Drugs that paralyze the ciliary body are termed **cycloplegics** (e.g., apraclonidine and dipivefrin) (Fig. 54-4).

The retinal layer of the eye is a thin delicate layer that contains light-sensitive receptors. It covers the choroid and is attached to the optic nerve near its center. The basic function of the retina is image formation via light-sensitive receptors called *rods* and *cones.* Both types of photoreceptors are located near the surface of the retina. **Rods** produce black-and-white vision, especially in low light, and **cones** are responsible for color vision (Fig. 54-5). The function of the attached optic nerve is to connect the retina with the visual center of the brain.

This chapter focuses on the drugs used to treat disorders of the eye, which can be divided into three major groups: antiglaucoma agents, mydriatics and cycloplegics, and antiinfective/antiinflammatory agents. In addition to the three principal types of drugs are the diagnostic products: enzymes, irrigating solutions, eye washes, and hyperosmolar preparations.

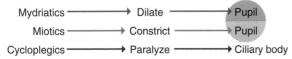

Fig. 54-4 Drug classes and their effects on pupil size.

ANTIGLAUCOMA DRUGS

The aqueous humor is a nourishing liquid that is produced by the ciliary body and flows from the posterior chamber (behind the iris) to the anterior chamber (in front of the iris). It is removed via the canal of Schlemm, which is located adjacent to the union of the sclera and cornea in the anterior chamber. When the normal flow and drainage of aqueous humor is inhibited, a serious ocular condition called glaucoma occurs. Figure 54-6 illus-

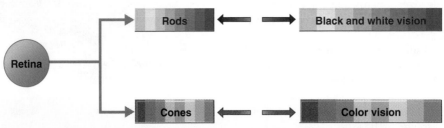

Fig. 54-5 Functions of rods and cones in relation to color vision.

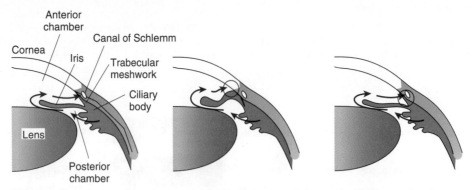

Fig. 54-6 Main structures of the eye and an enlargement of the canal of Schlemm showing an aqueous flow. (Modified from McKenry LM, Salerno E: *Mosby's pharmacology in nursing,* ed 21, St Louis, 2001, Mosby.)

trates the main structures of the eye and an enlargement of the canal of Schlemm showing aqueous flow.

Glaucoma is an eye disorder characterized by excessive intraocular pressure (IOP) created by abnormally elevated levels of aqueous humor. This occurs when the aqueous humor is not drained through the canal of Schlemm as quickly as it is formed. The accumulated aqueous humor creates a backward pressure that pushes the vitreous humor against the retina. Continued pressure on the retina destroys its neurons, leading to impaired vision and eventual blindness (Fig. 54-7). There are several categories of glaucoma that are classified according to underlying cause. The three main categories are primary glaucoma, secondary glaucoma, and congenital glaucoma. Table 54-1 lists the types of glaucoma and their characteristics.

Effective treatment of glaucoma involves reducing IOP either by increasing the drainage of aqueous humor or by decreasing the production of aqueous humor. Some drugs may do both. Drugs used to reduce IOP include the following:

- Parasympathomimetics, also called *cholinesterase inhibitors* (direct or indirect acting)
- Sympathomimetics
- Beta blockers
- Carbonic anhydrase inhibitors
- Osmotic diuretics.
- Prostaglandins

See Table 54-2 for a drug class comparison of aqueous humor effects.

PARASYMPATHOMIMETICS

Both the direct and indirect parasympathomimetic drugs cause miosis and pupillary constriction. These two types of ophthalmic agents work in different ways to *mimic* the PSNS neurotransmitter acetylcholine (ACh) and are thus referred to as parasympatho*mimetic* drugs. The direct-acting parasympathomimetic drugs are chemically related to ACh and can therefore mediate nerve impulse

transmission at all cholinergic or parasympathetic nerve sites. The indirect parasympathomimetic drugs indirectly stimulate the PSNS by inhibiting cholinesterase, the enzyme that normally inactivates ACh. This causes more ACh to be present at the PSNS receptor and potentiates the normal effects of ACh. The parasympathomimetics on the average lower intraocular pressure by 20% to 30%. Examples of ophthalmic drugs that fall into these two drug categories are found in Box 54-1.

Mechanism of Action

The direct-acting miotics are able to directly stimulate PSNS receptors because their structures closely resemble that of the PSNS neurotransmitter ACh. Direct-acting miotics are administered topically to the eye. This route of administration drastically limits systemic absorption of the drug by keeping the cholinergic effects localized to the site of administration in the eye. The cholinergic response produced by these drugs causes pupillary contraction (miosis), which leads to a reduction of IOP secondary to an increased outflow of aqueous humor (Fig. 54-8).

The indirect-acting miotics work by preventing ACh breakdown. They prevent ACh from being inactivated by inhibiting cholinesterase, which results in higher levels of ACh and allows ACh to remain at the receptor longer. The cholinergic response produced by these drugs causes miosis, which leads to reduced IOP (Fig. 54-9).

ACh is the endogenous mediator of nerve impulses in the PSNS. It stimulates cholinergic receptors. This results in several effects: miosis, vasodilation, contraction of ciliary muscles, and reduced IOP. The action of ACh is short lived. It is rapidly hydrolyzed by cholinesterases (acetylcholinesterase [AChE] and pseudocholinesterase) to choline and acetic acid. Direct-acting miotics have effects similar to those of ACh, but their actions are more prolonged (Fig. 54-10).

The indirect-acting miotics bind with and inactivate cholinesterases (AChE and pseudocholinesterase), thus

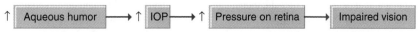

Fig. 54-7 How increased aqueous humor can result in impaired vision.

Glaucoma: Types and Characteristics

54-1

	Chronic Open-Angle	Acute Angle-Closure
Nature of angle	Large	Narrow
Age of onset and race	>30 yr African-American	>30 yr Caucasian
Major symptoms	Blurred vision	Blurred vision
	Occasional headaches	Severe headaches
		Eye pain
		Visual halos around lights
Treatment	Topical or systemic drugs	Topical or systemic drugs
	Surgery	Surgery

Antiglaucoma Drug Effects on Aqueous Humor

TABLE 54-2

Drug Class	Increased Drainage	Decreased Production
Direct parasympathomimetic	+++	+
Indirect parasympathomimetic (i.e., cholinesterase inhibitor)	+++	0
Sympathomimetic	++	+++
Beta blockers	+	+++
Carbonic anhydrase inhibitors	0	+++
Osmotic diuretics	0	+++
Prostaglandins	+++	++

Direct- and Indirect-Acting Parasympathomimetic Ophthalmic Drugs

BOX 54-1

DIRECT-ACTING	INDIRECT-ACTING
acetylcholine	demecarium
carbachol	echothiophate
pilocarpine	isofluorophate
	physostigmine

inhibiting hydrolysis of ACh. As a result ACh accumulates at cholinergic nerve endings. Indirect-acting agents that are organophosphates (echothiophate and isofluorophate) act by phosphorylating cholinesterase. This effect is irreversible. Pralidoxime, a cholinesterase reactivator, may reverse these effects and stimulate production of new cholinesterase enzymes by the body. This production of new enzymes may take days or even weeks.

Drug Effects

The drug effects of the miotics (direct and indirect) alter various eye muscles, IOP, aqueous humor, and vasodilation of blood vessels in and around the eye. The drug effects that alter the muscles of the eye result in contraction of the iris sphincter, which produces constriction of the pupil (miosis) and contraction of the ciliary muscle, resulting in spasm of accommodation.

The drug effects that alter the pressure within the eye reduce IOP in both normal and glaucomatous eyes. They do this by facilitating aqueous humor outflow by causing contraction of the ciliary muscle, thus widening the area from which this fluid escapes. IOP is also reduced by constriction of the pupil, which causes the iris to stretch and thus relieves blockage of the area where the fluid leaves the inner eye. This effect is less pronounced in individuals with dark eyes (brown or hazel) than in those with light eyes (blue) because the pigment absorbs the drugs and dark eyes have more pigment.

The drug effects of the miotics cause vasodilation of blood vessels of the conjunctiva, iris, and ciliary body, resulting in increased permeability of the blood aqueous barrier, which may lead to vascular congestion and ocular inflammation. This congestion and inflammation is more common with long-acting anticholinesterases (indirect miotics).

Therapeutic Uses

The direct- and indirect-acting miotics are used for open-angle glaucoma, angle-closure glaucoma, ocular surgery,

convergent strabismus, and ophthalmologic examinations. The miotics are used topically on the eye to reduce elevated IOP in the treatment of primary **open-angle glaucoma**. This reduction in IOP is the result of contraction of the ciliary muscle and widening of the exit route of the aqueous humor. **Acute (congestive) angle-closure glaucoma** may be relieved temporarily by pilocarpine or occasionally by carbachol to acutely decrease extremely high IOP.

Some of the miotic drugs may be used for ocular surgery. Pilocarpine, carbachol, and acetylcholine are used to reduce IOP and to protect the lens by causing miosis before certain types of laser surgery on the iris. Miotics may be used to counteract the mydriatic effects (dilation effects) of sympathomimetic agents such as hydroxyamphetamine and phenylephrine that are used for **ophthalmoscopic examinations**. Table 54-3 lists the miotic drugs and their indications.

Side Effects and Adverse Effects

Most of the side effects and adverse effects associated with the use of cholinergic and anticholinesterase drugs (miotics) are local and limited to the eye. There are, however, some systemic effects that can occur, especially if sufficient amounts of drug pass into the bloodstream. Some common side effects and adverse effects associated with the miotics are listed in Table 54-4.

The most common *ocular side effects* that may occur with use of miotic drugs are blurred vision and accommodative spasms. Other undesirable effects include conjunctivitis, lacrimation, twitching eyelids, poor low-light vision, and pain. Prolonged use can result in iris cysts, lens opacities, and rarely, retinal detachment.

Systemic effects that may occur with the use of miotic drugs are caused by PSNS stimulation. Cholinesterase inhibitors usually produce more pronounced effects than direct-acting agents. The most common side effects include bronchodilation, lacrimation, temporary stinging upon instillation, decreased night vision, nausea, vomiting, salivation, sweating, gastrointestinal (GI) stimulation, and urinary incontinence.

Activity

Toxicity and Management of Overdose

Occasionally toxic effects may develop after the use of topically applied miotic drugs. Toxicity produced by miotics is an extension of their systemic effects and is more common with prolonged use of high doses. Most severe

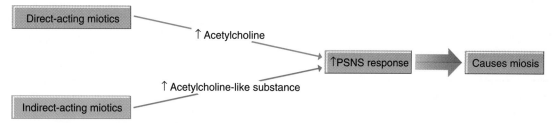

Fig. 54-8 The therapeutic effects of direct-acting parasympathomimetics on glaucoma.

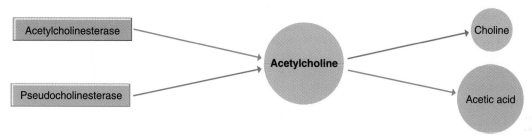

Fig. 54-9 Cholinergic response of miosis to parasympathomimetics.

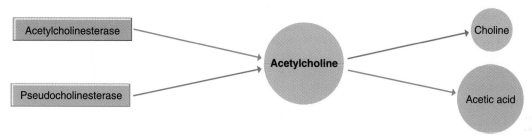

Fig. 54-10 Metabolism of acetylcholine by endogenous enzymes.

Miotics: Indications

Table 54-3

Miotic Agent	Indications
acetylcholine	Complete and rapid miosis after cataract lens extraction, iridectomy
carbachol	Open-angle glaucoma
demecarium	Accommodative estropia, obstructive aqueous humor outflow, open-angle glaucoma after iridectomy
echothiophate	Accommodative estropia, obstructive aqueous humor outflow, open- and closed-angle glaucoma after iridectomy
isoflurophate	Accommodative estropia, obstructive aqueous humor outflow, open-angle glaucoma after iridectomy
physostigmine	Open-angle glaucoma
pilocarpine	Open-angle glaucoma, secondary glaucoma after iridectomy, cyclo-plegic reversal

Miotics: Adverse Effects

Table 54-4

Body System	Side/Adverse Effect
Cardiovascular	Hypotension, bradycardia, or tachycardia
Central nervous system	Headache
Eye, ear, nose, throat	Visual blurring, myopia (nearsightedness), ciliary spasm, brow pain
Gastrointestinal	Nausea, vomiting, abdominal cramps, diarrhea
Respiratory	May precipitate asthma attacks

and prolonged effects are seen with long-acting anticholinesterases. Excessive PSNS effects are treated with 0.4 to 2 mg of atropine administered intramuscularly or intravenously for adults and 0.04 to 0.08 mg/kg administered intravenously or intramuscularly for children. If required, repeat doses can be given every 5 minutes intravenously and every 15 minutes intramuscularly. In addition, pralidoxime (Protapam) may be required to re-

verse paralysis induced by either of the organophosphate anticholinesterases (echothiophate and isoflurophate).

Interactions

Direct- and indirect-acting miotics are capable of interactions with several categories of drugs. The miotic drugs, when given with topical epinephrine, timolol, and carbonic anhydrase inhibitors, have additive lowering effects on IOP. Systemic cholinesterase inhibitors have additive effects when given with mitoic drugs. Indirect-acting miotics may potentiate the effects of anesthetic agents.

Dosages

For recommended dosages of miotic agents, see the dosages table on p. 860.

DOSAGES Selected Miotic Agents

agent	pharmacologic class	dosage range	purpose
acetycholine (Miochol-E)	Direct-acting	5-70 mg	Surgical miosis
demecarium (Humorsol) 0.125%, 0.25% solution	Indirect-acting	1-2 gtt/day	Glaucoma
echothiophate (Phospholine Iodide) 0.03%, 0.06%, 0.125%, 0.25% solution	Indirect-acting	2 gtt/day	Glaucoma
isoflurophate (Floropryl) 0.025% ophthalmic ointment	Indirect-acting	0.5 cm ribbon q8-72h	Glaucoma
physostigmine (Isopto Eserine) 0.25%, 0.5% solution 0.02% ophthalmic ointment	Indirect-acting	2 gtt up to 4 times/day 0.5 cm ribbon up to 3 times/day	Glaucoma
pilocarpine (Pilocar, Akarpine, IsoptoCarpine, Miocarpine) 0.25%, 0.5%, 1%, 2%, 3%, 4% solution 4% gel	Direct-acting	1-2 gtt q4-12h 1.5 cm ribbon/day hs	Glaucoma
pilocarpine insert (Ocusert Pilo) 20 μg/h, 40 μg/h	Direct-acting	Insert 1 wk	Glaucoma

gtt, Drop.

drug profiles

Direct-acting and indirect-acting miotics have a variety of uses. The principal use is that of relief of symptoms caused by glaucoma and increased IOP. The three most commonly used direct-acting miotics are acetylcholine, carbachol, and pilocarpine. These drugs have actions similar to those of ACh. The four commonly used indirect-acting miotics are demecarium, echothiophate, isoflurophate, and physostigmine. These agents work by preventing cholinesterase from breaking down ACh, allowing it to produce a prolonged PSNS response.

Since the safe use of miotics in pregnancy has not been established, many of the miotics are classified as pregnancy category C agents. Because of the potential risks of cholinesterase inhibition in general, the manufacturers of some anticholinesterase agents (e.g., demecarium and isoflurophate) state that the drugs are contraindicated in women who are or may become pregnant.

Direct-acting miotic drugs are contraindicated in patients who have shown a hypersensitivity reaction to them, those with acute inflammatory conditions in the anterior chamber, and those with pupillary block glaucoma. Indirect-acting miotics are contraindicated in patients who have shown a hypersensitivity reaction to them and in patients with acute inflammatory conditions and glaucoma associated with iridocyclitis. In addition, echothiophate is not suitable for treatment of most cases of closed-angle glaucoma.

DIRECT-ACTING MIOTICS
acetylcholine

Acetylcholine (Miochol-E) is a direct-acting parasympathomimetic agent that is used to produce miosis during ophthalmic surgery. It has very quick onset and may begin to work almost immediately. When used for ophthalmic indications, acetylcholine is administered directly into the anterior chamber of the eye before and after securing one or more sutures. It is available as a 20-mg powder for intraocular use only. Commonly recommended dosages for acetylcholine are listed in the dosages table above.

PHARMACOKINETICS

HALF-LIFE	ONSET	PEAK	DURATION
Short	Instant	Instant	10 min

pilocarpine

Pilocarpine (Ocusert Pilo, Pilopine HS, Isopto Carpine, Pilocar, and many others) is a direct-acting parasympathomimetic agent that is used as a miotic in the treatment of glaucoma. Unlike other direct-acting miotics (acetylcholine and carbachol), which have only one formulation and limited indications, pilocarpine has a variety of uses and is available in many different formulations and strengths.

Pilocarpine is available as an ocular system formulation that offers the advantage of less frequent dosing because it may only need to be administered once per week. This may be an advantage over ophthalmic solutions with shorter durations, particularly in patients with compliance problems.

Pilocarpine is also available as a gel, solution, and some combination solutions. Pilocarpine ocular system delivers 20 μg/hr for 7 days or 40 μg/hr for 7 days (Ocusert Pilo-20 and Ocusert Pilo-40). It is also available as a 4% gel and 0.25%, 0.5%, 1%, 2%, 3%, 4%, 5%, 6%, 7%, 8%, and 1% ophthalmic solutions. Commonly recommended dosages for pilocarpine are listed in the dosages table on p. 860.

PHARMACOKINETICS

HALF-LIFE	ONSET	PEAK	DURATION
Unknown	10-30 min	75 min	4-8 hr

INDIRECT-ACTING MIOTICS
echothiophate and isoflurophate
Echothiophate (Phospholine Iodide) and isoflurophate (Floropryl) act indirectly and are classified as long-acting anticholinesterase miotics. Structurally both of these agents are organophosphates, which work by phosphorylating the enzyme cholinesterase. This results in an irreversible inhibition of the enzyme. Because the enzyme is permanently inactivated and the patient must synthesize new enzyme to reverse the drug effects, these drugs are considered long acting.

Both drugs are indicated for the symptomatic treatment of glaucoma and convergent strabismus (crossed eyes). The potential for misuse and the consequences of this misuse are very harmful. For these reasons both of these drugs are available only by prescription. They are classified as pregnancy C drugs and are contraindicated in patients who have shown a hypersensitivity reaction to them and in those with uveitis. Echothiophate is available only in 0.03%, 0.06%, 0.125%, and 0.25% ophthalmic solutions. Isoflurophate is available only as a 0.025% ophthalmic ointment. Commonly recommended dosages for echothiophate and isoflurophate are listed in the dosages table on p. 860.

PHARMACOKINETICS

HALF-LIFE	ONSET	PEAK	DURATION
Long	10-30 min	30 min	1-4 wk

physostigmine
Physostigmine (Isopto Eserine, Isopto P-ES, Eserine Sulfate) and demecarium (Humorsol) are indirect-acting miotics that are classified as anticholinesterase inhibitors. Structurally both of these agents are carbamates. They inactivate cholinesterases by carbamylation; this inactivation of cholinesterase is reversible because the enzyme is not permanently inactivated and the patient does not have to synthesize new cholinesterase to reverse the drug effects.

These two agents are classified as pregnancy category C agents and are contraindicated in patients who have shown a hypersensitivity reaction to them and in those with inflammatory disease of the iris or ciliary body. Physostigmine is available as 0.25% and 0.5% ophthalmic solutions, and demecarium is available as 0.125% and 0.25% ophthalmic solutions. Commonly recommended dosages for physostigmine and demecarium are listed in the dosages table on p. 860.

PHARMACOKINETICS

HALF-LIFE	ONSET	PEAK	DURATION
Unknown	10-30 min	Variable	12-48 hr

SYMPATHOMIMETICS
Sympathomimetic drugs like brimonidine, apraclonidine, dipivefrin, and epinephrine are used for the treatment of glaucoma and ocular hypertension. Dipivefrin is the product of epinephrine. When instilled into the eye, it is hydrolyzed to epinephrine. Its advantage over epinephrine is that it has enhanced lipophilicity and can penetrate into the anterior chamber of the eye. On a weight basis, dipivefrin is 4 to 11 times as potent as epinephrine in reducing IOP and 5 to 12 times as potent as epinephrine in pupil dilation (mydriasis). Apraclonidine and brimonidine are structurally and pharmacologically related to clonidine. Apraclonidine is a relatively selective alpha$_2$ stimulant.

Because these drugs are sympathomimetic agents, they mimic the sympathetic neurotransmitters norepinephrine and epinephrine and stimulate the dilator muscle to contract. This stimulation results in increased pupil size (mydriasis) (Fig. 54-11). Dilation is seen within minutes of instillation of the ophthalmic drops and lasts for several hours, during which time the IOP is reduced.

Mechanism of Action
These agents reduce IOP in patients with normal IOP or in patients with elevated IOP, such as those with glaucoma. Dipivefrin 0.1% reduces mean IOP approximately 15% to 25%. The exact mechanism by which the sympathomimetic drugs lower IOP is unknown. They are believed to work by stimulating both α- and β_2-receptors, causing the dilator muscle to contract, resulting in mydriasis. During mydriasis there is an increase in aqueous humor outflow, resulting in a decrease in IOP. These effects appear to be dose dependent.

Apraclonidine reduces IOP 23% to 39% both peripherally and centrally. The centrally mediated effect is inhibition of adrenergic vasoconstriction in the eye. By stimulating α- and β_2-receptors, apraclonidine prevents constriction of the blood vessels of the eye and reduces pressure, resulting in reduced aqueous humor formation. Brimonidine works in a similar fashion to apraclonidine.

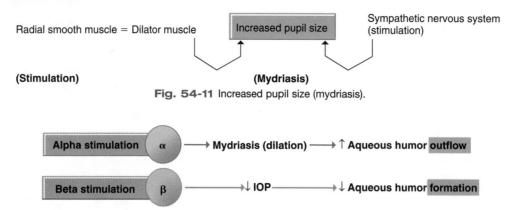

Fig. 54-11 Increased pupil size (mydriasis).

Fig. 54-12 Ocular effects of alpha (α) and beta (β) stimulation.

Drug Effects

The drug effects of dipivefrin and epinephrine are the result of both α- and β_2-stimulation, which causes both ocular and systemic effects. The ocular effects of these drugs are a decrease in IOP and an increase in aqueous humor outflow (Fig. 54-12). The decreased IOP is apparently the result of decreased aqueous humor fluid in the anterior chamber of the eye.

Dipivefrin is a more lipophilic agent and therefore has more localized effects in the eye. However, both dipivefrin and epinephrine can cause drug effects outside the eye. Because these two drugs mimic the effects of the SNS neurotransmitters, they can cause increased cardiovascular effects such as increased heart rate or blood pressure.

Therapeutic Uses

Both epinephrine and dipivefrin may be used to reduce elevated IOP in the treatment of chronic, open-angle glaucoma, either as initial therapy or as chronic therapy. Dipivefrin has been used to reduce IOP in other ocular conditions, including ocular hypertension and pseudoexfoliative, low-tension, and secondary glaucomas.

Apraclonidine is primarily used to inhibit perioperative IOP increases. Increases in IOP during ophthalmic surgery are usually mediated via increased catecholamine stimulation of the SNS. Apraclonidine stimulates the α_2-receptors, which oppose these effects, and thus corrects the surgery-induced changes in IOP. It has also been used in the treatment of open-angle glaucoma, but its effectiveness has not yet been established. Brimonidine is used to lower IOP in patient's with open-angle glaucoma or ocular hypertension.

Side Effects and Adverse Effects

The side effects and adverse effects of the sympathomimetic mydriatics are primarily limited to ocular effects; however, systemic effects are possible. Ocular side effects are transient and most commonly consist of burning, eye pain, and lacrimation. Other ocular effects are conjunctival hyperemia, localized melanin deposits in the conjunctiva, and released pigment granules from the iris.

The systemic effects associated with the use of sympathomimetic mydriatics are rare. They include cardiovascular effects such as extrasystoles, tachycardia, and hypertension. Other effects that may be noticed are headache and faintness.

Toxicity and Management of Overdose

Rare toxic reactions are primarily the result of an extension of the therapeutic and adverse effects of these drugs. The most significant are cardiac dysrhythmias. Discontinuation of the drugs usually alleviates the toxic symptoms.

Interactions

With sufficient topical absorption, sympathomimetic mydriatics have the potential to react with other drugs. Cardiac dysrhythmias are potentiated when mydriatic drugs are given with halogenated anesthetics, cardiac glycosides, thyroid hormones, or tricyclic antidepressants (TCAs).

Dosages

For recommended dosages of sympathomimetic agents see the dosages table on p. 863.

drug profiles

The two primary sympathomimetic agents are dipivefrin and epinephrine. Apraclonidine, brimonidine, and dexmedetomidine are three sympathomimetic drugs. They are not used as extensively as dipivefrin and epinephrine. Brimonidine works similarly to apraclonidine. It works by stimulating α_2-receptors. This inhibits increases in IOP. Dipivefrin and epinephrine are believed to work by stimulating both α- and β_2-receptors. This stimulation causes the dilator muscle to contract and results in mydriasis. During mydriasis there is an increase in aqueous humor outflow that results in a decrease in IOP.

Both epinephrine and apraclonidine are classified as pregnancy category C agents. Because of dipivefrin's lipophilicity and limited systemic absorption, it is classified as a pregnancy category B agent. Brimonidine is also classified as a pregnancy category B agent. These drugs are available only by prescription.

DOSAGES Selected Mydriatic Agents

agent	pharmacologic class	dosage range	purpose
apraclonidine 1% (Iopidine)	α_2-adrenergic	1 gtt 1 hr before and after surgery	Reduction of IOP for ocular surgery
dipivefrin 0.1% (Propine)	$\alpha-\beta$ adrenergic	1 gtt q12h	Open-angle glaucoma

gtt, Drop.

apraclonidine

Apraclonidine (Iopidine) is structurally and pharmacologically related to the α_2 stimulant clonidine. Apraclonidine is primarily used to inhibit perioperative IOP increases. Apraclonidine stimulates α_2-receptors, which inhibits increases in IOP that occur during ophthalmic surgery. Its use in the treatment of open-angle glaucoma remains to be established.

Apraclonidine is available as a 1% ophthalmic solution. Commonly recommended dosages for apraclonidine are listed in the dosages table above.

PHARMACOKINETICS			
HALF-LIFE	ONSET	PEAK	DURATION
8 hr	1 hr	3-5 hr	12 hr

dipivefrin

Dipivefrin (Propine) is a synthetic sympathomimetic miotic drug. It is a prodrug of epinephrine. The prodrug has little or no pharmacologic activity until hydrolyzed in the eye to two forms of epinephrine. These chemical alterations allow epinephrine to penetrate into the anterior chamber of the eye. The decrease in IOP is apparently the result of aqueous humor fluid outflow from the anterior chamber of the eye.

Dipivefrin is available as a 0.1% ophthalmic solution. Commonly recommended dosages for dipivefrin are listed in the dosages table above.

PHARMACOKINETICS			
HALF-LIFE	ONSET	PEAK	DURATION
1-3 hr	30 min	1 hr	12 hr

BETA-ADRENERGIC BLOCKERS

The antiglaucoma beta-adrenergic blockers that reduce IOP include selective β_1 and nonselective β_1 and β_2 blockers. These drugs are believed to work by reducing IOP through reducing aqueous humor formation and increasing its outflow. The most commonly used drugs in this drug class are listed in Table 54-5.

Mechanism of Action

The ophthalmic beta blockers reduce both elevated and normal IOP. They do this without affecting pupillary size

54-5 Glaucoma Therapy: Beta-Adrenergic Blockers

Class	Beta-Blockers
Selective beta-blocker (β_1)	betaxolol
Nonselective beta-blocker (β_1, β_2)	carteolol, levobunolol, metipranolol, timolol

or accommodation. They appear to reduce IOP by reducing aqueous humor formation. In addition, timolol may produce a minimal increase in aqueous outflow.

Drug Effects

The drug effects of the ophthalmic beta blockers are primarily limited to ocular effects; however, occasional systemic effects may occur. The primary ocular effect of ophthalmic beta blockers is reduced IOP by reducing aqueous humor production. They have little or no effect on accommodation, pupil size, and night vision.

The systemic effects are primarily those associated with the adrenergic blockers as discussed in Chapter 17, specifically systemic pulmonary and cardiovascular effects. Because these drugs are administered topically, few if any systemic effects are expected. These agents have not been shown to affect glucose metabolism as do some of the systemic adrenergic blockers.

Therapeutic Uses

Ophthalmic beta blockers are used to reduce elevated IOP in various conditions, including chronic open-angle glaucoma and ocular hypertension. They may also be used alone or in combination with a topical miotic (e.g., echothiophate iodide or pilocarpine), topical dipivefrin, and/or systemic carbonic anhydrase inhibitors. When used in combination these agents may have an additive IOP-lowering effect. They may also be used to treat some forms of angle-closure glaucoma.

Side Effects and Adverse Effects

The side effects and adverse effects of antiglaucoma beta blockers are primarily limited to ocular effects and limited systemic effects. The most common ocular effects are transient burning and discomfort. Other effects include blurred vision, pain photophobia, lacrimation, blepharitis, keratitis (inflammation of the cornea), and decreased corneal sensitivity. The systemic effects produced by beta blockers include headache, dizziness, cardiac irregularities, and bronchospasm.

Toxicity and Management of Overdose

Toxic reactions to beta blockers are rare and primarily involve the cardiovascular system. Symptoms include bradycardia, cardiac failure, hypotension, and bronchospasms. Treatment involves discontinuation of the drug and symptomatic treatment.

Interactions

With sufficient topical absorption, beta blockers can react with several categories of drugs. Ophthalmic beta blockers may have additive therapeutic and adverse effects when given with systemically administered beta blockers. This occurs when high doses of ophthalmic beta blockers are used and significant systemic absorption occurs. Verapamil, when used with ophthalmic beta blockers, can have additive adverse effects, resulting in asystole.

Dosages

For recommended dosages of beta-adrenergic blockers, see the dosages table below.

---

drug profiles

The ophthalmic beta-blocking drugs are betaxolol, carteolol, levobunolol, metipranolol, and timolol. The action of these drugs is reduction of IOP by decreased aqueous humor formation and an increase in outflow of aqueous humor.

These ophthalmic drugs are classified as pregnancy category C agents and are contraindicated in patients with bronchial asthma, cardiac failure, cardiogenic shock, obstructive breathing disorders, second- or third-degree atrioventricular (AV) block, and sinus bradycardia. They are also contraindicated in patients who have shown a hypersensitivity reaction to them. They are all available only by prescription.

betaxolol

Betaxolol (Betoptic, Betoptic S) is a β_1 selective beta blocker. It is structurally related to the systemic adrenergic blocker metoprolol (Lopressor) that is used primarily for cardiovascular disorders. Betax-

---

olol is one of the most potent and selective beta-blocking agents. Its ability to decrease aqueous humor formation and consequently IOP has made it an excellent agent for the treatment of ocular disorders such as open-angle glaucoma and ocular hypertension. Betaxolol is available as a 0.5% ophthalmic solution and a 0.25% ophthalmic suspension. Commonly recommended dosages for betaxolol are listed in the dosages table below.

PHARMACOKINETICS

HALF-LIFE	ONSET	PEAK	DURATION
Unknown	0.5-1 hr	2 hr	≥12 hr

timolol

Timolol (Timoptic, Timoptic Ocudose) may differ slightly from the other ophthalmic beta blockers in that it may increase the outflow of aqueous humor as well as its formation. Timolol is indicated for the treatment of open-angle glaucoma, ocular hypertension, secondary glaucoma, and glaucoma in aphakic eyes. It is available in 0.25% and 0.5% ophthalmic solutions as both a preservative-free and a preservative-containing product. Because some patients have had allergic reactions to benzalkonium chloride, one of the preservatives that is commonly in ocular products, the preservative-free products were developed. Commonly recommended dosages for timolol are listed in the dosages table below.

PHARMACOKINETICS

HALF-LIFE	ONSET	PEAK	DURATION
Unknown	15-30 min	1-5 hr	12-24 hr

CARBONIC ANHYDRASE INHIBITORS

Carbonic anhydrase inhibitors (CAIs) include acetazolamide, dichlorphenamide, dorzolamide, and methazolamide. Of these, dorzolamide (Trusopt) is the only CAI available in a topical formulation. Acetazolamide has been the most widely used of the CAIs. This may change with the convenience of the topically available dorzolamide. CAIs have many uses, but their use in oph-

---

DOSAGES Selected Beta-Adrenergic Blockers

agent	pharmacologic class	dosage range	purpose
betaxolol (Betoptic, Betoptic S) 0.25%, 0.5%	β_1-blocker	1 gtt bid	Open-angle glaucoma, ocular hypertension
timolol (Timoptic, Timoptic Ocudose) 0.25%, 0.5%	β_1–β_2–blocker	1 gtt bid	Open-angle glaucoma, ocular hypertension

gtt, Drop.

thalmic disorders is to decrease IOP. The prototype drug of the group, acetazolamide, is also used as an adjunct anticonvulsant and as treatment for acute mountain sickness. Their ophthalmic uses include treatment for open-angle, secondary, and angle-closure glaucoma as well as ocular hypertension.

Drug Effects

CAIs are administered orally as opposed to topically, with the exception of dorzolamide. The drug effects of CAIs are decreased IOP through reduced aqueous humor formation; increased renal excretion of water, bicarbonate, and potassium; and urinary alkalinization through decreased excretion of ammonia.

Therapeutic Uses

CAIs are used primarily in the treatment of glaucoma. Because they decrease IOP by reducing aqueous humor formation, they are excellent therapeutic agents in the treatment of such ocular disorders as open-angle glaucoma, secondary glaucoma, and closed-angle glaucoma before ocular surgery.

Side Effects and Adverse Effects

Since some of the CAIs are administered orally, they produce systemic side effects and adverse effects. Table 54-6 lists the most common such effects associated with CAIs. Dorzolamide is a CAI ophthalmic agent that has a structure resembling a sulfa antibiotic. For this reason, patients with sulfa allergies may also be allergic to this product.

Toxicity and Management of Overdose

Toxicity associated with the use of CAIs is rare. The mechanism by which these agents work predisposes the patient to possible acidotic states and electrolyte imbalances. These toxic reactions generally require only supportive care. This may include the restoration of electrolytes, especially potassium, and the administration of bicarbonate to correct the CAI—induced acidotic state.

Interactions

The systemic use of CAIs can result in several significant drug interactions. CAIs can cause hypokalemia and increase the likelihood of digitalis toxicity. Hypokalemia is also more likely to occur when they are coadministered with corticosteroids and diuretics. CAIs will increase renal excretion of lithium and decrease lithium's effects.

CAIs increase the drug effects of basic drugs as a result of decreased renal excretion.

Dosages

For recommended dosages of acetazolamide, see the dosages table below.

drug profiles

CAIs are the first class of ophthalmic drugs discussed thus far that can be given orally and produce therapeutic effects in the eye that are beneficial in the treatment of glaucoma. The CAIs include acetazolamide, dichlorphenamide, dorzolamide, and methazolamide. As mentioned previously, the most commonly used CAI is acetazolamide. Dorzolamide (Trusopt) is a new topically applied CAI that is gaining popularity. CAIs appear to work by decreasing the production of aqueous humor, which decreases IOP.

CAIs are classified as pregnancy category C agents and are contraindicated in patients with a history of hypersensitivity reactions to them or in patients with chronic noncongestive closed-angle glaucoma, marked kidney-liver disease, hyperchloremic acidosis, low sodium and potassium serum levels, and adrenal gland failure. All CAIs are available only by prescription. The prototype CAI, acetazolamide, is also used as an adjunct anticonvulsant and for treatment of acute mountain sickness. Their

Table 54-6 Carbonic Anhydrase Inhibitors: Adverse Effects

Body System	Side/Adverse Effect
Central nervous system	Drowsiness, confusion, paresthesias, seizures
Eyes, ears, nose, and throat	Transient myopia, tinnitus
Gastrointestinal	Anorexia, vomiting, diarrhea
Genitourinary	Polyurea, hematuria
Integumentary	Urticaria, rare photosensitivity
Metabolic	Acidotic states and electrolyte imbalance with long-term therapy

DOSAGES Acetazolamide

agent	pharmacologic class	dosage range	purpose
acetazolamide (Diamox)	Carbonic anhydrase inhibitor	*Pediatric* PO: 8-30 mg/kg/day divided q8h IM/IV: 5-10 mg/kg q6h *Adult* PO: 250 mg-1 g/day divided or 500 mg sequel bid IM/IV: 500 mg repeated in 2-4 hr if needed	Glaucoma

ophthalmic uses include open-angle, secondary, and angle-closure glaucoma.

acetazolamide

Acetazolamide (Diamox, AK-Zol) is a CAI that is primarily used in the treatment of glaucoma. It is available orally as 500-mg extended-release capsules and 125- and 250-mg tablets and parenterally as a 500-mg injection. Commonly recommended dosages for acetazolamide are listed in the dosages table on p. 865.

PHARMACOKINETICS

HALF-LIFE	ONSET	PEAK	DURATION
2.5-6 hr	1-1.5 hr	2-4 hr	8-12 hr

OSMOTIC DIURETICS

Osmotic agents may be administered either intravenously, orally, or topically to reduce IOP. The osmotic diuretics that are most commonly used for this purpose are glycerin and mannitol. Isosorbide and urea are two other less frequently used osmotic diuretics. These drugs create ocular hypotension by producing an osmotic gradient. This causes the blood to become hypertonic in the presence of intraocular fluids. The gradient forces the water from the aqueous and vitreous humors into the bloodstream causing a reduction of volume of intraocular fluid, which results in a decrease in IOP.

Mechanism of Action

Osmotic diuretics produce an increase in the osmolarity of the blood, causing it to become hypertonic. The hyperosmotic blood causes a shift of fluid from various isotonic extracirculatory fluids, especially from the cerebrospinal fluid and aqueous humor. Water via the osmotic gradient is removed, and the respective fluids in the brain and the eye are reduced in volume. This reduced volume of water decreases pressure on both the brain and the eye (Fig. 54-13).

Drug Effects

The drug effects of the osmotic diuretics are all related to their ability to extract fluid from certain spaces and shift it into the bloodstream. This action is important in the treatment of various ocular disorders because of the resultant reduction in IOP caused by the decreased volume of aqueous humor. Osmotic diuretics promote diuresis by increasing the osmolarity of the glomerular filtrate, which results in tubular reabsorption inhibition and an increase in the renal excretion of electrolytes.

Therapeutic Uses

The therapeutic effectiveness of the osmotic diuretics is the result of the production of hypertonic blood, which causes fluid extraction from various areas. In the brain this is beneficial for the treatment of altitude sickness. When fluid from the enclosed space of the skull is reduced, pressure is relieved and mountain sickness symptoms subside. In glaucoma, aqueous humor and vitreous humor are extracted from the anterior chamber of the eye and forced into the bloodstream. This reduces IOP.

The primary osmotic agents used in ocular disorders are glycerin and mannitol. They are used to treat acute glaucoma episodes and before or after ocular surgery to reduce IOP. Typically, glycerin is used first; if the treatment is unsuccessful, mannitol is tried. Isosorbide and urea are two other osmotic agents that may also be used in similar situations. They are usually used after glycerin or mannitol has failed.

Side Effects and Adverse Effects

The most frequent reactions to osmotic diuretic agents are nausea, vomiting, and headache. The most significant adverse effects are fluid and electrolyte imbalance. Other effects include possible irritation and thrombosis at the injection site. For a list of other possible side effects and adverse effects associated with the use of osmotic diuretics, see Table 54-7.

Toxicity and Management of Overdose

Toxic reactions are primarily a result of the hyperosmolarity of the blood. Hypovolemia caused by diuresis, cardiac dysrhythmias, and hyperosmolar nonketotic coma are the most significant toxic reactions. Treatment involves discontinuation of the drug and general symptomatic treatment.

Interactions

Increased lithium excretion caused by mannitol is the only significant drug interaction that has been reported.

Dosages

For recommended dosages of osmotic agents, see the dosages table on p. 867.

---

drug profiles

Osmotic diuretics are classified as pregnancy category C agents and are contraindicated in patients with pronounced anuria, acute pulmonary edema, cardiac decompensation, and severe dehydration.

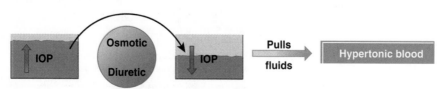

Fig. 54-13 Mechanism and ocular effects of osmotic diuretics.

They are also contraindicated in patients who have shown a hypersensitivity reaction to them.

glycerin

Glycerin (Osmoglyn, Ophthalgan) is an osmotic agent used orally to lower IOP or topically to reduce superficial corneal edema. Glycerin can be administered orally before iridectomy to reduce IOP in individuals with acute narrow-angle glaucoma. It is used preoperatively and postoperatively in conditions such as congenital glaucoma, retinal detachment, cataract extraction, and keratoplasty (corneal transplant). It may also be used in some secondary glaucomas.

Glycerin is administered orally as a 50% hyperosmotic solution (Osmoglyn). It is also available as an ophthalmic solution (Ophthalgan). Commonly recommended dosages for glycerin are listed in the dosages table below.

PHARMACOKINETICS

HALF-LIFE	ONSET	PEAK	DURATION
30-45 min	10-30 min	0.5-2 hr	4-8 hr

mannitol

Mannitol (Osmitrol) is used to reduce elevated IOP when the pressure cannot be lowered by other treatment. Mannitol has been shown to be effective in treatment of acute episodes of angle-closure, absolute, or secondary glaucoma and for lowering IOP before intraocular surgery. Mannitol does not penetrate the eye and may be used when irritation is present, unlike some of the other osmotic agents such as urea. Mannitol is available as 5%, 10%, 15%, 20%, and 25% parenteral injections. Commonly recommended dosages for mannitol are listed in the dosages table below.

PHARMACOKINETICS

HALF-LIFE	ONSET	PEAK	DURATION
1.5-2 hr	0.5-1 hr	0.5-1 hr	4-6 hr

PROSTAGLANDINS

Currently latanoprost (Xalatan) is the only agent in this new class of ophthalmic agents used to treat glaucoma.

Aqueous humor, a fluid made continuously by cells inside the eye, is necessary to maintain the shape of the eye and to nourish the lens and cornea. In most forms of glaucoma, aqueous humor is produced at a normal rate but exits the eye too slowly. Latanoprost is believed to act by increasing drainage of this fluid rather than by reducing its production as most current treatments do. This offers a physiologically attractive mechanism of action. Latanoprost has several positive features, including a single daily dosage regimen, a novel mechanism of action that enhances the IOP-lowering effect of contemporary agents, and a lack of systemic adverse effects. Latanoprost is available as a 0.005% ophthalmic solution and is contraindicated in patients who have had a hypersensitivity reaction to it.

Mechanism of Action

Latanoprost is a prodrug of a naturally occurring prostaglandin known as prostaglandin F2α. When this ester prodrug is administered it is converted to the prostaglandin F2α, which in turn reduces IOP. Prostaglandins reduce IOP primarily by increasing the outflow of IOP, not by decreasing its production. They are believed to increase the outflow of IOP by increasing uveoscleral outflow in addition to the usual exit through the trabecular meshwork. A single dose of latanoprost will lower IOP for 20 to 24 hours, allowing a single daily dosage regimen.

Table 54-7 Osmotic Diuretics: Adverse Effects

Body System	Side/Adverse Effect
Cardiovascular	Edema, thrombophlebitis, hypotension, hypertension, tachycardia, angina-like chest pains, fever, chills
Central nervous system	Dizziness, headache, convulsions, rebound increased intracranial pressure, confusion
Electrolytes	Fluid electrolyte imbalances, acidosis, electrolyte loss, dehydration
Eyes, ears, nose, throat	Loss of hearing, blurred vision, nasal congestion
Gastrointestinal	Nausea, vomiting, dry mouth, diarrhea
Genitourinary	Marked diuresis, urinary retention, thirst

DOSAGES Selected Osmotic Diuretics

agent	pharmacologic class	dosage range	purpose
glycerin (Osmoglyn, Ophthalgan)	Osmotic diuretic	PO: 1-2 g/kg 1-1.5 hr before surgery	Reduction of IOP
mannitol (Osmitrol)	Osmotic-diuretic	*Pediatric* IV: 1-2 g/kg by infusion or 30-60 min *Adult* IV: 1.5-2 g/kg by infusion over 30-60 min	Reduction of IOP

Drug Effects

The drug effects of latanoprost are primarily limited to effects on the eye. Very little if any latanoprost is absorbed into the circulation. The drug effect on the eye itself is that of decreasing IOP.

Therapeutic Effects

The therapeutic effects of latanoprost are decreased IOP in open-angle glaucoma and ocular hypertension. Prostaglandins are thought to lower IPO by increasing fluid outflow through the uveoscleral pathway in addition to the usual exit through the trabecular meshwork, a filter-like structure within the eye.

Side Effects and Adverse Effects

Latanoprost is well tolerated. Adverse effects reported in clinical trials included foreign body sensation, punctate epithelial keratopathy, stinging, conjunctival hyperemia, blurred vision, itching, and burning. In controlled clinical trials the incidence of these adverse effects was similar to those seen in patients treated with timolol. There is one usual side effect associated with latanoprost. Is some people with hazel, greenish, or bluish-brown eye color, their eyes will permanently turn brown, even if they stop using the medication. This side effect appears only to be cosmetic with no known ill effects on the eye. Caution should still be taken because long-term experience with this agent is lacking at this time. About 3% to 10% of patients treated with latanoprost have shown increased iris pigmentation after 3 to 4½ months of treatment. This iris color change does not affect IOP readings.

Interactions

No significant drug interactions have been reported with latanoprost.

OCULAR ANTIINFECTIVE DRUGS

Topical antiinfectives used for treating ocular infections include a wide range of antibacterial, antiviral, and antifungal drugs. Many of these drugs are also available for systemic administration. Caution should be used in deciding to use a topical antiinfective ophthalmic drug. In general, prophylactic use of antiinfective drugs is useless, wasteful, and potentially dangerous. Many of the inflammatory diseases seen in ophthalmology are caused by viruses or other agents that are not susceptible to any currently available antiinfective agents. The use of these agents in such situations is unwarranted.

Topically applied antiinfective drugs can cause sensitivity reactions. Symptoms associated with sensitivity reactions include stinging, itching, angioneurotic edema, urticaria, and dermatitis. Topical application of antiinfective drugs also interferes with growth of the normal bacterial flora of the eye, which may encourage growth of other more harmful organisms.

Any of the available systemically administered antibiotics are used at indicated times to treat infections of the eye. To avoid development of resistant strains of offending organisms and possible sensitization to common systemic antiinfectives, the antibiotic of choice is often administered topically rather than systemically.

The choice of a particular ophthalmic antiinfective drug should be based on the following:
- Clinical experience
- Sensitivity and characteristics of the organisms most likely to cause this infection
- The disease itself
- Sensitivity and response of the patient
- Laboratory results (cultures and sensitivities)

Some common eye infections that may require antibiotic therapy are listed in Box 54-2.

Mechanism of Action

The drugs used to treat infections of the eye work in a variety of ways to destroy the invading organism. The antimicrobial effects on susceptible organisms are primarily caused by inhibition of cell wall synthesis, inhibition of protein synthesis, or alteration of cell membrane permeability. Specific mechanisms of action can be found for the individual classes of antiinfectives in Chapter 36.

Drug Effects

The drug effects of the agents used to treat ocular infections are focused on the microorganism invading the eye. Some antiinfectives destroy the causative organism (**bactericidal**), whereas others simply inhibit the organism's

---

BOX 54-2 Common Ocular Infections

Infection	Description
Blepharitis	Inflammation of the eyelids.
Conjunctivitis	Inflammation of the conjunctiva, which is the mucous membrane lining the back of the lids and the front of the eye except the cornea. It may be bacterial or viral in nature and is often associated with common colds. When caused by *Haemophilus* organisms it is commonly called "pink eye." It is highly contagious but usually self-limiting.
Hordeolum (sty)	Acute localized infection of the eyelash follicles and the glands of the anterior lid; results in the formation of a small abscess or cyst.
Keratitis	Inflammation of the cornea caused by bacterial infection. Herpes simplex keratitis is caused by viral infection.
Uveitis	Infection of the uveal tract or the vascular layer of the eye, which includes the iris, ciliary body, and choroid.
Endophthalmitis	Inner eye structure inflammation caused by bacteria.

growth **(bacteriostatic),** allowing the body's immune system to fight the infection. Whatever the case, the final drug effect is elimination of the infecting organism.

Therapeutic Uses

The therapeutic effects of ocular antiinfectives vary depending on the individual antiinfective drug. The spectrum of bacteria that each drug kills is very specific to the individual agent. The therapeutic effect is elimination of ocular infections.

Side Effects and Adverse Effects

The most common side effects and adverse effects of ocular antibiotics are local and transient inflammation, burning, stinging, and drug hypersensitivity. Other such effects, toxicities, and drug interactions are specific for the individual antiinfectives and are therefore mentioned in the drug profiles.

Interactions

Ophthalmic agents undergo very little if any systemic absorption. For this reason, there are few drug interactions to mention for this category of agents. One possible interaction is the concurrent use of corticosteroids (e.g., dexamethasone). When used with ophthalmic antibiotics, the immunosuppression that may occur may make it more difficult to rid the eye of infection.

Dosages

For recommended dosages of ocular antiinfectives, see the dosages table below.

drug profiles

A variety of infections can occur in the eye; many are self-limiting (i.e., the body's own defense system

DOSAGES   Selected Ocular Antiinfective Agents

agent	pharmacologic class	dosage range	purpose
bacitracin (AK-Tracin)	Antibiotic: Polypeptide	Apply ointment 1-2 times/day	Bacterial infections
chlortetracycline (Aureomycin)	Antibiotic: Tetracycline	Apply ointment 1-2 times/day	Bacterial and chlamydial infection; apply once within 1 hr after delivery for ophthalmia neonatorum
chloramphenicol (Chloroptic)	Miscellaneous	Apply ointment or 1-2 gtt several times/day	Bacterial infections
ciprofloxacin (Ciloxan)	Fluroquinolone	2 gtt q15min for 6 hr followed by 2 gtt q30min for the remainder of the day; then 2 gtt qh on the second day followed by 2 gtt q4h for 12 more days	Bacterial keratitis
		1-2 gtt q2h while awake for 2 days followed by 1-2 gtt q4h while awake for 5 more days	Bacterial conjunctivitis
erythromycin (AK-Mycin)	Macrolide	Apply ointment several times/day	Bacterial and chlamydial infections; apply once within 1 hr after birth for ophthalmia neonatorum
gentamicin (Garamycin)	Aminoglycoside	Apply ointment or 1-2 gtt several times/day	Bacterial infections
natamycin (Natacyn)	Macrolide	1 gtt q1-2h for 3-4 days followed by 1 gtt q6-8h for 3-4 days	Fungal infections
polymyxin B	Antibiotic: Polypeptide	1-3 gtt several times/day	Bacterial infections
silver nitrate	Inorganic heavy metal salt	2 gtt after birth	Ophthalmia neonatorum
sulfacetamide (AK-Sulf, Bleph-10)	Sulfonamide	Apply ointment several times/day Solution: 1-3 gtt to lower conjunctival sac q2-3h	Bacterial infection Bacterial infection
tetracycline (Achromycin)	Antibiotic: Tetracycline	Apply ointment 2-4 times/day	Bacterial and chlamydial infections; apply ointment once within 1 hr after delivery for ophthalmia neonatorum
vidarabine (Vira-A)	Purine nucleoside	Apply ointment 5 times/day at 3-hr intervals	Viral infections

will fight them). They seldom result in harm. However, some infections require ocular antiinfectives in order to be eliminated. The most commonly used antiinfectives from the main antiinfective drug classes are discussed here.

AMINOGLYCOSIDES

Aminoglycosides are potent antiinfectives that destroy bacteria by interfering with protein synthesis in bacterial cells by binding to ribosomal subunits, which eventually leads to bacteria death. Because aminoglycosides kill bacteria, they are classified as bactericidal.

The three aminoglycosides that are used to treat ocular infections are gentamicin, neomycin, and tobramycin. They are classified as pregnancy category C agents and are contraindicated in patients who have shown a hypersensitivity reaction to them and in patients with vaccinia, varicella, mycobacterial or fungal infections of eye, and epithelial herpes simplex keratitis.

Side effects and adverse effects include swollen eyelids, mydriasis, and local erythema. Toxic reactions are rare because of poor topical absorption. Another possible toxic reaction is the overgrowth of nonsusceptible organisms, which can lead to eye infections that are resistant to treatment.

gentamicin

Gentamicin (Garamycin, Genoptic) is effective against a wide variety of gram-negative and gram-positive organisms. It is particularly useful against *Pseudomonas, Proteus,* and *Klebsiella* organisms. Gram-positive organisms that are effectively destroyed by gentamicin are staphylococci and streptococci that have developed resistance to other antibiotics. Gentamicin is available as an ophthalmic ointment and a solution. It is also available in combination with prednisolone as a suspension and an ointment. It is available as a 0.3% ophthalmic ointment and a 0.3% ophthalmic solution. Commonly recommended dosages are listed in the dosages table on p. 869.

PHARMACOKINETICS

HALF-LIFE	ONSET	PEAK	DURATION
Unknown	Variable	Immediate	6-12 hr

MACROLIDES

The antibacterial erythromycin is a bacteriostatic drug. In normal concentrations it will inhibit the growth of an organism but not destroy it. Erythromycin relies on the body's defense mechanisms to destroy the bacteria; however, in high concentrations it will become bactericidal. It is indicated for the treatment of neonatal conjunctivitis caused by *Chlamydia trachomatous* and for the prevention of eye infections in newborns that may be caused by *Neisseria gonorrhoea* or other susceptible organisms.

The two most commonly used agents in this antibiotic category are erythromycin ophthalmic ointment and natamycin ophthalmic suspension. Eye irritation is the only rare adverse reaction reported with these two antiinfectives.

erythromycin

Erythromycin (AK-Mycin, Ilotycin, Ocu-Mycin) is a macrolide antibiotic indicated for the treatment of various ophthalmic infections. It is classified as a pregnancy category C agent and is contraindicated in patients who have shown a hypersensitivity reaction to it and in patients with epithelial herpes, varicella, mycobacterial or fungal infections, and epithelial herpes simplex keratitis. It is available only as 0.5% strength ophthalmic ointment. Commonly recommended dosages are listed in the dosages table on p. 869.

PHARMACOKINETICS

HALF-LIFE	ONSET	PEAK	DURATION
Unknown	Variable	Immediate	Variable

natamycin

Natamycin (Natacyn) is an antifungal antibiotic that is structurally a macrolide antibiotic. It is related to the other antifungal agents amphotericin B and nystatin. It destroys fungi in the eye by binding to sterols in the fungal cell membrane, thus disrupting the protective capabilities of the cell, which results in cell death.

Natamycin is used topically in the treatment of blepharitis, conjunctivitis, and keratitis caused by susceptible fungi (*Candida* and *Aspergillus* spp.). The side effects and adverse effects associated with natamycin are limited to the eye and consist of temporary visual haze and overgrowth of nonsusceptible organisms. It is also classified as a pregnancy category C agent and is contraindicated in patients who have shown a hypersensitivity reaction to it. It is available as a 5% ophthalmic suspension. Commonly recommended dosages are listed in the dosages table on p. 869.

PHARMACOKINETICS

HALF-LIFE	ONSET	PEAK	DURATION
Unknown	Variable	Immediate	Variable

POLYPEPTIDES

Bacitracin and polymyxin B are polypeptide antibiotics. These drugs are rarely used systemically because of potent nephrotoxic effects. They are bactericidal antiinfectives that inhibit protein synthesis in susceptible organisms, which leads to cell death. They are most commonly used in the treatment of surface superficial infections caused by gram-positive bacteria.

Polypeptides are often used in combination with other antibiotics to broaden their spectrum of activity. Neosporin is a combination of bacitracin and gramicidin, neomycin, and polymyxin. Bacitracin is preferable to neomycin for topical use because fewer organisms are resistant to it, allergic reactions occur less frequently, and sensitization is avoided.

bacitracin

Bacitracin (AK-Tracin) is an ophthalmic antiinfective drug used to treat various eye infections. It is classified as a pregnancy category C agent and is contraindicated in patients who have shown a hypersensitivity reaction to it. It is available as a single-ingredient product and as a combination product with polymyxin or neomycin and polymyxin. These combinations were developed to make bacitracin a broad-spectrum antibiotic. Bacitracin is available as a 500-U/g ophthalmic ointment and as two combination ophthalmic ointments. Commonly recommended dosages are listed in the dosages table on p. 869.

PHARMACOKINETICS

HALF-LIFE	ONSET	PEAK	DURATION
Unknown	Variable	Immediate	Variable

QUINOLONES

Quinolone antibiotics are very effective broad-spectrum antibiotics. They are discussed in detail in Chapter 36. They are bactericidal, destroying a wide spectrum of organisms that are often very difficult to treat. There are currently three ophthalmic quinolones available ciprofloxacin, norfloxacin, and ofloxacin.

Quinolones are all classified as pregnancy category C agents and are contraindicated in patients who have shown a hypersensitivity reaction to them. Significant side effects and adverse effects include corneal precipitates during treatment for bacterial keratitis. Other reactions include corneal staining and infiltrates. Toxic reactions are limited because of poor topical absorption. Those that occur are usually taste disorders and nausea. There are no significant drug interactions.

ciprofloxacin

Ciprofloxacin (Ciloxan) is a synthetic quinolone antibiotic. It is available only by prescription. Although it is available in many systemic formulations, it is available only as a 0.3% ophthalmic solution in an ocular formulation. Ciprofloxacin is indicated in the treatment of bacterial keratitis and conjunctivitis caused by susceptible gram-positive and gram-negative bacteria. Commonly

recommended dosages are listed in the dosages table on p. 869.

PHARMACOKINETICS

HALF-LIFE	ONSET	PEAK	DURATION
1-2 hr	Variable	Immediate	Variable

SULFONAMIDES

Sulfonamides are synthetic bacteriostatic antibiotics that work by blocking the synthesis of folic acid in susceptible bacteria. Sulfacetamide sodium and sulfisoxazole are sulfonamides used to treat conjunctivitis and other ocular infections caused by susceptible bacteria.

The side effects and adverse effects are primarily limited to local reactions and include local irritation and stinging. Sulfonamide use can result in the overgrowth of nonsusceptible organisms. No significant topical toxic effects have been reported with their use. These ocular antiinfectives are classified as pregnancy category C agents and are contraindicated in infants under 2 months of age and in patients with varicella, vaccinia, viral disease, mycobacterial and fungal infections of the eye, and epithelial herpes simplex keratitis. They are also contraindicated in patients who have shown a hypersensitivity reaction to them. They are available in ophthalmic ointments, solutions, and suspensions.

sulfacetamide

Sulfacetamide (AK-Sulf, Bleph-10, Sodium Sulamyd, and many others) is the most commonly used ophthalmic sulfonamide antibacterial agent. It is available as a solution, ointment, and suspension in ophthalmic formulations. It is also used in combination with phenylephrine or prednisolone. It is aviailable as a 10% ophthalmic ointment and 10%, 15%, and 30% ophthalmic solutions. Commonly recommended dosages are listed in the dosages table on p. 869.

PHARMACOKINETICS

HALF-LIFE	ONSET	PEAK	DURATION
Unknown	Variable	Immediate	Variable

TETRACYCLINES

Tetracycline antibiotics are used topically to treat superficial infections of the cornea and conjunctiva. They are usually bacteriostatic rather than bactericidal. They are broad-spectrum antimicrobials. The administration of tetracyclines is recommended to prevent eye infections in newborns of mothers with gonorrheal infections. Topical tetracyclines rarely cause any side effects or adverse effects. They are better tolerated than silver nitrate and have a lower incidence of conjunctivitis and eye irritation. Presently there are three tetracycline-based ophthalmic preparations—chlortetracycline, oxytetracycline, and tetracycline.

tetracycline

The prototype tetracycline antibiotic is tetracycline (Achromycin). It is classified as a pregnancy category D agent and is contraindicated in patients who have shown a hypersensitivity reaction to it and in patients with varicella, vaccinia, mycobacterial or fungal infections of the eye, and epithelial herpes simplex keratitis. Tetracycline is available as a 1% ointment and suspension. Commonly recommended dosages are listed in the dosages table on p. 869.

PHARMACOKINETICS

HALF-LIFE	ONSET	PEAK	DURATION
Unknown	Variable	Immediate	Variable

MISCELLANEOUS OCULAR ANTIINFECTIVE AGENTS

Three other ophthalmic antiinfective drugs that are commonly used are chloramphenicol, silver nitrate, and zinc sulfate. These antiinfectives have been available for many years and remain very effective for susceptible organisms.

chloramphenicol

Chloramphenicol (Chloroptic, AK-Chlor, Ocu-Chlor) is a bacteriostatic antiinfective that works by preventing peptide bond formation and protein synthesis in a wide variety of gram-positive and gram-negative organisms. It is extremely useful in the treatment of superficial ocular infections. Side effects with the ophthalmic use of chloramphenicol are usually rare. As with most of the other ophthalmic antiinfectives, the most common side effects and adverse effects are burning and stinging upon instillation. Irreversible aplastic anemia has not been reported with the ophthalmic preparation of this drug. It is available as a 0.5% solution and a 1% ointment. Commonly recommended dosages are listed in the dosages table on p. 869.

PHARMACOKINETICS

HALF-LIFE	ONSET	PEAK	DURATION
Unknown	Variable	Immediate	Variable

silver nitrate

Silver nitrate is a topical antiinfective, astringent, and caustic agent. It also exhibits antiseptic and germicidal activity and works by inhibiting protein synthesis. It is not readily absorbed from mucous membranes and does not readily penetrate into tissues. It has had long-term use in newborns to prevent gonococcal infections of the eyes. This is required by law in many states. The U.S. Centers for Disease Control and Prevention (CDC) and the American Academy of Pediatrics (AAP) currently state that topical erythromycin or a topical tetracycline may be used as an alternative to 1% silver nitrate ophthalmic solution for prophylaxis of gonococcal ophthalmia neonatorum. Silver nitrate is classified as a pregnancy category C agent and is contraindicated in patients who have shown a hypersensitivity reaction to it. It is available as a 1% ophthalmic solution. Commonly recommended dosages are listed in the dosages table on p. 869.

PHARMACOKINETICS

HALF-LIFE	ONSET	PEAK	DURATION
Unknown	Variable	Immediate	Variable

ANTIVIRALS

There are four currently available antiviral ophthalmic agents—idoxuridine, trifluridine, vidarabine, and ganciclovir. Ganciclovir for cytomegalovirus (CMV) is in the form of an implant. The implant releases ganciclovir to the site of disease in the eye in which it is implanted. The Vitrasert implant of ganciclovir, surgically placed in the posterior of the eye, allows diffusion of the ganciclovir locally to the site of infection over an extended period of months. Implantation normally takes less than 1 hour, requires only local anesthesia, and is conducted in an outpatient setting.

Idoxuridine and trifluridine are both pyrimidine nucleosides; vidarabine is a purine nucleoside. These agents inhibit viral replication because their metabolites block viral DNA synthesis by inhibiting viral DNA polymerase. These three antiviral ophthalmic drugs destroy herpes simplex virus types 1 and 2, varicella-zoster, CMV, vaccinia, and hepatitis B virus. Of these agents, vidarabine has the broadest antiviral spectrum.

These antivirals are classified as pregnancy category C agents and are contraindicated in patients who have shown a hypersensitivity reaction to them. Significant side effects and adverse effects include secondary glaucoma, corneal punctate defects, uveitis, and stromal edema. The drugs exhibit no appreciable topical absorption, and no significant drug interactions have been reported.

vidarabine

Vidarabine (Vira-A) is an antiviral ophthalmic drug used in the treatment of epithelial herpes simplex keratitis and keratoconjunctivitis. It may also be useful in the treatment of vaccinia keratitis. Vidarabine is only available as a 3% ophthalmic ointment. Commonly recommended dosages are listed in the dosages table on p. 869.

PHARMACOKINETICS

HALF-LIFE	ONSET	PEAK	DURATION
Unknown	Variable	Immediate	Variable

ANTIINFLAMMATORY OPHTHALMIC AGENTS

Many of the same antiinflammatory drug classes that are used systemically may also be used ophthalmically to treat various inflammatory disorders and surgery-related pain and inflammation. Both nonsteroidal antiinflammatory drugs (NSAIDs) and corticosteroids are used ophthalmically as listed in Box 54-3.

Mechanism of Action

Corticosteroids and NSAIDs work by inhibiting the inflammatory response. However, they differ in the mechanisms of action. The corticosteroids and NSAIDs both act on enzymes involved in arachidonic acid metabolism. The corticosteroids work in a different area of the pathway than NSAIDs. Figure 54-14 illustrates where on this pathway corticosteroids and NSAIDs act.

When tissues are damaged their cell membranes release phospholipids as a part of the tissue-damaging process. These phospholipids are then broken down by several different enzymes and pathways that are collec-

tively referred to as the *arachidonic acid pathway*. Phospholipase is one of the first enzymes involved, and it is the enzyme that is inhibited by corticosteroids.

By preventing phospholipase from breaking down phospholipids, many of the inflammatory mediators or substances that cause inflammation and pain cannot be produced. This is the action of NSAIDs. However, they inhibit a different enzyme than corticosteroids. NSAIDs inhibit cyclooxygenase and, to a lesser extent, lipoxygenase. In doing so, they also prevent the production of many of the substances that cause inflammation and pain.

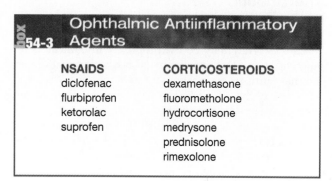

Box 54-3 Ophthalmic Antiinflammatory Agents

NSAIDS	CORTICOSTEROIDS
diclofenac	dexamethasone
flurbiprofen	fluorometholone
ketorolac	hydrocortisone
suprofen	medrysone
	prednisolone
	rimexolone

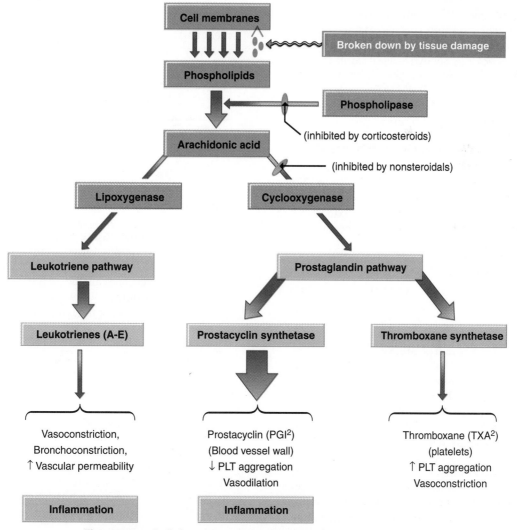

Fig. 54-14 Antiinflammatory action of corticosteroids and nonsteroidals.

Drug Effects

The drug effects of corticosteroids after topical application to the conjunctiva are primarily the inhibition of the inflammatory response to mechanical, chemical, or immunologic agents. NSAIDs exhibit antiinflammatory and analgesic activity (i.e., they decrease inflammation and relieve pain). This is believed to occur as a result of inhibition of the enzyme cyclooxygenase, which is the enzyme responsible for the production of prostaglandins and other inflammatory substances.

Therapeutic Uses

Corticosteroids and NSAIDs are applied topically for the symptomatic relief of many ophthalmic inflammatory conditions. They may be used topically in corneal, conjunctival, and scleral injuries from chemical, radiation, or thermal burns or penetration of foreign bodies. They are used during the acute phase of the injury process to prevent fibrosis and scarring that results in visual impairment. They should not be used for minor abrasions or wounds because they may suppress the eye's ability to resist bacterial, viral, or fungal infections. This adverse effect is more notable in corticosteroids than in NSAIDs. Consequently, NSAIDs are considered less toxic and are preferred as initial topical therapy.

Corticosteroids and NSAIDs may also be used prophylactically after ocular surgery, such as cataract extraction, glaucoma surgery, and corneal transplants, to prevent inflammation and scarring. NSAIDs are used in the symptomatic treatment of seasonal allergic conjunctivitis. They may also be used prophylactically before ocular surgery to prevent or reduce intraoperative miosis that may occur secondary to surgery-induced trauma.

Side Effects and Adverse Effects

The most common adverse effect of corticosteroids is transient burning or stinging on application. Since NSAIDs have the potential to cause increased bleeding, patients should be monitored closely. The extended use of corticosteroids may result in cataracts, increased IOP, and optic nerve damage.

Dosages

For recommended dosages of corticosteroid agents, see the dosages table on p. 875.

drug profiles

Corticosteroids and NSAIDs that are used to treat ophthalmic inflammatory disorders are discussed in Chapter 33 and Chapter 42, respectively. These ophthalmic formulations share many of the same characteristics of their systemic counterparts. However, the ophthalmic derivatives do have limited systemic absorption. Thus the majority of therapeutic and toxic effects are limited to the eye.

With the exception of diclofenac, which is classified as a pregnancy category B agent, NSAIDs are classified as pregnancy category C agents. They are contraindicated in patients who have shown a hypersensitivity reaction to them and in patients with epithelial herpes simplex keratitis. They are all available only by prescription as ophthalmic solutions.

Corticosteroid ophthalmic preparations are indicated for many of the same conditions as NSAIDs with a few exceptions. Many of these agents are also available in systemic formulations and are discussed in Chapter 33. Corticosteroids are classified as pregnancy category C agents and are contraindicated in patients with fungal and viral ocular infections and acute epithelial herpes simplex keratitis. Systemic reactions as a result of ophthalmic absorption and drug interactions with the ophthalmic corticosteroids are rare.

dexamethasone

Dexamethasone (AK-Dex, Decadron, and many others) is a synthetic corticosteroid that has many systemic and ophthalmic formulations. It is used to treat inflammation of the eye, eye lids, conjunctiva, and cornea, and it may also be used in the treatment of uveitis, iridocyclitis, allergic conditions, and burns and in removal of foreign bodies. Dexamethasone is available as an ophthalmic ointment and as a 0.1% suspension. It is also contained in many combination formulations with various antibiotics. Commonly recommended dosages are listed in the dosages table on p. 875.

PHARMACOKINETICS

HALF-LIFE	ONSET	PEAK	DURATION
Unknown	Variable	Immediate	Variable

flurbiprofen

Flurbiprofen (Ocufen Liquifilm) is an NSAID that is available as an ophthalmic drug. It is used to treat inflammatory ophthalmic conditions such as postoperative inflammation after a cataract extraction. It is also used to inhibit intraoperative miosis that may be induced by operative trauma and tissue injury. Flurbiprofen is available as a 0.03% ophthalmic solution. Commonly recommended dosages are listed in the dosages table on p. 875.

PHARMACOKINETICS

HALF-LIFE	ONSET	PEAK	DURATION
Unknown	2 hr	1-2 hr	Several hr

ketorolac

Ketorolac (Acular) is an NSAID that is available in many different formulations. It is the only parenteral NSAID and may be given either intravenously or intramuscularly. Ketorolac is available orally as well. Ketorolac is contraindicated in patients who have exhibited hypersensitivity to it. The ophthalmic formulation is used to reduce certain manifestations of ocular inflammation caused by trauma, such as ocular surgery, or inflammation secondary to external agents, such as allergens and bacteria. Ketorolac is available as a 0.5% ophthalmic solution. Commonly recommended dosages are listed in the dosages table above.

PHARMACOKINETICS

HALF-LIFE	ONSET	PEAK	DURATION
Unknown	Rapid	Immediate	4-6 hr

TOPICAL ANESTHETICS

Topical anesthetic ophthalmic drugs are used to prevent eye pain. This is beneficial during surgery, ophthalmic examinations, removal of foreign bodies, and any extremely painful procedure or condition. The two currently available topical anesthetics used for ophthalmic purposes are proparacaine and tetracaine. Anesthetic drugs are discussed in depth in Chapter 10.

Mechanism of Action

Local anesthetics stabilize the membranes of nerves, resulting in a decrease in the movement of ions into and out of the nerve endings. Without a change in the concentrations of these ions, a nerve impulse cannot be started or transmitted. Pain and many other sensory impulses are transmitted via nerves. When nerves are stabilized, as they are after application of topical anesthetics, they cannot transmit signals about painful stimuli to the brain.

Drug Effects

Usually the application of topical anesthetic drugs to the eye results in local anesthesia in less than 30 seconds. This drug effect of numbness or the absence of the ability to feel pain is beneficial in many circumstances.

Therapeutic Uses

Ophthalmic anesthetic drugs are used to produce ocular anesthesia for short corneal and conjunctival procedures.

They prevent pain during surgical procedures, such as removal of sutures and foreign bodies, and during certain painful ophthalmic examinations. The various procedures in which ophthalmic anesthetic drugs have been used are as follows:

- Tonometry
- Paracentesis
- Short procedures
- Gonioscopy
- Eye examinations of painful injuries
- Irrigation of painful injuries
- Removal of foreign bodies
- Removal of sutures
- Corneal scraping for diagnostic purposes

Side Effects and Adverse Effects

Side effects and adverse effects are rare with ophthalmic anesthetic agents and are limited to local effects such as stinging, burning, redness, and lacrimation. Some of the more common side effects and adverse effects are allergic contact dermatitis, softening and erosion of corneal epithelium, pupillary dilation, cycloplegia, conjunctival congestion and hemorrhage, and stromal edema.

Interactions

Because of limited systemic absorption and short duration of action, ophthalmic anesthetic agents have no significant drug interactions.

Dosages

Tetracaine is available as a 0.5% ophthalmic ointment and solution. The recommended dosage is application of 1.25 to 2.5 cm of the ointment or 1 to 2 drops of solution for local anesthesia as needed. Tetracaine is not intended for prolonged use.

drug profiles

Ophthalmic anesthetic drugs are a small class of the many available ophthalmic agents. There are currently only two drugs available to treat ophthalmic conditions that require an anesthetic—proparacaine and tetracaine. They are classified as mydriatic and cycloplegic agents. They dilate the pupil and paralyze the ciliary muscle, which prevents accommodation. Atropine is used for cycloplegic refraction and for iris and uveal tract inflammation. The usual dose (0.5% and 1%) for uveitis in children and adults is 1 to 2 drops or 0.3 to 0.5 cm of ointment two to three times daily. The adult dose for refraction is 1 drop (1% solution) 1 hour before the procedure.

tetracaine

Tetracaine (Pontocaine) is a local anesthetic of the ester type. It is used to numb the eye for cataract extraction, tonometry, gonioscopy, removal of foreign objects, corneal suture removal, and glaucoma surgery. Tetracaine begins to work in about 25 seconds and lasts for about 30 minutes. It is available in both a 0.5% ophthalmic ointment and solution.

PHARMACOKINETICS

HALF-LIFE	ONSET	PEAK	DURATION
Short	<30 sec	1-5 min	15-20 min

MISCELLANEOUS AGENTS

artificial tears

An array of OTC products is available to use as lubrication or moisture for the eyes. Artificial tears are isotonic and contain buffers for pH control. In addition they contain preservatives for microbial control and may contain viscosity agents for extended ocular activity. Selected OTC brand names include Cellafresh, Moisture Drops, Murine, Nutears, Lacrilube and Tears Plus.

atropine sulfate

Atropine sulfate solution 0.5%, 1.2%, and 3% and ophthalmic ointment 0.5% and 1% are used as mydriatic and cycloplegic agents. They dilate the pupil and paralyze the ciliary muscle, which prevents accommodation. Atropine is used for cycloplegic refraction and for iris and uveal tract inflammation. The usual dose (0.5% and 1%) for uveitis in children and adults is 1 to 2 drops or 0.3 to 0.5 cm of ointment two to three times a day. The adult dose for refraction is 1 drop (1% solution) 1 hour before the procedure.

cromolyn

Cromolyn sodium (Opticrom) is an antiallergic agent that inhibits the release of inflammation-producing mediators from sensitized inflammatory cells called *mast cells*. It is used in the treatment of vernol keratoconjunctivitis. The usual dose for children over 4 years of age and adults is 1 drop four to six times per day.

chymotrypsin

Chymotrypsin (Alpha Chymar, Catarese) is a proteolytic enzyme used as an aid in intracapsular lens extraction. Cataract extraction or removal is facilitated by injecting 0.2 to 0.5 ml of a freshly prepared solution behind the iris into the posterior chamber. Enzymatic activity dissolves the zonules that hold the lens so that it can be removed. After the procedure a miotic drug is administered to contract the pupil.

cyclopentolate

Cyclopentolate solution (Cyclogyl) 0.5%, 1%, and 2% is used as a diagnostic mydriatic and cycloplegic drug. The usual adult dose is 1 to 2 drops (0.5%, 1%, or 2%). This is repeated in 5 to 10 minutes if needed. The dose for children is the same as that for adults. Infants require 1 drop of the 0.5% solution.

fluorescein

Fluorescein sodium (AK-Fluor, Flu-Glo Strips) is an ophthalmic diagnostic dye used to identify corneal defects and to locate foreign objects in the eye. It is also used in fitting hard contact lenses. After instillation of fluorescein, various defects are highlighted. They are distinguished according to the following criteria:
- Corneal defects are colored bright green.
- Conjunctival lesions are colored yellow-orange.
- Foreign objects have a green halo around them.
- A contact lens that touches the cornea will appear black with ultraviolet light.

hyperosmolar sodium chloride

Hyperosmolar sodium chloride preparations (Adsorbonac, Muro 128 [2% and 5% solution], and Muro 128 ointment) are used to decrease corneal edema caused by osmotic pressure. These agents produce an osmotic gradient that draws fluid out of the cornea. They are available as ointments or solutions. One to two drops of 2% to 5% solution is applied every 3 to 4 hours. The 0.5% ophthalmic ointment is applied once daily.

nursing process

● Assessment

Before administering an ophthalmic agent per doctor's orders, the nurse should perform a baseline assessment of the eye and its structures to help document specific data about possible causes of the eye disorder and to measure success of treatment. Any redness, swelling, pain, tearing, eye discharge, decrease in visual acuity, or any other unusual symptoms should be noted, documented, and reported to the patient's physician. Hypersensitivity to the specific medication, contraindications and cautions, and preexisting diseases should also be noted and documented.

Specific contraindications and cautions to the use of *each* specific ophthalmic agent are as follows:

Parasympathomimetic agents or miotics (often used for glaucoma) are usually contraindicated in patients with bradycardia, hyperthyroidism, coronary artery disease, GI or urinary obstructive problems or disease, peptic ulcers, epilepsy or convulsive disorders, parkinsonism, and asthma. Cautious use with careful monitoring is recommended in patients who are pregnant or have hypertension or bronchial asthma. Baseline vital signs and an assessment of the respiratory system should be documented, and unusual (abnormal) findings should be reported to the physician.

Indirect-acting parasympathomimetics such as echothiophate iodide used for glaucoma are contraindicated in patients allergic to the drug or those with uveitis. Cautious use is recommended in patients with asthma, bradycardia, or peptic ulcer disease and in those who are pregnant.

The principal use of sympathomimetic ophthalmic agents is dilation of the eye before ophthalmic examination and related procedures. Dipivefrin is used in the treatment of open-angle glaucoma because the agent is converted to epinephrine, which acts to decrease aqueous humor production and increase outflow. Contraindications include patients with allergic reaction to the drugs and those with narrow-angle glaucoma. Cautious use is recommended in patients who are pregnant or breast-feeding and in patients with aphakia.

Beta-adrenergic blockers are contraindicated in patients who are allergic to these agents and in those who have chronic obstructive pulmonary disease (COPD), asthma, heart block, right pump failure, and congenital glaucoma.

CAIs should be administered cautiously in patients who have adrenocortical insufficiency because they are at higher risk for associated fluid and electrolyte disturbances. Cross allergies are possible in those individuals sensitive to sulfonamide drugs, such as thiazide diuretics and oral sulfonylureas and sulfonamide antibiotics, since they may be at risk for allergic reactions to CAIs. CAIs are contraindicated in patients with hyponatremia or hypokalemia or who have renal or liver dysfunction. In addition, it is important to question the patient about current medications because of the possibility of interactions with amphetamines, quinidine, mecamyaline, and methenamine. Baseline vital signs and an assessment of the patient's vision, IOP, serum electrolytes, urinalysis, and platelet and complete blood cell count (CBC) are also recommended before initiation of drug therapy.

Osmotic agents such as glycerin ophthalmic solution and glycerin oral solution are contraindicated in patients who have cardiac, renal, or hepatic disease because the sudden fluid volume shifts may precipitate circulatory overload and possible heart failure. The elderly patient may be subject to dehydration with these agents because of rapid fluid shifts and subsequent diuretic action. Blood sugar levels must be monitored more closely in patients who are diabetic and taking osmotic agents since glycerin has been found to cause transient hyperglycemia and glucosuria as a result of metabolism of glycerin to carbohydrates.

With the ophthalmic antibiotics, each drug carries its own contraindications or cautions. Chloramphenicol, erythromycin, tetracycline, neomycin, gentamicin, and tobramycin drops are contraindicated in patients who are allergic to the medication, and cautious use is recommended in patients who are pregnant or have antibiotic hypersensitivity.

Mydriatic agents, such as atropine, are contraindicated in patients with a history of severe reactions to atropine and should be used extremely cautiously in patients who have primary glaucoma. The dilation of the pupil results in narrowing of the canal of Schlemm and restriction of the drainage of intraocular fluids, which increases IOP that may result in precipitation of an acute glaucoma attack. It is also important to obtain and document baseline vital signs and vision status.

Sympathomimetic agents (epinephrine, phenylephrine, and tetrahydrozoline) cause mydriasis and help decrease the congestion of conjunctival blood vessels. These agents cause vasoconstriction, pupil dilation, relaxation of the ciliary muscle, an increase in the outflow of aqueous humor, and a decrease in aqueous humor formation. Most of these agents, as previously mentioned in this chapter, are used to treat wide-angle glaucoma secondary to uveitis or to produce mydriasis for ocular examination. It is important to remember contraindications and cautions to sympathomemetic use such as patients with coronary heart disease, angina, tachycardia, and hypertension. As with other ophthalmic agents, there is always the risk of systemic absorption, which can cause systemic effects and many drug interactions.

Antiviral agents are contraindicated during pregnancy. Antiseptics are rarely used because they do not completely sterilize the eye. There are limited cautions and contraindications with the use of antifungal agents because they are not systemically absorbed. Topical corticosteroid

---

case study **Glaucoma**

Ms. M.R., an 89-year-old patient with open-angle glaucoma, presents to the physician's office for her usual check-up. During the visit, the opthalmologist checks her intraocular pressure, which is elevated from her last check-up 6 weeks ago. During their discussion, Ms. M.R. tells the physician that she just has problems "getting the eye drops in" and so she often just "doesn't take the medicine." The physician has now decided to change her miotic drops to an oral agent, acetazolamide (Diamox) 250 mg tid, which is used with open angle glaucoma.

- Why is acetazolamide effective against glaucoma?
- What is a rationale for switching Ms. M.R. to the oral agent?
- What specific patient teaching tips should be shared with Ms. M.R. in written and oral forms?

For Answers see www.harcourthealth.com/MERLIN/Lilley/.

ophthalmic agents are contraindicated in patients with pyogenic infections or minor corneal abrasions. Ophthalmic steroids may also increase the incidence of fungal infections of the eye and are to be used only as directed with the advice of a physician. Antiinflammatory agents may also mask allergic reactions or hypersensitivity to other agents. Artificial tears and lubricants are usually safe, so there are no major contraindications or cautions to their use. Baseline vital signs and a visual assessment should be performed before starting therapy with any of these agents.

● Nursing Diagnoses

Nursing diagnoses associated with the use of ophthalmic agents include the following:
- Risk for infection related to eye disorder or possible noncompliance to therapy.
- Risk for injury related to possible improper use of medication.
- Acute pain related to eye disorder.
- Disturbed sensory perception related to eye disorder and side effects of medication.
- Deficient knowledge deficit related to lack of information about medication and disorder.

● Planning

Goals related to administration of ophthalmic medications include the following:
- Patient remains free of signs and symptoms of infection of the eye with therapy.
- Patient remains compliant to therapy.
- Patient remains free from self-injury related to side effects of therapy.
- Patient is without eye pain related to eye disorder.
- Patient regains normal visual patterns or preinfection or predisorder vision.

Outcome Criteria

Outcome criteria for the patient receiving ophthalmic agents include the following:
- Patient will state signs and symptoms of infection of the eye such as eye pain, drainage, redness, and decreased activity and report immediately to physician.
- Patient will state ways to become more compliant to therapy by taking medications as prescribed.
- Patient will minimize self-injury related to side effects of therapy such as a safe environment and assistance at home while experiencing decreased vision.
- Patient will minimize eye pain related to eye disorder with use of compresses or use of nonaspirin analgesics as ordered.
- Patient will show improvement in visual patterns with increased activity and tolerance to reading, activities of daily living, etc.

● Implementation

Since it is important to administer only clear solutions, the nurse should shake the medication vial before use. Any excess medication must be removed promptly and

pressure must be applied to the inner canthus for 1 minute to avoid systemic symptoms or side effects. Ointments should be applied as a thin layer. All ophthalmic agents should be administered in the conjunctival sac. Be sure to administer all eye medications as ordered and in the proper order if more than one medication is ordered by the physician. See an appropriate drug resource or handbook for specific instructions.

The following medications are discussed because of their special characteristics (all other agents and associated nursing implications are presented in Table 54-8). Atropine is an antidote for myotics and should be available. Echothiophate iodide, an indirect-acting parasympathomimetic agent, should be administered only after you carefully check the vial's concentration amount and after proper reconstitution of the powder.

Dipivefrin, a sympathomimetic and mydriatic, should be instilled as the previous agents with pressure to the lacrimal sac and inner canthus area for 1 minute. Although they have different mechanisms of action, beta-adrenergic blockers such as timolol maleate should be instilled as other optic agents.

Directions for antiviral ophthalmic preparations should be followed closely. The newer antiviral agent ganciclovir is in an implant form (Vitrasert) and should be given as ordered.

Topical anesthetics should be administered exactly as ordered for foreign body removal or treatment of eye injury. You should avoid repeated and continuous use because of the risk of delayed wound healing, possible corneal perforation, permanent corneal opacification, and visual loss. When used, the eye should be patched because of the loss of blink reflex.

With the prostaglandin agent latanoprost, there is one unusual side effect to emphasize to the patient. This ophthalmic agent permanently turns hazel, blue/brown, or green eyes to brown. There is no known injury to the eye associated with this color change. OTC tear solutions may be suggested by the health care provider. Examples include Hypotears and Lacri-lube.

Patient teaching tips for ophthalmic agents are presented on p. 881.

● Evaluation

Therapeutic responses to miotics include decreased aqueous humor of the eye with resultant decreased IOP and decreased signs, symptoms, and long-term effects associated with glaucoma. Possible side effects are included in the discussion of patient education.

Beta-adrenergic blockers, such as timolol maleate optic solution, have been therapeutic if there is a resultant decrease in IOP. Possible side effects include weakness, depression, anxiety, nausea, confusion, eye irritation, rash, bradycardia, hypotension, and dysrhythmias.

Therapeutic responses to antibiotic, antifungal, or antiviral ophthalmic agents include elimination of the infection and resolution of symptoms.

Therapeutic responses to ophthalmic anesthetic topical agents include healing of the eye without permanent

NURSING CARE PLAN Glaucoma

Ms. A.B. is at the physician's office today for instructions about self-administration of pilocarpine via Ocusert dosage form. Although 82 years old, she is healthy and all senses are intact. Her motor and cognition skills are intact with no deficits noted. She is eager to learn and has many questions regarding her glaucoma and associated care. She lives alone, but her 21-year-old niece helps her out quite a bit and has come with her today so that she may also learn how to help with this medication.

assessment	*Nursing Diagnosis*	Deficient knowledge related to new dosage technique for pilocarpine
	Subjective Data	Complaint of blurred vision, decreased vision acuity, and difficulty with "close up" vision
		Frequent headaches and eye pain
		States "I live all alone but I do pretty good."
	Objective Data	82-year-old woman who is having annual eye examination
		Increased IOP
		Good health otherwise and without significant medical problems
planning	*Goals*	Patient will remain compliant and have therapeutic response to pilocarpine Ocusert technique within 1 mo of therapy
	Outcome Criteria	Patient will demonstrate proper instillation technique of Ocusert dosage form before leaving physician's office as evidenced by:
		Proper technique and accurate skill of pulling down lid and inserting med
implementation		Patient teaching should include the following:
		• To insert the ocusert form of pilocarpine you must first wash your hands and then follow these instructions:
		• Pull down lower lid of eye.
		• Apply Ocusert med pouch into conjunctival sac.
		• Change weekly, but it is good to check each evening before bedtime.
		• If the med comes out then rinse it and reinsert as directed.
		• Teach a significant other, friend, or relative how to insert medication too, just in case the patient has any difficulty with the medication.
evaluation		Patient will show therapeutic response to medication regimen as evidenced by:
		• Decreased IOP
		• Decreased headaches and eye pain

Table 54-8 Ophthalmic Agents: Nursing Implications

Drug Group	Drug Examples	Nursing Implications
Beta-adrenergic blocking agents	timolol	Use nasolacrimal pressure to prevent possible systemic absorption as with all other topical ophthalmic solutions or ointments; monitor for bradycardia, heart block, and wheezing.
Carbonic anhydrase inhibitors (CAIs)	acetazolamide dichlorphenamide methazolamide	Administer as ordered and with meals if necessary to decrease GI upset; fluid volume should be monitored carefully; monitor affected eye closely for therapeutic effects; check for drug interactions.
Osmotic agents	mannitol urea glycerin	Mannitol use may result in digitalis toxicity when given concurrently; if crystallized, may dissolve in warm water; adequate hydration is important—up to 2000 ml/day;
		Urea, if given at a rate >4 ml/min may result in hemolysis and cerebral vasomotor symptoms; monitor fluid volume status closely; preparation and administration vary; read instructions carefully.
		Glycerin should be used with extreme caution; flavor with lemon or lime juice over cracked ice; monitor for signs of cerebral dehydration.

Continued

Ophthalmic Agents: Nursing Implications—cont'd

54-8

Drug Group	Drug Examples	Nursing Implications
Mydriatics and cycloplegics	atropine cyclopentolate	Atropine: Monitor for side effects such as irregular pulse, confusion, dry mouth, and fever; causes blurred vision and photosensitivity, so sunglasses should be worn outside until effect is gone. Cyclopentolate: Use with causion and give as ordered; same nursing management as with atropine.
Sympathomimetics	epinephrine phenylephrine hydroxyamphetamine tetrahydrozoline	Monitor for serious side effects that may occur if systemically absorbed, such as tachycardia and elevated blood pressure. With corticosteroid agents, report blurred vision or visual disturbances, eye pain, ptosis (lid drooping), or enlarged pupils.
Antiinfectives/ antiinflammatories		Prophylactic use is potentially dangerous and is not recommended; may cause local reactions such as redness, itching, edema, and dermatitis. Follow instructions for instillation.
Antibacterials	chloramphenicol erythromycin neomycin tetracycline gentamicin tobramycin sulfonamides	With chloramphenicol, monitor for drop in CBC, fever, sore throat, and unusual bleeding. With erythromycin, make sure to administer as ordered and apply only a thin ointment strip. With neomycin combination agents and tetracycline, be sure to follow instructions. Gentamicin and similar agents should be given as ordered. Cleanse eye with use of sulfonamide agents such as sulfacetamide and sulfisoxazole because they will be inhibited by purulent drainage or exudate; discard any darkened solution; may cause mild pain on instillation.
Antifungals	natamycin	May cause irritation of the eye.
Antivirals	idoxuridine trifluridine vidarabine	Notify physician if the patient complains of blurred vision, visual disturbances, or photosensitivity if not present before therapy; notify the physician about any blurred vision, eye irritations, or visual changes not previously experienced; apply as ordered and, if ointment, apply only a thin strip; always instill drops and ointments into conjunctival sac.
Antiseptics	silver nitrate	Used for gonococcal infections and may inactivate bacitracin if used concurrently; should leave in contact with sac for at least 3 sec; irrigation afterward not recommended.
Topical anesthetics	proparacaine tetracaine	These are not recommended for long-term use because they could lead to possible irreversible eye damage; eye should be patched until injury healed; CNS excitation and subsequent depression are potential systemic side effects if absorbed.
Artificial tears	lacrisert; Lacri-Lube, Duratears and Hypo Tears are ointment forms;	Instill as directed. Ocusert forms given daily.
Antiallergics	cromolyn sodium	Instill as ordered; therapeutic effects in 4 wk if given regularly.
Enzyme preparations	chymotrypsin	May result in postoperative glaucoma for about 1 wk, which can be reversed with parasympathomimetics.
Hyperosmolar preparations	sodium chloride ointment	Apply as ordered.
Nonsteroidal antiinflammatories	flurbiprofen suprofen diclofenac ketorolac	Use only as prescribed; solutions preferred for eye infections because ointments often decrease healing.
Ophthalmic surgery aids	sodium hyaluronate	Used to protect the eye from damage and to be given exactly as ordered.
Prostaglandin preparations	latanoprost	Instill as ordered; lowers IOP for 20-24 hours with one single dose; well tolerated; patients with hazel-colored eyes may experience permanent iris color change to brown, but this is not harmful to the patient.

damage and a decrease in symptoms associated with the damage. Side effects include CNS excitation if systemically absorbed, causing blurred vision, dizziness, tremors, nervousness, and restlessness. Drowsiness, dyspnea, and cardiac dysrhythmias may occur secondary to CNS depression.

Cromolyn sodium ophthalmic solution, if therapeutic, will lead to decreased allergic reactions such as decreased itching, tearing, redness, and eye discharge. Potential complications of this agent include hypersensitivity to it and swelling of the conjunctiva (chemosis).

---

patient teaching tips

Ophthalmic Agents

➤ Patients taking parasympathomimetic ophthalmic agents should be informed (with demonstrations) about the adequate procedure for instilling eye drops and for applying pressure to the inner canthus. Solutions and the eye dropper should be kept sterile. Long-term therapy is usually necessary, and compliance is important to prevent eye damage.

➤ Indirect parasympathomimetics, such as echothiphate iodide, should be given to patients only after they demonstrate adequate knowledge of the medication and technique for administration and after explanation of side effects associated with most direct- and indirect-acting agents (e.g., blurred vision, bronchospasm, nausea, vomiting, bradycardia, hypotension, and sweating). Patients should be informed that they may experience decreased night visual acuity, stinging sensation, dull ache, or tearing upon instillation and that they should call the physician if these symptoms worsen.

➤ Patients taking sympathomimetics, such as dipivefrin HCl and epinephrine, should be instructed on instillation procedure and told to report any stinging, burning, itching, lacrimation, or puffiness of the eye.

➤ Beta-adrenergic blocking agents such as timolol should be administered as any other optic agent, and pressure should be applied to the inner canthus for 1 full minute after administration. Patients should be encouraged to report any of the following symptoms to their physician: blurred vision, difficulty breathing, wheezing, sweating, flushing, or loss of sight.

➤ Patients should be encouraged to eat a high-potassium, low-sodium diet while taking carbonic anhydrase in-

hibitors and to drink at least 2 liters of fluid per day to reduce the risk of renal stone formation. Daily weights should be recorded, and patients should be informed of signs and symptoms of fluid and electrolyte imbalances.

➤ Patients taking osmotic agents should drink at least 2000 ml of fluid per day. Patients on glycerin should be informed that lying flat during and after the oral administration will help diminish any headache caused by cerebral dehydration.

➤ Patients taking atropine should be informed that the next dose should be omitted if they are experiencing dry mouth and tachycardia. Photosensitivity is an expected side effect; sunglasses will help ease the discomfort.

➤ With topical anesthetics, patients should not rub or touch the eye while it is numb because of possible eye damage. They should also wear a patch to protect the eye because of loss of blink reflex.

➤ Patients should take antiinfectives, antiinflammatory, and antibacterial ophthalmic solutions as prescribed and individual instructions followed. Increase in eye pain, discharge, and fever should be reported to the physician.

➤ Patients should take ophthalmic corticosteroids cautiously and not overuse or abuse them. The medication should not be stopped without consulting the physician because of the possibility of adverse reactions. Contact lenses should not be worn while taking these medications. All suspensions should be well mixed before use. Stinging is usually experienced after instillation of drops.

➤ Patients taking cromolyn sodium drops should not wear contact lenses until the medication has been discontinued.

POINTS TO REMEMBER

Antiglaucoma Drugs

• Glaucoma: disorder of the eye caused by inhibition of the normal flow and drainage of aqueous humor.
• Treatment: reduce IOP either by increasing aqueous humor drainage or decreasing its production.
• Drugs that increase aqueous humor drainage are direct parasympathomimetics, indirect parasympathomimetics, sympathomimetics, and beta blockers.
• Drugs that decrease aqueous humor production are sympathomimetics, beta blockers, carbonic anhydrase inhibitors, and osmotic diuretics.

Ocular Antiinfectives

• Treat bacterial, viral, and fungal infections of the eye.
• A large proportion of the inflammatory diseases seen in ophthalmology are caused by viruses.
• Common ocular infections include conjunctivitis, hordeolum (sty), keratitis, uveitis, and endophthalmitis.

Antiinflammatory Ophthalmic Agents

• Many of the same antiinflammatory drugs that are used systematically are used ophthalmically.
• Corticosteroids: used to inhibit inflammatory response to mechanical, chemical, or immunologic agents.

Topical Anesthetics
- Used to prevent pain to the eye.
- Beneficial during surgery, ophthalmic examinations, and removal of foreign bodies.
- Two currently available topical anesthetic drugs for ophthalmic use are proparacaine and tetracaine.

Nursing Considerations
- All ophthalmic preparations need to be administered *exactly* as ordered and using safe, accurate application or instillation technique.
- Report increase in symptoms, such as eye pain and drainage, to the physician immediately.
- Prostaglandin agents can change the color of the iris and may be of concern for the patient.

REVIEW QUESTIONS

1. Drugs that are indicated for patients with increased intraocular pressure in glaucoma include which of the following?
   a. Miotics
   b. Mydriatics
   c. Polypeptide drops
   d. Hypertonic saline instillations
2. Which of the following would occur if the ophthalmic solution dexamethasone is used with ophthalmic gentamicin ointment?
   a. Miosis
   b. Thorough healing
   c. Complete elimination of the infections
   d. Possible spread or worsening of the infection
3. Which of the following would be an appropriate patient teaching tip for administering ophthalmic timolol?
   a. Make sure to aim the tip of the bottle over the iris.

   b. Monitor for severe systemic reactions such as heart block.
   c. Administer the agent in the conjunctival sac as with all ophthalmic agents.
   d. Apply pressure to the inner canthus for 10 minutes after administration of the drug.
4. Atropine is contraindicated in patients with:
   a. Anemia.
   b. Polyuria.
   c. Diabetes.
   d. Glaucoma.
5. What is the antidote to the toxic effects of miotic agents?
   a. Atropine
   b. Dopamine
   c. Epinephrine
   d. Acetylcholine

For Answers see www.harcourthealth.com/MERLIN/Lilley/.

CRITICAL THINKING Activities

1. Describe the process of glaucoma and explain the value of treatment to preserve vision.
2. Develop a teaching plan for the elderly patient who is already vision-impaired and needs instructions for the daily administration of antiglaucoma ophthalmic drops.

3. Your patient has developed an infection and inflammation of the eye. What is the importance of using only the antibiotic agent before initiation of a corticosteroid ointment?

For Answers see www.harcourthealth.com/MERLIN/Lilley/.

bibliography

Albanese J, Nutz P: *Mosby's 2001 nursing drug reference and review cards*, St Louis, 2001, Mosby.

American Hospital Formulary Service: *AHFS drug information*, Bethesda, Md, 2000, American Society of Health-System Pharmacists.

Anderson PO, Knoben JE, Troutman WG: *Handbook of clinical drug data 1999-2000*, ed 9, New York, 1999, McGraw-Hill.

Johns Hopkins Hospital, Department of Pediatrics et al: *The Harriet Lane handbook*, ed 15, St Louis, 2000, Mosby.

Keen JH: *Critical care and emergency drug reference*, ed 3, St Louis, 1996, Mosby.

McEvoy GK: *AHFS drug information*, Bethesda, Md, 1998, American Society of Hospital Pharmacists.

McKenry LM, Salerno E: *Mosby's pharmacology in nursing*, ed 21, St Louis, 2001, Mosby.

Mosby's GenRx: a comprehensive reference for generic and brand drugs, ed 10, St Louis, 2000, Mosby.

DiPiro JT et al: *Pharmacotherapy: a pathophysiologic approach*, ed 4, New York, 1999, McGraw-Hill.

Skidmore-Roth L: *Mosby's 2001 nursing drug reference*, St Louis, 2001, Mosby.

United States Pharmacopeial Convention: *USP DI: drug information for the health care professional, vol. 1*, ed 20, Englewood, Colo, 2000, Micromedex.

Activity

Remember to check the **Online Worksheet** for additional learning opportunities: **www.harcourthealth.com/MERLIN/Lilley/**

Chapter 55

Otic Agents

www.harcourthealth.com/MERLIN/Lilley/

When you reach the end of this chapter, you should be able to do the following:

1 Describe the anatomy of the ear.

2 Cite the various ear disorders in the two categories of such disorders and explain their causes.

3 List the various types of otic preparations.

4 Discuss the mechanisms of action, dosage, cautions, contraindications and specific application techniques related to otic agents.

5 Discuss the nursing process as it relates to the administration of otic preparations.

6 Develop a nursing care plan that includes all phases of the nursing process as it relates to the administration of otic preparations.

Look for this symbol for topics covered in the **Online Worksheet**

drug profiles

carbamide peroxide, p. 886
chloramphenicol, p. 884
pramoxine and benzocaine, p. 885

glossary

Cerumen (se roo′ mən) A yellowish or brownish waxy excretion produced by vestigial apocrine sweat glands in the external ear canal. Also called *earwax.* (p. 885)

Otic agents (o′ tik) Drugs applied locally to treat inflammation of the external ear canal or to remove excess cerumen (earwax). Also called *otics.* (p. 884)

Otitis media (o ti′ tis med e ə) Inflammation or infection of the middle ear, a common affliction of childhood. It is often preceded by an upper respiratory tract infection. (p. 883)

Wax emulsifiers (e′ mul′ si fyers) Products that loosen and help in the removal of cerumen. (p. 885)

THE EAR AND EAR DISORDERS

The ear consists of three portions: the outer, middle, and inner ear. The outer, or external, ear is made up of the pinna (outer projecting part of the ear) and the external auditory meatus. The middle ear comprises the tympanic cavity, mastoid appendages (e.g., malleus, incus), and the auditory, or eustachian, tube. The inner ear is made up of such structures as the cochlea and semicircular canals. The ear and its associated structures are illustrated in Fig. 55-1.

The disorders of the ear can be categorized according to the portion of the ear affected. Those of the outer and middle ear are the ones pertinent to the discussion here because these are the disorders that are usually treated with the agents discussed in this chapter. In general the most common disorders of these portions of the ear are bacterial and fungal infections, inflammatory disorders that cause pain, and earwax accumulation. Such disorders tend to be self-limiting, and if treatment is needed, it is generally easy to accomplish. However, if problems persist or are left untreated, more serious problems such as hearing loss may eventuate.

External ear disorders are generally the result of physical trauma to the ear and consist of disorders such as lacerations or scrapes to the skin and localized infection of the hair follicles that usually results in the development of a boil. These are examples of the self-limiting types of disorders just mentioned. They are often minor and heal with time. Other more serious disorders may initially appear to be minor but, if left untreated, can become more serious. Such "minor" irritations are dermatitis of the ear, itching, local redness, weeping, or drainage, but they may be the result of inflammation caused by seborrhea, psoriasis, or contact dermatitis. They may also be the first signs of a more serious underlying disease process such as head trauma. Drainage, pain, and dizziness are sure indications of the need for prompt medical care.

By far the most common middle ear disorder is infection caused by various microorganisms, a condition commonly called **otitis media.** This disorder most commonly afflicts children and usually occurs after an upper

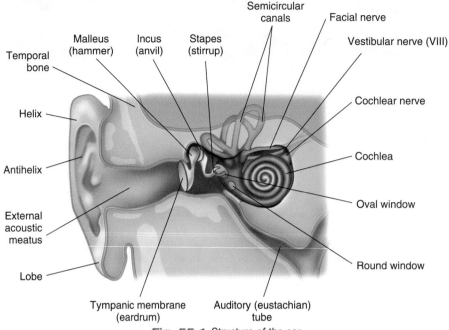

Temporal bone

Helix

Antihelix

External acoustic meatus

Lobe

Malleus (hammer)

Incus (anvil)

Stapes (stirrup)

Semicircular canals

Facial nerve

Vestibular nerve (VIII)

Cochlear nerve

Cochlea

Oval window

Round window

Tympanic membrane (eardrum)

Auditory (eustachian) tube

Fig. 55-1 Structure of the ear.

respiratory tract infection. It may also occur in adults, but it is then generally associated with trauma to the middle ear stemming from trauma to the tympanic membrane. Foreign objects and water sports are the usual sources of such trauma. Common symptoms of middle ear disorders such as otitis media are pain, fever, malaise, pressure, a sensation of fullness in the ears, and hearing loss. If left untreated, tinnitus (ringing in the ears), nausea, vertigo, and mastoiditis may occur. Hearing deficits and even hearing loss may eventuate if appropriate and prompt therapy is not started.

TREATMENT OF EAR DISORDERS

Some of the minor ailments that affect the outer ear can be treated with over-the-counter (OTC) medications, but persistent, painful conditions always require a physician's care. Middle ear disorders are rarely treated with OTC medications unless they are prescribed by a physician after referral. The drugs commonly used to treat the relatively minor disorders of the external and middle ear are called **otic agents** and are topically applied. They are listed as follows:
- Antibiotics
- Antifungals
- Local anesthetics
- Wax emulsifiers
- Antiinflammatory agents
- Steroids
- Local analgesics

More serious problems than those previously mentioned may require treatment with potent, systemically administered medications such as antimicrobial agents, analgesics, antiinflammatory drugs, and antihistamines. These medications have been discussed in earlier chapters.

ANTIBACTERIAL AND ANTIFUNGAL OTIC AGENTS

Many of the antibacterial and antifungal agents that are given systemically also come in topical formulations that are applied to the external ear; chloramphenicol and gentamicin are two commonly used ones. Several of these agents are also combined with steroids to take advantage of their additional antiinflammatory, antipruritic, and antiallergic drug effects. The antimicrobial drugs used as otic agents are effective in the treatment of mastoidectomy infections and infections of the external auditory canal. However, middle ear infections such as otitis media generally require treatment with systemically administered antibiotics.

drug profiles

chloramphenicol
Chloramphenicol (Chloromycetin Otic, Pentamycetin) has the advantage of possessing a very broad spectrum of activity. It is effective against *Staphylococcus aureus*, *Escherichia coli*, *Pseudomonas aeruginosa*, *Enterobacter aerogenes*, *Haemophilus influenzae*, and many others. It can cause adverse effects very similar to those caused by many of the topically applied antibiotics. These include burning, redness, rash, swelling, and other signs of topical irritation. Chloramphenicol is available as a 0.5% solution that is usually instilled in the ear. Two to three drops three times daily is the recommended dosage for both adults and children.

Table 55-1 Steroid and Antibiotic Combinations for Otic Use

Steroid	Antibiotic (dose/ml)	Trade Name
1% Hydrocortisone (solution)	5 mg of neomycin and 10,000 units of polymyxin B	Cortisporin Otic, Otocort
	10,000 units of polymyxin B	Otobiotic Otic, Pyocidine Otic
1% Hydrocortisone (suspension)	5 mg of neomycin and 10,000 units of polymyxin B	Cortisporin Otic, Otocort
	3.3 mg of neomycin and 3 mg of colistin	Coly-Mycin S Otic

ANTIBIOTIC AND STEROID COMBINATION PRODUCTS

The steroid most commonly used in combination with antibiotics is hydrocortisone, and it is added to reduce the inflammation and itching associated with ear infections. The antibiotics contained in the most popular combination products and the various trade names of these products are given in Table 55-1. These products are most commonly used for the treatment of bacterial infections of the external auditory canal caused by susceptible bacteria such as *S. aureus, E. coli, Klebsiella* spp., and others.

MISCELLANEOUS OTIC AGENTS

A wide variety of single-agent and combination-agent products are used to treat fungal and bacterial infections, inflammation, ear pain, and other minor or superficial problems of the external ear. An additional problem is the accumulation and eventual impaction of earwax, or **cerumen,** which can be the cause of many of these symptoms. Products that soften and help eliminate earwax are referred to as **wax emulsifiers** and are therefore also discussed with the miscellaneous agents.

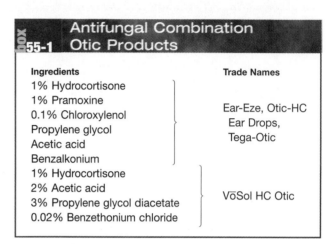

Box 55-1 Antifungal Combination Otic Products

Ingredients	Trade Names
1% Hydrocortisone 1% Pramoxine 0.1% Chloroxylenol Propylene glycol Acetic acid Benzalkonium	Ear-Eze, Otic-HC Ear Drops, Tega-Otic
1% Hydrocortisone 2% Acetic acid 3% Propylene glycol diacetate 0.02% Benzethonium chloride	VōSol HC Otic

drug profiles

ANTIFUNGAL AGENTS

Although fungal infections of the ear are uncommon, there are some otic agents that are available for their treatment. The agents contained in two commonly used antifungal combination products and the trade names of each are listed in Box 55-1. These combination products include drugs from several classes of agents—corticosteroids, local anesthetics, and topical antiseptics—and hence the therapeutic effect is a combination of the respective effects of the individual agents. They are used as antibacterial, antifungal, local anesthetic, and antiinflammatory otic drugs.

LOCAL ANESTHETIC AGENTS

Numerous otic combination products contain local anesthetic agents. Many common ear disorders are associated with some degree of pain and inflammation, and the numbing or anesthetic effect provided

by the local anesthetic makes it very beneficial in the relief of the pain. The same characteristics of the local anesthetics that were discussed in Chapter 10 apply to the topically applied local anesthetics used in these preparations.

pramoxine and benzocaine

One combination product that contains local anesthetics is mentioned in Box 55-1, and the local anesthetic it contains is pramoxine. Pramoxine is structurally similar to dyclonin and does not contain the usual ester or amide linkage of the procaine-type drugs. Besides its otic use, it is also applied topically for the temporary relief of the pain and itching associated with dermatoses, minor burns, anogenital pruritus or irritation, anal fissures, and hemorrhoids. Another local anesthetic otic agent that is used in combination with analgesics and emollients is benzocaine. This combination consists of the following:
- 1.4% benzocaine
- 5.4% antipyrine
- Glycerin
- Oxyquinoline sulfate

It may be used as an antiinflammatory, analgesic, or emollient. Common trade names for this combination product are Allergen Ear Drops, Auralgan Otic, and Auromid.

Benzocaine differs from pramoxine in that it is a local anesthetic of the ester type. It is also used for the temporary relief of pain and itching, either alone or in combination with other drugs. Side effects to these agents are rare and consist mostly of localized allergic reactions. They are typically seen after prolonged or repeated use.

WAX EMULSIFIERS

Wax, or cerumen, is a natural product of the ear and is produced by modified sweat glands in the auditory canal. However, it can occasionally build up and become impacted, resulting in pain and temporary deafness. The wax emulsifiers can loosen and help remove such impacted cerumen.

carbamide peroxide

One commonly used wax emulsifier is carbamide peroxide. It is customarily combined with other agents that work together to loosen and help remove cerumen. One such combination product contains the following:
• 6.5% carbamide peroxide
• Glycerin
• Propylene glycol

Trade names for combination products that contain these ingredients are Debrox Drops, Murine Ear Drops, and Auro Ear Drops.

As a source of hydrogen peroxide, carbamide peroxide slowly releases hydrogen peroxide and oxygen when exposed to moisture such as that on the skin or the mouth. This release of oxygen imparts a weak antibacterial action to the otic agent. In addition, the effervescence resulting from the release of oxygen has the mechanical effect of removing cerumen from inaccessible spaces such as the ear canal. Agents such as glycerin soften the cerumen, making it easier to remove.

---

nursing process

● Assessment

Before administering any of the otic preparations, the nurse should ensure that the patient's baseline hearing or auditory status is evaluated and the findings are documented. There should also be a thorough evaluation of the patient's symptoms, and any other related medical information should be elicited. Any drug and food allergies should be noted and documented. In addition, the nurse must understand the specific indication for or the intended use of the medication so that it can be given exactly as ordered. An understanding of the anatomy of the ear is important as well, especially as it relates to patients in different age groups. This understanding should extend to the specific administration technique used as well. Contraindications to the use of chloramphenicol otic preparations include hypersensitivity and eardrum perforation.

Drug hypersensitivity to hydrocortisone, neomycin sulfate, or polymyxin B sulfate would be a contraindication to the use of any of the individual agents or to any of the combination products containing these agents. A perforated eardrum would be a contraindication to the use of these agents as well.

● Nursing Diagnoses

Nursing diagnoses related to patients receiving otic agents include the following:
• Impaired verbal communication related to hearing loss stemming from damage from long-term ear disorders.
• Risk for injury related to symptoms of the ear disorder and possible vestibular dysfunction.
• Risk for infection related to inadequate treatment.
• Disturbed sensory perception related to complication from ear infections.
• Deficient knowledge related to lack of experience with otic drugs and their method of administration.

● Planning

Goals pertaining to patients receiving otic agents include the following:
• Patient regains normal patterns of hearing and communicating.
• Patient is free of discomfort and symptoms related to the ear disorder.
• Patient remains free of or experiences minimal signs and symptoms of ear infection with course of treatment.
• Patient is free of adverse reactions or side effects.
• Patient is free of complications associated with medication therapy.

Outcome Criteria

Outcome criteria for patients receiving otic agents include the following:
• Patient will openly verbalize feelings related to problems with communication (decreased hearing).
• Patient will report increased hearing loss and increased symptoms of ear pain, redness and swelling of the ear canal, and fever to the physician immediately.
• Patient will state measures to take to increase the effectiveness of the medication regimen such as accurate application or instillation.
• Patient will demonstrate accurate medication administration techniques.

● Implementation

Chloramphenicol drops should be instilled only after the ear has been thoroughly cleansed, all cerumen removed by irrigation, and the stopper cleaned with alcohol. Eardrops should generally be warmed to body temperature before instillation but not higher than the body temperature because this may affect the potency of the medication. Steroid and antibiotic combination otic preparations, wax emulsifiers, and ear-drying agents should all be administered according to these same guidelines. Wax emulsifiers should be administered according to manufacturer's guidelines or physician's orders.

See the box below for patient teaching tips.

● Evaluation

The therapeutic effects of the otic preparations include less pain, redness, and swelling in the ear; a reduction in fever and the WBC counts; and negative culture findings if previous culture has yielded positive findings. The ear canal should be watched for the occurrence of rash or contact dermatitis with a rash. Life-threatening reactions such as bone marrow suppression may occur in association with chloramphenicol use, but these are rare.

NURSING CARE PLAN Otitis Media

Karen, an 11 year old with otitis media, has been placed on cefaclor (Ceclor) 250 mg tid. She has tolerated cefaclor in the past, but her grandmother brought her into the physician's office and needs instructions for administration of the medicine because Karen's mother is out of town. Use of AuroEar drops has been recommended as well.

assessment	*Nursing Diagnosis*	Deficient knowledge related to needs for information about cefaclor and other otic drug administration.
	Subjective Data	"I don't remember much about how to take this medicine."
	Objective Data	Successful therapy before with cefaclor
		Grandmother caregiver for now; mother is out of town
planning	*Goals*	Patient and grandmother verbalize instructions associated with taking cefaclor before leaving physician's office.
	Outcome Criteria	Before leaving the physician's office, patient and grandmother:
		• State dosing times and amounts
		• State side effects of medication
		• State side effects to report to the physician
		• Demonstrate adequate technique for installing AuroEar drops as ordered
implementation		Patient education should include the following:
		• It is important to take medication exactly as prescribed and until all medication is gone.
		• Eating yogurt while on antibiotics will help maintain normal bacteria in the intestines and decrease diarrhea.
		• Contact the physician should you experience sore throat, bleeding, easy bruising, or joint pain.
		• Side effects to possibly expect include headache, dizziness, nausea, vomiting, diarrhea,* loss of appetite,* and rash.
		• AuroEar drops should be used daily.
		• Patient teaching on proper use of AuroEar drops with proper administration is needed.
evaluation		Patient will display the following therapeutic responses to cefaclor:
		• Decreased ear pain
		• Decreased fever
		Patient will experience minimal side effects, such as diarrhea.
		Patient's pain of the ear area will decrease with adequate response to cefaclor and with daily use of AuroEar drops.

*Most common side effects.

patient teaching tips

Otic Medications

➤ Patients should be instructed regarding chloramphenicol use. The patient should understand the frequency of dosing, its mechanism of action, and the technique of instillation. Patients should be encouraged to NOT touch the dropper to the ear. They should also be warned that dizziness may occur after its instillation, and so they may want to be supine when doing so.

➤ Patients should be told to administer eardrops at body temperature. This may be achieved by running warm water over the bottle, but they must be careful not to let water get into the bottle or to damage the label so that the directions are unreadable.

➤ In children older than 3 years of age and in adults, it is important to hold the pinna up and back during instillation of the eardrops. In children 3 years of age or younger, the pinna should be gently pulled down and back during instillation of the drug. A gentle massage of the area around the ear (anteriorly) can help promote access of the drops to the ear canal.

➤ Patients should lie on the side opposite the side of the affected ear for about 5 minutes after instillation of the

agent. If the patient prefers, a small cottonball may be inserted gently into the ear canal to keep the agent there, but it should not be forced into the ear or "jammed" down into the ear canal.

➤ Patients should be encouraged to show family members how to instill eardrops so that their assistance can be solicited if necessary.

➤ The eardrop solution and the placement of cotton balls in the ear may cause a seeming loss of hearing, but a loss of hearing not resulting from these factors may be due to the ear disorder.

POINTS TO REMEMBER

Pharmacologic Principles

- There are both antibacterial and antifungal otic agents.
- Most disorders of the ear are self-limiting.
- Many of the same antibacterial and antifungal agents that are given systemically can also be applied topically in the ear.
- Many of these antiinfective agents are combined with steroids to take advantage of their additional antiinflammatory, antipruritic, and antiallergic drug effects.

Local Anesthetic Otic Agents

- Many otic disorders are associated with some degree of pain and inflammation.
- Pramoxine and benzocaine are two commonly used anesthetic otic agents.

Wax Emulsifiers

- Wax, or cerumen, is a natural product of the ear.
- Wax is produced by modified sweat glands in the auditory canal.
- Emulsifying otic agents loosen and help remove this wax.
- Carbamine peroxide is a product commonly used for the removal of earwax.

Nursing Considerations

- Single agents and combination products are used to treat many ear conditions, and the nurse must know these indications and information about the drugs to ensure their safe use.
- Comfort and the potential for altered sensory integrity are major nursing diagnoses in patients receiving otic agents.

REVIEW QUESTIONS

1. Hydrocortisone ear drops are often used with otic antibiotics to:
   a. Reduce ear infection reoccurrence.
   b. Help with the inflammation and itching associated with the ear infection.
   c. Act as an antifungal agent, which is indicated for bacterial ear problems.
   d. Minimize the bacterial infection while softening and decreasing cerumen production.

2. For which of the following reasons is pramoxine added to an otic agent used to treat severe fungal ear infections?
   a. To soften the wax in the ear.
   b. To help with itching and inflammation.
   c. To enhance the effects of the antifungal agent.
   d. To anesthetize the area to help decrease the pain.

3. Chloramphenicol ear drops should be:
   a. Warmed to 106° F before using.
   b. Used only in severe fungal infections.

   c. Added to a cotton-tipped applicator for insertion.
   d. Used only after the removal of excessive cerumen.

4. Which of the following actions will help ensure that the ear medication will stay in the affected ear?
   a. There is nothing indicated for this.
   b. Stuff the ear canal tightly with cotton.
   c. Have the patient lie on the opposite side for about 5 minutes.
   d. Massage the outer ear canal for 10 minutes after instilling the ear drops.

5. Contraindications to the use of hydrocortisone ear drops include which of the following?
   a. Itching
   b. Inflammation
   c. Outer ear redness
   d. Severe ear infections

CRITICAL THINKING Activities

1. Develop a patient teaching plan for the caregiver who will be administering antibacterial and steroidal otic drops to a 3-year-old child.
2. Your pediatric patient's mother tells you that she does not understand why ear infections require treatment with antibiotics. She states, "We used home remedies when I was growing up." What information would you share with the patient's mother and why?
3. What is the indication for a wax emulsifier? Explain your answer.

For Answers see www.harcourthealth.com/MERLIN/Lilley/.

bibliography

Albanese J, Nutz P: *Mosby's 2001 nursing drug reference and review cards*, St Louis, 2001, Mosby.

Anderson PO, Knoben JE, Troutman WG: *Handbook of clinical drug data 1999-2000*, ed 9, New York, 1999, McGraw-Hill.

Drug facts and comparisons, St Louis, 1998, Facts and Comparisons.

Johns Hopkins Hospital, Department of Pediatrics et al: *The Harriet Lane handbook*, ed 15, St Louis, 2000, Mosby.

Keen JH: *Critical care and emergency drug reference*, ed 3, St Louis, 1996, Mosby.

McEvoy GK: *AHFS drug information*, Bethesda, Md, 2000, American Society of Hospital Pharmacists.

Mosby's GenRx: a comprehensive reference for generic and brand drugs, ed 10, St Louis, 2000, Mosby.

Skidmore-Roth L: *Mosby's 2001 nursing drug reference*, St Louis, 2001, Mosby.

Activity

Remember to check the **Online Worksheet** for additional learning opportunities: **www.harcourthealth.com/MERLIN/Lilley/**

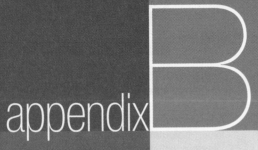

Pharmaceutical Abbreviations

ABBREVIATION	TRANSLATION
Drug Dosage	
cc	Cubic centimeter (equivalent to 1ml)
g or Gm	Gram
gr	Grain
gtt	Drop
L	Liter
lb	Pound
m	Minim
mEq	Milliequivalent
min	Minute
ml or mL	Milliliter
no	Number
qs	Quantity sufficient, as much as needed
ss	One half
oz	Ounce
tbsp	Tablespoon
tsp	Teaspoon
u or U	Unit
μg or mcg	Microgram
Drug Route	
AD	Right ear
AS	Left ear
AU	Both ears
ID	Intradermal
IM	Intramuscular
IV	Intravenous

ABBREVIATION	TRANSLATION
NG	Nasogastric
OD	Right eye
OS	Left eye
OU	Both eyes
PO	By mouth
SC or SQ	Subcutaneous
SL	Sublingual
Drug Administration	
aa	Of each
ac	Before meals
ad lib	As desired, freely
bid	Twice a day
h or hr	Hour
hs	Hour of sleep/at bedtime
noct	Night
NPO	Nothing by mouth
pc	After meals
prn	When needed
qd	Every day/once a day
qh	Every hour
qid	Four times a day
qod	Every other day
Rx	Prescribe/take
stat	Immediately
tid	Three times a day

disorders index

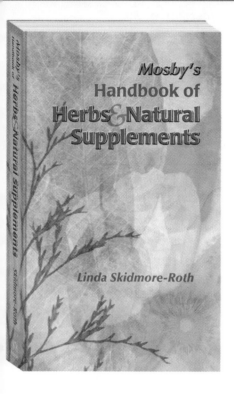

special features